AF653863

Textbook of

EMERGENCY CARDIOLOGY

Textbook of EMERGENCY CARDIOLOGY

Editors

Alan S Maisel MD
Professor of Medicine
Director, CCU and HF Program
Department of Medicine and Cardiology
VA Medical Center, University of California
San Diego, California, USA

W Frank Peacock MD FACEP FACC
Professor, Emergency Medicine
Associate Chair and Research Director
Baylor College of Medicine
Houston, Texas, USA

JAYPEE

JAYPEE BROTHERS MEDICAL PUBLISHERS
The Health Sciences Publisher
New Delhi | London

JAYPEE **Jaypee Brothers Medical Publishers (P) Ltd**

Headquarters
EMCA House
23/23-B, Ansari Road, Daryaganj
New Delhi 110 002, India
Landline: +91-11-23272143, +91-11-23272703
+91-11-23282021, +91-11-23245672
E-mail: jaypee@jaypeebrothers.com

Corporate Office
4838/24, Ansari Road, Daryaganj
New Delhi 110 002, India
Phone: +91-11-43574357
Fax: +91-11-43574314
E-mail: jaypee@jaypeebrothers.com

Overseas Office
J.P. Medical Ltd
83 Victoria Street, London
SW1H 0HW (UK)
Phone: +44 20 3170 8910
E-mail: info@jpmedpub.com

EU GPSR Authorised Representative
Logos Europe, 9 rue Nicolas Poussin
17000, La Rochelle, France
Phone: +33 (0) 6 67 93 73 78
E-mail: contact@logoseurope.eu

Website: www.jaypeebrothers.com
Website: www.jaypeedigital.com

Inquiries for bulk sales may be solicited at: jaypee@jaypeebrothers.com

Textbook of Emergency Cardiology / Alan S Maisel, W Frank Peacock

First Edition: 2021

Reprint: **2025**

ISBN: 978-93-86322-24-1

Printed in India

Contributors

Editors

Alan S Maisel MD
Professor of Medicine
Director, CCU and HF Program
Department of Medicine and Cardiology
Va Medical Center, University of California
San Diego, California, USA

W Frank Peacock MD FACEP FACC
Professor, Emergency Medicine
Associate Chair and Research Director
Baylor College of Medicine
Houston, Texas, USA

Contributing Authors

Boris Arbit MD
San Diego, California, USA

Kimberly C Atianzar MD
Seattle, Washington, USA

Denise D Barnard MD FACC
San Diego, California, USA

Daniel G Blanchard MD
San Diego, California, USA

Aaron M Brody MD MPH
Detroit, Michigan, USA

Cathleen MD Bury MD
Durham, North Carolina, USA

W Barton Campbell MD
Nashville, Tennessee, USA

Anna Marie Chang MD MSCE
Philadelphia, Pennsylvania, USA

Kay-Won Chang MD
San Diego, California, USA

Francesca R Civitarese DO
Dallas, Texas, USA

D Mark Courtney MD MS
Chicago, Illinois, USA

Lori B Daniels MD MAS FACC
La Jolla, California, USA

Nathan S Deal MD FACEP
Houston, Texas, USA

Jacqueline J Denysiak MD
Riverside, California, USA

Deborah B Diercks MD MSc
Dallas, Texas, USA

Jeremy Egnatios
San Diego, California, USA

Sutton R Fox MPH
San Diego, California, USA

Spencer C Greene MD MS FACEP FACMT
Houston, Texas, USA

Jonathan Harrison MD
San Diego, California, USA

Brian D Hoit MD
Cleveland, Ohio, USA

Judd E Hollander MD FACEP
Philadelphia, Pennsylvania, USA

Jillian B Horning MD
Dallas, Texas, USA

Michael S Jaung MD
Houston, Texas, USA

Caitlin M Kibbey MD
Dallas, Texas, USA

Joe T Kofoed MD
Dallas, Texas, USA

Nikola A Kozhuharov MD
Petersgraben, Basel, Switzerland

David E Krummen MD
San Diego, California, USA

Dick C Kuo MD
Houston, Texas, USA

Gautam G Lalani MD
San Diego, California, USA

Phillip D Levy MD MPH FACEP FAHA FACC
Detroit, Michigan, USA

Alexander T Limkakeng Jr MD MHSc FACEP
Durham, North Carolina, USA

Simon A Mahler MD MS
Winston-Salem, North Carolina, USA

Nicholas A Marston MD
San Diego, California, USA

Amal Mattu MD
Baltimore, Maryland, USA

Chadwick D Miller MD MS
Winston-Salem, North Carolina, USA

Christian Müller MD
Petersgraben, Basel, Switzerland

Silvia Navarin MD
Rome, Italy

Sean-Xavier Neath MD PhD FACEP
San Diego, California, USA

Matthew Noble MD
Portland, Oregon, USA

Edgardo Ordonez MD MPH FAAEM FACEP FACP
Houston, Texas, USA

Alex Pearce MD
San Diego, California, USA

Nicholas Phreaner MD
San Diego, California, USA

Ava E Pierce MD
Dallas, Texas, USA

Tyson Pillow MD FACEP
Houston, Texas, USA

Zubaid R Rafique MD FACEP
Houston, Texas, USA

Jayant K Raikhelkar MD
Chicago, Illinois, USA

Zaid Sabti MD
Petersgraben, Basel, Switzerland

Stephen Sanders
Atlanta, Georgia, USA

Amir A Schricker MD MS FACC FHRS
San Diego, California, USA

Navdeep S Sekhon MD FACEP
Houston, Texas, USA

Kevin S Shah MD
Los Angeles, California, USA

Samyut Shrestha MD
Petersgraben, Basel, Switzerland

Adam J Singer MD FACEP
Stony Brook, New York, USA

Lane M Smith MD PhD
Winston-Salem, North Carolina, USA

Salvatore Di Somma MD PhD
Rome, Italy

Semhar Z Tewelde MD
Baltimore, Maryland, USA

Martin Than MD
Christchurch, New Zealand

Traci L Thoureen MD MHS-CL MMCi FACEP
Durham, North Carolina, USA

Vaishal M Tolia MD MPH
San Diego, California, USA

Daniel C Walters MD
San Diego, California, USA

Nicholas W Wettersten MD
San Diego, California, USA

Joel R Wilson MD
Bellevue, Washington, USA

Darrin J Wong MD
San Diego, California, USA

Preface

We have been privileged to put together a state-of-the-art book called "*Textbook of Emergency Cardiology*." For this we assembled a team of co-authors that are superb researchers, clinicians, and teachers in the fields of cardiology and emergency medicine. This ensures that the readers will get a solid exposure with regard to current concepts in pathogenesis, diagnosis, and treatment of every cardiovascular emergency that "rolls into the emergency department or hospital." Thus, from medical or nursing student, to the intern or resident or fellow, and through to an experienced staff attending physician, this book should become a useful tool for everyday medical use.

Alan S Maisel

W Frank Peacock

Acknowledgments

I would like to thank my best mentors and best friends at work, Ralph Shabetai, whose memory lives with many, and Wilbur Lew, my chief and friend for many years. In the research field, I am indebted to Paul Insel and Scott Mader, and Steve Carter, my lab director for over 30 years. I thank my five children who have made being a father a joy and ongoing pleasure. Finally, my wife, Fran, thanks for the support over all these years.

Alan S Maisel

The best mentors may not even know the importance of their influence on the trajectory of an individual's professional career. For these I would like to acknowledge Bob Jesse, Jim Young, Johannes Holzmeister, Chuck Emerman, and Robert Weisenberger-Lipetz; three cardiologists, an emergency doctor, and a businessman, each of whom, in their own way, guided my trip into the world of emergency cardiology. And of course none of this happens without the support of one's family; my kids Ayla and Dakota, who put up with endless days of writing, and the tolerance of my wife Karina, who will never forget vacations with the laptop.

W Frank Peacock

Contents

Section 1: Cardiac Arrest

Section 2: Acute Myocardial Infarction and Acute Coronary Syndrome

Section 3: Acute Heart Failure

Section 4: Arrhythmias

PLATE 1

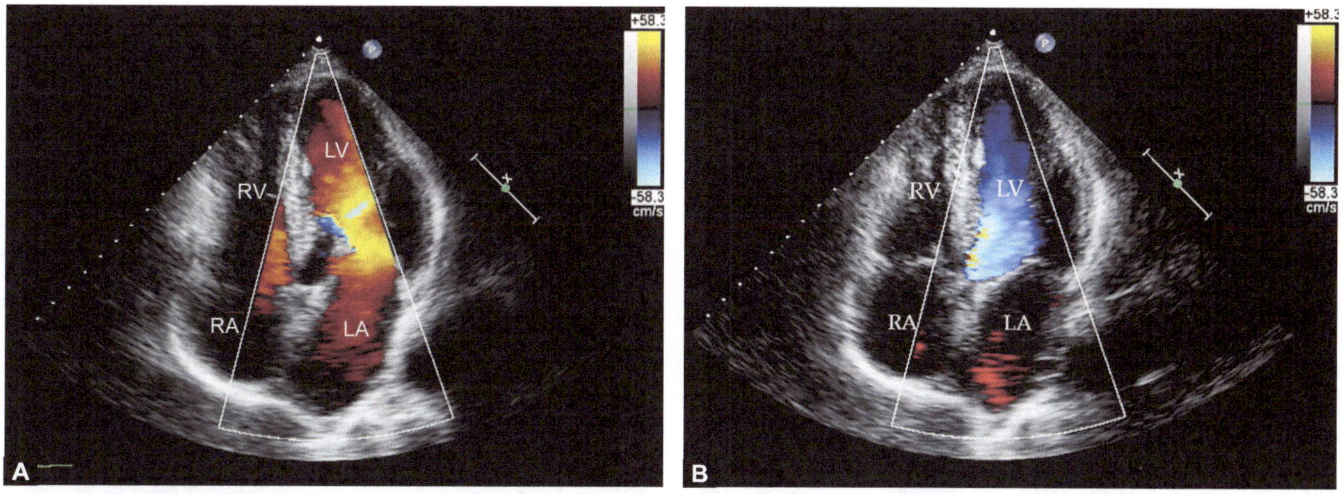

RV, right ventricle; LV, left ventricle; RA, right atrium; LA, left atrium.

FIG. 2: Apical four-chamber images with color-flow Doppler during diastole **(A)** and systole **(B)**. Red flow indicates movement towards the transducer (diastolic filling); blue flow indicates movement away from the transducer (systolic ejection) ***(Chapter 5)***

With permission from: DeMaria AN, Blanchard DG. Echocardiography. In: Fuster V, Walsh RA, Harrington R (Eds). Hurst's The Heart, 13th ed. New York, NY, USA: McGraw-Hill Medical Publishers; 2011. pp. 411-89.

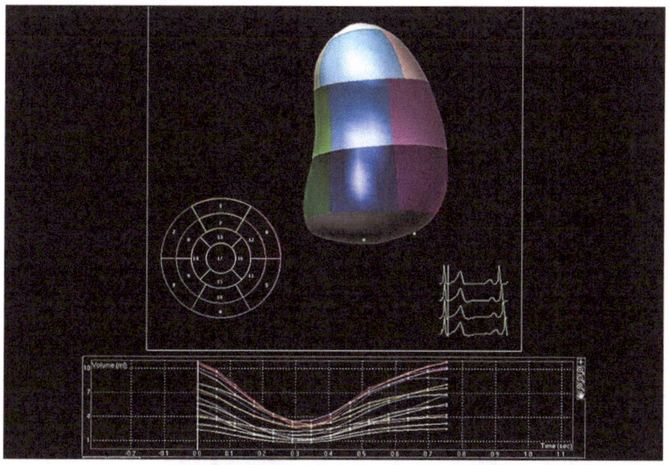

FIG. 6: Three-dimensional images of left ventricular wall motion with accompanying volume analysis ***(Chapter 5)***

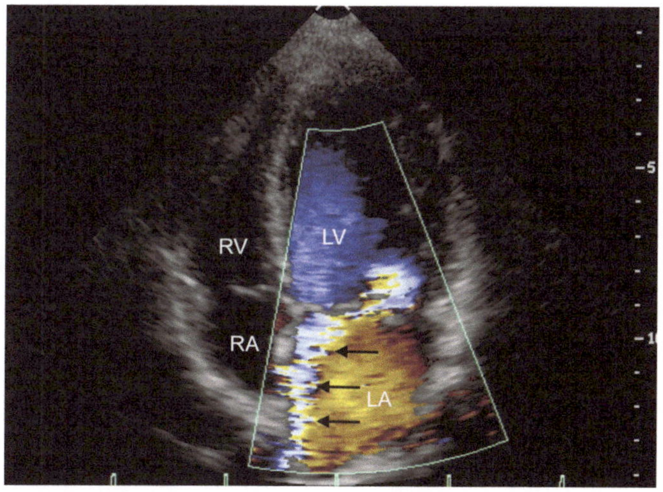

RV, right ventricle; LV, left ventricle; RA, right atrium; LA, left atrium.

FIG. 15: Apical four-chamber image of severe but eccentric mitral regurgitation. The left atrium is enlarged ***(Chapter 5)***

With permission from: DeMaria AN, Blanchard DG. Echocardiography. In: Fuster V, Walsh RA, Harrington R (Eds). Hurst's The Heart, 13th ed. New York, NY, USA: McGraw-Hill Medical Publishers; 2011. pp. 411-89.

PLATE 2

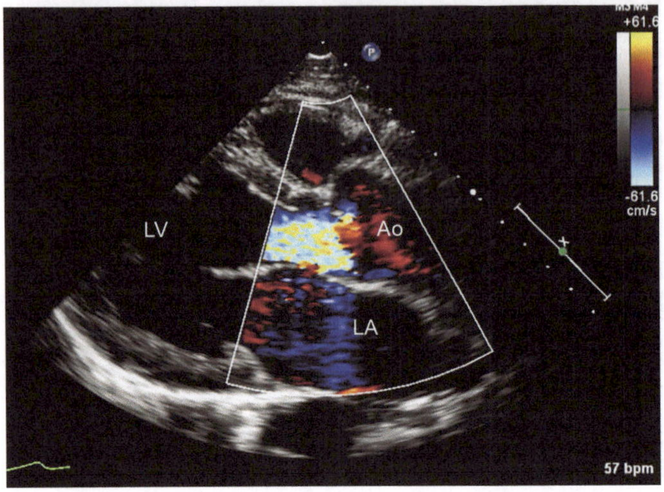

LV, left ventricle; Ao, aorta; LA, left atrium.

FIG. 17: Parasternal long-axis view with a wide jet of aortic regurgitation. The jet fills the width of the outflow tract, suggesting severe regurgitation ***(Chapter 5)***

With permission from: DeMaria AN, Blanchard DG. Echocardiography. In: Fuster V, Walsh RA, Harrington R (Eds). Hurst's The Heart, 13th ed. New York, NY, USA: McGraw-Hill Medical Publishers; 2011. pp. 411-89.

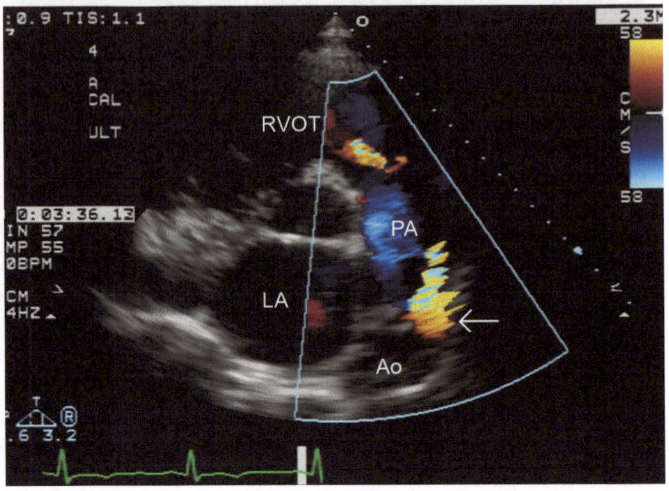

RVOT, right ventricular outflow tract; LV, LA, left atrium; PA, pulmonary artery; Ao, aorta.

FIG. 24: Parasternal short-axis view of a patent ductus arteriosus (arrow). Blood flow from the descending aorta (ascending aorta; in red) is seen entering the main pulmonary artery ***(Chapter 5)***

With permission from: DeMaria AN, Blanchard DG. Echocardiography. In: Fuster V, Walsh RA, Harrington R (Eds). Hurst's The Heart, 13th ed. New York, NY, USA: McGraw-Hill Medical Publishers; 2011. pp. 411-89.

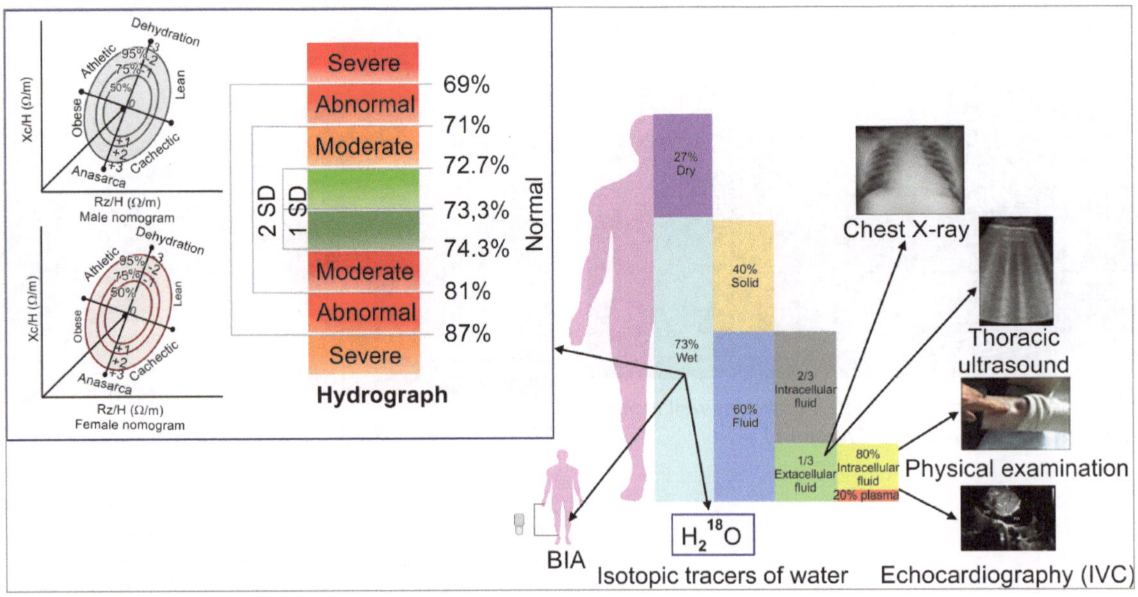

BIA, bioimpedence vector analysis; IVC, inferior vena cava.

FIG. 1: Methods for assessing congestion ***(Chapter 18)***

PLATE 3

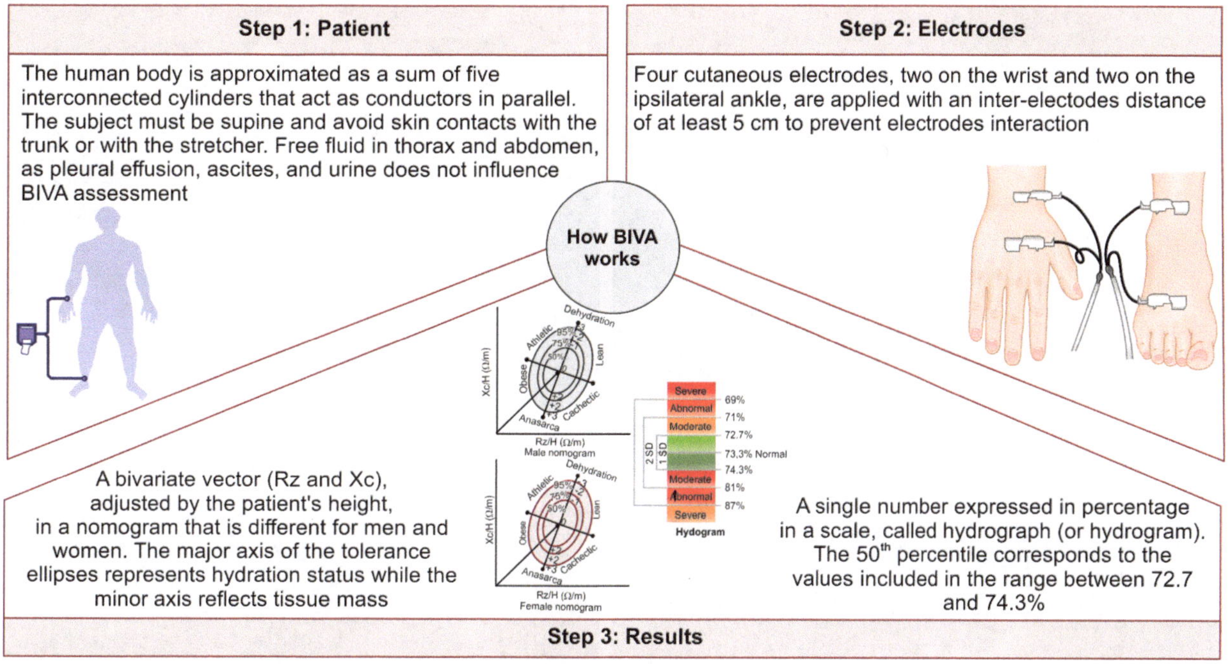

FIG. 2: Bioimpedance vector analysis measurement ***(Chapter 18)***

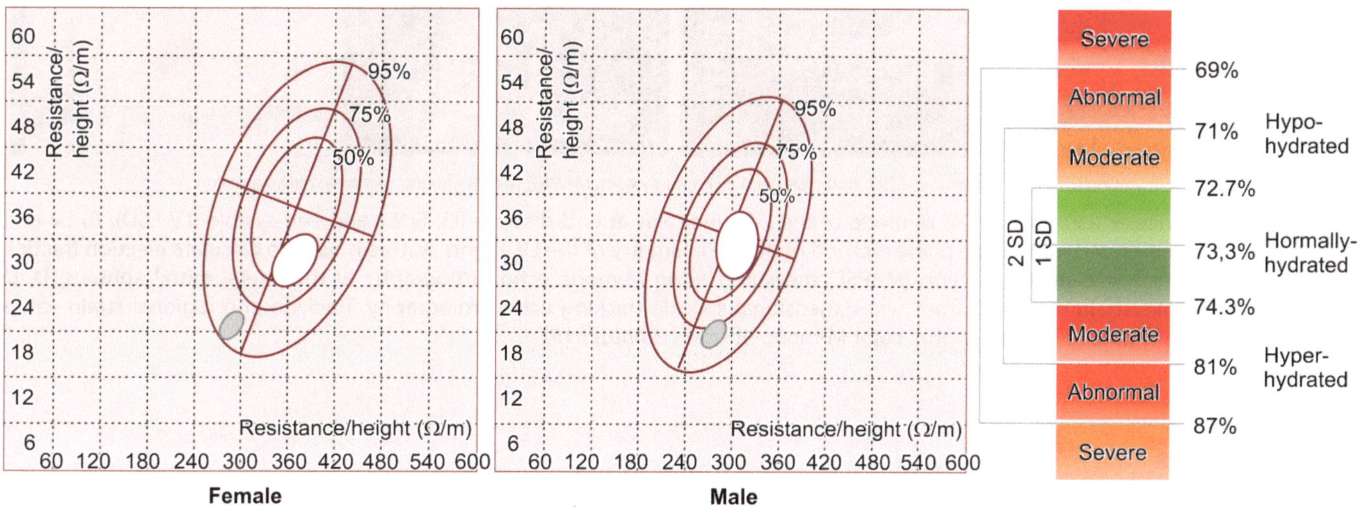

FIG. 3: Vectors' 95% confidence ellipses of congestive patients (gray) and control group (white) for female and for male[26] ***(Chapter 18)***

PLATE 4

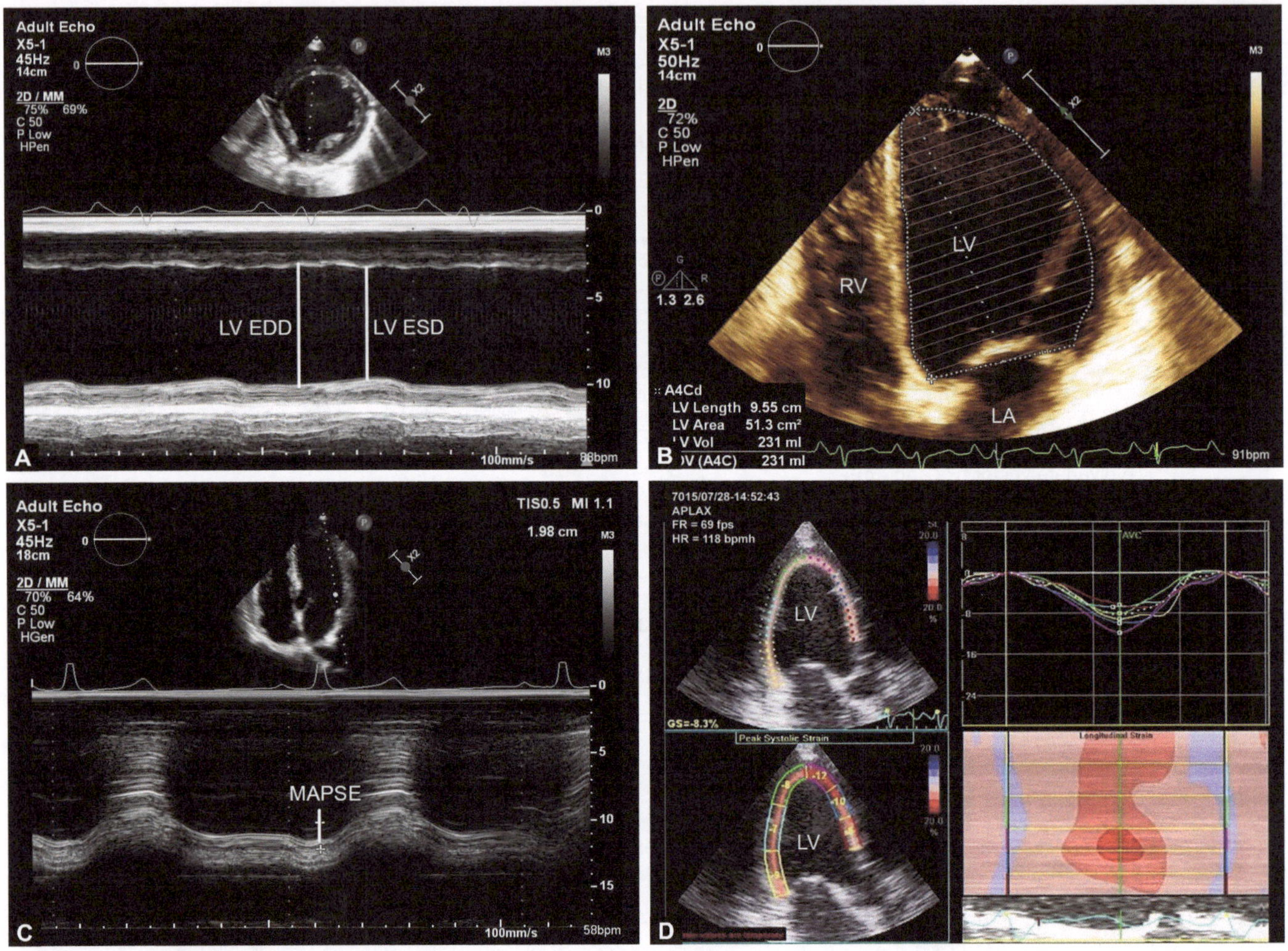

LA, left atrium; RV, right ventricle; LV, left ventricular; EDD, end-diastole; ESD, end-systole; MAPSE; mitral annular plane systolic excursion..

FIG. 1: Left ventricular (LV) function **A,** M-mode of the LV minor axis at end-diastole (LV EDD) and end-systole (LV ESD); **B,** LV end-diastolic volume measured from single plane method of discs. Planimetry of the LV at end-systole is used to calculate ejection fraction; **C,** Mitral annular plane systolic excursion (MAPSE) measured using M-mode echocardiography of the lateral mitral annulus; **D,** LV longitudinal systolic strain measured from two-dimensional speckle tracking echocardiography. Tracking and regional strain values (left), regional strain-time curves (top right), color M-mode of strain ***(Chapter 19)***

PLATE 5

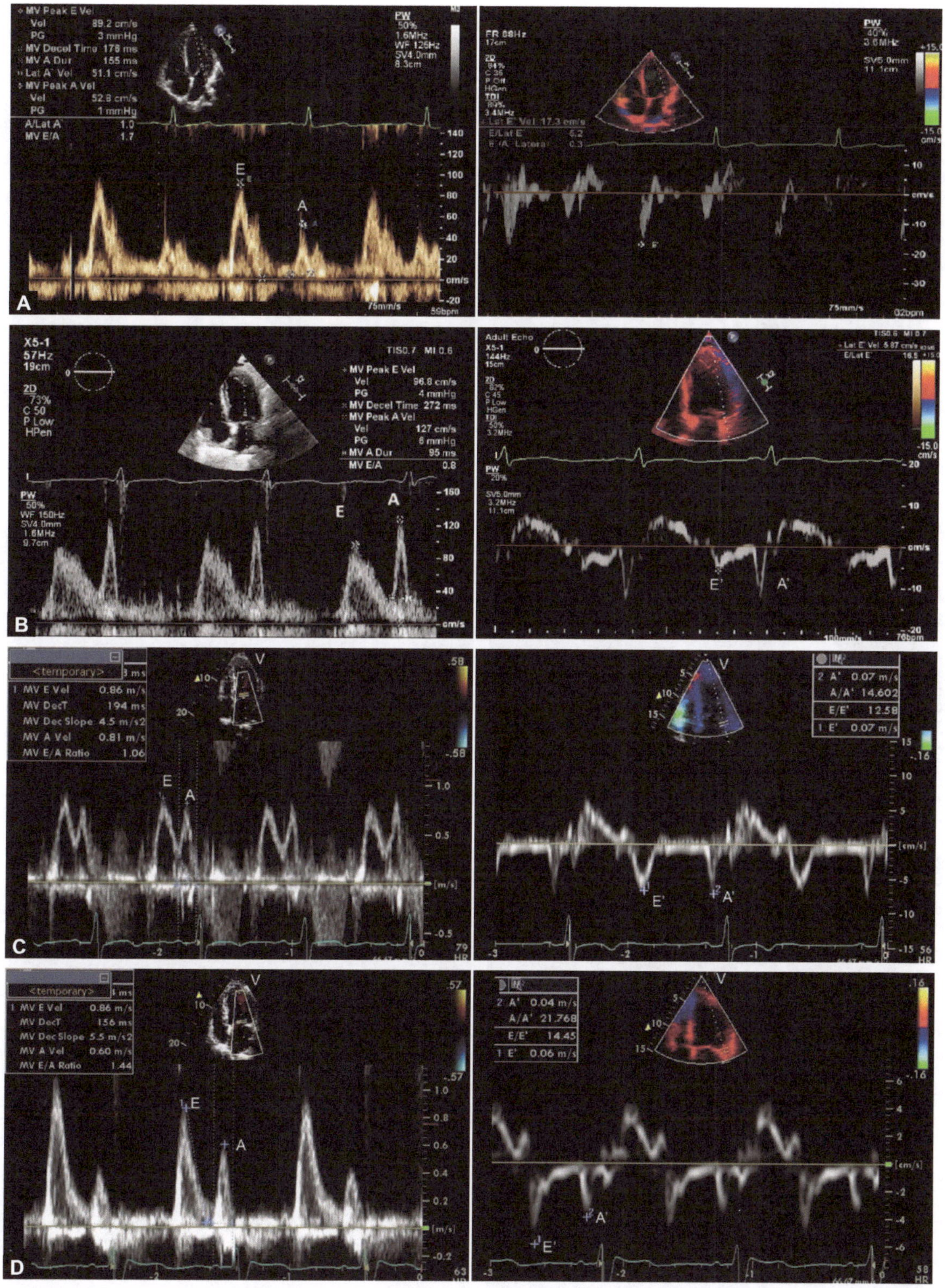

E, early diastolic transmitral flow velocity; A, late diastolic transmitral flow velocity; E′, early diastolic annular velocity; A′, late diastolic annular velocity.

FIG. 2: Transmitral flow (top) and mitral annular tissue velocities (bottom) from patients with **A,** normal diastolic function; **B,** impaired left ventricular (LV) relaxation or grade I diastolic dysfunction (DD); **C,** pseudonormal or grade II DD; and **D,** restrictive filling or grade III DD ***(Chapter 19)***

PLATE 6

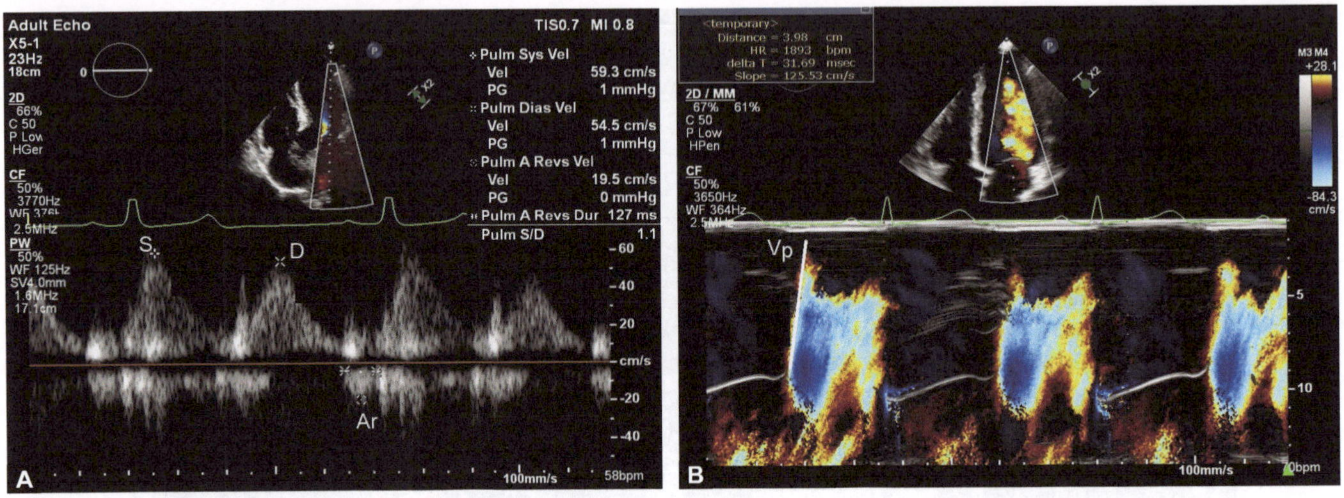

S, systolic PV velocity; D, diastolic PV velocity; Ar, reversed atrial systolic PV velocity.

FIG. 3: Ancillary parameters for grading diastolic dysfunction: **A,** pulmonary venous (PV) Doppler; **B,** flow propagation velocity (Vp) ***(Chapter 19)***

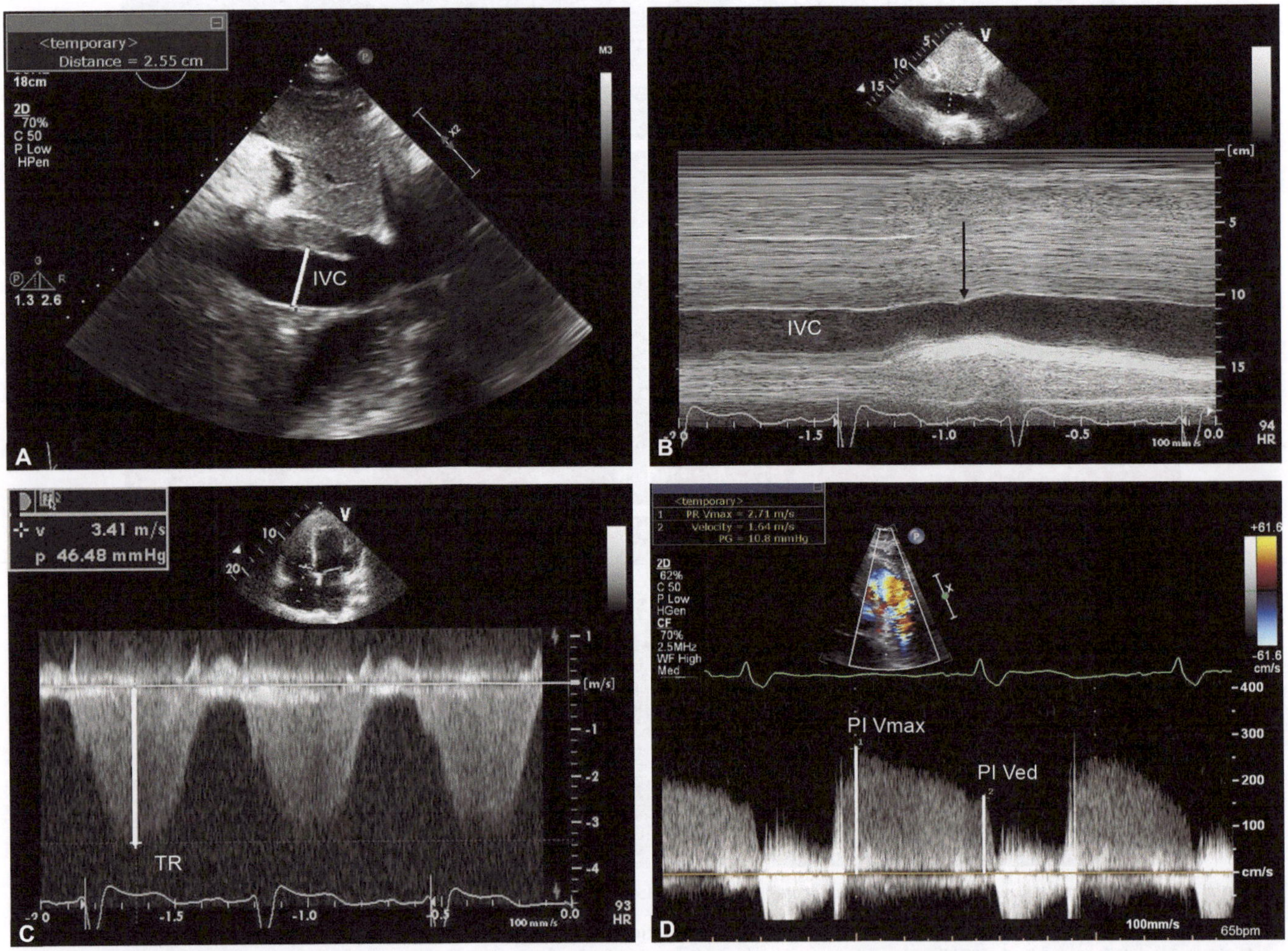

FIG. 4: Doppler-determined right heart pressures: **A,** two-dimensional of the inferior vena cava (IVC); **B,** M-mode of IVC with sniff (arrow); **C,** tricuspid regurgitation (TR) jet used to measure right ventricular (RV) and pulmonary artery (PA) systolic pressure; **D,** pulmonary insufficiency (PI) jet used to measure mean (from PI Vmax, the maximal PI velocity) and end-diastolic PA pressures (from PI Ved, the end-diastolic PI velocity) ***(Chapter 19)***

PLATE 7

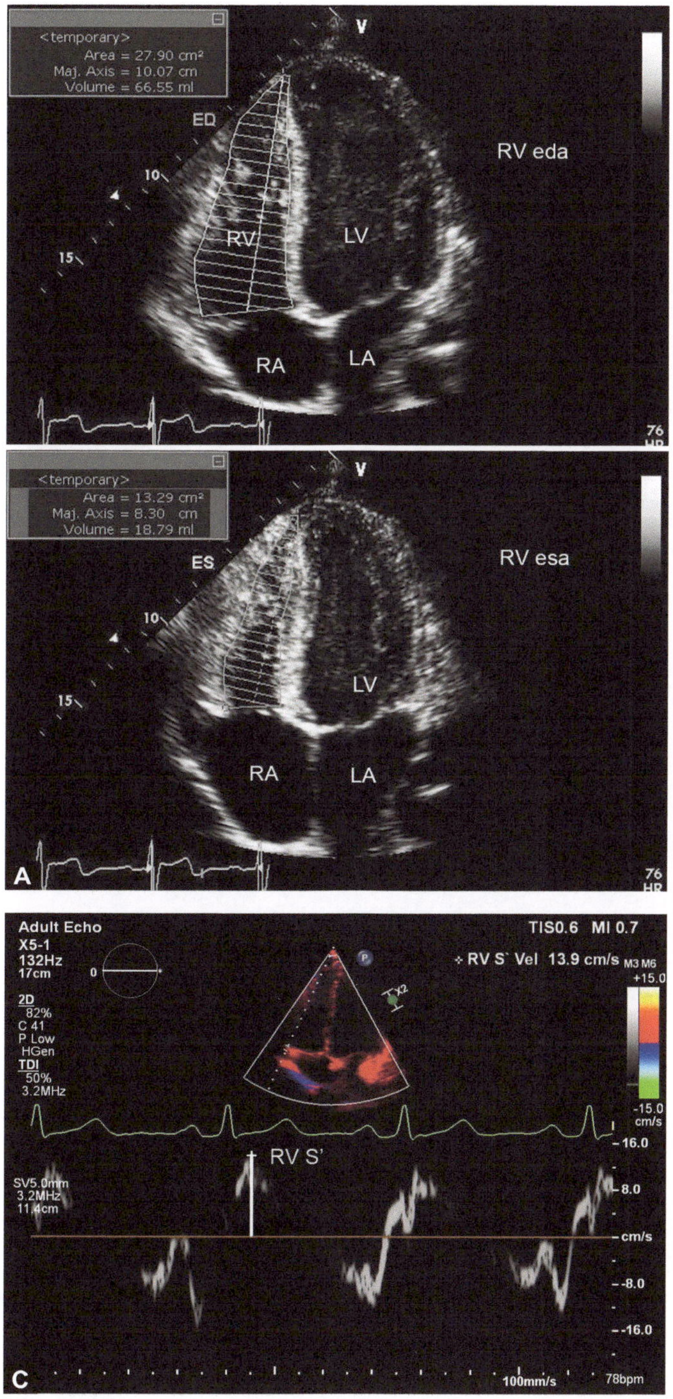

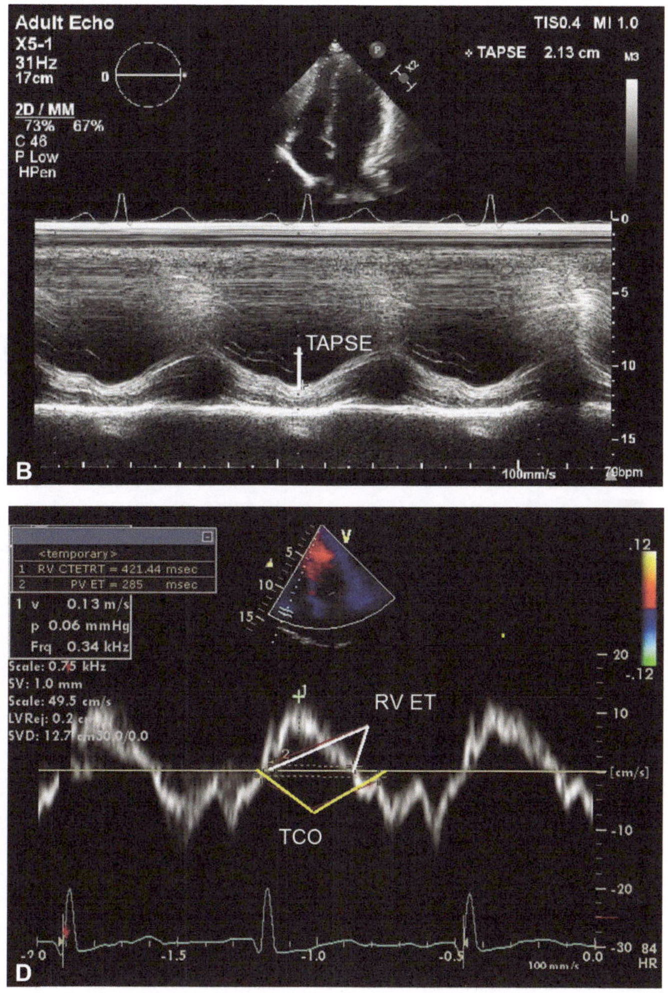

FIG. 6: Right ventricular (RV) functional measurements. **A,** Fractional area change (FAC) measured from RV end-diastolic (RV EDA) and end-systolic areas (RV ESA) in the RV focused view; **B,** tricuspid annular plane systolic excursion (TAPSE) measured from M-mode through the tricuspid lateral annulus; **C,** RV S′, the tricuspid annular systolic tissue velocity; and **D,** right ventricular index of myocardial performance (RIMP); measurements include RV ejection time (RVET) and tricuspid valve closure opening time (TCO). RIMP is calculated as (TCO – RVET)/RVET ***(Chapter 19)***

PLATE 8

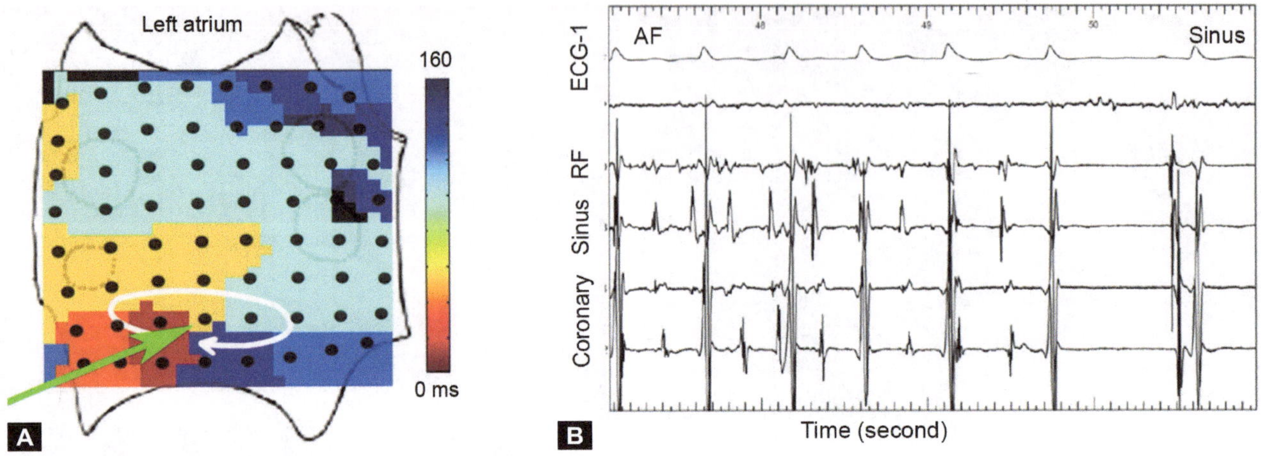

AF, atrial fibrillation; RF, radio frequency; ECG, electrocardiogram.

FIG. 3: Mapping and ablation of localized sources of atrial fibrillation (AF). **A,** Isochronal representation of left atrial electrical activation during AF shows a clockwise rotor (white circular arrow). **B,** Focal ablation at the site indicated by the green arrow terminated AF to sinus rhythm *(Chapter 28)*

SECTION 1

Cardiac Arrest

1

CHAPTER

Cardiac Resuscitation

Jillian B Horning, Caitlin M Kibbey, Joe T Kofoed, Deborah B Diercks

INTRODUCTION

Cardiac arrest has been defined as the cessation of cardiac mechanical activity confirmed by the absence of signs of circulation. Any arrest in an adult is presumed to be of cardiac etiology unless it is known, or likely to have been caused by another noncardiac cause as best determined by the healthcare provider.[1]

Despite important advances in prevention, cardiac arrest continues to affect thousands of individuals each year in both the prehospital and hospital environment. The American Heart Association (AHA) estimates that there were 359,400 adult out-of-hospital cardiac arrests (OHCA) in 2013, with an overall survival rate of 9.5%. This contrasts with the incidence of in-hospital cardiac arrest (IHCA) with an incidence of 209,000 in 2013 and a survival rate of 23.9% in adults.[2] This chapter reviews key components of adult cardiac resuscitation in the prehospital and hospital setting.

CARDIAC ARREST IN THE PREHOSPITAL SETTING

Emergency medical service (EMS) response to cardiac arrest usually begins with a layperson in the community and ends with the transfer of the patient to an emergency department. Over the last three decades, public health initiatives have attempted to improve the outcomes for OHCA. These efforts have focused on layperson education and recognition early activation of EMS, improving access to automated external defibrillation devices [automated external defibrillator (AED)] and increasing public education in cardiopulmonary resuscitation (CPR).[3,4] Due to these efforts, according to the AHA's update report in 2013, 79% of the lay public were confident that they knew what actions to take in a medical emergency, 98% recognized the function of an AED and 60% were familiar with CPR.[2]

Despite the general public familiarity with CPR and AEDs, several studies have shown that the translation of this knowledge into practice remains poor.[5-7] This is of particular importance as the majority of OHCA occur at a patient's home, and less than half of these arrests are witnessed by bystanders.[8]

One of the primary responsibilities of a layperson first responder is to call 911 and activate EMS immediately. Depending on the type of dispatch center contacted, there may be a trained EMS dispatcher who is able to provide bystanders with instructions prior to the arrival of an ambulance. Dispatchers are able to assist nontrained bystanders with recognizing cardiac arrest, providing CPR instructions and aiding with the location of an AED. The guidance provided by EMS dispatchers has been shown to nearly double the rate of bystander CPR.[9]

It is important to recognize that EMS providers have different levels of training and capabilities when treating patients following OHCA. Although differentiating between the various training levels of emergency medical technicians (EMTs) is not the focus of this chapter, medical providers should be aware that EMS systems will vary in the scope of life-saving interventions they are able to provide. These prehospital medical services will include a combination of basic life support (BLS), advanced cardiac life support (ACLS) and advanced airway management.[10] The level of training and care provided in the prehospital setting may have an impact on patient outcomes. Bakalos et al. performed a meta-analysis in 2011 comparing BLS and ACLS and showed an increase in survival for cardiac arrest patients who received ACLS level care in the prehospital setting [odds ratio (OR) = 1.47].[11]

Patient age, gender, initial cardiac rhythm, bystander CPR, and early defibrillation are all variables known to impact outcomes in out-of-hospital cardiac arrest.[12] A patient's socioeconomic status may also have an influence on outcomes. Vaillancourt et al. showed an association between socioeconomic status and rates of bystander CPR, with decreased likeliness of receiving bystander CPR associated with lower socioeconomic status.[13] In addition, a large emphasis has been placed on EMS scene response time for patients with OHCA. This emphasis is appropriate for patients experiencing OHCA due to association between survival rates and the time to arrive by EMS.[14] Even in the setting of a bystander witnessed arrest with initiation of bystander CPR, there is still a strong correlation between patient survival and EMS time of arrival.[15]

Regardless of the location of a cardiac arrest, the basic principles of early recognition, activation of EMS, and prompt decision-making will save lives. Cardiac arrest continues to be an active area of research and many of the accepted practices that were taught and adhered to a decade ago have undergone significant change. The remainder of this chapter will explore the principles and management approaches to optimally treat the cardiac arrest patient.

BASIC RESUSCITATION OF THE ADULT PATIENT

BASIC RESUSCITATION PRINCIPLES

While the resuscitation of a patient in cardiac arrest may seem complex, BLS skills remain the cornerstone of management. The key components that contribute to improved survival following cardiac arrest include immediate recognition of cardiac arrest, initiation of early and high quality chest compressions and rapid defibrillation.[16,17]

Recognition and Initial Management of Cardiac Arrest

The early recognition of cardiac arrest is a key step in initiating appropriate and timely treatment. Unfortunately, recognition is not always straightforward.[16] Cardiac arrest should be suspected when a patient is unresponsive and breathing is absent or is not normal.[18-20] The 2010 AHA guidelines deemphasize checking for breathing and using the pulse check as a mechanism to identify cardiac arrest.[16] Studies have shown that healthcare providers may be unable to accurately identify adequate or normal breathing in unresponsive victims and cannot reliably determine the presence or absence of a pulse.[21-23] Based on the 2010 AHA guidelines, if an adult suddenly collapses or is unresponsive, the healthcare provider should confirm unresponsiveness, activate the emergency response team and take no more than 10 seconds to check for a pulse. If a pulse is not definitely identified within that time period, the provider should immediately start chest compressions.[16]

Once cardiac arrest is recognized and CPR has been initiated, a coordinated team effort involving multiple healthcare personnel should ensue. This coordinated effort is most effective when a single individual (the team leader) is responsible for delegating specific tasks and maintaining an organized approach. Critical initial actions include placement of defibrillator pads and attachment to a cardiac monitor, rhythm identification, obtaining intravenous or intraosseous access, and airway management.

Chest Compressions

Once cardiac arrest has been recognized, the prompt initiation of effective chest compressions is a fundamental aspect of resuscitation.[24] Herlitz et al. demonstrated that even short delays in the initiation of CPR correlated with poor outcomes.[25] Reestablishing blood flow to the vital organs via CPR gives the medical team time to address the primary cause of arrest while improving the patient's chance of survival. The "2010 American Heart Association Guidelines for cardiopulmonary resuscitation and emergency cardiovascular care (AHA guidelines)" recommend the initiation of chest compressions before ventilation (which is illustrated in the acronym change from airway-breathing-circulation or ABC to circulation-airway-breathing or CAB). Chest compressions should be the highest priority when managing a patient in cardiac arrest.[16,26]

Additional studies show that chest compression only CPR provides an equivalent outcome, an equally beneficial outcome to patients in OHCA, and is easier for the untrained layperson to initiate in the field. This has inspired multiple education initiatives, including the "Hands Only CPR" campaign initiated by both the AHA and American Red Cross, and the SHARE (Save Hearts in Arizona Research and Education) program in Arizona.[27,28] Simplification of the arrest algorithm away from airway management with emphasis on compressions increases the likelihood that bystanders will provide life-saving measures to a patient outside of the hospital. Bystander CPR doubles or triples survival from witnessed cardiac arrest.[18]

Effective chest compressions improve the patient's chance of survival by increasing intrathoracic pressure via direct compression of the heart, which generates blood flow and oxygen delivery to the myocardium and brain.[16] Coronary perfusion pressure (CPP, aortic relaxation "diastolic" pressure minus right atrial relaxation "diastolic" pressure) during CPR correlates with both myocardial blood flow and return of spontaneous circulation (ROSC). While the monitoring of CPP during CPR is rarely available clinically, a reasonable surrogate is arterial relaxation (diastolic) pressure, which closely approximates aortic relaxation pressures during CPR in humans and can be measured using an arterial line. Although a specific target arterial relaxation pressure that optimizes the chance of ROSC has not been established, one should try to improve CPR quality, administering a vasopressor, or both if the arterial relaxation pressure is less than 20 mm Hg.[29]

The quality of CPR is a critical determinant of survival in cardiac arrest. Providers should focus on delivering high-quality chest compressions, which include providing chest compressions of adequate rate (at least 100 compressions per minute) and depth (at least 2 inches or 5 cm),[18] allowing complete chest recoil after each compression and minimizing interruptions.[16] Unfortunately, recent investigations have found that resuscitation performance frequently does not meet established guidelines. For instance, Wik et al. reported that 33% of chest compressions were too shallow and were being delivered only 48% of the time during OHCA resuscitations.[30] Abella et al. found similar deficiencies during in-hospital arrest care; 23% of chest compressions were with incorrect rates and 36% of chest compressions were too shallow.[31]

The importance of high-quality chest compressions cannot be overemphasized. Minimal interruption of chest compressions is a critically important element of CPR quality. Even short pauses in chest compressions decrease CPP, defibrillation success and survival.[16] Rescuer fatigue may lead to inadequate compression rates and/or depth and the person providing chest compressions should be changed every 2 minutes regardless of endurance (or after five cycles of compressions and ventilations at a ratio of 30:2) to ensure high-quality CPR.[16]

Manual versus Mechanical Chest Compressions

Chest compressions can be performed either manually or with the use of a mechanical device such as the LUCAS or a load-distributing band (LDB). These mechanical devices were developed to assist EMS personnel in delivering high-quality compressions, and studies have shown that these devices are as effective as manual compressions and safer for EMS personnel during transport. However, the majority of investigations have shown no improvement in patient outcomes with the use of these devices.[32-37] The largest randomized controlled trials (RCTs) show either no or minimal benefit in survival to hospital discharge and favorable neurologic outcomes; with one RCT demonstrating worse neurologic outcomes at hospital discharge in the LDB arm (in comparison to manual CPR).[30,38,39]

Given the equivocal results of research into the use of such devices, there are no clear recommendations for the replacement of manual CPR. However, the availability of such devices may be useful when consistent compressions may be difficult, for instance in a moving ambulance or in preparation for extracorporeal cardiopulmonary resuscitation [ECPR, also referred to as emergency department extracorporeal membrane oxygenation (ED ECMO)] or in locations with a shortage of personnel.[40] Providers should be familiar with the specific devices utilized in their region of practice in order to fully coordinate resuscitation efforts.

Rhythm Identification

The importance of rhythm identification in cardiac arrest cannot be overemphasized. The most reliable predictor of ROSC is the presence of a shockable rhythm. Shockable rhythms, include ventricular fibrillation (VF) and pulseless ventricular tachycardia (VT). Ventricular fibrillation is characterized by disorganized chaotic electrical activity whereas VT is characterized by an organized ventricular rhythm. Pulseless electrical activity (PEA) and asystole are nonshockable rhythms. Pulseless electrical activity is defined by an organized electrical rhythm associated with the absence of effective mechanical function. Asystole is characterized by the absence of electrical cardiac activity.[29] Of note, fine VF may appear similar to asystole in some leads. Orthogonal leads (lead I and aVF or lead II and aVL) should be monitored in order to differentiate these two rhythms.

The management algorithm for VF/VT and PEA/asystole is depicted in flowchart 1.

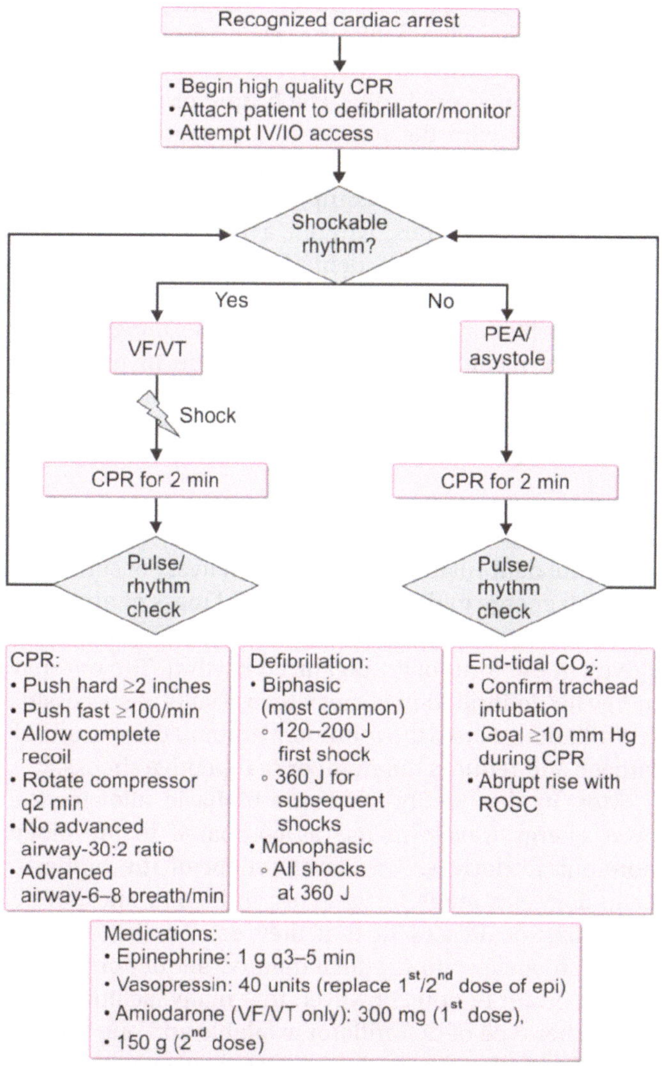

CPR, cardiopulmonary resuscitation; IO, intraosseous; IV, intravenous; PEA, pulseless electrical activity; ROSC, return of spontaneous circulation; VF, ventricular fibrillation; VT, ventricular tachycardia.

FLOWCHART 1: Management algorithm for shockable and nonshockable rhythms

DEFIBRILLATION

The most survivable rhythms in cardiac arrest are those responsive to defibrillation. These rhythms are typically identified as VT and VF. A study in the Annals of Emergency Medicine in 2010 showed that 23% of out-of-hospital arrests were found to be in either VF or VT.[41] Patients with IHCA are more likely to have an initial cardiac rhythm of PEA or asystole, but can progress to VF/VT during resuscitation attempts.[42] In patients found to have VF/VT, the rate of survival decreases by 3–4% every minute from the time of cardiac arrest to defibrillation. Deployment of public access AEDs in the out-of-hospital setting has significantly decreased the time to defibrillation delay, functionally removing the wait time of EMS call response.[43]

When VF/VT is identified on rhythm analysis, rapid defibrillation is essential to improving survival. The first provider who arrives to the patient should perform CPR via chest compressions while the second provider charges the defibrillator. Once the defibrillator is charged, CPR is momentarily paused during which time providers avoid direct contact with the patient in anticipation of shock delivery. The second provider should then administer a single shock and chest compressions are immediately resumed for 2 minutes, without a pause for a rhythm or pulse check. Even if defibrillation is successful, it is rare to appreciate a palpable pulse immediately after defibrillation and the delay in performing a pulse check may result in further insult to the myocardium if a perfusing rhythm has not been restored.[17] After 2 minutes, the sequence is repeated, beginning with a rhythm check.[16]

Waveform and Energy Level

Successful defibrillation requires the delivery of sufficient electrical energy to depolarize a critical mass of excitable cells simultaneously, restoring synchronized electrical activity in the form of an organized rhythm. The optimal energy for defibrillation is that which results in successful defibrillation, causes the minimum amount of myocardial damage and reduces the number of repetitive shocks.[16]

Most modern defibrillators are biphasic, allowing for lower energy waveform use as compared to the older monophasic devices. The development of the biphasic technology has made for ease of production and public availability of devices in that they are smaller, lighter, and often cheaper to produce than earlier defibrillators. It is important to note, however, that many facilities may have either type of defibrillator available and one should be familiar with distinguishing factors between the two in order to utilize them properly.[44]

The optimal initial energy dose using a biphasic device has not been determined. Based on an animal model, high-energy biphasic shocks (360 J) do not cause more cardiac damage or decrease cardiac function after prolonged VF when compared to low-energy biphasic shocks (150 J).[45] However, the 2010 AHA guidelines recommend a starting dose of 120–200 J using a biphasic defibrillator and escalating levels of energy for subsequent shocks. When using a monophasic defibrillator, both the initial and subsequent shocks should be performed using 360 J. Cardiopulmonary resuscitation should be reinitiated immediately following delivery of the shock and the pulse and rhythm checked after 2 minutes (or five cycles of chest compressions). There has been little evidence that resuming compressions after return of an organized rhythm prior to a pulse check will adversely affect patient outcome.[6] Table 1 displays the optimal recommended defibrillation energy doses, which varies depending on whether the device utilizes a monophasic or biphasic waveform.

TABLE 1: Defibrillation energy levels recommended for biphasic and monophasic defibrillators

Waveform	Defibrillation energy level (Joules)
Biphasic	120–200 J for initial shock, escalate energy level for subsequent shocks (maximum dose of 360 J)
Monophasic	360 J for initial and subsequent shocks

Automated External Defibrillators in the Prehospital Setting

Defibrillation is also an important component of the resuscitation of cardiac arrest patients by lay rescuers and involves the use of an AED in the prehospital setting. An AED is a reliable computerized device that analyzes the cardiac rhythm and uses voice and visual prompts to guide lay rescuers and healthcare professionals to safely deliver a shock if VF or VT is detected.[18] The use of these devices by laypersons has shown to increase the rate of survival in the out-of-hospital setting.[46]

Lay rescuers can be trained to safely and effectively use AEDs, which are increasingly available in public places and make it possible to defibrillate many minutes before the medical team arrives. Laypersons and first responders should continue CPR while applying an AED and follow the voice prompts immediately as they are received, which include resuming CPR immediately following defibrillation.

Special Circumstances

The optimal defibrillation technique involves delivery of current across the myocardium in the setting of minimal transthoracic impedance. Shock delivery can be impeded by multiple factors including body habitus, excessive body hair, medication patches, and the presence of a pacemaker or automatic implantable cardioverter-defibrillator (AICD). In these situations, the provider should aim to place the defibrillator pads in an optimal position to minimize transthoracic impedance. Transdermal medication patches may prevent adequate electrode contact and should be removed prior to electrode placement.[47] In heavily hirsute patients, it may be necessary to shave or remove hair prior to attachment. In cases of refractory VF or where excess tissue causes an increase in transthoracic impedance (e.g., morbid obesity) additional measures may need to be taken. There has been some research into the application of a second pair of defibrillator pads and delivering simultaneous shocks at maximum energy to increase current flow, but this has not shown any effect on survival outcomes.[48] Pacemakers and implantable cardioverter-defibrillators (ICDs) may be damaged during defibrillation if an electrode is placed and discharged directly over the device. In patients with an ICD or pacemaker, the defibrillator pads should be placed on the chest wall ideally at least 8 cm from the generator position. The anterior-posterior and anterior-lateral pad placements on the chest are acceptable.

AIRWAY MANAGEMENT

Providers in both the in-hospital and out-of-hospital settings often focus on early invasive airway management; however, current literature highlights the importance of other resuscitation actions.[49] Based on the 2010 AHA guidelines, the initiation of chest compressions are now recommended before ventilations (CAB rather than ABC).[16] This emphasis highlights the importance of chest compressions and emphasizes the fact that airway maneuvers should be performed quickly and efficiently so that interruptions in chest compressions are minimized.

Evidence to support the routine use of any specific approach to airway management during cardiac arrest is sparse.[17] No advanced airway intervention has been shown to increase survival to hospital discharge after cardiac arrest.[12,17,50] Endotracheal intubation was once considered the ideal approach to airway management during cardiac arrest.[17] There is increasing evidence that prolonged attempts at intubation are frequently associated with interruption of chest compressions, which may lead to decreased coronary and cerebral perfusion during this critical time period.[17,29] The optimal approach to airway management during cardiac arrest depends on the specific circumstances of the arrest and the experience of the provider.

The ventilation strategy during cardiac arrest depends on whether or not an advanced airway is present. The AHA guidelines recommend that CPR be performed in cycles of 30 compressions to 2 ventilations until an advanced airway is established. If two providers are present and a bag-valve-mask is being utilized, two breaths should be given following every 30 chest compressions. Once an advanced airway is in place, one breath should be given every 6–8 seconds (8–10 ventilations per min) while compressions are ongoing.[51] Chest compressions should not be paused in order to secure an airway unless absolutely necessary.

Airway Management in the Prehospital Setting

Recommendations for airway management and assisted ventilation during CPR vary based on the location, resources and level of training of providers on scene. The evidence for specific airway management strategies in cardiac arrest for EMS providers trained in advanced life support (ALS) remains elusive. There have been large conflicting studies showing both negative and positive associations with survival with the use of prehospital advanced airways.[52-55] A 2014 meta-analysis suggests that the current published literature contains too many confounders to draw any meaningful conclusions for the use of advanced airways during prehospital care, and additional prospective studies should be performed.[56]

Alternatives to Tracheal Intubation

The most basic approach to airway management during cardiac arrest is the use of bag-valve-mask ventilation. Bag-valve-mask ventilation is most effective when performed by two experienced providers. One rescuer opens the airway and seals the mask to the face while the other rescuer provides breaths by squeezing the bag. The provider should deliver ventilations during pauses in compressions and each breath should be delivered over 1 second with an adequate volume to produce visible chest rise.[16]

Supraglottic airway (SGA) devices such as the laryngeal mask airway (LMA), the esophageal-tracheal tube (combitube), and the laryngeal tube have been studied during vivo and manikin simulated CPR as an alternative to tracheal intubation. Contrary to endotracheal intubation, insertion of a SGA does not require visualization of the glottis, and therefore, these devices can be inserted without interruption of chest compressions.[29] Numerous studies have demonstrated that the SGA devices perform as well as, or better, than tracheal intubation with respect to successful insertion and/or time to insertion or to ventilation.[47] Based on the 2010 International Liaison Committee on Resuscitation (ILCOR) Consensus on Science and Treatment Recommendations, the insertion of an SGA is a reasonable alternative to endotracheal intubation and can be done successfully with minimal interruptions in chest compressions. Providers may consider extraglottic device use for airway management during cardiac arrest and as a rescue airway in a difficult or failed tracheal intubation.[47]

Timing of Advanced Airway Placement

The optimal timing of advanced airway placement in relation to other interventions during resuscitation from cardiac arrest, both in and out-of-hospital, is not well-defined.[47] Based on a study of approximately 25,000 IHCAs, earlier time to advanced airway placement (<5 min) was not associated with ROSC, but was associated with a slightly improved survival at 24 hours.[29,49] There are no prospective studies that directly assess whether early versus later airway placement during cardiac arrest has any effect on outcomes.

END-TIDAL CARBON DIOXIDE AND CAPNOGRAPHY

Capnography involves the continuous monitoring of the partial pressure of end-tidal carbon dioxide ($ETCO_2$), which is displayed graphically as a waveform and a number. Capnography is a direct measurement of lung ventilation, but also indirectly measures circulation. When ventilation is relatively constant, $ETCO_2$ correlates well with cardiac output during CPR.[29] For instance, during a state of low cardiac output (such as cardiac arrest), decreased pulmonary blood flow results in an abrupt decrease in $ETCO_2$.[57,58] During cardiac arrest, the level of $ETCO_2$ is determined entirely by the cardiac output generated by CPR.[59]

UTILITY OF CAPNOGRAPHY

Capnography is now considered the optimal method for monitoring the quality of chest compressions and identifying ROSC during cardiac arrest. Multiple studies have shown that persistently low $ETCO_2$ values (<10 mm Hg) during CPR in intubated patients correlate with a very low likelihood of achieving ROSC.[58,60-64] The height of the CO_2 waveform during CPR, which is a function of cardiac output during chest compressions, should be monitored.[59] A low $ETCO_2$ value (<10 mm Hg) during cardiac arrest indicates inadequate CPR and the provider should attempt to improve the quality of chest compressions.[60] In addition to monitoring the quality of CPR, capnography may be used to identify ROSC during cardiac arrest. Multiple studies have demonstrated that an abrupt increase in $ETCO_2$ values to levels of 35–40 during CPR suggests ROSC.[60,65-67] Based on the AHA expert panel recommendations, the provider should perform high-quality CPR and avoid excessive ventilation with a goal of achieving an $ETCO_2$ value greater than 20 mm Hg.[68]

Prediction of Outcome

Increasing data suggests that capnography may be used as an objective measure to predict outcome in cardiac arrest.[47,61,67] Levine et al. found that an $ETCO_2$ level less than 10 mm Hg measured 20 minutes after the initiation of ACLS accurately predicts death. At present, there is insufficient evidence to recommend a specific cutoff of $ETCO_2$ as a prognostic indicator during cardiac arrest.[47]

MEDICATION ADMINISTRATION

Drug administration is of secondary importance during cardiac arrest, with primary resuscitation efforts focused on basic CPR and early defibrillation. Only a few of the drugs used in the treatment of cardiac arrest are supported by evidence and no drug has been definitively shown to increase survival to hospital discharge in patients with cardiac arrest.[69]

While the management of VF/VT relies primarily on early defibrillation and the management of asystole/PEA on identifying a reversible cause of the arrest, the ACLS guidelines recommend the use of epinephrine (or vasopressin) and amiodarone as additional therapies within the cardiac arrest algorithms. The commonly used ACLS medications and drug doses are given in table 2.

Vasopressors

Epinephrine is the main drug utilized in cardiac arrest. Epinephrine has combined α-adrenergic and β-adrenergic effects and increases coronary and cerebral perfusion pressure during CPR primarily through its α-adrenergic properties (i.e., vasoconstriction). After beginning CPR and attempting defibrillation, providers should establish intravenous/intraosseous access and consider vasopressor administration. In patients with PEA or asystole, epinephrine 1 mg intravenous/intraosseous should be administered every 3–5 minutes during CPR while attempting to identify and correct reversible causes. The administration of one dose of vasopressin (40 units intravenous/intraosseous) may replace either the first or second dose of epinephrine. In cases of VF/VT, there is inadequate evidence regarding the optimal number of CPR cycles and defibrillation attempts that should be performed prior to initiation of drug therapy. Based on expert consensus, the AHA recommends the administration of a vasopressor if VF/VT persists after the first or second defibrillation attempts.[69]

TABLE 2: Advanced cardiac life support medications and recommended drug doses

Vasopressors	Antiarrhythmics
Epinephrine 1 mg IV/IO q3–5 min	Amiodarone 300 mg IV/IO initial dose, then 150 mg IV/IO for subsequent dose
Vasopressin 40 units IV/IO (may replace 1st or 2nd dose of epinephrine)	Lidocaine 1–1.5 mg/kg IV/IO initial dose, may be given additional 0.5–0.75 mg/kg (maximum of 3 mg/kg)

IV, intravenous; IO, intraosseous.

Some studies have indicated that vasopressin improves coronary artery perfusion pressure compared to epinephrine,[70] and in rats it has been shown to be associated with less neuronal apoptosis. [71] There has been no evidence to date that vasopressin compared to epinephrine improves patient based outcomes. In addition, one randomized trial using a combination of epinephrine, vasopressin, and steroids showed improved neurologic outcomes when used during CPR, however, further studies are needed to validate these findings.[72]

Antiarrhythmics

There is no evidence that any antiarrhythmic drug given during cardiac arrest increases survival to hospital discharge. Amiodarone has been shown to increase short-term survival to hospital admission when compared with placebo or lidocaine.[69] The Resuscitation Outcomes Consortium-Amiodarone, Lidocaine or Placebo Study (ROC-ALPS) is an ongoing double-blinded randomized trial comparing the effectiveness of amiodarone, lidocaine and placebo in OHCA due to shock-refractory VF/VT.[71]

When VF/VT persists after two or three shocks and administration of a vasopressor, the provider should consider administration of amiodarone (initial dose of 300 mg intravenous/intraosseous, subsequent dose of 150 mg intravenous/intraosseous). If amiodarone is not available or if the provider encounters refractory VF/VT, lidocaine may be considered. In the setting of torsades de pointes associated with a long QT interval, the provider should consider administration of magnesium 1–2 g intravenously.[69]

The most commonly recommended vasopressors and antiarrhythmics are illustrated in table 2.

ASSESSMENT AND TREATMENT OF REVERSIBLE CAUSES OF CARDIAC ARREST

When a primary electrical cause for cardiac arrest is identified, definitive treatment is generally directed at reversing the electrical abnormality (i.e., defibrillation). In contrast, when a nonelectrical cause of cardiac arrest is being managed (i.e., PEA/asystole), medical providers should recall the H's and T's to identify the most common reversible causes of cardiac arrest. Pulseless electrical activity is often caused by reversible conditions and can be treated successfully if these conditions are identified and corrected, otherwise the prognosis is poor.[73]

H's

If ***hypoxia*** is the suspected etiology of cardiac arrest, the provider must ensure that the patient's airway is patent and there is adequate chest rise and bilateral breath sounds with ventilation. The placement of an advanced airway should be considered to ensure adequate oxygenation and ventilation during CPR.

If cardiac arrest is associated with extreme volume loss, ***hypovolemia*** should be suspected. In this case, management should consist of intravenous/intraosseous crystalloid administration and consideration of a blood transfusion if severe blood loss is suspected (for instance, gastrointestinal bleeding or rupture of an aortic aneurysm).[47]

Hyperkalemia, ***hypokalemia***, ***hypoglycemia***, and other electrolyte abnormalities are detected by lab tests or suggested by the patient's medical history. Targeted therapy in these situations is aided immensely by clinical history and availability of rapid lab results through point-of-care testing or blood gas analysis. ***Hyperkalemia*** is the most common electrolyte disorder associated with cardiopulmonary arrest and should be suspected in any patient with a wide-complex arrhythmia. Immediate initial therapy consists of administration of either calcium gluconate or calcium chloride to stabilize the cardiac membrane. Other temporizing measures aimed at shifting potassium intracellularly include intravenous insulin, sodium bicarbonate and albuterol. Definitive treatment with hemodialysis should be considered once the patient is stabilized. If ***hypoglycemia*** is suspected, 1 ampule of 50% dextrose should be administered or 1 mg of intramuscular glucagon if intravenous access has not been obtained.

Acidosis (***hydrogen ions, H+***) is a frequent cause of cardiac arrest and is associated with a variety of clinical conditions, including septic shock, diabetic ketoacidosis, renal failure causing uremia, and ingestion of toxic agents or drug overdose, such as, aspirin, ethylene glycol and other alcohols, tricyclic antidepressants, or isoniazid. When acidosis is suspected, serum alkalinization with sodium bicarbonate may be considered while the underlying cause of the acidosis is identified and definitively addressed. In select cases, hemodialysis may be warranted once the patient has been stabilized.

Hypothermia should be considered in all drowning cases or when history suggests an environmental exposure. The hypothermic patient may be unresponsive to drug therapy and attempted electrical pacing and defibrillation. In cardiac arrest patients with severe hypothermia (core temperature <30°C), active internal rewarming is the recommended modality to raise the core temperature. Techniques for rewarming include administration of warmed, humidified oxygen, warmed intravenous fluids, peritoneal lavage with warmed fluids, pleural lavage with warm saline via chest tubes, and extracorporeal rewarming with partial bypass and cardiopulmonary bypass.[69] Patients who suffer a cardiac arrest as a result of hypothermia should not be pronounced dead until they are rewarmed.

T's

Tension pneumothorax may be the primary cause of cardiac arrest and the diagnosis is made clinically (i.e., tracheal deviation, absent breath sounds). If suspected, tension pneumothorax should be managed with emergent needle decompression, followed by tube thoracostomy.

*Cardiac **tamponade*** can be difficult to diagnose in the setting of cardiac arrest because the traditional clinical features of Beck's triad (elevated jugular venous pressure, muffled heart sounds and hypotension) may not be evident. However, the increasing use of bedside ultrasound is making the diagnosis of cardiac tamponade much more reliable.[73] When tamponade is suspected, immediate pericardiocentesis should be performed, preferably with ultrasound guidance.

Acute pulmonary ***thrombosis*** and coronary ***thrombosis*** are common causes of cardiac arrest. Routine use of thrombolytic therapy is not recommended in cardiac arrest.[29] However, when cardiac arrest is due to known or suspected massive pulmonary embolism (PE), empiric fibrinolytic therapy should be considered.[17] A reasonable treatment regimen for presumed massive PE in the setting or cardiac arrest is alteplase (tPA) 0.6–1.0 mg/kg bolus (maximum dose of 100 mg).[74,75] Some studies suggest that resuscitative efforts following thrombolytic administration should be continued for a minimum of 30 minutes, or until ROSC is achieved, in order to allow time for the medication to have an effect. Acute myocardial infarction should be strongly considered in cases of refractory VF/pulseless VT. Reperfusion strategies including immediate percutaneous coronary intervention (PCI) or thrombolysis should be considered once the patient has been stabilized.

A variety of ***toxins***, including medications and illicit drugs, can precipitate cardiac arrest. Some of the more common agents include tricyclic antidepressants (TCAs), digoxin, β-blockers and calcium channel blockers. Cardiac arrest due to toxicity should be managed based on the standard ACLS algorithm. In the majority of cases, there are no unique antidotes or toxin-specific interventions that are recommended during the management of cardiac arrest. Once ROSC is achieved, the provider should consider administration of specific antidotes when indicated and urgent consultation with a medical toxicologist or certified regional poison center is recommended.[76]

The most common H's and T's contributing to cardiac arrest are listed in table 3, along with the recommended treatment interventions that should be considered in these specific scenarios.

TABLE 3: Reversible causes of cardiac arrest (H's and T's) and treatment considerations

H's and T's	Treatment considerations
Hyperkalemia	• Calcium chloride/gluconate 2 g IV (cardiac membrane stabilization) • Additional therapy ○ Regular insulin 10 units/D50 1 ampule ○ Albuterol 10–20 mg (nebulized) ○ Consider hemodialysis once patient stabilized
Hypoglycemia	• D50 1 ampule • Glucagon 1 mg IM (if IV access has not been obtained)
Tension pneumothorax	• Needle decompression with 14 g angiocatheter in 2nd intercostal space, midclavicular line follow by tube thoracostomy
Cardiac tamponade	• Pericardiocentesis ± ultrasound guidance • 18 g spinal needle and 20–60 cc syringe • Subxiphoid approach, aim towards left shoulder and aspirate while advancing needle
Pulmonary embolism	• tPA 0.6–1.0 mg/kg IV bolus (100 mg maximum dose)
Myocardial infarction	• ≤67 kg: tPA 15 mg IV over 1–2 min, then 0.75 mg/kg IV over 30 min (max 50 mg), then 0.5 mg/kg IV over next 60 min (max 30 mg) • >67 kg: tPA 15 mg IV over 1–2 min, then 50 mg over 30 min, then 35 mg over final 60 min (100 mg total over 1.5 h)

IV, intravenous; IO, intraosseous; tPA, tissue plasminogen activator.

ADDITIONAL ADJUNCTS

Once cardiac arrest has been identified and emergency response services have been activated, the medical team is then tasked with resuscitating the patient using a variety of interventions. The most common interventions are those addressed in the ACLS pathway provided by the AHA. Though traditional ACLS algorithms have been in place for many years, additional diagnostic and therapeutic adjuncts are gaining popularity and are becoming increasingly available to medical practitioners within the hospital setting, including bedside echocardiography and ECMO.

Ultrasound

The appropriate application and interpretation of bedside ultrasound can aid the provider in identifying many of the potentially reversible causes of cardiac arrest while guiding potentially life-saving therapeutic interventions.[73] Echocardiography can be used to identify diastolic collapse of the right ventricle in cases of cardiac tamponade and can also provide evidence of a massive PE by demonstrating right ventricular dilatation or McConnell's sign (akinesis of the right ventricular mid-wall with sparing of the apex).[77] In cases of cardiac tamponade, pericardiocentesis should be performed using ultrasound to guide the optimal approach. In addition, ultrasound can be used to rapidly identify a pneumothorax, which is suggested when lung sliding is absent.

Ultrasound can also assist the provider in making the decision to terminate resuscitative measures in the setting of cardiac arrest. Emergency physicians who are trained in ultrasound may use it during pulse checks to determine the presence or absence of cardiac activity. Based on a meta-analysis examining the accuracy of focused echo as a prognostic tool during cardiac arrest, only 2.4% of patients with cardiac standstill on ultrasound will go on to achieve ROSC.[78] These findings suggest that, while not perfect, the absence of cardiac motion on ultrasound can be used in conjunction with other clinical findings when making the decision to terminate resuscitation efforts.

Extracorporeal Membrane Oxygenation

Another promising technology in development is the use of ECMO in the emergency department (also known as ED ECMO or ECPR). In ECPR, a large bore catheter is placed in femoral vein using ultrasound guidance, allowing blood flow into a portable device that removes carbon dioxide and adds oxygen, then returns the oxygenated blood to the patient through a catheter in the femoral artery. It is thought to be most applicable to the arresting patient in whom the underlying cause is likely to be reversible by a specific intervention such as PCI or coronary artery bypass grafting (CABG) and for whom traditional ACLS interventions remain ineffective. In an initial study, five of eight patients who underwent successful ED ECMO survived with good neurological outcome.[79] Despite these promising results, use of the technique is limited due to cost of equipment as well as availability of trained personnel in both the ED and ICU settings.

CARDIAC ARREST IN SPECIAL SITUATIONS

CARDIAC ARREST ASSOCIATED WITH PREGNANCY

Maternal cardiac arrest during pregnancy is particularly challenging due to the concurrent management of two critically ill patients, the mother and unborn baby. The provider should focus on maternal resuscitation, as maternal survival offers the best hope for survival of the fetus.[76] The standard ACLS algorithm should be followed; however, there are several important considerations that should be taken into account when managing cardiac arrest in pregnancy.

Patient Positioning

The positioning of the pregnant patient during cardiac arrest is of the utmost importance in ensuring high-quality CPR. The gravid uterus causes compression of the inferior vena cava (IVC), which may impede venous return and reduce cardiac output. Left uterine displacement (LUD) is recommended after 20 weeks gestation or if the uterus is palpable at or above the umbilicus in order to minimize IVC compression.[76] Left uterine displacement is optimally performed by the provider using two hands from the left side of the patient to pull the uterus leftward and upward. Another approach is to have the provider apply displacement from the right side of the patient by pushing with one or both hands, although this is technically more difficult to perform adequately. Tilting the patient 30° to the left can also be used to provide LUD; however, this position may affect the quality of chest compressions.[76]

Perimortem Cesarean Delivery

The decision to proceed with perimortem cesarean delivery (PMCD) should occur within minutes of the cardiac arrest. The healthcare team should actively prepare for expedited delivery as soon as maternal cardiac arrest is recognized and the obstetric and neonatal teams should be activated. At 25 weeks gestation, the best chance of infant survival occurs when delivery is performed no more than 5 minutes after the onset of cardiac arrest. Providers should continue CPR and attempt to make the incision within 4 minutes from the start of cardiac arrest if ROSC has not been achieved.[76] Discussion of this procedure is beyond the scope of this text. Although definitive evidence is lacking, PMCD may provide the best option to improve the chance of ROSC and maternal survival.[80-82]

CARDIAC ARREST AND LEFT VENTRICULAR ASSIST DEVICES

Left ventricular assist devices (LVADs) are surgically implanted mechanical devices used for the treatment of advanced heart failure. They can be used as a bridge to either recovery, cardiac transplantation or as long-term destination therapy.[83] As the number of patients with LVADs increases each year, an understanding of the optimal resuscitative strategy of this patient population becomes increasingly important.[84]

Left ventricular assist devices patients possess a unique physiology and anatomy, which makes the management of the LVAD patient in cardiac arrest particularly challenging and complex. An in-depth discussion of LVAD anatomy, physiology and a comprehensive guide to device interrogation is beyond the scope of this text. One unique difference in newer generation LVADs is that the patient will often not have a palpable peripheral pulse, as continuous-flow LVADs have largely replaced pulsatile-flow devices. This difference makes determination of an "arrest state" difficult in the LVAD population and following the standard outline of ACLS may be problematic in these patients.[84]

The initiation of chest compressions in LVAD patients is controversial. Many guidelines, both prehospital and inhospital, recommend against performing chest compressions on a patient with an LVAD. Fears of cannula dislodgment or damage to the outflow conduit are the primary concerns in this subset of patients. However, there is now a growing body of evidence that supports the safe initiation of chest compressions in LVAD patients with the newer generation devices. A recently published small retrospective case series reported on eight LVAD patients that received CPR; none of the eight patients receiving chest compressions had cannula dislodgment.[84]

Numerous institutions have developed their own protocols for the management of critically ill LVAD patients; however, none have been validated or certified by the AHA. More research is needed to determine the safety and efficacy of chest compressions in the arresting LVAD patient.

THERAPEUTIC HYPOTHERMIA

In patients found to have an initial cardiac rhythm amenable to defibrillation and ROSC has been achieved, studies have suggested that targeted postresuscitation hypothermia may improve neurological outcome and survival to discharge.[85] Use of postresuscitative hypothermia is thought to slow cellular metabolism and production of free radicals amongst other harmful byproducts formed during resuscitation. The AHA recommends initiation of induced hypothermia in patients with ROSC following witnessed VT/VF arrests that remain comatose within 1–2 hours of arrest. Use of chilled intravenous fluid, ice packs, and cooling blankets may be used to obtain a target core temperature of 32–34°C, typically by bladder catheter. Hypothermia is maintained for 12–24 hours prior to rewarming.[86] Several studies have looked at the initiation of patient cooling in the prehospital environment and have proven that patient temperature can be lowered by varying interventions. None of these studies, however, showed an improvement in survival to hospital discharge, favorable neurological outcome at hospital discharge, or rearrest.[87]

Studies regarding the use of targeted hypothermia following arrest with an initial rhythm of PEA/asystole have been inconclusive, some revealing minimal benefit, others harmful effects, and still more showing no benefit at all.[88]

TERMINATION OF RESUSCITATION EFFORTS

While the goal of resuscitation is the ROSC, attempts will be unsuccessful in a majority of cases and a decision must be made to terminate all efforts and pronounce the patient deceased. While this may be routine for many emergency physicians within the hospital setting, EMS guidelines regarding resuscitation of patients at the scene are making it more likely that one may be called upon to pronounce a termination in the field without ever having seen the patient.

The National Association of Emergency Medical Services Physicians (NAEMSP) published a position statement in 2000 stating that the termination of resuscitation should be considered in patients who meet the following criteria: arrest unwitnessed by EMS, absence of a shockable rhythm and inability to obtain ROSC prior to transport.[89,90] Following institution of those guidelines, additional studies have shown a 0.09% survival rate in patients meeting all three of the NAEMSP termination criteria.

Though there are no similar guidelines explicitly recommended for inhospital termination, many of the same principles apply. The easiest factor in consideration, and the one least likely to be available at time of arrest, is the presence of a do not resuscitate (DNR) directive. In cases where a DNR directive is in place, resuscitation efforts should immediately cease in conjunction with the patient's previously documented preference. In all patients for whom a DNR directive is not available, efforts should persist until a medical power of attorney or legal next of kin requests cessation or a decision to terminate is made.

Several studies have shown relative consistency amongst providers in regards to factors taken into consideration when determining whether or not to terminate resuscitation efforts. These factors commonly include comorbidities, "down time" prior to CPR and duration of resuscitative efforts, cardiac rhythm of asystole or PEA, normothermia, and age of the patient. Absence of brainstem reflexes is also a factor taken into consideration, though found to be used less reliably amongst providers.[91,92]

It is difficult to identify purely objective endpoints for termination of resuscitation efforts during adult cardiac arrest. The most reliable objective criteria are an end-tidal CO_2 measurement of less than 10 mm Hg throughout resuscitation and cardiac standstill on echocardiography. In all but one of the studies reviewed, 100% of patients with end-tidal measurements of less than 10 mm Hg failed to achieve ROSC.[61,63,64] Bedside, echocardiography is dependent in part on the skill of the provider, but studies have shown that less than 2.4% of patients with documented akinesia on examination progress to ROSC.[78]

General consensus amongst providers is that the decision to stop resuscitation is the result of careful consideration of many of the above factors and a degree of personal preference, though efforts continue to study more reliable objective criteria.

CONCLUSION

Emergency medicine providers must maintain familiarity and competence with basic ACLS guidelines as they are the only interventions known to improve survival in cardiac arrest. Though research continues into interventions that may improve outcomes, the data clearly has shown that early recognition and EMS activation, uninterrupted high quality chest compressions, early defibrillation, and postresuscitation care are the cornerstone of ACLS. Success in resuscitating patients with cardiac arrest is rarely attributable to the presence of a competent emergency physician; efforts must include a community awareness and access to AEDs, timely EMS response and a well-trained support team of nurses, technicians and respiratory therapists within the hospital.

REFERENCES

1. Jacobs I, Nadkarni V, Bahr J, Berg RA, Billi JE, Bossaert L, et al. Cardiac arrest and cardiopulmonary resuscitation outcome reports: update and simplification of the Utstein templates for resuscitation registries: a statement for healthcare professionals from a task force of the International Liaison Committee on Resuscitation (American Heart Association, European Resuscitation Council, Australian Resuscitation Council, New Zealand Resuscitation Council, Heart and Stroke Foundation of Canada, InterAmerican Heart Foundation, Resuscitation Councils of Southern Africa). Circulation. 2004;110(21):3385-97.
2. Go AS, Mozaffarian D, Roger VL, Benjamin EJ, Berry JD, Borden WB, et al. Executive summary: heart disease and stroke statistics--2013 update: a report from the American Heart Association. Circulation. 2013;127(1):143-52.
3. Smith SC, Hamburg RS. Automated external defibrillators: time for federal and state advocacy and broader utilization. Circulation. 1998;97(13):1321-4.
4. Abella BS, Aufderheide TP, Eigel B, Hickey RW, Longstreth WT, Nadkarni V, et al. Reducing barriers for implementation of bystander-initiated cardio-pulmonary resuscitation: a scientific statement from the American Heart Association for healthcare providers, policymakers, and community leaders regarding the effectiveness of cardiopulmonary resuscitation. Circulation. 2008;117(5):704-9.
5. McNally B, Robb R, Mehta M, Vellano K, Valderrama AL, Yoon PW, et al. Out-of-hospital cardiac arrest surveillance—Cardiac Arrest Registry to Enhance Survival (CARES), United States, October 1, 2005—December 31, 2010. MMWR Surveill Summ. 2011;60(8):1-19.
6. Johnson MA, Grahan BJ, Haukoos JS, McNally B, Campbell R, Sasson C, et al. Demographics, bystander CPR, and AED use in out-of-hospital pediatric arrests. Resuscitation. 2014;85(7):920-6.
7. Nishi T, Takei Y, Kamikura T, Ohta K, Hashimoto M, Inaba H. Improper bystander-performed basic life support in cardiac arrests managed with public automated external defibrillators. Am J Emerg Med. 2015;33(1):43-9.
8. Chugh SS, Jui J, Gunson K, Stecker EC, John BT, Thompson B, et al. Current burden of sudden cardiac death: multiple source surveillance versus retrospective death certificate-based review in a large U.S. community. J Am Coll Cardiol. 2004;44(6):1268-75.
9. Lerner EB, Rea TD, Bobrow BJ, Acker JE, Berg RA, Brooks SC, et al. Emergency medical service dispatch cardiopulmonary resuscitation prearrival instructions to improve survival from out-of-hospital cardiac arrest: a scientific statement from the American Heart Association. Circulation. 2012;125(4):648-55.
10. NHTSA. National EMS Scope of Practice Model. 2006.
11. Bakalos G, Mamali M, Komninos C, Koukou E, Tsantilas A, Tzima S, et al. Advanced life support versus basic life support in the pre-hospital setting: a meta-analysis. Resuscitation. 2011;82(9):1130-7.
12. Stiell IG, Wells GA, Field B, Spaite DW, Nesbitt LP, De Maio VJ, et al. dvanced cardiac life support in out-of-hospital cardiac arrest. N Engl J Med. 2004;351(7):647-56.
13. Vaillancourt C, Lui A, De Maio VJ, Wells GA, Stiell IG. Socioeconomic status influences bystander CPR and survival rates for out-of-hospital cardiac arrest victims. Resuscitation. 2008;79(3):417-23.
14. Gold LS, Fahrenbruch CE, Rea TD, Eisenberg MS. The relationship between time to arrival of emergency medical services (EMS) and survival from out-of-hospital ventricular fibrillation cardiac arrest. Resuscitation. 2010;81(5):622-5.
15. Nehme Z, Andrew E, Bernard S, Smith K. Comparison of out-of-hospital cardiac arrest occurring before and after paramedic arrival: epidemiology, survival to hospital discharge and 12-month functional recovery. Resuscitation. 2015;89:50-7.
16. Berg RA, Hemphill R, Abella BS, Aufderheide TP, Cave DM, Hazinski MF, et al. Part 5: adult basic life support: 2010 American Heart Association Guidelines for Cardiopulmonary Resuscitation and Emergency Cardiovascular Care. Circulation. 2010;122(18 Suppl 3):S685-705.
17. Nolan JP, Hazinski MF, Billi JE, Boettiger BW, Bossaert L, de Caen AR, et al. Part 1: Executive summary: 2010 International Consensus on Cardiopulmonary Resuscitation and Emergency Cardiovascular Care Science With Treatment Recommendations. Resuscitation. 2010;81 Suppl 1:e1-25.
18. Koster RW, Sayre MR, Botha M, Cave DM, Cudnik MT, Handley AJ, et al. Part 5: Adult basic life support: 2010 International consensus on cardiopulmonary resuscitation and emergency cardiovascular care science with treatment recommendations. Resuscitation. 2010;81(Suppl 1):e48-70.
19. Berdowski J, Beekhuis F, Zwinderman AH, Tijssen JG, Koster RW. Importance of the first link: description and recognition of an out-of-hospital cardiac arrest in an emergency call. Circulation. 2009;119(15):2096-102.
20. Culley LL, Clark JJ, Eisenberg MS, Larsen MP. Dispatcher-assisted telephone CPR: common delays and time standards for delivery. Ann Emerg Med. 1991;20(4):362-6.
21. Lapostolle F, Petrovic T, Alhéritière A, Agostinucci JM, Adnet F. Life signs in "dead" patients. Resuscitation. 2012;83(7):e164.
22. Moule P. Checking the carotid pulse: diagnostic accuracy in students of the healthcare professions. Resuscitation. 2000;44(3):195-201.
23. Nyman J, Sihvonen M. Cardiopulmonary resuscitation skills in nurses and nursing students. Resuscitation. 2000;47(2):179-84.
24. Travers AH, Rea TD, Bobrow BJ, Edelson DP, Berg RA, Sayre MR, et al. Part 4: CPR overview: 2010 American Heart Association Guidelines for Cardiopulmonary Resuscitation and Emergency Cardiovascular Care. Circulation. 2010;122(18 Suppl 3):S676-84.
25. Herlitz J, Bång A, Alsén B, Aune S. Characteristics and outcome among patients suffering from in hospital cardiac arrest in relation to whether the arrest took place during office hours. Resuscitation. 2002;53(2):127-33.
26. Sutton RM, Nadkarni V, Abella BS. "Putting it all together" to improve resuscitation quality. Emerg Med Clin North Am. 2012;30(1):105-22.
27. Hüpfl M, Selig HF, Nagele P. Chest-compression-only versus standard cardio-pulmonary resuscitation: a meta-analysis. Lancet. 2010;376(9752):1552-7.
28. Hong DY, Park SO, Lee KR, Baek KJ, Shin DH. A different rescuer changing strategy between 30:2 cardiopulmonary resuscitation and hands-only cardiopulmonary resuscitation that considers rescuer factors: a randomised cross-over simulation study with a time-dependent analysis. Resuscitation. 2012;83(3):353-9.
29. Neumar RW, Otto CW, Link MS, Kronick SL, Shuster M, Callaway CW, et al. Part 8: adult advanced cardiovascular life support: 2010 American Heart Association Guidelines for Cardiopulmonary Resuscitation and Emergency Cardiovascular Care. Circulation. 2010;122(18 Suppl 3):S729-67.
30. Wik L, Kramer-Johansen J, Myklebust H, Sørebø H, Svensson L, Fellows B, et al. Quality of cardiopulmonary resuscitation during out-of-hospital cardiac arrest. JAMA. 2005;293(3):299-304.
31. Abella BS, Alvarado JP, Myklebust H, Edelson DP, Barry A, O'Hearn N, et al. Quality of cardiopulmonary resuscitation during in-hospital cardiac arrest. JAMA. 2005;293(3):305-10.
32. Ikeno F, Kaneda H, Hongo Y, Sakanoue Y, Nolasco C, Emami S, et al. Augmentation of tissue perfusion by a novel compression device increases neurologically intact survival in a porcine model of prolonged cardiac arrest. Resuscitation. 2006;68(1):109-18.

33. Duchateau FX, Gueye P, Curac S, Tubach F, Broche C, Plaisance P, et al. Effect of the AutoPulse automated band chest compression device on hemodynamics in out-of-hospital cardiac arrest resuscitation. Intensive Care Med. 2010;36(7):1256-60.
34. Timerman S, Cardoso LF, Ramires JA, Halperin H. Improved hemodynamic performance with a novel chest compression device during treatment of in-hospital cardiac arrest. Resuscitation. 2004;61(3):273-80.
35. Halperin HR, Paradis N, Ornato JP, Zviman M, Lacorte J, Lardo A, et al. Cardiopulmonary resuscitation with a novel chest compression device in a porcine model of cardiac arrest: improved hemodynamics and mechanisms. J Am Coll Cardiol. 2004;44(11):2214-20.
36. Brooks SC, Hassan N, Bigham BL, Morrison LJ. Mechanical versus manual chest compressions for cardiac arrest. Cochrane Database Syst Rev. 2014;2:CD007260.
37. Perkins GD, Lall R, Quinn T, Deakin CD, Cooke MW, Horton J, et al. Mechanical versus manual chest compression for out-of-hospital cardiac arrest (PARAMEDIC): a pragmatic, cluster randomised controlled trial. Lancet. 2015;385(9972):947-55.
38. Wik L, Olsen JA, Persse D, Sterz F, Lozano M, Brouwer MA, et al. Manual vs. integrated automatic load-distributing band CPR with equal survival after out of hospital cardiac arrest. The randomized CIRC trial. Resuscitation. 2014;85(6):741-8.
39. Hallstrom A, Rea TD, Sayre MR, Christenson J, Anton AR, Mosesso VN, et al. Manual chest compression vs use of an automated chest compression device during resuscitation following out-of-hospital cardiac arrest: a randomized trial. JAMA. 2006;295(22):2620-8.
40. Biondi-Zoccai G, Abbate A, Landoni G, Zangrillo A, Vincent JL, D'Ascenzo F, et al. An updated systematic review and meta-analysis on impedance threshold devices in patients undergoing cardiopulmonary resuscitation. Heart Lung Vessel. 2014;6(2):105-13.
41. Rea TD, Cook AJ, Stiell IG, Powell J, Bigham B, Callaway CW, et al. Predicting survival after out-of-hospital cardiac arrest: role of the Utstein data elements. Ann Emerg Med. 2010;55(3):249-57.
42. Meaney PA, Nadkarni VM, Kern KB, Indik JH, Halperin HR, Berg RA. Rhythms and outcomes of adult in-hospital cardiac arrest. Crit Care Med. 2010;38(1):101-8.
43. Link MS, Atkins DL, Passman RS, Halperin HR, Samson RA, White RD, et al. Part 6: electrical therapies: automated external defibrillators, defibrillation, cardioversion, and pacing: 2010 American Heart Association Guidelines for Cardiopulmonary Resuscitation and Emergency Cardiovascular Care. Circulation. 2010;122(18 suppl 3):S706-19.
44. Cummins RO, Hazinski MF, Kerber RE, Kudenchuk P, Becker L, Nichol G, et al. Low-energy biphasic waveform defibrillation: evidence-based review applied to emergency cardiovascular care guidelines: a statement for healthcare professionals from the American Heart Association Committee on Emergency Cardiovascular Care and the Subcommittees on Basic Life Support, Advanced Cardiac Life Support, and Pediatric Resuscitation. Circulation. 1998;97(16):1654-67.
45. Walcott GP, Melnick SB, Killingsworth CR, Ideker RE. Comparison of low-energy versus high-energy biphasic defibrillation shocks following prolonged ventricular fibrillation. Prehosp Emerg Care. 2010;14(1):62-70.
46. Hazinski MF, Idris AH, Kerber RE, Epstein A, Atkins D, Tang W, et al. Lay rescuer automated external defibrillator ("public access defibrillation") programs: lessons learned from an international multicenter trial: advisory statement from the American Heart Association Emergency Cardiovascular Committee; the Council on Cardiopulmonary, Perioperative, and Critical Care; and the Council on Clinical Cardiology. Circulation. 2005;111(24):3336-40.
47. Deakin CD, Morrison LJ, Morley PT, Callaway CW, Kerber RE, Kronick SL, et al. Part 8: Advanced life support: 2010 International Consensus on Cardiopulmonary Resuscitation and Emergency Cardiovascular Care Science with Treatment Recommendations. Resuscitation. 2010;81 Suppl 1:e93-e174.
48. Cabanas JG, Myers JB, Williams JG, De Maio VJ, Bachman MW. Double Sequential External Defibrillation in Out-of-Hospital Refractory Ventricular Fibrillation: A Report of Ten Cases. Prehosp Emerg Care. 2015;19(1):126-30.
49. Wong ML, Carey S, Mader TJ, Wang HE, American Heart Association National Registry of Cardiopulmonary Resuscitation Investigators. Time to invasive airway placement and resuscitation outcomes after inhospital cardiopulmonary arrest. Resuscitation. 2010;81(2):182-6.
50. Holmberg M, Holmberg S, Herlitz J. Low chance of survival among patients requiring adrenaline (epinephrine) or intubation after out-of-hospital cardiac arrest in Sweden. Resuscitation. 2002;54(1):37-45.
51. Cave DM, Gazmuri RJ, Otto CW, Nadkarni VM, Cheng A, Brooks SC, et al. Part 7: CPR techniques and devices: 2010 American Heart Association Guidelines for Cardiopulmonary Resuscitation and Emergency Cardiovascular Care. Circulation. 2010;122(18 suppl 3):S720-8.
52. Hasegawa K, Hiraide A, Brown DF. Prehospital airway management for out-of-hospital cardiac arrest--reply. JAMA. 2013;309(18):1889-90.
53. Hanif MA, Kaji AH, Niemann JT. Advanced airway management does not improve outcome of out-of-hospital cardiac arrest. Acad Emerg Med. 2010;17(9):926-31.
54. McMullan J, Gerecht R, Bonomo J, Robb R, McNally B, Donnelly J, et al. Airway management and out-of-hospital cardiac arrest outcome in the CARES registry. Resuscitation. 2014;85(5):617-22.
55. Wang HE, Szydlo D, Stouffer JA, Lin S, Carlson JN, Vaillancourt C, et al. Endotracheal intubation versus supraglottic airway insertion in out-of-hospital cardiac arrest. Resuscitation. 2012;83(9):1061-6.
56. Fouche PF, Simpson PM, Bendall J, Thomas RE, Cone DC, Doi SA. Airways in out-of-hospital cardiac arrest: systematic review and meta-analysis. Prehosp Emerg Care. 2014;18(2):244-56.
57. Domsky M, Wilson RF, Heins J. Intraoperative end-tidal carbon dioxide values and derived calculations correlated with outcome: prognosis and capnography. Crit Care Med. 1995;23(9):1497-503.
58. Wayne MA, Levine RL, Miller CC. Use of end-tidal carbon dioxide to predict outcome in prehospital cardiac arrest. Ann Emerg Med. 1995;25(6):762-7.
59. Kodali BS, Urman RD. Capnography during cardiopulmonary resuscitation: Current evidence and future directions. J Emerg Trauma Shock. 2014;7(4):332-40.
60. Pokorná M, Necas E, Kratochvíl J, Skripský R, Andrlík M, Franek O. A sudden increase in partial pressure end-tidal carbon dioxide (P(ET)CO(2)) at the moment of return of spontaneous circulation. J Emerg Med. 2010;38(5):614-21.
61. Grmec S, Klemen P. Does the end-tidal carbon dioxide (EtCO2) concentration have prognostic value during out-of-hospital cardiac arrest? Eur J Emerg Med. 2001;8(4):263-9.
62. Kolar M, Krizmaric M, Klemen P, Grmec S. Partial pressure of end-tidal carbon dioxide successful predicts cardiopulmonary resuscitation in the field: a prospective observational study. Crit Care. 2008;12(5):R115.
63. Levine RL, Wayne MA, Miller CC. End-tidal carbon dioxide and outcome of out-of-hospital cardiac arrest. N Engl J Med. 1997;337(5):301-6.
64. Ahrens T, Schallom L, Bettorf K, Ellner S, Hurt G, O'Mara V, et al. End-tidal carbon dioxide measurements as a prognostic indicator of outcome in cardiac arrest. Am J Crit Care. 2001;10(6):391-8.
65. Sehra R, Underwood K, Checchia P. End tidal CO2 is a quantitative measure of cardiac arrest. Pacing Clin Electrophysiol. 2003;26(1 Pt 2):515-7.
66. Garnett AR, Ornato JP, Gonzalez ER, Johnson EB. End-tidal carbon dioxide monitoring during cardiopulmonary resuscitation. JAMA. 1987;257(4):512-5.
67. Falk JL, Rackow EC, Weil MH. End-tidal carbon dioxide concentration during cardiopulmonary resuscitation. N Engl J Med. 1988;318(10):607-11.
68. Meaney PA, Bobrow BJ, Mancini ME, Christenson J, de Caen AR, Bhanji F, et al. Cardiopulmonary resuscitation quality: [corrected] improving cardiac resuscitation outcomes both inside and outside the hospital: a consensus statement from the American Heart Association. Circulation. 2013;128(4):417-35.
69. ECC Committee, Subcommittees and Task Forces of the American Heart Association. 2005 American Heart Association Guidelines for Cardiopulmonary Resuscitation and Emergency Cardiovascular Care. Circulation. 2005;112(24 Suppl):IV1-203.
70. Youngquist ST, Shah A, McClung C, Thomas JL, Rosborough JP, Niemann JT. Does prearrest adrenergic integrity affect pressor response? A comparison of epinephrine and vasopressin in a spontaneous ventricular fibrillation swine model. Resuscitation. 2011;82(2):228-31.
71. Kudenchuk PJ, Brown SP, Daya M, Morrison LJ, Grunau BE, Rea T, et al. Resuscitation Outcomes Consortium-Amiodarone, Lidocaine or Placebo Study (ROC-ALPS): Rationale and methodology behind an out-of-hospital cardiac arrest antiarrhythmic drug trial. Am Heart J. 2014;167(5):653-9.e4.
72. Mentzelopoulos SD, Malachias S, Chamos C, Konstantopoulos D, Ntaidou T, Papastylianou A, et al. Vasopressin, steroids, and epinephrine and neurologically favorable survival after in-hospital cardiac arrest: a randomized clinical trial. JAMA. 2013;310(3):270-9.
73. Price S, Uddin S, Quinn T. Echocardiography in cardiac arrest. Curr Opin Crit Care. 2010;16(3):211-5.
74. Prom R, Dull R, Delk B. Successful alteplase bolus administration for a presumed massive pulmonary embolism during cardiopulmonary resuscitation. Ann Pharmacother. 2013;47(12):1730-5.

75. Janata K, Holzer M, Kürkciyan I, Losert H, Riedmüller E, Pikula B, et al. Major bleeding complications in cardiopulmonary resuscitation: the place of thrombolytic therapy in cardiac arrest due to massive pulmonary embolism. Resuscitation. 2003;57(1):49-55.
76. Vanden Hoek TL, Morrison LJ, Shuster M, Donnino M, Sinz E, Lavonas EJ, et al. Part 12: cardiac arrest in special situations: 2010 American Heart Association Guidelines for Cardiopulmonary Resuscitation and Emergency Cardiovascular Care. Circulation. 2010;122(18 Suppl 3):S829-61.
77. Sosland RP, Gupta K. Images in cardiovascular medicine: McConnell's Sign. Circulation. 2008;118(15):e517-8.
78. Blyth L, Atkinson P, Gadd K, Lang E. Bedside focused echocardiography as predictor of survival in cardiac arrest patients: a systematic review. Acad Emerg Med. 2012;19(10):1119-26.
79. Bellezzo JM, Shinar Z, Davis DP, Jaski BE, Chillcott S, Stahovich M, et al. Emergency physician-initiated extracorporeal cardiopulmonary resuscitation. Resuscitation. 2012;83(8):966-70.
80. Katz V, Balderston K, DeFreest M. Perimortem cesarean delivery: were our assumptions correct? Am J Obstet Gynecol. 2005;192(6):1916-20; discussion 1920-1.
81. Katz VL. Perimortem cesarean delivery: its role in maternal mortality. Semin Perinatol. 2012;36(1):68-72.
82. Zdolsek HJ, Holmgren S, Wedenberg K, Lennmarken C. Circulatory arrest in late pregnancy: caesarean section a vital decision for both mother and child. Acta Anaesthesiol Scand. 2009;53(6):828-9.
83. Harris C, Croce B, Xie A. Ventricular assist devices. Ann Cardiothorac Surg. 2014;3(5):546.
84. Shinar Z, Bellezzo J, Stahovich M, Cheskes S, Chillcott S, Dembitsky W. Chest compressions may be safe in arresting patients with left ventricular assist devices (LVADs). Resuscitation. 2014;85(5):702-4.
85. Arrich J, Holzer M, Havel C, Mullner M, Herkner H. Hypothermia for neuroprotection in adults after cardiopulmonary resuscitation. Cochrane Database Syst Rev. 2012;9:CD004128.
86. Peberdy MA, Callaway CW, Neumar RW, Geocadin RG, Zimmerman JL, Donnino M, et al. Part 9: post–cardiac arrest care: 2010 American Heart Association Guidelines for Cardiopulmonary Resuscitation and Emergency Cardiovascular Care. Circulation. 2010;122(18 suppl 3):S768-86.
87. Diao M, Huang F, Guan J, Zhang Z, Xiao Y, Shan Y, et al. Prehospital therapeutic hypothermia after cardiac arrest: a systematic review and meta-analysis of randomized controlled trials. Resuscitation. 2013;84(8): 1021-8.
88. Sandroni C, Cavallaro F, Antonelli M. Therapeutic hypothermia: is it effective for non-VF/VT cardiac arrest? Crit Care. 2013;17(2):215.
89. Millin MG, Khandker SR, Malki A. Termination of resuscitation of nontraumatic cardiopulmonary arrest: resource document for the National Association of EMS Physicians position statement. Prehosp Emerg Care. 2011;15(4):547-54.
90. Bailey ED, Wydro GC, Cone DC. Termination of resuscitation in the prehospital setting for adult patients suffering nontraumatic cardiac arrest. National Association of EMS Physicians Standards and Clinical Practice Committee. Prehosp Emerg Care. 2000;4(2):190-5.
91. Horsted TI, Rasmussen LS, Lippert FK, Nielsen SL. Outcome of out-of-hospital cardiac arrest--why do physicians withhold resuscitation attempts? Resuscitation. 2004;63(3):287-93.
92. Mohr M, Bahr J, Schmid J, Panzer W, Kettler D. The decision to terminate resuscitative efforts: results of a questionnaire. Resuscitation. 1997;34(1):51-5.

2
CHAPTER
Postcardiac Arrest Syndrome and Therapeutic Hypothermia

Nathan S Deal

INTRODUCTION

Medical history is full of attempts to understand the physiology of cardiac arrest and to identify maneuvers that could assist in the restoration of blood flow. This early work has evolved into the familiar chest compressions used today as part of cardiopulmonary resuscitation. Despite the success of CPR, our understanding of cardiac arrest physiology remained limited and robust post-arrest therapies were largely absent. However, in the last couple of decades, the field of post-arrest management has blossomed with the advent of therapeutic hypothermia. Today, therapeutic hypothermia, provides patients with the opportunity to survive cardiac arrest with meaningful neurologic recovery.

CARDIAC ARREST INCIDENCE AND SURVIVAL

It is estimated that out-of-hospital cardiac arrest (OHCA) affects roughly 325,000 patients per year in the United States,[1,2] with another 210,000 patients suffering cardiac arrest while hospitalized.[3] Despite advances in the area of intra-arrest resuscitation, out-of-hospital, nontraumatic cardiac arrest survival to hospital discharge remains low, estimated to be 10.6% nationally.[4] Those patients who do survive are often burdened with neurologic impairment due to the hypoxic insult endured during the arrest. Postarrest neurologic function is often classified using the Cerebral performance category (CPC) system (Table 1), with overall survival with a CPC score of 1 or 2 as low as 8.3% of patients.

Cardiac arrest survival data may be further delineated based on intermediate goals along the path towards survival to hospital discharge, including return of spontaneous circulation (ROSC), and survival to hospital admission.[6] Sustained ROSC in the prehospital arena, estimated at approximately 30%, has been demonstrated to have the greatest correlation with survival [odds ratio (OR ≥35)].[7] Less than 1% of patients with no prehospital ROSC survived to discharge.[8] This declining survival data suggests that while patients may survive the acute emergency of cardiac arrest, irreversible damage sustained during the event, and/or ongoing cardiovascular collapse results in further mortality (Fig. 1).

The incidence of cardiac arrest, with such a high overall mortality, paired with the additional neurologic impair-

TABLE 1: Cerebral Performance Category Scale[5]

CPC 1	Good cerebral performance: Conscious, alert, able to work, might have mild neurologic or psychological deficit
CPC 2	Moderate cerebral disability: Conscious, sufficient cerebral function for independent activities of daily life. Able to work in sheltered environment
CPC 3	Severe cerebral disability: Conscious, dependent on others for daily support because of impaired brain function. Ranges from ambulatory state to severe dementia or paralysis
CPC 4	Coma or vegetative state: Any degree of coma without the presence of all brain death criteria. Unawareness, even if appears awake (vegetative state) without interaction with environment; may have spontaneous eye opening and sleep/awake cycles. Cerebral unresponsiveness
CPC 5	Brain death: Apnea, areflexia, EEG silence, etc.

CPC, cerebral performance category; EEG, electroencephalogram.

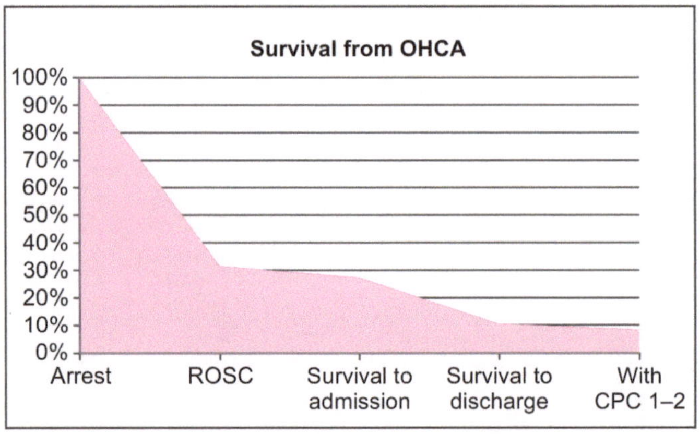

ROSC, return of spontaneous circulation; CPC, Cerebral Performance Category.

FIG. 1: Data from Cardiac Arrest Registry to Enhance Survival (CARES) Summary Report. 31,127 out-of-hospital cardiac arrest patients, 01/01/13 – 12/31/13. mycares.net ment faced by those who do survive has engendered a great deal of research into the pathophysiology of ischemic/hypoxic injury.

PATHOPHYSIOLOGY MODEL OF ISCHEMIC/HYPOXIC INJURY

It was recognized early in cardiac arrest research that even minutes of ischemia and hypoxia can result in deleterious effects throughout the body.[9,10] Subsequent reperfusion compounds this injury, and is attributed to a multifactorial process that includes cell membrane injury,[11] calcium dysregulation,[12] resulting in mitochondria-mediated ROS formation,[13] and subsequent cellular apoptosis.[14] These mechanisms affect multiple organ systems, but are most pronounced in the central nervous system. It is this injury to the brain that accounts for two-thirds of the mortality and a significant amount of morbidity in the postarrest patient.[15]

Recognizing the significance of ischemia/reperfusion pathology and the continued cellular death occurring in this phase, the American Heart Association renewed focus on the support of the postarrest patient. In 2010, a new link in the chain of survival was added, specifically focusing on the support required to aid in the recovery of these patients (Fig. 2).[16]

EMERGENCE OF THERAPEUTIC HYPOTHERMIA

To date, limited therapies have been demonstrated to be effective in minimizing the deleterious effects seen following cardiac arrest.[17] Two landmark studies, published in 2002, introduced the utility of therapeutic hypothermia (TH) in postarrest survivors.[18,19] In these studies, patients who experienced OHCA, and whose initial rhythm was identified as a nonperfusing ventricular arrhythmia (ventricular fibrillation and ventricular tachycardia in one study, and only ventricular fibrillation in the other), and who experienced ROSC were rapidly cooled to a target temperature of 32–34°C.

Recognition and activation of the emergency response system
Immediate high-quality CPR
Rapid defibrillation
Basic and advanced emergency medical services
Advanced life support and postarrest care

ACLS, advanced cardiac life support; CPR, cardiopulmonary resuscitation.

FIG. 2: American Heart Association 2015 Out-of-Hospital-Cardiac-Arrest (OHCA) Chain of Survival

This hypothermia was maintained for 12–24 hours before the patient was rewarmed to 37°C. These patients were compared to a similar cohort of patients in which no active temperature management was initiated.

Using survival to hospital discharge as an endpoint of the studies, both groups were able to demonstrate a significant improvement in the patients receiving hypothermia. In addition, neurologic recovery, measured by a CPC score of 1 or 2 also was substantially higher in patients receiving hypothermia. Subsequent analysis of these two studies plus one similar study of OHCA survivors reviewed survival with good neurologic outcome data at 6 month postarrest and found significant improvement in the hypothermia cohorts. Based on this analysis, it is calculated that the number needed to treat (NNT) patients with OHCA with TH to result in one more survivor with good neurologic outcome is six.[20]

A variety of mechanisms have been proposed to explain the remarkable improvement exhibited by TH.[21] Therapeutic hypothermia results in reduction of global cerebral metabolism and oxygen demand, likely reducing the overall production of ROS.[22] Excitatory neurotransmitter release is blunted by TH and may limit the excitotoxicity seen in cerebral ischemia.[23,24] Proapoptotic pathways are also blunted with the application of TH.[25,26] Global inflammatory markers are also suppressed following the application of TH.[27] The body's response to ischemia/reperfusion injury is complex, with cellular damage resulting from a collection of metabolic pathways. While TH should be viewed as a blunt tool for this complicated biochemical process, its success in improving neurologic survival is profound.

Inclusion of Asystole and Pulseless Electrical Activity Patients

Initial work focused on TH for the treatment of OHCA patients in whom initial rhythm analysis demonstrated ventricular fibrillation/ventricular tachycardia (VF/VT). Subsequent work attempted to determine what benefit this therapy could provide to patients with asystole or pulseless electrical activity (PEA) as the initial nonperfusing rhythm. Some institutions have included all OHCA patients, including asystole and PEA patients, in their TH protocols with demonstrated improvements in all cohorts.[28,29]

A meta-analysis of 12 nonrandomized control trials using TH for asystole and PEA patients demonstrates statistically significant improvement in survival to hospital discharge.[30] Only sparse data exists from randomized control trials with few patients enrolled. While the data cautiously demonstrates a trend towards long-term improvement in survival,[31,32] the small numbers of patients prevent any conclusive statements from being made. Based primarily on the observational data, the most recent AHA recommendations state that TH may be considered for patients suffering from OHCA with asystole or PEA.[17]

TIME TO TARGET TEMPERATURE

Most data evaluating the speed with which cardiac arrest survivors should be cooled is based on work in animal models.[33-38] By reaching the goal temperature of 33°C within 4 hours of arrest, animal models demonstrated improved outcomes compared to normothermic controls. However, this benefit was absent if cooling was delayed more than 8 hours.[39] This work in animal models supports the need for rapid cooling in postarrest survivors.

Additional analysis of human cardiac arrest data has provided mixed results regarding the conclusions of earlier animal work in which a delay in initiation of hypothermia and delays in achieving the desired target temperature resulted in worsening outcomes for patients. In a registry-based study of approximately 1,000 OHCA patients, treated with TH by a variety of modalities, time to initiation of TH (mean of 90 min) and time to target temperature (mean of 260 min) were not associated with any difference in patient outcome.[40]

However, additional data in human survivors supports the conclusion that time to target temperature is critical. On study of 49 consecutive OHCA patients, it demonstrated time to target temperature (mean of 410 min) as an independent predictor of good outcome.[41] In a more recent study of 172 OHCA patients receiving TH, each 30 minute delay in time to target temperature resulted in a 17% increase in poor neurologic outcome.[42] Based on a wealth of animal models and complementary human data, many experts recommended that TH be initiated as quickly as possible, although this continues to be an area of continued investigation.

Target Temperature: 32–34°C

Initial identification of a target temperature between 32°C and 34°C was guided primarily by earlier work in animal models. For this reason, initial studies[18,19] used this range for early human trials. Subsequent work has investigated whether very mild hypothermia of 36°C is sufficient to achieve the desired benefits. In one large, multicenter trial, patients were randomized to a goal temperature of 33°C versus 36°C and demonstrated no difference in overall outcomes.[43] However, in this study, the mean time to achieving the target temperature in the 33°C cohort was roughly 8 hours. Any beneficial effect that may have been conferred in this 33°C cohort may have been blunted by the delay in time to target temperature.[44] The optimal target temperature remains an active area of research.

Following cardiac arrest, it has been noted that patients frequently develop hyperthermia if no active temperature management in performed.[18] It is thought that this hyperthermia is a result of the global inflammation that occurs following ischemia/reperfusion injury.[45] This hyperthermia may be exhibited soon after the arrest or a few days later, requiring continued vigilance and intervention as needed.

THERAPEUTIC HYPOTHERMIA PROTOCOLS AND METHODOLOGY

Since the publication of successful TH trials in 2002, this therapy for OHCA patients has experienced continued adoption. Institutions have taken the parameters outlined in early trials and adapted them to their own environments, with the creation of predetermined TH protocols being critical in improving adoption and implementation rates.[46,47] Some centers have augmented their protocols by creating specialized response teams to support primary care providers in the use of this therapy.[48]

Hypothermia treatment protocols differ from institution to institution but the overarching principles remain consistent.[49] Patients suffering from OHCA who achieve ROSC are cooled to a target temperature of 32–34°C as quickly as possible. Once the patient's temperature reaches the target range, hypothermia is maintained for 24 hours before rewarming. The rewarming phase occurs much more slowly with a goal rewarming rate no faster than 0.25–0.5°C per hour.

Multiple temperature management modalities have been developed since the advent of TH. Initial studies used externally applied cold packs or a device that circulated cold air over the patient to achieve the desired temperature.[18,19] Since that time, additional techniques have been developed that allow for greater control of the patient's temperature. In an endovascular approach, a catheter is placed within the central vasculature and chilled saline is circulated in a closed-loop system within the catheter. Blood passing over the catheter is rapidly cooled and this technique has been shown to safely, accurately and quickly reduce the patient's core temperature. External cooling modalities including ice-water immersion, circulation of cold air, and surface cooling devices have been described. The use of adhesive pads that are cooled using circulating water is commonly referenced and also has demonstrated rapid and accurate temperature management.[51] Additional modalities including cooling helmets,[52] and intranasal cooling devices[53] have been described but are less commonly used when compared to surface or endovascular methods (Box 1).

BOX 1 Sample therapeutic hypothermia criteria and protocol developed primarily from University of Chicago Medical Center Protocol

Sample therapeutic hypothermia criteria

Inclusion criteria (all must apply)

- Cardiac arrest (any rhythm)
- Return of spontaneous circulation (ROSC)
- Comatose
    - Does not open eyes to pain
    - Does not follow commands
- Age ≥18 years old

Absolute contraindications

- Refractory shock
    - Mean arterial pressure (MAP) <65 mm Hg despite fluids and vasoactive agents
- Life-threatening coagulopathy or uncontrollable bleeding
    - Disseminated intravascular coagulation
    - Severe thrombocytopenia, liver failure
    - Vaso-occlusive disease (e.g., Hgb-SS)
- End-stage terminal illness

Relative contraindications

- Refractory ventricular arrhythmia
    - Ventricular tachycardia, ventricular fibrillation
- Pregnancy
    - Obstetrics/gynecology consultation recommended
- Significant preexisting neurologic impairment

Sample therapeutic hypothermia protocol

Target temperature: 32–34°C

- General principles
    - Proper sedation should be titrated for a Richmond Agitation Sedation score of –4 or –5
    - Oxygenation and ventilation techniques should be focused on minimizing hypoxia while also avoiding unnecessarily high oxygen concentrations
    - Cardiovascular support with fluid administration, vasoactive, medications or mechanical support e.g., intra-aortic balloon pump, should be targeted to a MAP ≥65 mm Hg
- Induction phase
    - Cooling should be initiated, as quickly as possible, following ROSC
    - Apply ice packs to axilla, groin, and neck
    - Chilled intravenous saline or chilled nasogastric saline lavage may be considered
    - Primary maintenance modality (e.g., endovascular, surface cooling) should be applied promptly
- Maintenance phase
    - Continuous monitoring of core temperature should be continued with appropriate temperature probes (e.g., bladder, orogastric/nasogastric)
    - Once target temperature range is reached, it should be maintained for 24 h
- Rewarming phase
    - Rewarming should occur no faster than 0.25–0.5°C per hour
    - Once 37°C has been achieved, temperature management should continue to prevent rebound hyperthermia

NEUROCOGNITIVE RECOVERY AND PROGNOSTICATION

Due to the complex global injury process that occurs and the multifactorial manner in which TH supports cardiac arrest survivors, early signs of meaningful neurologic recovery may take several days to manifest. Providers are often motivated to provide family members with some kind of prognostication of patient recovery early on in the treatment period. In one study, greater than 50% of patients were given a "poor or grave" prognosis while undergoing TH, with roughly one-fifth of these patients surviving with good neurologic outcomes.[54] Additional work suggested that neurologic examinations to assess for meaningful recovery may be inaccurate if performed before 72 hours after TH has been completed.[55] For this reason, it is recommended that any prognostication be cautiously withheld until at least 3 days after the completion of the TH protocol (Table 2).

TABLE 2: General guidelines for therapeutic hypothermia

What is the goal temperature?	Between 32°C and 34°C
How fast should the patient be cooled?	As fast as possible
How long should the patient remain at the target temperature?	24 h
What modality should I use to maintain hypothermia?	Many modalities have been shown to be effective with the most common strategies using endovascular or surface cooling approaches
How quickly can I rewarm the patient?	No faster than 0.25–0.5°C per hour
Can patients with an initial rhythm of asystole or PEA benefit from TH?	Yes, while the potential benefit for VF/VT patients is greater, asystole and PEA can be included
When should the care team begin to prognosticate long-term recovery?	No earlier than 72 h after the completion of the hypothermia protocol

PEA, pulseless electrical activity; TH, therapeutic hypothermia; VF, ventricular fibrillation; VT, ventricular tachycardia.

REGIONAL SYSTEMS OF POSTARREST CARE

Recognizing the many resources that postarrest patients require for optimal care, the multidisciplinary team that must be assembled to provide that care and the technical challenges associated with postarrest therapies, there is ongoing interest in the development of postarrest treatment centers. These regional centers would be structured in a similar fashion to the regional centers for other high-acuity, time-sensitive diseases such as trauma, ST-segment elevation myocardial infarction (STEMI) and stroke.

Initial work using the Nationwide Inpatient Sample, a large United States-based database, demonstrated varying survival data in patients suffering cardiac arrest based on hospital factors. It was found that large, urban, academic hospitals demonstrated substantially improved survival.[56] Building on these data, a few communities have developed cardiac arrest centers of excellence, in which TH as well as complementary cardiac interventions [percutaneous coronary intervention (PCI), automated implantable cardioverter defibrillator placement, intra-aortic balloon pump, etc.] are available. Transport of OHCA patients to these centers, paired with other improvements in cardiac arrest care has demonstrated improved patient survival.[57]

In Japan, hospitals may be designated as critical care medical centers in which the therapies discussed herein are available. In a large registry of approximately 10,000 OHCA patients transported to various facilities, it was demonstrated that neurologically favorable survival was substantially higher if a patient was transported to a critical care-designated facility.[58] With the documented success of centers specializing in the care of cardiac arrest patients, it is anticipated that more communities will begin to develop regional systems akin to the framework currently used from trauma, STEMI, and stroke to further improve the medical care provided to postarrest patients.

AREAS OF FUTURE RESEARCH

While the last 10–15 years has brought a considerable amount of interest and investigation into the field of cardiac arrest and postarrest therapy, a great deal of questions remain. Currently, there is great interest in determining the optimal temperature to which patients should be cooled during TH. While cooler temperatures may be more effective in blunting the global inflammation and ROS-associated damage that characterizes postarrest pathophysiology, cooler temperatures present their own side effects and technical limitations. This field of optimal target temperature is expected to receiving increasing interest in the upcoming years.

In addition to defining the optimal temperature target, investigators are also examining the link between the time to target temperature. Analogous to other life-saving, time-sensitive therapies, like PCI in STEMI and tissue plasminogen activator (tPA) in stroke, it is expected that TH will have the greatest impact when provided as quickly as possible. Attempts to correlate time to hypothermia and long-term outcomes have produced mixed results and for that reason, studies including larger patient cohorts are underway.

Closely related to the question of the timing of hypothermia is the possibility of prehospital initiation of cooling. Assuming that there is advantage to providing this therapy as quickly as possible, interest exists in initiating cooling by paramedics and first-responders. A small collection of studies has begun to look at the feasibility of this with limited results. Barriers to successful implementation include provider training and familiarity with the intervention, decisions on which cooling modalities can be successfully used in a prehospital setting and the anticipated manpower needed to initiate and maintain this treatment. Studies in large emergency medical service agencies are in process to further investigate the feasibility of prehospital hypothermia.

A critical and overarching concern for many cardiac arrest and hypothermia researchers is the great complexity associated with postarrest physiology. As described earlier, a multitude of cellular changes occur in the postarrest setting, ultimately cascading towards cell death. The ability to further parse these biochemical and cellular pathways and to understand which are most relevant will be critical in development of better therapies. While TH remains the most successful intervention for postarrest survivors, it is, in its essence, a blunt tool. As complex as is the cellular response to ischemia/reperfusion injury,[45] the effect of hypothermia is just of multifaceted and opaque. Better understanding at the cellular level of the processes involved may lead to more targeted interventions aimed at the central biochemical pathways.

CONCLUSION

Affecting over 300,000 patients in the United States each year, OHCA is associated with significant mortality and morbidity. The complex biochemical pathways that are associated with the ischemia/reperfusion injury of this disease are collectively known as the postcardiac arrest syndrome. Although few interventions exist for this disease, TH has proven to reduce mortality and allow for a greater degree of meaningful neurologic recovery. Several modalities including endovascular and surface cooling techniques exist but most institutions in the United States follow a similar framework for the TH protocols. Patients with any initial rhythm can be cooled to a targeted temperature of 32–34°C, as rapidly as possible, and maintained at this level for 24 hours. Support for the postarrest patient is increasing, being provided as regional centers that specialize in this complex care. Because of this therapy, a growing community of cardiac arrest survivors exists. With a great deal of research still needed to further develop this therapy and other interventions for postcardiac arrest syndrome, this field represents an exciting area of discovery.

REFERENCES

1. Mozaffarian D, Benjamin EJ, Go AS, Arnett DK, Blaha MJ, Cushman M, et al. Heart disease and stroke statistics--2015 update: a report from the American Heart Association. Circulation. 2015;131(4):e29-322.
2. Nichol G, Thomas E, Callaway CW, Hedges J, Powell JL, Aufderheide TP, et al. Regional variation in out-of-hospital cardiac arrest incidence and outcome [published correction appears in JAMA. 2008;300:1763]. JAMA. 2008;300:1423-31.
3. Merchant RM, Yang L, Becker LB, Berg RA, Nadkarni V, Nichol G, et al. Incidence of treated cardiac arrest in hospitalized patients in the United States. Crit Care Med. 2011;39:2401-6.
4. Centers for Disease Control and Prevention. 2013 Cardiac Arrest Registry to Enhance Survival (CARES) National Summary Report. Available from: https://mycares.net/sitepages/uploads/2014/2013CARESNationalSummaryReport.pdf.
5. Safar P. Resuscitation after brain ischemia. In: Grenvik A, Safar P (Eds). Brain Failure and Resuscitation. New York: Churchill Livingstone; 1981. pp. 155-84.
6. Weil MH, Tang W. CPR: Resuscitation of the Arrested Heart. Philadelphia: W.B. Saunders Co.; 1999.
7. Sasson C, Rogers MA, Dahl J, Kellermann AL. Predictors of survival from out-of-hospital cardiac arrest: a systematic review and meta-analysis. Circ Cardiovasc Qual Outcomes. 2010;3:63-81.
8. Drennan IR, Lin S, Sidalak DE, Morrison LJ. Survival rates in out-of-hospital cardiac arrest patients transported without prehospital return of spontaneous circulation: an observational cohort study. Resuscitation. 2014;85(11):1488-93.
9. Weisfeldt ML, BeckerLB. Resuscitation after cardiac arrest: a 3-phase time-sensitive model. JAMA. 2002;288(23):3035-8.
10. Nolan JP, Neumar RW, Adrie C, Aibiki M, Berg RA, Bottiger BW, et al. Post-cardiac arrest syndrome: Epidemiology, pathophysiology, treatment, and prognostication. A Scientific Statement from the International Liaison Committee on Resuscitation; the American Heart Association Emergency Cardiovascular Care Committee; the Council on Cardiovascular Surgery and Anesthesia; the Council on Cardiopulmonary, Perioperative, and Critical Care; the Council on Clinical Cardiology; the Council on Stroke. Resuscitation. 2008;79:350-79.
11. Vanden Hoek TL, Shao Z, Li C, Zak R, Schumacker PT, Becker LB. Reperfusion injury in cardiac myocytes after simulated ischemia. Am J Physiol. 1996;270:H1334-41.
12. Kristián T, Siesjö BK. Calcium in ischemic cell death. Stroke. 1998;29: 705-18.
13. Loor G, Kondapalli J, Iwase H, Chandel NS, Waypa GB, Guzy RD, et al. Mitochondrial oxidant stress triggers cell death in simulated ischemia-reperfusion. Biochim Biophys Acta. 2011;1813(7):1382-94.
14. Vanden Hoek TL, Qin Y, Wojcik K, Li CQ, Shao ZH, Anderson T, et al. Reperfusion, not simulated ischemia, initiates intrinsic apoptosis injury in chick cardiomyocytes. Am J Physiol Heart Circ Physiol. 2003;284(1):H141-50.
15. Laver S, Farrow C, Turner D, Nolan J. Mode of death after admission to an intensive care unit following cardiac arrest. Intensive Care Med. 2004;30:2126-8.
16. Field JM, Hazinski MF, Sayre MR, Chameides L, Schexnayder SM, Hemphill R, et al. Part 1: executive summary: 2010 American Heart Association Guidelines for Cardiopulmonary Resuscitation and Emergency Cardiovascular Care. Circulation. 2010;122:S640-56.
17. Peberdy MA, Callaway CW, Neumar RW, Geocadin RG, Zimmerman JL, Donnino M, et al. Part 9: post-cardiac arrest care: 2010 American Heart Association Guidelines for Cardiopulmonary Resuscitation and Emergency Cardiovascular Care. Circulation. 2010;122:S768-86.
18. Hypothermia after Cardiac Arrest Study Group. Mild therapeutic hypothermia to improve the neurologic outcome after cardiac arrest. N Engl J Med. 2002;346:549-56.
19. Bernard SA, Gray TW, Buist MD, Jones BM, Silvester W, Gutteridge G, et al. Treatment of comatose survivors of out-of-hospital cardiac arrest with induced hypothermia. N Engl J Med. 2002;346:557-63.
20. Holzer M, Bernard SA, Hachimi-Idrissi S, RoineRO, SterzF, Müllner M, et al. Hypothermia for neuroprotection after cardiac arrest: Systematic review and individual patient data meta-analysis. Crit Care Med. 2005;33(2):414-8.
21. González-Ibarra FP, Varon J, López-Meza EG. Therapeutic hypothermia: critical review of the molecular mechanisms of action. Front Neurol. 2011;2:4.
22. Sakoh M, Gjedde A. Neuroprotection in hypothermia linked to redistribution of oxygen in brain. Am J Physiol Heart Circ Physiol. 2003;285(1):H17-25.
23. Illievich UM, Zornow MH, Choi KT, Scheller MS, Strnat MA. Effects of hypothermic metabolic suppression on hippocampal glutamate concentrations after transient global cerebral ischemia. Anesth Analg. 1994;78:905-11.
24. Ooboshi H, Ibayashi S, Takano K, Sadoshima S, Kondo A, Uchimura H, et al. Hypothermia inhibits ischemia-induced efflux of amino acids and neuronal damage in the hippocampus of aged rats. Brain Res. 2000;884:23-30.
25. Bargonetti J, Manfredi JJ. Multiple roles of the tumor suppressor p53. Curr Opin Oncol. 2002;14:86-91.
26. Ji X, Luo Y, Ling F, Stetler RA, Lan J, Cao G, et al. Mild hypothermia diminishes oxidative DNA damage and pro-death signaling events after cerebral ischemia: a mechanism for neuroprotection. Front Biosci. 2007;12:1737-47.
27. Deng H, Han HS, Cheng D, Sun GH, Yenari MA. Mild hypothermia inhibits inflammation after experimental stroke and brain inflammation. Stroke. 2003; 34(10):2495-501.
28. Sunde K, Pytte M, Jacobsen D, Mangschau A, Jensen LP, Smedsrud C, et al. Implementation of a standardised treatment protocol for post resuscitation care after out-of-hospital cardiac arrest. Resuscitation. 2007;73:29-39.
29. Busch M, Soreide E, Lossius HM, Lexow K, Dickstein K. Rapid implementation of therapeutic hypothermia in comatose out-of-hospital cardiac arrest survivors. Acta Anaesthesiol Scand. 2006;50:1277-83
30. Kim YM, Yim HW, Jeong SH, Klem ML, Callaway CW. Does therapeutic hypothermia benefit adult cardiac arrest patients presenting with non-shockable initial rhythms?: A systematic review and meta-analysis of randomized and non-randomized studies. Resuscitation. 2012;83(2): 188-96.
31. Hachimi-Idrissi S, Zizi M, Nguyen DN, Schiettecate J, Ebinger G, Michotte Y, et al. The evolution of serum astroglial S-100 beta protein in patients with cardiac arrest treated with mild hypothermia. Resuscitation. 2005;64(2): 187-92.
32. Laurent I, Adrie C, Vinsonneau C, Cariou A, Chiche JD, Ohanessian A, et al. High-volume hemofiltration after out-of-hospital cardiac arrest: a randomized study. J Am Coll Cardiol. 2005;46(3):432-7.
33. Busto R, Dietrich WD, Globus MY, Ginsberg MD. Postischemic moderate hypothermia inhibits CA1 hippocampal ischemic neuronal injury. Neurosci Lett. 1989;101:299-304.
34. Kuboyama K, Safar P, Radovsky A, Tisherman SA, Stezoski SW, Alexander H. Delay in cooling negates the beneficial effect of mild resuscitative cerebral hypothermia after cardiac arrest in dogs: a prospective, randomized study. Crit Care Med. 1993;21(9):1348-58.
35. Markgraf CG, Clifton GL, Moody MR. Treatment window for hypothermia in brain injury. J Neurosurg. 2001;95(6):979-83.
36. Alam HB, Chen Z, Honma K, Koustova E, Querol RI, Jaskille A, et al. The rate of induction of hypothermic arrest determines the outcome in a Swine model of lethal hemorrhage. J Trauma. 2004;57(5):961-9.
37. Shao ZH, Chang WT, Chan KC, Wojcik KR, Hsu CW, Li CQ, et al. Hypothermia-induced cardioprotection using extended ischemia and early reperfusion cooling. Am J Physiol Heart Circ Physiol. 2007;292(4):H1995-2003.
38. Zhao H, Steinberg G. Limited Therapeutic Time Windows of Mild-to-Moderate Hypothermia in a Focal Ischemia Model in Rat. Stroke Res Treat. 2011;2011:131834
39. Che D, Li L, Kopil CM, Liu Z, Guo W, Neumar RW. Impact of therapeutic hypothermia onset and duration on survival, neurologic function, and neurodegeneration after cardiac arrest. Crit Care Med. 2011;39(6):1423-30.
40. Nielsen N, Hovdenes J, Nilsson F, Rubertsson S, Stammet P, Sunde K, et al. Outcome, timing and adverse events in therapeutic hypothermia after out-of-hospital cardiac arrest. Acta Anaesthesiol Scand. 2009;53(7):926-34.
41. Wolff B, Machill K, Schumacher D, Schulzki I, Werner D. Early achievement of mild therapeutic hypothermia and the neurologic outcome after cardiac arrest. Int J Cardiol. 2009;133(2):223-8.
42. Sendelbach S, Hearst MO, Johnson PJ, Unger BT, Mooney MR. Effects of variation in temperature management on cerebral performance category scores in patients who received therapeutic hypothermia post cardiac arrest. Resuscitation. 2012;83(7):829-34.
43. Nielsen N, Wetterslev J, Cronberg T, Erlinge D, Gasche Y, Hassager C, et al. Targeted temperature management at 33°C versus 36°C after cardiac arrest. N Engl J Med. 2013;369(23):2197-206.
44. Peacock WF, Deal NS. Is time to cooling target temperature important? Crit Pathw Cardiol. 2014;13(2):82-3.
45. Adrie C, Adib-Conquy M, Laurent I, Monchi M, Vinsonneau C, Fitting C, et al. Successful cardiopulmonary resuscitation after cardiac arrest as a "sepsis-like" syndrome. Circulation. 2002;106(5):562-8.
46. RittenbergerJC, Guyette FX, Tisherman SA, DeVita MA, Alvarez RJ, Callaway CW. Outcomes of a hospital-wide plan to improve care of comatose survivors of cardiac arrest. Resuscitation. 2008;79(2):198-204.

47. Sunde K, Pytte M, Jacobsen D, Mangschau A, Jensen LP, Smedsrud C, et al. Implementation of a standardized treatment protocol for post resuscitation care after out-of-hospital cardiac arrest. Resuscitation. 2007;73(1):29-39.
48. Deal NS, Sharp WW, Orbelyan GA, Borak MH, Friant J, Shah AP, et al. The emergency cardiac arrest response team (eCART): a novel strategy for improving therapeutic hypothermia utilization following out-of-hospital cardiac arrest. Resuscitation. 2014;85(12):1775-8.
49. Center for Resuscitation Science. University of Pennsylvania. (2014). Hypothermia Protocols. [online] Available from: https://www.med.upenn.edu/resuscitation/hypothermia/protocols.shtml [Accessed Jan, 2016].
50. Gillies MA, Pratt R, Whiteley C, Borg J, Beale RJ, Tibby SM. Therapeutic hypothermia after cardiac arrest: a retrospective comparison of surface and endovascular cooling techniques. Resuscitation. 2010;81(9):1117-22.
51. Shinada T, Hata N, Yokoyama S, Kobayashi N, Tomita K, Shirakabe A, et al. Usefulness of a surface cooling device (Arctic Sun®) for therapeutic hypothermia following cardiac arrest. J Cardiol. 2014;63(1):46-52.
52. Hachimi-Idrissi S, Corne L, Ebinger G, Michotte Y, Huyghens L. Mild hypothermia induced by a helmet device: a clinical feasibility study. Resuscitation. 2001; 51(3):275-81.
53. Castren M, Nordberg P, Svensson L, Taccone F, Vincent J-L, Desruelles D, et al. Intra-arrest transnasal evaporative cooling: a randomized, prehospital, multicenter study (PRINCE: Pre-ROSC IntraNasal Cooling Effectiveness). Circulation. 2010;122(7):729-36.
54. Perman SM, Kirkpatrick JN, Reitsma AM, Gaieski DF, Lau B, Smith TM, et al. Timing of neuroprognostication in post-cardiac arrest therapeutic hypothermia. Crit Care Med. 2012;40(3):719-24.
55. Al Thenayan E, Savard M, Sharpe M, Norton L, Young B. Predictors of poor neurologic outcome after induced mild hypothermia following cardiac arrest. Neurology. 2008;71(19):1535-7.
56. Carr BG, Goyal M, Band RA, Gaieski DF, Abella BS, Merchant RM, et al. A national analysis of the relationship between hospital factors and post-cardiac arrest mortality. Intensive Care Med. 2009;35(3):505-11.
57. Lurie K, Steinkamp J, Lick C, Aufderheide T, Sayre M, White L, et al. Take Heart AmericaTM: a community-based sudden cardiac arrest survival initiative is saving lives by implementing the most highly recommended 2005 American Heart Association resuscitation guidelines. Circulation. 2008;118:S1464.
58. Kajino K, Iwami T, Daya M, Nishiuchi T, Hayashi Y, Kitamura T, et al. Impact of transport to critical care medical centers on outcomes after out-of-hospital cardiac arrest. Resuscitation. 2010;81(5):549-54.

3 CHAPTER Biomarkers in Acute Care

Kevin S Shah, Vaishal M Tolia

INTRODUCTION

In the emergency department (ED), rapid diagnostic testing is an integral part of decision making. In this chapter, we will review the role of biomarkers as a critical part of this evolving arena. Biomarkers can serve many different roles including identifying risk, diagnosing, staging, prognostication, and assessing response to therapy. In the ED, the primary role of the biomarkers will be for diagnostic testing. The accuracy of a biomarker is determined by its sensitivity (detection of disease when disease is truly present) and its specificity (recognition of absence of disease when disease is truly absent) at various cutpoints.[1] Additionally, with the biomarkers discussed, it is critical to incorporate a Bayesian approach, specifically incorporating pretest probability to estimate the post-test probability of disease. No test should be used alone in isolation in clinical decision making; one should always be incorporated with the entire patient evaluation to maximize clinical utility.

CHEST PAIN

Chest pain accounts for approximately 5–10% of all presentations to the ED.[2] Our ability to assess for cardiac ischemia and acute coronary syndrome (ACS) as the etiology of presenting chest pain is evolving. We rely primarily on clinical risk factors, description of chest pain, electrocardiogram (ECG) testing, and cardiac biomarkers. Biomarker testing is a staple in the initial evaluation of patients presenting with chest pain and a part of the joint American College of Cardiology and American Heart Association guidelines.[3] We will briefly review traditional markers that have fallen out favor, evolving markers with improving assays, and novel biomarkers whose clinical utility is still being refined.

Creatine Kinase-Myocardial Band

Creatine kinase-myocardial band (CK-MB) is a measurement of the myocardial band (MB) subtype of creatine kinase (CK). In the early 1990s, CK-MB was the biochemical marker of choice for the diagnosis of acute myocardial infarction (AMI). It is elevated approximately 4–6 hours after symptom onset in the setting of AMI and returns to normal in 48–72 hours. The test itself is a two-step process requiring determination of total CK and measurement of the MB fraction. The MB fraction is more specific for myocardial damage than serum CK. More recently, given the rise of higher sensitive troponin assays, the utility and cost of CK-MB in routine clinical testing has come in to question.[4,5] Experts have advocated that clinical care may be simplified and cost and confusion may be reduced if CK-MB is no longer routinely used.[6] Current guidelines state that CK-MB testing is no longer necessary in the routine evaluation of chest pain.

Troponin

Cardiac troponin (cTn) is a protein whose primary function is to control the interaction between myosin and actin. Troponin is made up of three subunits (C, I, and T). The term "cTn" refers to either TnT or TnI or to both. Cardiac troponin is released from myocardial cells in the setting of injury, typically sequelae of cellular necrosis. cTn is the most specific cardiac biomarker in current clinical practice.

In AMI, contemporary cTn begins to rise to detectable concentrations 3–4 hours after the onset of ACS. Cardiac troponin levels remain elevated typically for 7–10 days after initial insult. Cardiac troponin is then cleared by the reticuloendothelial system and broken down and eventually renally cleared. The guideline definition of AMI (type 1) is as follows: a rising or falling pattern of cTn concentrations with at least one value above the 99th percentile limit of a normal reference population, in the setting of a patient with clinical evidence of myocardial ischemia. This clinical evidence includes either symptoms of ischemia, ECG changes representing ischemia or imaging evidence of damaged myocardium.[3] The importance of a dynamic rise and fall of cTn in the diagnosis of AMI is important, since many conditions may cause a rise in cTn.

BOX 1 Alternate etiologies for troponin elevation

Causes of troponin elevation

- Acute respiratory distress syndrome
- Aortic dissection
- Cardiac contusion
- Cardioversion or radio-frequency ablation
- Chemotherapy
- Congestive heart failure
- Endocarditis
- Septic shock
- Stroke
- Strenuous exercise
- Pulmonary embolism
- Peri/myocarditis
- Renal failure

Given the increased sensitivity of cTn for detection of myocardial damage, it is by no means a specific biomarker for AMI. Although cTn usually indicates myocardial cell necrosis, its detection in the blood does not indicate the cause of necrosis. Alternate etiologies for troponin elevation are listed in box 1.[7]

Nonischemic causes include direct myocardial injury from trauma or electrical cardioversion, myocardial wall stretch, toxins, infection or inflammation as in myocarditis, infiltrative disease, and sepsis. Renal failure and neurologic injury, including acute ischemic stroke and subarachnoid hemorrhage, can also cause cTn elevation. Ischemic (but nonthrombotic) causes of elevation include supply and demand imbalances in coronary blood flow seen with tachycardia, hypotension, or anemia. Cardiac troponin release has also been observed in circumstances of physiologic stress in the absence of myocardial necrosis; i.e., in marathon runners. Cardiac troponin elevation signifies myocardial damage and ischemia/necrosis; and while cTn represents the most sensitive biomarker we have for AMI in clinical practice, we will review the next generation of cTn: the high-sensitivity assay.

High-sensitivity Troponin

Use of a new generation of high-sensitivity cTn (hs-cTn) assays is common in Europe and arriving in the United States. Improved analytical performance of hs-cTn assays increases their clinical ability to detect small amounts of myocardial damage and to precisely identify small increases in cTn concentrations.[8,9] Single baseline values have improved sensitivity compared to contemporary assays. With increased sensitivity and decreased specificity as compared to conventional troponin, the major advantage of hs-cTn will be in earlier diagnosis/detection of myocardial ischemia.[10] In fact, in hospitalized patients, hs-cTn is found greater than 99th percentile in over 75% of patients aged more than 70 years old.[9]

In practice and AMI diagnosis, serial measurements will be important in order to establish the kinetics of hs-cTn in the absence of high clinical suspicion for ACS. At least two measurements of hs-cTn are necessary to verify a kinetic pattern; this is required to comply with the Universal Definition of Myocardial Infarction.[10,11] The precise use of these assays has yet to be determined in that if the absolute versus relative rise in hs-cTn will need to be determined to find the optimal cutoffs for clinical use.[12] Some studies have demonstrated the potential for a single baseline measurement of an hs-cTn may be used to rule out AMI if low cut off values are used and early presenters are excluded.[13,14] Similarly, other studies have prospectively analyzed the potential for a 1- or 2-hour "rule-out" algorithm using hs-cTn.[15,16] Larger-scale prospective studies will likely be undertaken to develop specific management algorithms, which may vary between assays, but the use of hs-cTn as a part of chest pain evaluation will undoubtedly replace contemporary cTn use.

There is emerging data with regards to the prognostic value of elevated hs-cTn. In all-comers with chest pain, elevated hs-cTn is associated with increased incidence of death, MI, and heart failure 1 year later.[17] In addition to diagnosis of AMI, hs-cTn has a risk stratification role in acute pulmonary embolism (PE) evaluation. An elevated hs-cTn in the setting of acute PE has prognostic information and is associated with increased short-term mortality.[18] While proving to be an extremely sensitive marker for AMI, hs-cTn in the ED setting may also prove to be a risk stratification marker for cardiovascular disease and potentially impact triage strategies given its tremendous ability to detect myocardial damage.

Copeptin

Copeptin is a novel biomarker, which is a measurement of the c-terminal part of the vasopressin prohormone.[19] It is secreted along with arginine-vasopressin from the neurohypophysis and quantitates endogenous stress level in multiple medical conditions. Its role as a biomarker is still evolving, but has found value as a nonspecific stress response indicator. In elderly patients presenting to the ED, copeptin on presentation are associated with mortality up to 1 year out from initial presentation.[20] Similar outcomes show reliable prognostication of adverse outcomes in a heterogeneous group of patients with nonspecific complaints.[21,22]

The rationale for utilizing copeptin as a "rule-out" marker in ACS is simple. Since it is a nonspecific stress marker, it has little specificity but significant sensitivity for AMI. Its kinetics have demonstrated an early rise in the setting of AMI, within the first few hours, earlier than contemporary cTn. An increase in copeptin concentrations after AMI was first reported by Khan.[19] Many studies have shown the ability to improve the negative predictive value (NPV) for ACS rule-out when copeptin is combined with cTn.[23-25] Incorporation of this study has led many to believe that copeptin combined with cTn may facilitate rapid discharge from the ED.[26,27] Some studies have shown the value may not necessarily add clinical value, except in the situation of "early presenters".[28] Most analyses incorporating copeptin use a contemporary cTn assay; the use of copeptin in conjunction with hs-cTn will need to be evaluated in prospective studies.[29]

From a prognostic and risk stratification standpoint, copeptin has demonstrated to be a significant predictor of events in ACS, chest pain, and even all-comers to the ED. In chest pain, those with elevated copeptin have been found to have increased incidence of 30-, 60- and 180-day mortality.[24,30,31] Similar prognostic data was found for prediction of death and HF admission in those with ACS.[19,31,32] Since copeptin is a nonspecific stress indicator, recognition of its ability to identify patients who are high risk for future events may eventually lead to further diagnostic testing or closer follow-up upon discharge in these patients.

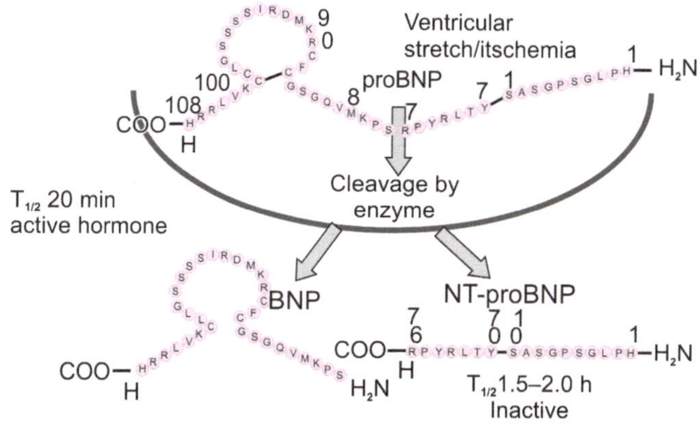

NT-proBNP, N-terminal prohormone-B-type natriuretic peptide.

FIG. 1: Prohormone-B-type natriuretic peptide (proBNP) is cleaved into NT-proBNP and BNP in circulation

DYSPNEA

Acute dyspnea in the ED has a broad differential diagnosis including etiologies ranging from pulmonary, cardiac, hematologic, metabolic, neuromuscular, and psychogenic. In terms of the utility of biomarkers, we will review the commonly in-practice biomarkers including natriuretic peptides (NPs) and D-dimer. Additionally, we will briefly discuss the novel biomarkers of HF, cardiac fibrosis, infection, and inflammation.

Natriuretic Peptides

The NPs are active hormones secreted from cardiac myocytes in response to wall stretch and volume overload.[33] B-type natriuretic peptide (BNP) and A-type natriuretic peptide (ANP) both exist in circulation with the former being produced primarily from ventricular myocyte and the latter from atrial tissue. Prohormone BNP (ProBNP) is secreted in response to cardiac myocyte stretch and is cleaved in circulation to BNP and N-terminal proBNP (NT-proBNP) (Fig. 1). The physiological effects of the NPs include diuresis, vasodilation, and natriuresis.[34] Knowledge of the circumstances in which NPs are elevated has been captured and integrated in the use of diagnostic medicine.

In patients presenting with shortness of breath, elevated NPs have a significant role in their ability to diagnose decompensated HF as the cause of dyspnea.[35] B-type natriuretic peptide and NT-proBNP are primarily used in clinical practice for this purpose. The Breathing Not Properly trial demonstrated that BNP less than 100 pg/mL had a high sensitivity for ruling out decompensated HF and more than 400 pg/mL had reasonable specificity for the same diagnosis.[36] Additionally, the REDHOT trial demonstrated a disconnect between perceived severity of HF and confirmation with BNP.[37] The ProBNP Investigation of Dyspnea in the Emergency Department (PRIDE) study demonstrated similar results showing NT-proBNP plus clinical judgment as superior to clinical judgment alone to diagnose HF; additionally, specific age-specific cutoffs were determined with this study.[38]

When BNP is interpreted, it should be noted that reduced levels are found in obese patients with HF.[39] Additionally, those with renal dysfunction and older age have elevated NP levels compared to those with preserved renal function and younger ages. Finally, HF with reduced ejection fraction (EF) has greater NPs than preserved EF. Flowchart 1 demonstrates an algorithm to use BNP in the evaluation of dyspnea to diagnose HF. A novel assay exists to measure the precursor to ANP, mid regional pro-ANP (MR-proANP), which has comparable diagnostic accuracy with BNP.[40] MR-proANP is as useful as BNP for HF diagnosis and may provide additional clinical utility when BNP is difficult to interpret.

ST2 Biomarker

ST2 is a novel biomarker that has been shown in animal models to represent physiologic stress on the ventricle, directly linked to myocardial fibrosis, hypertrophy, and ventricular dysfunction that are seen in acute and chronic HF.[41-43] ST2 is a member of the interleukin (IL)-1 family and can be found in two forms: (i) ST2L, which is a transmembrane receptor and (ii) sST2, which is a soluble decoy receptor and is detectable in serum. Interleukin-33 is the ligand for ST2 and functions to reduce fibrosis and hypertrophy in strained tissue. Excess sST2 or abnormal signaling of ST2 leads to remodeling seen in HF. In the clinical setting, symptomatic HF patients from either chronic or acute decompensation can correlate disease severity with the concentration of ST2, and it can also independently predict the increased risk of complications. ST2 levels can be useful in post-MI patients to predict development of ventricular dysfunction along with an

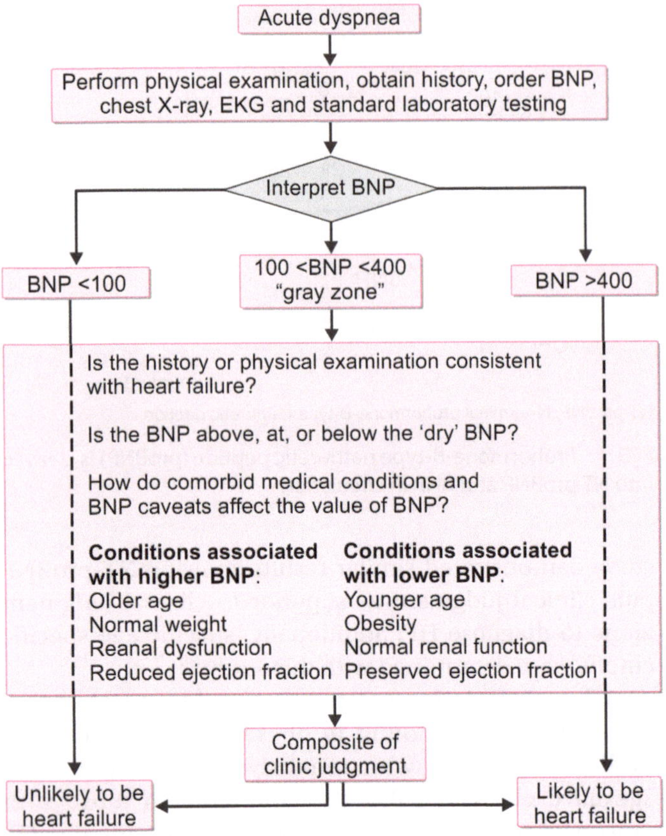

BNP, B-type natriuretic peptide; EKG, electrocardiogram.

FLOWCHART 1: Utilization of B-type natriuretic peptide in evaluation of dyspnea

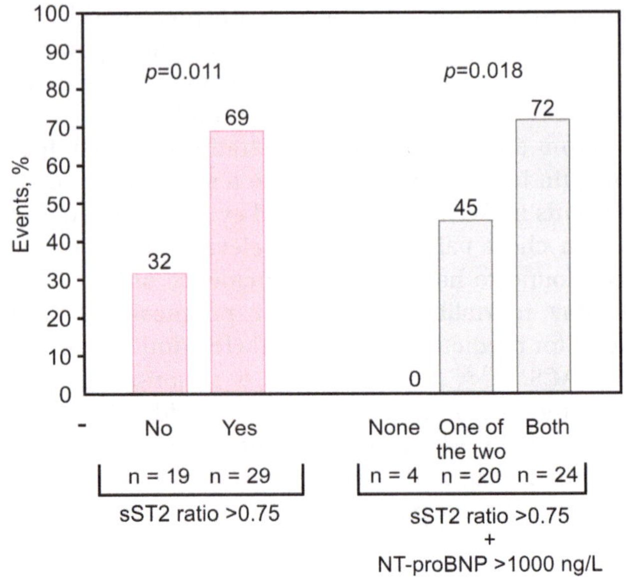

NT-proBNP, N-terminal prohormone-B-type natriuretic peptide.

FIG. 2: Bar Graphs showing events according to sST2 ration more than 0/75 along and in combination with N-terminal prohormone-B-type natriuretic peptide concentration more than 1,000 ng/L (at week 2)

With permission from: Bayes-Genis A, Pascual-Figal D, Januzzi JL, Maisel A, Casas T, Valdés Chávarri M, et al. Soluble ST2 monitoring provides additional risk stratification for outpatients with decompensated heart failure. Rev Esp Cardiol. 2010;63(10):1171-8.

increased risk of cardiac events and mortality.[42,43] Most of the ST2 data has been reported in patients with chronic HF; however ED patients who present with a complaint of dyspnea have a higher risk of death at 1 year when found to have elevated ST2 levels.[43] Further study of acute HF patients revealed that there are strong symptom and biochemical correlates with ST2 due to its role in stretch of the myocardium and in the acute setting has a similar and complementary role to that of the natriuretic peptides. Using natriuretic peptides, clinical data, and serial ambulatory monitoring of ST2, adverse events were higher in those whose biomarkers did not improve at the 2 week mark making the prognostic value of ST2 as a complement to current practice a significant one (Fig. 2).[44] One of the proposed advantages of ST2 over natriuretic peptides is that it is not altered by impaired renal glomerular filtration, obesity, or extremes of age.[45] ST2 has an adjunctive role to current biomarkers and clinical decision rules in the diagnosis, management, and prognostication of patients with acute and chronic HF.

D-dimer

One of the more commonly used and controversial biomarker tests used in the acute care setting is the D-dimer. It is a cross-linked product of fibrin degradation during the fibrinolysis of clots. It is normally not detected in human blood testing except when active coagulation is occurring for a variety of reasons. Detection is dependent on the binding of a monoclonal antibody to a source on the D-Dimer fragment. The primary use for the D-dimer in the acute care setting is when clinicians are evaluating for venous thromboembolic disease (VTE). Traditionally, low pretest probability (<15–20% likelihood) combined with a negative D-dimer effectively reduces the probability of thrombotic disease, such as deep vein thrombosis or PE, to acceptably low levels less than 1% and, thus, obviating the need for further testing.[46] Thus, the D-dimer possesses a very high NPV with high sensitivity, but positive values require further testing due to the poor specificity. Newer assays, such as the Hemosil D-dimer HS 500, uses a latex enhanced turbidimetric immunoassay, which preserved the sensitivity and specificity for all pretest probability except for high probabilities in which the D-dimer should not be utilized.[47] A novel approach to the use of the D-dimer that emerged about 10 years ago and one that continues to be discussed is that in the cases of patients being evaluated for chest pain with the desire to rule out an acute aortic dissection. Several pooled studies and meta-analyses show D-dimer to have a sensitivity of 94–97%.[48] However, other studies have reported a high false-negative rate of up to 18%, thus diminishing the utility of the D-dimer for aortic dissection evaluation.[49] Further exploration needs to be undertaken to look at various pretest probability combined with threshold value of a standardized D-dimer in order for clinical utility in D-dimer to be beneficial in the acute setting as it is to exclude VTE in the present day.

Mid-Regional pro-Adrenomedullin

Adrenomedullin (ADM) is an amino acid peptide that causes prolonged vasodilation through nitric oxide production and levels are correlated with the severity of HF and LV systolic dysfunction. Measuring levels of ADM are difficult due to its short plasma half-life. However, ADM has a larger precursor peptide known as mid-regional pro-ADM (MR-proADM), which is measurable and may have an impact as a biomarker for acute HF. Theoretically, the levels of MR-proADM correlate with those of ADM but this molecule is more stable and measurable.[50] *In vivo*, ADM has the effect of afterload reduction and increase in cardiac output by causing both potent diuresis and vasodilation. There is also a thought that ADM functions to inhibit cell growth and hypertrophy of cardiac myocytes, thus preventing remodeling leading to further ventricular dysfunction. Measurement of serum MR-proADM has independent prognostic value of adverse events on ST segment elevation myocardial infarction (STEMI) patients discharged from the hospital.[51] Combining this value with established biomarkers, such as NT-proBNP, provide complementary information and help in deciding which patients need more aggressive investigation and therapy after reperfusion of the acute MI. More recently, the study of MR-proADM on STEMI patients was extended to include patients with non-STEMI with the data suggesting that admission levels may help to identify which patients would benefit from early revascularization.[52] In the acute care setting, the Biomarkers in Acute HF (BACH) trial evaluated ED patients presenting with dyspnea as the chief complaint. Higher median levels of MR-proADM were predictive of death at 90 days in the subgroup of these patients that were diagnosed with acute HF. Combining with another biomarker, copeptin, the utility of predicting major adverse cardiac events (MACE) in these patients at 14 days, thus being more relevant to the emergency physician. In other studies, MR-proADM combined with other biomarkers in a "multimarker panel" can help in predicting rehospitalization and mortality at 30 and 90 days for ED patients with acute dyspnea particularly with serial panel assessment both at admission and 72 hours after hospitalization.[53] Mid-regional pro-ADM is a complex biomarker that has utility both in the acute setting for evaluation and prognostication in patients with acute dyspnea when combined with other biomarkers. It also can help to provide information on the risk of poor outcomes in patients with acute MI. Biomarkers, such as MR-proADM, can aid in the risk stratification of patients with acute HF and can help acute care physicians to make a proper diagnosis and disposition as well as the cardiologist choosing in whom to tailor a more aggressive future diagnostic and treatment plan.

Procalcitonin

Early identification of patients with severe sepsis has become a strong point of emphasis for the surviving sepsis campaign as well as increasing standards and regulations most hospital systems are being held to. The complaint of acute dyspnea in the ED setting provides a challenge for providers trying to differentiate respiratory disease, acute infection and congestive HF as the underlying cause of symptomatology. Early recognition for sepsis and acute HF[54] can be beneficial in reducing mortality from the condition as treatment can begin more rapidly and aggressively. Procalcitonin (PCT) is the prehormone of calcitonin, and in cases of systemic inflammation can be produced in a variety of extrathyroid tissue. Procalcitonin rises early in cases of systemic infection, which can help to guide therapy. In patients with acute dyspnea, elevated PCT levels can reduce the time to antibiotic administration and lead the clinician to treat the sepsis in accordance to the established operational guidelines. Procalcitonin is a biomarker more of a state than a condition. Elevated levels suggest infection and systemic inflammatory response syndrome (SIRS) to sepsis spectrum of illness, but not one in particular.[55] It does, however, have some use in particular clinical scenarios. In patients with suspected meningitis, elevated PCT levels had a positive predictive value for bacterial meningitis versus aseptic meningitis.[56] In specific infectious disease etiologies, PCT use helped to differentiate between a serious bacterial infection or the absence of one and effectively reduced the ED use of antibiotics. In combination with the NT-proBNP, PCT can be a helpful biomarker at the point of triage to help differentiate the acute patient complaining of dyspnea between HF and sepsis.

CONCLUSION

In the ED, the role of biomarkers continues to evolve. Traditional markers, such as troponin and NPs, have mainstay roles in the evaluation of ACS and HF. Novel markers including copeptin, ST2, MR-proADM, and PCT continue to be investigated for their diagnostic and prognostic niche in an environment where rapid and accurate decision making is fundamental. Multimarker strategies with higher precision, which provide therapy-guiding decision paths, will need to be validated to help optimize strategies for the future of cardiac emergency cardiology.

REFERENCES

1. Vasan RS. Biomarkers of cardiovascular disease: molecular basis and practical considerations. Circulation. 2006;113(19):2335-62.
2. Owens PL, Barrett ML, Gibson TB, Andrews RM, Weinick RM, Mutter RL. Emergency department care in the United States: A profile of national data sources. Ann Emerg Med. 2010;56:150-65.
3. Amsterdam EA, Wenger NK, Brindis RG, Casey DE Jr, Ganiats TG, Holmes DR Jr, et al. 2014 AHA/ACC Guideline for the Management of Patients With Non-ST-Elevation Acute Coronary Syndromes: A Report of the American College of Cardiology/American Heart Association Task Force on Practice Guidelines. J Am Coll Cardiol. 2014;64(24):e139-228.
4. Singh G, Baweja PS. Creatine kinase-MB: the journey to obsolescence. Am J Clin Pathol. 2014;141(3):415-9.
5. Melanson SF, Lewandrowski EL, Januzzi JL, Lewandrowski KB. Reevaluation of myoglobin for acute chest pain evaluation: would false-positive results on "first-draw" specimens lead to increased hospital admissions? Am J Clin Pathol. 2004;121(6):804-8.
6. Saenger AK, Jaffe AS. Requiem for a heavyweight: the demise of creatine kinase-MB. Circulation. 2008;118(21):2200-6.
7. Agewall S, Giannitsis E, Jernberg T, Katus H. Troponin elevation in coronary vs. non-coronary disease. Eur Heart J. 2011;32(4):404-11.
8. Thygesen K, Mair J, Giannitsis E, Mueller C, Lindahl B, Blankenberg S, et al. How to use high-sensitivity cardiac troponins in acute cardiac care. Eur Heart J. 2012;33(18):2252-7.
9. Stein GY, Alon D, Korenfeld R, Fuchs S. Clinical implications of high-sensitivity cardiac troponin measurements in hospitalized medical patients. PLoS One. 2015;10(1):e0117162.
10. Al-Saleh A, Alazzoni A, Al Shalash S, Ye C, Mbuagbaw L, Thabane L, et al. Performance of the high-sensitivity troponin assay in diagnosing acute myocardial infarction: systematic review and meta-analysis. CMAJ Open. 2014;2(3):E199-207.
11. Thygesen K, Alpert JS, Jaffe AS, Simoons ML, Chaitman BR, White HD, et al. Third universal definition of myocardial infarction. Eur Heart J. 2012;33(20):2551-67.
12. Apple FS, Morrow DA. Delta cardiac troponin values in practice: are we ready to move absolutely forward to clinical routine? Clin Chem. 2012;58(1):8-10.
13. Zhelev Z, Hyde C, Youngman E, Rogers M, Fleming S, Slade T, et al. Diagnostic accuracy of single baseline measurement of Elecsys Troponin T high-sensitive assay for diagnosis of acute myocardial infarction in emergency department: systematic review and meta-analysis. BMJ. 2015; 350:h15.
14. Kelly AM, Klim S. Does undetectable troponin I at presentation using a contemporary sensitive assay rule out myocardial infarction? A cohort study. Emerg Med J. 2015;32(10):760-3.
15. Reichlin T, Cullen L, Parsonage WA, Greenslade J, Twerenbold R, Moehring B, et al. Two-hour Algorithm for Triage Toward Rule-out and Rule-in of Acute Myocardial Infarction Using High-sensitivity Cardiac Troponin T. Am J Med. 2015;128(4):369-79.
16. Reichlin T, Schindler C, Drexler B, Twerenbold R, Reiter M, Zellweger C, et al. One-hour rule-out and rule-in of acute myocardial infarction using high-sensitivity cardiac troponin T. Arch Intern Med. 2012;172(16):1211-8.
17. Aldous SJ, Richards M, Cullen L, Troughton R, Than M. Diagnostic and prognostic utility of early measurement with high-sensitivity troponin T assay in patients presenting with chest pain. CMAJ. 2012;184(5):E260-8.
18. Lankeit M, Jimenez D, Kostrubiec M, Dellas C, Hasenfuss G, Pruszczyk P, et al. Predictive value of the high-sensitivity troponin T assay and the simplified pulmonary embolism severity index in hemodynamically stable patients with acute pulmonary embolism: a prospective validation study. Circulation. 2011;124(24):2716-24.
19. Khan SQ, Dhillon OS, O'Brien RJ, Struck J, Quinn PA, Morgenthaler NG, et al. C-terminal provasopressin (copeptin) as a novel and prognostic marker in acute myocardial infarction: Leicester Acute Myocardial Infarction Peptide (LAMP) study. Circulation. 2007;115(16):2103-10.
20. Iversen K, Gøtze JP, Dalsgaard M, Nielsen H, Boesgaard S, Bay M, et al. Risk stratification in emergency patients by copeptin. BMC Med. 2014;12:80.
21. Nickel CH, Messmer AS, Geigy N, Misch F, Mueller B, Dusemund F, et al. Stress markers predict mortality in patients with nonspecific complaints presenting to the emergency department and may be a useful risk stratification tool to support disposition planning. Acad Emerg Med. 2013;20(7):670-9.
22. Nickel CH, Ruedinger J, Misch F, Blume K, Maile S, Schulte J, et al. Copeptin and peroxiredoxin-4 independently predict mortality in patients with nonspecific complaints presenting to the emergency department. Acad Emerg Med. 2011;18(8):851-9.
23. Afzali D, Erren M, Pavenstädt HJ, Vollert JO, Hertel S, Waltenberger J, et al. Impact of copeptin on diagnosis, risk stratification, and intermediate-term prognosis of acute coronary syndromes. Clin Res Cardiol. 2013;102(10):755-63.
24. Maisel A, Mueller C, Neath SX, Christenson RH, Morgenthaler NG, McCord J, et al. Copeptin helps in the early detection of patients with acute myocardial infarction: primary results of the CHOPIN trial (Copeptin Helps in the early detection Of Patients with acute myocardial INfarction). J Am Coll Cardiol. 2013;62(2):150-60.
25. Reichlin T, Hochholzer W, Stelzig C, Laule K, Freidank H, Morgenthaler NG, et al. Incremental value of copeptin for rapid rule out of acute myocardial infarction. J Am Coll Cardiol. 2009;54(1):60-8.
26. Keller T, Tzikas S, Zeller T, Czyz E, Lillpopp L, Ojeda FM, et al. Copeptin improves early diagnosis of acute myocardial infarction. J Am Coll Cardiol. 2010;55(19):2096-106.
27. Lipinski MJ, Escárcega RO, D'Ascenzo F, Magalhães MA, Baker NC, Torguson R, et al. A systematic review and collaborative meta-analysis to determine the incremental value of copeptin for rapid rule-out of acute myocardial infarction. Am J Cardiol. 2014;113(9):1581-91.
28. Sukul D, Bonaca MP, Ruff CT, Kosowsky J, Conrad M, Murphy SA, et al. Diagnostic performance of copeptin in patients with acute nontraumatic chest pain: BWH-TIMI ED chest pain study. Clin Cardiol. 2014;37(4):227-32.
29. Raskovalova T, Twerenbold R, Collinson PO, Keller T, Bouvaist H, Folli C, et al. Diagnostic accuracy of combined cardiac troponin and copeptin assessment for early rule-out of myocardial infarction: a systematic review and meta-analysis. Eur Heart J Acute Cardiovasc Care. 2014;3(1):18-27.
30. Thelin J, Borna C, Erlinge D, Öhlin B.. The combination of high sensitivity troponin T and copeptin facilitates early rule-out of ACS: a prospective observational study. BMC Cardiovasc Disord. 2013;13(1):42.
31. Reinstadler SJ, Klug G, Feistritzer HJ, Mayr A, Harrasser B, Mair J, et al. Association of copeptin with myocardial infarct size and myocardial function after ST segment elevation myocardial infarction. Heart. 2013;99(20):1525-9.
32. Sanchez M, Llornes P, Herrero P, Martín-Sanchez FJ, Piñera P, Miró Ò, et al. The utility of copeptin in the emergency department as a predictor of adverse outcomes in non-ST-elevation acute coronary syndrome: the COPED-PAO study. Emerg Med J. 2014;31(4):286-91.
33. Nakagawa O, Ogawa Y, Itoh H, Suga S, Komatsu Y, Kishimoto I, et al. Rapid transcriptional activation and early mRNA turnover of brain natriuretic peptide in cardiocyte hypertrophy. Evidence for brain natriuretic peptide as an "emergency" cardiac hormone against ventricular overload. J Clin Invest. 1995;96(3):1280-7.
34. Hall C. Essential biochemistry and physiology of (NT-pro)BNP. Eur J Heart Fail. 2004;6(3):257-60.
35. Maisel A, Mueller C, Adams K Jr, Anker SD, Aspromonte N, Cleland JG, et al. State of the art: Using natriuretic peptide levels in clinical practice. Eur J Heart Fail. 2008;10(9):824-39.
36. Maisel AS, Krishnaswamy P, Nowak RM, McCord J, Hollander JE, Duc P, et al. Rapid measurement of B-type natriuretic peptide in the emergency diagnosis of heart failure. N Engl J Med. 2002;347(3):161-7.
37. Maisel A, Hollander JE, Guss D, McCullough P, Nowak R, Green G, et al. Primary results of the Rapid Emergency Department Heart Failure Outpatient Trial (REDHOT). A multicenter study of B-type natriuretic peptide levels, emergency department decision making, and outcomes in patients presenting with shortness of breath. J Am Coll Cardiol. 2004;44(6):1328-33.
38. Januzzi JL Jr, Camargo CA, Anwaruddin S, Baggish AL, Chen AA, Krauser DG, et al. The N-terminal Pro-BNP investigation of dyspnea in the emergency department (PRIDE) study. Am J Cardiol. 2005;95(8):948-54.
39. Mehra MR, Uber PA, Park MH, Scott RL, Ventura HO, Harris BC, et al. Obesity and suppressed B-type natriuretic peptide levels in heart failure. J Am Coll Cardiol. 2004;43(9):1590-5.
40. Maisel A, Mueller C, Nowak R, Peacock WF, Landsberg JW, Ponikowski P, et al. Mid-region pro-hormone markers for diagnosis and prognosis in acute dyspnea: results from the BACH (Biomarkers in Acute Heart Failure) trial. J Am Coll Cardiol. 2010;55(19):2062-76.
41. Shah RV, Januzzi JL Jr. ST2: a novel remodeling biomarker in acute and chronic heart failure. Curr Heart Fail Rep. 2010;7(1):9-14.
42. Bhardwaj A, Januzzi JL Jr. ST2: a novel Biomarker for Heart Failure. Expert Review of Molecular Diagnostics. 2010;10(4):459-64.
43. Januzzi JL Jr, Peacock WF, Maisel AS, Chae CU, Jesse RL, Baggish AL, et al. Measurement of the interleukin family member ST2 in patients with acute

dyspnea: results from the PRIDE (Pro-Brain Natriuretic Peptide Investigation of Dyspnea in the Emergency Department) study. J Am Coll Cardiol. 2007;50(7): 607-13.

44. Bayes-Genis A, Pascual-Figal D, Januzzi JL, Maisel A, Casas T, Valdés Chávarri M, et al. Soluble ST2 monitoring provides additional risk stratification for outpatients with decompensated heart failure. Rev Esp Cardiol. 2010; 63(10):1171-8.
45. Rehman SU, Mueller T, Januzzi JL Jr. Characteristics of the novel interleukin family biomarker ST2 in patients with acute heart failure. J Am Coll Cardiol. 2008;52(18):1458-65..
46. Wells PS, Anderson DR, Rodger M, Forgie M, Kearon C, Dreyer J, et al. "Evaluation of D-dimer in the diagnosis of suspected deep-vein thrombosis". N Engl J Med. 2003;349(13):1227-35.
47. Legnani C, Cini M, Scarvelis D, Toulon P, Wu JR, Palareti G. Multicenter evaluation of a new quantitative highly sensitive D-dimer assay, the Hemosil® D-dimer HS 500, in patients with clinically suspected venous thromboembolism. Thromb Res. 2010;125(5):398-401.
48. Sodeck G, Domanovits H, Schillinger M, Ehrlich MP, Endler G, Herkner H, et al. D-dimer in ruling out acute aortic dissection: a systematic review and prospective cohort study. Eur Heart J. 2007;28(24):3067-75.
49. Paparella D, Malvindi PG, Scrascia G, de Ceglia D, Rotunno C, Tunzi F, et al. D-dimers are not always elevated in patients with acute aortic dissection. J Cardiovasc Med (Hagerstown). 2009;10(2):212-4.
50. Potocki M, Ziller R, Mueller C. Mid-regional pro-adrenomedullin in acute heart failure: a better biomarker or just another biomarker? Curr Heart Fail Rep. 2012;9(3):244-51.
51. Khan SQ, O'Brien RJ, Struck J, Quinn P, Morgenthaler N, Squire I, et al. Prognostic value of midregional pro-adrenomedullin in patients with acute myocardial infarction. J Am Coll Cardiol. 2007;49(14):1525-32.
52. Dhillon O, Khan SQ, Narayan HK, Ng KH, Struck J, Quinn PA, et al. Prognostic value of mid regional pro-adrenomedullin levels taken on admission and discharge in non-ST elevation myocardial infarction. 2010;56(2):125-33.
53. Travaglino F, Russo V, De Berardinis B, Numeroso F, Catania P, Cervellin G et al. Thirty and ninety days mortality predictive value of admission and in-hospital procalcitonin and mid-regional pro-adrenomedullin testing in patients with dyspnea. Results from the VERyfing DYspnea trial. Am J Emerg Med. 2014;32(4):334-41.
54. Ray P, Birolleau S, Lefort Y, Becquemin MH, Beigelman C, Isnard R, et al. Acute respiratory failure in the elderly: etiology, emergency diagnosis and prognosis. Crit Care. 2006;10(3):R82.
55. Gaini S, Koldkjaer OG, Pedersen C, Pedersen SS. Procalcitonin, lipopolysaccharide-binding protein, interleukin-6 and C-reactive protein in community-acquired infections and sepsis: a prospective study. Crit Care. 2006;10(2):R53.
56. Viallon A, Zeni F, Lambert C, Pozzetto B, Tardy B, Venet C, et al. High sensitivity and specificity of serum procalcitonin levels in adults with bacterial meningitis. Clin Infect Dis. 1999;28(6):1313-6.

4 CHAPTER

Electrocardiography in the Emergency Department

Semhar Z Tewelde, Amal Mattu

"Using experience, knowledge, and insight... we can anticipate dangers, opportunities, and take steps to avoid hazards."

—Suzuki

INTRODUCTION

The era of unaided history taking and physical examination to diagnose an illness has long vanished. The practice of medicine in the 21st century has been transformed with the advent of modern technology, genomics, and rampant research. Medicine is no longer based on anecdote and scientific theory, but is based on "evidence". Conclusive data that is derived from Randomized Clinical Trials (RCTs), observational and retrospective studies are now applied to patients. Nevertheless certain innovative ideas and discoveries of the 18th, 19th and 20th centuries remain indispensible tools in medicine. Willem Einthoven's discovery of the electrocardiogram (ECG) is one that is an essential part of the evaluation of countless, if not all patients.[1] The objective of this chapter is to describe the role and importance of the ECG as it relates to emergency department (ED) evaluations, as well as discuss some of the ongoing challenges for integrating ECG in contemporary medicine.

The evaluation of the undifferentiated patient normally occurs in the ED. In the ED, an ECG is frequently obtained in triage, prior to any assessment by a healthcare provider based on chief complaint (i.e., weakness, chest pain, shortness of breath), vital sign abnormalities (i.e., bradycardia/tachycardia), or protocol. Although acquiring an ECG is most often thought about in patients with suspected acute coronary syndrome (ACS), there is widespread utility for the ECG as a screening tool for other clinical conditions. As a diagnostic tool it is superb, unlike many others, it is rapid, noninvasive, and cost-effective. Modern-day ECG equipment has algorithm-based computer analysis and automated interpretation that is then given to the ordering physician for approval. Manufacturers of different ECG machines have differing algorithms for ECG interpretation.[2] Not surprisingly, the accuracy of algorithms also differs. Unfortunately, many healthcare providers do not examine the ECG and merely rely on the computer's analysis, hence errors occur.[3] One study comparing nine computer algorithms with eight cardiologists found that overall the percent of correct classifications of computer programs was 69.7% compared to 76.3% for the cardiologists.[4] It is useful to have insight into the reliability and hazards of computer interpretation to assess the value of these results. The American Heart Association (AHA)/American College of Cardiology (ACC) recommends, "computer-based interpretation of the ECG as an adjunct to the electrocardiographer, and all computer-based reports require physician over reading. Accurate individual templates should be formed in each lead before final feature extraction and measurement used for diagnostic interpretation."[3] Healthcare providers at different levels of training and expertise are expected to interpret ECGs. Therefore, high-quality and continual education is required for the novice ECG interpreter to become skilled. A medical evaluation normally consists of a brief history and examination followed by the necessary diagnostic studies, laboratory and imaging. The necessary number of studies in the emergent setting can be plentiful, leading to delays in diagnose and treatment, potentially detrimental to patient outcomes. Attaining ECG proficiency in analysis can be immediately elucidating and life-saving. Proper reading of ECGs should be systematic and thorough, as taught by the various texts. Electronic ECG analysis should only serve as a supplement and certainly is not a substitute to ECG interpretation.[5]

INTERPRETATION AUTHORITY

Cardiologists are considered the authority in ECG interpretation because they are presumed to spend a more significant amount of time dedicated to ECG interpretation as a core component of their training than other specialists. The ACC/AHA criterion for competency in ECG interpretation requires successful completion of: cardiology board certification, 500 ECG interpretations under the supervision of a cardiologist or an ECG certifying examination for those not board certified in cardiology.[6] Despite interpreting ECGs with high accuracy in acute care settings that require intervention without assistance, having read in excess of 500 ECGs under attending supervision and comprehensive training throughout residency; emergency medicine physicians are not considered equally accomplished by cardiology counterparts. Recent studies have raised doubts about whether all cardiologist and only cardiologist should be dubbed the expert. Eken et al., Kuhn et al., Schaffer et al., Todd et al., and Westdrop et al. have all found high rates of agreement in ECG reading when comparing emergency medicine to cardiology.[7-11]

CLINICAL CONDITIONS

Acute Coronary Syndrome

Heart disease is the leading cause of death in the United States. As such any person with symptoms of chest pain, dyspnea, jaw or neck pain, weakness, fatigue, or syncope is recommended emergent evaluation for ACS. The greatest threat for patients and physicians alike is ST elevation myocardial infarction (STEMI) resulting in myocardial necrosis. Hence, patients with the aforementioned symptoms should receive an ECG in less than 10 minutes of arrival to the ED.[12] In the prehospital setting, an ECG should be transmitted electronically while en route to the ED by emergency medical services (EMS), if feasible.[13] The earliest ECG changes preceding ST elevation and Q-waves are hyperacute T-waves (Fig. 1) that are broad based and asymmetrically peaked.[14] Electrocardiogram criteria for STEMI based on the 2013 ACA/AHA guidelines and universal task force are:

- New ST elevation at the J-point in at least two contiguous leads of greater than or equal to 2 mm in men or greater than or equal to 1.5 mm in women in leads V2–V3 (Fig. 2), and/or greater than or equal to 1 mm in other contiguous chest or limb leads
- Multilead ST-depression with coexistent ST elevation in aVR (Fig. 3)
- ST-depression in greater than or equal to 2 precordial leads (V1–V4) (Fig. 4).[15]

If any of the above criteria are met, the emergency physician (EP) should initiate activation for cardiac catheterization and emergent percutaneous coronary intervention (PCI). In addition to primary reperfusion therapy while in the ED adjunctive antiplatelet agents are typically administered, specifically aspirin

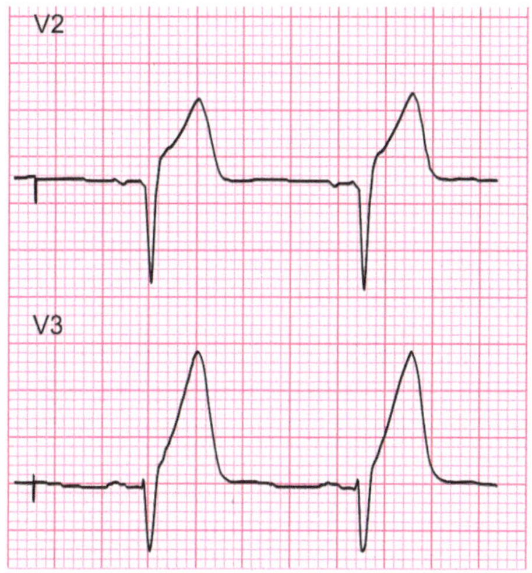

FIG. 1: Hyperacute T-waves

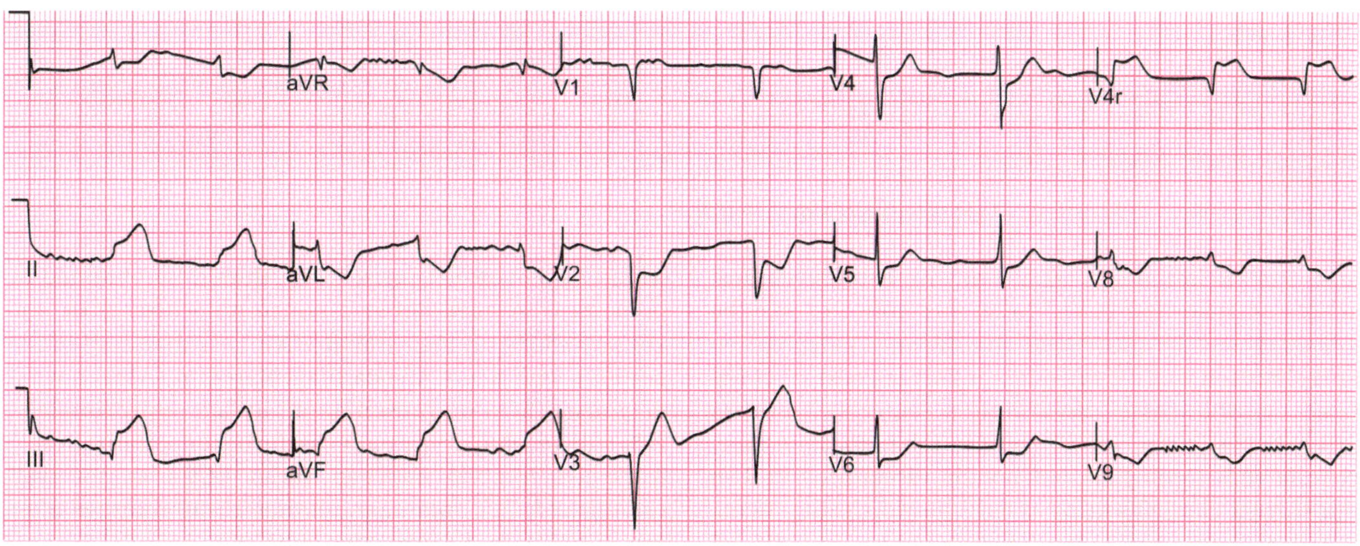

FIG. 2: Inferior and right ventricular ST elevation myocardial infarction

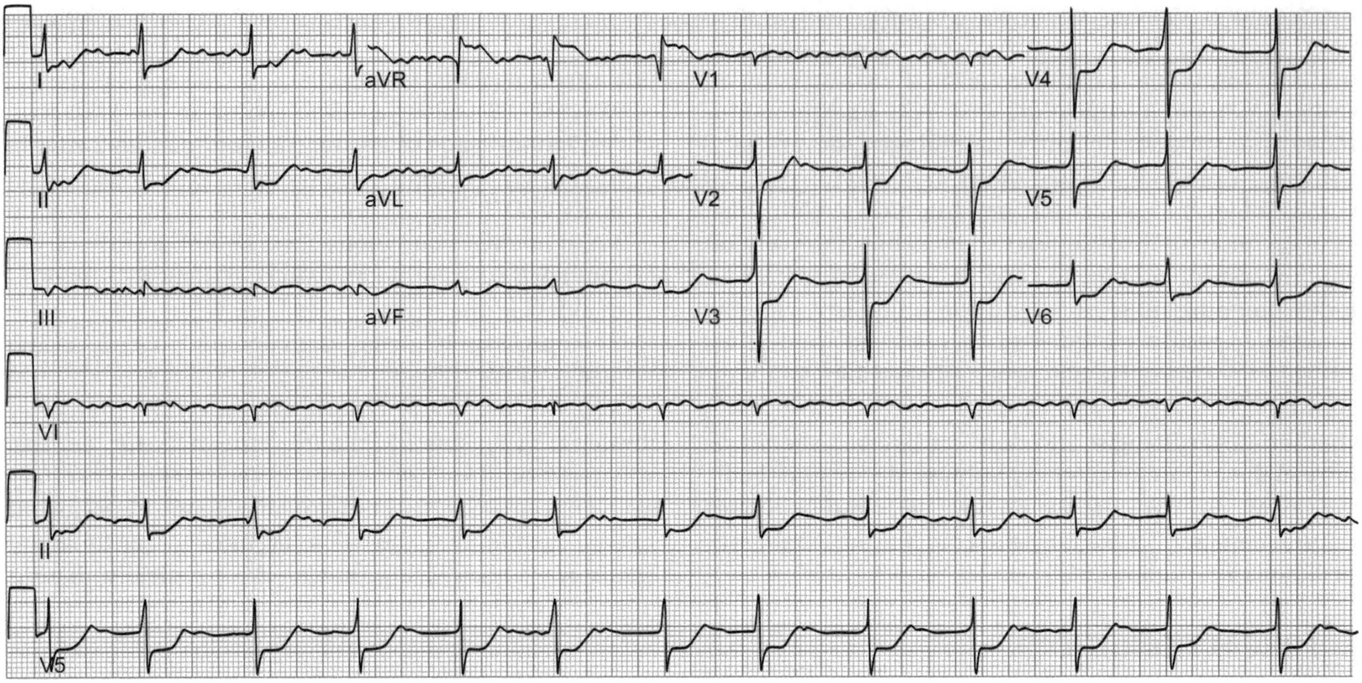

FIG. 3: Diffuse ST-depressions with ST elevation aVR

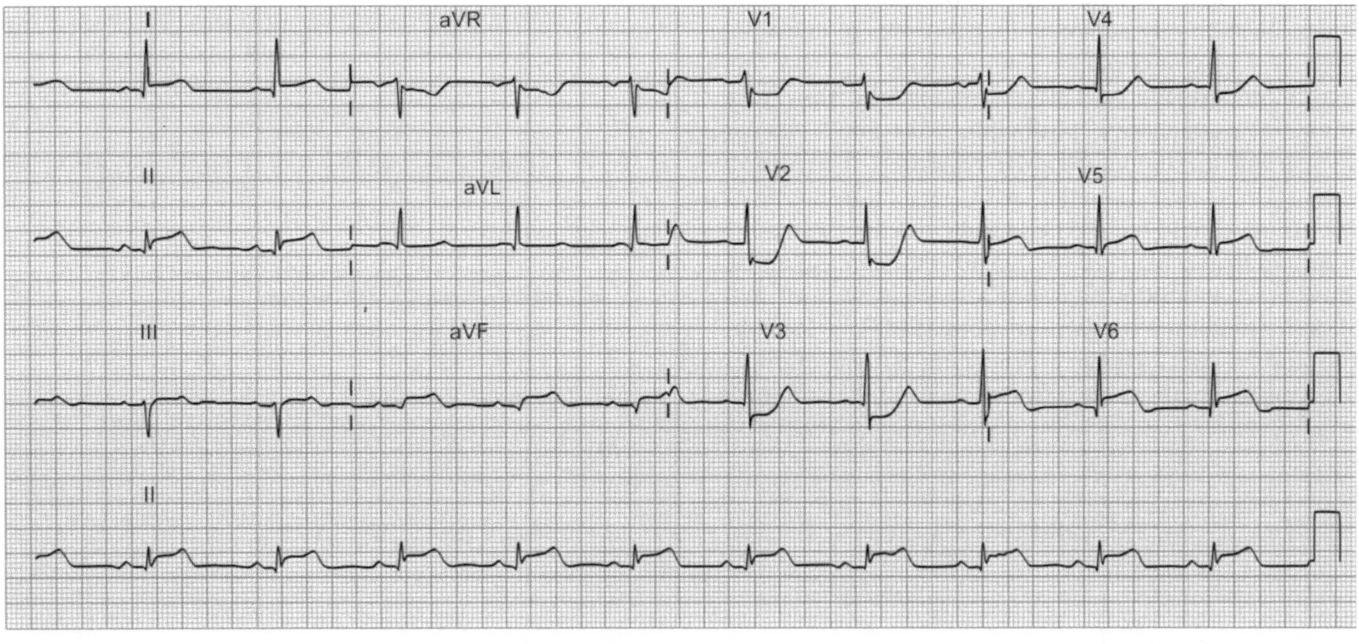

FIG. 4: Inferolateral and posterior ST elevation myocardial infarction

and P2Y12 inhibitors. However, in certain clinical scenarios, deferring P2Y12 inhibitors until PCI may be advantageous in those with multilead ST-depression and elevation in aVR since it is highly suggestive of left main or triple-vessel disease often requiring coronary artery bypass surgery.[16] ST elevation that does not meet criteria (0.5–1 mm) should not be discounted and in the correct clinical setting should be worrisome. Acute coronary syndrome is dynamic in nature and the EP should anticipate that with worsening ischemia the ECG would also evolve.[17] Serial ECGs should be obtained in patients who have either a concerning history or any abnormalities on their initial ECG. Less than half of ED patients with acute myocardial infarction (AMI) have a diagnostic ECG on presentation, in fact approximately, 20% will develop injury patterns during hospitalization.[18] An exact interval between serial ECGs is not well established, but obtaining another 15–30 minutes after presentation or during active chest pain is judicious and recommended.

The prior STEMI guidelines (2004) considered a new left bundle branch block (LBBB) a STEMI equivalent and suggested those patients undergo emergent cardiac catheterization, however, the frequency of false catheterization and inappropriate fibrinolytic therapy has led to recent removal of this recommendation.[19] Diagnosis of STEMI in patients with baseline ECG abnormalities, LBBB or ventricular paced rhythms, is fraught with difficulty. Despite this change, the astute clinician will apply Sgarbossa's criteria (Fig. 5) to identify patients who may require immediate PCI that would otherwise go unnoticed by both computer analysis and inexperienced ECG interpreters. Sgarbossa's criteria rely on consideration of three parameters: (i) concordant ST elevation greater than 1 mm in a lead with a positive QRS-complex, (ii) concordant ST-depression greater than 1 mm in precordial leads (V1–V3), and (iii) excessive discordant ST elevation greater than 5 mm in a lead with a negative QRS-complex.[20] These findings only need to be positive in a single lead for concern and emergent cardiology consultation is necessary. Concordant ST elevation is considered the most specific finding, followed by precordial ST-depression and excessive discordance. A total score of greater than or equal to 3 is reported to have 90% specificity for AMI.[19,21]

Early revascularization has led to a dramatic decline in STEMI, but over the prior decade there have been increasing rates of unstable angina (UA) and non-ST elevation myocardial infarction (NSTEMI).[22] The rate of morbidity and mortality is also exponentially rising in this subset. Unlike STEMI these two forms of ACS are based solely on history and cardiac biomarkers since ECG abnormalities may not be present. A normal ECG does not exclude ACS and can occur in approximately 1–6% of patients.[17] Certain ECG patterns, ST-depression (Fig. 3), and T-wave flattening or inversions (Fig. 6) greater than or equal to 0.5 mm at the J-point in two contiguous leads are suggestive of myocardial ischemia.[23] Electrocardiogram changes should always be interpreted in conjunction with a complete history since several other medical conditions can cause similar ECG abnormalities. ST-depressions can be diffuse or focal. When diffuse, it may represent subendocardial ischemia or as previously discussed STEMI when in conjunction with elevation in aVR.[15,24] Focal ST-depression is more concerning for "reciprocal changes" that are secondary to impending or subtle existing ST elevation.[24] This is commonly seen in the inferior and high lateral leads. An acute inferior infarct is frequently preceded by a single T-wave inversion in aVL, with or without ST-depressions.[25] Similarly inferior ST-depression is regularly seen prior to a high lateral infarct (Fig. 7).[26] Inversions of T-waves in lead III, aVR, and V1 are normal variants and should not alone be considered pathological.[27] Likewise T-wave inversions in the right precordial leads (V1–V3) of adolescents (juvenile T-wave pattern) are also normal and may continue to be present

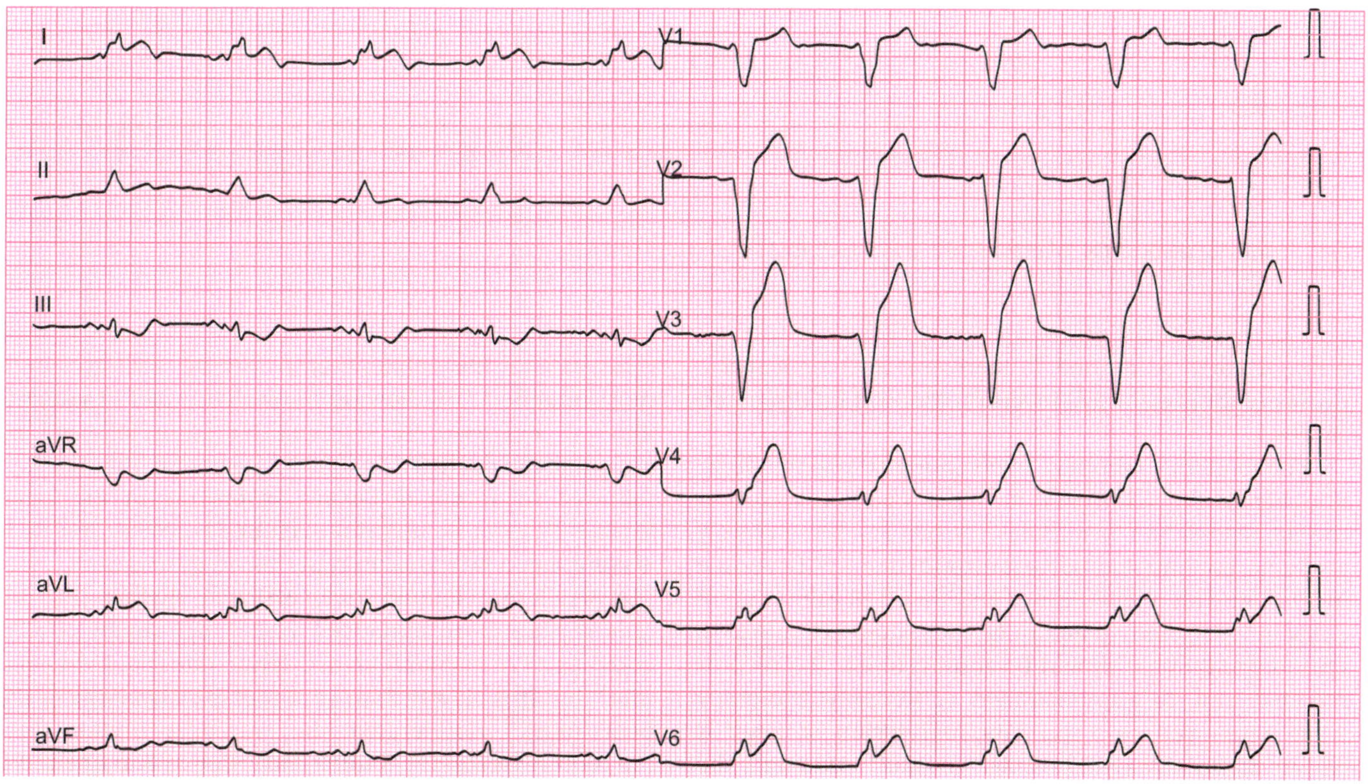

FIG. 5: Sgarbossa criteria—concordance (I-aVL and V5-V6)

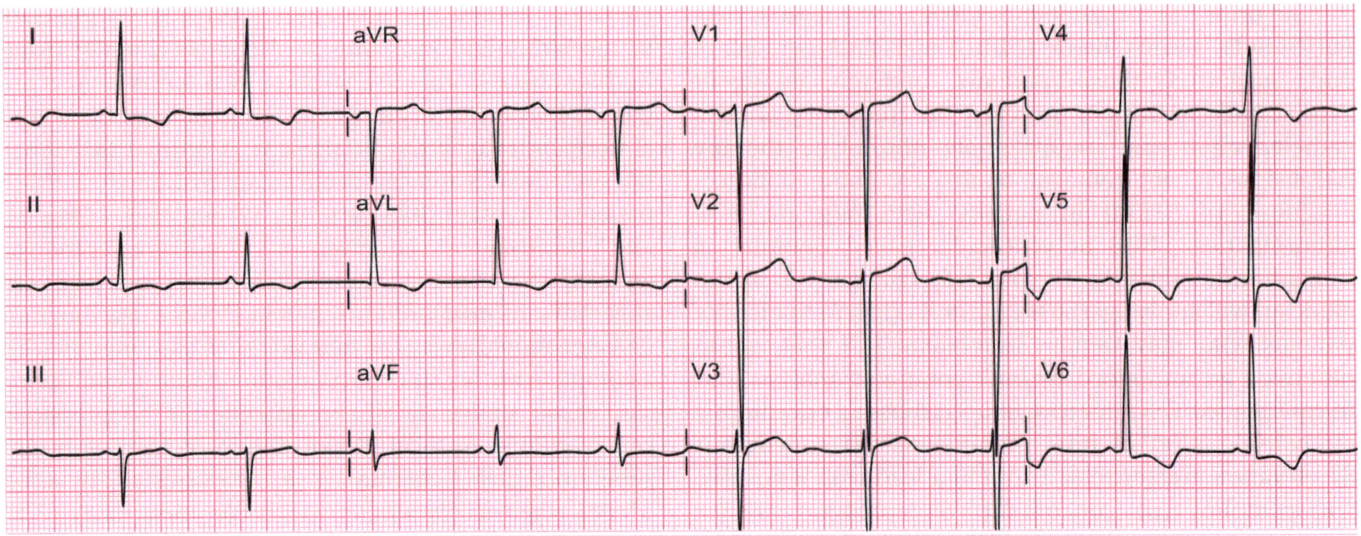

FIG. 6: T-wave inversions

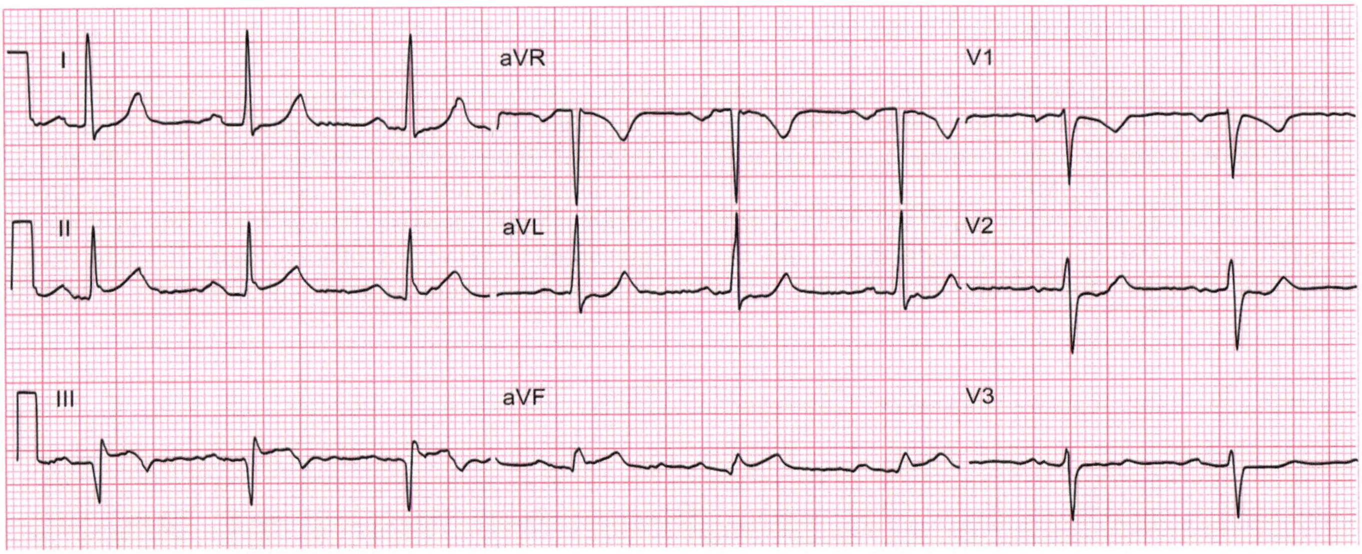

FIG. 7: Inferior myocardial infarction with lateral reciprocal changes (I and aVL)

through early adulthood.[28] There are also noncardiac causes of diffuse T-wave inversion that will be discussed shortly.

Percutaneous coronary intervention is essential first-line therapy for STEMI and the ideal time to reperfusion should be less than 90 minutes.[15] When PCI is not readily available, patients should be transported to a PCI-capable institution with a goal time of less than 120 minutes.[15] If delay in PCI is anticipated to be more than 120 minutes, fibrinolytic therapy should be administered. The recommended time to administration of fibrinolytic therapy when employed as a primary reperfusion strategy is within 30 minutes of hospital arrival.[15] Although the electrocardiographic effects of reperfusion have been well documented, prior to the advent of PCI, the expected changes after fibrinolytic therapy are not well-known to most providers.[29] Following fibrinolytics half of patients develop increased ST segment elevation followed by a significant decrease in the ST segment; this is often followed by terminal T-wave inversions in the same leads.[30] Patency of the prior occluded coronary vessels is accompanied by transient reperfusion arrhythmias, most specifically accelerated idioventricular rhythm (Fig. 8). This rhythm is an enhanced ventricular rhythm (QRS-complex ≥120 ms) with an accelerate rate (50–110 beats/min), but it is slower than ventricular tachycardia (<120 beats/min).[31] Accelerated idioventricular rhythm does not require treatment. Studies have shown that treatment of the rhythm with antiarrhythmic agents have led to hemodynamic decompensation.[32]

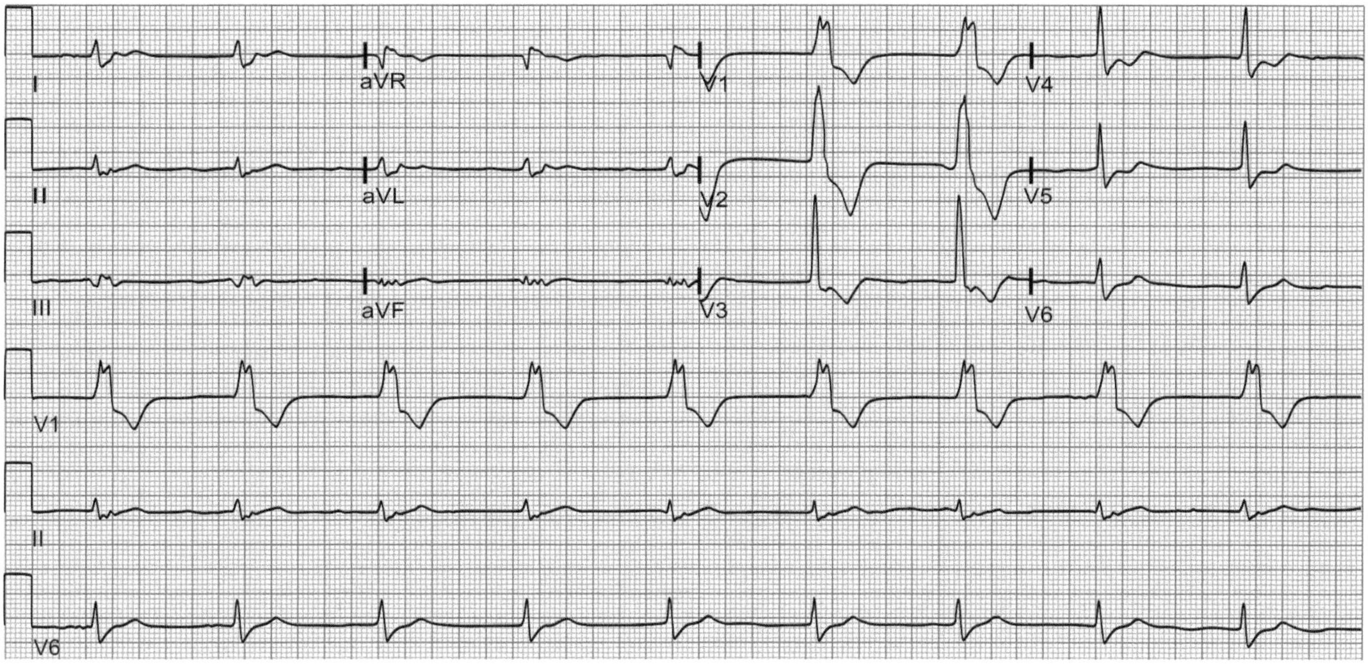

FIG. 8: Accelerated idioventricular rhythm (AIVR)

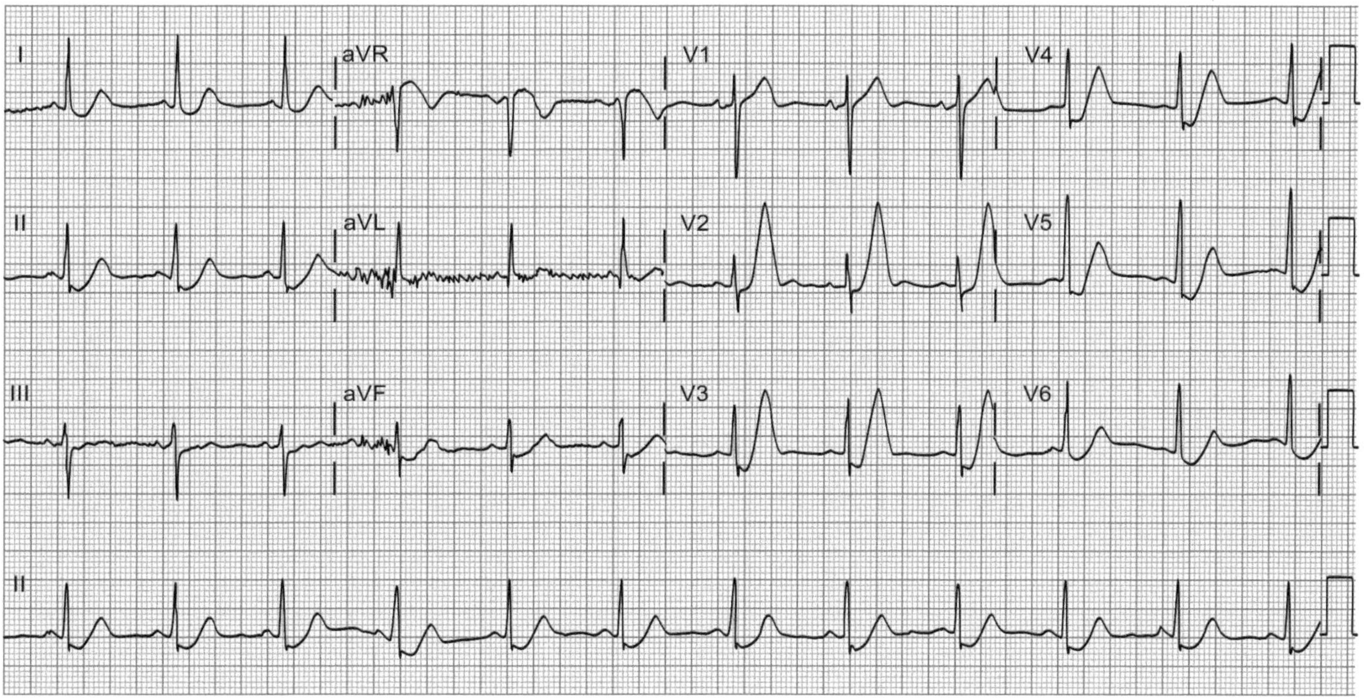

FIG. 9: De Winter T-waves

ST Elevation Myocardial Infarction Equivalents

Emergency department physicians must be well versed in the less discussed, yet ominous ECG patterns that exist. If unidentified in the acute evaluation, these patients are at great risk for myocardial necrosis and subsequent sequel. A novel ECG finding is the de Winter T-wave (Fig. 9), which is notorious for its upsloping ST segment depression greater than or equal to 1 mm with tall symmetrically peaked T-waves in the precordial leads.[33] This is seen in approximately 2% of acute proximal left anterior descending artery (LAD) occlusions.[33] When compared to classic STEMIs, these patients are younger males with a higher incidence of hyperlipidemia.[33] A history of chest pain and de Winter changes should be considered an

STEMI equivalent and cardiology should be consulted for emergent reperfusion therapy, despite its lack of mention in the 2013 STEMI guidelines. Equally worrisome, but less emergent when identified are Wellens' wave. Gerson and colleagues first described it as an inverted U-wave, but Wellens and colleagues coined Wellens syndrome in 1982.[34] The characteristic ECG findings are resultant of a subacute proximal LAD occlusion with reperfusion of the myocardium. These affects alter the T-wave morphology. Unlike patients with de Winter, these patients may be chest pain free on initial evaluation. However, they are at high risk (75%) for development of infarction in the coming days to week.[35] These patients require catheterization urgently in contrast to the more emergent de Winter pattern. There are two distinct morphologies that have been described by Wellens: (i) type 1 (Fig. 10) deep symmetrically inverted T-waves, and (ii) type 2 (Fig. 11) biphasic T-waves with an initial positive then negative deflection.[35] The abnormalities are classically in leads V2–V3, but may extend from V1 to V6. When these patients undergo provocative testing, complete occlusion of the already critically stenotic LAD can occur leading to STEMI or even cardiac arrest.[35] Therefore, stress is not recommended and can be considered a relative contraindication. A less recognized ECG irregularity to ponder is lack of T-wave inversion in V1. Healthy young adults normally have an inverted T-wave in lead V1 and when upright, it should be considered abnormal. When the T-wave is also tall, especially if it is larger than the T-wave in V6, it may be hyperacute and is suspicious for ischemia.[36] The former is referred to as loss of precordial T-wave balance. One study revealed that 84% of patients with an upright V1 T-wave had severe atherosclerotic disease of the circumflex or right coronary artery.[37] In the presence of left ventricular hypertrophy (LVH), LBBB, or misplaced precordial leads, an upright T-wave in V1 is expected and should not alone be a cause for concern.

ST Elevation Myocardial Infarction Mimics

A small number of medical conditions exist that also display ST segment elevation, but are not STEMI. Pericarditis (Fig. 12) or myopericarditis remains one of the most frequently reported diseases that mimic an STEMI. It occurs from inflammation of the pericardium, often causing pericardial fluid accumulation—pericardial effusion. The presentation can be similar to an AMI described by patients as chest pain, with or without a pleuritic component, and dyspnea. The chest pain is usually precordial or retrosternal with referred pain to the trapezius ridge, neck, or shoulder. Other associated symptoms include low-grade fever, cough and tachypnea. When present, a friction rub is thought to be pathognomonic for pericarditis. The ECG is often described by diffuse concave ST segment elevation with no reciprocal depressions (except aVR and V1).[38] Diffuse PR-depression with PR-elevation in aVR, may be seen, but is not obligatory for the diagnosis.[38,39] The ST segment elevation should not be greater in lead III than

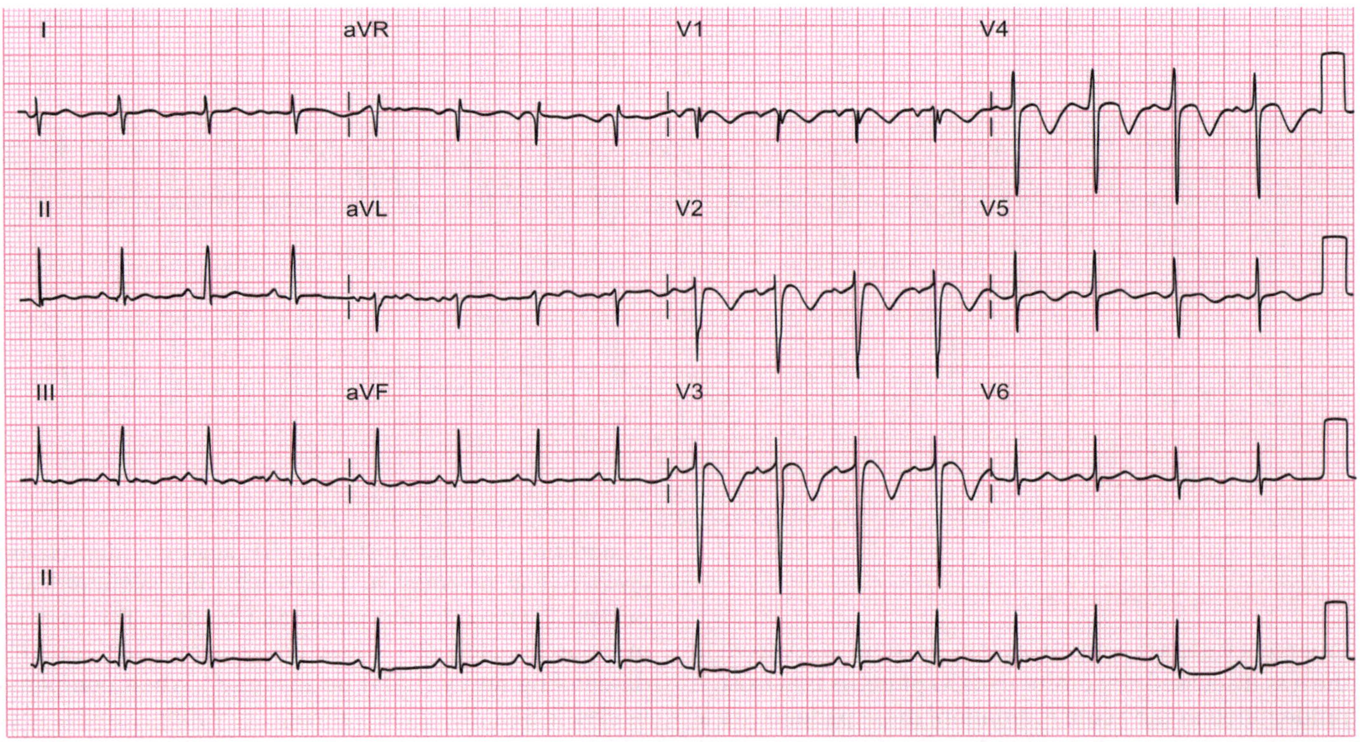

FIG. 10: Wellens (Type 1)

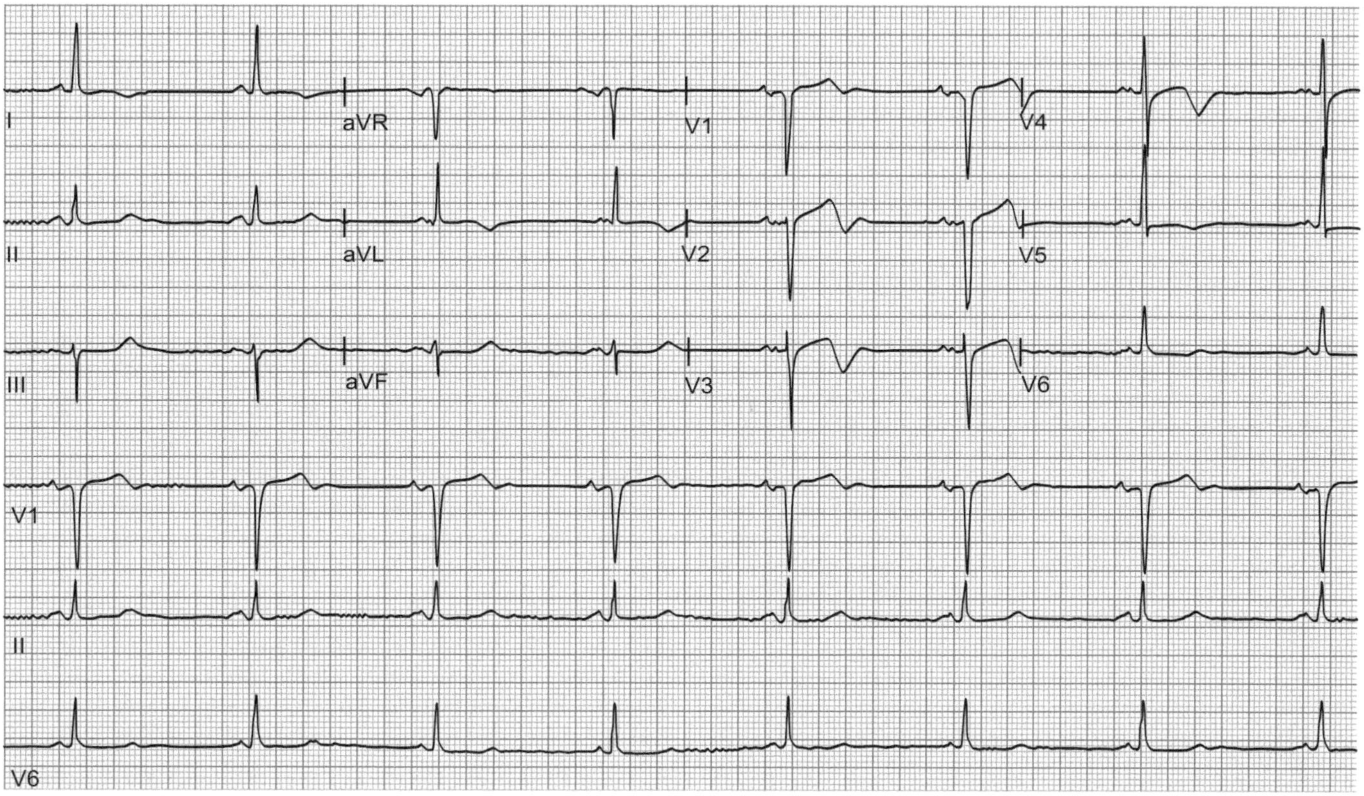

FIG. 11: Wellens (Type 2)

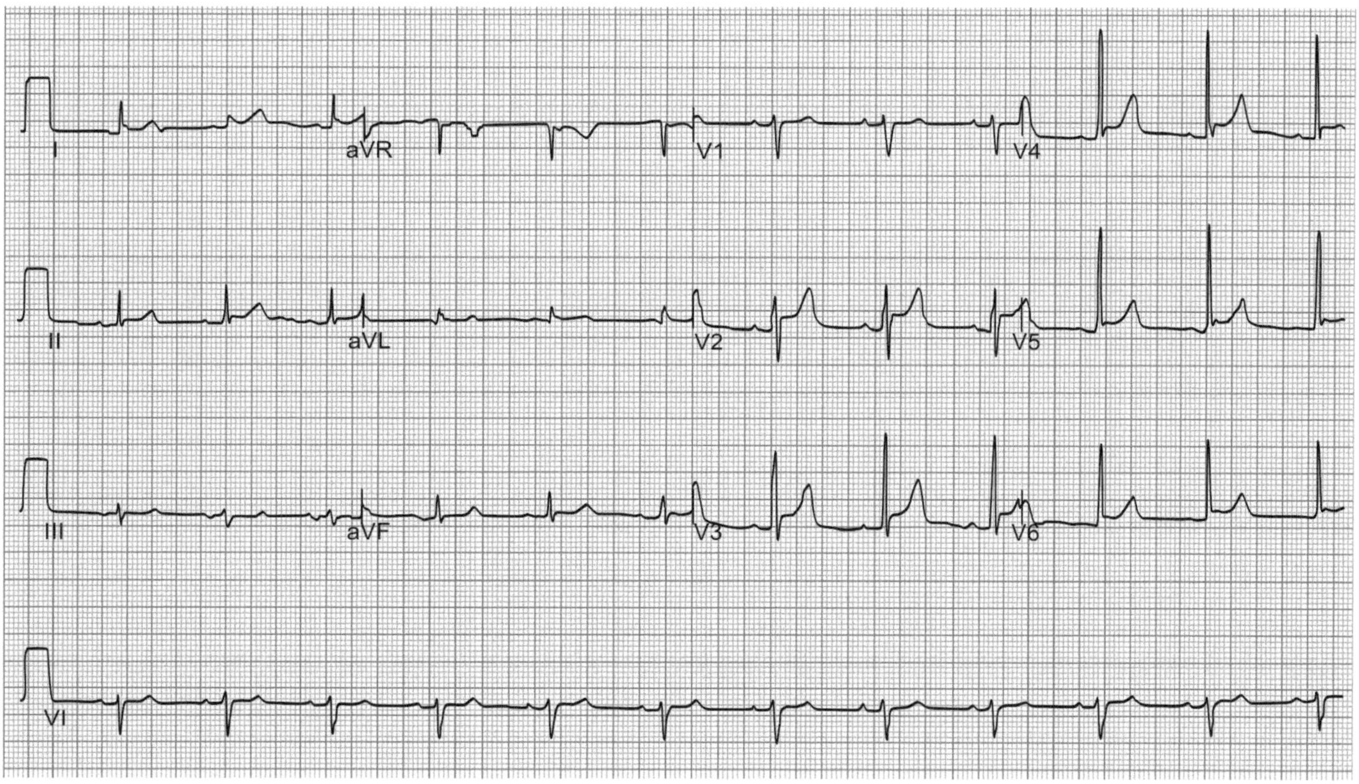

FIG. 12: Pericarditis

lead II and if present is much more likely a diagnosis of STEMI.[40] Diffuse ST elevation is the first of the classically described four stages of pericarditis. The second stage is normalization of the ST segment, followed by flattening or inversion in T-waves and the final stage is normalization. This occurs over days to weeks in contrast to the acute evolution seen in STEMI. A second clinical condition that impersonates STEMI is benign early repolarization (BER). BER (Fig. 13) is most commonly seen in young healthy patients. The ST segment elevation is concave up and typically limited to the precordial leads, although it can be diffuse.[39] There is a characteristic "fish-hook" appearance with T-wave prominence.[40] Just as with pericarditis there should never be reciprocal changes in BER, but unlike pericarditis the ECG remains stable over time. In BER, the degree of ST elevation is modest compared to the T-wave. The ST segment to T segment ratio is less than 0.25 and that ratio in pericarditis is greater than 0.25.[39] Formation of a ventricular aneurysm can occur following an anterior AMI if a significant part of myocardium is injured. The effect of a left ventricular aneurysm (LVA) on an ECG is ST elevations in the anterior leads that can be concave or convex in morphology.[41] Emergency department evaluation of patients without a prior documented ECG or known history of AMI can lead to concern for STEMI in patients who actually have LVA. Unlike STEMI, the ST elevations of LVA are only seen in the precordial leads and a Q or QS-waves are typically seen given their prior infarct. Additionally, the T-waves are small in amplitude when compared to the QRS-complex unlike the hyperacute T-waves seen in STEMI.[42] Benign early repolarization and LVA ECG findings are stable and do not change over time. Left ventricular hypertrophy (Fig. 14) results from increased afterload generally secondary to hypertension. This is often the most difficult imitator to differentiate from STEMI, particularly when prior ECGs are not available for comparison. The ECG irregularities that can be seen with LVH include: large LV voltages, ST elevation in right precordial leads (V1–V3) with discordant deep S-waves, large R-wave amplitude in left sided leads (III, aVR, V4–V6), strain pattern (ST-depression and T-wave inversions), left axis deviation, prominent U-waves and delayed repolarization in the lateral leads.[43] Numerous criteria exist to assist in the diagnosis of LVH, none of which are unflawed. The most used are the Sokolow-Lyon, Cornell, and Romhilt-Estes criteria. The Sokolow-Lyon is

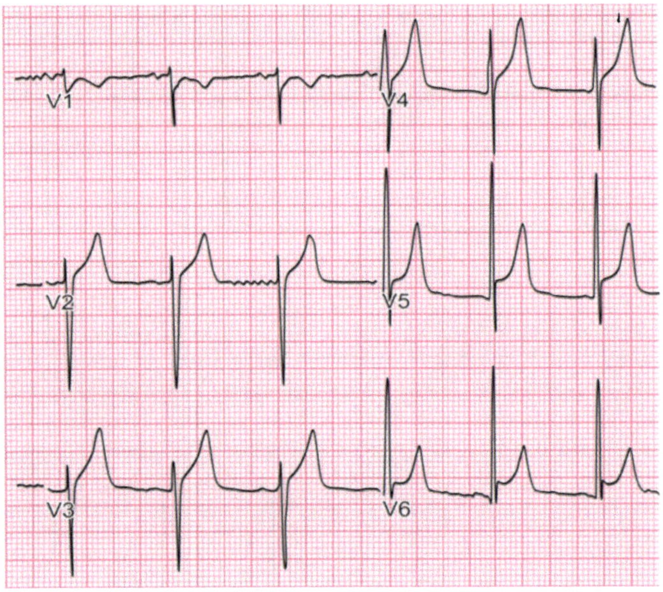

FIG. 13: Benign early repolarization

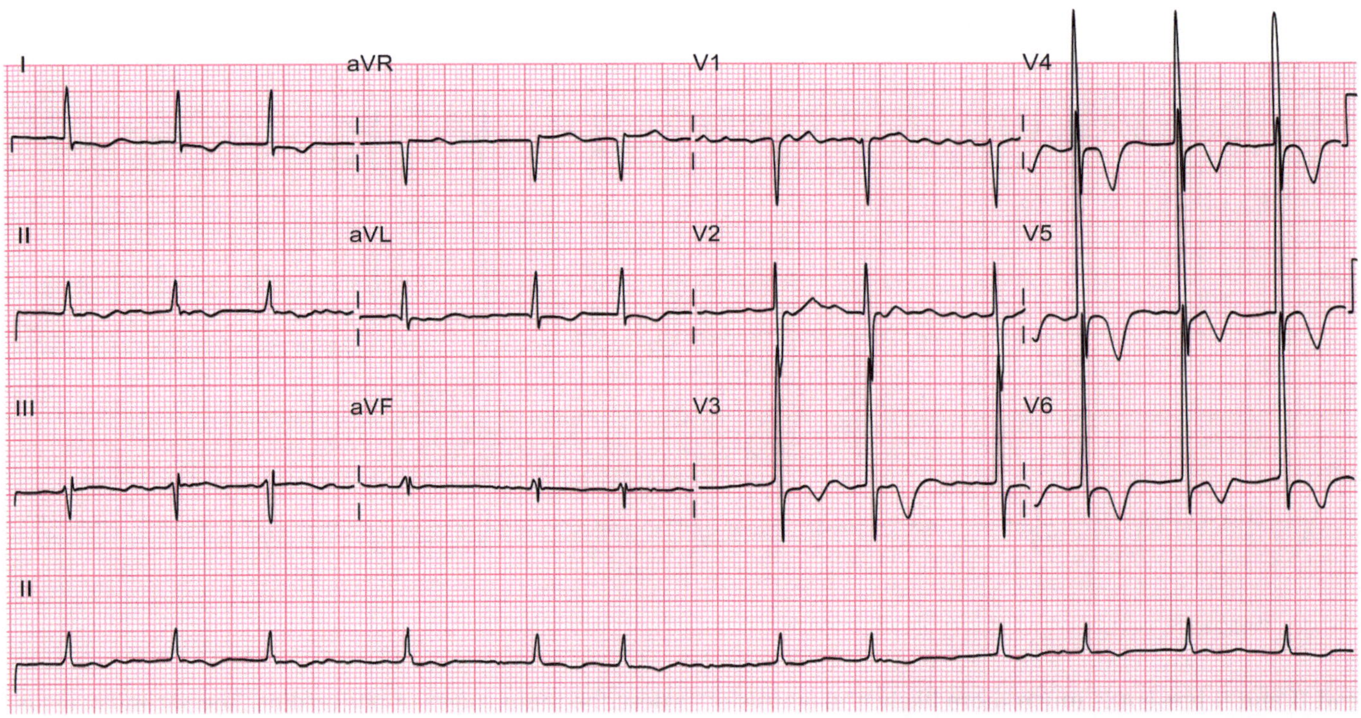

FIG. 14: Atrial fibrillation with left ventricular hypertrophy

positive for LVH if the S-wave in V1 plus the R-wave in V5 or V6 is greater than or equal to 35 mm or the R-wave in aVL is greater than or equal to 11 mm.[44] Left ventricular hypertrophy based on the Cornell voltage criteria is present if there is an S-wave in V3 plus the R-wave in aVL greater than 28 mm in men and greater than 20 mm in women. The Romhilt-Estes criteria is based on a scoring system and considered diagnostic if there is a calculated score of greater than 5 points and probable for a score of 4 points. Three points are given if any of the following are present on ECG: R or S in limb leads greater than 20 mm, S in V1 or V2 greater than or equal to 30 mm, R in V5 or V6 greater than or equal to 30 mm, ST-T vector opposite the QRS-complex without digitalis, or a negative terminal P-wave in V1 indicting left atrial enlargement.[45] Left axis deviation is given two points.[45] A QRS-duration greater than 90 ms, delayed intrinsicoid deflection in V5 or V6, or ST-T vector opposite QRS-complex with digitalis are all given one point.[45] Of the above-mentioned criteria, the most specific is thought to be the Romhilt-Estes.[46,47] Ultimately, echocardiography is the principal method to diagnose LVH measuring the thickness of the heart; however, an ECG is often used as a screening examination. For ED providers, LVH is the most common cause of false activation of the catheterization laboratory, but to date no criteria exist that can safely differentiate this mimic from STEMI.[48] Utilization of medical records, prior ECGs, and history is vital in this often-encountered clinical dilemma. Other causes of ST segment elevation are paced rhythms and LBBB, but most providers rarely confuse them for STEMI. A bundle branch block refers to abnormal electrical cardiac conduction. Electrical activity in a healthy heart classically starts at the sinoatrial (SA) nodes and propagates through the atria to the atrioventricular (AV) node then down to the bundle of His and divides into the left and right bundles branches. The bundles branches can become injuries for various reasons and not allow for proper electrical activity. When the QRS-complex is greater than 120 ms, a bundle branch is present.[49] An LBBB is present when the QRS is widened and there are also QS or rS complex in V1 and an R wave in V6.[49] The T-wave should also be opposite the terminal deflection of the QRS-complex and this is termed appropriate discordance.[49] Electrocardiogram appearance of a paced patient is dependent on the pacing mode, device threshold and native electrical activity. A chapter dedicated to pacing is found in this book.

Electrical/Structural Disorders

Young healthy patients have good cardiopulmonary reserve and despite serious illness can appear to have normal vital signs and benign physical examinations. Their ECGs are usually normal. A unique population of adolescents and young adults must be considered when acutely evaluating patients with transient or nonspecific symptoms (i.e., near-syncope, dizziness, or lightheadedness). Often their ECGs will be read as "normal" by computer analysis and inexperienced ECG interpreters, which is falsely reassuring and unfortunate. Of those discharged, a minority will return after suffering cardiac death secondary to a dysrhythmia. Emergency department physicians must always scrutinize the ECG of seemingly young healthy patients with transient symptoms given the risk of arrhythmogenic disorders, which are often discovered in this age group. Monogenic cardiac diseases are caused by rare mutations in single genes changing the electrical or structural substrate of the myocardium. It is a significant cause of sudden cardiac death (SCD). Approximately, 500,000 people die of SCD per year in the United States, of them approximately 5% are from a primary electrical disease, approximately 10–15% are from an inherited cardiomyopathy, and greater than 80% are from coronary artery disease (CAD) and its sequel.[50] Long QT syndrome (LQTS) (Fig. 15) is the most frequent of the electrical disorders and is characterized by prolongation of the QT interval greater than approximately 440 ms for men and approximately 460 ms for woman.[51] Long QT syndrome is usually diagnosed after a person has a cardiac event, but may be diagnosed earlier if carefully screened. Symptoms

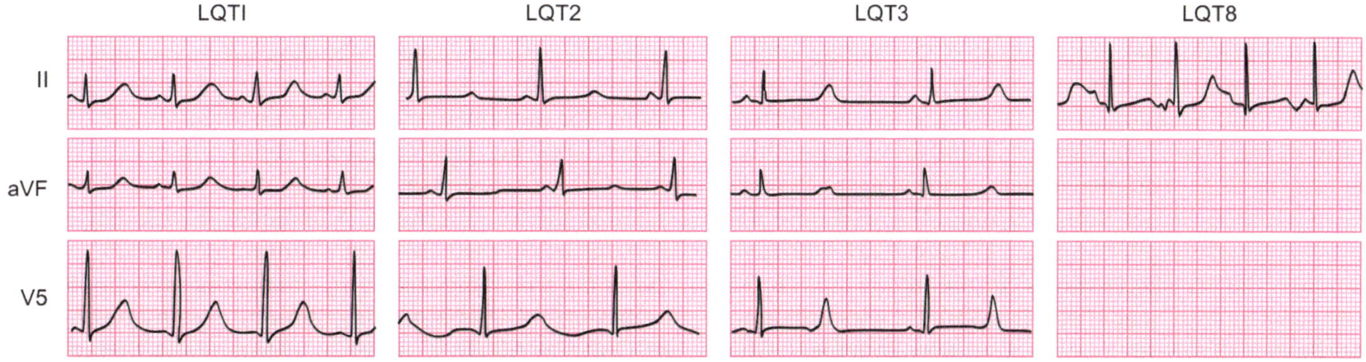

FIG. 15: Long QT syndrome

include dizziness, light-headedness, and near-syncope. A presumptive first time seizure in an adolescent or young adult with no prior history should alter the ED provider to consider syncope. The latter is challenging because the event may have not been witnessed and myoclonus is frequently confused for seizures. If a screening ECG is not obtained, LQTS or another arrhythmogenic disease may go undiagnosed. Long QT syndrome is caused by mutations in the genes for cardiac calcium, potassium, or sodium channels. Long QT syndrome and other acquired causes of QT prolongation can lead to torsade de pointes (TdP). Torsade de pointes is more common when the QT interval is greater than 500 ms.[52] It is a form of polymorphic ventricular tachycardia, which itself can also lead to SCD.[53] Fortunately, episodes of TdP are usually self-terminating in patients with LQTS; only about 4–5% of cardiac events are fatal.[52] Long QT syndrome patients who are symptomatic (i.e., syncope, dysrhythmias, or cardiac arrest) are usually started on β-blockers and will require implantable cardioverter-defibrillator (ICD). An electrical disorder that is increasingly being recognized as a culprit in SCD is Brugada syndrome. It is a channelopathy that is caused by an alteration in the cardiac action potential.[54] There are several described pathophysiological theories attributed to this disease, but none is clearly elucidated. Symptoms range from asymptomatic to SCD, but certain clinical situations have been reported to unmask or exacerbate the ECG patterns of Brugada syndrome. Examples are fever, electrolyte imbalance, alcohol, illicit substances, and some medications.[55] There are three described ECG patterns in Brugada syndrome (Fig. 16); (i) coved ST elevation with an inverted T-wave in leads V1–V2, (ii) saddleback ST elevation, and (iii) minimal ST elevation.[56] In the appropriate clinical setting, a screening ECG analyzed by a skilled interpreter can be lifesaving. Like LQTS, this disorder easily results in SCD and the only known effective treatment is with ICD placement.

The inherited structural diseases unlike the electrical disorders show more variable presentations, but do also carry a higher incidence of SCD than that of the general population. Hypertrophic cardiomyopathy (HCOM) is a familial disease causing myocardial hypertrophy. Two variants exist: (i) an obstructive and (ii) a nonobstructive type. It is the number one cause of SCD in young athletes with an estimated annual mortality of approximately 1–2%.[57] Complications of HCOM are on a spectrum ranging anywhere from asymptomatic to congestive heart failure or SCD. Younger patients, particularly children, have a much higher mortality rate. The well-described ECG findings of HCOM (Fig. 17) are LVH with deep narrow "dagger like Q-waves" in the lateral (I, aVL, V5–V6) and inferior leads (II, III, aVF).[58] Echocardiogram findings of HCOM include: LVH, atrial enlargement, small ventricular cavity, decreased midaortic flow, and partial systolic closure of aortic valve.[59] Treatment is dictated by degree of disease manifestations and symptomatology. Management may include pharmacological agents such as β-blockers and/or a surgical approach. Arrhythmogenic right ventricular dysplasia (ARVD) is an inherited cardiomyopathy characterized by structural and functional abnormalities. It is not easily identified and often found postmortem. There is increasing evidence of its contribution in SCD of young adults. There is fatty-fibrotic infiltrate primarily in the right ventricle, but it can also occur in the left ventricle.[57] The former leads to ventricular dilation and dysfunction. Like HCOM, the symptoms range from asymptomatic, to heart failure, and SCD. Some patients have completely normal ECGs making the diagnosis perplexing. In patients with concerning history, other diagnostic testing can be perused despite a normal ECG. As the diseases progresses ECG changes can be more notable. The criterion for AVRD (Fig. 18) is complex and involves major and minor findings.[60] Having two major criteria, or one major plus two minor criteria, or four minor makes a definite diagnosis.[60] A probable diagnosis is met when there is one major criterion plus one minor or three minor criteria alone.[60] A possible diagnosis is made when there is either one major or two minor criteria.[60] The major diagnostic ECG findings are: inverted T-waves in the absence of a right bundle branch block (RBBB) with a low amplitude signal between the end of the QRS complex and T-wave (epsilon wave) in the precordial leads (V1–V3). The minor ECG manifestations include: inverted T-waves in V1–V2 or in V4–V6 in the absence of RBBB, or inverted T-waves in V1–V4 in the presence of an RBBB, or an interventricular conduction delay of greater than or equal to 110 ms, or a prolonged S-wave upstroke greater than or equal to 55 ms. Sustained or paroxysmal episodes of ventricular tachycardia with LBBB morphology and superior axis meet major arrhythmogenic criteria. The former findings with an RV outflow configuration and an inferior axis meet minor criteria.[61] Diagnostic imaging studies are also divided into the major/minor criteria. An echocardiogram with regional RV akinesia, dyskinesia, or aneurysm plus an abnormal outflow tract size or volume meets major criteria as does magnetic resonance image showing the former or an angiography showing the same. The minor imaging criteria are the same as stated earlier, but the values for outflow tract and volume are different. Tissue biopsy showing greater fibrous replacement is a major criterion versus those with less myocyte replacement meeting the minor criteria. A first degree with diagnostic criteria or known autopsy confirming ARVD meets major criteria compared to an unknown family history of premature SCD is a minor criterion. Treatment of both HCOM and ARVD is aimed at symptomatic therapy for heart failure and ICD placement for SCD.

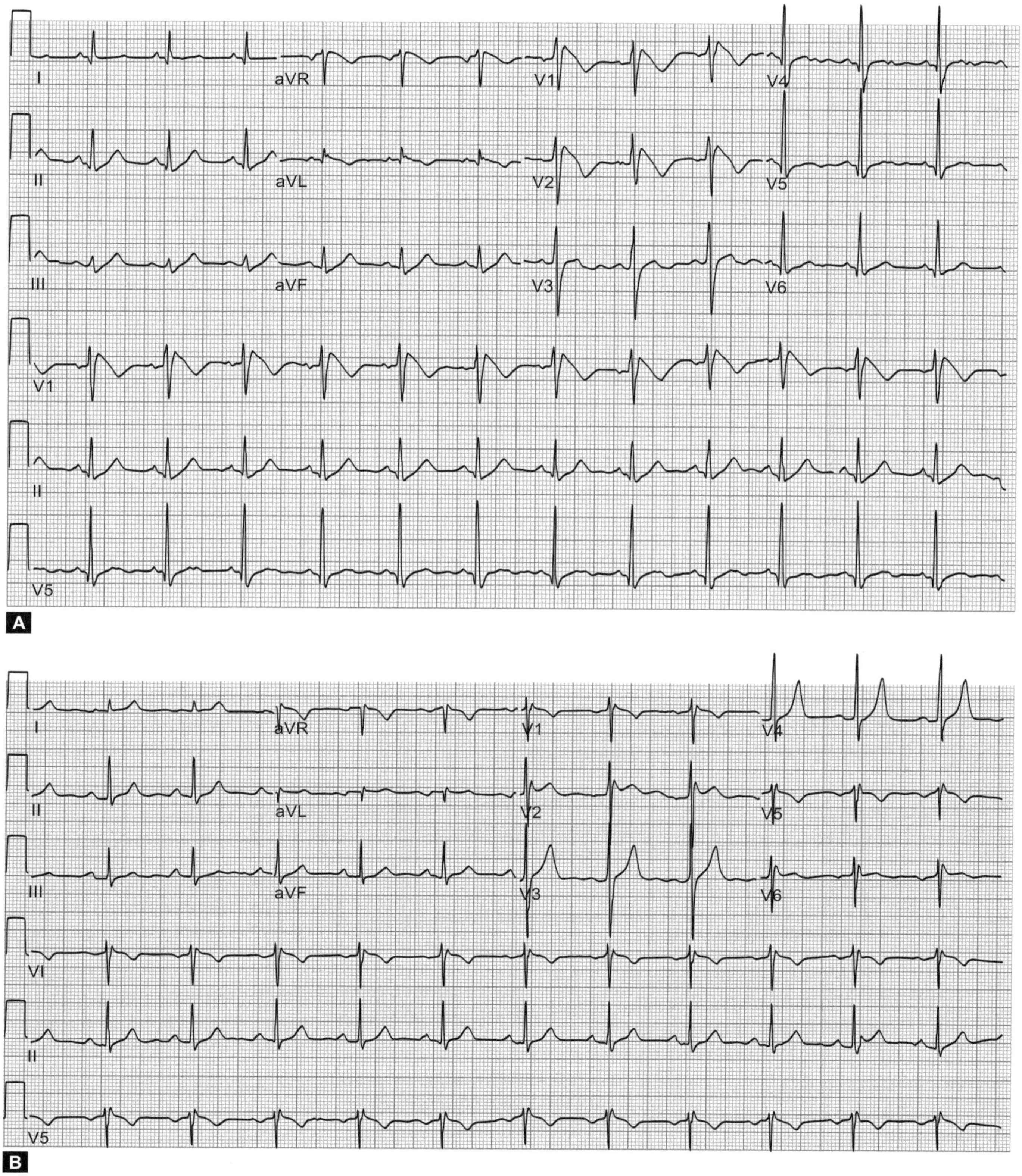

FIG. 16: **A,** Brugada (Type I) and **B,** Brugada (Type 2)

Wolff-Parkinson-White (WPW) syndrome is caused by congenitally abnormal conductive cardiac tissue between the atria and the ventricles that provides a pathway for a reentrant circuit.[62] The accessory atrioventricular (AV) connection bypasses the AV node and His-bundle. The accessory pathway can conduct faster than the AV node and cause ventricular preexcitation that manifests on the ECG (Fig. 19) with a short PR interval (<120 ms),

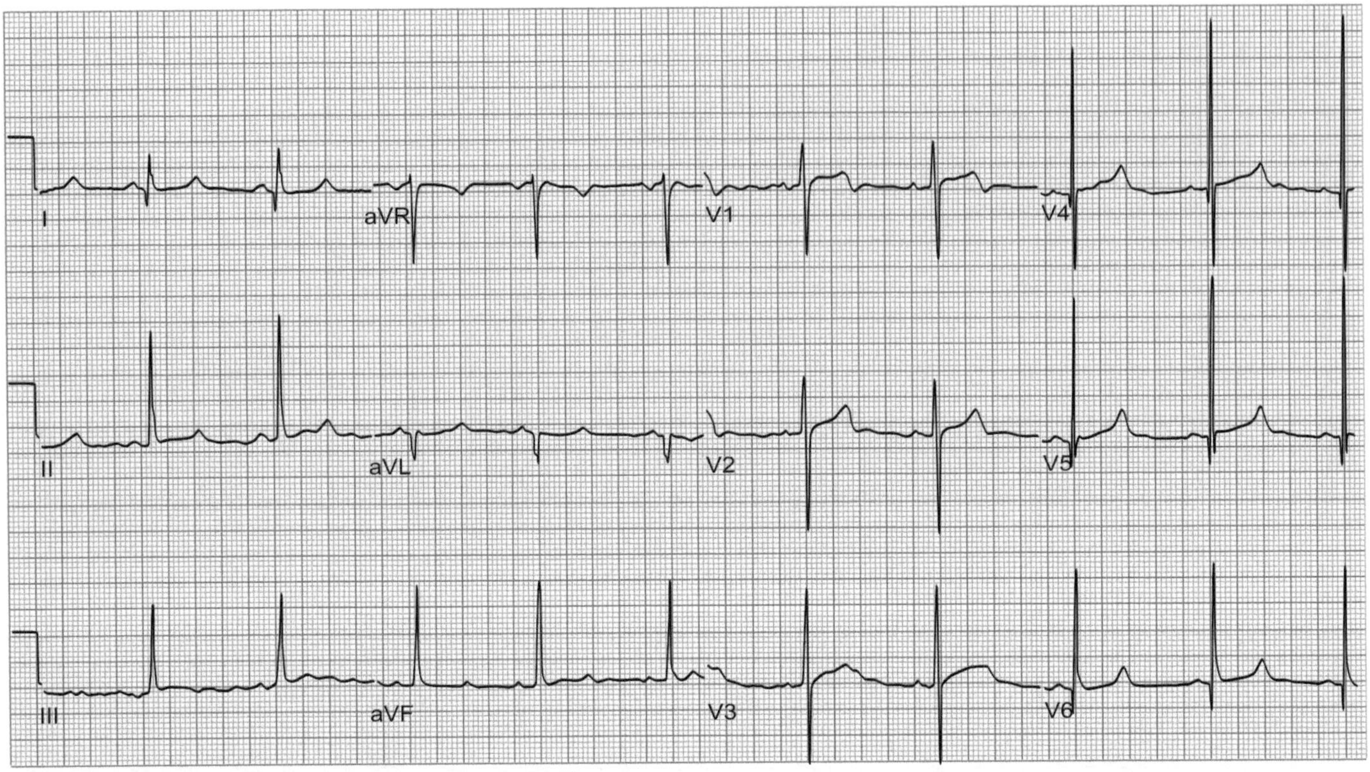

FIG. 17: Hypertrophic cardiomyopathy

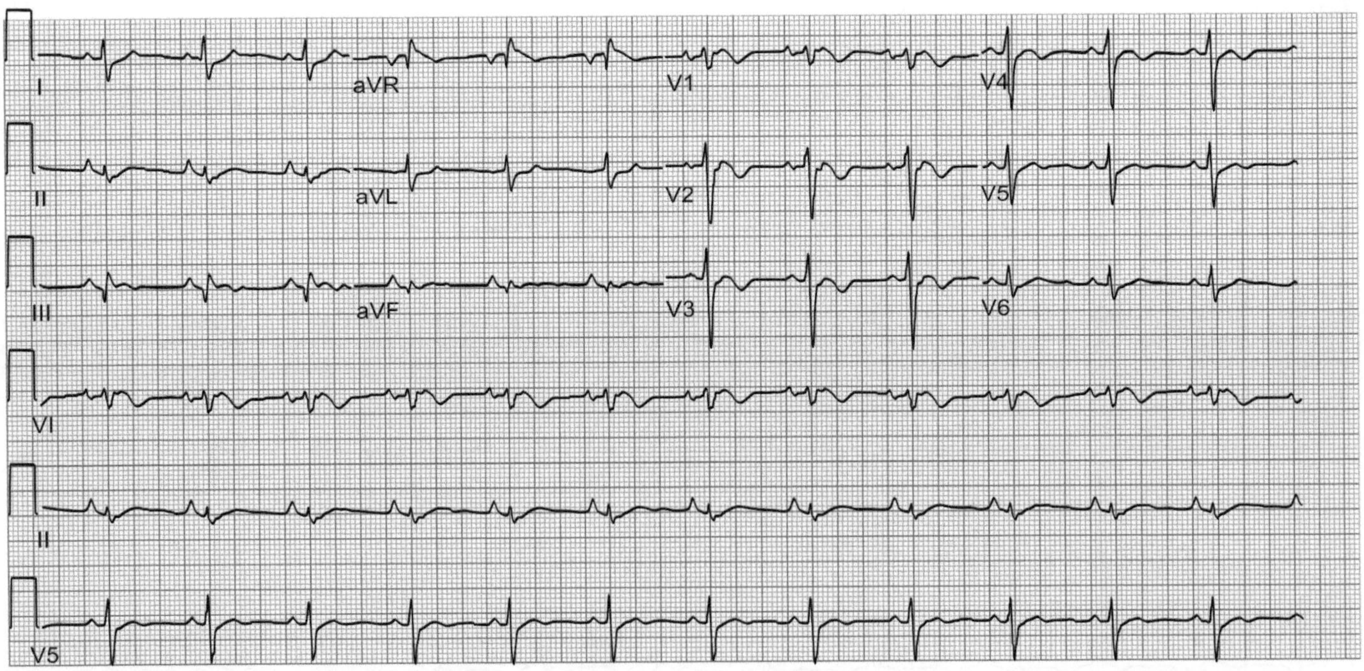

FIG. 18: Arrhythmogenic right ventricular dysplasia (ARVD)

a slurred upstroke of the QRS complex (δ wave), and a prolonged QRS (>120 ms).[62] Most patients with WPW syndrome have otherwise structurally normal hearts. A small percentage of cases are familial and associated with structural abnormalities. Wolff-Parkinson-White syndrome may present at any time from childhood to midlife and severity can vary from chest pain to syncope. Patients can develop symptomatic arrhythmias over time, which can be prevented with elective radiofrequency ablation. In the acute setting, patients presenting with a tachydysrhythmias are at risk for clinical decompensation and treatment must be based on the hemodynamics and ECG findings. If the patient has any alteration in sensorium, ischemic chest pain, pulmonary edema,

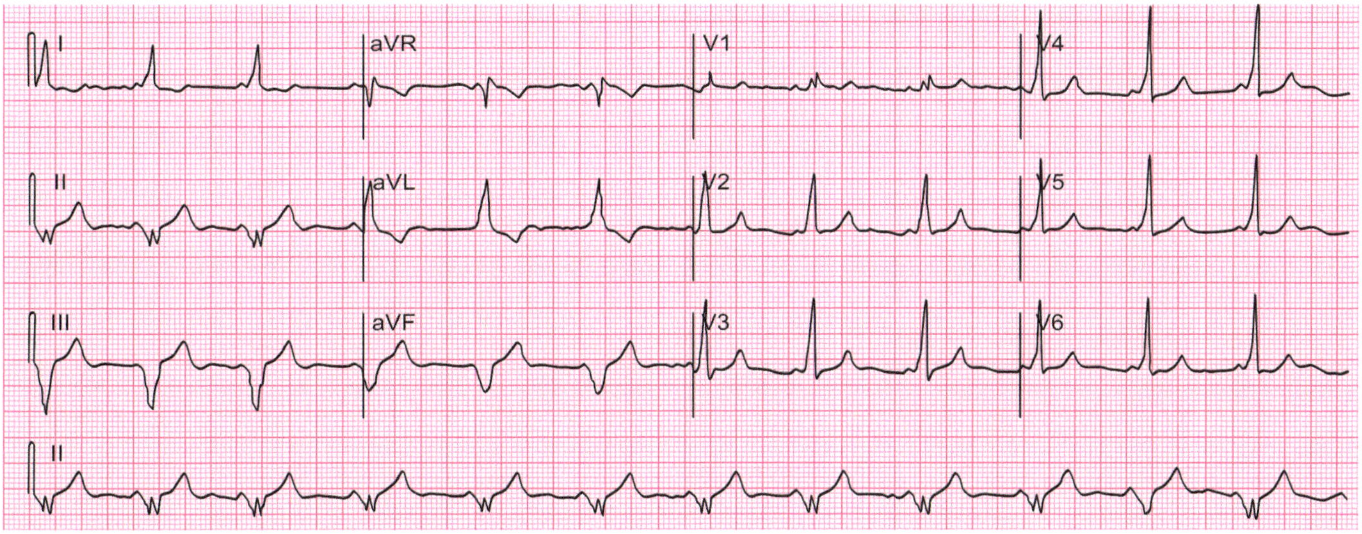

FIG. 19: Wolff-Parkinson-White syndrome

and/or hypotension direct—current cardioversion is necessary. If atrial flutter or fibrillation occurs in those with WPW they are at increased risk of tachydysrhythmias due to accelerated conduction across the bypass tract. These patients typically have an ECG with an extremely fast rate which is irregularly irregular although given the rapid rate may deceitfully appear regular with varying QRS complexes.[63] Emergent treatment is either cardioversion or intravenous procainamide/ibutilide.[63] Agents such as adenosine, β or calcium channels blockers, and digoxin all are AV nodal blockers that cause worsening of the dysthymias and may lead to cardiac arrest.[63] Those with a family history of dysrhythmias have a worse prognosis, but only a minority is at risk of SCD.

Special Considerations

Many conditions can produce electrolyte abnormalities causing varying degrees of symptomology for patients. Laboratory studies often lag behind the initial ED assessment. A screening ECG and expert interpretation can alert the ED physician to critical abnormalities that require swift intervention. Of all electrolytes, hyperkalemia is most known to cause abnormal heart and skeletal muscle function by lowering the resting action potential, preventing repolarization, and ultimately leading to muscle paralysis. The classic ECG findings for hyperkalemia are peaked T-waves, lengthening of the QRS and PR intervals, flattening or disappearance of the P-wave, and a sinusoidal wave prior to cardiac arrest (Fig. 20).[64] Differentiating T-waves can be challenging. A broad based and asymmetric T-wave is more consistent with a hyperacute wave and infarction whereas a narrow based and symmetric T-wave is more suggestive of hyperkalemia. Hyperkalemia is a known cause of very wide QRS complexes, bizarre rhythms, and high-grade AV blocks, yet it is commonly forgotten.[65] The typical algorithm for bradydysrhythmias such as atropine, pacing, and pharmacological agents (i.e., dobutamine, epinephrine, isoproterenol) often fails. Therapy must be directed at potassium shifting and ultimately excretion. The ECG findings of hyperkalemia are unique, but many other electrolytes deficiencies cause nonspecific ECG changes. Hypokalemia, hypomagnesemia, and hypocalcemia, in addition to nonelectrolyte conditions, produce a prolonged QT-complex.[66] Hypokalemia unlike other electrolytes has QT prolongation as the result of fusion of the T and U waves (Fig. 21). Electrocardiogram abnormalities seen with more profound hypokalemia, ST segment depression, T-wave flattening or inversion, prolonged PR-interval, and increased P wave amplitude are often confused for ischemia.[67] Severe hypokalemia can result in ventricular ectopy and life-threatening dysrhythmias. Hypokalemia is associated with hypomagnesemia, which further increases the risk of malignant dysrhythmias.[68] Hypocalcemia is distinct from the other electrolytes causing QT-prolongation because it specifically lengthens the ST-portion as opposed to the T wave.[69] The all ECG irregularities mentioned, resolve with electrolyte repletion.

An Osborn wave (J-wave) is a positive deflection at the J-point and is most prominent in the precordial leads. It is characteristically seen in hypothermia, but is also associated with hypercalcemia, some medications and neurological insults. Hypothermia (Fig. 22) whether environmental or secondary to an underlying medical problem (i.e., endocrine dysfunction) causes the same ECG manifestations, sinus bradycardia, prolongation of the P, QRS, and QT complexes.[70] The severity of the hypothermia is directly related to the prolongation and presence of J waves. Hypercalcemia can cause Osborn waves, but its effects on the QT interval are far more

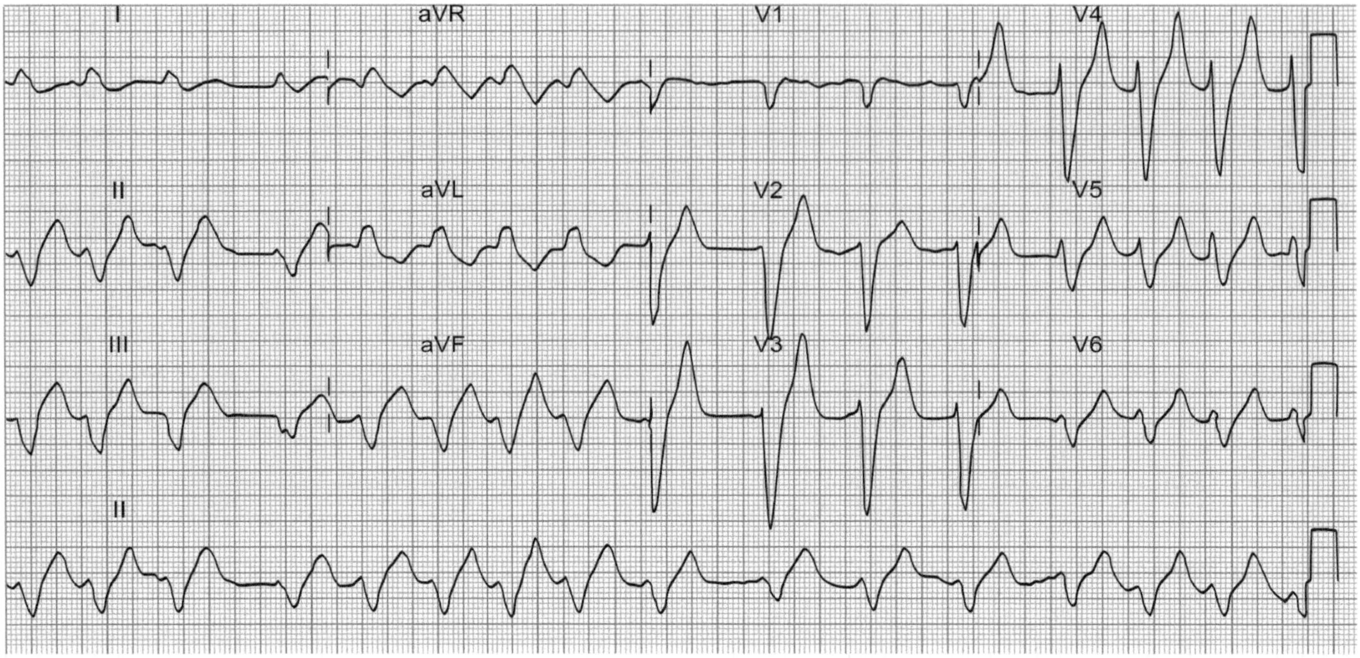

FIG. 20: Hyperkalemia

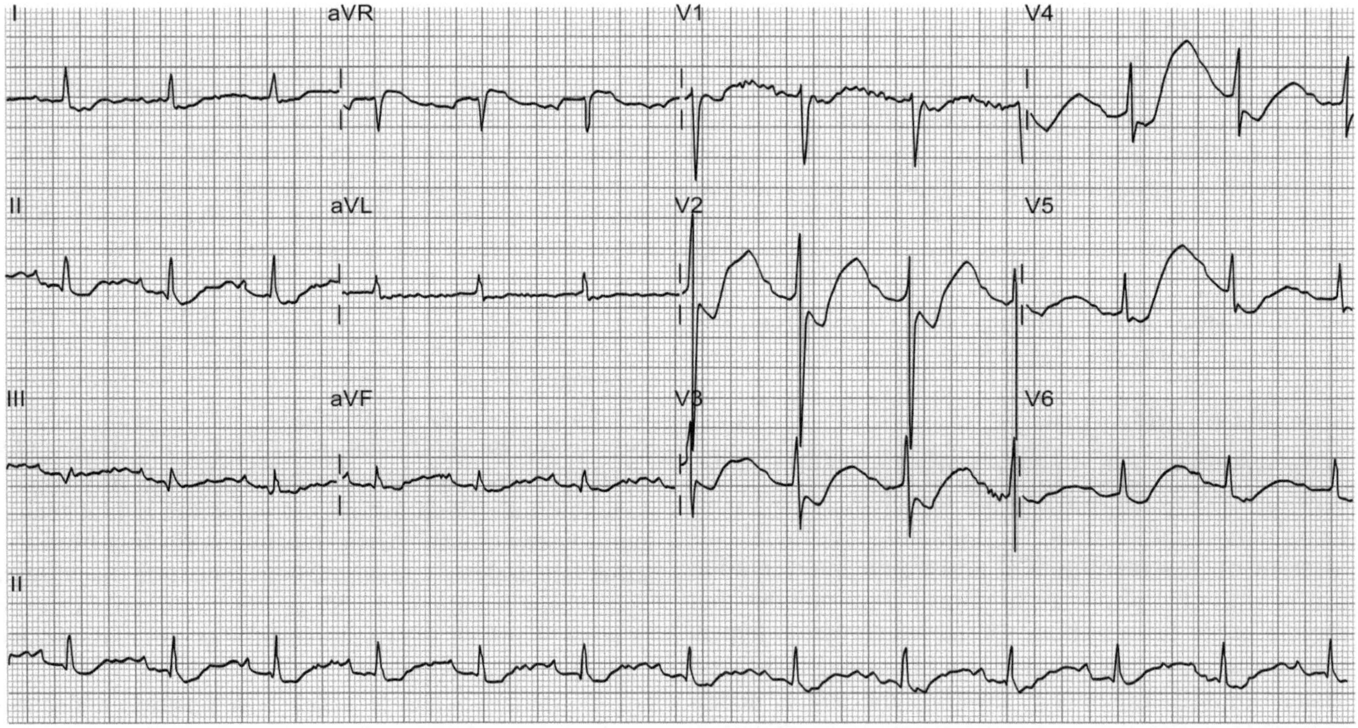

FIG. 21: Hypokalemia

worrisome. Hypercalcemia produces a short QT (Fig. 23) that can cause ventricular ectopy and arrest if severe.[71] Few things are associated with a short QT interval besides hypercalcemia, arrhythmogenic disease and digitalis toxicity.[72] Short QT syndrome (SQTS) like LQTS is a disease of the electrical system of the heart. It is thought to be the result of a short refractory period and transmural dispersion of repolarization. Short QT syndrome is associated with paroxysmal atrial, syncope, ventricular fibrillation, and SCD.[72] The ECG characteristics are a QT interval less than 300 ms that does not change with heart rate, tall peaked T-waves, and a structurally normal heart.[72] Treatment for SQTS as with all the other congenital disorders is ICD placement.

Any patient who presents to the ED with an altered sensorium is routinely placed on continuous cardio-

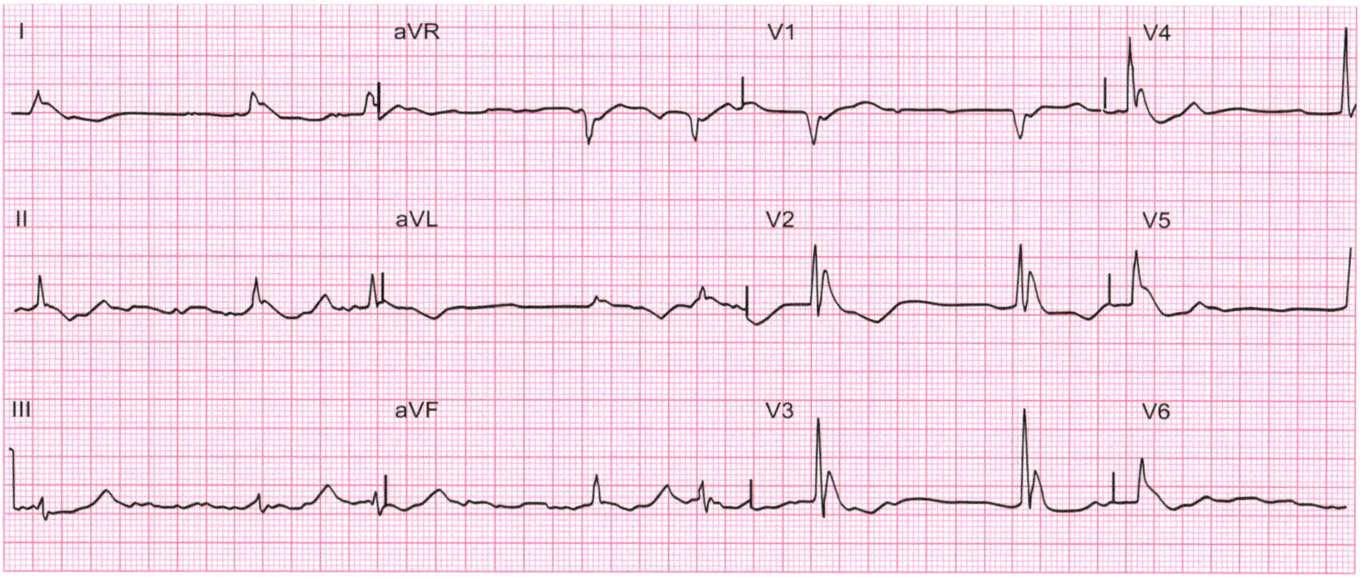

FIG. 22: Hypothermia

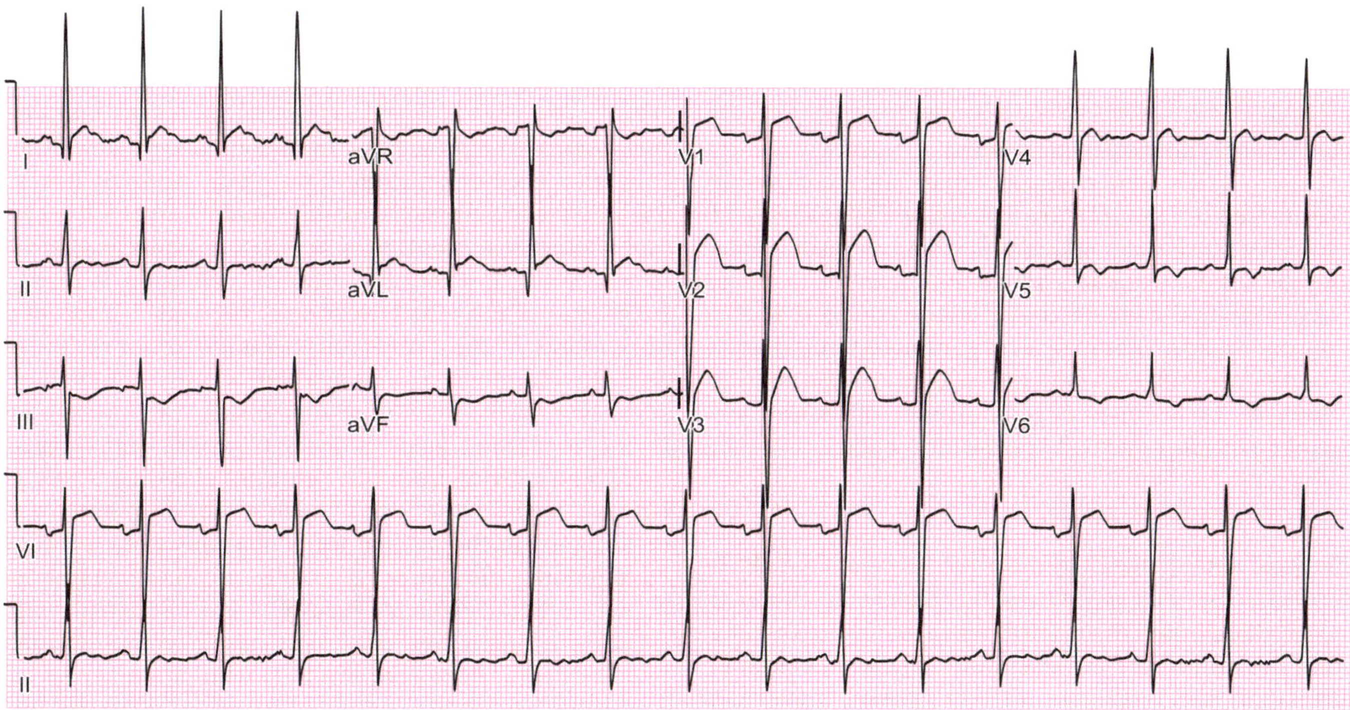

FIG. 23: Hypercalcemia

pulmonary monitoring and vital signs including glucose are obtained. Immediately after, if not simultaneously an ECG should be obtained. If diffuse T-wave inversions are observed, the diagnosis of cardiac ischemia is likely, however, T-waves that are diffuse and large with increased amplitude can also be indicative of other lethal non-cardiac conditions. Cerebral T waves (Fig. 24) are seen because of increased intracranial pressure (ICP).[73] Increased ICP can also cause QT interval prolongation and ST segment elevation or depression.[73] If the patient is not able to give an appropriate history, imaging of the head is important.

Two rapidly deteriorating processes that are associated with distinct ECG abnormalities and are always screened for in the ED are pulmonary embolism (PE) and cardiac tamponade. The ECG may reveal sinus tachycardia, inferior and right precordial T-waves inversions, RBBB (incomplete and complete), right heart strain, right axis deviation, and S1Q3T3 pattern or sinus tachycardia; low voltage, and electrical alternans, respectively.[74,75]

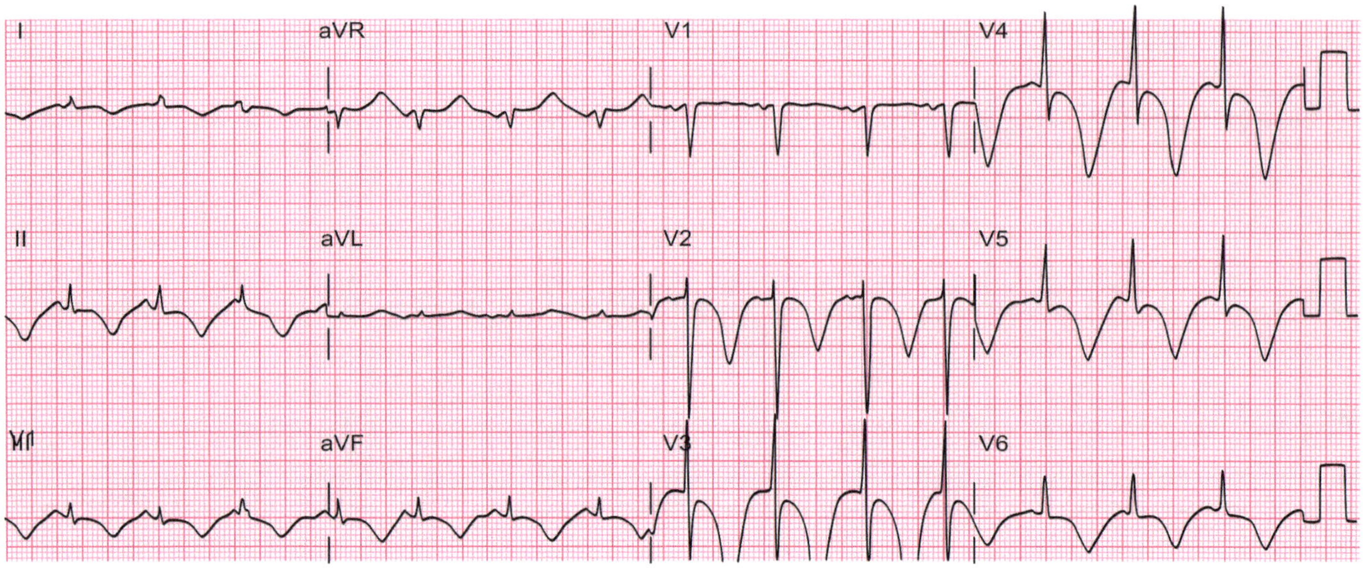

FIG. 24: Cerebral T-waves

Both these topics are discussed at length in subsequent chapters; however, an ECG is always obtained in patients with complaints of chest pain or dyspnea. These two harbingers of death can be presumptively diagnosed and acted upon if clinical decline ensues.

Other ECG abnormalities that are commonly encountered in the ED are dysrhythmias (tachy and brady), AV blocks, and effects of cardiotoxic medications (tricyclic antidepressants, antipsychotics, antihistamines, anticonvulsants, calcium and β-blockers, digoxin and antiarrhythmics). These are all of paramount importance since they are lethal, but when identified are also curable if done so in a timely fashion. These topics are also discussed in subsequent chapters of this book.

Electrode Misplacement

The inadvertent misplacement of any of the ECG electrodes can lead to unforeseen changes on the ECG and misdiagnosis.[76] Right-left reversal involves switching either the arm or the leg electrodes. The most common mistakes in ECG reading result from reversal of the right to left. This is frequently seen when the right arm and left arm electrodes are reversed. The key findings seen after arm reversal includes: inverted P-QRS-T-waves in lead I, an upright P-QRS-T in lead aVR (opposite the expected inversions of these waveforms in a normal ECG tracing), and a QRS vector in lead I that does not match that of lead V6.[77] Similarly, dextrocardia is known to cause inversion of the P-QRS-T complex in lead I; however, it will also exhibit a lack of normal precordial R-wave progression from leads V1–V6. Reversal in the arm leads will not affect the precordial leads. Lead reversal involving one side, either right arm with right leg or left arm with left leg, can result in several changes. The aberration that is most noticed is a flat line in one of the three limb leads (occurs in the lead II when there is right arm with right leg reversal).[77] Unlike the right-sided reversal between the arm and leg, the reversal of the left arm and leg is quite difficult to detect in the absence of a prior ECG. Even comparison with prior ECG may not be revealing of the error. An indicator of left-sided lead reversal is an abnormal P-wave. A P-wave that is smaller in lead II than in lead I, or biphasic P wave in lead III with a terminal positive deflection is highly suggestive of left-sided electrodes reversal.[78] Improper positioning of the precordial electrodes may result in poor R-wave progression suggestive of prior infarction or silent myocardial infarction. The typically ECG transition in the precordial leads is R-wave growth and S-wave regression moving from the rightward chest leads to the leftward leads.[76] The lack of such a pattern points to a disturbance in the normal leads placement of electrical conduction. The latter is called a pseudoinfarction pattern.[76] If the patient's history is not consistent with myocardial infarction, electrode misplacement should be considered. Repeating the ECG with attentiveness to precordial electrode positioning will usually resolve the abnormalities. Electrocardiogram irregularities from electrode misplacement can simulate clinical diseases and lead to misdiagnosis and inappropriate treatment, thus electrode misplacement patterns must be considered and recognized by all ED providers.

CONCLUSION

Patients with serious illnesses frequently come to the ED with a myriad of complaints that must be critically analyzed by the ED physician. In the majority of clinical presentations, an ECG is obtained to assess if any identifiable impending emergency is identifiable.

Utilization of the ECG should not be limited to cardiac complaints given its widespread clinical applicability. Highlighted in this chapter are several crucial ECG manifestation, which if undiagnosed could result in improper treatment or unfortunate premature demise of patients. The task of ECG scrutiny and mastery belongs to every ED physician and we should rise to the challenge. Rendering it to computer-based analysis or other colleagues, including cardiologists, who are not immediately and always available, without clinical context, and not exposed to as many ECGs in their daily practice is imprudent and regretful.

REFERENCES

1. Barold SS. Willem Einthoven and the birth of clinical electrocardiography a hundred years ago. Card Electrophysiol Rev. 2003;7(1):99-104.
2. Yong CM, Froelicher V, WagnerG. The electrocardiogram at a crossroads. Circulation. 2013;128(1):79-82.
3. Mason JW, Hancock EW, Gettes LS, Bailey JJ, Childers R, Deal BJ, et al. Recommendations for the standardization and interpretation of the electrocardiogram: part II: electrocardiography diagnostic statement list a scientific statement from the American Heart Association Electrocardiography and Arrhythmias Committee, Council on Clinical Cardiology; the American College of Cardiology Foundation; and the Heart Rhythm Society Endorsed by the International Society for Computerized Electrocardiology. J Am Coll Cardiol. 2007;49(10):1128-35.
4. Willems JL, Abreu-Lima C, Arnaud P, van Bemmel JH, Brohet C, Degani R, et al. The diagnostic performance of computer programs for the interpretation of electrocardiograms. N Engl J Med. 1991;325(25):1767-73.
5. Estes NA. Computerized interpretation of ECGs: supplement not a substitute. Circ Arrhythm Electrophysiol. 2013;6(1):2-4.
6. Kadish AH, Buxton AE, Kennedy HL, Knight BP, Mason JW, Schuger CD, et al. ACC/AHA clinical competence statement on electrocardiography and ambulatory electrocardiography: A report of the ACC/AHA/ACP-ASIM task force on clinical competence (ACC/AHA Committee to develop a clinical competence statement on electrocardiography and ambulatory electrocardiography) endorsed by the International Society for Holter and noninvasive electrocardiology. Circulation. 2001;104(25):3169-78.
7. Eken C, Goksu E, Eray O, Yalcinkaya S. The consistency of emergency physicians' and cardiologists' ECG interpretation and likelihood classification of chest pain patients. Int J Clin Pract. 2006;60(10):1194-7.
8. Kuhn M, Morgan MT, Hoffman JR Quality assurance in the emergency department: evaluation of the ECG review process. Ann Emerg Med. 1992;21(1):10-5.
9. Todd KH, Hoffman JR, Morgan MT. Effect of cardiologist ECG review on emergency department practice. Ann Emerg Med. 1996;27(1):16-21.
10. Westdrop EJ, Gratton MC, Watson WA. Emergency department interpretation of electrocardiograms. Ann Emerg Med. 1992;21(5): 541-4.
11. Wathen JE, Rewers AB, Yetman AT, Schaffer MS. Accuracy of ECG interpretation in the pediatric emergency department. Ann Emerg Med. 2005;46(6):507-11.
12. Takakuwa KM, Burek GA, Estepa AT, Shofer FS. A method for improving arrival-to-electrocardiogram time in emergency department chest pain patients and the effect on door-to-balloon time for ST-segment elevation myocardial infarction. Acad Emerg Med. 2009;16(10):921-7.
13. Ting HH, Krumholz HM, Bradley EH, Cone DC, Curtis JP, Drew BJ, et al. Implementation and integration of prehospital ECGs into systems of care for acute coronary syndrome: a scientific statement from the American Heart Association Interdisciplinary Council on Quality of Care and Outcomes Research, Emergency Cardiovascular Care Committee, Council on Cardiovascular Nursing, and Council on Clinical Cardiology. Circulation. 2008;118(10):1066-79.
14. Mattu A, Brady WJ, Perron AD, Robinson DA. Prominent R wave in lead V1: electrocardiographic differential diagnosis. Am J Emerg Med. 2001;19(6):504-13.
15. O'Gara PT, Kushner FG, Ascheim DD, Casey DE, Chung MK, de Lemos JA, et al. 2013 ACCF/AHA guideline for the management of ST-elevation myocardial infarction: executive summary: a report of the American College of Cardiology Foundation/American Heart Association Task Force on Practice Guidelines: developed in collaboration with the American College of Emergency Physicians and Society for Cardiovascular Angiography and Interventions. Catheter Cardiovasc Interv. 2013;82(1):E1-27.
16. Nough H, Jorat MV, Varasteravan HR, Ahmadieh MH, Tavakkolian N, Sheikhvatan M. The value of ST-segment elevation in lead aVR for predicting left main coronary artery lesion in patients suspected of acute coronary syndrome. Rom J Intern Med. 2012;50(2):159-64.
17. Turnipseed SD, Trythall WS, Diercks DB, Laurin EG, Kirk JD, Smith DS, et al. Frequency of acute coronary syndrome in patients with normal electrocardiogram performed during presence or absence of chest pain. Acad Emerg Med. 2009;16(6):495-9.
18. Challa PK, Smith KM, Conti CR. Initial presenting electrocardiogram as determinant for hospital admission in patients presenting to the emergency department with chest pain: a pilot investigation. Clin Cardiol. 2007;30(11):558-61.
19. Cai Q, Mehta N, Sgarbossa EB, Pinski SL, Wagner GS, Califf RM, et al. The left bundle-branch block puzzle in the 2013 ST-elevation myocardial infarction guideline: from falsely declaring emergency to denying reperfusion in a high-risk population. Are the Sgarbossa Criteria ready for prime time? Am Heart J. 2013;166(3):409-13.
20. Sgarbossa EB, Pinski SL, Barbagelata A, Underwood DA, Gates KB, Topol EJ, et al. Electrocardiographic diagnosis of evolving acute myocardial infarction in the presence of left bundle-branch block. GUSTO-1 (Global Utilization of Streptokinase and Tissue Plasminogen Activator for Occluded Coronary Arteries) Investigators. N Engl J Med. 1996;334(8):481-7.
21. Maloy KR, Bhat R, Davis J, Reed K, Morrissey R. Sgarbossa Criteria are Highly Specific for Acute Myocardial Infarction with Pacemakers. West J Emerg Med. 2010;11(4):354-7.
22. McManus DD, Gore J, Yarzebski J, Spencer F, Lessard D, Goldberg RJ. Recent trends in the incidence, treatment, and outcomes of patients with STEMI and NSTEMI. Am J Med. 2011;124(1):40-7.
23. Amsterdam EA, Wenger NK, Brindis RG, Casey DE, Ganiats TG, Holmes DR,et al. 2014 AHA/ACC Guideline for the Management of Patients with Non-ST-Elevation Acute Coronary Syndromes: a report of the American College of Cardiology/American Heart Association Task Force on Practice Guidelines. J Am Coll Cardiol. 2014;64(24):e139-228.
24. Pollehn T, Brady WJ, Perron AD, Morris F. The electrocardiographic differential diagnosis of ST segment depression. Emerg Med J. 2002;19(2): 129-35.
25. Mittal CM, Aslam N, Mohan B, Tandon R, Sood N, Wander GS. Spontaneous closure of post-myocardial infarction ventricular septal rupture. Tex Heart Inst J. 2011;38(5):596-7.
26. Barrabes JA, Figueras J, Moure C, Cortadellas J, Soler-Soler J. Prognostic significance of ST segment depression in lateral leads I, aVL, V5 and V6 on the admission electrocardiogram in patients with a first acute myocardial infarction without ST segment elevation. J Am Coll Cardiol. 2000;35(7):1813-9.
27. Channer K, Morris F. ABC of clinical electrocardiography: Myocardial ischaemia. BMJ. 2002;324(7344):1023-6.
28. Papadakis M, Basavarajaiah S, Rawlins J, Edwards C, Makan J, Firoozi S, et al. Prevalence and significance of T-wave inversions in predominantly Caucasian adolescent athletes. Eur Heart J. 2009;30(14):1728-35.
29. Doevendans PA, Gorgels AP, van der Zee R, Partouns J, Bär FW, Wellens HJ. Electrocardiographic diagnosis of reperfusion during thrombolytic therapy in acute myocardial infarction. Am J Cardiol. 1995;75(17):1206-10.
30. Engels W, Van Bilsen M, De Groot MJ, Lemmens PJ, Willemsen PH, Reneman RS, et al. Ischemia and reperfusion induced formation of eicosanoids in isolated rat hearts. Am J Physiol. 1990;258(6 Pt 2):H1865-71.
31. Gorgels AP, Vos MA, Letsch IS, Verschuuren EA, Bär FW, Janssen JH, et al. Usefulness of the accelerated idioventricular rhythm as a marker for myocardial necrosis and reperfusion during thrombolytic therapy in acute myocardial infarction. Am J Cardiol. 1988;61(4):231-5.
32. Delewi R, Remmelink M, Meuwissen M, van Royen N, Vis MM, Koch KT, et al. Acute haemodynamic effects of accelerated idioventricular rhythm in primary percutaneous coronary intervention. EuroIntervention. 2011;7(4):467-71.
33. de Winter RJ, Verouden NJ, Wellens HJ, Wilde AA, Interventional Cardiology Group of the Academic Medical Center. A new ECG sign of proximal LAD occlusion. N Engl J Med. 2008;359(19):2071-3.
34. Movahed MR. Wellens' syndrome or inverted U-waves? Clin Cardiol. 2008;31(3): 133-4.

35. Mead NE, O'Keefe KP Wellen's syndrome: An ominous EKG pattern. J Emerg Trauma Shock. 2009;2(3):206-8.
36. Unluer EE, Pınar A, Bozdemir H, Bayata S, Unlüer S, Yavaşi O. Red Flags in Electrocardiogram for Emergency Physicians: Remembering Wellens' Syndrome and Upright T wave in V(1). West J Emerg Med. 2012;13(2):160-2.
37. Haines DE, Raabe DS, Gundel WD, Wackers FJ. Anatomic and prognostic significance of new T-wave inversion in unstable angina. Am J Cardiol. 1983;52(1):14-8.
38. Rathore S, Dodds PA. Diagnosing chest pain: characteristic ECG changes in acute pericarditis. Heart. 2007;93(9):1063.
39. Bhardwaj R, Berzingi C, Miller C, Hobbs G, Gharib W, Beto RJ, et al. Differential diagnosis of acute pericarditis from normal variant early repolarization and left ventricular hypertrophy with early repolarization: an electrocardiographic study. Am J Med Sci. 2013;345(1):28-32.
40. Rossello X, Wiegerinck RF, Alguersuari J, Bardají A, Worner F, Sutil M, et al. New electrocardiographic criteria to differentiate acute pericarditis and myocardial infarction. Am J Med. 2014;127(3):233-9.
41. Madias JE, Ashtiani R, Agarwal H, Narayan VK, Win M, Sinha A. Diagnosis of ventricular aneurysm and other severe segmental left ventricular dysfunction consequent to a myocardial infarction in the presence of right bundle branch block: ECG correlates of a positive diagnosis made via echocardiography and/or contrast ventriculography. Ann Noninvasive Electrocardiol. 2005;10(1):53-9.
42. Smith SW. T/QRS ratio best distinguishes ventricular aneurysm from anterior myocardial infarction. Am J Emerg Med. 2005;23(3):279-87.
43. Hancock EW, Deal BJ, Mirvis DM, Okin P, Kligfield P, Gettes LS, et al. AHA/ACCF/HRS recommendations for the standardization and interpretation of the electrocardiogram: part V: electrocardiogram changes associated with cardiac chamber hypertrophy: a scientific statement from the American Heart Association Electrocardiography and Arrhythmias Committee, Council on Clinical Cardiology; the American College of Cardiology Foundation; and the Heart Rhythm Society. Endorsed by the International Society for Computerized Electrocardiology. J Am Coll Cardiol. 2009;53(11):992-1002.
44. Palmieri V, Okin PM, de Simone G, Bella JN, Wachtell K, Gerdts E, et al. Electrocardiographic characteristics and metabolic risk factors associated with inappropriately high left ventricular mass in patients with electrocardiographic left ventricular hypertrophy: the LIFE Study. J Hypertens. 2007;25(5):1079-85.
45. Morrison I, Clark E, Macfarlane PW. Evaluation of the electrocardiographic criteria for left ventricular hypertrophy. Anadolu Kardiyol Derg. 2007; 7(Suppl 1):159-63.
46. Vandenberg BF, Romhilt DW. Electrocardiographic diagnosis of left ventricular hypertrophy in the presence of bundle branch block. Am Heart J. 1991;122(3 Pt 1):818-22.
47. Vandenberg B, Sagar K, Paulsen W, Romhilt D. Electrocardiographic criteria for diagnosis of left ventricular hypertrophy in the presence of complete right bundle branch block. Am J Cardiol. 1989;63(15):1080-4.
48. Shamim S, McCrary J, Wayne L, Gratton M, Bogart DB. Electrocardiograhic findings resulting in inappropriate cardiac catheterization laboratory activation for ST-segment elevation myocardial infarction. Cardiovasc Diagn Ther. 2014; 4(3):215-23.
49. Da Costa D, Brady WJ, Edhouse J. Bradycardias and atrioventricular conduction block. BMJ. 2002;324(7336):535-8.
50. Kaltman JR, Thompson PD, Lantos J, Berul CI, Botkin J, Cohen JT, et al. Screening for sudden cardiac death in the young: report from a national heart, lung, and blood institute working group. Circulation. 2011;123(17):1911-8.
51. Morita H, Wu J, Zipes DP. The QT syndromes: long and short. Lancet. 2008; 372(9640):750-63.
52. Khan IA. Twelve-lead electrocardiogram of torsades de pointes. Tex Heart Inst J. 2001;28(1):69.
53. Kirchhof P, Franz MR, Bardai A, Wilde AM. Giant T-U waves precede torsades de pointes in long QT syndrome: a systematic electrocardiographic analysis in patients with acquired and congenital QT prolongation. J Am Coll Cardiol. 2009;54(2):143-9.
54. Vorobiof G, Kroening D, Hall B, Brugada R, Huang D. Brugada syndrome with marked conduction disease: dual implications of a SCN5A mutation. Pacing Clin Electrophysiol. 2008;31(5):630-4.
55. Antzelevitch C, Brugada P, Brugada J, Brugada R. Brugada syndrome: from cell to bedside. Curr Probl Cardiol. 2005;30(1):9-54.
56. Bayes de Luna A, Brugada J, Baranchuk A, Borggrefe M, Breithardt G, Goldwasser D, et al. Current electrocardiographic criteria for diagnosis of Brugada pattern: a consensus report. J Electrocardiol. 2012;45(5):433-42.
57. Kim L, Devereux RB, Basson CT. Impact of genetic insights into mendelian disease on cardiovascular clinical practice. Circulation. 2011;123(5): 544-50.
58. Kelly BS, Mattu A, Brady WJ. Hypertrophic cardiomyopathy: electrocardiographic manifestations and other important considerations for the emergency physician. Am J Emerg Med. 2007;25(1):72-9.
59. Musat D, Sherrid MV. Echocardiography in the treatment of hypertrophic cardiomyopathy. Anadolu Kardiyol Derg. 2006;6(Suppl 2):18-26.
60. Marcus FI, McKenna WJ, Sherrill D, Basso C, Bauce B, Bluemke DA, et al. Diagnosis of arrhythmogenic right ventricular cardiomyopathy/dysplasia: proposed modification of the Task Force Criteria. Eur Heart J. 2010;31(7):806-14.
61. Cox MG, van der Smagt JJ, Wilde AA, Wiesfeld AC, Atsma DE, Nelen MR, et al. New ECG criteria in arrhythmogenic right ventricular dysplasia/cardiomyopathy. Circ Arrhythm Electrophysiol. 2009;2(5):524-30.
62. Brembilla-Perrot B, Yangni N'da O, Huttin O, Chometon F, Groben L, Christophe C, et al. Wolff-Parkinson-White syndrome in the elderly: clinical and electrophysiological findings. Arch Cardiovasc Dis. 2008;101(1):18-22.
63. January CT, Wann LS, Alpert JS, Calkins H, Cigarroa JE, Cleveland JC, et al. 2014 AHA/ACC/HRS guideline for the management of patients with atrial fibrillation: a report of the American College of Cardiology/American Heart Association Task Force on Practice Guidelines and the Heart Rhythm Society. J Am Coll Cardiol. 2014;64(21):e1-76.
64. Levis JT. ECG diagnosis: hyperkalemia. Perm J. 2013;17(1):69.
65. Webster A, Brady W Morris F. Recognising signs of danger: ECG changes resulting from an abnormal serum potassium concentration. Emerg Med J. 2002;19(1):74-7.
66. Diercks DB, Shumaik GM, Harrigan RA, Brady WJ, Chan TC. Electrocardiographic manifestations: electrolyte abnormalities. J Emerg Med. 2004;27(2):153-60.
67. Levis JT. ECG diagnosis: hypokalemia. Perm J. 2012;16(2):57.
68. Efstratiadis G, Sarigianni M, Gougourelas I. Hypomagnesemia and cardio-vascular system. Hippokratia. 2006;10(4):147-52.
69. RuDusky BM. ECG abnormalities associated with hypocalcemia. Chest. 2001;119(2):668-9.
70. Levis JT. ECG Diagnosis: Hypothermia. Perm J. 2010;14(3):73.
71. Gardner JD, Calkins JB, Garrison GE. ECG diagnosis: The effect of ionized serum calcium levels on electrocardiogram. Perm J. 2014;18(1):e119-20.
72. Patel C, Yan GX, Antzelevitch C. Short QT syndrome: from bench to bedside. Circ Arrhythm Electrophysiol. 2010;3(4):401-8.
73. Bailey WB, Chaitman BR. Images in clinical medicine. Electrocardiographic changes in intracranial hemorrhage mimicking myocardial infarction. N Engl J Med. 2003;349(6):561.
74. Levis JT. ECG Diagnosis: Pulmonary Embolism. Perm J. 2011;15(4):75.
75. Friedman HS, Gomes JA, Tardio AR, Haft JI. The electrocardiographic features of acute cardiac tamponade. Circulation. 1974;50(2):260-5.
76. Stevenson WG, Maisel WH. Electrocardiography artifact: what you do not know, you do not recognize. Am J Med. 2001;110(5):402-3.
77. Batchvarov VN, Malik M, Camm AJ. Incorrect electrode cable connection during electrocardiographic recording. Europace. 2007;9(11):1081-90.
78. Abdollah H, Milliken JA. Recognition of electrocardiographic left arm/left leg lead reversal. Am J Cardiol. 1997;80(9):1247-9.

5

CHAPTER

Echocardiography

Darrin J Wong, Daniel G Blanchard

INTRODUCTION

Echocardiography (Echo) utilizes ultrasound (US) energy to evaluate cardiac structures and function. Echocardiography has evolved into a technique that can image the heart in both two- and three-dimensions (2D and 3D) and that can be performed from the chest wall or from the esophagus.[1,2] In addition, Doppler examination augments the standard 2D imaging by measuring blood flow velocity and has become an essential component of the complete echocardiographic evaluation. Doppler ultrasound technology includes pulsed-wave (PW), continuous-wave (CW) and 2D color-flow imaging. The field of cardiac ultrasound continues to grow rapidly, recent clinical additions include tissue Doppler imaging and real-time 3D echocardiography.[3]

PHYSICS AND PRINCIPLES

Ultrasound is sonic energy with a frequency greater than 20,000 Hz. Ultrasound waves are created with a rapidly alternating electrical current that aligns and polarizes a piezoelectric crystal within a transducer. This crystal also generates an electrical signal when struck by reflected ultrasound waves. The frequency, at which ultrasound waves are created, is dependent on the thickness of the piezoelectric crystal (or transducer size). Like light, ultrasound can be focused into a beam that obeys the usual laws of reflection and refraction. An ultrasound beam travels straight through tissue of homogeneous density but part of the beam's energy is reflected when it encounters an interface of different acoustic impedance.

The transducer rapidly alternates between sending and receiving the ultrasound energy and the reflected energy can then be used to construct an image of the heart.[1]

Velocity of sound through soft tissue is relatively constant (~1,540 m/s). Thus, distance between the transducer and an object can be measured by calculating the time needed to send and receive the reflected ultrasound wave. Computers can assess reflections from multiple structures simultaneously and display them on a screen as a one-dimensional (1D) image. If the ultrasound beam is then electronically swept rapidly across a sector, a 2D image is generated.

DOPPLER ECHOCARDIOGRAPHY

Two-dimensional and three-dimensional ultrasound provide a wealth of information about cardiac structure and function, but essentially no direct data on blood flow direction or velocity. Doppler echocardiography can image blood flow and velocity by detecting the change in frequency of reflected ultrasound waves off of a moving objects (red blood cells in this case). The frequency of the reflected wave is proportional to the object's velocity and direction. The velocity of the moving object can be calculated using the Doppler equation:

$$v = f_d \times c/[2f_0 \times (\text{Cos } \theta)]$$

Where v is the velocity of red blood cells under examination, f_d is the Doppler frequency shift recorded, f_0 is the transmitted frequency and c is the velocity of sound.[4] The angle "θ" is the angle between the ultrasound beam and the direction of blood flow (so if the ultrasound beam is parallel to blood flow, the angle is 0° and Cos θ is 1). This angle is extremely important, and should be as close to 0° as possible. If θ is more than 20°, significant errors in velocity calculations will occur.[5]

The so-called "spectral" Doppler tracings plot velocity as the Y-axis and time as the X-axis. The spectral display shows blood flow direction and velocity. Blood flow towards the transducer is displayed above the "zero" line and flow away from the transducer is below the line. For example, figure 1 shows a typical spectral Doppler tracing of blood flow through the mitral valve (MV) during diastole. The normal flows of early filling (E) and late filling from atrial contraction (A) are easily visualized (in this case, the transducer is in the apical position).

There are three basic forms of Doppler flow imaging: (i) PW, (ii) CW, and (iii) color-flow Doppler. Pulsed-wave Doppler uses a method called "range gating" to analyze flow at specific depths of the heart and blood vessels. The received signal is dictated by depth as represented by a specific wait time before the transducer samples the reflected US. This capability is useful for assessment of local flow disturbances, but is limited by a phenomenon called "aliasing" (more complete discussions of range gating and aliasing is given by Nishimura et al. and Bom et al.).[5,6] The normal velocity of flow through the tricuspid valve (TV) is 0.3–0.7 m/s and 0.6–0.9 m/s through the pulmonary artery. Normal flow velocity through the MV is 0.6–1.3 m/s and 1.0–1.7 m/s through the left ventricular outflow tract (LVOT). Furthermore, PW Doppler has been used to assess left ventricle (LV) diastolic function and can help to predict LV diastolic pressure. The left ventricular end-diastolic pressure has important hemodynamic implications and can help in direct therapeutic interventions. A full discussion of this topic is addressed by DeMaria and Blanchard, and Zile and Brutsaert.[1,7]

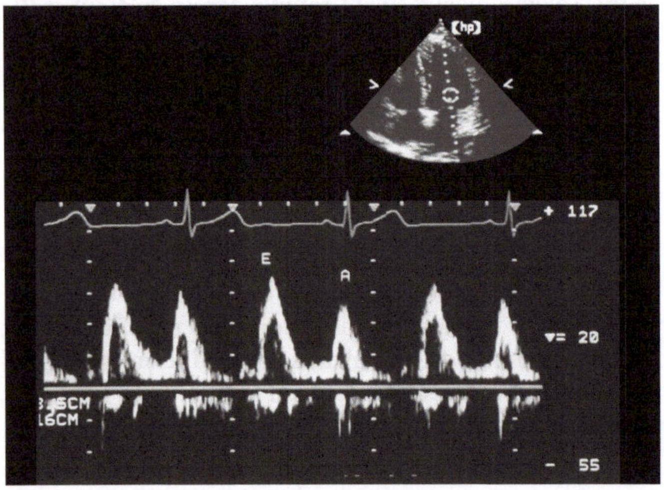

FIG. 1: Normal pulsed-wave Doppler tracing from the left ventricular inflow tract displays the early rapid filling and atrial contraction phases of diastolic flow. The transducer is in the apical position, and the sample volume is at the mitral leaflet tips

With permission from: DeMaria AN, Blanchard DG. Echocardiography. In: Fuster V, Walsh RA, Harrington R (Eds). Hurst's The Heart, 13th ed. New York, NY, USA: McGraw-Hill Medical Publishers; 2011. pp. 411-89.

Color-flow imaging is an extension of PW Doppler that samples multiple volumes along multiple beam paths. Each velocity is then assigned a color to create a color "map" of real-time blood flow that is superimposed onto the 2D image. By convention, blood flow moving towards and away from the transducer is coded red and blue, respectively (Fig. 2). Very high-velocity flow is assigned a speckled color. Color-flow Doppler is an essential tool for both screening and semiquantitation of valvular narrowing (stenosis) and leakage (regurgitation).

Unlike PW Doppler, CW Doppler records all blood flow velocities encountered along the Doppler ultrasound beam. Unlike PW Doppler, CW Doppler can successfully record very high-flow velocities but there is some uncertainty in the location (depth).

FLUID DYNAMICS: CONTINUITY AND BERNOULLI EQUATIONS

Two of the most important equations in clinical echocardiography are the continuity equation and the modified Bernoulli equation.

The "continuity equation" states that the rate at which mass enters a closed system is equal to that of the rate at which mass will leaves it.

$$A_1V_1 = A_1V_2$$

The continuity equation is commonly used to calculate aortic valve area (AVA) in aortic stenosis (AS). The variables are the area of the LVOT, the diameter of the LVOT, the peak systolic velocity in the LVOT (measured

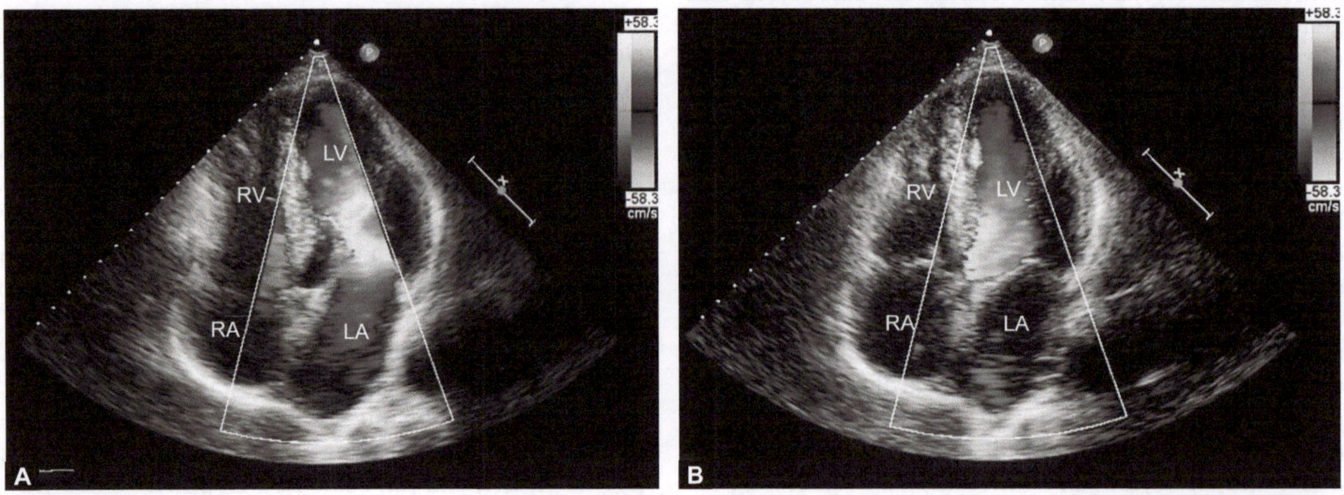

RV, right ventricle; LV, left ventricle; RA, right atrium; LA, left atrium.

FIG. 2: Apical four-chamber images with color-flow Doppler during diastole **(A)** and systole **(B)**. Red flow indicates movement towards the transducer (diastolic filling); blue flow indicates movement away from the transducer (systolic ejection) ***(For color version, see Plate 1)***

With permission from: DeMaria AN, Blanchard DG. Echocardiography. In: Fuster V, Walsh RA, Harrington R (Eds). Hurst's The Heart, 13th ed. New York, NY, USA: McGraw-Hill Medical Publishers; 2011. pp. 411-89.

by PW Doppler) and the peak velocity through the stenotic aortic valve (AV) orifice (measured by CW Doppler). The AVA is equal to the cross-sectional area of the LVOT times the flow velocity of the LVOT divided by the peak velocity through the AV orifice.[8,9]

Therefore,

$A_{LVOT} V_{LVOT} = A_{AV} V_{AV}$.

Since $A_{LVOT} = \pi(d/2)^2$,

Then $A_{AV} = [\pi(d/2)^2 \times V_{LVOT}]/V_{AV}$.

The "modified Bernoulli equation" states that the pressure gradient across a discrete stenosis (i.e., narrowing) in the heart or vasculature is related to the velocity through the stenosis and can be estimated as:

Pressure gradient = 4 × [(Stenotic orifice velocity)^2 – (Proximal velocity)^2].

If the proximal velocity is less than 1.5 m/s then this term can be ignored. Thus, the pressure gradient across a discrete stenosis is 4 times the square of the peak velocity through the stenotic orifice. This equation is used to calculate pressure gradients across any flow-limiting orifice, but is particularly helpful in the assessment of AV stenosis.[8] In addition, the modified Bernoulli equation can be used to estimate pressure gradients across the TV and MV. This is clinically helpful for assessment of pulmonary artery pressure, as the peak right ventricular and pulmonary artery pressure equals 4 times [peak tricuspid regurgitation (TR) velocity]^2 plus the right atrial pressure (which can be estimated on physical examination).

TWO-DIMENSIONAL ECHOCARDIOGRAPHY: STANDARD EXAMINATION

An ultrasound beam can image the heart in 2D from a number of areas on the chest wall and abdomen. The American Society of Echocardiography standardized the echocardiographic examination by recommending three orthogonal imaging planes: (i) the long-axis plane (parallel to the long axis of the LV), (ii) the short-axis plane (perpendicular to the long axis of the LV), and (iii) the four-chamber plane (view from the apex, perpendicular to the short axis) (Fig. 3).[2] The long- and short-axes relate to the positioning of the heart and not of the entire body. These three planes can be imaged in four basic transducer positions: (i) parasternal, (ii) apical, (iii) subcostal, and (iv) suprasternal (Fig. 4).

From the parasternal positions, the transducer is placed in the left third or fourth intercostal space next to the sternum and can be angled to obtain views of the

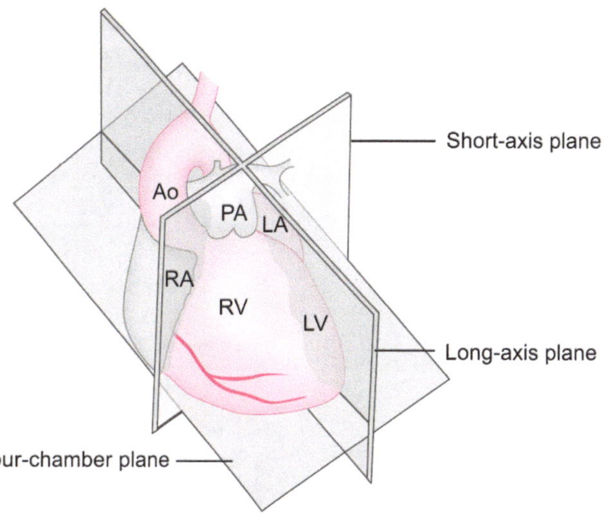

Ao, aorta; PA, pulmonary artery; RA, right atrium; LA, left atrium; RV, right ventricle; LV, left ventricle.

FIG. 3: The three basic tomographic imaging planes used in echocardiography: Long-axis plane, short-axis plane, and four-chamber plane

With permission from: DeMaria AN, Blanchard DG. Echocardiography. In: Fuster V, Walsh RA, Harrington R (Eds). Hurst's The Heart, 13th ed. New York, NY, USA: McGraw-Hill Medical Publishers; 2011. pp. 411-89.

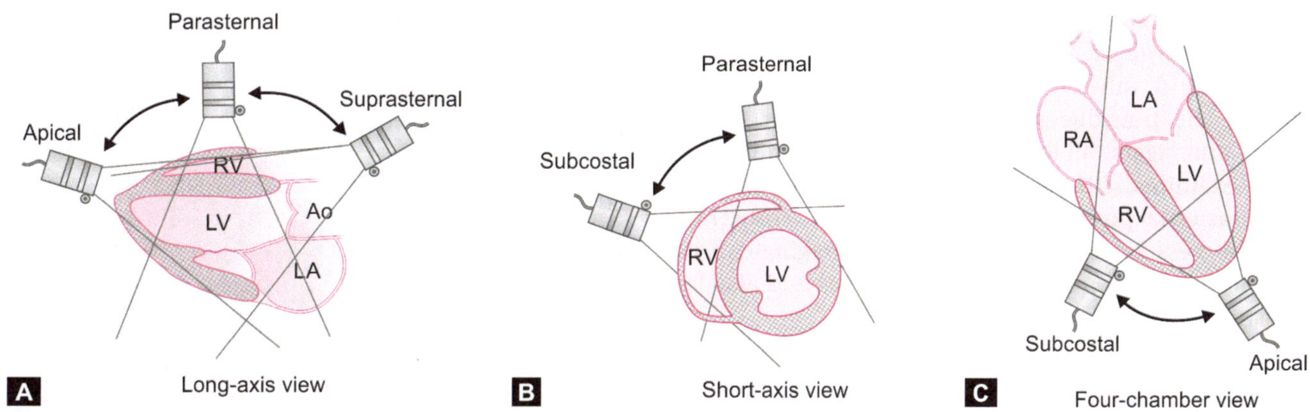

RV, right ventricle; LV, left ventricle; Ao, aorta; LA, left atrium; RA, right atrium.

FIG. 4: Visualization of the heart's basic tomographic imaging planes by various transducer positions. The long-axis plane **(A)** can be imaged in the parasternal, suprasternal, and apical positions; the short-axis plane **(B)** in the parasternal and subcostal positions; and the four-chamber plane **(C)** in the apical and subcostal positions

With permission from: DeMaria AN, Blanchard DG. Echocardiography. In: Fuster V, Walsh RA, Harrington R (Eds). Hurst's The Heart, 13th ed. New York, NY, USA: McGraw-Hill Medical Publishers; 2011. pp. 411-89.

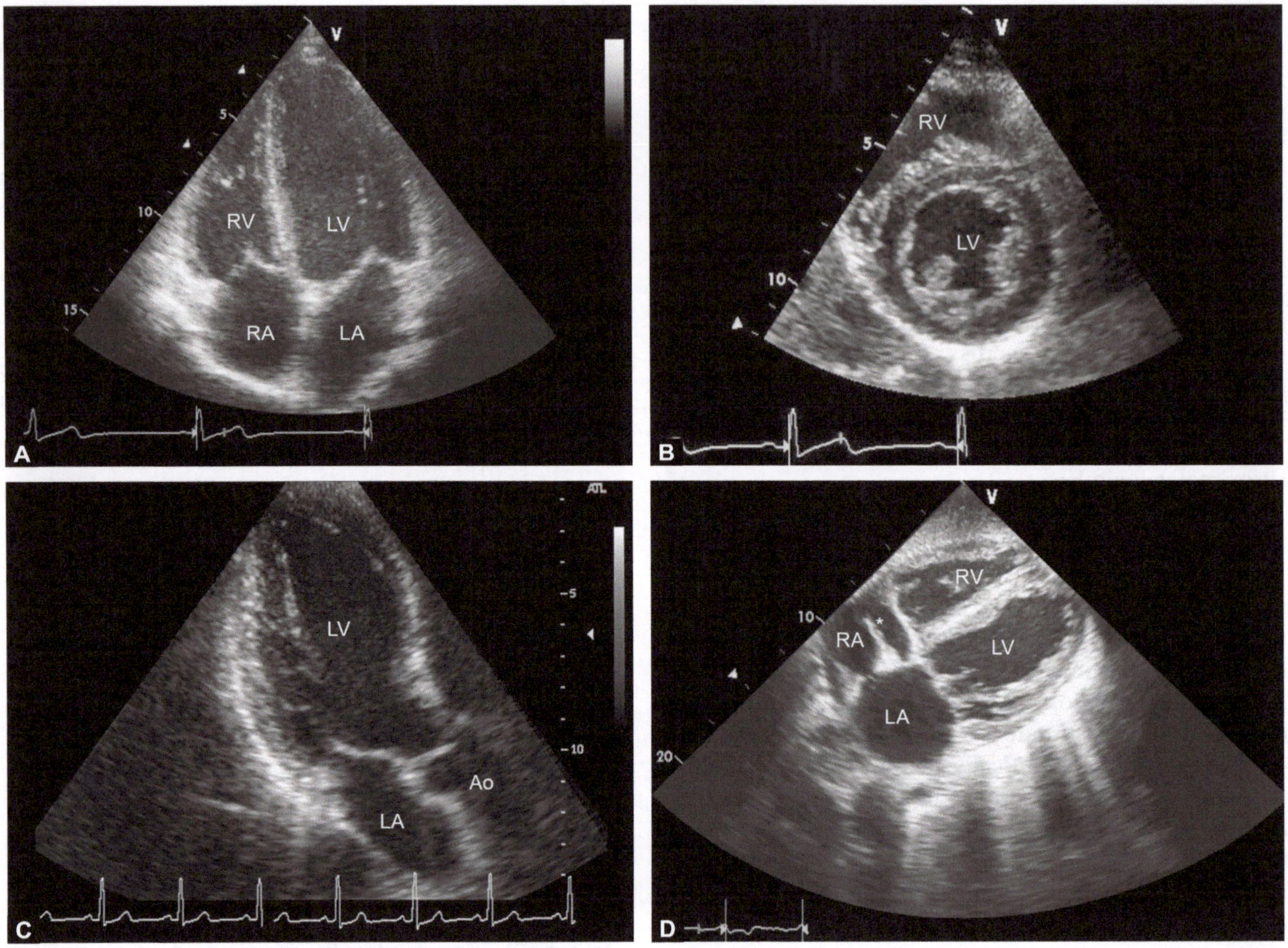

RV, right ventricle; LV, left ventricle; LA, left atrium; RA, right atrium; Ao, aorta.

FIG. 5: **A,** Two-dimensional (2D) image of the heart in the parasternal long-axis view. The cardiac chambers correlate with the diagram in Figure 2A; **B,** Short-axis plane through the heart at the level of the papillary muscle; **C,** 2D image of the apical four-chamber plane, and **D,** 2D image of the apical two-chamber plane

With permission from: DeMaria AN, Blanchard DG. Echocardiography. In: Fuster V, Walsh RA, Harrington R (Eds). Hurst's The Heart, 13th ed. New York, NY, USA: McGraw-Hill Medical Publishers; 2011. pp. 411-89.

cardiac valves and myocardial function (Fig. 5). From the apical position, the transducer is placed on the left lateral chest wall on the apical impulse and all cardiac chambers and valves are imaged. From the subcostal position, the transducer is placed just inferior to the xiphoid and, again, all four cardiac chambers and valves can be examined. The transducer can also be placed in the suprasternal position to image the thoracic aorta (AO) and great vessels. In selected cases, 3D imaging can be useful for calculation of ventricular volumes and also for assessment of valvular function (Fig. 6).[3]

By employing these imaging planes and transducer positions, full visualization of cardiac structures is possible in the great majority of cases. Image quality depends on transducer frequency, instrument settings, and tissue penetration. Image quality is limited by severe obesity, emphysema, or chest wall deformities. Echocardiography is a well-accepted method to evaluate cardiac contraction (systole) and relaxation (diastole).

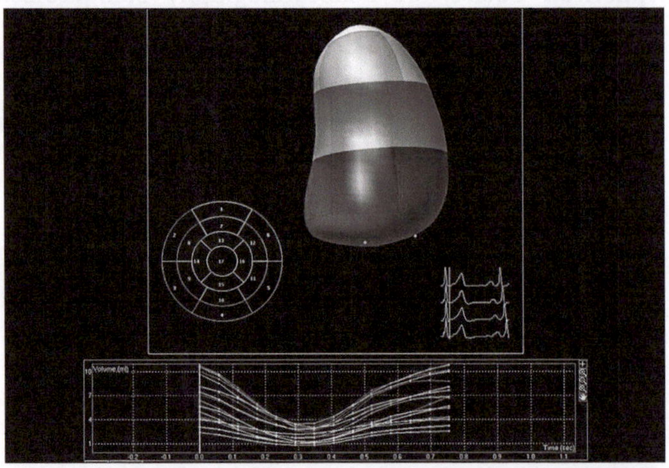

FIG. 6: Three-dimensional images of left ventricular wall motion with accompanying volume analysis ***(For color version, see Plate 1)***

Assessments of cardiac contractility and regional ventricular dysfunction correlate well with those made with other imaging techniques (e.g., computed tomography and magnetic resonance imaging).

TRANSESOPHAGEAL AND CONTRAST ECHOCARDIOGRAPHY

Occasionally, transthoracic echocardiography (TTE) does not provide adequate ultrasound images. As mentioned prior, this can happen because of obesity, but can also occur during assessment of posterior cardiac structures, prosthetic cardiac valves, the thoracic aorta, and small intracardiac infections or clots. Transesophageal echocardiography (TEE) is ideal for imaging this structure because the esophagus is adjacent to the left atrium (LA) and thoracic aorta.[10] Transesophageal echocardiography is performed by a physician trained in echocardiography using a small and directable ultrasound transducer that is embedded into the tip of an endoscope. The endoscope is then passed through a patient's mouth and down the esophagus.

Transesophageal echocardiography images can be recorded from a variety of positions within the esophagus and stomach. The views are dependent upon the patient's anatomy and relationships between the esophagus and the heart (Fig. 7). There are several specific instances in which TEE is particularly useful, including evaluation of:

- Cardiac anatomy when transthoracic imaging is suboptimal (especially with MV anatomy and congenital heart disease)
- Intracardiac infection (i.e., bacterial endocarditis)
- Prosthetic valve function
- Intracardiac clots and other sources of emboli
- Aortic dissection or trauma (Fig. 8).[11]

Contrast echocardiography has grow dramatically in the last several years and has two basic types. The first is intravenous injection of saline that is agitated to produce microbubbles. The bubbles are very echogenic and opacify the right heart. However, they do not survive long enough to pass through the pulmonary vasculature. Thus, if microbubbles are seen in the left heart, an intracardiac shunt is present (Figs 9A and B). The second type of intravenous contrast is an emulsion of albumin microshells with a dense perfluorocarbon gas inside. These bubbles do pass through the pulmonary vessels, and

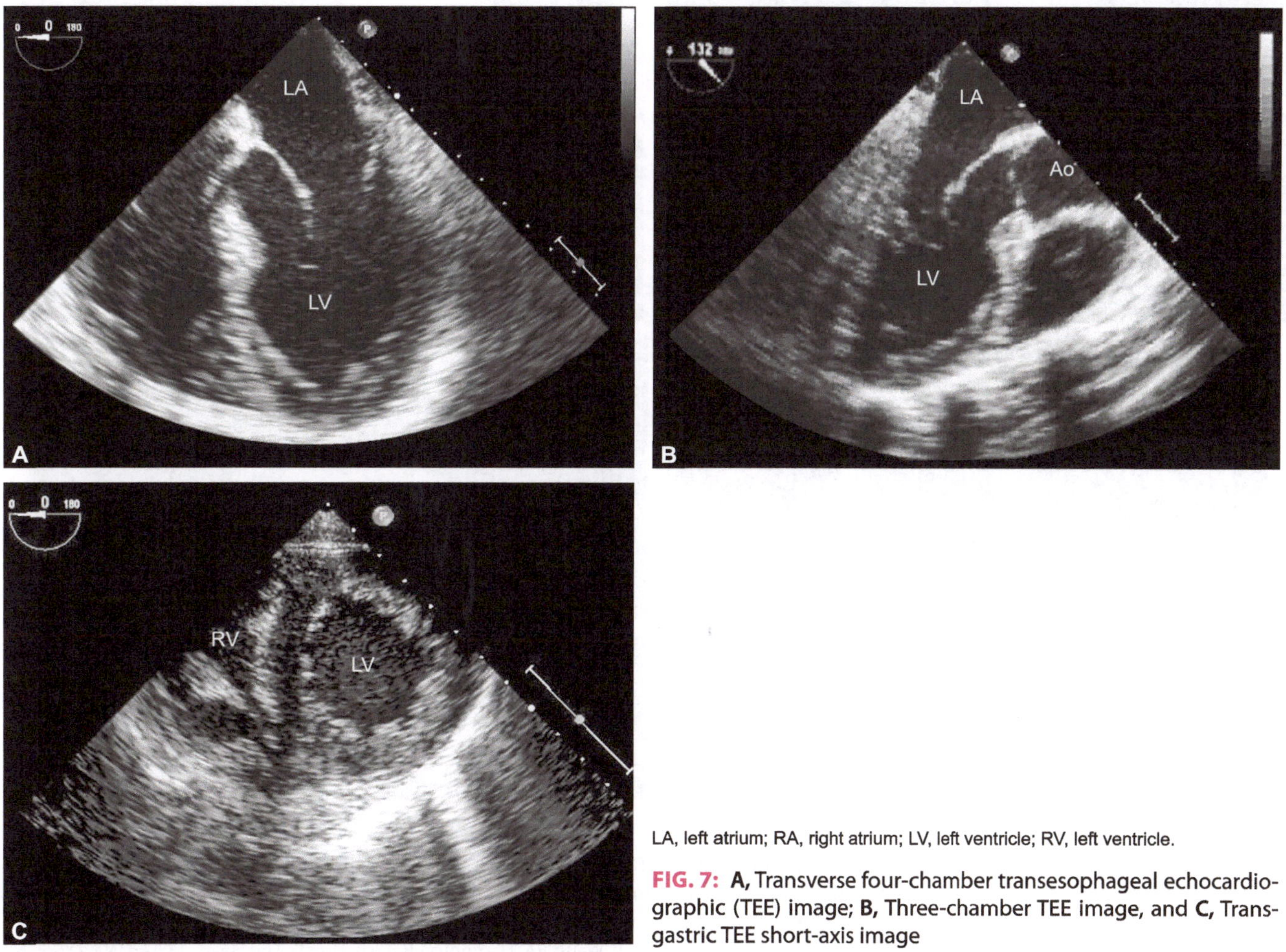

LA, left atrium; RA, right atrium; LV, left ventricle; RV, left ventricle.

FIG. 7: **A,** Transverse four-chamber transesophageal echocardiographic (TEE) image; **B,** Three-chamber TEE image, and **C,** Transgastric TEE short-axis image cause the LV chamber to turn white (instead of the usual black) on echocardiography imaging. This technique can markedly enhance LV endocardial definition and improve overall quality of the examination (Fig. 9C).

ISCHEMIC HEART DISEASE

Echocardiography is an important technique in evaluating inadequate myocardial blood flow (i.e., ischemia) as well as permanent damage to the myocardium (infarction). Left ventricle ischemia quickly produces decreased systolic contraction (hypokinesis) of the involved ventricular segment. If coronary flow is not restored, permanent damage occurs with resulting absent systolic contraction (akinesis) and scarring of the affected myocardium. If the region of hypokinetic myocardium is identified, the blocked or narrowed coronary artery can be inferred.[12] Echocardiography

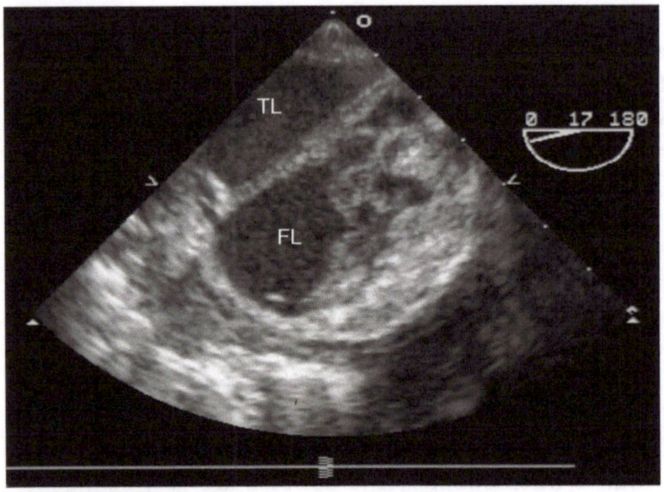

TL, true lumen; FL, false lumen.

FIG. 8: Transesophageal echocardiographic image of the descending thoracic aorta showing a dissection within the vessel

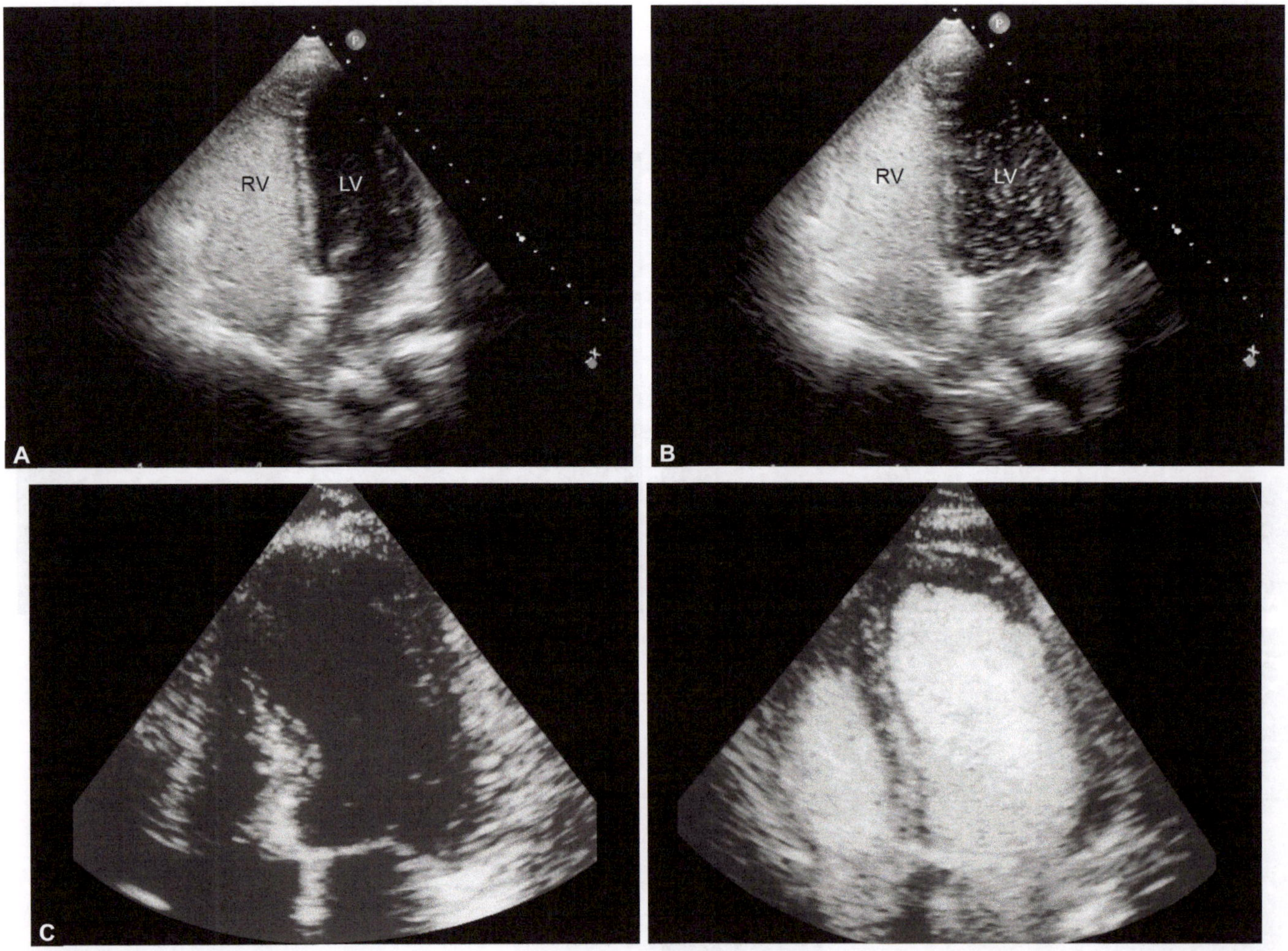

RV, right ventricle; LV, left ventricle.

FIG. 9: **A,** Microbubble injection with contrast filling right ventricle; **B,** Microbubbles in the left ventricle (LV) two heartbeats later, demonstrating the presence of an interatrial shunt; and **C,** Apical four-chamber images of the LV before (upper) and after (below) intravenous injection of echocardiography contrast, demonstrating the markedly improved endocardial definition with echocardiography contrast

With permission from: DeMaria AN, Blanchard DG. Echocardiography. In: Fuster V, Walsh RA, Harrington R (Eds). Hurst's The Heart, 13th ed. New York, NY, USA: McGraw-Hill Medical Publishers; 2011. pp. 411-89.

can detect these abnormalities, along with chronicity of ischemic disease, as evidenced by LV size, thickness, and depression of overall systolic contraction.

Stress Echocardiography

Echocardiography can be combined with stress testing (exercise or pharmacologic) to induce ischemia and diagnose blockages or narrowings in the coronary arteries.[13] In this technique, 2D-image cine-loops at rest and under stress are placed side-by-side on a computer monitor. In normal cases, the LV myocardium thickens more vigorously with exercise. Exercise-induced segmental hypokinesis or impaired wall thickening strongly suggests transient ischemia. As discussed previously, the affected coronary artery can often be predicted with echocardiographic imaging. Multiple wall motion abnormalities and LV enlargement with stress are seen in cases of severe stenoses in multiple coronary arteries and widespread ischemia.

Myocardial Infarction

Although, echocardiography is not a part of the diagnostic criteria for acute coronary syndromes (unstable angina, non-ST-elevation myocardial infarction and ST-elevation myocardial infarction), it may provide assistance with clinical decision-making. Nondiagnostic ECGs may be augmented with echocardiography, as diastolic and systolic dysfunctions occur prior to ECG changes in the setting of acute coronary syndromes. Wall motion abnormalities indicate coronary disease and myocardial ischemia, but this finding does not necessarily differentiate acute versus old changes.

CARDIOMYOPATHIES

Cardiomyopathies are primary abnormalities of the myocardium. These diseases are separated into three categories: (i) dilated cardiomyopathy (DCM), (ii) hypertrophic cardiomyopathy (HCM), and (iii) restrictive cardiomyopathy (RCM). Echocardiography plays an important role in diagnosis, providing information on cavity size, ventricular wall thickness, valvular function, and overall contractility.

Dilated Cardiomyopathy

Typical echocardiographic findings in DCM include enlargement of all four cardiac chambers and marked LV dilation. The etiology is varied, but may be due to viral infection, nutritional deficiencies, metabolic disorders, toxins or drugs, neuromuscular disease, or stress. The standard echocardiographic windows will assist in the quick evaluation of the cardiac chambers. The LV walls are often thin and by definition, hypocontractile (Fig. 10). Because the LV is dilated, the mitral annulus is also dilated, and resultant mitral regurgitation (MR) occurs frequently.[14] Myocardial relaxation (diastole) is often abnormal in DCM, and severe diastolic dysfunction portends a very poor prognosis. Elevated LV filling pressures can be estimated with echocardiography, and may assist in clinical care.

A recently described disorder, "takotsubo" cardiomyopathy, mimics the echocardiographic findings of a large myocardial infarction, but coronary angiography is normal. The echocardiogram is characterized by the appearance of apical "ballooning" (Fig. 11). This acute cause of LV dysfunction often occurs after a stressful event and is seen more often in women. Left ventricle contractile function generally improves within a few weeks.

Hypertrophic Cardiomyopathy

Hypertrophic cardiomyopathy is generally an inherited disease with marked growth and thickening of the LV myocardium (i.e., hypertrophy). The first and fundamental echocardiographic abnormality is severe, often asymmetric LV hypertrophy.[15] Classically, the interventricular septum is involved more extensively than other areas, but the hypertrophy may also be concentric or apical. Asymmetric septal hypertrophy leads to another classic feature of HCM, i.e., systolic anterior motion (SAM) of the MV, which causes dynamic obstruction of the LVOT during systole (Fig. 12). This obstruction usually occurs during mid-to-late systole, and can be best visualized in the parasternal long-axis view.[1] Furthermore, LV systolic

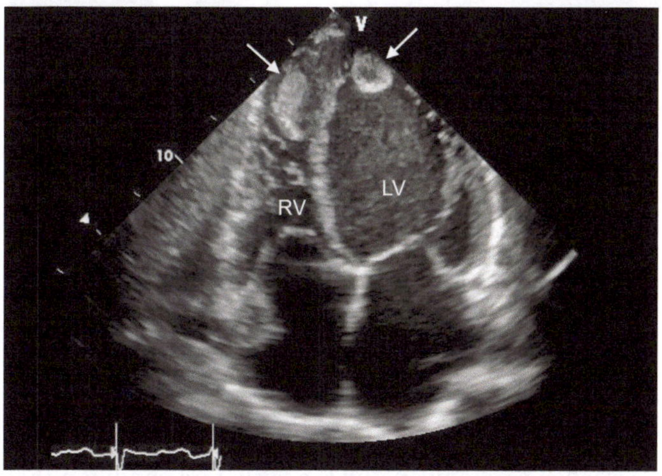

RV, left ventricle; RV, right ventricle.

FIG. 10: Apical four-chamber view in a case of dilated cardiomyopathy. Diffuse thinning and hypokinesis of left ventricular contractile function is present. Apical thrombi are present in the apices of both the right ventricle and left ventricle (arrows)

With permission from: DeMaria AN, Blanchard DG. Echocardiography. In: Fuster V, Walsh RA, Harrington R (Eds). Hurst's The Heart, 13th ed. New York, NY, USA: McGraw-Hill Medical Publishers; 2011. pp. 411-89.

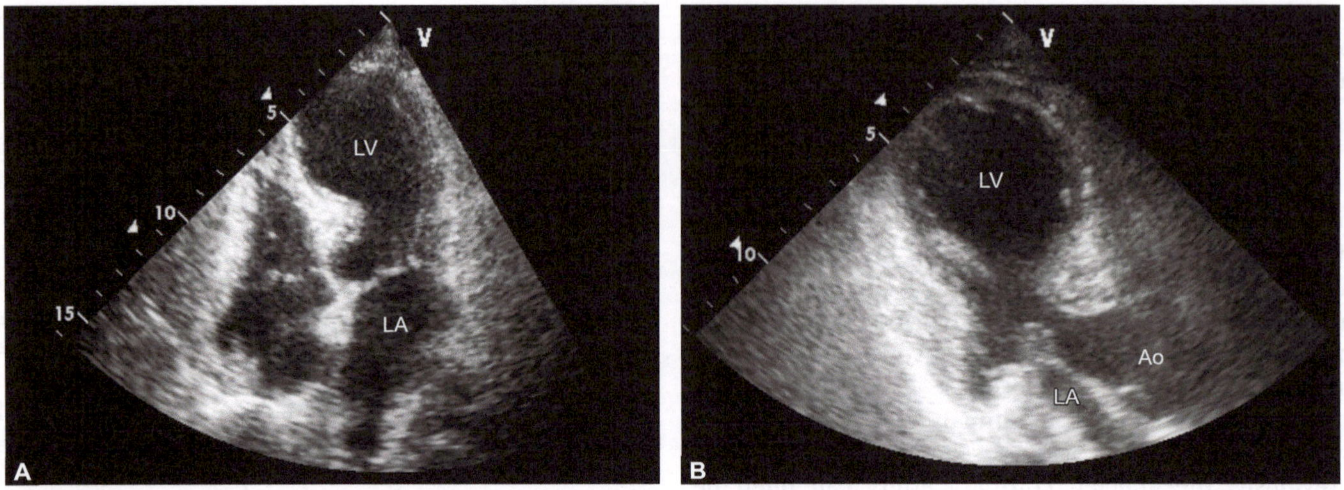

LV, left ventricle; LA, left atrium; Ao, aorta.

FIG. 11: Takotsubo cardiomyopathy, demonstrating apical ballooning during systole

With permission from: DeMaria AN, Blanchard DG. Echocardiography. In: Fuster V, Walsh RA, Harrington R (Eds). Hurst's The Heart, 13th ed. New York, NY, USA: McGraw-Hill Medical Publishers; 2011. pp. 411-89.

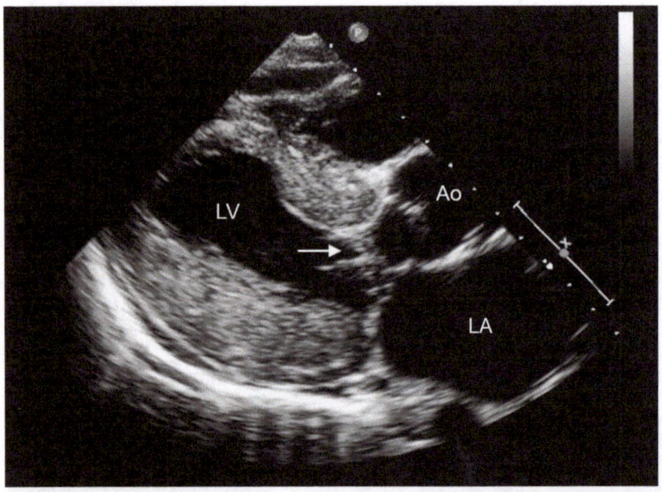

LV, left ventricle; LA, left atrium; Ao, aorta.

FIG. 12: Parasternal long-axis view of hypertrophic cardiomyopathy. Marked left ventricle hypertrophy is present, as well as systolic anterior motion of the anterior mitral leaflet (arrow)

With permission from: DeMaria AN, Blanchard DG. Echocardiography. In: Fuster V, Walsh RA, Harrington R (Eds). Hurst's The Heart, 13th ed. New York, NY, USA: McGraw-Hill Medical Publishers; 2011. pp. 411-89.

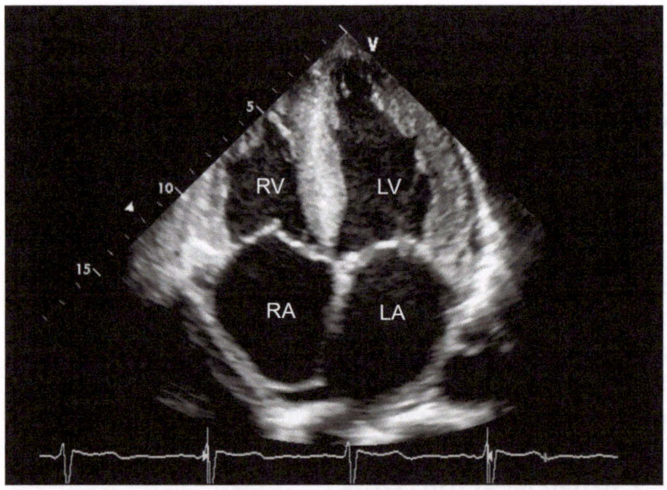

RV, right ventricle; LV, left ventricle; RA, right atrium; LA, left atrium.

FIG. 13: Apical four-chamber view of cardiac amyloid. There is severe thickening of the myocardium as well as biatrial enlargement

With permission from: DeMaria AN, Blanchard DG. Echocardiography. In: Fuster V, Walsh RA, Harrington R (Eds). Hurst's The Heart, 13th ed. New York, NY, USA: McGraw-Hill Medical Publishers; 2011. pp. 411-89.

function is often preserved while diastolic function is impaired.

Restrictive Cardiomyopathy

Restrictive cardiomyopathy is a fairly rare condition that is characterized on echocardiography by a generalized increase in LV wall thickness in the absence of cavity dilation, severe biatrial enlargement and severe LV diastolic dysfunction.[16] Restrictive cardiomyopathy may be idiopathic (i.e., unexplained) or secondary to infiltrative diseases, such as hemochromatosis. The most common cause of RCM in the United States, however, is amyloidosis, which causes biventricular hypertrophy and diffuse thickening of the interatrial septum and cardiac valves (Fig. 13). Although ejection fraction is often normal, diastolic dysfunction is common, and portends a grim prognosis.

Mechanical Support

Left ventricular assist devices (LVADs) are used in end-stage heart failure to augment cardiac output prior to transplant bridge to transplantation therapy or indefinitely until cardiac function returns (destination therapy). The current generation of LVADs provides cardiac output through continuous flow. Blood flow exits through the cardiac apex via a cannula and returns to circulation at the level of the ascending aorta. Optimization of LVAD function is often based on echocardiographic imaging. Thus, it is important to note several parameters while evaluating the LVAD such as LVAD type, mode, and pump speed; LV dimensions and volumes; the motion of the AV; and flow into and out of the LVAD through the apical cannula and into the ascending aorta. Notable LVAD complications that may be detected by echocardiography are thrombus formation and pericardial tamponade.

VALVULAR HEART DISEASE

The two main problems that occur with cardiac valves are: (i) stenosis (where the valve is restricted and does not open normally) and, (ii) regurgitation (where the valve does not close properly and therefore allows backflow of blood). In this regard, valvular regurgitation is synonymous with insufficiency.

Mitral Valve

Detection of mitral stenosis (MS) was one of the earliest applications of cardiac US. Mitral stenosis is usually caused by rheumatic heart disease, and is characterized by tethering and fibrosis of the mitral leaflets. The leaflets are abnormally thickened (often more at the tips than the base or midsections) and display characteristic "doming" during diastole (Fig. 14). In the parasternal short-axis view, the commissural fusion produces a "fish-mouth" appearance at the mitral orifice.[17] Doppler examination reveals abnormally high diastolic flow velocity through the MV and often detects coexistent MR.

Mitral stenosis leads to chronic LA pressure overload and as a result enlarges the chamber gradually over time. This enlargement increases the risk of atrial fibrillation as well as atrial thrombus and systemic emboli. Echocardiography is particularly useful in quantifying the severity of MS. The MV orifice area can be directly measured via planimetry in the parasternal short-axis view. When properly done, this technique is accurate and correlates well with other imaging modalities. The second commonly used technique is the "pressure half-time" method[18] which usually correlates well with the planimetry method. The pressure half-time method relies on the concept that the rate of pressure decline across an orifice directly correlates with the area of the mitral orifice.

Mitral regurgitation can occur in multiple settings, including MV disease, DCM, myocardial infarction, and bacterial infection (endocarditis). Echocardiography is very sensitive for detecting MR, but quantification is more difficult. In the setting of MR, there is often concomitant thickened, abnormal MV leaflets. The direction and shape of a regurgitant jet may denote anatomic disease; abnormalities in the posterior leaflet often result in anteriorly directed regurgitant jets; abnormalities in the anterior leaflet often result in posteriorly regurgitant jets; and mitral valvular dilation often results in a central regurgitant jet. Color-flow Doppler is currently the best echocardiographic method to semiquantitate MR. Color-flow imaging shows a jet of blood flow in the LA during systole, and the size of this color jet correlates roughly with MR severity.[19] Eccentrically directed MR, however, may produce a misleadingly small cross-sectional area on ultrasound imaging (Fig. 15). Volumetric analysis with PW Doppler can also be used to calculate regurgitant volumes and effective regurgitant orifice area, but the accuracy of this technique is limited. Finally, the LA and

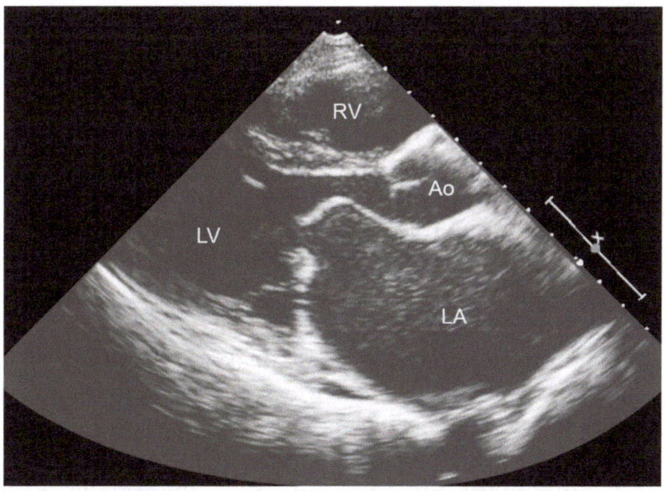

RV, right ventricle; LV, left ventricle; Ao, aorta; LA, left atrium.

FIG. 14: Parasternal long-axis view of mitral stenosis. The left atrium is enlarged, mitral opening is limited, and "doming" of the anterior mitral leaflet is present

With permission from: DeMaria AN, Blanchard DG. Echocardiography. In: Fuster V, Walsh RA, Harrington R (Eds). Hurst's The Heart, 13th ed. New York, NY, USA: McGraw-Hill Medical Publishers; 2011. pp. 411-89.

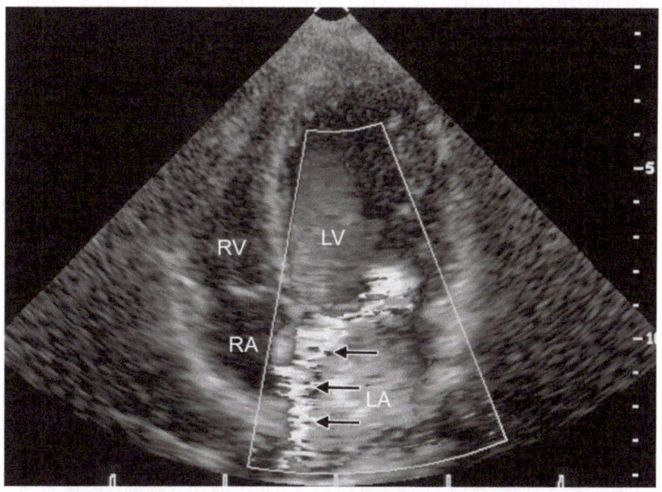

RV, right ventricle; LV, left ventricle; RA, right atrium; LA, left atrium.

FIG. 15: Apical four-chamber image of severe but eccentric mitral regurgitation. The left atrium is enlarged ***(For color version, see Plate 1)***

With permission from: DeMaria AN, Blanchard DG. Echocardiography. In: Fuster V, Walsh RA, Harrington R (Eds). Hurst's The Heart, 13th ed. New York, NY, USA: McGraw-Hill Medical Publishers; 2011. pp. 411-89.

the LV are often enlarged because of the volume overload of the left heart in the setting of severe MR.

Aortic Valve

The normal, thin leaflets of the AV are usually well seen with echocardiography. The prevalence of acquired (calcific) AS increases with age. The valve leaflets are calcified and thickened, and their motion is markedly restricted (Fig. 16). Standard 2D imaging accurately detects AS, but does not quantify it well.

Doppler imaging generally provides an accurate quantification method for AS. Continuous-wave Doppler can measure the peak velocity of blood flow through the AV. The peak gradient can then be calculated using the modified Bernoulli equation [peak gradient = 4 × (peak velocity)^2]. The AV orifice area is then calculated via the continuity equation, as described above. These calculations correlate well with values obtained from other imaging techniques, and are valid as long as the LVOT flow velocity is less than 1.5 m/s.[9]

Many patients with AS often have coexisting valvular disease. Of these, aortic regurgitation (AR) and MR may be present. Furthermore, the response of the LV to chronic AS and pressure overload is eventual, concentric hypertrophy.

Significant AR is usually seen in the presence of an abnormal AV. Although 2D imaging can provide clues to the existence of AR, the Doppler examination is more helpful and easily detects the abnormal flow. As with MR, color-flow Doppler is a quick screening tool that detects AR with nearly 100% sensitivity. Quantitation of AR, however, is more difficult.

There are several echocardiographic methods for semiquantitation of AR. The most commonly used technique utilizes color-flow imaging. Severity of AR can be estimated by the diameter of the color jet in the LVOT (Fig. 17). Mild AR usually has a jet diameter less than 25% of the outflow tract diameter, while a severe AR color jet often occupies more than 75% of the outflow tract during diastole. Findings with moderate AR fall between these.

Although echocardiographic assessment of AS is quantitative and generally accurate, assessment of AR is semiquantitative at best. Therefore, clinical correlation is essential. Despite these limitations, echocardiography is a useful and convenient noninvasive method to evaluate AV disease.

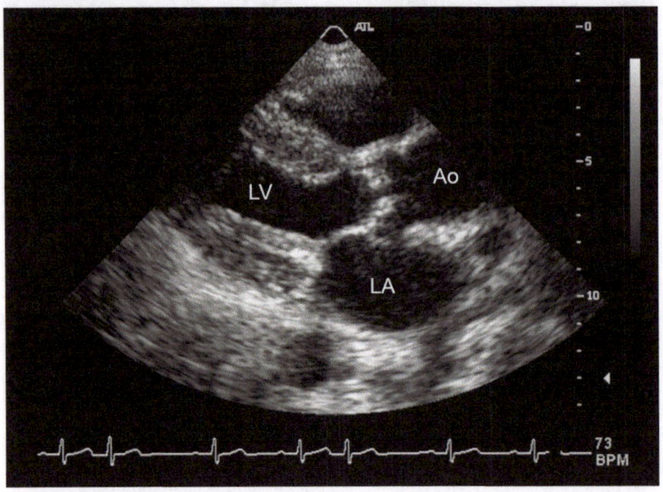

LV, left ventricle; Ao, aorta; LA, left atrium.

FIG. 16: Parasternal long-axis view demonstrates a thickened, stenotic aortic valve

With permission from: DeMaria AN, Blanchard DG. Echocardiography. In: Fuster V, Walsh RA, Harrington R (Eds). Hurst's The Heart, 13th ed. New York, NY, USA: McGraw-Hill Medical Publishers; 2011. pp. 411-89.

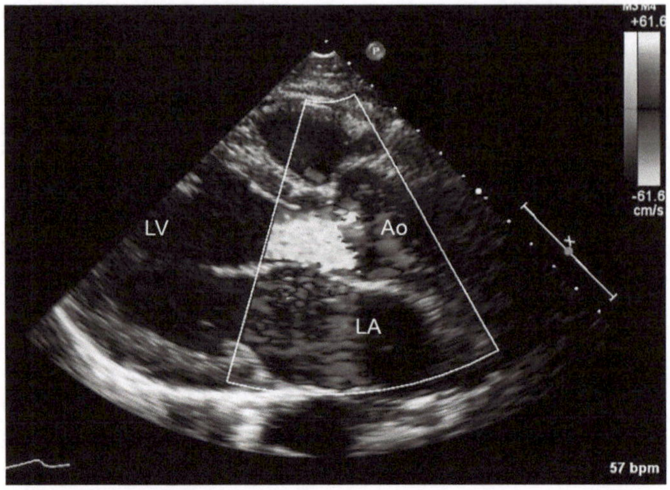

LV, left ventricle; Ao, aorta; LA, left atrium.

FIG. 17: Parasternal long-axis view with a wide jet of aortic regurgitation. The jet fills the width of the outflow tract, suggesting severe regurgitation ***(For color version, see Plate 2)***

With permission from: DeMaria AN, Blanchard DG. Echocardiography. In: Fuster V, Walsh RA, Harrington R (Eds). Hurst's The Heart, 13th ed. New York, NY, USA: McGraw-Hill Medical Publishers; 2011. pp. 411-89.

Right-sided Valvular Disease and Pulmonary Hypertension

Two-dimensional echocardiography can detect abnormalities of the right-sided heart valves (TV and pulmonic valve). Similar to AR and MR, color-flow Doppler imaging can detect and semiquantify TR and pulmonic regurgitation. Measurement of the peak TR velocity by CW Doppler can be used to estimate peak systolic pulmonary artery and right ventricular pressures (via the modified Bernoulli equation, as discussed earlier).

The 2D findings associated with right heart overload and pulmonary hypertension (i.e., abnormally high blood pressure in the pulmonary arteries) include enlargement of the right ventricle (RV) and right atrium (RA), dilation of the pulmonary arteries, flattening of the interventricular septum, and thickening of the right ventricular myocardium (Fig. 18). Doppler examination may also reveal moderate-to-severe TR.

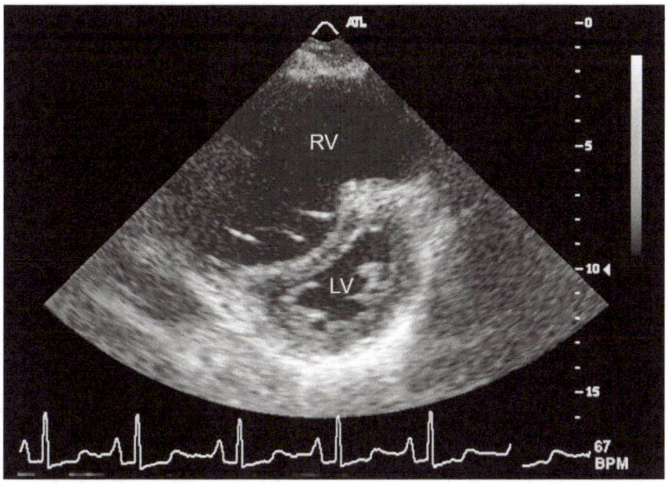

RV, right ventricle; LV, left ventricle.

FIG. 18: Parasternal short-axis view in severe pulmonary hypertension, showing right ventricle (RV) enlargement as well as displacement of the interventricular septum towards the left (due to RV pressure overload)

With permission from: DeMaria AN, Blanchard DG. Echocardiography. In: Fuster V, Walsh RA, Harrington R (Eds). Hurst's The Heart, 13th ed. New York, NY, USA: McGraw-Hill Medical Publishers; 2011. pp. 411-89.

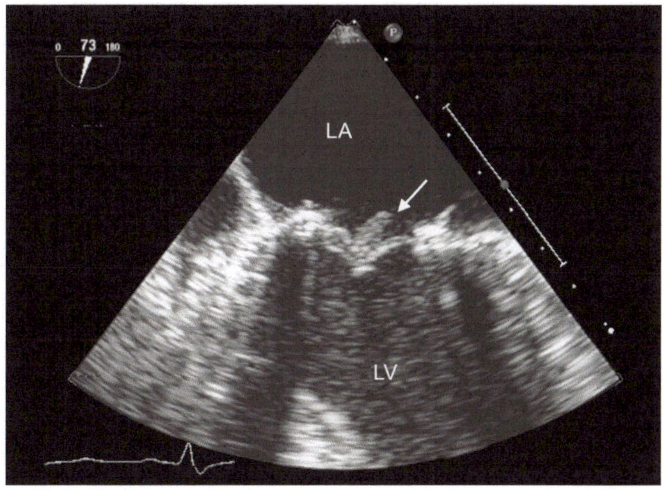

LA, left atrium; LV, left ventricle.

FIG. 19: Transesophageal echocardiographic image of an infected vegetation (arrow) attached to a repaired mitral valve

With permission from: DeMaria AN, Blanchard DG. Echocardiography. In: Fuster V, Walsh RA, Harrington R (Eds). Hurst's The Heart, 13th ed. New York, NY, USA: McGraw-Hill Medical Publishers; 2011. pp. 411-89.

INFECTIVE ENDOCARDITIS

In infective endocarditis, a bacterial infection is present on one or more cardiac valves. Echocardiography is an integral part of the diagnosis and management of this disorder. Although the diagnosis remains a clinical one, echocardiographic detection of valvular vegetations (infected masses) is a strong predictor of the disease. The major criteria for diagnosis include persistent bacteremia with a typical organism and echocardiographic findings of an endocardial infection. An infective valvular vegetation is shown in figure 19. Transthoracic echocardiography detects these with reasonable sensitivity, although approximately 20% of patients with proven endocarditis may have unremarkable TTE findings. Vegetations can occur anywhere on the valvular leaflet, but they most often occur at the coaptation point. Transesophageal echocardiography is more sensitive and specific than TTE for detecting valve infections, and is also better in diagnosing valvular abscesses and prosthetic valve endocarditis.[20] In low-risk patients with good quality images, TTE remains a quick and easy way to rule out endocarditis. Echocardiography also helps to visualize other abnormalities associated with endocarditis, such as valvular regurgitation, pericardial effusion, and intracardiac fistulae.

DISEASES OF THE AORTA

Evaluation of the aorta by echocardiography is a routine part of a standard examination. Imaging includes evaluation from the aortic annulus to the proximal abdominal aorta.

Aortic Dissection and Aneurysm

Aortic dissection is a disease entity most associated with severe hypertension and the Marfan syndrome. In this disorder, the wall of the aorta suddenly tears, separating the inner and outer layers of the aortic wall. Patients often experience severe, ripping chest pain when this occurs. This tear, and the false channel it produces, often propagates down the distal vessel. Finding the location of dissection is imperative for management. If the dissection involves the ascending aorta, it is a surgical emergency, and any delay in treatment may lead to frank aortic rupture, acute AR, cardiac tamponade, and death. Distal aortic dissection (i.e., involving only the descending aorta), however, can usually be treated medically.

Echocardiography has fundamentally changed the diagnostic approach to suspected aortic dissection. Transthoracic echocardiography is a reasonably accurate screening tool for ascending aortic dissection, but is not sensitive for detecting descending aortic dissection. Diagnostic findings include a dilated aorta with a linear, mobile echogenic signal in the lumen which represents the dissection flap. Furthermore, color-flow Doppler imaging may reveal normal flow in the true lumen and slow flow in the false channel. Although TTE is sometimes helpful, TEE is a diagnostic procedure of choice for aortic dissection (Fig. 8).[11] It provides better image quality than TTE, with sensitivity and specificity similar to those of computed tomography. Additionally, TEE has the advantage of being portable. Echocardiography is also an excellent screening tool for aortic aneurysms. Like aortic dissections, aneurysms can occur in patients with hypertension as well as patients with Marfan syndrome or

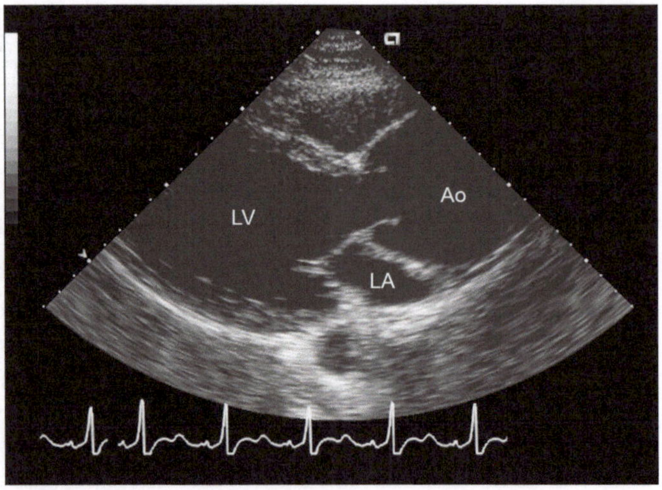

LV, left ventricle; LA, left atrium; Ao, aorta.

FIG. 20: Parasternal long-axis image demonstrating a large aneurysm of the ascending aorta

With permission from: DeMaria AN, Blanchard DG. Echocardiography. In: Fuster V, Walsh RA, Harrington R (Eds). Hurst's The Heart, 13th ed. New York, NY, USA: McGraw-Hill Medical Publishers; 2011. pp. 411-89.

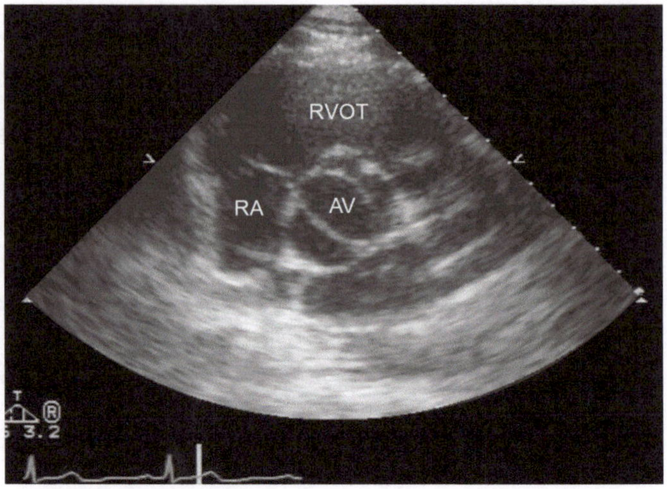

RVOT, right ventricular outflow tract; RA, right atrium; AV, aortic valve.

FIG. 21: Parasternal short-axis image of a bicuspid aortic valve

With permission from: DeMaria AN, Blanchard DG. Echocardiography. In: Fuster V, Walsh RA, Harrington R (Eds). Hurst's The Heart, 13th ed. New York, NY, USA: McGraw-Hill Medical Publishers; 2011. pp. 411-89.

congenital bicuspid AV. Measurements in aortic diameter are generally accurate and reproducible (Fig. 20).

CONGENITAL HEART DISEASE

There are several congenital heart diseases that can be found in adult and only a few will be discussed in this text. A few common congenital heart defects include bicuspid AV, intra- and extracardiac shunts, including ventricular septal defect (VSD), atrial septal defect (ASD), and patent ductus arteriosus (PDA).

Bicuspid Aortic Valve

The most common congenital heart defect in adults involves the AV. The normal AV is tricuspid in anatomy, but in 1–2% of the human population, a congenitally bicuspid AV is present at birth. A physician may suspect a bicuspid AV because of a systolic murmur, and echocardiography is the most expedient method for definitive diagnosis (Fig. 21). A bicuspid AV increases the likelihood of both AV stenosis and AR later in life. There is also an association with ascending aortic aneurysm, congenital narrowing of the descending thoracic aorta (aortic coarctation), and aortic dissection.

Ventricular Septal Defects

Ventricular septal defects can occur in several segments of the interventricular septum. The majority of VSDs in adults occurs in the perimembranous portion of the septum. Inlet (atrioventricular canal), trabecular or muscular and outlet (supracristal) defects are much more rare (Fig. 22). Small muscular VSDs may close spontaneously during childhood. Although large VSDs are often visible on 2D imaging alone, color-flow Doppler imaging is essential for detection of small defects.[21] Most VSDs in adults result in small flow volume. In larger VSDs with significant flow volume, associated findings include cardiac enlargement. Other associated 2D and Doppler findings include RV pressure overload, mitral and tricuspid valvular regurgitation, coexistent ASD, and AR (particularly with supracristal VSD).

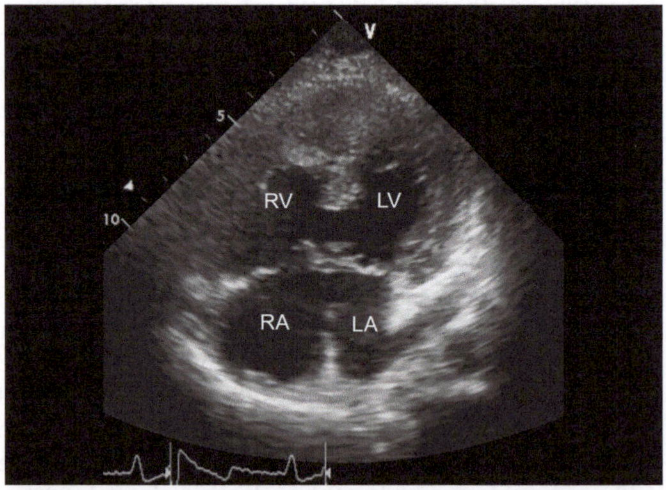

RV, right ventricular; LV, left ventricular; RA, right atrium; LA, left atrium.

FIG. 22: Apical four-chamber view of a large atrioventricular canal type of ventricular septal defect

With permission from: DeMaria AN, Blanchard DG. Echocardiography. In: Fuster V, Walsh RA, Harrington R (Eds). Hurst's The Heart, 13th ed. New York, NY, USA: McGraw-Hill Medical Publishers; 2011. pp. 411-89.

Atrial Septal Defect

There are three main types of ASDs, including (i) ostium secundum, (ii) ostium primum, and (iii) sinus venosus

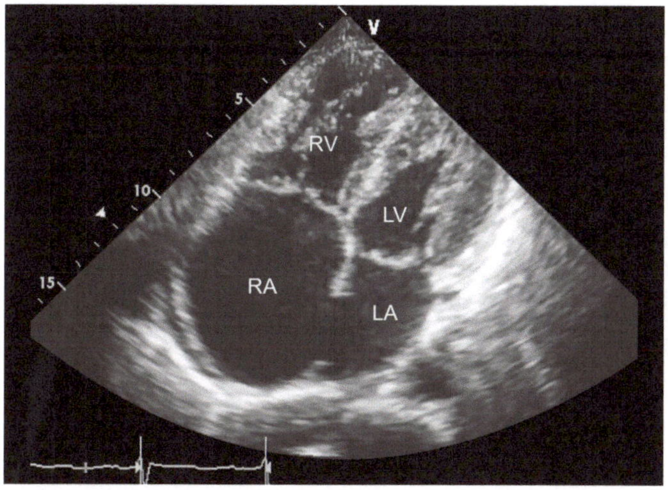

RV, right ventricular; LV, left ventricular; RA, right atrium; LA, left atrium.

FIG. 23: Apical four-chamber view of an ostium secundum atrial septal defect. The right heart is larger than the left, suggesting a significant shunt volume

With permission from: DeMaria AN, Blanchard DG. Echocardiography. In: Fuster V, Walsh RA, Harrington R (Eds). Hurst's The Heart, 13th ed. New York, NY, USA: McGraw-Hill Medical Publishers; 2011. pp. 411-89.

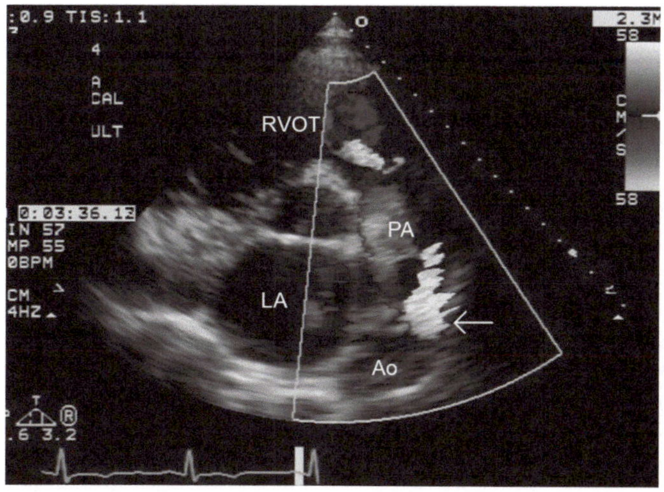

RVOT, right ventricular outflow tract; LV, LA, left atrium; PA, pulmonary artery; Ao, aorta.

FIG. 24: Parasternal short-axis view of a patent ductus arteriosus (arrow). Blood flow from the descending aorta (ascending aorta; in red) is seen entering the main pulmonary artery ***(For color version, see Plate 2)***

With permission from: DeMaria AN, Blanchard DG. Echocardiography. In: Fuster V, Walsh RA, Harrington R (Eds). Hurst's The Heart, 13th ed. New York, NY, USA: McGraw-Hill Medical Publishers; 2011. pp. 411-89.

defects. The first two types are easily seen with TTE, but sinus venosus defects can be difficult to detect without TEE because of their posterior position in the interatrial septum.[22] The most common defect, ostium secundum, is distinguished by absence of tissue in the mid portion of the interatrial septum (Fig. 23). The absence of any septal tissue interposed between the defect and the base of the interventricular septum suggests an ostium primum defect. Sinus venosus ASDs are seen in the superior and posterior portions of the interatrial septum. These are often associated with abnormal drainage of one or more pulmonary veins into the RA instead of the LA. Additional 2D findings seen in ASD with a significant left-to-right shunt include right atrial and RV enlargement and flattening of the interventricular septum. Doppler interrogation often demonstrates blood flow though the ASD defect.

Patent Ductus Arteriosus

Patent ductus arteriosus is an abnormal connection between the distal portion of the aortic arch and the pulmonary artery. This connection is normal in utero, and facilitates delivery of oxygenated blood from the mother to the fetus' systemic circulation. However, this shunt should close early after birth. A persistent PDA may manifest as dilated LA and LV due to chronic volume overload. The 2D imaging may detect a persistent PDA, but color Doppler examination is more likely to detect the high-velocity diastolic flow coming into the pulmonary artery from the aorta (Fig. 24).[23] A large PDA, like a large VSD and ASD, should be closed either surgically or percutaneously, as right heart failure will otherwise eventually occur.

PERICARDIAL DISEASE

The pericardium is a thin membrane that envelops the heart and is composed of two layers reflected onto each other—the visceral and parietal pericardium. The pericardium serves as a barrier to infection and reduces friction with the surrounding structures. In certain disease states, the pericardium can become inflamed (pericarditis) or filled with fluid (pericardial effusion). Pericarditis is a clinical diagnosis, but there are echocardiographic clues, such as pericardial thickening and/or an effusion. However, the echocardiogram may also appear normal. Echocardiography is a reliable tool for detecting a pericardial effusion as well as cardiac tamponade with high sensitivity and specificity. On echocardiographic imaging, pericardial fluid is identified as a "dark" or Echo-free space surrounding the heart with separation between the two layers of the pericardium (Fig. 25). Pericardial effusions may be concentric or loculated, and can vary significantly in size. Multiple fibrinous strands in the pericardial effusion increase the likelihood of infection, hemorrhage, or cancer.

Cardiac tamponade occurs when the pressure within the pericardial space exceeds the diastolic pressure within the cardiac chambers and subsequently impedes blood flow into the heart. This manifests as tachycardia, low blood pressure, and in severe cases, cardiogenic shock. Not all pericardial effusions lead to cardiac

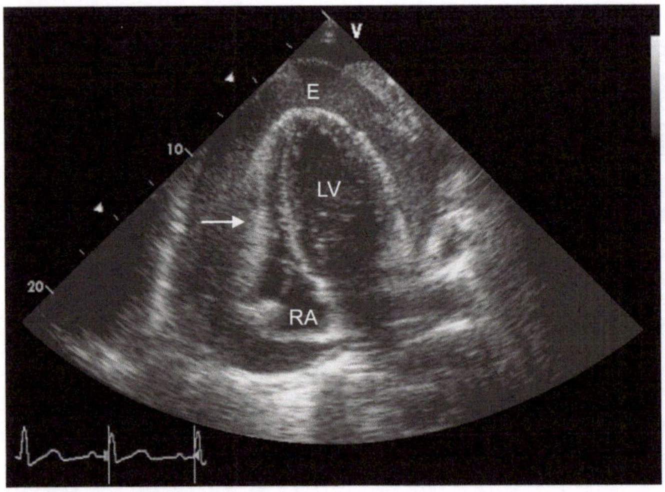

LV, left ventricle; RA, right atrium.

FIG. 25: Apical four-chamber image of a large pericardial effusion. The right ventricular wall buckles towards the left ventricle during diastole (arrow), suggesting cardiac tamponade

With permission from: DeMaria AN, Blanchard DG. Echocardiography. In: Fuster V, Walsh RA, Harrington R (Eds). Hurst's The Heart, 13th ed. New York, NY, USA: McGraw-Hill Medical Publishers; 2011. pp. 411-89.

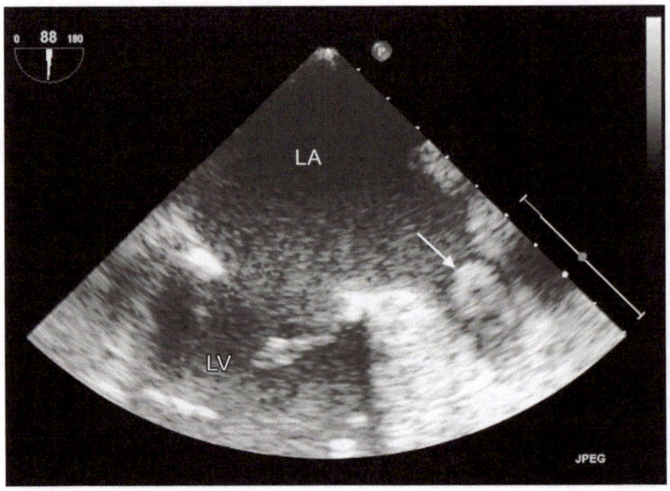

LA, left atrium; LV, left ventricle.

FIG. 26: Transesophageal echocardiographic image of a thrombus in the left atrial appendage (arrow)

With permission from: DeMaria AN, Blanchard DG. Echocardiography. In: Fuster V, Walsh RA, Harrington R (Eds). Hurst's The Heart, 13th ed. New York, NY, USA: McGraw-Hill Medical Publishers; 2011. pp. 411-89.

tamponade, and it depends on the rate and volume of fluid accumulated within the pericardial space. Doppler imaging is quite accurate for the diagnosis of cardiac tamponade.[24] Doppler signals at the RV and LV inflow show enhanced RV and reduced LV diastolic filling with inspiration but reversal of this pattern during expiration.

CARDIAC MASSES

Echocardiography is one of the procedures of choice to detect intracardiac thrombi, vegetations, and tumors. It can also detect intracardiac foreign bodies, including pacemaker leads and intracardiac catheters.

Thrombi

The most common intracardiac masses in patients with heart disease or heart failure are thrombi (clots) due to low flow or static blood. Although clots can occur in any of the four cardiac chambers, right-sided clots are much more rare. Left ventricle thrombi are most likely to occur with apical wall motion abnormalities due to local myocardial injury. Left atrium thrombi often occur in atrial fibrillation and MV disease. These may lead to stroke or other embolic events if they dislodge and leave the heart.[25] Transthoracic echocardiography is sensitive and specific for detecting LV thrombi, but not especially sensitive for detecting LA thrombi. Transthoracic echocardiography is the imaging modality of choice for detecting LA thrombi (Fig. 26). The echocardiographic appearance of thrombi is quite variable.

Tumors

Other causes of intracardiac masses include benign and malignant tumors, which can be primary or metastatic. Nonprimary cardiac tumors are up to 20 times more common than primary cardiac tumors and 75% are metastases from lung, breast, and hematologic cancers. These malignancies often involve the pericardium and present as pericardial effusions; direct myocardial involvement is less common.

Most primary cardiac tumors are benign. Myxomas are the most common primary cardiac tumors, and mostly occur in the LA arising from the fossa ovalis.[26] On 2D imaging, these tumors often appear irregular in shape, gelatinous, and heterogeneously echogenic (Fig. 27). Papillary fibroelastoma is a less common benign primary cardiac tumor, which arises from valves, and tends to embolize systemically. These may appear like vegetations; but unlike vegetations, fibroelastomas usually appear on the more distal side of the valve. Malignant tumor masses are rare, but are often seen in the RA as well as the pericardial space. Transesophageal echocardiography is superior to TTE for the detection of intracardiac masses, particularly those in posterior cardiac structures (e.g., the LA).

CONCLUSION

Echocardiography is an essential tool in clinical cardiology. It is an ubiquitous examination and can be performed by either sonographers or physicians. It

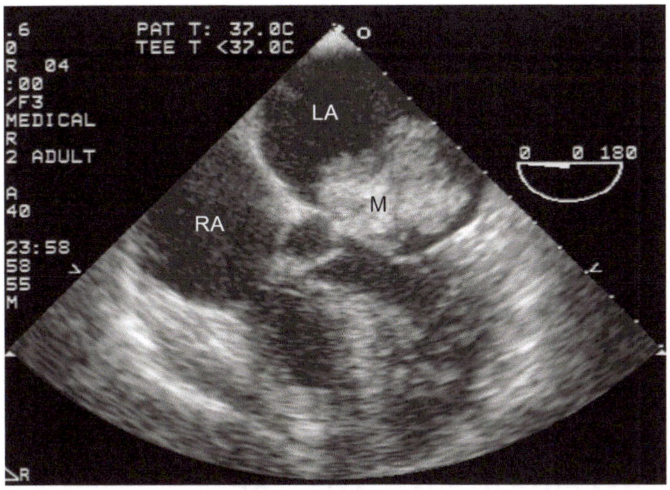

LA, left atrium; RA, right atrium.

FIG. 27: Transesophageal echocardiographic image of a large myxoma in the left atrium

With permission from: DeMaria AN, Blanchard DG. Echocardiography. In: Fuster V, Walsh RA, Harrington R (Eds). Hurst's The Heart, 13th ed. New York, NY, USA: McGraw-Hill Medical Publishers; 2011. pp. 411-89.

provides a quick assessment of cardiac structure and function. In the emergency room setting, it can provide simple answers to common clinical scenarios such as heart failure, suspected acute coronary syndrome, pericardial effusions, and valvular disease. Ultimately, echocardiography provides emergency medicine providers with key data that can be acted on emergently and/or relayed to a cardiologist to help make clinical decisions in the acute care setting.

REFERENCES

1. DeMaria AN, Blanchard DG. Echocardiography. In: Fuster V, Walsh RA, Harrington R (Eds). Hurst's The Heart, 13th edition. New York, NY, USA: McGraw-Hill Medical Publishers; 2011. pp. 411-89.
2. Henry WL, DeMaria A, Gramiak R, King DL, Kisslo JA, Popp RL, et al. Report of the American Society of Echocardiography: nomenclature and standards in two-dimensional echocardiography. Circulation. 1980;62(2):212-7.
3. Lang RM, Tsang W, Weinert L, Mor-Avi V, Chandra S. Valvular heart disease. The value of 3-dimensional echocardiography. J Am Coll Cardiol. 2011;58(19):1933-44.
4. Burns PN. The physical principles of Doppler and spectral analysis. J Clin Ultrasound. 1987;15(9)567-90.
5. Nishimura RA, Miller FA Jr, Callahan MJ, Benassi RC, Seward JB, Tajik AJ. Doppler echocardiography: theory, instrumentation, technique, and application. Mayo Clin Proc. 1985;60(5):321-43.
6. Bom K, de Boo J, Rijsterborgh H. On the aliasing problem in pulsed Doppler cardiac studies. J Clin Ultrasound. 1984;12(9):559-67.
7. Zile MR, Brutsaert DL. New concepts in diastolic dysfunction and diastolic heart failure: Part I. Circulation. 2002;105(11):1387-93.
8. Hegrenaes L, Hatle L. Aortic stenosis in adults. Noninvasive estimation of pressure differences by continuous wave Doppler echocardiography. Br Heart J. 1985;54(4):396-404.
9. Richards KL, Cannon SR, Miller JF, Crawford MH. Calculation of aortic valve area by Doppler echocardiography: a direct application of the continuity equation. Circulation. 1986;73(5):964-9.
10. Daniel WG, Mugge A. Transesophageal echocardiography. N Engl J Med. 1995;332(19):1268-79.
11. Blanchard DG, Kimura BJ, Dittrich HC, DeMaria AN. Transesophageal echocardiography of the aorta. JAMA. 1994;272(7):546-51.
12. Segar DS, Brown SC, Sawada SC, Ryan T, Feigenbaum H. Dobutamine stress echocardiography: correlation with coronary lesion severity as determined by quantitative angiography. J Am Coll Cardiol. 1992;19(6):1197-202.
13. Quinones MA, Verani MS, Haichin RM, Mahmarian JJ, Suarez J, Zoghbi WA. Exercise echocardiography versus T1-201 single photon emission computerized tomography in evaluation of coronary artery disease. Analysis of 292 patients. Circulation. 1992;85(3):1026-31.
14. Shah PM. Echocardiography in congestive or dilated cardiomyopathy. J Am Soc Echocardiogr. 1988;1(1):20-30.
15. Wigle ED, Rakowski H, Kimball BP, Williams WG. Hypertrophic cardiomyopathy: clinical spectrum and treatment. Circulation. 1995;92(7):1680-92.
16. Picano E, Pinamonti B, Ferdeghini EM, Landini L, Slavich G, Orlandini A, et al. Two-dimensional echocardiography in myocardial amyloidosis. Echocardiography. 1991;8(2):253-62.
17. Glover MU, Warren SE, Vieweg WV, Ceretto WJ, Samtoy LM, Hagan AD. M-mode and two-dimensional echocardiographic correlation with findings at catheterization and surgery in patients with mitral stenosis. Am Heart J. 1983; 105(1):98-102.
18. Hatle L, Angelsen B, Tromsdal A. Noninvasive assessment of atrioventricular pressure half-time by Doppler ultrasound. Circulation. 1979;60(5):1096-104.
19. Spain MG, Smith MD, Grayburn PA, Harlamert EA, DeMaria AN. Quantitative assessment of mitral regurgitation by Doppler color flow imaging: angiographic and hemodynamic correlations. J Am Coll Cardiol. 1989;13(3):585-92.
20. Yvorchuk KJ, Chan KL. Application of transthoracic and transesophageal echocardiography in the diagnosis and management of infective endocarditis. J Am Soc Echocardiogr. 1994;7(3 Pt 1):294-308.
21. Linker DT, Rossvoll O, Chapman JV, Angelsen BA. Sensitivity and speed of color Doppler flow mapping compared with continuous wave Doppler for the detection of ventricular septal defects. Br Heart J. 1991;65(4):201-3.
22. Shub C, Dimopoulos IN, Seward JB, Callahan JA, Tancredi RG, Schattenberg TT, et al. Sensitivity of two-dimensional echocardiography in the direct visualization of atrial septal defect utilizing the subcostal approach: experience with 154 patients. J Am Coll Cardiol. 1983;2(1):127-35.
23. Liao PK, Su WJ, Hung JS. Doppler echocardiographic flow characteristics of isolated patent ductus arteriosus: better delineation by Doppler color flow mapping. J Am Coll Cardiol. 1988;12(5):1285-91.
24. Appleton CP, Hatle LK, Popp RL. Cardiac tamponade and pericardial effusion: respiratory variation in transvalvular flow velocities studied by Doppler echocardiography. J Am Coll Cardiol. 1988;11(5):1020-30.
25. Haugland JM, Asinger RW, Mikeil FL, Elsperger J, Hodges M. Embolic potential of left ventricular thrombi: detection by two-dimensional echocardiography. Circulation. 1984;70(4):588-98.
26. Reynen K. Cardiac myxomas. N Engl J Med. 1995;333(24):1610-7.

6
CHAPTER Magnetic Resonance Imaging

Kimberly C Atianzar, Joel R Wilson

INTRODUCTION

Cardiovascular disease is the number one reason for inpatient admission from the emergency department (ED),[1] accounting for approximately 4 million hospitalizations annually.[2] Imaging plays an important role in the triage of patients presenting with cardiovascular complaints in the ED. Cardiovascular magnetic resonance imaging (CMRI) is helpful in a subset of these patients, particularly in the evaluation of patients presenting with chest pain. The spectrum of potential etiologies for undifferentiated chest pain is broad, but cardiovascular causes include stable or unstable angina, non-ST elevation segment myocardial infarction (NSTEMI), ST segment myocardial infarction, myocarditis, pericarditis, and acute aortic syndromes such as dissection. Patients with intermediate pretest probability for coronary artery disease will often undergo noninvasive imaging to further risk stratification, which can be accomplished using CMRI.

Cardiovascular magnetic resonance imaging has several advantages over other imaging modalities. Stress testing with CMRI provides more accurate information about coronary perfusion, global and regional ventricular function, and presence and extent of myocardial fibrosis (e.g., prior myocardial infarction) than do single photon emission computed tomography (SPECT) or echocardiographic stress studies. Unlike nuclear studies, Cardiovascular magnetic resonance imaging uses no ionizing radiation, and unlike echocardiography, imaging planes are unhindered by acoustic windows. CMR provides excellent delineation of cardiovascular anatomy. It is considered a gold standard modality for measuring myocardial volumes, mass and ejection fraction. It also has the ability to characterize tissue, including differentiating acute or chronic infarct from normal myocardium. Importantly, in chronic myocardial infarctions, CMRI can determine myocardial viability. Although aortic pathology is more frequently initially evaluated by computed tomography (CT) in the ED, it can also be readily assessed with CMRI using contrast and noncontrast techniques.

MAGNETIC RESONANCE IMAGING IN EVALUATION OF POSSIBLE ACUTE CORONARY SYNDROME

Patients initially presenting to the ED with acute chest pain are typically immediately evaluated for STEMI. If this is determined to be unlikely on the basis of initial electrocardiogram and clinical grounds, additional diagnoses must be considered. Although cardiac enzymes are sensitive for NSTEMI diagnoses, these assays may require between 4 hours and 12 hours for serially monitored cardiac enzymes to be definitive. Patients at intermediate or high risk for acute coronary syndrome are usually admitted to the hospital for inpatient care and evaluation, while lower risk patients are often either discharged or are managed in chest pain observation units where they are typically referred for further diagnostic testing.

Stress testing is generally most useful for patients with chest pain and intermediate pretest probability of coronary artery disease. Stress testing using CMRI is reliable, cost effective, accurate, and has been well validated for use in the ED setting.[3-7] Cardiovascular magnetic resonance imaging stress can be performed using either dobutamine in a manner analogous to dobutamine stress echocardiography, or more commonly using first-pass myocardial perfusion imaging with gadolinium contrast agent administered during a vasodilator challenge (Fig. 1). With protocols in place for ED triage of patients using vasodilator stress CMRI, images can be available for rapid interpretation, qualitatively as well as quantitatively.

There are several important advantages to using CMRI as a stress modality.

- Sensitivity and specificity of stress testing with CMRI is superior to that of dobutamine stress echocardiography and vasodilator SPECT for identifying obstructive coronary artery disease[8,9]
- Cardiovascular magnetic resonance imaging stress tests contain additional information about cardiac function and localization and characterization of myocardial pathology. Therefore, CMRI is especially well suited to characterize ischemic heart disease:

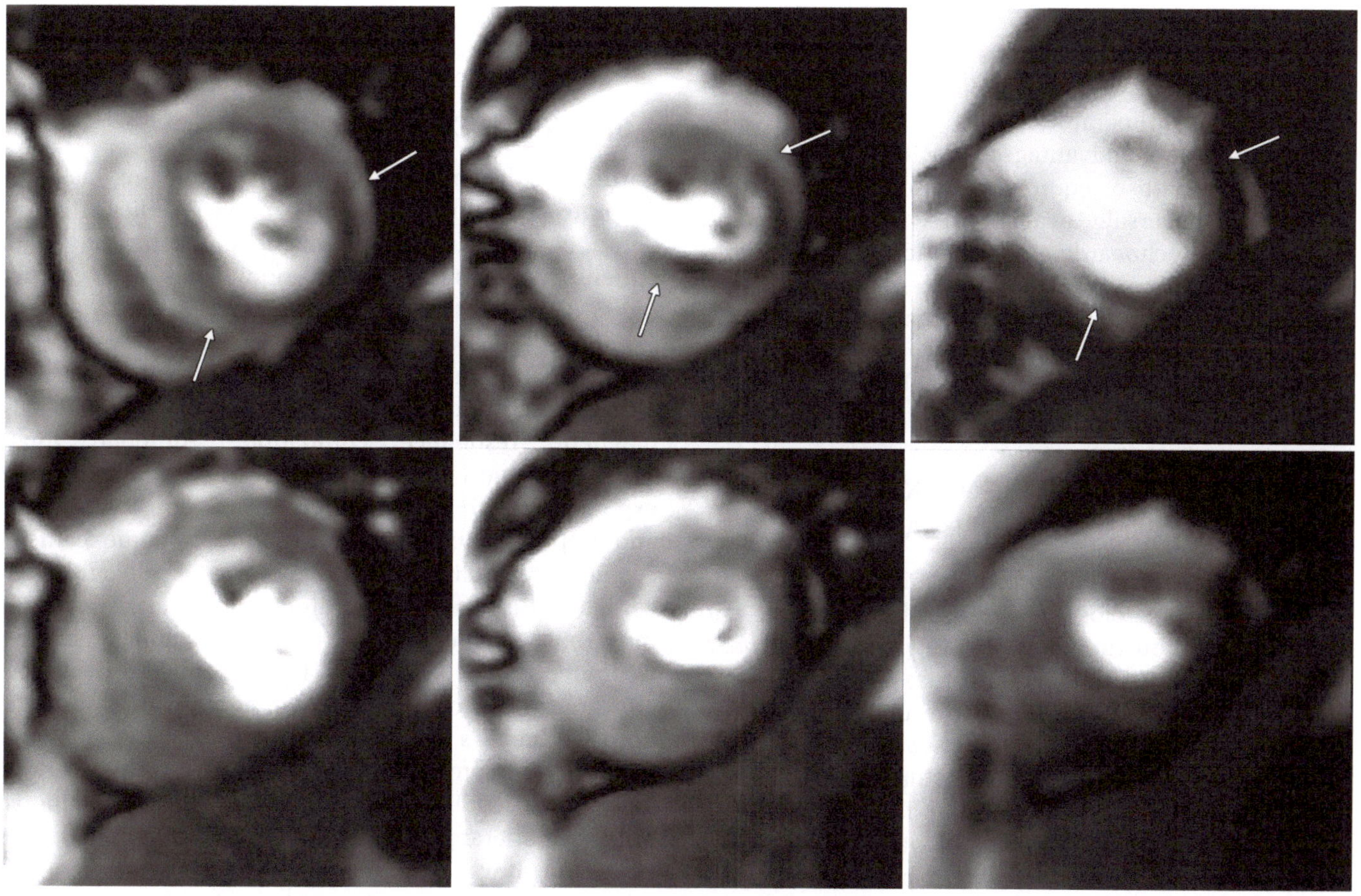

FIG. 1: Abnormal cardiovascular magnetic resonance imaging vasodilator stress test: First pass gadolinium myocardial perfusion during rest (bottom row) and vasodilator stress (top row) in three short-axis slices (base, mid and apex) in a patient presenting with angina. (Note darker regions of myocardium in the inferior to anterolateral wall in stress perfusion images (arrows) indicating a perfusion defect)

- Cardiovascular magnetic resonance imaging can distinguish acute from chronic myocardial infarction. In acute myocardial infarction, it can help to identify the infarct-related artery[8,9] (Fig. 2)
- Cardiovascular magnetic resonance imaging is the gold standard for diagnosis of chronic myocardial infarction using a technique called late gadolinium enhancement. Chronic myocardial infarction is underdiagnosed, particularly in the elderly, and undiagnosed myocardial infarction leads to less aggressive medical management[10-12]
- Cardiovascular magnetic resonance imaging is well validated as a tool to evaluate myocardial viability and is routinely assessed during vasodilator stress myocardial perfusion CMRI protocols. Thus, when ischemic heart disease is identified, CMRI can provide information about optimal revascularization strategies
- A CMRI-focused diagnostic algorithm for triage of intermediate to high risk patients presenting to the ED with chest pain can lead to faster discharge from hospital, fewer invasive coronary angiograms, and marginal cost savings out to 1 year relative to a standard-of-care approach.[5-7]

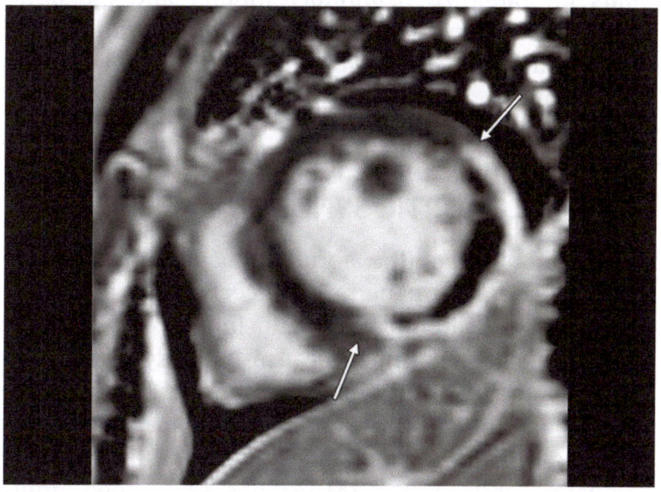

FIG. 2: Late gadolinium enhancement of an acute myocardial infarct: Midventricular short-axis slice showing acute myocardial infarction of the inferior and inferolateral walls (arrows). The black region surrounded by the white enhanced myocardium represents microvascular obstruction. [This finding indicates that there is a low likelihood of functional recovery of myocardium following revascularization (nonviable territory)]

- In addition to evaluating for ischemic heart disease, CMRI provides information about causes of chest pain other than ischemia. For example, CMRI can readily identify myocarditis, pericardial effusions, and pericarditis with greater diagnostic certainty than using echocardiography.

Despite these advantages, CMRI requires local specialized expertise required to perform and interpret and is not universally available. As with nuclear and transthoracic echocardiography studies, CMRI does not currently have adequate spatial resolution for direct visualization of coronary artery plaques in routine clinical practice. However, delineation of coronary arteries is typically sufficient to exclude anomalies of origin and course.

CARDIOVASCULAR MAGNETIC RESONANCE IMAGING IN HEART FAILURE

Cardiovascular magnetic resonance imaging is useful in determining etiology of systolic heart failure and infiltrative cardiomyopathies, quantifying valvular heart disease, and evaluating cardiac masses among other indications. A full discussion of the utility of CMRI in chronic heart failure is beyond the scope of this chapter. Despite this well-established role in diagnosis, prognosis and management of chronic heart failure, CMRI has a limited role for management of patients presenting to the ED in acute heart failure. In patients with poor sonographic windows, systolic function can be rapidly assessed by CMRI with a focused noncontrast study. Although images are typically acquired during breath-holds to minimize respiratory motion and maximize spatial and temporal resolution, lower resolution real time acquisitions are possible for patients unable to hold their breath.

MAGNETIC RESONANCE IMAGING IN ACUTE AORTIC SYNDROMES

Acute pathology of the aorta or major branches can include dissection, penetrating ulcer, pseudoaneurysm, intramural hematoma, traumatic injury, postoperative complication, or aortitis. Because of ready availability, ease of operation, and rapid scan times, CT is generally the modality of choice when evaluating for acute aortic pathology. Magnetic resonance imaging (MRI)/magnetic resonance angiography (MRA) has established utility in serial monitoring of chronic aortopathy as it avoids repeated ionizing radiation exposure. However, the thoracic aorta is usually partially evaluable on stress CMRI studies, so incidental aortic pathology is sometimes noted. The standard CMRI protocol can also be modified to include MRA in cases where there is sufficient clinical suspicion of aortic pathology. Magnetic resonance imaging/MRA of the aorta is also valuable to further assess findings from CT; for example, to help define whether edema is present to suggest aortitis.

SAFETY AND TOLERABILITY

Cardiovascular magnetic resonance imaging has few absolute contraindications. The most significant consideration is avoiding ferromagnetic interactions with patient implants or patient-monitoring devices and the MRI. Patients need to be screened for magnetic resonance compatibility of all implanted devices for the MRI field strength being employed. Peripheral and coronary stents and prosthetic joints are usually magnetic resonance compatible. Although long-considered contraindications to MRI, there is increasing experience with scanning patients with pacemakers and implanted cardiac defibrillators at some centers. Secondly, gadolinium chelates are usually used in cardiac MRI unless contraindications exist. Patients must have adequate renal function (stable creatinine clearance above 30 mg/mL, for example) to avoid the life-threatening complication of nephrogenic systemic fibrosis. There is no strong evidence that patients with allergy to iodinated contrast agents are at any greater risk of allergy to gadolinium agents than to other medications. Mild-to-moderate reactions, such as rash and shortness of breath, have been reported in approximately 1 in 5,000 patients.[31] Severe anaphylactic reactions occur less often than with iodinated agents, at a rate of about 1 in 250,000–300,000 patients.[31] Finally, claustrophobia is relatively common and may require premedication with an anxiolytic, although claustrophobia severe enough to preclude CMRI is relatively rare (<5%).

CONCLUSION

The best established role for CMRI in the ED is as a stress modality in the triage of chest pain in patients with intermediate pretest probability. Otherwise, CMRI typically plays a supporting or troubleshooting role, for example, in cases, where initial imaging leaves diagnostic uncertainty.

REFERENCES

1. National Center for Health Statistics. (2007-10). Number of discharges from short-stay hospitals, by first-listed diagnosis and age: United States. [online] Available from: http://www.cdc.gov/nchs/nhds/nhds_tables.html. [Accessed July, 2016].
2. Healthcare Cost and Utilization Project, Statistical Brief #2. (2003). Reasons for Being Admitted to the Hospital through the Emergency Department. [online] Available from: http://www.hcup-us.ahrq.gov/reports/statbriefs/sb2.jsp. [Accessed July, 2016].
3. Kwong RY, Schussheim AE, Rekhraj S, Aletras AH, Geller N, Davis J, et al. Detecting acute coronary syndrome in the emergency department with cardiac magnetic resonance imaging. Circulation. 2003;107(4):531-7.

4. Ingkanisorn WP, Kwong RY, Bohme NS, Geller NL, Rhoads KL, Dyke CK, et al. Prognosis of negative adenosine stress magnetic resonance in patients presenting to an emergency department with chest pain. J Am Coll Cardiol. 2006;47(7):1427-32.
5. Miller CD, Hwang W, Hoekstra JW, Case D, Lefebvre C, Blumstein H, et al. Stress cardiac magnetic resonance imaging with observation unit care reduces cost for patients with emergent chest pain: a randomized trial. Ann Emerg Med. 2010;56(3):209-19.e2.
6. Miller CD, Hwang W, Case D, Hoeskstra JW, Lefebvre C, Blumstein H, et al. Stress CMR imaging observation unit in the emergency department reduces 1-year medical care costs in patients with acute chest pain: a randomized study for comparison with inpatient care. JACC Cardiovasc Imaging. 2011;4(8):862-70.
7. Miller CD, Case LD, Little WC, Mahler SA, Burke GL, Harper EN, et al. Stress CMR reduces revascularization, hospital readmission, and recurrent cardiac testing in intermediate-risk patients with acute chest pain. JACC Cardiovasc Imaging. 2013;6(7):785-94.
8. Greenwood JP, Maredia N, Younger JF, Brown JM, Nixon J, Everett CC, et al. Cardiovascular magnetic resonance and single-photon emission computed tomography for diagnosis of coronary heart disease (CE-MARC): a prospective trial. Lancet. 2012;379(9814):453-60.
9. Nagel E, Lehmkuhl HB, Bocksch W, Klein C, Vogel U, Frantz E, et al. Noninvasive diagnosis of ischemia-induced wall motion abnormalities with the use of high-dose dobutamine stress MRI: comparison with dobutamine stress echocardiography. Circulation. 1999;99(6):763-70.
10. Abdel-Aty H, Zagrosek A, Schulz-Menger J, Taylor AJ, Messroghli D, Kumar A, et al. Delayed enhancement and T2-weighted cardiovascular magnetic resonance imaging differentiate acute from chronic myocardial infarction. Circulation. 2004;109(20):2411-6.
11. Cury RC, Shash K, Nagurney JT, Rosito G, Shapiro MD, Nomura CH, et al. Cardiac magnetic resonance with T2-weighted imaging improves detection of patients with acute coronary syndrome in the emergency department. Circulation. 2008;118(8):837-44.
12. Schelbert EB, Cao JJ, Sigurdsson S, Aspelund T, Kellman P, Aletras AH, et al. Prevalence and prognosis of unrecognized myocardial infarction determined by cardiac magnetic resonance in older adults. JAMA. 2012;308(9):890-6.

7

CHAPTER

Coronary Computed Tomography Angiography

Anna Marie Chang, Judd E Hollander

INTRODUCTION

Nature of the Problem

More than 5 million patients are evaluated in the emergency department (ED) annually for chest pain, the great majority of which are not found to have a cardiac cause for their symptoms.[1,2] At an estimated cost of over $10 billion annually,[3,4] reducing hospital admissions and overall costs of care through improved risk stratification and better diagnostic testing of patients with potential acute coronary syndrome represents a critical focus for saving healthcare dollars.

Patient History and Physical Examination

The tools most readily available to guide disposition of the patient with chest pain are the patient's age and sex, history of coronary artery disease (CAD) or its risk factors, and the chest pain characteristics. Usually, an initial 12-lead electrocardiogram (ECG) is added as well. Despite the fact that cardiac risk factors have prognostic value in population-based studies of asymptomatic patients, they have been shown to be very poor predictors of acute myocardial infarction (AMI), acute coronary syndrome (ACS), and 30-day cardiovascular events in symptomatic patients, especially in those patients over the age of 40.[5,6] In the group of patients over 65 years of age, they essentially perform no better than the flip of a coin.

The initial 12-lead ECG has low sensitivity for AMI,[7] and a single set of biochemical markers also has poor sensitivity.[1,8] As none of these tools used alone is a reliable predictor of ACS and "low risk is not no risk", observation unit strategies incorporate serial ECGs and cardiac injury markers over a 6- to 12-hour period. In the era of higher sensitivity troponin assays, routine use of serial ECGs in asymptomatic patients probably has no value. The likelihood that an ECG becomes diagnostic of ischemia in an asymptomatic patient without a troponin elevation is exceedingly small.

A negative evaluation without evidence of myocardial infarction (MI) or ischemia is typically followed by a confirmatory study to exclude inducible ischemia, the absence of which permits patient discharge.[9] Given the concerns nationwide of ED crowding, protocols that reduce length of stay and eliminate potentially avoidable admissions (or prolonged periods of observation) are widely needed.

CORONARY COMPUTED TOMOGRAPHY ANGIOGRAPHY

Based on available literature, coronary computed tomography angiography (CCTA) identifies ED patients with potential ACS who are at low risk for cardiovascular events, thereby safely allowing early discharge.

PROTOCOL

In most institutions, a low-dose noncontrast ECG-triggered acquisition is performed through the entire chest for the purpose of calcium scoring and evaluation of lung abnormalities. This is typically followed by a weight-based intravenous injection of 80–120 mL of nonionic iodinated contrast with bolus tracking in the descending aorta. After a scan delay, an ECG-gated acquisition from the pulmonary artery bifurcation through the inferior heart border is performed. Studies should be interpreted by radiologists or cardiologists with subspecialty cardiovascular imaging training (American College of Cardiology/American Heart Association level 3 training) on dedicated three-dimensional workstations using axial, multiplanar reformatted and thin-slab maximum-intensity projection images in an interactive display. Image data are reconstructed at multiple phases of the cardiac cycle, postprocessed and analyzed on independent workstations. The degree of any observed stenosis can be measured with an electronic caliper by comparing the lumen diameter with the diameter of a proximal reference segment.

DIAGNOSTIC ACCURACY

Coronary computed tomography angiography has been found to be comparable to invasive angiography, in several large studies and meta-analyses. Technological improvement has increased sensitivity of detection of coronary artery stenosis from 84% for 4-slice computed tomography (CT) to 83% for 16-slice CT and 93% for 64-slice CT, with concurrent specificities of 93%, 96% and 96%, respectively.[10] A systematic review of 41 studies totaling 2,515 patients indicated a sensitivity of 95% and specificity of 85% for detection of CAD in all types of scanners combined.[11] A report by the European Society of Cardiology and the European Council of Nuclear Cardiology describing a pooled analysis of 800 patients found a sensitivity of 89% [95% confidence interval (CI) = 87–90] with a specificity of 96% (95% CI = 96–97) in 64-slice CT.[12]

Budoff et al. compared the diagnostic accuracy of CCTA to invasive coronary angiography (ICA) in 230 patients. On a per-patient basis, the sensitivity, specificity, positive predictive value, and negative predictive value to detect greater than or equal to 50% stenosis were 95%, 83%, 64%, and 99%, respectively.[13] Miller et al. also compared the accuracy of CCTA to ICA and found similar results in 291 patients.[14] Further examples of large studies comparing 64-slice CCTA to ICA are shown in table 1. These sensitivities and specificities translate to a high negative predictive value for the low-to-intermediate risk patient in the ED.

Meijboom et al. evaluated the diagnostic utility of those found at high, intermediate and low pretest risk of CAD. They found that in the low pretest probability group, a negative CCTA was present in 75% of the patients.[23] The negative predictive value of CCTA to exclude significant CAD was excellent in these patients, reducing the estimated post-test probability to zero and concluded that these patients would not need further downstream diagnostic tests. On the other hand, they found that CCTA was of limited clinical value in the evaluation of the high estimated pretest probability group.

Calcium Score

The role of coronary artery calcium score (CACS) alone, or in combination with angiography, remains the subject of some debate. The American College of Cardiology Foundation (ACCF)/American Heart Association (AHA) 2007 clinical expert consensus document on coronary artery calcium scoring by computed tomography evaluated six published reports in 27,622 patients, none of which were symptomatic ED patients.[24] The relative risk for MI or death over 3–5 years was 4.3-fold increased for any measurable calcium as compared with a CACS of zero. Patients without detectable calcium (or a CACS of zero) have a very low rate of CHD death or MI (0.4%) within this time frame. In contradiction, Gottlieb et al. evaluated 291 patients who were undergoing CCTA and ICA, of whom most (95%) patients were at intermediate to high probability of obstructive CAD. A total of 72 patients had CACS = 0, among whom 14 (19%) had at least one greater than or equal to 50% stenosis.[25] This holds true among the low-risk population as well. Chang et al. found that in patients with a CACS = 0, 23.5% of patients still had CAD (4/17).[26] Within the COroNary computed tomography angiography evaluation For clinical outcomes: an InteRnational Multicenter (CONFIRM) registry, over 5,000 patients had a CACS = 0, yet 16% of these patients still had evidence of CAD on CCTA. Those with CAD despite a CACS = 0 had higher rates of MI and revascularization at 90 days.[27] And thus, freedom from CACS does not appear to provide enough information to effectively risk stratify patients in the ED for acute events.

30-DAY EVENTS

It has been well established that a cardiac catheterization known to be negative predicts a low risk of adverse events. Patients documented to have a less than 25% stenosis or a past normal coronary arteriogram have a less than

TABLE 1: Studies of 64-slice coronary computed tomography angiography diagnostic properties

Author	Number of patients	Sensitivity	Specificity	PPV	NPV
Pugliese[15]	35	100	90	96	100
Leschka[16]	67	94	97	87	99
Raff[17]	70	95	90	93	93
Nikolaou[18]	72	97	79	96	Not reported
Ropers[19]	84	96	91	98	83
Maffei[20]	177	100	98	92	100
Miller[14]	291	83	91	92	81
Meijboom[21]	360	99	64	86	97
Hoffman[22]	368	100	54	17	100

NPV, negative predictive values; PPV, positive predictive values.

TABLE 2: Studies of 64-slice coronary computed tomography angiography used in the emergency department disposition of patients based on their results

Authors	Number of patients	Follow-up time (months)	Number discharged	Event rate in those with maximal stenosis <50%
Gallagher[31]	99	6	88	0%
Rubinshtein[32]	58	12	32	0%
Takakuwa[33]	197	1	133	0%
Hollander[34]	568	1	476	0%

2% risk of MI over the next decade.[28] Repeat cardiac catheterizations over a 9-year-later period have shown that approximately 90% of patients do not develop CAD.[29] Recent cardiac catheterization with normal or minimally diseased vessels almost eliminates the possibility of an ACS. Since CCTA correlates well with catheterization, it makes sense that negative CCTA results should be similarly predictive.

It has been well demonstrated that a negative CCTA (defined as maximal stenosis < 50% in all vessels) predicts freedom from 30-day MI, coronary revascularization, and cardiovascular death (Table 2). In a recent meta-analysis of studies of 1,559 patients with symptoms suggestive of ACS that presented to ED, the sensitivity was 93.3%, specificity was 89.9%, positive predictive value was 48.1%, and negative predictive value was 99.3% for 30-day cardiovascular events.[30]

The American College of Radiology Imaging Network (ACRIN-PA) 4,005 multicenter trial randomized 1,370 patients to either CCTA or traditional care. Patients with a negative CCTA (<50% maximal stenosis) were free from cardiac death or MI at 30 days (upper limit of 95% CI = 0.57%). Additionally, a CCTA-based strategy doubled the discharge rate (50% vs. 23%) and shortened length of stay (18 vs. 25 h) while identifying more patients with coronary disease (9 vs. 3%), while simultaneously reducing the likelihood of a negative catheterization.[35] Similarly, the Rule Out Myocardial Infarction/Ischemia Using Computer Assisted Tomography (ROMICAT)-II study was a multicenter randomized controlled trial comparing the effectiveness of CCTA evaluation versus standard evaluation.[36] Patients who received CT evaluation had shorter length of stay, and were more likely to be discharged from the ED (47 vs. 12%). Overall, there were no differences in clinical adverse events between the two groups, and no undetected ACS at 28 days.

These data support the recommendations that patients with a maximal stenosis of less than 50% can be safely discharged home from the ED.

LONGER TERM EVENTS

Hollander et al. evaluated 588 low-risk patients who received CCTA in the ED. Of the 481 patients with a less than 50% stenosis in any vessel who also did not have depressed left ventricular function, 53 patients (11%) were rehospitalized and 51 patients (11%) received further diagnostic testing (stress or catheterization) over the subsequent year. There was only one death (0.2%) and no AMI during this time period.[37] Hadamitzky et al. enrolled 1,256 consecutive patients with suspected CAD undergoing 64-slice CCTA and observed them prospectively for the occurrence of cardiac death, MI, or unstable angina requiring hospitalization. In the 802 patients without any stenosis greater than 50%, only one case of unstable angina occurred during the initial 90 days. Within a median of 18 months, there were only four events in these 802 patients whereas there were 17 events in the 348 patients with obstructive CAD.[38]

Two other studies focused on low-to-intermediate risk chest pain patients. The ROMICAT trial reported 2-year outcomes for their cohort. Of 368 patients who presented to the ED with acute chest pain, negative initial troponin and a nonischemic ECG, 333 patients (90.5%) had a median follow-up period of 23 months. Contrast-enhanced 64-slice CT was obtained during index hospitalization. Overall, at the end of the follow-up period, 25 patients (6.8%) experienced 35 events (no cardiac deaths, 12 MIs, and 23 revascularizations). Cumulative probability of 2-year events increased across CT strata for CAD but none occurred in patients without disease (no CAD = 0%; nonobstructive CAD = 4.6%; obstructive CAD = 30.3%).[39]

In a cohort of 227 patients, 96 patients had no CAD and 76 had nonobstructive CAD on CCTA. At 2.3-year follow-up, there were no cardiovascular events in the no CAD group and two events in the nonobstructive CAD group. On the other hand, in the 55 patients with disease, 11 patients (20%) had a cardiovascular event during the time interval.[40] Abdulla et al. conducted a meta-analysis that included 5,675 patients who were mostly intermediate-to-high risk in 10 studies with mean follow-up of 21 months. Of these patients, 2,045 (36%) patients had a normal CCTA, 2,068 (36%) had nonobstructive CAD and 1,562 (28%) had obstructive CAD. Overall, 331 (5.8%) had cardiac death, nonfatal MI, and revascularization. The event rate was 0.5% in patients with normal CTA, 3.5% in nonobstructive CAD and 16% in obstructive CAD.[41]

Large, multicenter studies are also being completed to further research in CCTA. The CONFIRM registry screened 27,125 CCTA patients at 12 participating centers. Clinical information was available for over 14,000 patients, with 13,966 (99.3%) patients having mean follow-up of 22.5 months. All-cause mortality (271 deaths) occurred in 0.6% of patients without coronary atherosclerosis, 1.9% of patients with nonobstructive CAD, 2.9% of patients with non-high-risk CAD and 4.9% for patients with high-risk CAD.[42,43] The PROspective Multicenter Imaging Study for Evaluation of Chest Pain (PROMISE) trial was a 2-year multicenter randomized clinical trial that enrolled over 10,000 patients to evaluate the 2-year incidence of death, MI, major complications from cardiovascular procedures or testing, unstable angina hospitalizations, and comparing CCTA to stress testing. There was no difference in death, MI, hospitalizations for unstable angina, or major procedural complication.[44] In addition, the CTA strategy was also associated with lower incidence of invasive cardiac catheterization showing no obstructive CAD.

DO WE EVEN NEED SERIAL BIOMARKERS/OBSERVATION?

Hollander et al. examined 568 low-risk [thrombolysis in myocardial infarction (TIMI) score = 0–2][45] chest pain patients in the ED, and of these, 285 received CCTA without serial cardiac biomarkers, of whom 214 (75%) were discharged to home after testing.[34] Those who had immediate CCTA in the ED had a median length of stay of 7.1 hours compared to 20.8 hours for those who had serial marker testing in the observation unit. Of those with a negative evaluation, no patient suffered an adverse cardiovascular event at 30 days.[34] Although this is a small cohort, it suggests that serial cardiac biomarker testing is not necessary for the evaluation of these chest pain patients, further reducing length of stay.

COST

Coronary computed tomography angiography is associated with decreased length of stay and decreased costs. Khare et al. used computer-based modeling and found that an evaluation utilizing CCTA dominated (less costly and more effective) both observation unit plus stress echocardiography and observation unit plus stress ECG strategies.[46] Chang et al. compared four strategies in the evaluation of chest pain in the ED: (i) immediate CCTA; (ii) CCTA after observation unit care; (iii) stress test in the observation unit versus (iv) care by inpatient medical team and found that median costs were less and length of stay was shorter. The diagnosis of CAD was similar, but fewer patients had 30-day death, MI, or readmissions in the CCTA groups.[47] Goldstein et al. conducted a randomized trial of patients allocated to CCTA (n = 361) or myocardial perfusion imaging (MPI; n = 338) as the index noninvasive test.[48] The CCTA group had a 54% reduction in time to diagnosis compared with stress tests. Costs of care were 38% lower compared with standard (median $2,137 vs. $3,458). The two diagnostic strategies had no difference in major adverse cardiac events after normal index testing.

One study found higher costs associated with CCTA utilization. Shreibati et al. used a 20% sample of Medicare beneficiaries and compared functional imaging to CCTA in costs and subsequent health service utilization. Computed tomography angiography was associated with an increased likelihood of subsequent cardiac catheterization (22.9 vs. 12.1%), percutaneous coronary intervention (7.8 vs. 3.4%), and coronary artery bypass graft surgery (3.7 vs. 1.3%). Computed tomography angiography was also associated with higher total healthcare spending ($4,200) but no difference in all-cause mortality.[49] However, this study only focused on outpatient claims in elderly patients with a higher pretest likelihood of disease and not the typical low-to-intermediate risk patients evaluated in the ED.

AREAS OF UNKNOWN

Although it is established that patients with CAD on CCTA are at increased risk for cardiovascular events at 30 days and up to 2 years, there are no clear guidelines for the evaluation of low-to-intermediate risk ED patients with CAD detected by CCTA, especially those with greater than 50% stenosis in any vessel. Weustink et al. recommend that in patients with a low (<20%) pretest probability of disease, negative stress test, or CCTA results have no need for further testing. In patients with an intermediate (20–80%) pretest probability, a positive CCTA result suggests the need to proceed with ICA where a negative result would then not require any further testing. Physicians could proceed directly with ICA in patients with a high (>80%) pretest probability.[50] However, most patients in this study had a stress test if diagnosed with obstructive CAD, so it is unclear how this translates to clinical practice. In the study by Hollander et al., very few patients with less than 50% stenosis on CCTA received further diagnostic testing and none were reported to have positive stress testing.[34,35] It is unlikely that patients with less than 70% lesions would have ischemia in response to a stress test, and thus, the logic of performing this test in these patients is unclear.

Furthermore, it is unclear what the downstream medical management of patients with nonobstructive disease on CCTA should be. Most observational studies show an increased use of antiplatelet and lipid-lowering agents in those who are found to have both nonobstructive and obstructive disease.[51-53] In a recent Scottish trial, patients undergoing CCTA had improved angina stability and frequency at 6 weeks compared to standard care.[54] Although not statistically significant, CTA was associated with a 38% reduction in coronary heart disease (CHD) death and MI over a median of 1.7 years, as patients received more preventive and antianginal treatment.

RADIATION

When 64-slice CCTA was first utilized, retrospectively gated techniques were used with high doses of radiation. Using then-current dose protocols, Einstein et al. "calculated" relative risk of cancer for men and women evaluated with CCTA and believed that there was four-fold increase in the lifetime attributable risk of cancer incidence associated with radiation exposure.[55] Synchronization to the ECG can be performed in three ways: (i) "retrospective gating" where the X-ray tube is at full current throughout a spiral scan resulting in increased radiation exposure; (ii) as "dose-modulated" spiral scan where the tube current is reduced outside the diastolic window during which cardiac motion is reduced; and (iii) prospective gating (step-and-shoot) axial scan where slices are acquired only in diastole and summated together to form a volume of data. Prospective gating is becoming more frequently used, as it results in high-quality images at the lowest possible radiation dose, but requires adequate patient preparation and heart rate control to avoid artifacts.[56] New studies and techniques now report that radiation using the prospective gating method can decrease radiation dose to 2–4 mSv.[57] This radiation dose is much lower than the estimated radiation dose of 7 mSv for a rest-only technetium-99m MPI or 24 mSv for a dual isotope study.[58]

Furthermore, in those with a negative CCTA, there may be less downstream testing. At a single academic institution during a 10-year period, 1,097 patient records were evaluated. A total of 344 patients (31.4%) received cumulative estimated effective dose from all medical sources of more than 100 mSv, and multiple MPI studies were performed in 424 patients (38.6%), for whom cumulative estimated effective dose was 121 mSv.[59] Thus, if CCTA can decrease future testing, as indicated by some studies, and given that the overall cumulative radiation dose is of concern, CCTA may be beneficial relative to nuclear imaging.

OTHER IMAGING MODALITIES

Triple Rule-out

Coronary computed tomography angiography has a limited capacity to diagnose noncardiac causes of chest pain arising from sources outside the anatomic window it interrogates. Technical advances in cardiac CT and intravenous contrast injection protocols have made a "triple rule-out" protocol feasible, which can effectively image the coronary, aortic and pulmonary arterial beds, to exclude CAD, aortic dissection and pulmonary embolism as causes of acute chest pain. Takakuwa et al. in 197 patients found that over 30 days no further diagnostic testing was performed in 133 (76%) of 175 of patients with none or mild coronary disease on triple rule-out scans. Three cases of pulmonary embolism were found, and one case of aortic dissection.[33]

Rogers et al. randomized patients to receive a comprehensive cardiothoracic CT or a CCTA in 59 patients. No significant difference was found in the median length of stay, rate of hospital discharge without additional imaging, costs of care, or the number of revisits between the dedicated and comprehensive arms, respectively. Radiation dosages were similar between the two arms.[60] Madder et al. identified patients who underwent triple rule-out or CCTA at two hospitals in Michigan; 272 patients had triple rule-out and 1,796 patients had CCTA performed. Pulmonary embolism was identified in only 1.1% of triple rule-out and 0.2% of cardiac CT examinations, and there were no aortic dissections.[61] At 90 days, there were no differences in death, ACS, PE or aortic dissection diagnosis, or major differences in downstream resource utilization. Burris et al., with 12,834 patients in an observational study, found that when compared to CCTA, triple rule-out scans were more likely to detect pulmonary embolism and aortic dissection; however, the provider selection (decision as to which test to order in any specific patient) may account for this difference, rather than anything specific with the tests.[62] Given that the radiation dose and intravenous contrast dose is higher[61] in these triple rule-out scans, it does not seem to provide enough additional information to warrant the examination in the majority of patients. Additionally, although it is known that triple rule-out scans perform similarly to CCTA with respect to diagnosis of CAD, there is no data comparing diagnostic accuracy of triple rule-out scan with CT pulmonary angiography or CT aortography.[63,64]

Coronary Computed Tomography Angiography with Perfusion Stress

One of the major critiques of CCTA is that it does not provide information on the physiologic significance of coronary luminal stenosis. A greater than or equal to 50% coronary luminal stenosis identified by CCTA is a poor predictor of ACS. Thus, the best noninvasive diagnostic test for evaluating chest pain in the ED would be a test that can measure both presence of CAD and myocardial ischemia in patients. Bezerra et al. conducted a subset analysis from the ROMICAT trial of 35 subjects who had chest pain and ICA; 22 of the patients were diagnosed with ACS. The sensitivity and specificity of myocardial perfusion defects for ACS were 86% (95% CI = 64–96%) and 62% (95% CI = 32–85%). Adding myocardial perfusion defects and regional wall motion abnormality to the assessment for significant stenosis (>50%) resulted in a higher sensitivity of 91% (69–98%) and specificity of 85% (54–97%) and a significantly increased overall diagnostic accuracy when compared with assessment for stenosis.[65]

A recent review of the literature shows sensitivity ranges from 79–97% and specificity from 72–98% depending on the scanner type, reference standard, studied population and whether analysis is per patient, segment, or territory. Most studies have been completed on intermediate-to-high risk patients.[66] However, given that none of these studies had more than 47 patients, more data are needed for this technology. The CORE320 (Coronary Artery Evaluation Using 320-Row Multidetector CT Angiography) study compared the diagnostic capability of the combination of quantitative 320-CCTA and quantitative perfusion imaging to the combination of conventional coronary angiography and single photon emission computed tomography (SPECT) MPI at the patient level. In 381 patients, the area under the curve for combined CCTA and perfusion was 0.87 for the prediction of a 50% or greater stenosis by ICA with perfusion imaging, which was more predictive than CCTA alone.[67]

Coronary Computed Tomography Angiography with Fractional Flow Reserve

Fractional flow reserve (FFR) is a measurement of the ratio of the mean coronary pressure distal to a coronary stenosis to the mean aortic pressure during maximal coronary blood flow. An FFR less than 0.8 indicates hemodynamically significant ischemia that may need revascularization.[68] Using biomechanical engineering and flow mechanics, it is possible to calculate the FFR based on CCTA images. In the Determination of Fractional Flow Reserve by Anatomic Computed Tomographic Angiography (DeFACTO) study, the authors compared the diagnostics performance of CCTA with FFR versus CCTA alone for ischemia and found improved diagnostic accuracy, although it did not reach its prespecified endpoint. However, the performance characteristics suggest a low false-negative rate if FFR was used in addition to CCTA to identify ischemia-causing intermediate stenosis lesions.[69] Furthermore, processing these images take about 6 hours per case. Thus, more studies are needed for this technology.

Cardiovascular Magnetic Resonance Imaging

A full discussion of cardiovascular magnetic resonance (CMR) is beyond the scope of this chapter. Cardiovascular magnetic resonance allows a comprehensive evaluation of myocardial function, perfusion and morphology in patients with CAD. In a recent meta-analysis that compared CT to CMR, the authors found that for ruling out CAD, CT was more accurate than CMR. In a total of 19 studies, the mean sensitivity for CMR was 87% and specificity was 70% for the detection of CAD.[70] In cardiovascular disease, MRI has been proven to be a reliable and well-tolerated tool and is useful post-ACS to focus on remodeling or for diagnoses of diseases such as myocarditis. However, in the setting of acute chest pain in the ED, rapid diagnosis is required to ensure instant therapy, and thus CMR may not be the examination of choice.[71]

CONCLUSION

Coronary computed tomography angiography has been used with increasing frequency as part of evaluation of chest pain in the ED. In the appropriate low-to-intermediate risk group of patients, it appears to be an excellent evaluation strategy safely and efficiently allowing for the rapid discharge of patients home.

REFERENCES

1. Fesmire FM, Hughes AD, Fody EP, Jackson AP, Fesmire CE, Gilbert MA, et al. The Erlanger chest pain evaluation protocol: a one-year experience with serial 12-lead ECG monitoring, two-hour delta serum marker measurements, and selective nuclear stress testing to identify and exclude acute coronary syndromes. Ann Emerg Med. 2002;40(6):584-94.
2. Blomkalns AL, Gibler WB. Chest pain unit concept: rationale and diagnostic strategies. Cardiol Clin. 2005;23(4):411-21, v.
3. Gibler WB, Runyon JP, Levy RC, Sayre MR, Kacich R, Hattemer CR, et al. A rapid diagnostic and treatment center for patients with chest pain in the emergency department. Ann Emerg Med. 1995;25(1):1-8.
4. Roberts RR, Zalenski RJ, Mensah EK, Rydman RJ, Ciavarella G, Gussow L, et al. Costs of an emergency department-based accelerated diagnostic protocol vs hospitalization in patients with chest pain. JAMA. 1997;278(20):1670-6.
5. Marsan RJ, Shaver KJ, Sease KL, Shofer FS, Sites FD, Hollander JE. Evaluation of a clinical decision rule for young adult patients with chest pain. Acad Emerg Med. 2005;12(1):26-31.
6. Han JH, Lindsell CJ, Storrow AB, Luber S, Hoekstra JW, Hollander JE, et al. The role of cardiac risk factor burden in diagnosing acute coronary syndromes in the emergency department setting. Ann Emerg Med. 2007;49(2):145-52, 152.e1.
7. Fesmire FM, Percy RF, Wears RL, MacMath TL. Initial ECG in Q wave and non-Q wave myocardial infarction. Ann Emerg Med. 1989;18(7):741-6.
8. Fesmire FM, Christenson RH, Fody EP, Feintuch TA. Delta creatine kinase-MB outperforms myoglobin at two hours during the emergency department identification and exclusion of troponin positive non-ST-segment elevation acute coronary syndromes. Ann Emerg Med. 2004;44(1):12-9.
9. Amsterdam EA, Kirk JD, Bluemke DA, Diercks D, Farkouh ME, Garvey JL, et al. Testing of low-risk patients presenting to the emergency department with chest pain: a scientific statement from the American Heart Association. Circulation. 2010;122(17):1756-76.
10. Vanhoenacker PK, Heijenbrok-Kal MH, Van Heste R, Decramer I, Van Hoe LR, Wijns W, et al. Diagnostic performance of multidetector CT angiography for assessment of coronary artery disease: meta-analysis. Radiology. 2007; 244(2):419-28.
11. Janne d'Othée B, Siebert U, Cury R, Jadvar H, Dunn EJ, Hoffmann U. A systematic review on diagnostic accuracy of CT-based detection of significant coronary artery disease. Eur J Radiol. 2008;65(3):449-61.
12. Schroeder S, Achenbach S, Bengel F, Burgstahler C, Cademartiri F, de Feyter P, et al. Cardiac computed tomography: indications, applications, limitations, and

training requirements: report of a Writing Group deployed by the Working Group Nuclear Cardiology and Cardiac CT of the European Society of Cardiology and the European Council of Nuclear Cardiology. Eur Heart J. 2008;29(4):531-56.

13. Budoff MJ, Dowe D, Jollis JG, Gitter M, Sutherland J, Halamert E, et al. Diagnostic performance of 64-multidetector row coronary computed tomographic angiography for evaluation of coronary artery stenosis in individuals without known coronary artery disease: results from the prospective multicenter ACCURACY (Assessment by Coronary Computed Tomographic Angiography of Individuals Undergoing Invasive Coronary Angiography) trial. J Am Coll Cardiol. 2008;52(21):1724-32.
14. Miller JM, Rochitte CE, Dewey M, Arbab-Zadeh A, Niinuma H, Gottlieb I, et al. Diagnostic performance of coronary angiography by 64-row CT. N Engl J Med. 2008;359(22):2324-36.
15. Pugliese F, Mollet NRA, Runza G, van Mieghem C, Meijboom WB, Malagutti P, et al. Diagnostic accuracy of non-invasive 64-slice CT coronary angiography in patients with stable angina pectoris. Eur Radiol. 2006;16(3):575-82.
16. Leschka S, Alkadhi H, Plass A, Desbiolles L, Grünenfelder J, Marincek B, et al. Accuracy of MSCT coronary angiography with 64-slice technology: first experience. Eur Heart J. 2005;26(15):1482-7.
17. Raff GL, Gallagher MJ, O'Neill WW, Goldstein JA. Diagnostic accuracy of noninvasive coronary angiography using 64-slice spiral computed tomography. J Am Coll Cardiol. 2005;46(3):552-7.
18. Nikolaou K, Knez A, Rist C, Wintersperger BJ, Leber A, Johnson T, et al. Accuracy of 64-MDCT in the diagnosis of ischemic heart disease. AJR Am J Roentgenol. 2006;187(1):111-7.
19. Ropers D, Rixe J, Anders K, Küttner A, Baum U, Bautz W, et al. Usefulness of multidetector row spiral computed tomography with 64- x 0.6-mm collimation and 330-ms rotation for the noninvasive detection of significant coronary artery stenoses. Am J Cardiol. 2006;97(3):343-8.
20. Maffei E, Seitun S, Martini C, Palumbo A, Tarantini G, Berti E, et al. CT coronary angiography and exercise ECG in a population with chest pain and low-to-intermediate pre-test likelihood of coronary artery disease. Heart. 2010;96(24):1973-9.
21. Meijboom WB, Meijs MFL, Schuijf JD, Cramer MJ, Mollet NR, van Mieghem CA, et al. Diagnostic accuracy of 64-slice computed tomography coronary angiography: a prospective, multicenter, multivendor study. J Am Coll Cardiol. 2008;52(25):2135-44.
22. Hoffmann U, Bamberg F, Chae CU, Nichols JH, Rogers IS, Seneviratne SK, et al. Coronary computed tomography angiography for early triage of patients with acute chest pain: the ROMICAT (Rule Out Myocardial Infarction using Computer Assisted Tomography) trial. J Am Coll Cardiol. 2009;53(18):1642-50.
23. Meijboom WB, van Mieghem CAG, Mollet NR, Pugliese F, Weustink AC, van Pelt N, et al. 64-slice computed tomography coronary angiography in patients with high, intermediate, or low pretest probability of significant coronary artery disease. J Am Coll Cardiol. 2007;50(15):1469-75.
24. Greenland P, Bonow RO, Brundage BH, Budoff MJ, Eisenberg MJ, Grundy SM, et al. ACCF/AHA 2007 clinical expert consensus document on coronary artery calcium scoring by computed tomography in global cardiovascular risk assessment and in evaluation of patients with chest pain: a report of the American College of Cardiology Foundation Clinical Expert Consensus Task Force (ACCF/AHA Writing Committee to Update the 2000 Expert Consensus Document on Electron Beam Computed Tomography). Circulation. 2007;115(3):402-26.
25. Gottlieb I, Miller JM, Arbab-Zadeh A, Dewey M, Clouse ME, Sara L, et al. The absence of coronary calcification does not exclude obstructive coronary artery disease or the need for revascularization in patients referred for conventional coronary angiography. J Am Coll Cardiol. 2010;55(7):627-34.
26. Chang AM, Le J, Matsuura AC, Litt HI, Hollander JE. Does coronary artery calcium scoring add to the predictive value of coronary computed tomography angiography for adverse cardiovascular events in low-risk chest pain patients? Acad Emerg Med. 2011;18(10):1065-71.
27. Villines TC, Hulten EA, Shaw LJ, Goyal M, Dunning A, Achenbach S, et al. Prevalence and severity of coronary artery disease and adverse events among symptomatic patients with coronary artery calcification scores of zero undergoing coronary computed tomography angiography: results from the CONFIRM (Coronary CT Angiography Evaluation for Clinical Outcomes: An International Multicenter) registry. J Am Coll Cardiol. 2011;58(24):2533-40.
28. Pitts WR, Lange RA, Cigarroa JE, Hillis LD. Repeat coronary angiography in patients with chest pain and previously normal coronary angiogram. Am J Cardiol. 1997;80(8):1086-7.
29. Papanicolaou MN, Califf RM, Hlatky MA, McKinnis RA, Harrell FE, Mark DB, et al. Prognostic implications of angiographically normal and insignificantly narrowed coronary arteries. Am J Cardiol. 1986;58(13):1181-7.
30. Takakuwa KM, Keith SW, Estepa AT, Shofer FS. A meta-analysis of 64-section coronary CT angiography findings for predicting 30-day major adverse cardiac events in patients presenting with symptoms suggestive of acute coronary syndrome. Acad Radiol. 2011;18(12):1522-8.
31. Gallagher MJ, Ross MA, Raff GL, Goldstein JA, O'Neill WW, O'Neil B. The diagnostic accuracy of 64-slice computed tomography coronary angiography compared with stress nuclear imaging in emergency department low-risk chest pain patients. Ann Emerg Med. 2007;49(2):125-36.
32. Rubinshtein R, Halon DA, Gaspar T, Jaffe R, Goldstein J, Karkabi B, et al. Impact of 64-slice cardiac computed tomographic angiography on clinical decision-making in emergency department patients with chest pain of possible myocardial ischemic origin. Am J Cardiol. 2007;100(10):1522-6.
33. Takakuwa KM, Halpern EJ. Evaluation of a "triple rule-out" coronary CT angiography protocol: use of 64-section CT in low-to-moderate risk emergency department patients suspected of having acute coronary syndrome. Radiology. 2008;248(2):438-46.
34. Hollander JE, Chang AM, Shofer FS, McCusker CM, Baxt WG, Litt HI. Coronary computed tomographic angiography for rapid discharge of low-risk patients with potential acute coronary syndromes. Ann Emerg Med. 2009;53(3):295-304.
35. Litt HI, Gatsonis C, Snyder B, Singh H, Miller CD, Entrikin DW, et al. CT angiography for safe discharge of patients with possible acute coronary syndromes. N Engl J Med. 2012;366(15):1393-403.
36. Hoffmann U, Truong QA, Schoenfeld DA, Chou ET, Woodard PK, Nagurney JT, et al. Coronary CT angiography versus standard evaluation in acute chest pain. N Engl J Med. 2012;367(4):299-308.
37. Hollander JE, Chang AM, Shofer FS, Collin MJ, Walsh KM, McCusker CM, et al. One-year outcomes following coronary computerized tomographic angiography for evaluation of emergency department patients with potential acute coronary syndrome. Acad Emerg Med. 2009;16(8):693-8.
38. Hadamitzky M, Distler R, Meyer T, Hein F, Kastrati A, Martinoff S, et al. Prognostic value of coronary computed tomographic angiography in comparison with calcium scoring and clinical risk scores. Circ Cardiovasc Imaging. 2011;4(1):16-23.
39. Schlett CL, Banerji D, Siegel E, Bamberg F, Lehman SJ, Ferencik M, et al. Prognostic value of CT angiography for major adverse cardiac events in patients with acute chest pain from the emergency department: 2-year outcomes of the ROMICAT trial. JACC Cardiovasc Imaging. 2011;4(5):481-91.
40. Carrigan TP, Nair D, Schoenhagen P, Curtin RJ, Popovic ZB, Halliburton S, et al. Prognostic utility of 64-slice computed tomography in patients with suspected but no documented coronary artery disease. Eur Heart J. 2009;30(3):362-71.
41. Abdulla J, Asferg C, Kofoed KF. Prognostic value of absence or presence of coronary artery disease determined by 64-slice computed tomography coronary angiography A systematic review and meta-analysis. Int J Cardiovasc Imaging. 2011;27(3):413-20.
42. Min JK, Dunning A, Lin FY, Achenbach S, Al-Mallah MH, Berman DS, et al. Rationale and design of the CONFIRM (COronary CT Angiography EvaluatioN For Clinical Outcomes: An InteRnational Multicenter) Registry. J Cardiovasc Comput Tomogr. 2011;5(2):84-92.
43. Chow BJW, Small G, Yam Y, Chen L, Achenbach S, Al-Mallah M, et al. Incremental prognostic value of cardiac computed tomography in coronary artery disease using CONFIRM: COroNary computed tomography angiography evaluation for clinical outcomes: an InteRnational Multicenter registry. Circ Cardiovasc Imaging. 2011;4(5):463-72.
44. Douglas PS, Hoffmann U, Patel MR, Mark DB, Al-Khalidi HR, Cavanaugh B, et al. Outcomes of anatomical versus functional testing for coronary artery disease. N Engl J Med. 2015;372(14):1291-300.
45. Pollack CV, Sites FD, Shofer FS, Sease KL, Hollander JE. Application of the TIMI risk score for unstable angina and non-ST elevation acute coronary syndrome to an unselected emergency department chest pain population. Acad Emerg Med. 2006;13(1):13-8.
46. Khare RK, Courtney DM, Powell ES, Venkatesh AK, Lee TA. Sixty-four-slice computed tomography of the coronary arteries: cost-effectiveness analysis of patients presenting to the emergency department with low-risk chest pain. Acad Emerg Med. 2008;15(7):623-32.

47. Chang AM, Shofer FS, Weiner MG, Synnestvedt MB, Litt HI, Baxt WG, et al. Actual financial comparison of four strategies to evaluate patients with potential acute coronary syndromes. Acad Emerg Med. 2008;15(7): 649-55.
48. Goldstein JA, Chinnaiyan KM, Abidov A, Achenbach S, Berman DS, Hayes SW, et al. The CT-STAT (Coronary Computed Tomographic Angiography for Systematic Triage of Acute Chest Pain Patients to Treatment) trial. J Am Coll Cardiol. 2011;58(14):1414-22.
49. Shreibati JB, Baker LC, Hlatky MA. Association of coronary CT angiography or stress testing with subsequent utilization and spending among medicare beneficiaries. JAMA. 2011;306(19):2128-36.
50. Weustink AC, Mollet NR, Neefjes LA, Meijboom WB, Galema TW, van Mieghem CA, et al. Diagnostic accuracy and clinical utility of noninvasive testing for coronary artery disease. Ann Intern Med. 2010;152(10):630-9.
51. Øvrehus KA, Bøtker HE, Jensen JM, Munkholm H, Johnsen SP, Nørgaard BL. Influence of coronary computed tomographic angiography on patient treatment and prognosis in patients with suspected stable angina pectoris. Am J Cardiol. 2011;107(10):1473-9.
52. LaBounty TM, Devereux RB, Lin FY, Weinsaft JW, Min JK. Impact of coronary computed tomographic angiography findings on the medical treatment and control of coronary artery disease and its risk factors. Am J Cardiol. 2009;104(7):873-7.
53. Chow BJW, Small G, Yam Y, Chen L, McPherson R, Achenbach S, et al. Prognostic and therapeutic implications of statin and aspirin therapy in individuals with nonobstructive coronary artery disease results from the CONFIRM (Coronary CT Angiography EvaluatioN For Clinical Outcomes: An InteRnational Multicenter registry) registry. Arterioscler Thromb Vasc Biol. 2015;35(4):981-9.
54. SCOT-HEART investigators. CT coronary angiography in patients with suspected angina due to coronary heart disease (SCOT-HEART): an open-label, parallel-group, multicentre trial. Lancet. 2015;385(9985):2383-91.
55. Einstein AJ, Henzlova MJ, Rajagopalan S. Estimating risk of cancer associated with radiation exposure from 64-slice computed tomography coronary angiography. JAMA. 2007;298(3):317-23.
56. Earls JP. How to use a prospective gated technique for cardiac CT. J Cardiovasc Comput Tomogr. 2009;3(1):45-51.
57. Fink C, Krissak R, Henzler T, Lechel U, Brix G, Takx RA, et al. Radiation dose at coronary CT angiography: second-generation dual-source CT versus single-source 64-MDCT and first-generation dual-source CT. AJR Am J Roentgenol. 2011;196(5):W550-7.
58. Einstein AJ. Radiation risk from coronary artery disease imaging: how do different diagnostic tests compare? Heart. 2008;94(12):1519-21.
59. Einstein AJ, Weiner SD, Bernheim A, Kulon M, Bokhari S, Johnson LL, et al. Multiple testing, cumulative radiation dose, and clinical indications in patients undergoing myocardial perfusion imaging. JAMA. 2010;304(19): 2137-44.
60. Rogers IS, Banerji D, Siegel EL, Truong QA, Ghoshhajra BB, Irlbeck T, et al. Usefulness of comprehensive cardiothoracic computed tomography in the evaluation of acute undifferentiated chest discomfort in the emergency department (CAPTURE). Am J Cardiol. 2011;107(5):643-50.
61. Madder RD, Raff GL, Hickman L, Foster NJ, McMurray MD, Carlyle LM, et al. Comparative diagnostic yield and 3-month outcomes of "triple rule-out" and standard protocol coronary CT angiography in the evaluation of acute chest pain. J Cardiovasc Comput Tomogr. 2011;5(3):165-71.
62. Burris AC, Boura JA, Raff GL, Chinnaiyan KM. Triple Rule Out Versus Coronary CT Angiography in Patients With Acute Chest Pain: Results From the ACIC Consortium. JACC Cardiovasc Imaging. 2015;8(7):817-25.
63. Ayaram D, Bellolio MF, Murad MH, Laack TA, Sadosty AT, Erwin PJ, et al. Triple rule-out computed tomographic angiography for chest pain: a diagnostic systematic review and meta-analysis. Acad Emerg Med. 2013;20(9):861-71.
64. Hollander J, Chang AM. Triple Rule Out CTA Scan or the Right Test for the Right Patient. JACC Cardiovasc Imaging. 2015;8(7):826-7.
65. Bezerra HG, Loureiro R, Irlbeck T, Bamberg F, Schlett CL, Rogers I, et al. Incremental value of myocardial perfusion over regional left ventricular function and coronary stenosis by cardiac CT for the detection of acute coronary syndromes in high-risk patients: a subgroup analysis of the ROMICAT trial. J Cardiovasc Comput Tomogr. 2011;5(6):382-91.
66. Ko BS, Cameron JD, DeFrance T, Seneviratne SK. CT stress myocardial perfusion imaging using Multidetector CT—A review. J Cardiovasc Comput Tomogr. 2011;5(6):345-56.
67. Rochitte CE, George RT, Chen MY, Arbab-Zadeh A, Dewey M, Miller JM, et al. Computed tomography angiography and perfusion to assess coronary artery stenosis causing perfusion defects by single photon emission computed tomography: the CORE320 study. Eur Heart J. 2014;35(17):1120-30.
68. De Bruyne B, Pijls NHJ, Kalesan B, Barbato E, Tonino PA, Piroth Z, et al. Fractional flow reserve–guided PCI versus medical therapy in stable coronary disease. N Engl J Med. 2012;367(11):991-1001.
69. Min JK, Leipsic J, Pencina MJ, Berman DS, Koo BK, van Mieghem C, et al. Diagnostic accuracy of fractional flow reserve from anatomic CT angiography. JAMA. 2012;308(12):1237-45.
70. Schuetz GM, Zacharopoulou NM, Schlattmann P, Dewey M. Meta-analysis: noninvasive coronary angiography using computed tomography versus magnetic resonance imaging. Ann Intern Med. 2010;152(3):167-77.
71. Hunold P, Bischoff P, Barkhausen J, Vogt FM. Acute chest pain: the role of MR imaging and MR angiography. Eur J Radiol. 2012;81(12):3680-90.

8 CHAPTER

Clinical Evaluation of Chest Pain

Matthew Noble, Anna Marie Chang

INTRODUCTION

Chest pain currently represents the second most common chief complaint of patients presenting to emergency departments (EDs) in the United States (~5.4%).[1] Evaluating chest pain can be clinically challenging, considering the wide range of severity associated with underlying causes, the array of diagnostic tests and tools available, and the potential harm to a patient from an insufficient or inappropriate work-up. Additionally, while the tools for evaluating chest pain continue to evolve and improve, translating these new tests and imaging studies into an updated yet meaningful and efficient clinical evaluation within the time and resource constraints faced by ED providers can be a complicated and often confusing task.

Much of what will be covered in this chapter is explored in more detail in other chapters. As such, the goal of this chapter is limited to a practical and up-to-date approach to evaluating the adult patient with nontraumatic, undifferentiated chest pain in the ED.

Statistically, 1 in every 20 ED patients will have a chief complaint of chest pain. Emergency department providers face a unique challenge to first rule out life-threatening conditions associated with patients' chief complaints, after which a broader evaluation can be undertaken that balances thoroughness with efficiency. Eliciting historical information and physical examination findings can help a provider prioritize a differential diagnosis, order appropriate lab and imaging tests, and reach treatment and management decisions. This chapter will mirror this clinical approach, with a discussion of life-threatening conditions, pertinent history and physical examination, building a differential diagnosis, focused testing for each potential diagnosis, and a brief consideration of patient disposition.

A basic understanding of test characteristics is invaluable to clinicians. Generally speaking, unless a definitive diagnosis can be made, the ED provider often focuses his or her efforts on being able to effectively eliminate diagnoses from the differential. This is best accomplished with negative results to tests that have high sensitivities for a particular condition, which then rules out that condition. Conversely, when the pretest probability of a patient having a particular diagnosis is high, the provider should then look for confirmatory tests with high specificity, in order to rule in that diagnosis. Adept application of specialized tests with an informed awareness of their sensitivities and specificities allows the ED provider to confidently navigate an otherwise challenging chief complaint.

THE FIRST 10 MINUTES

In every adult patient with undifferentiated chest pain, the ED physician must first be able to recognize life-threatening causes, including myocardial infarction (MI), cardiac tamponade, tension pneumothorax, acute aortic dissection (AAD), massive pulmonary embolism (PE), myocarditis, and mediastinitis. Some of these and other etiologies of chest pain will be explored later in the chapter (Flowchart 1).

Within the first 10 minutes of arrival to the ED, patients complaining of chest pain should have their vital signs measured and an electrocardiogram (ECG) performed. Unstable vital signs must be addressed, following advanced cardiac life support algorithms, after which focused diagnostic tests and imaging should be considered. Point-of-care ultrasound is quickly becoming an indispensible tool for the ED provider.

For hypoxic and/or tachypneic patients, the ED provider should check breath sounds and trachea position to evaluate for pneumothorax, including tension pneumothorax and the potential need for emergent needle decompression thoracostomy. Bedsides, ultrasound may also be useful in determining presence or absence of pneumothorax, and can often be performed more rapidly and more reliably than a portable chest radiograph.

For tachycardic patients, the ED provider should first assess the patient's mental status and distal perfusion before considering the potential benefit of interventions to reduce heart rate.

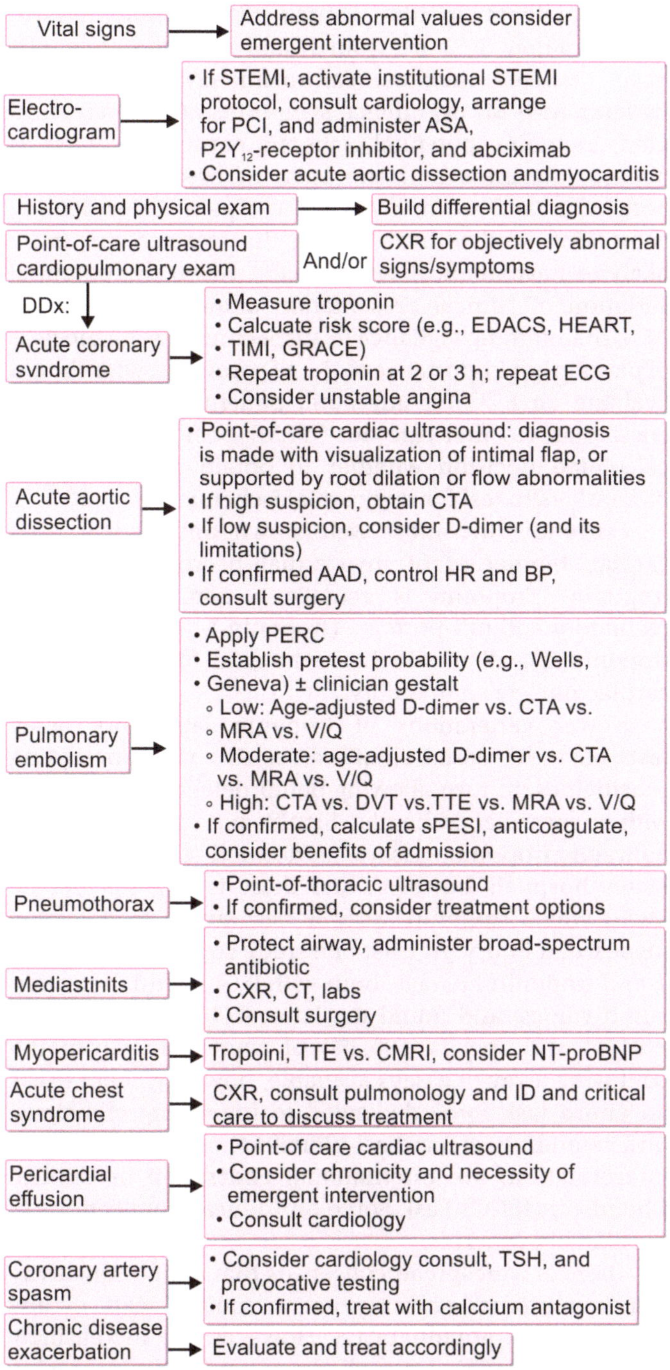

AAD, acute aortic dissection; ASA, aspirin; BP, blood pressure; CMRI, cardiac magnetic resonance imaging; CT, computed tomography; CTA, computed tomography angiography; CXR, chest X-ray; DDx, differential diagnosis, DVT, deep vein thrombosis; ECG, electrocardiogram; HR, heart rate; ID, infectious disease; MRA, magnetic resonance angiography; NT-proBNP, N-terminal pro-brain natriuretic peptide; PCI, percutaneous coronary intervention; PERC, PE rule-out criteria, sPESI, simplified Pulmonary Embolism Severity Index; STEMI, ST elevation myocardial infarction; TSH, thyroid stimulating hormone; TTE, transthoracic echocardiogram; V/Q, ventilation-perfusion scintigraphy.

FLOWCHART 1: Algorithmic approach to the clinical evaluation of undifferentiated chest pain in the emergency department

For hypotensive patients, the ED provider should strongly consider bedside cardiac ultrasound to evaluate for pericardial effusion and cardiac tamponade including evidence of right heart strain and a general assessment of cardiac volume, motion and ejection fraction, as well as possible obstructive shock from a pneumothorax. If needed, immediate treatment of cardiogenic shock should be undertaken, possibly including intravenous fluids, vasopressors, early consultation with an intensivist and/or transfer to a critical care unit. Emergent pericardiocentesis may be indicated.

Fever should prompt consideration for the need of early implementation of treatment for sepsis including but certainly not limited to causes such as pneumonia or endocarditis.

Acute ischemic changes on a patient's ECG should prompt activation of the catheterization laboratory and consultation with an interventional cardiologist.

HISTORY AND PHYSICAL

Pertinent historical features to be ascertained by the ED provider in patients complaining of chest pain include the timing and context of onset of pain, location, severity, history of similar pain, associated symptoms (dyspnea, diaphoresis, nausea/vomiting), positional versus nonpositional quality, and exertional versus nonexertional characteristics. Pertinent past medical history includes heart disease (such as prior MIs, prior bypass grafting or stent placement, history of transplant, anticoagulant or antiplatelet medication use), history of pulmonary diseases (chronic obstructive pulmonary disease, asthma), history of thromboembolic diseases or events (deep venous thrombosis, PE), and history of malignancy and other relevant medical conditions such as diabetes mellitus, hypertension, hyperlipidemia, sickle cell disease, Marfan syndrome, and pregnancy. Pertinent elements of the social history include stimulant use (cocaine, methamphetamine) and tobacco use. Family history of cardiac arrest or sudden nontraumatic death at a young age may also be important.

The physical examination of an adult patient with undifferentiated chest pain is relatively insensitive, but may be specific. A complete cardiac examination (with particular attention to rate, rhythm, and the presence or absence of murmur or rub) should be performed, as well as palpation of pulses in distal extremities, assessing for the presence of jugular venous distention, a complete pulmonary examination (evaluating for breath sounds and their symmetry, crackles, wheezing), relevant findings on skin examination (such as diaphoresis), a targeted abdominal examination, and if suggested by history, the presence of leg swelling or pain in the popliteal region.

Once historical and physical examination data have been gathered, the ED provider should consider a differential diagnosis, upon which further testing should be based. The remainder of this chapter will consider several potential diagnoses and a focused evaluation of each.

ACUTE CORONARY SYNDROME

Acute coronary syndrome (ACS) is generally defined as rupture of atherosclerotic plaques with subsequent thrombus formation and ischemia within coronary arteries. Since the extent of ischemia exists on a continuum, it may be reversible and relieved by rest, or it may be permanent and cause myocardial necrosis and infarction.

The most recent third universal definition of MI distinguishes five types of MIs. The development of more sensitive and specific cardiac biomarkers and diagnostic imaging techniques now allows for detection of very small amounts of myocardial injury or necrosis. There has also been advancement in imaging and treatment such that it has become necessary to distinguish conditions that may cause MI. Briefly, type 1 is a spontaneous infarction, type 2 is secondary to an ischemic imbalance, type 3 relates to death when biomarker values are unavailable, type 4a is related to percutaneous coronary intervention (PCI), type 4b is related to stent thrombosis, and type 5 is related to coronary artery bypass grafting.[2]

Early detection of MI in the ED improves patient outcomes, and relies primarily on the ECG and biomarkers of myocardial necrosis as diagnostic tests. ST segment elevation myocardial infarction (STEMI) represents 25–40% of MI presentations and is detected from the ECG.[3] Non-ST segment elevation myocardial infarction (NSTEMI) also signifies myocardial injury or necrosis, as evidenced by elevated biomarkers but in the absence of ECG changes.

Reperfusion therapy is the recommended treatment for patients with STEMI. According to the 2013 American College of Cardiology Foundation and American Heart Association Task Force on Practice Guidelines,[3] there is level A evidence to support both reperfusion therapy for all patients with STEMI within 12 hours of symptom onset as well as PCI as the recommended method of reperfusion. Level B evidence supports transfer of patients with STEMI from any non-PCI-capable hospital to a PCI-capable hospital, or initiation of fibrinolytic therapy (within 30 minutes of hospital arrival, in the absence of contraindications) for STEMI patients at non-PCI-capable institutions when transfer time to PCI-capable facility exceeds 120 minutes. Level B evidence supports administration of aspirin (162–325 mg) before primary PCI (Class I recommendation), and a loading dose of a $P2Y_{12}$-receptor inhibitor (clopidogrel 600 mg or prasugrel 60 mg or ticagrelor 180 mg) as early as possible (Class I recommendation), as well as administration of intravenous GP IIb/IIIa receptor antagonist (such as abciximab) to patients for whom PCI is intended (Class IIb recommendation). These guidelines should be discussed in advance with cardiologists and a protocol should be enacted at each institution for treatment of STEMI. Regional protocols and quality improvement initiatives have been shown to reduce door-to-reperfusion times.[4]

Of patients in the United States with STEMI, approximately 30% are women and approximately 23% have diabetes mellitus. Approximately one-third of patients with MI experience symptoms other than chest pain, including potential ischemic equivalents such as nausea, dizziness and shortness of breath.[3] Although both men and women have chest pain as presenting complaint, studies have shown that women are more likely to have atypical symptoms.[5-7] Given the potential variation of clinical presentation among patients with ACS, maintaining vigilance in suspecting this diagnosis is of paramount importance to the ED provider, who should evaluate an ECG for any adult patient complaining of chest pain (to first rule out STEMI), before reaching a calculated decision whether to obtain cardiac serum biomarkers to test for myocardial ischemia.

Currently, the most well-known and widely used cardiac biomarker of myocardial necrosis is cardiac troponin. Troponin is actually a complex of three regulatory subunit proteins (troponin I, troponin C and troponin T), all of which are integral for skeletal and cardiac muscle contractility.

Newer generations of troponin laboratory assay tests have decreased cutoff values that yield increasing sensitivities, in turn allowing better detection of patients with myocardial ischemia. Significant variability exists between troponin assays performed in the United States hospitals however, and there is ongoing debate about which troponin assay is best suited to detecting myocardial injury. At least one study compared troponin T and troponin I assays, both with 0.04 ng/mL detection cutoff values, and found the latter to be more sensitive (90.7%) and specific (90.2%) of acute MI.[8] Given the confusing array of assays available, however, there exists an entire task force dedicated to improving clinicians' understanding of cardiac biomarker assays and their interpretation, the International Federation of Clinical Chemistry (IFCC) Task Force on Clinical Applications of Cardiac Bio-Markers.

There is widespread consensus that a high sensitivity troponin biomarker assay be an integral part of any evaluation for potential ACS. However, the increasingly sensitive troponin assays have created increasing potential for positive results, in which elevated levels may be seen in patients not actually suffering a MI. Conditions other than ACS that may elevate serum troponin levels include myocardial injury related to supply-demand imbalance (including arrhythmia, aortic dissection, severe anemia, coronary spasm), as well as injury not related to myocardial ischemia (including cardiac contusion, myocarditis, rhabdomyolysis with cardiac involvement, cardiotoxic agents), and multifactorial injury (such as heart failure, sepsis, renal failure, severe PE, infiltrative disease, strenuous exercise).[2] Thus, although troponins are the best biomarker to detect myocardial injury, not all detectable myocardial injury originates from ACS.

Furthermore, the majority of patients presenting to EDs complaining of chest pain are not ultimately diagnosed with ACS. As such, and given the unique time demands of the ED in which prolonged assessments can cause crowding and adverse patient outcomes, there is significant interest in developing risk stratification scores and diagnostic protocols which can reliably classify patients without ischemic ECG changes or positive initial cardiac biomarkers as acceptably "low-risk" for acute MI and thus safe for discharge without further emergent testing.

Although historical features are neither reliable nor sufficient to predict for or against ACS, some patient-reported characteristics of chest pain may be helpful to clinicians trying to form pretest probabilities. Generally, pains that are stabbing, pleuritic, positional or reproducible by palpation have lower likelihood ratios for ACS or MI (0.2–0.3). Meanwhile, pain that radiates to one or both shoulders or is precipitated by exertion (likelihood ratios 2.3–4.7) makes ACS a more likely diagnosis.[9] Nitroglycerin has no diagnostic utility, as neither a response to nitroglycerin nor the lack thereof is useful in differentiating the etiology of a patient's chest pain.[10]

While solitary historical factors are not predictive, there may be diagnostic utility in composite risk scores. One simple risk score that is frequently used is the thrombolysis in myocardial infarction (TIMI) risk score, a 7-item clinical assessment tool derived from trials of patients with unstable angina. The TIMI score includes age older than or equal to 65, aspirin use in the last 7 days, at least two angina episodes within the last 24 hours, ST changes of at least 0.5 mm in contiguous leads, known coronary artery disease (CAD) with stenosis greater than or equal to 50%, elevated cardiac serum biomarker, and at least three cardiac risk factors. Thrombolysis in myocardial infarction is one of several scores that have been prospectively validated to correlate with (and thus predict) outcome for patients presenting to EDs with undifferentiated chest pain. However, even with TIMI risk score zero, there remains a 1.7% risk of 30-day adverse events including MI, revascularization, and death.[11]

In patients with known ACS, multiple other composite risk scores exist including PURSUIT (Platelet Glycoprotein IIb/IIIa in Unstable Angina: Receptor Suppression Using Integrilin Therapy), GRACE (Global Registry of Acute Coronary Events), and FRISC (Fracture and Immobilization Score). Global Registry of Acute Coronary Events, which includes age, heart rate, blood pressure, serum creatinine, presence of cardiac arrest at admission, ST segment deviation on ECG, elevated cardiac enzymes and signs/symptoms (of congestive heart failure, pulmonary edema and cardiogenic shock), has been validated to estimate mortality risk for patients with confirmed ACS.[12,13] However, these may have less utility in the undifferentiated patient in the ED.

Several risk scores have been developed specifically for the undifferentiated ED patient. The HEART score (which includes history, ECG, age, risk factors, troponin) has been validated to estimate risk of ACS to suggest the need for intervention in some patients.[14,15] In one study, HEART score compared favorably to TIMI and GRACE.[15] Others applaud HEART for its superior applicability to ED patients, predictability and simplicity.[16] More recently, the Emergency Department Assessment of Chest Pain Score (EDACS) was developed in Australia. The EDACS is a composite score designed specifically for undifferentiated patients presenting to the ED with potential ACS and includes age, sex, known CAD or greater than or equal to 3 risk factors, and signs/symptoms (diaphoresis, radiation to arm or shoulder, worsened by inspiration, reproducible by palpation). The score was 99% sensitive for 30-day adverse cardiac events. The major difference between this score and some others are that nonemergent vascularization was not considered within the definition of major adverse cardiac event (MACE).[17]

There is increasingly consistent validation of multiple accelerated diagnostic protocols (ADPs), which incorporate reassuring patient historical features, a nonischemic ECG and negative serial troponins (often performed at narrow time intervals), that yield high sensitivities to detect populations of patients at acceptably low-risk for ACS. These patients may then be safely discharged from the ED without further testing for ACS.

In the Asia-Pacific Evaluation of Chest Pain Trial (ASPECT), the authors were able to use a refined ADP [which consisted of low TIMI score, nonischemic ECG, and high sensitivity cardiac troponin T (hs-cTnT)] to identify patients at acceptably low-risk of 30-day ACS. With TIMI = 0, this ADP had a sensitivity of 99% and identified 15% of patients suitable for discharge; including patients with TIMI = 1 allowed 20% of patients to be discharged, with sensitivity of 97%.[18]

Data show that up to 23% of patients who were found to have acute MI had initially normal troponins,[19] which suggests limited utility of single biomarker measurements at time of presentation to the ED. Some research suggests that in patients presenting with chest pain of less than 8 hours duration, diagnostic accuracy as measured by troponins within 3 hours is not improved with extension of serial troponin measurements to 6 hours.[20] Therefore, many guidelines still recommend serial testing of cardiac troponins, most commonly at time of presentation and again 3 hours later.[21,22] Some studies support measuring the difference between troponin results between time of arrival and 2 hours; when this difference is less than 30%, both the sensitivity and negative predictive value (NPV) of the tests appear to increase to 100%.[23] Initial efforts to increase this delta troponin difference to 50% have revealed some missed cases of ACS.[24]

In the Accelerated Diagnostic Protocol to Assess Patients With Chest Pain Symptoms Using Contemporary Troponins as the Only Biomarker (ADAPT) trial, an ADP using a nonischemic ECG, TIMI score = 0, and negative troponin I measurements at 0 and 2 hours had sensitivity of 99.7%, NPV of 99.7%, and specificity 23.4%, and classified 20% of patients as low risk for ACS.[25] The authors also compared this accelerated approach to a "standard-care pathway", in which patients presenting to the ED had troponins drawn at 0 and 6–12 hours after presentation. The 2-hour accelerated approach resulted in 19.3% of patient being discharged within 6 hours, compared to 11.0% in the standard group.[26]

Using nonischemic ECG and negative measurements at 0 and 2 hours of high sensitivity cardiac troponin I (hs-TnI) with cutoffs of less than or equal to 26.2 ng/L, another ADP evaluated 30-day risk for MACE for patients in the ED. With TIMI score of 0, sensitivity of this ADP was 100%, specificity 23.1%, and NPV was 100%, and 19.6–25.3% of patients were classified as low risk with 0% MACE. With TIMI score of less than or equal to 1, sensitivity was 99.2%, specificity was 48.7%, and NPV 99.7%, classifying 38.6–41.5% of patients as low risk with 0.8% 30-day MACE.[27]

Another ADP used a nonischemic ECG plus a TIMI score less than or equal to 1, as well as hs-cTnT at time 0 and again at 2 hours. When the hs-cTnT was normal for both measurements, the ADP showed between 97% and 100% sensitivity and 99% and 100% NPV for MACE within 30 days. Practically, this ADP approach meant early identification of 35–40% of patients as extremely low risk and thus safely dischargeable.[28]

An ADP using EDACS criteria plus nonischemic ECG and negative troponins at 0 and 2 hours showed sensitivity 99–100%, specificity 49.9–59.0% and classified 42.2–51.3% of patients as low-risk.[17]

Chest radiograph is often obtained in patients complaining of chest pain, including those for whom providers are considering a diagnosis of ACS. While there are many valid reasons to get chest X-rays, which are traditionally part of STEMI protocols, several studies have invited criticism of the utility of chest radiography in suspected ACS.

One retrospective study evaluated 760 ED patients who had a chest radiograph performed as part of an evaluation for suspected ACS. Of these patients, 12% had a clinically significant chest X-ray. Canadian ACS guidelines were then applied to this cohort and showed a sensitivity of 80%, a specificity of 50%, a positive predictive value (PPV) of 18% and an NPV of 95%. If these guidelines had been applied to the study population a priori, the number of chest radiographs performed would have been reduced by 47%. Unfortunately, the authors do not report the number or percentage of clinically significant chest X-rays that would have been missed if the guidelines had been applied.[29] In another study of 130 adult patients in whom ACS was suspected and a chest X-ray was obtained, only 5 patients (<4%) had a clinically significant radiographic abnormality.[30]

One study of 1,650 patients attempted to establish a clinical decision rule for predicting chest radiograph abnormality in nontrauma patients presenting to the ED. While these patients were not necessarily evaluated for chest pain or possible ACS, the authors suggest a 10-item set of clinical signs and symptoms that have 95% sensitivity, 40% specificity, 25% PPV, and 98% NPV for detecting clinically significant radiographic abnormalities. These criteria were age older than or equal to 60, temperature greater than or equal to 38°C, oxygen saturation less than 90%, respiratory rate greater than 24, hemoptysis, rales, diminished breath sounds, a history of alcohol abuse, or tuberculosis, or thromboembolic disease.[31]

In adult patients presenting to the ED with chest pain and possible ACS, one group has derived a refined clinical decision rule with 100% sensitivity, 11.5% specificity, 6.7% PPV, and 100% NPV for radiographic abnormality requiring intervention. These criteria included no shortness of breath, no history of smoking, no abnormalities on lung auscultation, and age younger than 55 years.[32]

In patients experiencing chest pain without ECG changes suggestive of STEMI, the ED provider should be aware that further diagnostic testing may reveal abnormalities. As testing can lead to more testing, these imaging abnormalities often prompt further investigation, including invasive evaluation such as cardiac catheterization. However, this course of testing and evaluation may not necessarily improve outcomes, such as patient risk for MI. In a recent large retrospective analysis, "compared with no testing, exercise electrocardiography, myocardial perfusion scintigraphy, and coronary computed tomography angiography were associated with significantly higher odds of cardiac catheterization and revascularization procedures without a concomitant improvement in the odds of experiencing an MI".[33]

Historically common practice among ED providers is to recommend patients with intermediate risk of CAD but negative work-up for acute ischemia undergo further cardiac risk stratification following their ED visit. In a cohort of patients admitted from the ED to an observation unit for further risk stratification, the rate of positive stress tests was about 11%, suggesting that 3.3% of patients with positive stress tests would be missed if they were instead discharged directly from the ED with a plan for further outpatient risk stratification.[34] However, some studies suggest that only 42–70% of patients referred for an outpatient stress test following their ED visit for chest pain actually have this test performed, with less than 10% of stress testing completed within 72 hours following discharge from the ED.[34,35]

In addition, routine follow-up provocative stress testing may generate only a very small therapeutic yield, with significant numbers of false positives. One study redemonstrated that approximately 11% of patients undergoing stress testing had findings consistent with coronary ischemia. However, of these patients, half had confirmed obstructive disease and half had false positive stress test results, and less than 1% of patients who underwent coronary angiography for positive stress test results had lesions that were amenable to positive benefits of revascularization.[36] More recently, coronary computed tomography angiography (CTA) has been utilized in low-to-intermediate chest pain patients presenting to the ED. Early studies showed high correlation with cardiac catheterization results and increased sensitivity and specificity compared to stress testing. In most studies, approximately 50% of patients with chest pain and low-to-intermediate risk had no CAD (defined as less than 50% stenosis in any vessel) on coronary CTA and no evidence of ACS. In addition, when coronary CTA is positive for plaque and stenosis, the specificities for ACS remained low (54% and 87%, respectively).[37] This may create situations in which patients not actually suffering from ACS but with positive CTA findings are subjected to additional invasive testing, with associated costs and risks. Further research is necessary for this technology, and how to incorporate data that includes both structure and flow.

Thus, it is important for physicians to understand pretest probability and use appropriate diagnostic testing. Furthermore, physicians should take into account patient preferences, and allow patients to participate in shared decision-making regarding further testing.

PULMONARY EMBOLISM

Pulmonary embolism is venous thromboembolism located in the pulmonary vasculature, and the estimated annual incidence of PE is 23–69 cases per 100,000 people.[38] The majority of PEs are thought to originate as deep vein thrombosis (DVT) of the legs, with subsequent embolism to pulmonary arteries.

There is a spectrum of clinical severity associated with PEs, which is determined almost entirely by size and location of the embolus. Subsegmental emboli may be an incidental and asymptomatic finding, whereas a massive (or saddle) PE may cause rapid and significant oxygen desaturation, right heart failure (cor pulmonale), hypotension, and cardiogenic shock. While the full critical care management of massive PE is beyond the scope of this chapter, the general principles of treatment include fibrinolysis (unfractionated heparin vs. tissue plasminogen activator) and/or surgical thrombectomy, with concurrent supportive care to prevent full hemodynamic collapse. Judicious intravenous fluids are necessary, as excess fluid administration may exacerbate right ventricular wall stress, shift the interventricular septum further into the left ventricle and worsen left ventricular filling and function. Vasopressors are frequently required; dobutamine and dopamine increase cardiac output and may decrease pulmonary vascular resistance, and norepinephrine increases both cardiac output and systemic vascular resistance.[39]

Detecting submassive, segmental, and subsegmental PE presents a significant challenge for the ED physician. Of course, not everyone who presents to the ED complaining of chest pain needs to be evaluated for PE. Establishing a pretest probability is a vital first step in determining whether to pursue evaluation for PE, given its paramount importance in selecting the appropriate diagnostic test as well as interpreting those test results. To establish a pretest probability, providers may rely on their clinical impression (gestalt), or they may use structured clinical prediction rules, and the optimal choice of approach has been the subject of numerous studies.

An earlier meta-analysis reviewing 16 studies with 8,300 patients found similar accuracy between clinician gestalt and clinical prediction rules (simplified Wells, extended Wells, Geneva) in determining low, moderate or high pretest probability for PE.[40] The authors ultimately advocated for the use of clinical decision rules, although they did not identify any of the rules as superior. A more recent meta-analysis of 52 studies and 55,000 patients also examined clinician gestalt and clinical decision rules for diagnosing PE. Gestalt showed 85% sensitivity and 51% specificity, compared to 84% sensitivity and 58% specificity with the Wells rule using cutoff value of less than 2, 60% sensitivity and 80% specificity with the Wells rule using cutoff of 4, 84% sensitivity and 50% specificity with the Geneva rule, and 91% sensitivity and 37% specificity with the revised Geneva rule.[41] These authors also advocated for the use of clinical decision rules over clinician gestalt, but again did not identify any one particularly superior rule.

Once a pretest probability has been established, there are various methods to reliably confirm or exclude PE. A 2005 meta-analysis, including 48 studies and 11,000 patients (in which the prevalence of PE was approximately 30%), summarized the diagnostic yield of multiple testing modalities for different pretest probabilities.[42] When the pretest probability of PE is low, a sufficiently low (<5%) posttest probability of excluding PE—and therefore confidently avoiding further testing—can be achieved with negative test results for any one of the following: quantitative D-dimer assays (<500 μg/L), CTA, magnetic resonance angiography (MRA), or ventilation/perfusion (V/Q) lung scan. Importantly, neither a negative echocardiography result nor a negative lower extremity venous ultrasound result alone would be sufficient to rule-out PE, even in patients with low pretest probability. In patients with a moderate pretest probability for PE, negative D-dimer assay results, normal (or near-normal) V/Q scan or a combination of negative CTA plus negative venous ultrasonography (but not either one independently) were each sufficient to exclude PE. When pretest probability is high, positive test results of any one of the following can confidently support the diagnosis of PE: CTA, lower extremity venous ultrasonography, echocardiography, MRA, or positive V/Q scan.

Pulmonary angiography remains the gold standard to confirm PE,[43] although CTA has shown 90–95% specificity for detecting PE.[44,45] Given its widespread availability and rapid interpretability, CTA is often employed as the go-to methodology for evaluating PE in the ED, especially when compared to the other imaging options of lower extremity venous ultrasound, echocardiogram, MRA or V/Q scan. Computed tomography angiography has only about 75–90% sensitivity;[44,45] however, it can be a costly and time-consuming test that exposes patient to the risks of ionizing radiation and intravenous contrast dye. Therefore, the ED provider should remain motivated to employ tests with higher sensitivities, many of which are simpler, faster and safer than CTA, to exclude PE from the differential.

Occasionally, ED providers may be able to confidently avoid testing entirely. The pulmonary embolism rule-out criteria (PERC) are a set of historical factors and clinical presentation characteristics, including age younger than 50 years, pulse less than 100, SaO_2 greater than or equal to 95%, no hemoptysis, no exogenous estrogen use, no surgery or trauma requiring hospitalization within the past 4 weeks, no history of venous thromboembolism, and no unilateral leg swelling. Combining low-suspicion clinician gestalt with fulfillment of PERC yields a diagnostic sensitivity of 97% and reduces the probability of venous thromboembolism to below 2%.[46] When PERC is unattainable but pretest probability is still low or moderate, D-dimer has become a popular choice for ruling out PE, since it is the easiest, fastest, safest, and cheapest of the aforementioned diagnostic tests. Systematic review data suggest that the sensitivity of D-dimer for PE is consistently around 95%.[47]

Some clinical situations invite modification of D-dimer interpretation including older patients since studies have suggested that D-dimer levels increase with age.[48,49] Data from a multicenter, multinational, prospective ADJUST-PE (age-adjusted D-dimer cutoff levels to rule out pulmonary embolism) study suggest that using an age-adjusted D-dimer cutoff value (of age × 10 in patients 50 years or older, as compared to the conventional cutoff of <500 μg/L) increased the proportion of patients in whom PE could be confidently excluded, without any additional false-negatives and with maintaining a sufficiently low likelihood of subsequent clinically significant venous thromboembolism.[49]

For confirmed PE diagnosis, anticoagulants remain the mainstay of treatment. Deep vein thrombosis and PE patients generally require 3 months of anticoagulant therapy after which the ongoing risks of venous thromboembolism versus bleeding must be weighed before additional anticoagulation is indicated.[50] Traditionally, initial parenteral anticoagulants have been used concurrently with oral vitamin K antagonists in an overlapping manner. Several new direct oral anticoagulants now expand the treatment options and may offer improved safety profiles, including factor Xa inhibitors (rivaroxaban, apixaban, edoxaban), as well as a direct thrombin inhibitor (dabigatran).[51] Rivaroxaban and apixaban alone, and dabigatran and edoxaban after parenteral anticoagulant induction, have been shown to be noninferior to enoxaparin/warfarin for the prevention of recurrent venous thromboembolism. And in comparison to enoxaparin/warfarin, the risk of major bleeding seems to be similar with dabigatran and edoxaban, and significantly reduced with rivaroxaban and apixaban.[52]

There are some additional subtleties of test results that may add prognostic information and thus guide treatment decisions. In patients with PE, right ventricle dilation as detected by CTA is associated with increased 30-day mortality [odds ratio (OR) 2.08], and 3-month mortality (OR 4.65), as well as death from PE (OR 7.35).[53]

Clinical decision-making matrices may also provide useful prognostic information for major adverse events such as death. The Pulmonary Embolism Severity Index (PESI) score divides patients with confirmed PEs into five risk classes. This PESI matrix includes the following risk factors: age, male sex, history of cancer, history of heart failure, history of chronic lung disease, pulse greater than or equal to 110, systolic blood pressure (SBP) less than 100, relative risk (RR) greater than or equal to 30, temperature less than 36°C, altered mental status (AMS), and arterial oxyhemoglobin saturation less than 90%. From the original PESI score, a simplified PESI (sPESI) score was developed, including age older than 80, history of cancer, chronic cardiopulmonary disease, pulse greater than or equal to 110, SBP less than 100, and arterial oxyhemoglobin saturation less than 90%. The sPESI matrix divides patient into either low risk (zero factors) or high risk (≥1 factors). For 30-day mortality, when compared to PESI, sPESI showed increased sensitivity, decreased specificity, similar PPV, improved NPV, similar positive likelihood ratio, and improved negative likelihood ratio.[54] The sPESI score has also been shown to have similar prognostic accuracy and clinical utility, with greater ease of use, as compared to the original PESI score,[54] as well as potentially greater accuracy of short- and long-term survival prediction compared to the European Society of Cardiology model.[55]

Traditionally, patients with newly diagnosed PE are hospitalized and started on treatment. Looking forward, however, patients with hemodynamically stable PE may be increasingly managed on an outpatient basis, including discharge from ED. Wells et al. suggest that the decision to treat patients with acute PE as outpatients should be based on clinical severity and prognosis.[50]

Conflicting studies have examined initial outpatient versus inpatient treatment of PE. One study raised concern that patients treated initially as outpatients were less likely to initiate vitamin K antagonist therapy, compared to patients admitted to the hospital (hazard ratios 0.75 and 1.81, respectively).[56] However, if patients are compliant with their therapy, as in another study of 344 patients with low-risk PESI classification who were treated with 5 days of enoxaparin plus oral anticoagulation, there may be similar rates of recurrent venous thromboembolism, major bleeding, and death.[57] A 2014 Cochrane review was unable to assess the efficacy and safety of outpatient versus inpatient treatment of acute PE in terms of overall mortality, recurrent PE, and major bleeding due to the low quality of available evidence.[38] Given the increasing demands on United States hospitals, it is reasonable to expect future studies that explore the possibility of outpatient PE management.

Since most PEs originate in the legs, one valid clinical question is whether healthcare providers should be concerned with possible PE in asymptomatic patients with confirmed lower extremity DVT. One study evaluated the incidence and prognosis of asymptomatic PE in patients with demonstrated lower limb DVT. In these 103 hospitalized patients, all without symptoms of PE, 66% were found to have PE by CTA. Iliac and femoral DVTs were most likely to be associated with asymptomatic PE. D-dimer (above 578 ng/mL cutoff) showed good sensitivity but low specificity to identify patients with known DVT who also had asymptomatic PE. Importantly, diagnosis of asymptomatic PE incurred higher hospital costs, and in the absence of symptoms, there appeared to be no significant recurrence rate of thromboembolic events and "no short- or long-term clinical or therapeutic consequences" from these asymptomatic PEs.[58]

AORTIC DISSECTION

While the incidence of AAD is thought to be low (3.5 cases per 100,000 people per year),[59] Acute aortic dissection is the most common form of acute aortic syndrome, followed by intramural hematoma and penetrating aortic ulcer.[60] Acute aortic dissection is a very serious condition with early mortality rates of 18–25%.[61] And early diagnosis is critical, since within the first several hours, mortality rates increase at up to 1% per hour.[62]

Two AAD classification systems are based on anatomic location of the dissection: DeBakey type I (ascending aorta with extension to at least the aortic arch), DeBakey type II (ascending aorta only), and DeBakey type III (descending aorta distal to left subclavian artery); or Stanford A (ascending aorta including DeBakey types I and II) and Stanford B (descending aorta). Dissections involving the proximal or ascending aorta (i.e., Stanford A) represent the majority of AAD.[63]

According to the International Registry of Aortic Dissections,[64] 95% of AAD occurs in patients over 40 years of age. The most common risk factor for AAD is a history of hypertension (present in up to 70% of patients), although it is important to remember that many patients with AAD are normotensive at presentation. Other risk factors include connective tissue diseases, cardiac disorders (such as coarctation, bicuspid aortic valve and Turner's syndrome), trauma, and stimulant use (especially cocaine and methamphetamine). In patients with AAD below 40 years of age, as many as 50% have a history of Marfan syndrome.

The pain of AAD is classically maximal at onset, in contrast to the crescendo characteristic of ischemic chest pain. The pain of AAD also typically follows an anatomic distribution, according to the part of the aorta involved; proximal/ascending AAD is accompanied by anterior chest pain, whereas distal/descending AAD is accompanied by posterior chest or back pain.[65] Type A dissections are more commonly accompanied by hypotension.[66] Most patients with AAD endorse "tearing" or "ripping" pain, but a significant proportion of presentations may be painless. This poses a particularly difficult challenge for the ED physician, who must remain vigilant to evaluate for AAD.

Although they are often first-line diagnostic tests, chest radiographs lack adequate sensitivity to diagnose AAD, especially with dissections involving the descending aorta. Multidetector-row computed tomography (CT) remains the imaging modality of choice and approaches 100% sensitivity and specificity.[67] Astute point-of-care ultrasonographers may be able to detect dilation of the aortic root, or even an intimal flap, which is highly specific of AAD and allows a rapid diagnosis.

Some studies have suggested a possible role for using D-dimer biomarker assays to help identify AAD. In a 2007 systematic review, D-dimer testing showed high sensitivity (97%) and low negative likelihood ratio (0.06) for AAD. Using D-dimer cutoff of less than 0.1 μg/mL had an NPV of 100% and excluded AAD in all cases.[68] A 2011 meta-analysis suggested negative D-dimer assay results (with 500 ng/mL cutoff) had 97% sensitivity and 96% NPV for identifying AAD, with specificity of 56% and PPV of 60%. The authors conclude that "plasma

D-dimer less than 500 ng/mL is a useful screening tool to identify patients who do not have AAD ... and may thus be used to identify subjects who are unlikely to benefit from further aortic imaging".[69] A 2015 meta-analysis of the use of D-dimer assays to detect AAD showed similar results, reporting a sensitivity of 94.5% and specificity of 69.1%, and concluded that "D-dimer levels are best used for ruling out acute aortic dissection in patients with low likelihood of the disease".[70]

However, the most recent American College of Emergency Physicians clinical policy on AAD offered a solitary Level C recommendation to "do not rely on D-dimer alone to exclude the diagnosis". The clinical policy cites selection bias and variation in methodology among the studies included in meta-analyses and identifies multiple conditions which may lead to falsely negative D-dimer results in patients with proven AAD, such as chronicity of the dissection, time from symptom onset, presence of thrombosis or intramural hematoma, short length of dissection, and young age of patient. Finally, the policy suggests that because of its lack of specificity, "routinely" testing patients for D-dimer elevations may inadvertently lead to harm including radiation exposure and increased cost.[63]

For the ED physician evaluating undifferentiated chest pain and relying on imaging and/or biomarker tests with high sensitivities, using D-dimer to either rule out the condition or prompt additional evaluation in the form of CTA may be tempting, but the search for better and more specific tests continues. Several such assays and biomarker targets are being explored and show promise, including smooth muscle myosin heavy chain, calponin, soluble elastin fragments and transforming growth factor β.[61]

If a dissection is proximal and involves coronary arteries, AAD may be accompanied by acute MI. Acute aortic dissection may also masquerade as acute stroke if the dissection interrupts cerebral blood supply. These situations can present particular challenges for the ED provider, with significant danger to miss a diagnosis of AAD in a case where enough convincing evidence for an acute MI or stroke has already become available. It is important for providers to resist early closure bias.

The primary focus of treatment for AAD is to stop extension of the dissection, with efforts targeted to reduce blood pressure and heart rate to as low as possible while still maintaining normal mental status. Early surgical consultation is vital, and surgical intervention has been shown to reduce mortality rates in type A (but probably not type B) dissections.[71,72]

PNEUMOTHORAX

Pneumothorax is an abnormal collection of air in the pleural space and may present spontaneously, as an iatrogenic complication, or in the context of blunt or penetrating trauma.

Primary spontaneous pneumothorax (PSP) is defined as a first pneumothorax in people without known underlying lung disease and without an inciting event such as trauma. Primary spontaneous pneumothorax is most common in men (6:1 male:female ratio), between the age of 20 and 40 years, who are tall and thin, and often smokers. These patients may have subclinical lung damage or disease, such as pleural blebs, often associated with a history of tobacco use. In fact, the risk for PSP is approximately 20 times higher for smokers, and up to 100 times higher for heavy smokers.[73] Targeted questioning of a patient's medical and social history may help inform a clinician as to the risk factors and likelihood for pneumothorax.

Pneumothorax is almost always accompanied by pulmonary symptoms, such as shortness of breath, tachypnea, distant or absent breath sounds, decreased tactile fremitus, and/or respiratory distress. As mentioned previously, tension pneumothorax is accompanied by respiratory distress and unilateral breath sounds, may be associated with tracheal deviation or hypotension, and should be treated immediately if clinically suspected.

Ultrasound has consistently outperformed chest radiograph in the diagnosis of pneumothorax, with sensitivity between 82 and 91% and specificity 98 and 99%. A 2011 meta-analysis reported sensitivity of 88% and specificity of 99% for ultrasound in diagnosing pneumothorax, compared to 52% and 100%, respectively, for chest radiograph.[74] In a 2012 systematic review of 570 articles, including a final cohort of 1,000 total patients, ultrasound was 91% sensitive and 98% specific for pneumothorax, compared to 50% sensitivity and 99% specificity of chest radiograph. The authors conclude that ultrasound is "superior" to chest radiograph for diagnosing pneumothorax.[75] A 2013 meta-analysis of 601 articles reached the same conclusion that with a sensitivity of 79% and specificity of 98% (compared to 40% and 99%, respectively, with chest radiograph) ultrasonography is more accurate for detection of pneumothorax.[76] Subgroup analysis showed that patients with traumatic injuries had significantly higher heterogeneity of sensitivity, suggesting that an evaluation of the undifferentiated but nontraumatic patient in the ED may benefit even more from ultrasonography. When studies were limited to those in which the diagnosing provider used a high-frequency linear probe (compared to a convex array probe), the sensitivity for diagnosing pneumothorax with ultrasonography increased to 82%.

It seems reasonable to utilize ultrasound alone for diagnosing pneumothorax in a patient presenting with chest pain and some degree of respiratory involvement. However, chest radiograph may still be needed for quantification of size of the pneumothorax. Chest

X-rays are also typically more amenable to durable communication with other healthcare providers, given the ease of radiograph reproducibility.

Treatment of PSP involves a spectrum of options, ranging from watchful waiting with or without supplemental oxygen, to simple aspiration, to thoracostomy (pigtail catheter vs. chest tube) and finally to invasive video-assisted thoracoscopic surgery (VATS). Some providers, particularly in Europe, may be starting to favor initial outpatient management of PSP, even for large pneumothoraxes. In one French retrospective study that also cites other smaller pilot studies, approximately 80% of patients were successfully treated as outpatients using a smaller pigtail catheter rather than chest tube without hospital admission.[77]

MEDIASTINITIS

Mediastinitis refers to inflammation or infection of the mediastinum, can be acute or chronic, and is usually precipitated by intimal disruption of the esophagus. Causes include iatrogenic injury (such as cardiothoracic surgery, upper endoscopy, bronchoscopy, or even endotracheal intubation), forceful vomiting, trauma (including swallowed foreign bodies), malignancy, sarcoidosis, tuberculosis, and radiation-induced injury. Bacterial infection associated with mediastinitis poses a significant health risk. When the infection descends from the head or neck into the mediastinum, this potentially lethal condition is known as descending necrotizing mediastinitis.

In addition to chest pain, symptoms of acute mediastinitis often include dyspnea and fever. Patients will generally appear ill, and may endorse recent vomiting or surgical intervention (such as median sternotomy or endoscopy). Mediastinitis is a clinical diagnosis, although inflammatory markers such as white blood cell count, C-reactive protein and erythrocyte sedimentation rate are often elevated. While chest radiographs may be revealing, the imaging modality of choice remains CT of the chest (and often also of the neck).[78]

Acute infectious mediastinitis may be associated with polymicrobial flora, and given the potential clinical severity of infection, initial broad-spectrum antibiotic therapy is indicated. Prompt attention to securing a patient's airway is also vital, and any evidence of septic shock at time of presentation should guide resuscitative efforts. Emergent surgical consultation is necessary, as debridement is often required.

Other conditions involving the esophagitis, including gastroesophageal reflux or esophageal spasm or pill-associated esophagitis, may present as chest pain. A more reassuring clinical presentation, as well as corroborative history, is typically helpful in considering these less severe diagnoses.

MYOPERICARDITIS

Pericarditis is inflammation of the pericardium and is classically described as pleuritic positional chest pain accompanied by ECG changes and a friction rub on physical examination. Relying on this classic textbook presentation of pericarditis almost assuredly leads providers to miss the diagnosis. One retrospective analysis suggested that of patients ultimately diagnosed with pericarditis, most (90%) presented complaining of chest pain and 52% complained of dyspnea. Physical examination findings varied significantly, with tachycardia being the most common (although in only one-third of patients), followed by tachypnea and fever. Only 4% of patients had an audible friction rub on examination. Electrocardiogram changes were similarly unreliable—42% had diffuse ST elevation and 21% had PR depression. Both chest pain and ECG changes were there in 52% of patients.[79]

Myocarditis is inflammation of the myocardium, and is usually caused by a viral infection, most notably parvovirus B19. Less commonly, myocarditis, may be caused by Lyme disease, *Trypanosoma cruzi* infection, hypersensitivity reaction to medications or an autoimmune condition. Myocarditis may have a variety of clinical presentations, which vary by severity of disease, ranging between transient mild symptoms to dilated cardiomyopathy to heart failure to ventricular dysrhythmias to sudden cardiac death. A definitive diagnosis of myocarditis is made via myocardial biopsy, although other less-invasive diagnostic modalities are typically employed. These include ECG, biomarkers (such as serum troponin), echocardiogram, and cross-sectional imaging such as cardiac magnetic resonance imaging (CMRI).[80,81] Due to the difficulty of establishing a diagnosis of myocarditis, it is almost certainly underdiagnosed in the ED setting.

One study evaluated diagnostic data for patients with an ultimate diagnosis of myocarditis, as made by CMRI. Of the 41 patients included in the study, 90% presented with chest pain, over 50% with dyspnea and viral prodrome, and only 15% with fever. Serum troponin levels were elevated in 85% of patients. Out of the patients, 75% had abnormal ECGs, although the abnormalities were widely variable and included ST segment elevation (39%) or abnormal QRS (29%).[82]

Ultrasound and CMRI have shown good sensitivity for making the diagnosis of myocarditis.[80,81] Cardiac magnetic resonance imaging also seems to yield promising prognostic information. According to recent studies, abnormal CMRI showed statistically significant ability to predict MACEs (including cardiac death, sudden cardiac death, firing of implanted cardiac defibrillator, and worse New York Heart Association status) among patients with clinically suspected myocarditis, independent of their clinical symptoms.[83,84] In addition, there seems to be good correlation between both troponin and creatine kinase with late gadolinium enhancement (LGE) on CMRI, which is the primary abnormal finding in patients with myocarditis. In contrast, C-reactive protein does not seem to show statistically significant correlation with abnormal LGE on CMRI.[84] Cardiac magnetic resonance imaging may have some limitations, however, as its sensitivity to detect infarct-like clinical presentations is high, but low for cardiomyopathy and very low for arrhythmic clinical presentations of myocarditis.[85]

It can be difficult to differentiate between myopericarditis and STEMI based solely on ECG changes such as ST elevation. One study found that PR depression in any ECG lead has high sensitivity (88%) but lower specificity (78%) for myopericarditis. When differentiating myopericarditis from STEMI, PR depression in both precordial and limb ECG leads had 97% PPV for myopericarditis.[86] Other investigators have concluded that "patients with acute STEMI, but not those with acute pericarditis, show prolongation of the QRS complex and shortening of the QT interval in ECG leads with ST segment elevation".[87]

In addition to ECG, biomarkers may be helpful in differentiating between myopericarditis and STEMI. At least one small study found statistically significant differences between elevation of N-terminal pro-brain natriuretic peptide (NT-proBNP) levels, with myocarditis having the largest elevation, followed by STEMI, and with the least significant and least frequent elevation in pericarditis.[88]

ACUTE CHEST SYNDROME

Acute chest syndrome, which is a vaso-occlusive crisis of the pulmonary vasculature, is the most lethal complication of sickle cell disease, with a mortality rate of about 12%.[89,90] The diagnostic criteria for acute chest syndrome include a new infiltrate on chest radiograph and one or more new pulmonary symptoms, including fever, cough, sputum production, dyspnea, or hypoxia.[91] Of these, fever is the most common.[92]

As acute chest syndrome is historically thought to be triggered by pulmonary infections, empiric antibiotics are generally indicated. However, clinicians should also consider fat emboli as the source of the vaso-occlusive inciting event,[91] especially in patients not undergoing hydroxyurea therapy.[93] Inhaled bronchodilators may be useful, but there exists very little, if any, data to support or refute this practice.[94]

When considering a diagnosis of acute chest syndrome, the ED physician should institute supportive care and strongly consider consultation with pulmonary, infectious disease, and if necessary critical care specialists. Exchange transfusion is often indicated, especially in patients with new oxygen requirements or respiratory failure. Importantly, treatment with intravenous fluids should generally be limited to patients with hypotension, in order to avoid the risks of iatrogenic pulmonary edema. Additional therapies may be beneficial but have not yet been studied in enough detail to achieve recommendation status, including bronchoscopy, inhaled nitric oxide, and steroids.

PERICARDIAL EFFUSION

Abnormal accumulation of fluid within the pericardium can be caused by many disease entities including malignancy, trauma, acute pericarditis, end-stage renal disease, acute MI, cardiac surgery, and tuberculosis. In 1935, Dr Claude Beck proposed a clinical triad of signs for acute pericardial tamponade including the presence of jugular venous distention, hypotension, and diminished heart sounds. Relying on this triad of clinical signs is insensitive in correctly identifying tamponade, however, as they are present in approximately only 54%, 28%, and 22% of cases, respectively.[95] A meta-analysis of the diagnostic modalities for identifying tamponade revealed the highest sensitivity for echocardiography (97%), compared to chest radiograph (81%) and EKG changes (66%) such as low QRS voltage, tachycardia, PR depression, and morphologic changes to the P, QRS, T, or ST segments.[95]

While tamponade remains a clinical diagnosis, it appears that point-of-care ultrasonography can and should play an important role in confirming the diagnosis. A consensus statement released by the American Society of Echocardiography and the American College of Emergency Physicians supports focused cardiac ultrasound as having high sensitivity and specificity of detecting pericardial effusion, and suggests that it should remain a reliable first-line approach to making the diagnosis.[96] Additionally, point-of-care ultrasound has shown high sensitivity for detecting the size of an effusion, when present.[97] Even novice trainees show excellent sensitivity, specificity, and negative and positive predictive values in diagnosing pericardial effusion by bedside ultrasonography.[98]

Medical management of pericardial effusion is dictated primarily by the underlying etiology including any inflammatory component. Tamponade frequently requires pericardiocentesis. Whether to drain a non-tamponade pericardial effusion depends on the chronicity and etiology of the effusion,[99] and if it does not need to be done emergently in the ED, can be discussed further with cardiology.

PRINZMETAL'S ANGINA

Coronary artery spasm (CAS) may present as acute chest pain in patients otherwise at low risk of CAD, but may play an important role in syndromes of myocardial ischemia such as acute infarction, stable and unstable angina, and even sudden cardiac death. The pathophysiology of CAS remains a poorly understood phenomenon, but is very likely multifactorial in its etiology. The ED provider should have a heightened suspicion for CAS in patients presenting with angina at rest at early morning hours, young female tobacco users or any patient presenting following cocaine use.[100,101] A definitive diagnosis is usually made with coronary angiography, occasionally with provocative testing (such as ergonovine). Testing thyroid function should be done for all patients with CAS, as concurrent thyrotoxicosis carries more severe clinical and angiographic presentations in patients with CAS than normal thyroid function.[102] Treatment relies on calcium antagonists, and although recurrent episodes of angina may occur, the general prognosis is reassuringly benign.[103]

DISPOSITION

Most patients who present to the ED with undifferentiated chest pain are usually discharged, following reassuring testing. Patients with concerning positive test results will generally be admitted and managed on an inpatient basis. However, there are large numbers of patients, some with significant risk factors or non-negative testing, for whom a diagnosis remains unclear but potentially serious. These patients often require admission for further evaluation and potential intervention.

Increasing numbers of EDs have observation units, to which patients may be admitted for continued monitoring, serial testing, and further risk stratification. As described earlier, in many patients for whom diagnostic testing has revealed low risk for ACS, prolonged observation unit stays may be unnecessary. However, many other patients may benefit from short-term admission for observation. Conditions that are amenable to observation unit admission include pneumothorax being treated with supplemental oxygen and requiring repeat imaging for confirmation of improvement/resolution of pneumothorax, patients with acute chest syndrome or pericarditis requiring pain management, patients with PE requiring initiation of treatment, or treatment of clinically significant acute exacerbations of chronic conditions not severe enough to warrant admission to an inpatient service.

Given the seemingly inherent diagnostic uncertainty in patients presenting to the ED with undifferentiated chest pain, those who can safely be discharged should nonetheless be apprised by the ED provider of the risks of unforeseen complications. While an accurate estimate of statistical risk of MACE is difficult to ascertain, there seems to be widespread consensus that even with entirely negative testing during an ED encounter, the risk of subsequent adverse events is not zero. Patients should routinely be cautioned about this nonzero risk, as well as clear indications to follow up with a primary care provider or cardiologist or to return to the ED. Patients should be engaged in this decision-making process. And when possible, honest discussions about providers' inabilities to be medically certain about a diagnosis may be invaluable to facilitating patients' understanding.

CONCLUSION

Emergency Department providers face unique challenges in evaluating hemodynamically stable adult patients presenting with undifferentiated chest pain. In every patient, vital signs and an ECG should be evaluated. Priority should be given to first ruling out the potentially life-threatening causes of chest pain, as well as initiating any emergently indicated treatments or interventions. Thereafter, a patient's past medical history, history of presenting illness, and physical examination should guide the ED provider's construction of a differential diagnosis. Providers should estimate a patient's pretest probability for any of the differential diagnoses, and use biomarker tests and imaging studies in a targeted fashion to revise and adjust their pretest probabilities. Providers may then either arrive at a diagnosis and initiate appropriate treatment and disposition, or reasonably reassure themselves and their patients against the need for further emergent evaluation.

REFERENCES

1. US Centers for Disease Control and Prevention (2010). National Hospital Ambulatory Medical Care Survey: 2010 Emergency Department Summary Tables. [online] Available from: http://www.cdc.gov/nchs/data/ahcd/nhamcs_emergency/2010_ed_web_tables.pdf. [Accessed February, 2016].
2. Thygesen K, Alpert JS, Jaffe AS, Simoons ML, Chaitman BR, White HD, et al. Third universal definition of myocardial infarction. J Am Coll Cardiol. 2012;60(16):1581-98.
3. American College of Emergency Physicians, Society for Cardiovascular Angiography and Interventions, O'Gara PT, Kushner FG, Ascheim DD, Casey DE, et al. 2013 ACCF/AHA guideline for the management of ST-elevation myocardial infarction: a report of the American College of Cardiology Foundation/American Heart Association Task Force on Practice Guidelines. J Am Coll Cardiol. 2013;61(4): 485-510.
4. Ting HH, Rihal CS, Gersh BJ, Haro LH, Bjerke CM, Lennon RJ, et al. Regional systems of care to optimize timeliness of reperfusion therapy for ST-elevation myocardial infarction: the Mayo Clinic STEMI Protocol. Circulation. 2007;116(7):729-36.
5. Milner KA, Funk M, Richards S, Wilmes RM, Vaccarino V, Krumholz HM. Gender differences in symptom presentation associated with coronary heart disease. Am J Cardiol. 1999;84(4):396-9.
6. Gupta M, Tabas JA, Kohn MA. Presenting complaint among patients with myocardial infarction who present to an urban, public hospital emergency department. Ann Emerg Med. 2002;40(2):180-6.
7. Khan NA, Daskalopoulou SS, Karp I, Eisenberg MJ, Pelletier R, Tsadok MA, et al. Sex differences in acute coronary syndrome symptom presentation in young patients. JAMA Intern Med. 2013;173(20):1863-71.
8. Keller T, Zeller T, Peetz D, Tzikas S, Roth A, Czyz E, et al. Sensitive troponin I assay in early diagnosis of acute myocardial infarction. N Engl J Med. 2009;361(9):868-77.

9. Swap CJ, Nagurney JT. Value and limitations of chest pain history in the evaluation of patients with suspected acute coronary syndromes. JAMA. 2005;294(20):2623-9.
10. Diercks DB, Boghos E, Guzman H, Amsterdam EA, Kirk JD. Changes in the numeric descriptive scale for pain after sublingual nitroglycerin do not predict cardiac etiology of chest pain. Ann Emerg Med. 2005;45(6):581-5.
11. Chase M, Robey JL, Zogby KE, Sease KL, Shofer FS, Hollander JE. Prospective validation of the Thrombolysis in Myocardial Infarction Risk Score in the emergency department chest pain population. Ann Emerg Med. 2006;48(3):252-9.
12. Fox KAA, Dabbous OH, Goldberg RJ, Pieper KS, Eagle KA, Van de Werf F, et al. Prediction of risk of death and myocardial infarction in the six months after presentation with acute coronary syndrome: prospective multinational observational study (GRACE). BMJ. 2006;333(7578):1091.
13. Elbarouni B, Goodman SG, Yan RT, Welsh RC, Kornder JM, Deyoung JP, et al. Validation of the Global Registry of Acute Coronary Event (GRACE) risk score for in-hospital mortality in patients with acute coronary syndrome in Canada. Am Heart J. 2009;158(3):392-9.
14. Six AJ, Backus BE, Kelder JC. Chest pain in the emergency room: value of the HEART score. Neth Heart J. 2008;16(6):191-6.
15. Backus BE, Six AJ, Kelder JC, Bosschaert MA, Mast EG, Mosterd A, et al. A prospective validation of the HEART score for chest pain patients at the emergency department. Int J Cardiol. 2013;168(3):2153-8.
16. Backus B, Six A, Kelder J, Gibler W, Moll F, Doevendans P. Risk scores for patients with chest pain: evaluation in the emergency department. Curr Cardiol Rev. 2011;7(1):2-8.
17. Than M, Flaws D, Sanders S, Doust J, Glasziou P, Kline J, et al. Development and validation of the Emergency Department Assessment of Chest pain Score and 2 h accelerated diagnostic protocol. Emerg Med Australas. 2014;26(1):34-44.
18. Aldous SJ, Richards MA, Cullen L, Troughton R, Than M. A new improved accelerated diagnostic protocol safely identifies low-risk patients with chest pain in the emergency department. Acad Emerg Med. 2012;19(5):510-6.
19. Hoeller R, Rubini Giménez M, Reichlin T, Twerenbold R, Zellweger C, Moehring B, et al. Normal presenting levels of high-sensitivity troponin and myocardial infarction. Heart. 2013;99(21):1567-72.
20. Diercks DB, Peacock WF, Hollander JE, Singer AJ, Birkhahn R, Shapiro N, et al. Diagnostic accuracy of a point-of-care troponin I assay for acute myocardial infarction within 3 hours after presentation in early presenters to the emergency department with chest pain. Am Heart J. 2012;163(1):74-80.e4.
21. Thygesen K, Mair J, Giannitsis E, Mueller C, Lindahl B, Blankenberg S, et al. How to use high-sensitivity cardiac troponins in acute cardiac care. Eur Heart J. 2012;33(18):2252-7.
22. Hamm CW, Bassand J-P, Agewall S, Bax J, Boersma E, Bueno H, et al. ESC Guidelines for the management of acute coronary syndromes in patients presenting without persistent ST-segment elevation: The Task Force for the management of acute coronary syndromes (ACS) in patients presenting without persistent ST-segment elevation of the European Society of Cardiology (ESC). Eur Heart J. 2011;32(23):2999-3054.
23. Scharnhorst V, Krasznai K, van't Veer M, Michels R. Rapid detection of myocardial infarction with a sensitive troponin test. Am J Clin Pathol. 2011;135(3):424-8.
24. Sajeev JK, New G, Roberts L, Menon SK, Gunawan F, Wijesundera P, et al. High sensitivity troponin: Does the 50% delta change alter clinical outcomes in chest pain presentations to the emergency room? Int J Cardiol. 2015;184:170-4.
25. Than M, Cullen L, Aldous S, Parsonage WA, Reid CM, Greenslade J, et al. 2-Hour accelerated diagnostic protocol to assess patients with chest pain symptoms using contemporary troponins as the only biomarker: the ADAPT trial. J Am Coll Cardiol. 2012;59(23):2091-8.
26. Than M, Aldous S, Lord SJ, Goodacre S, Frampton CMA, Troughton R, et al. A 2-hour diagnostic protocol for possible cardiac chest pain in the emergency department: a randomized clinical trial. JAMA Intern Med. 2014;174(1):51-8.
27. Cullen L, Mueller C, Parsonage WA, Wildi K, Greenslade JH, Twerenbold R, et al. Validation of high-sensitivity troponin I in a 2-hour diagnostic strategy to assess 30-day outcomes in emergency department patients with possible acute coronary syndrome. J Am Coll Cardiol. 2013;62(14):1242-9.
28. Meller B, Cullen L, Parsonage WA, Greenslade JH, Aldous S, Reichlin T, et al. Accelerated diagnostic protocol using high-sensitivity cardiac troponin T in acute chest pain patients. Int J Cardiol. 2015;184:208-15.
29. Goldschlager R, Roth H, Solomon J, Robson S, Green J, Green S, et al. Validation of a clinical decision rule: chest X-ray in patients with chest pain and possible acute coronary syndrome. Emerg Radiol. 2014;21(4):367-72.
30. Ng JJ, Taylor DM. Routine chest radiography in uncomplicated suspected acute coronary syndrome rarely yields significant pathology. Emerg Med J. 2008;25(12):807-10.
31. Rothrock SG, Green SM, Costanzo KA, Fanelli J-M, Cruzen ES, Pagane JR. High yield criteria for obtaining non-trauma chest radiography in the adult emergency department population. J Emerg Med. 2002;23(2):117-24.
32. Poku JK, Bellamkonda-Athmaram VR, Bellolio MF, Nestler DM, Stiell IG, Hess EP. Failure of prospective validation and derivation of a refined clinical decision rule for chest radiography in emergency department patients with chest pain and possible acute coronary syndrome. Acad Emerg Med. 2012;19(9):E1004-10.
33. Foy AJ, Liu G, Davidson WR, Sciamanna C, Leslie DL. Comparative effectiveness of diagnostic testing strategies in emergency department patients with chest pain: an analysis of downstream testing, interventions, and outcomes. JAMA Intern Med. 2015;175(3):428-36.
34. Madsen T, Mallin M, Bledsoe J, Bossart P, Davis V, Gee C, et al. Utility of the emergency department observation unit in ensuring stress testing in low-risk chest pain patients. Crit Pathw Cardiol. 2009;8(3):122-4.
35. Milano P, Carden DL, Jackman KM, Rongkavilit A, Groves K, Tyndall J, et al. Compliance with outpatient stress testing in low-risk patients presenting to the emergency department with chest pain. Crit Pathw Cardiol. 2011;10(1):35-40.
36. Hermann LK, Newman DH, Pleasant WA, Rojanasarntikul D, Lakoff D, Goldberg SA, et al. Yield of routine provocative cardiac testing among patients in an emergency department-based chest pain unit. JAMA Intern Med. 2013;173(12):1128-33.
37. Hoffmann U, Bamberg F, Chae CU, Nichols JH, Rogers IS, Seneviratne SK, et al. Coronary computed tomography angiography for early triage of patients with acute chest pain: the ROMICAT (Rule Out Myocardial Infarction using Computer Assisted Tomography) trial. J Am Coll Cardiol. 2009;53(18):1642-50.
38. Yoo HH, Queluz TH, El Dib R. Outpatient versus inpatient treatment for acute pulmonary embolism. Cochrane Database Syst Rev. 2014;11:CD010019.
39. Kucher N, Goldhaber SZ. Management of massive pulmonary embolism. Circulation. 2005;112(2):e28-32.
40. Chunilal SD, Eikelboom JW, Attia J, Miniati M, Panju AA, Simel DL, et al. Does this patient have pulmonary embolism? JAMA. 2003;290(21):2849-58.
41. Lucassen W, Geersing G-J, Erkens PMG, Reitsma JB, Moons KGM, Büller H, et al. Clinical decision rules for excluding pulmonary embolism: a meta-analysis. Ann Intern Med. 2011;155(7):448-60.
42. Roy PM, Colombet I, Durieux P, Chatellier G, Sors H, Meyer G. Systematic review and meta-analysis of strategies for the diagnosis of suspected pulmonary embolism. BMJ. 2005;331(7511):259.
43. Harvey RT, Gefter WB, Hrung JM, Langlotz CP. Accuracy of CT angiography versus pulmonary angiography in the diagnosis of acute pulmonary embolism: evaluation of the literature with summary ROC curve analysis. Acad Radiol. 2000;7(10):786-97.
44. Hogg K, Brown G, Dunning J, Wright J, Carley S, Foex B, et al. Diagnosis of pulmonary embolism with CT pulmonary angiography: a systematic review. Emerg Med J. 2006;23(3):172-8.
45. Safriel Y, Zinn H. CT pulmonary angiography in the detection of pulmonary emboli: a meta-analysis of sensitivities and specificities. Clin Imaging. 2002; 26(2):101-5.
46. Kline JA, Courtney DM, Kabrhel C, Moore CL, Smithline HA, Plewa MC, et al. Prospective multicenter evaluation of the pulmonary embolism rule-out criteria. J Thromb Haemost. 2008;6(5):772-80.
47. Stein PD, Hull RD, Patel KC, Olson RE, Ghali WA, Brant R, et al. D-dimer for the exclusion of acute venous thrombosis and pulmonary embolism: a systematic review. Ann Intern Med. 2004;140(8):589-602.
48. Tardy B, Tardy-Poncet B, Viallon A, Lafond P, Page Y, Venet C, et al. Evaluation of D-dimer ELISA test in elderly patients with suspected pulmonary embolism. Thromb Haemost. 1998;79(1):38-41.
49. Righini M, Van Es J, Den Exter PL, Roy PM, Verschuren F, Ghuysen A, et al. Age-adjusted D-dimer cutoff levels to rule out pulmonary embolism: the ADJUST-PE study. JAMA. 2014;311(11):1117-24.
50. Wells PS, Forgie MA, Rodger MA. Treatment of venous thromboembolism. JAMA. 2014;311(7):717-28.
51. Piovella F, Iosub DI. Acute pulmonary embolism: risk assessment, risk stratification and treatment options. Clin Respir J. 2015. [Epub ahead of print].
52. Cohen AT, Dobromirski M, Gurwith MM. Managing pulmonary embolism from presentation to extended treatment. Thromb Res. 2014;133(2):139-48.
53. Becattini C, Agnelli G, Germini F, Vedovati MC. Computed tomography to assess risk of death in acute pulmonary embolism: a meta-analysis. Eur Respir J. 2014;43(6):1678-90.

54. Jiménez D, Aujesky D, Moores L, Gómez V, Lobo JL, Uresandi F, et al. Simplification of the pulmonary embolism severity index for prognostication in patients with acute symptomatic pulmonary embolism. Arch Intern Med. 2010;170(15):1383-9.
55. Kilic T, Gunen H, Gulbas G, Hacievliyagil SS, Ozer A. Prognostic role of simplified Pulmonary Embolism Severity Index and the European Society of Cardiology Prognostic Model in short- and long-term risk stratification in pulmonary embolism. Pak J Med Sci. 2014;30(6):1259-64.
56. Tagalakis V, Patenaude V, Kahn SR, Suissa S. Treatment patterns of venous thromboembolism in a real-world population: the Q-VTE study cohort. Thromb Res. 2014;134(4):795-802.
57. Aujesky D, Roy PM, Verschuren F, Righini M, Osterwalder J, Egloff M, et al. Outpatient versus inpatient treatment for patients with acute pulmonary embolism: an international, open-label, randomised, non-inferiority trial. Lancet. 2011;378(9785):41-8.
58. García-Fuster MJ, Fabia MJ, Furió E, Pichler G, Redon J, Forner MJ, et al. Should we look for silent pulmonary embolism in patients with deep venous thrombosis? BMC Cardiovasc Disord. 2014;14:178.
59. Clouse WD, Hallett JW, Schaff HV, Spittell PC, Rowland CM, Ilstrup DM, et al. Acute aortic dissection: population-based incidence compared with degenerative aortic aneurysm rupture. Mayo Clin Proc. 2004;79(2):176-80.
60. Clough RE, Nienaber CA. Management of acute aortic syndrome. Nat Rev Cardiol. 2015;12(2):103-14.
61. Listijono DR, Pepper JR. Current imaging techniques and potential biomarkers in the diagnosis of acute aortic dissection. JRSM Short Rep. 2012;3(11):76.
62. Braverman AC. Acute aortic dissection: clinician update. Circulation. 2010; 122(2):184-8.
63. American College of Emergency Physicians Clinical Policies Subcommittee (Writing Committee) on Thoracic Aortic Dissection, Diercks DB, Promes SB, Schuur JD, Shah K, Valente JH, et al. Clinical policy: critical issues in the evaluation and management of adult patients with suspected acute nontraumatic thoracic aortic dissection. Ann Emerg Med. 2015;65(1):32-42.e12.
64. Information for Patients from the International Registry of Aortic Dissections. Aortic Dissection. [online] Available from: http://www.iradonline.org/about.html#incidence [Accessed February, 2016].
65. Tsai TT, Trimarchi S, Nienaber CA. Acute aortic dissection: perspectives from the International Registry of Acute Aortic Dissection (IRAD). Eur J Vasc Endovasc Surg. 2009;37(2):149-59.
66. Tsai TT, Bossone E, Isselbacher EM, Nienaber CA, Evangelista A, Fang J, et al. Clinical characteristics of hypotension in patients with acute aortic dissection. Am J Cardiol. 2005;95(1):48-52.
67. Abbas A, Brown IW, Peebles CR, Harden SP, Shambrook JS. The role of multidetector-row CT in the diagnosis, classification and management of acute aortic syndrome. Br J Radiol. 2014;87(1042):20140354.
68. Sodeck G, Domanovits H, Schillinger M, Ehrlich MP, Endler G, Herkner H, et al. D-dimer in ruling out acute aortic dissection: a systematic review and prospective cohort study. Eur Heart J. 2007;28(24):3067-75.
69. Shimony A, Filion KB, Mottillo S, Dourian T, Eisenberg MJ. Meta-analysis of usefulness of d-dimer to diagnose acute aortic dissection. Am J Cardiol. 2011;107(8):1227-34.
70. Cui JS, Jing ZP, Zhuang SJ, Qi SH, Li L, Zhou JW, et al. D-dimer as a biomarker for acute aortic dissection: a systematic review and meta-analysis. Medicine (Baltimore). 2015;94(4):e471.
71. Hagan PG, Nienaber CA, Isselbacher EM, Bruckman D, Karavite DJ, Russman PL, et al. The International Registry of Acute Aortic Dissection (IRAD): new insights into an old disease. JAMA. 2000;283(7):897-903.
72. Fattori R, Cao P, De Rango P, Czerny M, Evangelista A, Nienaber C, et al. Interdisciplinary expert consensus document on management of type B aortic dissection. J Am Coll Cardiol. 2013;61(16):1661-78.
73. Bense L, Eklund G, Wiman LG. Smoking and the increased risk of contracting spontaneous pneumothorax. Chest. 1987;92(6):1009-12.
74. Ding W, Shen Y, Yang J, He X, Zhang M. Diagnosis of pneumothorax by radiography and ultrasonography: a meta-analysis. Chest. 2011;140(4):859-66.
75. Alrajhi K, Woo MY, Vaillancourt C. Test characteristics of ultrasonography for the detection of pneumothorax: a systematic review and meta-analysis. Chest. 2012;141(3):703-8.
76. Alrajab S, Youssef AM, Akkus NI, Caldito G. Pleural ultrasonography versus chest radiography for the diagnosis of pneumothorax: review of the literature and meta-analysis. Crit Care. 2013;17(5):R208.
77. Voisin F, Sohier L, Rochas Y, Kerjouan M, Ricordel C, Belleguic C, et al. Ambulatory management of large spontaneous pneumothorax with pigtail catheters. Ann Emerg Med. 2014;64(3):222-8.
78. Tintinalli JE, Stapczynski JS, Ma OJ, Cline DM, Cydulka RK, Meckler GD (Eds). Tintinalli's Emergency Medicine: A Comprehensive Study Guide, 7th edition. New York: McGraw-Hill; 2011.
79. Gleason M, Kolb J, Miley M. 363: Pericarditis: Incidence and Clinical Presentation. Ann Emerg Med. 2007;50(3, Suppl):S113.
80. Shauer A, Gotsman I, Keren A, Zwas DR, Hellman Y, Durst R, et al. Acute viral myocarditis: current concepts in diagnosis and treatment. Isr Med Assoc J. 2013;15(3):180-5.
81. Magnani JW, Dec GW. Myocarditis current trends in diagnosis and treatment. Circulation. 2006;113(6):876-90.
82. Jhamnani S, Fuisz A, Lindsay J. The spectrum of electrocardiographic manifestations of acute myocarditis: an expanded understanding. J Electrocardiol. 2014;47(6):941-7.
83. Schumm J, Greulich S, Wagner A, Grün S, Ong P, Bentz K, et al. Cardiovascular magnetic resonance risk stratification in patients with clinically suspected myocarditis. J Cardiovasc Magn Reson. 2014;16:14.
84. Mewton N, Dernis A, Bresson D, Zouaghi O, Croisille P, Flocard E, et al. Myocardial biomarkers and delayed enhanced cardiac magnetic resonance relationship in clinically suspected myocarditis and insight on clinical outcome. J Cardiovasc Med (Hagerstown). 2015;16(10):696-703.
85. Francone M, Chimenti C, Galea N, Scopelliti F, Verardo R, Galea R, et al. CMR sensitivity varies with clinical presentation and extent of cell necrosis in biopsy-proven acute myocarditis. JACC Cardiovasc Imaging. 2014;7(3):254-63.
86. Porela P, Kytö V, Nikus K, Eskola M, Airaksinen KEJ. PR depression is useful in the differential diagnosis of myopericarditis and ST elevation myocardial infarction. Ann Noninvasive Electrocardiol. 2012;17(2):141-5.
87. Rossello X, Wiegerinck RF, Alguersuari J, Bardají A, Worner F, Sutil M, et al. New electrocardiographic criteria to differentiate acute pericarditis and myocardial infarction. Am J Med. 2014;127(3):233-9.
88. Bentancur AG, Sela B, Agranat O, Kuperstein R, Matetzky S. 92: Comprehensive Study of Myocarditis in the Emergency Department (COSMED III): Elevated N-terminal proBNP Differentiates Acute Myocarditis and Acute Ischemia from Acute Pericarditis in the Emergency Department. Ann Emerg Med. 2007;50(3, Suppl):S30.
89. Traill LM, Barton MA. (2008). Focus On: Acute Chest Syndrome – The Critical Cough. [online] ACEP News. Available from: http://www.acep.org/Clinical—Practice-Management/Focus-On--Acute-Chest-Syndrome—The-Critical-Cough/ [Accessed February, 2016].
90. Platt OS, Brambilla DJ, Rosse WF, Milner PF, Castro O, Steinberg MH, et al. Mortality in sickle cell disease. Life expectancy and risk factors for early death. N Engl J Med. 1994;330(23):1639-44.
91. Walters MC, Nienhuis AW, Vichinsky E. Novel therapeutic approaches in sickle cell disease. Hematology Am SocHematol Educ Program. 2002;10-34.
92. Siddiqui AK, Ahmed S. Pulmonary manifestations of sickle cell disease. Postgrad Med J. 2003;79(933):384-90.
93. Johnson CS. (1995). Sickle Cell Disease: The Acute Chest Syndrome, 1995 [online]. Available from: http://sickle.bwh.harvard.edu/acutechest.html [Accessed February, 2016].
94. Knight-Madden JM, Hambleton IR. Inhaled bronchodilators for acute chest syndrome in people with sickle cell disease. Cochrane Database Syst Rev. 2014;8:CD003733.
95. Jacob S, Sebastian JC, Cherian PK, Abraham A, John SK. Pericardial effusion impending tamponade: a look beyond Beck's triad. Am J Emerg Med. 2009;27(2):216-9.
96. Labovitz AJ, Noble VE, Bierig M, Goldstein SA, Jones R, Kort S, et al. Focused cardiac ultrasound in the emergent setting: a consensus statement of the American Society of Echocardiography and American College of Emergency Physicians. J Am Soc Echocardiogr. 2010;23(12):1225-30.
97. Pepi M, Muratori M. Echocardiography in the diagnosis and management of pericardial disease. J Cardiovasc Med (Hagerstown). 2006;7(7):533-44.
98. Bustam A, Noor Azhar M, Singh Veriah R, Arumugam K, Loch A. Performance of emergency physicians in point-of-care echocardiography following limited training. Emerg Med J. 2014;31(5):369-73.
99. Sagristà-Sauleda J, Mercé AS, Soler-Soler J. Diagnosis and management of pericardial effusion. World J Cardiol. 2011;3(5):135-43.
100. Vandergoten P, Benit E, Dendale P. Prinzmetal's variant angina: three case reports and a review of the literature. Acta Cardiol. 1999;54(2):71-6.
101. Keller KB, Lemberg L. Prinzmetal's angina. Am J Crit Care. 2004;13(4): 350-4.
102. Lee SY, Yu CW, Choi YJ, Choi RK, Park JS, Lee HJ, et al. A comparison of clinical features of coronary artery spasm with and without thyrotoxicosis. Coron Artery Dis. 2014;25(2):125-32.
103. Hung MJ, Hu P, Hung MY. Coronary artery spasm: review and update. Int J Med Sci. 2014;11(11):1161-71.

9

CHAPTER

Syncope

Sean-Xavier Neath

INTRODUCTION

"Syncope", while a frequently used term in emergency medicine and cardiology, is not a discrete disease state or a definitive diagnosis. Rather, syncope is a symptom characterized by a period of transient loss of consciousness (TLOC) that is short in duration, typically self-limited and characteristically due to a spontaneously reversible inadequacy of cerebral nutrient flow. Nonmedical terms that frequently indicate syncope include faint, collapse, swoon, "pass out", "fall out" and other regional variations depending on vernacular. The most common causal factor for syncope is cerebral hypoperfusion due to transient hypotension. Syncope has many possible precipitating causes. However, the principal etiologies may be classified into three categories:

- Reflex (neutrally mediated)
- Orthostatic
- Cardiovascular disorders.

Delineating the underlying etiology in a given patient is often challenging but is important, since syncope, while frequently benign from a mortality perspective in most cases, has a tendency to recur and may leave the affected individual subject to risk of physical injury and diminished quality of life.[1]

EPIDEMIOLOGY

From the perspective of the clinician practicing emergency medicine, it is important to place the evaluation of syncope in the much larger framework of "transient total loss of consciousness" in order to more broadly explore the differential diagnosis for a patient presenting with this type of symptom.[2] Transient loss of consciousness can be precipitated directly by trauma; this type of TLOC is not discussed further in this chapter. While it is true that trauma can occur during syncope due to the loss of postural tone, this is a secondary event. The evaluation for secondary trauma remains an important component of the emergency clinician's workup but the reader is referred to other sources for these guidelines. Additionally, there are nontraumatic causes of TLOC (such as epileptic seizure). These syncope-mimics are discussed in a later section of this chapter.

Transient loss of consciousness is a rather frequent clinical presentation in emergency departments (EDs). However, since syncope is only one of several reasons for TLOC, estimates of the frequency of syncope that are based on TLOC occurrences are really only an approximation. Since TLOC/syncope events are short-lived, the traditional epidemiological metrics such as "prevalence" and "incidence" are actually not very useful in describing this particular disease state. Sheldon and colleagues have advocated measuring other indices such as cumulative event rate or cumulative incidence to provide a more meaningful portrait of syncope.[3]

Most epidemiological reports indicate an apparent bimodal distribution of syncope incidence over a broad age range.[4] Peaks occur in adolescence and in older years. Data derived from several studies reveal a potential cumulative incidence varying from 7 to 40% by age 80 years.[5] Certain subpopulations have a higher frequency of syncope. Older individuals and patients with structural heart disease are at the highest risk. In certain conditions such as valvular aortic stenosis and dilated cardiomyopathy syncope has been clearly associated with increased mortality risk. While syncope remains of great concern in many other conditions [such as hypertrophic cardiomyopathy (HCM) and the channelopathies], the relation of syncope to increased mortality is more controversial.[6] Neurally mediated syncope and syncope in the absence of structural heart disease is associated with much lower sudden death risk. The relationships between age and types of syncope usually encountered by the clinician are depicted in figure 1.

Nomenclature aside, approximately 1–5% of all visits to the ED are related to syncope with annual healthcare costs for syncope-related admissions estimated at $4.2 in the United States.[7]

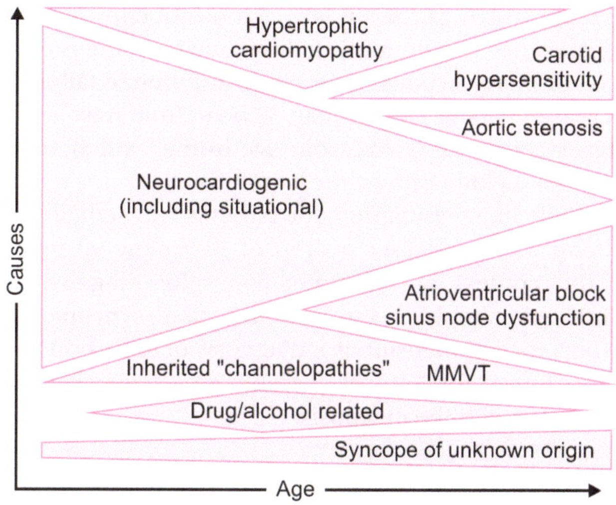

MMVT, monomorphic ventricular tachycardia.

FIG. 1: Relationship between the age of patient and the types of syncope

With permission from: Pavri BB. Handbook of Syncope: A Concise Clinical Approach. New Delhi: Jaypee Brothers Medical Publishers (P) Ltd; 2014.

INITIAL EVALUATION, DIAGNOSIS AND RISK STRATIFICATION

The initial evaluation of patient with potential syncope in the ED should include basic resuscitation (the so-called "ABCs") and the evaluation for immediate life-threatening causes. When syncope is considered in the differential, it is important to keep these three broad categories of syncope in mind:

1. Reflex (neutrally mediated)
2. Orthostatic
3. Cardiovascular disorders.

The patient history, physical examination, and diagnostic testing are geared toward ensuring that serious etiologies from all three branches have been considered and ruled-out.

History

Historical questions should be asked of both the patient and any dependable eyewitnesses. The responding paramedical team may also have insights into the surroundings and the patient appearance/behavior in the immediate postincident period. If it seems that the patient may be confabulating or trying to fill in gaps with guesses, it is important to be aware of the potential effect on the accuracy of the history.

Historical questions that should be asked about the circumstances surrounding the TLOC are listed in table 1.

Key elements of the past medical history and family history:

- Prior cardiac disease
- Neurological history (Parkinsonism, epilepsy, narcolepsy)
- Metabolic disorders (diabetes, etc.)
- Medication (antihypertensive, antianginal, antidepressant agent, antiarrhythmic, diuretics, and QT-prolonging agents) A list of medications most frequently associated with syncope in the elderly is provided in table 2
- Prior episodes: A history of syncopal episodes may be of value. A single episode or multiple episodes over many years suggest a benign etiology. Several episodes over a short period of time in someone with no history of syncope suggest a more significant cause, such as dysrhythmia
- Family history: A family history of unexplained sudden death or early cardiovascular disease (in younger first-degree relatives) places patients at increased risk for cardiac syncope[8]
- Associated injury: Acute loss of consciousness may result in significant injury or events that predispose to injury. Motor vehicle accidents, hip fractures, and subdural hematomas can result following syncope. Emergency clinicians should assess the patient for

TABLE 1: Historical questions that should be asked about the circumstances surrounding a transient loss of consciousness

Question	Responses that may point toward certain etiologies
What position was the patient in?	Supine, sitting, standing
What activity was the patient performing at the time?	Exertion, changing position, urination, defecation, coughing, swallowing
What factors might have predisposed the patient to the event?	Crowded or warm places, prolonged standing, postprandial period, fear, intense pain, neck movements
Was there a "prodrome" associated with the event?	Nausea, vomiting, chills, sweating, aura, pain in neck or shoulders, blurred vision, dizziness
How did the patient fall over?	Hit the ground quickly, slumping, assisted to chair or ground
Was this TLOC associated with any sort of accident?	Atraumatic, following trauma, trauma occurred during fall
What happened after the TLOC?	Prompt resumption of normal behavior, confusion, nausea, vomiting, sweating, muscle aches, skin color, chest pain, palpitations, urinary or fecal incontinence, tongue biting

TLOC, transient loss of consciousness.

TABLE 2: Drugs commonly used in the elderly that predispose to syncope[4]

ACE inhibitors	Hydralazine	Tricyclic antidepressants
Calcium blockers	Nitrates	Ethanol
Phenothiazines	MAO-inhibitors	Diuretics
Bromocriptine	α-blockers	Ganglionic blocking agents
Opiates	β-blockers	Sildenafil citrate

ACE, angiotensin converting enzyme; MAO, monoamine oxidase

potential injuries. Although patients with prodromal symptoms have less risk of death and other adverse outcomes following syncope, there is no evidence they have less risk of acute injury from syncope (e.g., from falls). Such patients may ignore warning signs and may be just as likely to incur injury as patients without a prodrome.

Physical Examination

The key elements of the physical examination include vital signs, focused cardiac and neurologic examinations, as well as attention to any specific complaints that either predated, or resulted from, the TLOC. The physical examination can be a useful diagnostic tool in this disease state.[9]

Vital Signs

Transient hypotension or bradycardia occurs during most syncopal events. Abnormal vital signs typically return to normal by the time of evaluation in the ED. Persistently abnormal vital signs are concerning and must be investigated for another reversible etiology. Discrepancies between upper extremities in pulse or blood pressure (BP) may reflect aortic dissection or subclavian steal syndrome, prompting appropriate workup for these etiologies. Low patient oxygen saturation or tachypnea may be a sign of comorbid heart failure (HF), pulmonary embolism, or pneumonia.

Orthostatic vital signs should be obtained. The patient should be supine for 5 minutes before the initial set is obtained. Vital signs are retaken after the patient has been standing for 3 minutes and compared with initial measurements. The following changes are considered abnormal and may reflect hypovolemia or autonomic dysfunction.

Postural (orthostatic) hypotension is diagnosed when, within 2–5 minutes of quiet standing (after a 5-minute period of supine rest), one or both of the following is present:[10]

- At least a 20 mm Hg fall in systolic pressure
- At least a 10 mm Hg fall in diastolic pressure.

Normally, the heart rate (HR) rises immediately on standing. The absence of an appropriate reflex-induced increase in HR as the BP falls is a useful clinical clue to the presence of autonomic failure; however, the presence of a HR increase does not exclude autonomic failure. An increase in HR of greater than 30 beats/min may actually suggest postural tachycardia syndrome, which usually does not include orthostatic hypotension.

While many asymptomatic patients will actually meet criteria for orthostasis, a drop of BP below 90 mm Hg in the context of symptoms is useful diagnostically. Clinicians should keep in mind that syncope from orthostatic hypotension is a diagnosis of exclusion in the ED, reserved for low-risk patients who have symptoms consistent with the diagnosis.

Cardiac Examination

Auscultation of the heart may reveal a rate that is either abnormal or irregular (e.g., atrial fibrillation). The clinician should listen for murmurs, specifically for aortic and mitral stenosis. Extra heart sounds, either an S3 or S4, can often be heard in patients with HF but may be difficult to auscultate in the noisy environment of EDs. Findings on cardiac examination suggesting structural heart disease should be further investigated.

Lung Examination

Auscultation of the lungs may reveal abnormal sounds (e.g., crackles, wheezes) consistent with HF or other pathology.

Neurologic Examination

Patients with syncope by definition return to baseline neurologic function. A thorough examination should be done to identify any subtle focal abnormality suggestive of stroke.

Head and Neck Examination

Clinicians should listen for a carotid bruit. Murmurs of aortic stenosis may also radiate to the neck. Examine the neck for elevated jugular venous pressure, a possible sign of HF. Lacerations to the lateral aspect of the tongue are suggestive of seizure.

Certain authors suggest that carotid massage be performed as part of the evaluation of syncope, others feel this test lacks sufficient sensitivity and specificity to play a meaningful diagnostic role in the ED. Caution is advised when considering whether to perform carotid massage in patients with potential carotid artery disease.

Rectal Examination

A rectal examination with a stool guaiac test can potentially identify a patient with gastrointestinal bleed, which can present with syncope as its inciting feature.

Injury Assessment and General Examination

The emergency clinician should perform a secondary trauma survey looking for evidence of occult or distracting injuries. Common injuries associated with falls following syncope include facial fractures, hips fractures, wrist fractures, and subdural hematomas.

Diagnosis of Syncope and Differential Diagnosis of Syncope

Life-threatening Conditions

The primary responsibility of the emergency clinician is first to assess whether an immediate life-threatening cause of TLOC is present and, second, to provide appropriate management and disposition of the patient with TLOC. The most important immediate life-threatening causes to consider are: cardiac syncope, blood loss, pulmonary embolism, and subarachnoid hemorrhage. Other conditions, such as seizure, stroke, and head injury, while not meeting the technical definition of syncope should also be considered during the initial assessment of TLOC.

Common Conditions

Cardiac Syncope

Cardiac causes are the most common life-threatening conditions associated with syncope. They include arrhythmia, ischemia, structural/valvular abnormalities (e.g., aortic stenosis), cardiac tamponade and pacemaker malfunction.

Studies of short-term and 1-year outcomes following syncope found patients with cardiac syncope to be at significant risk for sudden death.[11] Patients with syncope and a history of HF are at even greater risk.[12]

Hemorrhage

Large blood loss, particularly acute severe hemorrhage, can manifest as syncope. Potential causes of such hemorrhage include: polytrauma, gastrointestinal bleeding, ruptured aortic aneurysm, ruptured ovarian cyst, ruptured ectopic pregnancy, and ruptured spleen.

Pulmonary Embolism

Hemodynamically significant pulmonary embolism is an uncommon but frequently discussed cause of syncope.

Subarachnoid Hemorrhage

Patients presenting with syncope following a headache require evaluation for a possible subarachnoid hemorrhage.

Syncope Mimics

Episodes that may be confused with syncope include disorders where there may be some change in patient's status but there is typically not a transient, but total, loss of consciousness.

Seizures

Seizures are the probable cause in 5–15% of apparent syncopal episodes.[13] They can mimic syncope, especially when the seizure is atypical and not associated with tonic-clonic movements, the seizure is not observed, or a complete history cannot be obtained.

Metabolic or Toxic Abnormalities

Metabolic or toxic abnormalities, such as hypoglycemia and hepatic encephalitis, are rarely associated with a rapid onset or offset. However, if a patient does not recall the history surrounding the event or if the event was unwitnessed, distinguishing coma from syncope can be difficult.

Anaphylaxis

Anaphylaxis is an acute, potentially lethal, multisystem syndrome resulting from the sudden release of mast cell and basophil-derived mediators into the circulation. Anaphylaxis typically presents with a combination of cutaneous, respiratory and cardiovascular symptoms. However, it may also present as an isolated sudden decrease in BP, leading to presyncope or collapse, without accompanying respiratory or cutaneous symptoms.

Transient Ischemic Attacks

While carotid artery transient ischemic attacks (TIAs) can cause specific transient neurologic disturbances, they do not cause TLOC.[14] A complete loss of consciousness would require substantial loss of brain stem function or of a very large portion of the cerebral cortex. Vertebrobasilar TIAs might be expected to cause TLOC more often than do carotid TIAs, but loss of consciousness would not be the sole symptom in this case. The clinician should search for other posterior circulation symptoms (e.g., vertigo, imbalance) that accompanied the event and, if present, these would support a vertebrobasilar TIA.

Mechanical Falls

Mechanical falls are a common cause of ED visits. A clear history from a cogent patient (ideally with corroboration by bystanders) is critical in determining whether syncope or presyncope caused a fall. If there are discrepancies in the history, or discordant injuries based on reported mechanism, clinicians tend to broaden the workup to examine for cardiac or neurologic factors which may have contributed to the fall.

Migraine Syndromes

Migraine syndromes, particularly basilar migraines, may present with symptoms that are similar to syncope such as loss of conscious, ataxia, or vertigo. Loss of consciousness is usually longer than several seconds. In addition, patients generally have other neurologic symptoms, as well as headache and nausea. Persistent headache is not a feature of syncopal episodes. There is a high frequency of syncope in patient who suffer from migraines, but the migraines and syncopal attacks do not appear to occur at the same times.[15]

Hyperventilation

Hyperventilation is usually associated with emotional stress. The patient may complain of chest pain, chest tightness, and shortness of breath. In addition, symptoms may include lightheadedness, paresthesias, and visual disturbances. Carpopedal spasms are frequently reported by hyperventilating patients who mistake this side effect of hyperventilation alkalosis with stroke or seizure.

Narcolepsy

Patients with narcolepsy may have cataplexy, emotionally triggered muscle weakness with collapse that may mimic syncope. However, they also have other features that indicate a disorder of sleep-wake control (such as chronic daytime sleepiness, hypnagogic hallucinations) or sleep paralysis.

Drug-induced loss of consciousness. Drugs of abuse and alcohol may cause a TLOC, but generally these patients manifest signs of toxicity, and do not spontaneously and rapidly return to normal neurologic function immediately after regaining consciousness.

Psychogenic Syncope

Psychogenic syncope is syncope in the absence of HR or BP alterations. Anxiety and panic disorders can cause situational syncope. Emergency clinicians must be cautious when attributing syncope to psychiatric causes.[16] Patients with hypoxia, inadequate cerebral perfusion, or other medical conditions may appear confused or anxious and may demonstrate abnormal behavior. Patients with psychiatric syncope are generally young, without cardiac disease and complain of multiple episodes. Hysteria/conversion disorder is most common in adolescent patients. These events typically occur in the presence of an audience, lack hemodynamic (HR, BP) or autonomic (sweating, pallor) changes, may be prolonged, and rarely result in injury. Patients may describe the event in a calm indifferent manner. They may disclose details of the event that indicate no loss of consciousness.

Emergency Department Approach and Risk Stratification

When evaluating potential syncope patients, it is recommended that emergency clinicians keep three questions in mind:[17]

- Is this true syncope or does some other serious condition account for the patient's loss of consciousness (e.g., stroke, seizure, head injury)?
- If this is true syncope, is there a clear life-threatening cause?
- If this is true syncope and the cause is not clear, is the patient at high risk for near-term complications, is cardiac disease present?

Emergency clinicians are frequently unable to determine a definitive diagnosis in a significant number of patients who present to the ED with syncope. In such instances, using risk stratification to guide management and disposition represents the best possible approach. Using risk factors identified in previously conducted syncope surveys can help clinicians determine patient risk and appropriate disposition. While individual studies may be limited by such factors as the size of the cohort, the number of adverse events, and the definition of an event, a consistent theme emerges: patients with an abnormal electrocardiogram (ECG) on presentation or a history of heart disease, particularly structural heart disease (e.g., chronic heart failure), are at greater risk for adverse outcomes.[18]

Risk stratification tools should be used to assist clinical judgment, but should not replace it.[19] When applying such tools, clinicians must be careful to include only patients for whom the clinical decision rules are appropriate.[20] Patients with significant comorbidities who may not be reflective of the study population represented in the risk stratification tool study would not be appropriate subjects for an algorithmic approach.

Diagnostic Tests

Electrocardiogram

While it is true that practice guidelines suggest that all patients presenting with syncope receive an ECG, the initial ECG is usually nondiagnostic in patients with TLOC/syncope. Only approximately 2–7% of ECGs in this setting reveal a significant abnormality.[21] However, when abnormal, the ECG may disclose an arrhythmia associated with a high likelihood of syncope, or an abnormality (e.g., conduction system disease, long QT, pre-excitation), which may predispose to arrhythmia development and syncope. Moreover, any abnormality of the baseline ECG is an independent predictor of cardiac syncope or increased mortality, suggesting the need for pursuing evaluation for cardiac causes in these patients. Equally important, a normal ECG is associated with a low risk of cardiac syncope as the cause, with a few possible exceptions, for example, in case of syncope due to a paroxysmal supraventricular tachyarrhythmia or certain poorly characterized channelopathies.

Syncope Biomarkers

Laboratory Evaluation

Routine laboratory screening seldom aids in syncope management but may be important in the workup of undifferentiated TLOC. Hypoglycemia may rarely explain an acute syncopal event, but should be performed on all patients with altered mental status. Clinicians should obtain other tests based on clinical circumstance. Electrolytes may be beneficial in critically ill patients or patients thought to have electrolyte abnormalities from volume loss or diuretic use. In patients with active bleeding or suspected anemia, a hematocrit should be obtained, and coagulation studies may be useful. A hematocrit less than 30 increases the risk of adverse short-term events in patients with syncope.[22] A urine pregnancy test should be performed in any female of childbearing age.

Brain natriuretic peptide (BNP) or proBNP measurements appear to be predictive of those at risk for adverse outcomes following syncope.[5] One prospective observational study found that a single BNP level greater than 300 pg/mL in the setting of syncope is associated with increased risk of unfavorable outcome, another study has looked at the serial rise of N-terminal (NT) proBNP over 6 hours as a marker to predict arrhythmogenic syncope as compared to a matched vasovagal cohort.

Other biomarkers of neurohormonal stress may provide additional insight and risk stratification for patients with TLOC and syncope. Fedorowski and et al. have shown in preliminary work that the levels of mid-regional-pro-atrial natriuretic peptide (MR-proANP) and C-terminal pro-endothelin-1 (CT-proET-1) are markedly changed in common forms of syncope, suggesting the mechanistic and measurable neurohormonal pathways in syncopal attacks.[23]

Additional diagnostic testing is based on the results of the initial evaluation. There is currently no single significantly sensitive or specific diagnostic test to evaluate syncope other than the clinical evaluation. A variety of tests, mostly cardiologic, can be used in the evaluation of the patient with syncope. The 2009 European Society of Cardiology (ESC) guidelines recommend the following testing strategy:

- Carotid sinus massage in patients above 40 years old
- Echocardiogram when there is previous known heart disease or data suggestive of structural heart disease or syncope secondary to cardiovascular cause
- Immediate ECG monitoring when there is a suspicion of arrhythmic syncope
- Orthostatic challenge (lying to standing orthostatic test or head-up tilt testing) when syncope is related to the standing position or there is suspicion of a reflex mechanism
- Other less specific tests, such as neurological evaluation or blood tests, are indicated only when there is suspicion of nonsyncopal TLOC.

Carotid Sinus Massage

Carotid sinus hypersensitivity, which is responsible for the carotid sinus syndrome, can be demonstrated by careful carotid sinus massage. The 2009 ESC guidelines recommend carotid sinus massage in patients over an age of 40 years with syncope of unknown etiology after the initial evaluation. Carotid sinus massage should be avoided in patients with history of TIA or stroke within the past 3 months and in patients with carotid bruits (except if carotid Doppler studies excluded significant stenosis).

Carotid sinus massage may be considered diagnostic if syncope is reproduced together with asystole longer than 3 seconds and/or a fall in systolic BP greater than 50 mm Hg.

Orthostatic Challenge

The 2009 ESC syncope guidelines describe two methods for assessing the response to change in posture from supine to erect—active standing and tilt testing. Changing from supine to upright position produces a displacement of blood from the thorax to the lower limbs that leads to a decrease in venous return and cardiac output (CO). In the absence of compensatory mechanisms, a fall in BP may lead to syncope.

Active Standing

"Active standing" is frequently referred to as "orthostatic vital signs". Orthostatic BP measurement is performed with the patient standing after at least 5 minutes of lying supine. Blood pressure should be measured each minute in the standing position for 3 minutes or more (or as long as the patient tolerates) until the BP nadir is reached.

Tilt Testing

Tilt testing is commonly performed for the evaluation of syncope, although the test has limited specificity, sensitivity, and reproducibility. Tilt testing enables the reproduction of a neurally mediated reflex in laboratory settings. Blood pooling and decrease in venous return due to orthostatic stress and immobilization trigger the reflex. The final effect, hypotension and usually concomitant HR slowing, is related to impaired vasoconstrictor capability followed by sympathetic withdrawal and vagal overactivity. The clinical situation corresponding to tilt testing is reflex syncope triggered by prolonged standing. However, this test can also be positive in patients with other forms of reflex syncope and in patients with sick sinus syndrome.

Echocardiography

Increasingly available in many EDs, echocardiography is helpful in determining the presence of structural heart disease. Echocardiography can show valvular anomalies, wall motion abnormalities, elevated pulmonary pressure (seen in pulmonary embolism), and pericardial effusions. It is most useful in patients with a history of cardiac disease or abnormal ECG findings. Emergency clinicians are becoming more proficient with limited bedside echocardiography with the potential for increasing initial diagnostic yields in syncope workups.[24] Echocardiography plays an important role in risk stratification on the basis of left ventricular ejection fraction (LVEF). In the presence of structural heart disease, other tests to evaluate a cardiac cause of syncope should be performed. In some cases (e.g., aortic stenosis, cardiac tamponade, and atrial myxoma), echocardiography can identify the cause of syncope in some patients sufficiently so that no further diagnostic testing may be needed.

Electrocardiographic Monitoring (Noninvasive and Invasive)

Electrocardiographic monitoring is a procedure for diagnosing intermittent bradyarrhythmias and tachyarrhythmias. Currently several systems of ECG ambulatory monitoring are available: conventional ambulatory Holter monitoring, inhospital monitoring, event recorders, external or implantable loop recorders (ILRs), and remote (i.e., at home) telemetry.

Inhospital Monitoring

Inhospital monitoring (telemetry) is warranted when the patient is at high risk for a life-threatening arrhythmia. A period of ECG monitoring may be of value in patients with clinical features or ECG abnormalities suggesting arrhythmic syncope, especially if the monitoring has begun immediately after syncope. Although in such circumstances, the diagnostic yield of ECG monitoring may be only as high as 16%,[25] it is justified by the need to avoid immediate risk to these high-risk patients.

Clinical or ECG features suggesting an arrhythmic syncope:[2]

- Syncope during exertion or supine
- Palpitations at the time of syncope
- Family history of sudden death
- Nonsustained ventricular tachycardia (VT)
- Bundle branch block (QRS duration >0.12 s)
- Sinus bradycardia (<50 beats/min) or sinoatrial block in the absence of negatively chronotropic medications or physical/endurance training
- Preexcited QRS complexes
- Prolonged or short QT interval
- Right bundle branch block pattern with ST-elevation in leads V1–V3 (Brugada syndrome)
- Negative T waves in right precordial leads, epsilon waves, and ventricular late potentials suggestive of arrythmogenic right ventricular dysplasia (ARVD).

Remote Telemetry/Holter Monitoring (Outpatient)

Ambulatory (Holter) electrocardiography is a noninvasive test most frequently used to evaluate cardiac rhythm abnormalities. Ambulatory ECG has also been used for assessing pacemaker and implantable cardioverter-defibrillator function, evidence of myocardial ischemia, late potentials, and HR variability.[26]

Ambulatory ECG monitoring is available in several forms:

- Traditional Holter monitors store 24–48 hours of data and require offline analysis after the patient returns the device
- Newer ambulatory monitors can transmit data via telephone or internet for immediate clinician review
- Implantable loop recorders are placed subcutaneously and can provide continuous monitoring for months to years.

Ambulatory ECG monitoring is generally performed for the evaluation of unexplained syncope, near syncope, or dizziness, or for the evaluation of unexplained recurrent palpitations. Diagnostic yields from 24-hour ambulatory ECG in unselected populations are low. There is still some controversy as to whether the diagnostic yield can be improved by increased duration of use such as provided by external loop recorders[2] or perhaps by more selective choice of patients (e.g., those with syncope and loss of consciousness rather than simple dizziness, or patients with very frequently occurring symptoms).

In patients with syncope of uncertain origin, ILRs allow for continuous ECG monitoring to detect cardiac arrhythmias for months to years, which may increase the likelihood of identifying a cause of syncope.

Implantable Loop Recorder

The ILR is a subcutaneous monitoring device for the detection of cardiac arrhythmias. Such a device is typically implanted in the left pectoral region and stores events when the device is activated automatically according to programmed criteria or manually with magnet application. This device can be useful in the evaluation of palpitations or syncope of undetermined etiology, particularly when symptoms are infrequent (e.g., less than once per month). In patients with unexplained syncope and a recurrence during an extended period of follow-up, the ILR revealed or contributed to establishing the mechanism of syncope in the vast majority of patients. Moreover, the proportion of patients with an ILR-guided diagnosis increased over time and was still growing at the end of the follow-up period, implying that more patients could potentially get a diagnosis before the end of ILR battery life.[27]

Exercise Stress Testing

Although exercise-induced syncope is infrequent,[2] exercise testing should be performed in patients who have experienced episodes of syncope during or shortly after exertion, especially if an echocardiogram does not suggest structural abnormalities. Careful ECG and BP monitoring should be performed during both the test and the recovery phase as syncope can occur during or immediately after exercise. Syncope occurring during exercise may be due to cardiac causes, whereas syncope occurring after exercise is almost invariably due to a reflex mechanism. There are no data supporting an indication for exercise testing in a general population with syncope absent exertional symptoms.

Psychiatric Evaluation

"Functional" attacks of syncope conditions that resemble to known somatic conditions are found but without a plausible psychological mechanism. Two types of patients have to be included in the differential diagnosis of TLOC. In both, patients are nonresponsive and do not show normal motor control, implying that falls are common. In one type, gross movements resemble epileptic seizures; these attacks have been described as "pseudoepilepsy", or "pseudoseizures". In the other type, there are no gross movements, so the attacks resemble syncope or longer lasting loss of consciousness. These attacks have been described as "psychogenic syncope", "pseudosyncope", "syncope of psychiatric origin", and "medically unexplained syncope". Note that the latter two terms are inconsistent with the definition of syncope because there is no cerebral hypoperfusion in these cases of functional TLOC.

The frequency of such attacks is not known, as they vary with the setting. Functional TLOC mimicking epilepsy occurs in 15–20% of cases in specialized epilepsy clinics and in up to 6% in syncope clinics.[28] Identification and treatment of psychogenic pseudosyncope is complex and benefit from expert clinical consultation and modalities such as video electroencephalogram (EEG) monitoring.[29]

Pseudosyncope usually lasts longer than syncope; patients may lie on the floor for many minutes. Other clues are a high frequency including numerous attacks in a day, and lack of a recognizable trigger. Injury does not exclude functional TLOC as trauma can occur in pseudoseizures. The eyes are usually open in epileptic seizures and syncope but are usually closed in functional TLOC.

Neurological Evaluation

Autonomic Failure

In autonomic failure (ANF), the autonomic nervous system (ANS) cannot cope with physiological demands, which is then expressed as orthostatic hypotension. The 2009 ESC guidelines described three categories of ANF.[2] Primary ANF comprises degenerative neurological disease such as pure ANF, multiple system atrophy, Parkinson's disease, and Lewy body dementia.[30] Secondary ANF involves autonomic damage by other diseases such as diabetes mellitus, amyloidosis, and various polyneuropathies. Drug-induced orthostatic hypotension is the most frequent cause of orthostatic hypotension; drugs commonly causing orthostatic hypotension include the antihypertensives, diuretics, tricyclic antidepressants, phenothiazines, and alcohol. While in primary and secondary ANF, the dysfunction is due to structural damage to the ANS (either central or peripheral), in drug-induced orthostatic hypotension, the failure is an interruption of normal function.

Referral for neurological evaluation should be considered in primary ANF. Warning signs are early impotence and disturbed micturition, and later Parkinsonism and ataxia. Referral in secondary ANF and drug-induced orthostatic hypotension depends on which physician treats the underlying disease.

Neurological Tests

Interictal EEGs will be normal in syncope.[31] An interictal normal EEG cannot rule out epilepsy, and should be interpreted in the clinical context. When uncertain, it is better to postpone the diagnosis of epilepsy than incorrectly diagnose it.

An EEG is not recommended when syncope is the most likely cause of TLOC, but when epilepsy remains high in the differential diagnosis after initial evaluation is completed, it can be considered. An EEG, especially a video-monitored EEG, may be useful to establish psychogenic pseudosyncope, if recorded during a provoked attack in the appropriate setting.

TREATMENT

The principal goals of treatment for patients with syncope are to prolong survival, limit physical injuries, and prevent recurrences.

Treatment of Reflex Syncope and Orthostatic Intolerance

Evidence for effectiveness of therapy of neurally mediated syncope has historically been weak.[32] Limited randomized controlled trials have been undertaken, especially in terms of evaluating physical maneuvers and drug therapy options. Moya has reviewed the evidence behind various syncope therapies,[33] commenting that reflex syncope is a benign condition, with a good prognosis in terms of survival. Only patients with recurrent and/or severe episodes tend to benefit from specific treatment. At first, nonpharmacologic measures should be attempted such as providing information about the benign status of their condition, helping in identifying and avoiding triggers, optimizing water ingestion, counterpressure maneuvers in those patients with prodromal symptoms, as well as tilt training to the extent it proves effective. Drug therapy has generally not showed any beneficial effect in patients with reflex syncope, with the possible exception of β-blockers in patients older than 42 years.

Cardiac pacing may be effective when a dominant cardioinhibitory reflex is documented (the best example being carotid sinus syndrome), but the coexistence of a vasodepressor reflex accounts for the failure of pacing to prevent all symptoms in some cases. On the other hand, no predictably effective therapies for the vasodepressor reflex yet exist. Even physical counter maneuvers, which are probably the most effective among current acute treatments, often fail to abort the attack because the patients are unable to activate them with sufficient force, or at all. This limitation most frequently happens when prodromes are absent or are of very short duration and in older patients because they have diminished muscle strength and difficulty reacting rapidly.

Orthostatic Hypotension and Orthostatic Intolerance Syndromes

Orthostatic intolerance syndromes are a frequent cause of syncope and near-syncope. The most common form is orthostatic hypotension. Some individuals may be asymptomatic while others are more disabled by their symptoms. Orthostatic hypotension can be quite serious in the elderly in whom it may be responsible for triggering falls with potential for serious injury. Orthostatic hypotension in the young is much less often serious than it is in the elderly. On the other hand, postural orthostatic tachycardia syndrome (POTS) occurs more frequently in younger than in older individuals, and can interfere with quality of life. With the exception of eliminating inciting drugs, treatment in most cases of orthostatic hypotension focuses on symptom relief rather than cure. The overall strategy must address improving venous return to the heart in both orthostatic hypotension and POTS. Additionally, in POTS patients, it is important to diminishing adrenergic hyperactivity. However, while the goals are clear and now widely accepted, they are often difficult to accomplish and the treatment approach must be adapted to each individual. Higher ranking treatment recommendations currently include—the maintenance of adequate hydration and salt intake, the use of midodrine as adjunctive therapy if needed, and the use of fludrocortisone as adjunctive therapy is needed.[2]

Cardiac Arrythmias as the Primary Cause of Syncope

Sinus Node Dysfunction and Atrioventricular Conduction System Disease

Pacemakers are indicated in patients with certain symptomatic bradyarrhythmias caused by sinus node dysfunction and in those with frequent, prolonged sinus pauses. Patients with third-degree or complete atrioventricular (AV) block benefit from pacemaker placement, as do those with type II second-degree AV block because of the risk of progression to complete AV block[34] or as a consequence of abnormal sinus node recovery time (SNRT). Biventricular pacing should be considered in those patients with an indication for pacing due to AV block and depressed LVEF, HF, and prolonged QRS duration.[35]

Paroxysmal Supraventricular and Ventricular Tachycardias

In patients with paroxysmal AV nodal reentrant tachycardia, AV reciprocating tachycardia, or typical atrial flutter associated with syncope, catheter ablation is the first choice treatment.[2] In these supraventricular dysrhythmia patients, the role of drug therapy is limited to being a bridge to ablation or when ablation has failed. In patients with syncope associated with atrial fibrillation or atypical left atrial flutter, the decision should be individualized. In syncope from torsades de pointes, a search for drugs which prolong the QT interval should be undertaken and these medications discontinued. Catheter ablation or drug therapy should be considered in patients with syncope due to VT in the setting of a normal heart or of heart disease with mild cardiac dysfunction. An implantable cardioverter defibrillator (ICD) is indicated in patients with syncope and depressed cardiac function, and VT or fibrillation without correctable cause.[36,37] Although in these patients, ICD may not prevent syncopal recurrences, the benefit will be in risk reduction for sudden coronary death (SCD).

Syncope Secondary to Structural Cardiac or Cardiovascular Disease

In patients with syncope secondary to structural cardiac disease, including congenital heart disease malformations or acquired cardiopulmonary disease, care should be taken to identify and treat the underlying existing disease. Similarly, the existence of structural heart disease does not mean that a search should be abandoned for other potential causes of the patient's syncope. Some of these patients have typical reflex syncope, but in others, such as those with inferior myocardial infarction or aortic stenosis, the underlying cardiac disease may play a role in triggering or potentiating a reflex mechanism.[2] In addition, in many of these patients, the underlying cardiac disease is the background for the supraventricular or ventricular arrhythmia that causes syncope. Treatment of syncope associated with structural heart disease varies with the type of abnormality. In patients with syncope secondary to severe aortic stenosis or atrial myxoma, surgical treatment of the underlying disease is indicated. In patients with syncope secondary to acute cardiovascular disease, such as myocardial infarction or pericardial tamponade, treatment should be directed to the underlying process. In HCM, specific treatment of the arrhythmia is usually warranted; in most of these patients, an ICD should be implanted to prevent SCD.

In syncope associated with myocardial ischemia, coronary revascularization and/or medical management is clearly the first-line strategy.

Unexplained Syncope in Patients with High Risk of Sudden Cardiac Death

In patients at high risk of SCD, a disease-specific treatment is warranted in order to reduce the risk of death and of life-threatening events, even if the exact mechanism of syncope is still unknown or uncertain at the end of a complete workup. In these patients, the goal of treatment is primarily the reduction of mortality risk.

It is important to bear in mind, however, that even if an effective specific treatment of the underlying disease is found, patients may remain at risk of recurrence of syncope. For example, ICD-treated patients may remain at risk for fainting because only the SCD risk is being addressed and not the cause of syncope.

The majority of adult patients with syncope in whom there is concern regarding underlying structural heart disease will have evidence of coronary artery disease or nonischemic dilated cardiomyopathy. This is a clear sign of risk of sudden death attributed to the risk of ventricular arrhythmia. In most cases, the risk of SCD due to ventricular arrhythmia is proportional to the severity of left ventricular dysfunction, which currently guides ICD management although with varying degrees of evidence for the ischemic versus nonischemic cardiomyopathy.[38] Syncope is a major risk factor for sudden death in HCM and other inherited cardiomyopathies, and should lead to consideration of implantation of an ICD.

Arrhythmogenic right ventricular cardiomyopathy (ARVC) is a leading cause of ventricular arrhythmia and sudden death in young individuals, and can be challenging to diagnose. Exercise may be a precipitant of ventricular arrhythmias leading to exertional syncope, and may also contribute to the progression of disease.[39]

The "channelopathies" refer to a group of inherited arrhythmia syndromes that result from mutations in genes encoding proteins that form or regulate ion channels. The currently identified channelopathies known to cause syncope and sudden death include long QT syndrome (LQTS), short QT syndrome (SQTS), Brugada syndrome and catecholaminergic polymorphic ventricular tachycardia (CPVT).[39] In contrast to the majority of patients with syncope who often have a benign prognosis, syncope as a result of a channelopathy carries a poor prognosis. Additionally, the identification of these disorders allows for the institution of treatments, such as ICD, which can be highly effective at reducing the risk of both syncope and mortality.[40]

SPECIAL POPULATIONS

Syncope in the Elderly

The most common causes of syncope in the elderly are orthostatic hypotension, reflex syncope, especially carotid sinus sensitivity and cardiac arrhythmias. Different forms may often coexist in a patient, making diagnosis difficult.[2] Hospitalization related to orthostatic hypotension increases progressively with age. Medication effects and atrial fibrillation are large contributors to orthostatic hypotension in the elderly. Following orthostatic hypotension in frequency, cardioinhibitory carotid sinus syndrome is the cause of symptoms in up to 20% of elderly patients with syncope.[41]

One-third of individuals over 65 years are taking three or more prescribed medications, which may cause or contribute to syncope. Stopping these medications will reduce recurrences of syncope and falls.[42] Medication history should include the time relationship with onset of syncope.

The utility of an eyewitness to a patient's potential TLOC is especially important in the elderly for two reasons. Firstly, problems with balance and gait, coupled with slow reflexes are frequently present in the elderly. When combined with subtle hemodynamic changes, the patient may fall but actually not have had a complete loss of consciousness. Secondly, cognitive impairment frequently present in the elderly may blunt the patient's ability to correctly recall details of falls and/or syncope.[43]

Syncope in Pediatric Patients

Although the etiology of syncopal events in children is usually benign, syncope can also occur as the result of more serious disease with the potential for sudden death, especially in the context of structure heart disease or conduction defects.[44] Many of the serious etiologies of childhood syncope are similar to their adult counterparts and include the inherited cardiomyopathies and channelopathies.

Other common conditions that cause syncope include vasovagal syncope, breath-holding spells, and orthostatic hypotension.[45] Syncope mimics are similar to those in adults but also include breath-holding spells. Breath-holding spells typically occur in children 6–24 months of age and are triggered by an emotional insult, such as pain, anger, or fear. The spells may be cyanotic or pallid. The cyanotic variety begins with breath holding, followed by cyanosis and loss of consciousness. In a pallid spell, loss of consciousness occurs before breath holding. Brief posturing or tonic-clonic motor activity may occur with either cyanotic or pallid spells.[45] The clinical course for children with breath-holding spells is generally benign. Spells typically stop by 5 years of age. Some of these children go on to develop vasovagal syncope. Breath-holding spells may represent a variation of vasovagal (neurocardiogenic) syncope. Autonomic dysfunction appears to play a role in both cyanotic and pallid breath-holding spells.

Syncope in Pregnant Patients

Physiological changes of pregnancy may predispose pregnant women to syncope more frequently than nonpregnant women.[46] Syncope and presyncopal symptoms are so common that they are often considered a normal part of pregnancy; however, the casual assumption that loss of consciousness is a normal manifestation of pregnancy is not justifiable. Most cases of syncope in pregnancy are caused by neurocardiogenic or postural syncope. However, structural heart disease and associated arrhythmias may present for the first time in pregnancy due to some of the hemodynamic changes which occur during pregnancy.[47] In general, the indications for temporary and permanent pacing during pregnancy are similar to those in the overall population.[48] Many of the medications used for the control of dysrhythmias have been used effectively in pregnant patients but the reader is requested to consult current pharmacy and obstetrical professionals to optimize the benefits versus risks equation for the mother and fetus.

SAFE DISPOSITION OF THE PATIENT WITH SYNCOPE

Diagnostic and Management Algorithms and Their Limitations

There have been multiple attempts to derive syncope prediction tools to guide clinician decision-making. Despite being extensively promulgated, they are not widely adopted, partly because of their lack of sensitivity and specificity. Current prediction tools do not tend to show better sensitivity, specificity or prognostic yield compared with clinical judgment in predicting short-term serious outcome after syncope. A recent systematic review by leading syncope researchers strengthens the evidence that current prediction tools should not be strictly used in clinical practice.[14]

Admission versus Discharge and Follow-Up

If the physician's risk assessment indicates that a patient may be at risk for significant dysrhythmia or sudden death and that observation might detect that event and enable an intervention, admission to a monitored area in the hospital is often considered. Problematic is the definition of short-term outcome, which is subjective and not clearly defined. Which patients will benefit from a 24–48-hour hospital admission or observation unit admission is not adequately described in the medical literature, nor has the value of admission in preventing a later adverse outcome been demonstrated.[21] However, it should be clear that the absence of such data does not quell liability concerns of treating emergency physicians, particularly in regions with a higher rate of malpractice litigation. The risk management of syncope patients can be a frequently source of contention between emergency physicians and the admitting physicians. Some syncope experts[49] have advocated the concept of a syncope service or team. Some evidence shows that a designated syncope unit may improve diagnostic yield, reduce hospital admissions, and reduce total length of hospital stay without affecting recurrent syncope and all-cause mortality when compared with current standard care.

Socioeconomic and Legal Issues in Syncope Management in the Emergency Department

Socioeconomic and Legal Considerations in Syncope

Reporting requirements by clinicians who have evaluated patients with a suspected loss of consciousness vary by jurisdiction. Additionally, various additional reporting concerns may arise depending upon the particular occupation or activities of a patient with syncope.

Syncope and Driving

Driving risks presented by a patient with an episode of syncope need to be individualized. It is important to realize that there is not only the risk to patient but of course to others also when a patient operating a motor vehicle loses consciousness.

The suspected (or proven) cause of syncope, the effectiveness of treatment performed (and thus the subsequent risk of recurrence after treatment) and the type of driving done by the patient (commercial trucks or buses versus passenger car) determine the risk profile of that particular patient resuming driving.[4]

Syncope and Flying

The operation of aircraft is tightly regulated. Clinicians should contact the appropriate authorities in their geographic areas. Typically, patients with conditions requiring pacemakers and ICDs face stringent restrictions that usually prevent them from flying an aircraft.

Syncope and the Athlete

The underlying cause of syncope is the critical factor for clinicians' recommendations about return to play (or cessation of play) for the athlete. Most syncope in the young athlete is of benign etiology. When sudden cardiac death occurs during sports, it is usually related to cardiac dysrhythmias.[50] High-intensity, competitive sports appear to have the highest risk associated with syncope in those with predisposing underlying etiologies such as ARVD,

CPVT, hypertrophic cardiomyopathy, most congenital forms of LQTSs, SQTS, Brugada syndrome, and any patient requiring an ICD. On the other hand, athletes with a clear diagnosis of vasovagal syncope have an excellent prognosis, and after appropriate institution of therapeutic measures, do not necessarily require restriction from sports.[4]

CONCLUSION

Syncope is a form of TLOC with associated loss of postural tone, resulting from a brief period of inadequacy of cerebral nutrient flow. Myriad disease states can lead to syncope. The causes of syncope can be grouped into three major categories based upon mechanism, these are:

- Reflex/neurally mediated
- Orthostatic
- Cardiovascular.

The identification of true syncope, and the determination of whether there is the potential for a life-threatening cause for the episode, presents a challenge to the emergency clinician. A careful history is critical in elucidating cause and potential risks. Most of the additional testing for underlying etiology is done for suspected subtypes of cardiovascular syncope. The key role played by emergency clinicians is in sorting out true syncope from the multiple "mimics" of syncope (some of which can also be life-threatening) and determining an appropriate risk stratification plan. The emergency management process in syncope goes beyond the decision to admit versus discharge and includes multiple stages of evaluation to ensure that the appropriate disposition is being made and that life-threatening underlying causes are determined as quickly as possible.

REFERENCES

1. Iwai S. Syncope: an evidence-based approach. In: Stergiopoulos K, Brown DL (Eds). Evidence-Based Cardiology Consult. London: Springer; 2014. pp. 553-63.
2. Task Force for the Diagnosis and Management of Syncope, European Society of Cardiology (ESC), European Heart Rhythm Association (EHRA), Heart Failure Association (HFA), Heart Rhythm Society (HRS), Moya A, et al. Guidelines for the diagnosis and management of syncope (version 2009). Eur Heart J. 2009;30(21):2631-71.
3. Solbiati M, Sheldon RS. Epidemiology of vasovagal syncope. In Alboni P, Furlan R (Eds). Vasovagal Syncope. Switzerland: Springer; 2015. pp. 41-9.
4. Pavri BB. Handbook of Syncope: A Concise Clinical Approach. New Delhi: Jaypee Brothers Medical Publishers (P) Ltd; 2014.
5. Colman N, Nahm K, Ganzeboom K, Shen W, Reitsma J, Linzer M, et al. Epidemiology of reflex syncope. Clin Auton Res. 2004;14(Suppl 1):9-17.
6. Brignole M, Benditt DG. Syncope: An Evidence-Based Approach. London: Springer-Verlag; 2011.
7. Sun BC, Emond JA, Camargo CA. Direct medical costs of syncope-related hospitalizations in the United States. Am J C. 2005;95(5):668-71.
8. Holmegard HN, Benn M, Kaijer M, Haunsø S, Mehlsen J. Prevalence of family history in patients with reflex syncope. J Clin Neurosci. 2013;20(5):692-6.
9. Lizer M, Yang EH, Estes NA, Wang P, Vorperian VR, Kapoor WN. Diagnosing syncope. Part I. Value of history, physical examination, and electrocardiography: Clinical Efficacy Assessment Project of the American College of Physicians. Ann Intern Med. 1997;126(12):989-96.
10. Freeman R, Wieling W, Axelrod FB, Benditt DG, Benarroch E, Biaggioni I, et al. Consensus statement on the definition of orthostatic hypotension, neurally mediated syncope and the postural tachycardia syndrome. Auton Neurosci. 2011;161(1):46-8.
11. Soteriades ES, Evans JC, Larson MG, Chen MH, Chen L, Benjamin EJ, et al. Incidence and prognosis of syncope. N Engl J Med. 2002;347(12):878-85.
12. Middlekauff HR, Stevenson WG, Stevenson LW, Saxon LA. Syncope in advanced heart failure: high risk of sudden death regardless of origin of syncope. J Am Coll Cardiol. 1993;21(1):110-6.
13. Olshansky B. (2015). Pathogenesis and etiology of syncope. [online] Available from http://www.uptodate.com/contents/pathogenesis-and-etiology-of-syncope. [Accessed February, 2016].
14. Benditt DG, Adkisson WO. Evaluating transient-loss of consciousness and suspected neurally mediated reflex syncope. In: Sra JS, Akhtar M, Natale A, Wilber DJ (Eds). Practical Electrophysiology. Minneapolis: Cardiotext Publishing; 2014. pp. 147-62.
15. Thijs RD, Kruit MC, van Buchem MA, Ferrari MD, Launer LJ, van Dijk JG. Syncope in migraine: the population-based CAMERA study. Neurology. 2006;66(7):1034-7.
16. Kanjwal K, Kanjwal Y, Karabin B, Grubb BP. Psychogenic syncope? A cautionary note. Pacing Clin Electrophysiol. 2009;32(7):862-5.
17. McDermott D, Quinn J. (2015). Approach to the adult patient with syncope in the emergency department. [online] Available from http://www.uptodate.com/contents/approach-to-the-adult-patient-with-syncope-in-the-emergency-department. [Accessed February, 2016].
18. Puppala VK, Dickinson O, Benditt DG. Syncope: classification and risk stratification. J Cardiol. 2014;63(3):171-7.
19. Costantino G, Casazza G, Reed M, Bossi I, Sun B, Del Rosso A, et al. Syncope risk stratification tools vs clinical judgment: an individual patient data meta-analysis. Am J Med. 2014;127(11):1126.e13-25.
20. Serrano LA, Hess EP, Bellolio MF, Murad MH, Montori VM, Erwin PJ, et al. Accuracy and quality of clinical decision rules for syncope in the emergency department: a systematic review and meta-analysis. Ann Emerg Med. 2010;56(4):362-73.e1.
21. Huff JS, Decker WW, Quinn JV, Perron AD, Napoli AM, Peeters S, et al. Clinical policy: critical issues in the evaluation and management of adult patients presenting to the emergency department with syncope. Ann Emerg Med. 2007;49(4):431-44.
22. Quinn JV, Stiell IG, McDermott DA, Sellers KL, Kohn MA, Wells GA. Derivation of the San Francisco Syncope Rule to predict patients with short-term serious outcomes. Ann Emerg Med. 2004;43(2):224-32.
23. Fedorowski A, Burri P, Struck J, Juul Möller S, Melander O. Novel cardiovascular biomarkers in unexplained syncopal attacks: the SYSTEMA cohort. J Intern Med. 2013;273(4):359-67.
24. Chiu DT, Shapiro NI, Sun BC, Mottley JL, Grossman SA. Are echocardiography, telemetry, ambulatory electrocardiography monitoring, and cardiac enzymes in emergency department patients presenting with syncope useful tests? A preliminary investigation. J Emerg Med. 2014;47(1):113-8.
25. Croci F, Brignole M, Alboni P, Menozzi C, Raviele A, Del Rosso A, et al. The application of a standardized strategy of evaluation in patients with syncope referred to three syncope units. Europace. 2002;4(4):351-5.
26. Crawford MH, Bernstein SJ, Deedwania PC, DiMarco JP, Ferrick KJ, Garson A. ACC/AHA Guidelines for Ambulatory Electrocardiography. A report of the American College of Cardiology/American Heart Association Task Force on Practice Guidelines (Committee to Revise the Guidelines for Ambulatory Electrocardiography). Developed in collaboration with the North American Society for Pacing and Electrophysiology. J Am Coll Cardiol. 1999;34(3):912-48.
27. Edvardsson N, Frykman V, van Mechelen R, Mitro P, Mohii-Oskarsson A, Pasquié J-L, et al. Use of an implantable loop recorder to increase the diagnostic yield in unexplained syncope: results from the PICTURE registry. Europace. 2011;13(2):262-9.
28. Benbadis SR, Chichkova R. Psychogenic pseudosyncope: an underestimated and provable diagnosis. Epilepsy Behav. 2006;9(1):106-10.
29. Tannemaat MR, Thijs RD, van Dijk JG. Managing psychogenic pseudosyncope: Facts and experiences. Cardiol J. 2014;21(6):658-64.
30. Freeman R. Clinical practice. Neurogenic orthostatic hypotension. N Engl J Med. 2008;358(6):615-24.

31. Abubakr A, Wambacq I. The diagnostic value of EEGs in patients with syncope. Epilepsy Behav. 2005;6(3):433-4.
32. Brignole M. Randomized clinical trials of neurally mediated syncope. J Cardiovasc Electrophysiol. 2003;14(Suppl 9):S64-9.
33. Moya A. Therapy for Syncope. Cardiol Clin. 2015;33(3):473-81.
34. Denay KL, Johansen M. Common questions about pacemakers. Am Fam Physician. 2014;89(4):279-82.
35. Tracy CM, Epstein AE, Darbar D, DiMarco JP, Dunbar SB, Ellenbogen KA, et al. 2012 ACCF/AHA/HRS Focused Update of the 2008 Guidelines for Device-Based Therapy of Cardiac Rhythm Abnormalities: a report of the American College of Cardiology Foundation/American Heart Association Task Force on Practice Guidelines and the Heart Rhythm Society. [corrected]. Circulation. 2012;126(14):1784-800.
36. European Heart Rhythm Association, Heart Rhythm Society, Zipes DP, Camm AJ, Borggrefe M, Buxton AE, et al. ACC/AHA/ESC 2006 guidelines for management of patients with ventricular arrhythmias and the prevention of sudden cardiac death: a report of the American College of Cardiology/American Heart Association Task Force and the European Society of Cardiology Committee for Practice Guidelines (Writing Committee to Develop Guidelines for Management of Patients With Ventricular Arrhythmias and the Prevention of Sudden Cardiac Death). J Am Coll Cardiol. 2006;48(5):e247-346.
37. Pedersen CT, Kay GN, Kalman J, Borggrefe M, Della-Bella P, Dickfeld T, et al. EHRA/HRS/APHRS expert consensus on ventricular arrhythmias. Europace. 2014;16(9):1257-83.
38. Arnar DO. Syncope in patients with structural heart disease. J Intern Med. 2013;273(4):336-44.
39. Herman A, Bennett MT, Chakrabarti S, Krahn AD. Life threatening causes of syncope: Channelopathies and cardiomyopathies. Auton Neurosci. 2014;184: 53-9.
40. Yousuf O, Chrispin J, Tomaselli GF, Berger RD. Clinical management and prevention of sudden cardiac death. Circ Res. 2015;116(12):2020-40.
41. McIntosh SJ, Lawson J, Kenny RA. Clinical characteristics of vasodepressor, cardioinhibitory, and mixed carotid sinus syndrome in the elderly. Am J Med. 1993;95(2):203-8.
42. van der Velde N, van den Meiracker AH, Pols HA, Stricker BHC, van der Cammen TJ. Withdrawal of fall-risk-increasing drugs in older persons: effect on tilt-table test outcomes. J Am Geriatr Soc. 2007;55(5):734-9.
43. Martin TP, Hanusa BH, Kapoor WN. Risk stratification of patients with syncope. Ann Emerg Med. 1997;29(4):459-66.
44. Gillette P, Garson A. Sudden cardiac death in the pediatric population. Circulation. 1992;85(1 Suppl):I64-9.
45. Salerno JC, Coleman B. (2016). Causes of syncope in children and adolescents. [online] Available from http://www.uptodate.com/contents/causes-of-syncope-in-children-and-adolescents. [Accessed February, 2016].
46. Yarlagadda S, Poma PA, Green LS, Katz V. Syncope during pregnancy. Obstet Gynecol. 2010;115(2 Pt 1):377-80.
47. Poppas A, Larson L. Syncope and arrhythmias. In: Rosene-Montella K, Keely E, Lee R, Barbour L (Eds). Medical Care of the Pregnant Patient (ACP Women's Health Series), 2nd edition. Philadelphia, PA: American College of Physicians; 2008. pp 334-9.
48. Harris L, Yap S-C, Silversides C. (2015). Maternal conduction disorders and bradycardia during pregnancy. [online] Available from http://www.uptodate.com/contents/maternal-conduction-disorders-and-bradycardia-during-pregnancy. [Accessed February, 2016].
49. Brignole M, Hamdan MH. New concepts in the assessment of syncope. J Am Coll Cardiol. 2012;59(18):1583-91.
50. Hastings JL, Levine BD. Syncope in the athletic patient. Prog Cardiovasc Dis. 2012;54(5):438-44..

10

CHAPTER

Clinical Evaluation of Palpitations

Jeremy Egnatios, Nicholas A Marston

INTRODUCTION

The evaluation of palpitations, a chief complaint often described as a "racing heart" or extra beats, is one of the most common presentations in the clinical setting. Previous literature has reported that palpitations may account for more than 6% of all outpatient and urgent care visits.[1-3] The etiology of the palpitations can vary drastically, from completely benign to significant cardiac disease requiring emergent medical attention. Palpitations are not considered an independent risk factor of morbidity or mortality;[4] however, certain causes can be life-threatening. The differential for palpitations is broad and requires a comprehensive history, and physical examination before determining the extent of workup warranted.

EPIDEMIOLOGY

Palpitations can present in individuals of any age, race, gender, or socioeconomic status. Women present with palpitations more commonly than men, leading to increased enrollment in clinical studies which can cause challenges when drawing conclusions in men. Additionally, women are more likely to be diagnosed with noncardiac causes, specifically higher rates of anxiety-related palpitations. This trend can lead to overgeneralization in women as they are more likely to have a missed diagnosis compared to men. In contrast, males present less often with palpitations but have a higher likelihood of cardiac etiology.[2,3,5] Figure 1 summarizes these epidemiological considerations.

Palpitations	• Females > Males • Ages 21–65 years most common age range
Noncardiac causes	• Females > Males • Those with history of psychiatric disease
Cardiac causes	• Cardiac comorbidities • Males > Females
Most likely to have missed diagnosis	• Females > Males • Those with a history of psychiatric disease

FIG. 1: Brief summary of epidemiological considerations

INITIAL EVALUATION

Initial evaluation of a patient with palpitations requires examination of vital signs and qualitative assessment of hemodynamic and cardiopulmonary stability. Proper perfusion to the vital organs is particularly important in assessing severity and is often measured through surrogate means such as mentation, urine output, and temperature or color of the extremities. In the emergency setting, it is appropriate to screen all patients presenting with palpitations with an electrocardiogram (ECG) and standard vital signs under continuous monitoring.[6] Prior to any additional workup, perhaps the most important aspect of an initial evaluation of a patient with palpitations is the identification of risk factors associated with significant morbidity or mortality. Dizziness, confusion, syncope, or pounding in neck veins are all concerning for more serious pathology and may warrant hospital admission.[7] Additionally, males with prior cardiac disease and young African Americans with new onset palpitations are also at increased risk for serious etiologies.[8] On examination, the presence of a new murmur or extra heart sound in a patient with palpitations should also be taken into account. Prior to forming the differential and ordering extensive testing, this thorough history and examination will guide your level of suspicion and tailor your workup (Fig. 2).

DIFFERENTIAL DIAGNOSIS

The differential for palpitations can be divided into cardiac and noncardiac causes. A detailed history regarding duration, intensity, frequency, mode of onset, aggravating agents or other, lifestyle, prior cardiac history, and other comorbidities are all important in the consideration of cardiac etiology.[5] Unfortunately, determination of origin

Red flag symptoms
- Dizziness
- Near or true syncope
- Confusion
- Young adult with new onset palpitations

Red flag findings
- Significant neck pulsations
- Jugular venous distension
- Prolonged QTc on ECG
- Early repolarization pattern on ECG

Medical history
- Men with history of prior cardiac disease
- African Americans
- Family history of sudden death or genetic cardiac disease

ECG, electrocardiography; Prolonged QTc, corrected QT segment interval (>440 ms) early repolarization in (>0.1 mV) inferior or (>0.2 mV) lateral leads.

FIG. 2: A brief summary of characteristics associated with increased morbidity and mortality that warrant urgent evaluation

is often complicated by poor description of episodes; including variable perception of the palpitations and inaccurate patient history, most notably for etiologies that are paroxysmal in nature.

While the literature is conflicting, cardiac disease appears to be the most common cause for those complaining of recurrent palpitations. One prospective study regarding patients presenting to the emergency department or a medical clinic with palpitations found that the most common etiology was a cardiac origin (43%), followed by anxiety disorders (31%). Given its high occurrence, any patient presenting with a complaint of palpitations warrants initial suspicion for a cardiac origin.[2]

Only a few characteristics have been verified to increase the likelihood ratio (LR) of a cardiac origin over another. Age, history of prior cardiac disease, and male gender are all related to increased likelihood of palpitations secondary to cardiac disease. For example, a reported history of heart disease increases cardiac likelihood by 2.0. Males are also more likely to present with cardiac-related dysfunction (LR varies in literature between 2.6 and 3.2) with the greatest increase in likelihood seen in patients older than 60 years of age.[2,3,5,9]

Several other factors have been identified in smaller studies and should be considered but interpreted with caution. Of highest significance, a patient reporting a pounding sensation of the neck veins has a much greater likelihood of the palpitations being a result of a cardiac origin. Interestingly, physician observed neck pulsations does not have as strong of an association but still increases the likelihood of cardiac etiology by 2–3 times.[5] The reported duration of the episode is also related to a diagnosis of cardiac origin with episodes lasting longer than 5 minutes having a 50% increased likelihood.[10] Finally, palpitation episodes that occur at work or are affected by sleep are twice as likely to be caused by cardiac origin.[9] Table 1 summarizes these signs and symptoms that are associated with increased likelihood of cardiac disease.

Along with cardiac and psychiatric etiologies, other causes can be associated with palpitations. Hemodynamic instability, symptomatic anemia, and pulmonary abnormalities leading to hypoxia should all be considered as well. Disturbances in homeostatic concentrations of potassium, calcium, magnesium, blood glucose, or thyroid hormone can also present with palpitations; as can various toxic exposures and environmental influences including prescription and illicit drugs.[6-11]

INITIAL ARRHYTHMIA WORKUP

Electrocardiogram

The ECG is the best initial study in the evaluation of palpitations, however, may only be helpful if obtained during the symptomatic episode. Of the possible cardiac concerns, arrhythmia is most likely to be associated with ambiguous symptoms such as palpitations, dizziness, or presyncope. While identification of specific ECG findings related to an arrhythmia is crucial, it is important to consider other causative cardiac processes

TABLE 1: Findings associated with increased likelihood of cardiac disease

Finding	Positive LR (95% CI)	Negative LR (95% CI)	Limitations and considerations
Regular rapid-pounding sensation in neck[5,6]	177 (25–1,251)	0.07 (0.03–0.19)	n = 40, no report on baseline health parameters, population characteristics, or criteria for diagnosis of arrhythmia. All patients had normal ejection fraction
Episode duration greater than 5 min[2]	1.52 (1.25–1.85)	Not significant	n = 190, majority White females, presenting to the emergency department
Episode at work[9]	2.17 (1.19–3.96)	0.7 (0.53–0.93)	n = 139, patients prescreened by general practitioner
Episode affected by sleeping[9]	2.29 (1.33–3.94)	Not significant	
Previous diagnosis of panic disorder[5]	Not significant	1.3 (1.10–1.53)	n = 40, diagnosis solely by 24 h ambulatory ECG, DSMIII criteria of panic disorder

CI, confidence interval; LR, likelihood ratio; DSMIII, 3rd edition of the American Psychiatric Association's Diagnostic and Statistical Manual of Mental Disorders.

when reviewing the ECG as well (ischemia, pericardial disease, etc.).

Arrhythmias can be secondary to other cardiopulmonary pathology such as decompensated heart failure, pulmonary embolism, and myocardial infarction. It is important to consider these causes while working up the patient. If the palpitations are associated with chest pain and diaphoresis, especially in the setting of cardiovascular risk factors, acute myocardial infarction should be ruled out with serial ECGs and cardiac enzymes.[12] Patients with known or possible heart failure should be evaluated for an acute decompensating episode with a combination of physical examination, imaging, and laboratory values.[13] Pulmonary embolism can be evaluated through risk scores such as the Well's criteria and ultimately a computed tomography scan of the chest with contrast if necessary.[14]

Echocardiogram

If history or physical examination reveals any significant suspicion for a potential structural abnormality, an echocardiogram should be ordered. Any young patient or African American with palpitations should have an increased pretest probability for a structural abnormality. Current joint guidelines by the American Heart Association (AHA), American College of Cardiology (ACC), and the European Heart Rhythm Society (ESC) guidelines state the need for special consideration for several groups including young patients presenting with palpitations, patients with a history of myocardial infarction, or those at risk for cardiomyopathy.[15] Still, mitral valve prolapse remains the most frequent structural abnormality associated with palpitations and is common in the general population.[16] In pediatric patients, congenital heart disease is relatively common and occurs in close to 1% of all births.[17] All of these structural considerations highlight the importance of a careful physical examination to best select which patients require an echocardiogram.

Ambulatory Cardiac Monitoring

Four variations of ambulatory ECG modalities are currently in use. Holter monitors, event recorders, continuous recorders, and implantable recorders are all tools available for outpatient monitoring of patients with palpitations and arrhythmias.[18]

Holter Monitors

Holter monitors have been the standard for prolonged (24–72 h) ECG monitoring in the ambulatory patient, with a diagnostic yield reportedly between 15 and 39%.[19] Traditionally, monitoring has been reserved for patients with symptomatic complaints (palpitations, dizziness, syncope) consistent with a potential cardiac etiology. They are relatively cheap compared to other continuous monitoring devices and are a good first line in healthy subjects with low pretest probability of cardiac disease.

Holter monitors do carry a risk of false positives which may have clinical significance. Device misplacement or malfunction are related to a high number of artifacts on recorders[20] but abnormalities can be found even when used appropriately. One historical study conducted on medical students revealed a substantial amount of abnormal rhythms and arrhythmias in healthy young males with no complaint, suspicion, or indication of heart malfunction. This high rate of abnormal rhythms has been replicated in other healthy populations as well.[21,22] To reduce these false positives, the Holter monitor is ideally combined with a symptom diary to help ensure that the Holter findings are temporally in sync with the patient's symptoms.[23]

Event Recorders

Event recorders are diagnostic tools that are worn for a longer period of time in hopes of capturing less common events. Event recorders are categorized as either looping or nonlooping symptom monitors. Looping event recorders are able to repeatedly store cardiac activity for short periods ("looping" over its previous recording) and only permanently store data once activated by the patient. This would allow ECG data to be retained from the time leading up to the event, even if the patient did not activate the device until after symptom onset. Symptom recorders, on the other hand, only record ECG data starting when the patient activates the device. This may miss valuable ECG data near the beginning of the episode.

Event recorders with memory looping have a diagnostic yield varying from 30 to 84% for patients with palpitations. A higher yield rate was found when looping time was long enough to record preevent symptoms (64–84%). Symptom recorders, however, showed a much narrower range with a diagnostic yield of 23–42%. A major caveat to these findings is the lack of designation of clinically relevant arrhythmias. For studies that only included rates of significant arrhythmias, the yield was only about half of what it was when all arrhythmias were included.[19]

Another difference between the looping and nonlooping event recorders is cost. The technical cost of an event recorder is at least triple that of Holter monitoring and should be considered when deciding on a device.[24] In general, event recorders have superior diagnostic ability than a simple Holter monitor due to patient activation, but cost of testing should be addressed.[25]

Continuous Recorders

Continuous recorders are similar to event recorders in that they allow for prolonged monitoring with enhanced ability to capture ECG activity surrounding a symptomatic event. Real time observation of cardiac activity can be achieved with software analysis included in continuous recorders. Physicians can set the parameters such that abnormal or dangerous rhythms will trigger an alert to seek medical attention. As expected, real time continuous monitoring systems are considerably more expensive than traditional monitoring, nearly 10 times the technical cost of Holter monitoring, and about three times more expensive than event monitoring.[19]

Implantable Event Recorders

Implantable recorders compose the final major variation of ECG monitoring available for a patient with palpitations. These devices require a simple, minimally invasive procedure and allow for long-term (up to 1 year) monitoring. The majority of patients will not require such extensive monitoring and this option may be best reserved for monitoring of therapy in a known arrhythmia. It is not clear how the diagnostic ability of implantable recorders compares to other devices as it is not typically the initial diagnostic study.

Electrophysiology Studies

Electrophysiology studies are beyond the scope of this chapter, but do make up a definitive way to diagnose and locate arrhythmias. These studies are performed immediately prior to any ablative therapy.

REACHING A DIAGNOSIS: CARDIAC CAUSES

A suspected cardiac etiology can have a fairly set algorithm in regards to workup and diagnosis. First, it is important to rule out life-threatening presentations such as ventricular tachycardia (VT). Any patient unresponsive at presentation with an ambiguous ECG should be considered for VT until determined otherwise.[13] Information taken from history and physical examination can raise suspicion as to the type of arrhythmia present, however, cardiac monitoring is typically required to confirm. Multiple studies have reported arrhythmias as the primary diagnosis ranging from 30 to 60% of all patients presenting with palpations.[2,3,26]

Once an abnormal ECG is identified, classification by rate, QRS duration, and rhythm can quickly narrow your differential for any arrhythmia. Bradycardia and heart block rarely cause the sensation of palpitations or racing heart, so this discussion will focus on tachycardias. When evaluating a tachycardia, a key distinction to make is whether it is of ventricular or supraventricular origin. The QRS duration can be helpful in making this determination and if it is narrow (<120 ms) then we can be confident that it is supraventricular in origin. If the QRS complex is wide (>120 ms), a life-threatening ventricular rhythm is much higher on our differential and requires immediate attention. In the case of supraventricular narrow complex tachycardias, we can next look to rhythm (regularity and atrial activity) to narrow the diagnosis. Atrial fibrillation (AF), atrioventricular (AV) nodal or accessory pathway re-entrant tachycardia are the most common arrhythmias in this category.

Tachycardias

Regular Interval Narrow Complex Tachycardia

Supraventricular tachycardia (SVT) is a nonspecific term often used to describe regular interval narrow complex tachycardias. It is the most common type of arrhythmia associated with palpitations and has an incidence and prevalence of 35 cases per 100,000 person years and 2.25 per 1,000, respectively.[27] Supraventricular tachycardia usually results from a re-entry mechanism and can either occur at the AV node through retrograde travel or through an accessory pathway. Atrioventricular nodal re-entry tachycardia (AVnRT) is twice as common as that mediated by an accessory pathway, and accounts for nearly 60% of the SVT cases.[27] The SVT normally presents with a narrow QRS complex (<120 ms), however, a wide QRS complex is possible and referred to as SVT with aberrancy.[28,29] Because SVT can often present in the setting of an acute myocardial infarction, cardiac enzymes, such as troponins and creatine kinase-MB, should be ordered in the appropriate clinical scenario.[30]

Atrioventricular Nodal Re-entry Tachycardias

Atrioventricular nodal re-entry tachycardias is most often paroxysmal with acute onset and cessation; however, some experience persistent tachycardia or episodic onset following emotional or pharmacological stimuli. Associated symptoms may include pulsatile neck veins or a sensation of chest pounding, both of which have a high association with AVnRT. Other associated symptoms vary, but include diaphoresis, angina, dyspnea, feeling of anxiousness, or less commonly syncope or dizziness.[27] Women have a greater predisposition for developing AVnRTs, with some evidence demonstrating a 2:1 ratio of female to male predominance. High progesterone and low estrogen appears to be partially responsible for this observation as higher rates are seen in the premenstrual period leading up to menses.[31] Finally, it is important to note that panic disorder and paroxysmal SVT frequently overlap regarding presentation and it is important to fully consider both before determining a diagnosis.[32]

Atrioventricular nodal re-entry tachycardia most commonly presents with a heart rate between 100 and 200 beats/min. Given the presence of a secondary circuit within the AV node, two different conduction speeds are often noted on ECG. One pathway has fast conduction with a long refractory period, while the other has a slower conduction speed with shorter refractory period. In a classic presentation, the fast conduction pathway is retrograde in direction, while the slow pathway is anterograde. Electrocardiogram is likely to show a diminished upright p wave with a retrograde p′ wave seen following the QRS complex. This may be difficult to see due the more prominent ventricular depolarization. Identification of p′ waves are best discerned in V1, and in many cases leads II, III, and aVF.

Atroventricular Re-entry Tachycardias

Atrioventricular re-entry tachycardia (AVRT) is a type of SVT that occurs due to an accessory bundle of muscle tissue capable of conduction. Atrioventricular re-entry tachycardia is second only to AVnRT as most prevalent type of SVT. Like AVnRT, AVRT produces rates in the 100–200 beats/min range, and the two cannot be distinguished by examination.

Atrioventricular re-entry tachycardia includes Wolff-Parkinson-White (WPW) syndrome, a classic example that often presents with palpitations or syncopal episodes. Men appear to be several times more likely to have WPW syndrome, however, there does not appear to be any genetic predisposition that would explain this discrepancy.[31] Wolff-Parkinson-White syndrome can cause a malignant arrhythmia capable of sudden death, a phenomenon that can occurs about 0.15% per patient year.[33] Incidence and first presentation of WPW syndrome is more likely at a younger age, however, its total prevalence appears between 0.68 and 1.74 per 1,000 persons.[34] The WPW syndrome often presents with AF and can lead to potential fatal arrhythmias with time. While no conclusive predictors have been found, decompensation to ventricular fibrillation may be more common in males, especially the young and elderly.[35] Young male patients with palpitations and a family history of arrhythmia should have a very high index of suspicion for AVRT and WPW syndrome. On ECG, a shortened PR interval and slurred upstroke of the QRS known as a "delta wave" are present and represent ventricular pre-excitation due to the accessory pathway.

Atrial Tachycardia and Multifocal Tachycardia

Atrial tachycardia accounts for about 10% of SVT arrhythmias and may have one or more foci. Like the other causes of SVT, a rate of 100–200 beats/min should raise suspicion but an ECG is required to differentiate them. In atrial tachycardia, p waves are present but do not arise from the sinus node. This is more evident in multifocal atrial tachycardia, where three or more different p-wave morphologies can be seen, representing the different atrial foci contributing to the rhythm. Multifocal atrial tachycardia is more common in patients of increasing age, especially those with pulmonary disease such as chronic obstructive pulmonary disease (COPD).[36]

Atrial Fibrillation

Atrial fibrillation is one of the most common arrhythmias seen in clinical practice and often presents with nonspecific symptoms such as palpitations, dyspnea, or presyncope. The ECG is notable for an irregularly irregular rhythm with no organized atrial activity. Atrial fibrillation is increasingly common with age, and is associated with hypertension and diabetes. Men are more commonly afflicted, however, the incidence is increasing in women. Heart failure and valvular heart disease are also associated with AF, as is smoking.[37] Atrial fibrillation increases the risk of stroke, sudden death, and early mortality in all populations, and thus, appropriate identification and management is crucial.[38,39]

Atrial Flutter

Atrial flutter (AFL) is another common arrhythmia with an incidence of 88 cases per 100,000 person years. Like AF, AFL increases in incidence with age and is more prevalent in men by a factor of more than two. Heart failure, COPD, and valvular disease are all associated with AFL.[34] On ECG, flutter waves are present and appear in a "saw-tooth" pattern at approximately 300 beats/min. Classically, ventricular conduction occurs in a 2:1 conduction pattern leading to heart rates near 150. However, ventricular conduction can be variable leading to 3:1 or 4:1 conduction with rates in the 75–100 beats/min range. In general, AFL and AF should be seriously considered in any patient with advanced age and new onset palpitations.

Wide QRS Complex Tachycardias

Ventricular Tachycardia

Wide QRS complexes suggest delayed conduction throughout the myocardium of the ventricles rather than throughout the His-Purkinje system. This can occur in a bundle branch block or in the setting of a ventricular rhythm. In the setting of a wide-complex tachycardia, VT must be the presumed diagnosis due to its life-threatening nature. Ventricular tachycardia is typically a monomorphic, wide QRS rhythm that frequently does not provide organ perfusion. Ventricular tachycardia can also be polymorphic, known as torsade de pointes.

Premature Ventricular Contractions

Premature ventricular contractions (PVCs) are a common finding in patients with and without palpitations. Cardiac history and frequency of PVCs are the two most important factors in management of these patients. In a patient without cardiac risk factors and an otherwise normal ECG, PVCs are typically considered benign. However, frequent PVCs may justify outpatient cardiology consultation and prolonged runs of multiform PVCs may require inpatient observation. In patients with heart disease, PVCs should also be considered more carefully as they may represent concerning conduction abnormalities.[40-43] Although controversial, there is a growing body of literature to suggest that even in patients without prior cardiac disease, frequent or repetitive ventricular contractions are associated with increased morbidity, mortality, and even sudden cardiac death. Infrequent premature beats, on the other hand, are common in the population and can be considered benign in a healthy asymptomatic individual.[41,44-48]

Bradyarrhythmias

Pure bradyarrhythmias are unlikely to be described with palpitations, racing heart, or a similar descriptor. Therefore, the majority of bradyarrhythmias are beyond the scope of this chapter. However, one bradyarrhythmia that will be discussed is tachycardia-bradycardia syndrome, or commonly, sick sinus syndrome (SSS).

Sick Sinus Syndrome

Sick sinus syndrome is a relatively uncommon cardiac pathology with an incidence known to increase with age. The typical patient with SSS is an elderly White individual with large body habitus. Cardiovascular evaluation may reveal a long QRS interval, right bundle branch block, or low normal resting heart rate. In the general population, incidence is rare with 8 cases per 10,000 person years. Age carries the greatest relative risk for SSS estimated at 1.7 (95% confidence interval = 1.47–2.05) per every 5 years aging.[49] When captured fully on ECG, SSS is identified by episodic tachycardia followed by intermittent sinus pauses or prolonged AV block with slow ventricular rates. Sick sinus syndrome can also be associated with SVTs such as AF or AFL. Any sinus pause lasting more than 3 seconds should have high suspicion for SSS.[50]

Structural Cardiac Disease

Structural abnormalities, such as valvular disease or congenital abnormalities, can lead to palpitations. While less common than arrhythmias, structural abnormalities must be ruled out if clinical suspicion exists as they have potential for significant morbidity and mortality in this population. Abnormalities, such as aortic insufficiency, mitral valve prolapse, congenital or acquired long QT syndrome, and congenital or acquired left ventricular hypertrophy, are important pathology address during medical history.

Given the variation in presentation, few factors have consistently been found to have predictive value of cardiac origin in causing palpitations. The European Society of Cardiology recommends possible hospital admission if a patient presenting for palpitations has associated symptoms of syncope, a confirmed or suspected history of prior (structural or anatomical) cardiac disease, a family history of sudden death, or history of arrhythmia.[7]

REACHING A DIAGNOSIS: NONCARDIAC CAUSES

The differential for noncardiac-related causes of palpitations is broad and requires consideration beyond the more common cardiac etiologies. A psychiatric cause of palpitations is the most common alternative diagnosis to a cardiac origin and can be challenging to diagnose.[2,51,52] Multiple studies have observed an elevated rate of psychiatric disease in patients with frequent healthcare utilization related to palpitations without increased rates of arrhythmia.[53,54] However, it has also been reported that arrhythmias frequently mimic anxiety disorder resulting in misdiagnosis. Therefore, thorough cardiac workup should be considered prior to a psychiatric diagnosis.[32,53]

Palpitations can also be associated with a variety of underlying medical conditions. Anemia, hypoxemia, electrolyte imbalance, thyroid disease, hypoglycemia, and pheochromocytoma should all be considered in a patient with palpitations. Luckily, relatively inexpensive routine blood tests can be used to screen for many of these causes.

Finally, palpitations can occur through a variety of exposures, toxins, supplements, and drugs, both prescribed and illicit. For example, alcohol, tobacco, and caffeine are three commonly abused substances in the United States that are all associated with palpitations.[55] This highlights the importance of doing a thorough social history and medication review. For a summary of the noncardiac differential diagnosis for palpitations, see table 2.

TABLE 2: Noncardiac differential

Psychiatric	Exposure/Toxins	Metabolic	Iatrogenic	Hemodynamic
• Generalized anxiety • Panic disorder • Depression	• Ethanol • Smoking • Caffeine • Cocaine • Amphetamine • Weight loss supplements	• Potassium abnormality • Calcium irregularity • Magnesium irregularity • Hypoglycemia • Thyroid disease • Adrenal excess	• Sympathomimetics • Phosphodiesterase type 5 inhibitor • Digitalis • Phenothiazine • β-agonists	• Anemia • Hypoxemia • Hypovolemia

CONCLUSION

Palpitations are a common complaint of patients seeking medical attention and are often associated with cardiac disease. While women are more likely to present with palpitations, men appear to be more likely to have an underlying cardiac etiology. Regardless of gender, a history of cardiac disease increases the likelihood of cardiac-related palpitations. Arrhythmias are the most common cardiac abnormality associated with palpitations and are often detected in young adults and elderly populations.

Several characteristics of the symptomatic episode can suggest cardiac etiologies and can be used to narrow the differential. For example, pulsation of the jugular vein as described by the patient or a witness can support an underlying arrhythmia. Other factors such as duration of episode, description of the sensation, or certain environmental triggers leading up to the episode are important as well. In the absence of these more concerning symptoms or other medical abnormalities, anxiety and other psychogenic causes should be considered as they are the second most common cause of palpitations.

When cardiac etiology is suspected, the workup should focus on whether the underlying abnormality is purely an arrhythmia, or if there is a structural component. This workup can be done in the inpatient or outpatient setting depending on severity and clinical suspicion. All patients should receive a resting ECG along with longer term cardiac monitoring depending on location. The decision of which monitoring device to use depends on the symptom frequency and availability of the study. If the physical examination or other components of the initial assessment suggest a structural abnormality, an echocardiogram may be performed as well. Wall motion abnormalities, defects in cardiac development, or most commonly, valvular abnormalities can all cause arrhythmias presenting as palpitations.

In young and otherwise healthy individuals, the sensations of palpitations are often the result of benign PVCs. If persistent, palpitations in young adults may be due to a SVT such as AV nodal or re-entry tachyarrhythmias. In older patients with more medical problems, AF, AFL, and multifocal atrial tachycardia become more likely. Less often, serious ventricular arrhythmias can occur and represent medical emergencies that require immediate attention.

While suspicion for a cardiac etiology should lead to the workup outlined earlier, it may also be necessary to investigate other causes of palpitations. The majority of these causes can be investigated through simple laboratory studies. Complete blood count, a metabolic panel with electrolytes and blood glucose, serum thyroid stimulating hormone level, and urine toxicology studies could all help explain an episode of palpitations in the right clinical setting.

REFERENCES

1. Kroenke K, Arrington ME, Mangelsdorff AD. The prevalence of symptoms in medical outpatients and the adequacy of therapy. Arch Intern Med. 1990;150(8):1685-9.
2. Weber BE, Kapoor WN. Evaluation and outcomes of patients with palpitations. Am J Med. 1996;100(2):138-48.
3. Lok NS, Lau CP. Prevalence of palpitations, cardiac arrhythmias and their associated risk factors in ambulant elderly. Int J Cardiol. 1996;54(3):231-6.
4. Knudson MP. The natural history of palpitations in a family practice. J Fam Pract. 1987;24(4):357-60.
5. Thavendiranathan P, Bagai A, Khoo C, Dorian P, Choudhry NK. Does this patient with palpitations have a cardiac arrhythmia? JAMA. 2009;302(19):2135-43.
6. Brugada P, Gursoy S, Brugada J, Andries E. Investigation of palpitations. Lancet. 1993;341(8855):1254-8.
7. Brignole M, Hamdan MH. New concepts in the assessment of syncope. J Am Coll Cardiol. 2012;59(18):1583-91.
8. Zimetbaum P, Josephson ME. Evaluation of patients with palpitations. New Engl J Med. 1998;338(19):1369-73.
9. Summerton N, Mann S, Rigby A, Petkar S, Dhawan J. New-onset palpitations in general practice: assessing the discriminant value of items within the clinical history. Fam Pract. 2001;18(4):383-92.
10. Kalantzis N, Papanikolaou IS, Giannakoulopoulou E, Alogari A, Kalantzis C, Papacharalampous X, et al. Capsule endoscopy; the cumulative experience from its use in 193 patients with suspected small bowel disease. Hepatogastroenterology. 2005;52(62):414-9.
11. Sedaghat-Yazdi F, Koenig PR. The teenager with palpitations. Pediatr Clin North Am. 2014;61(1):63-79.
12. Karras DJ, Kane DL. Serum markers in the emergency department diagnosis of acute myocardial infarction. Emerg Med Clin North Am. 2001;19(2):321-37.
13. Zipes DP, Camm AJ, Borggrefe M, Buxton AE, Chaitman B, Fromer M, et al. ACC/AHA/ESC 2006 guidelines for management of patients with ventricular arrhythmias and the prevention of sudden cardiac death: a report of the American College of Cardiology/American Heart Association Task Force and the European Society of Cardiology Committee for Practice Guidelines (Writing Committee to Develop Guidelines for Management of Patients With Ventricular Arrhythmias and the Prevention of Sudden Cardiac Death). J Am Coll Cardiol. 2006;48(5):e247-346.
14. Yetgin GO, Aydin SA, Koksal O, Ozdemir F, Mert DK, Torun G. Clinical probability and risk analysis of patients with suspected pulmonary embolism. World J Emerg Med. 2014;5(4):264-9.
15. Cheitlin MD, Armstrong WF, Aurigemma GP, Beller GA, Bierman FZ, Davis JL, et al. ACC/AHA/ASE 2003 guideline update for the clinical application of echocardiography--summary article: a report of the American College of Cardiology/American Heart Association Task Force on Practice Guidelines (ACC/AHA/ASE Committee to Update the 1997 Guidelines for the Clinical Application of Echocardiography). J Am Coll Cardiol. 2003;42(5):954-70.
16. Freed LA, Levy D, Levine RA, Larson MG, Evans JC, Fuller DL, et al. Prevalence and clinical outcome of mitral-valve prolapse. N Engl J Med. 1999;341(1):1-7.
17. Øyen N, Poulsen G, Boyd HA, Wohlfahrt J, Jensen PK, Melbye M. Recurrence of congenital heart defects in families. Circulation. 2009;120(4):295-301.
18. Wexler RK, Pleister A, Raman S. Outpatient approach to palpitations. Am Fam Physician. 2011;84(1):63-9.
19. Hoefman E, Bindels PJ, van Weert HC. Efficacy of diagnostic tools for detecting cardiac arrhythmias: systematic literature search. Neth Heart J. 2010;18(11):543-51.
20. Guirguis E. Holter monitoring. Can Fam Physician. 1987;33:985-92.
21. Brodsky M, Wu D, Denes P, Kanakis C, Rosen KM. Arrhythmias documented by 24 hour continuous electrocardiographic monitoring in 50 male medical students without apparent heart disease. Am J Cardiol. 1977;39(3):390-5.
22. Sobotka PA, Mayer JH, Bauernfeind RA, Kanakis C, Rosen KM. Arrhythmias documented by 24-hour continuous ambulatory electrocardiographic monitoring in young women without apparent heart disease. Am Heart J. 1981;101(6):753-9.
23. Barrett PM, Komatireddy R, Haaser S, Topol S, Sheard J, Encinas J, et al. Comparison of 24-hour Holter monitoring with 14-day novel adhesive patch electrocardiographic monitoring. Am J Med. 2014;127(1):95.e11-7.
24. Zimetbaum P, Goldman A. Ambulatory arrhythmia monitoring: choosing the right device. Circulation. 2010;122(16):1629-36.
25. Rolfe A, Burton C. Reassurance after diagnostic testing with a low pretest probability of serious disease: systematic review and meta-analysis. JAMA Intern Med. 2013;173(6):407-16.

26. Giada F, Gulizia M, Francese M, Croci F, Santangelo L, Santomauro M, et al. Recurrent unexplained palpitations (RUP) study comparison of implantable loop recorder versus conventional diagnostic strategy. J Am Coll Cardiol. 2007;49(19):1951-6.
27. Link MS. Clinical practice. Evaluation and initial treatment of supraventricular tachycardia. N Engl J Med. 2012;367(15):1438-48.
28. Gula LJ, Skanes A, Krahn AD, Klein GJ. Novel approach to diagnosis of a wide-complex tachycardia. J Cardiovasc Electrophysiol. 2004;15(4):466-9.
29. Kappos KG, Andrikopoulos GK, Tzeis SE, Manolis AS. Wide-QRS-complex tachycardia with a negative concordance pattern in the precordial leads: Are the ECG criteria always reliable? Pacing Clin Electrophysiol. 2006;29(1):63-6.
30. Zoni Berisso M, Ferroni A, De Caro E, Carratino L, Mela GS, Vecchio C. Clinical significance of supraventricular tachyarrhythmias after acute myocardial infarction. Eur Heart J. 1986;7(9):743-8.
31. Villareal RP, Woodruff AL, Massumi A. Gender and cardiac arrhythmias. Tex Heart Inst J. 2001;28(4):265-75.
32. Lessmeier TJ, Gamperling D, Johnson-Liddon V, Fromm BS, Steinman RT, Meissner MD, et al. Unrecognized paroxysmal supraventricular tachycardia. Potential for misdiagnosis as panic disorder. Arch Intern Med. 1997;157(5): 537-43.
33. Lu CW, Wu MH, Chen HC, Kao FY, Huang SK. Epidemiological profile of Wolff-Parkinson-White syndrome in a general population younger than 50 years of age in an era of radiofrequency catheter ablation. Int J Cardiol. 2014;174(3):530-4.
34. Granada J, Uribe W, Chyou PH, Maassen K, Vierkant R, Smith PN, et al. Incidence and predictors of atrial flutter in the general population. J Am Coll Cardiol. 2000;36(7):2242-6.
35. Pappone C, Vicedomini G, Manguso F, Baldi M, Pappone A, Petretta A, et al. Risk of malignant arrhythmias in initially symptomatic patients with Wolff-Parkinson-White syndrome: results of a prospective long-term electrophysiological follow-up study. Circulation. 2012;125(5):661-8.
36. Colucci RA, Silver MJ, Shubrook J. Common types of supraventricular tachycardia: diagnosis and management. Am Fam Physician. 2010;82(8): 942-52.
37. Kannel WB, Wolf PA, Benjamin EJ, Levy D. Prevalence, incidence, prognosis, and predisposing conditions for atrial fibrillation: population-based estimates. Am J Cardiol. 1998;82(8A):2N-9N.
38. Benjamin EJ, Wolf PA, D›Agostino RB, Silbershatz H, Kannel WB, Levy D. Impact of atrial fibrillation on the risk of death: the Framingham Heart Study. Circulation. 1998;98(10):946-52.
39. Scardi S, Mazzone C. [Impact of chronic atrial fibrillation on cardiovacular mortality]. Ital Heart J Suppl. 2000;1(9):1117-22.
40. Qureshi W, Shah A, Salahuddin T, Soliman EZ. Long-term mortality risk in individuals with atrial or ventricular premature complexes (results from the Third National Health and Nutrition Examination Survey). Am J Cardiol. 2014;114(1):59-64.
41. Jouven X, Zureik M, Desnos M, Courbon D, Ducimetière P. Long-term outcome in asymptomatic men with exercise-induced premature ventricular depolarizations. N Engl J Med. 2000;343(12):826-33.
42. Inohara T, Kohsaka S, Okamura T, Watanabe M, Nakamura Y, Higashiyama A, et al. Long-term outcome of healthy participants with atrial premature complex: a 15-year follow-up of the NIPPON DATA 90 cohort. PLoS One. 2013;8(11):e80853.
43. Lin CY, Chang SL, Lin YJ, Lo LW, Chung FP, Chen YY, et al. Long-term outcome of multiform premature ventricular complexes in structurally normal heart. Int J Cardiol. 2014;180:80-5.
44. Cheriyath P, He F, Peters I, Li X, Alagona P, Wu C, et al. Relation of atrial and/or ventricular premature complexes on a two-minute rhythm strip to the risk of sudden cardiac death (the Atherosclerosis Risk in Communities [ARIC] study). Am J Cardiol. 2011;107(2):151-5.
45. Ataklte F, Erqou S, Laukkanen J, Kaptoge S. Meta-analysis of ventricular premature complexes and their relation to cardiac mortality in general populations. Am J Cardiol. 2013;112(8):1263-70.
46. Morshedi-Meibodi A, Evans JC, Levy D, Larson MG, Vasan RS. Clinical correlates and prognostic significance of exercise-induced ventricular premature beats in the community: the Framingham Heart Study. Circulation. 2004;109(20):2417-22.
47. Lee V, Hemingway H, Harb R, Crake T, Lambiase P. The prognostic significance of premature ventricular complexes in adults without clinically apparent heart disease: a meta-analysis and systematic review. Heart. 2012;98(17):1290-8.
48. Messineo FC. Ventricular ectopic activity: prevalence and risk. Am J Cardiol. 1989;64(20):53J-56J.
49. Jensen PN, Gronroos NN, Chen LY, Folsom AR, deFilippi C, Heckbert SR, et al. Incidence of and risk factors for sick sinus syndrome in the general population. J Am Coll Cardiol. 2014;64(6):531-8.
50. Adan V, Crown LA. Diagnosis and treatment of sick sinus syndrome. Am Fam Physician. 2003;67(8):1725-32.
51. Barsky AJ, Cleary PD, Coeytaux RR, Ruskin JN. Psychiatric disorders in medical outpatients complaining of palpitations. J Gen Intern Med. 1994;9(6):306-13.
52. Barsky AJ, Cleary PD, Coeytaux RR, Ruskin JN. The clinical course of palpitations in medical outpatients. Arch Intern Med. 1995;155(16):1782-8.
53. Chignon JM. [Cardiovascular pathology and panic disorder]. Can J Psychiatry. 1993;38(2):127-33.
54. Barsky AJ, Cleary PD, Sarnie MK, Ruskin JN. Panic disorder, palpitations, and the awareness of cardiac activity. J Nerv Ment Dis. 1994;182(2):63-71.
55. Abbott AV. Diagnostic approach to palpitations. Am Fam Physician. 2005; 71(4):743-50.

SECTION 2

Acute Myocardial Infarction and Acute Coronary Syndrome

11 CHAPTER Acute Coronary Syndrome: Diagnosis of Acute Myocardial Infarction and Acute Coronary Syndrome

Francesca R Civitarese, Ava E Pierce, Deborah B Diercks

ACUTE CORONARY SYNDROME: DEFINITIONS AND CRITERIA

One of the most common presenting complaints in the emergency department (ED) is "chest pain". Given the complex anatomy and extensive list of potential diagnosis contained within this topic, emergency physicians face the task of distinguishing the benign etiologies from the critical. Initial screening and management of cardiac etiologies is crucial and evolving, and as an emergency medicine practitioner, you are responsible for being an expert in cardiac diagnosis and management.

Presentation

Classically, cardiac chest pain is substernal or left-sided, radiating to the back, jaw, shoulder, abdomen, or arm, brought on by exertion and relieved by rest. Discomfort caused by cardiac etiologies is generally not exacerbated by movement of the chest wall muscles or by inspiration, and typically not sharp or highly localized.[1]

It can be described as "crushing", pressure-like, or squeezing. Associated symptoms include diaphoresis, nausea, vomiting, lightheadedness, shortness of breath, or even syncope. In some populations, particularly women, diabetics, minority populations, and the elderly, the presentation can vary widely from this textbook presentation, and can present very subtly, making the diagnosis complex. These atypical presentations include epigastric pain, unexplained indigestion, belching, referred pain, nausea, exertional shortness of breath, or fatigue.[2,3]

Certain social and historical risk factors increase the probability that the patient could be suffering from ischemic cardiac disease, including smoking, hyperlipidemia, family history, hypertension, and diabetes. Diabetes and chronic renal disease are considered "risk equivalents" to coronary artery disease (CAD).[4] However, in the acute chest pain, patient risk factors alone are not predictive of the diagnosis of acute coronary syndrome (ACS), particularly in the ED setting.

Chest Pain in Women

Patients with atypical presentations can be one of the most challenging obstacles to making a diagnosis of ACS in the ED. Atypical presentations have been studied based on gender, age, and medical risk factors. Atypical symptoms, which women are more likely to experience, can include "burning" sensations, reproducible discomfort on palpation of the chest wall, pain with a pleuritic component, epigastric pain or indigestion-like symptoms, unexplained shortness of breath, or even lack of chest pain at all with pain identified near the jaw, arm, or back.[5-9]

There are many theories as to why women present differently than male patients in ACS. Women typically present at older ages than males, which may lead to perceived differences in symptomatology. Additionally, women have a higher risk of hypercoagulability secondary to estrogen-related issues, than males, particularly if they are taking oral contraceptives. Cardiac anatomy, diameter of the lumen of cardiac vessels, cardiac output, and collateral circulation also vary amongst women in comparison to men.[10] Atherosclerotic plaques in women have been found to contain more lipid-laden foam cells, making them more susceptible to rupture.[11]

In a review of 39 studies analyzing gender differences in acute myocardial infarction (AMI), they found women presented at older ages than men, had greater risk of both long- and short-term mortality, and tended to have different risk factor profiles than male patients. Women, in their review and consistent with previous literature, tended to have higher rates of diabetes, depression, heart failure, and renal failure than males.[12]

In a study retrospectively analyzing 325 ST segment elevation myocardial infarction (STEMI) patients (23.1% female, 76.9% male), Biava et al. found that the women tended to present at older ages than the male patients (age 71.8 ± 11.7 vs. age 62.5 ± 12.6 years), presented more frequently in renal failure, had higher rates of hemodynamic impairment, sustained more major arrhythmias (8% vs. 2.8%) and had a higher inhospital overall mortality rate (14.7% vs. 4.8%) and cardiac death rates (12% vs. 2%) than male patients.[13]

Once a patient has been identified as potentially having cardiac-related chest pain, the patient should have been connected to a cardiac monitor, their vital signs assessed and an electrocardiogram (ECG) conducted within 10 minutes of arrival in the ED, if it has not already been done in the prehospital or triage setting. After these critical actions have been taken, it allows you some time, barring any abnormal initial findings or unstable vital signs, to investigate the pain further.

Some important and concerning physical examination findings, in addition to history components and underlying risk factors, include evidence of mitral regurgitation or a new murmur on cardiac examination, evidence of pulmonary edema or rales, a third heart sound, and jugular venous distention (JVD). Additionally, it should be noted if the patient is hypotensive, tachycardiac, or diaphoretic.[14]

Acute Coronary Syndrome

Acute coronary syndrome essentially functions as a term to encompass the spectrum of ischemic myocardial disease. There are several subcategories, with varying degrees of severity and morbidity/mortality, and include angina, unstable angina (UA), non-ST segment elevation myocardial infarction (NSTEMI) and STEMI.

Acute coronary syndrome typically results from instability or progression of atherosclerotic plaques that place myocardial tissue at risk of decreased perfusion or ultimate infarction, however, can also be attributable to coronary vasospasm, dissection, and coronary artery inflammation, amongst other diagnoses.[15]

Stable Angina

Stable angina is classically defined as chest pain, brought on by exertion, relieved by rest. The symptoms are unchanged from prior episodes in character, frequency, or duration. Additionally, similar levels of exertion provoke the pain.[15]

Unstable Angina

Unstable Angina is acute chest pain and is often brought on by exertion, worsening in frequency, character, duration, or with lesser exertion required to provoke a similar response than prior episodes. Unstable angina can also occur at rest or be a new onset of severe angina (<2 months) with no prior episodes of similar chest pain. Prolonged angina at rest (>20 min) is also considered UA. No ST elevations are initially found on ECG, but the ECG may exhibit signs of ischemia such as ST depressions, T-wave inversions, and flattened T-waves. This diagnosis is differentiated from NSTEMI by cardiac biomarkers such as troponin.[15,16]

ST Segment Elevation Myocardial Infarction/ ST Segment Elevation Acute Coronary Syndrome

Patients with an STEMI can present with typical acute chest pain for more than 20 minutes with ST elevations in an anatomical pattern noted on ECG. The STEMI can present atypically in some populations, with angina equivalent symptoms in addition to or even in the absence of chest pain. The distinguishing factor here is evidence of ST elevations on the ECG. These symptoms with cardiac biomarker elevation in the absences of ST elevations are designated NSTEMI.[15]

Prinzmetal's Angina

Prinzmetal's angina is the result of acute coronary vasospasm, which can manifest chest pain that occurs suddenly or at rest in a young patient, often associated with use of methamphetamines or cocaine. Interestingly, in these patients, less than 2% develop true ACS.[17]

INITIAL MANAGEMENT AND DIAGNOSIS

Electrocardiogram: Accuracy, Use, and Applications

Electrocardiogram interpretation is a critical skill for the emergency physician. Fortunately, the ECG is easily obtained, inexpensive, and noninvasive. It is one of the most useful tests and can provide a great deal of information on a variety of chief complaints, the most prominent of which is chest pain, but also include palpitations, syncope, toxidromes, or overdoses, hypotension and shortness of breath.

Often, ECGs are obtained either prehospital, or as the patient arrives in the ED, as STEMI is a time-dependent diagnosis and time to reperfusion of the ischemic cardiac tissue is critical. Door-to-ECG time recommendations are currently to have it obtained within 10 minutes, with increased risk of poor clinical outcomes in STEMI patients in which this acquisition is delayed.[18,19]

Electrocardiogram: Lead Placement

Typically a 12-lead ECG lead is used for initial testing. Additional leads are most commonly placed when there is suspicion for right ventricular (RV) infarction or for posterior infarction. The lead used for right ventricle evaluation is called V4R, and is placed in the same location as V4, but on the right side of the chest.

The posterior leads are placed on the left side of the body on the back and are designated V7, V8, and V9. They provide direct imaging of the posterior wall of the left ventricle. V8 is typically positioned at the inferior tip of the scapula on the left. V9 is halfway between this lead and the vertebral column at the midline, on the left.

Electrocardiogram and Cardiac Anatomy

When diagnosing ACS and evaluating the ECG for ischemia or infarction, the emergency physician should be aware of the regions of the heart represented on the ECG. In an ischemic event, the vessel and subsequent region of the heart that is affected can greatly impact management during the initial resuscitation period.

Table 1 depicts the lead on the ECG, and correlating region of the heart, as well as the classic responsible vessel for supplying that region.[20]

Electrocardiogram and Expected Reciprocal Changes with Ischemia

One of the crucial ECG findings to note when evaluating the patient for ACS is the presence of reciprocal changes (Table 2). The reciprocal changes represent the territories at the "ischemic penumbra" of the heart. They are the regions of the heart directly abutting the ischemic tissue anatomically, which may be at risk for larger areas of infarction without adequate and timely reperfusion. It does appear that after reperfusion, those with reciprocal changes on the initial ECG seem to have a better potential for myocardial salvage.[21-24]

Electrocardiogram and Injury Patterns

There is often a progression of ECG abnormalities in the setting of ACS. Ischemia or infarct can be heralded by hyperacute T-waves, T-wave inversions, or ST depressions. The most important pattern to recognize is the ST elevation.

ST Elevations/ST Segment Elevation Myocardial Infarction Criteria

The ST elevations are perhaps the most ominous finding while investigating a patient with ongoing chest pain suspicious for ACS.

The STEMIs frequently occur when there is an atherosclerotic plaque rupture and abrupt cessation of blood flow to the downstream myocardial tissue, producing infarction. Of the greater than 900,000 patients experiencing myocardial infarction (MI) each year, approximately one-third cases present with ST elevations. Slow growing progressive occlusions do not typically progress to total occlusion resulting in STEMI, likely due to the development of collateral vessels that have grown over time to accommodate for the decreased flow through the problem vessel. Often, lipid-laden nonobstructive plaques with inflammatory cells and macrophages are more prone to rupture, thus occluding the distal vessel and creating MIs.[25]

The morphology of the ST segments was investigated by Nable et al. in the setting of diagnosing acute STEMI in a patient sample of 171 STEMI patients. They investigated the differences between concave and nonconcave ST segment morphologies. Of the patients with nonconcave

TABLE 1: Electrocardiogram leads with associated cardiac vessels and anatomical vascular territory

I (LV Lateral wall), L Circumflex artery	• aVR	• V1 (septal/LV anterior wall) LAD	• V4 (LV Anterior wall) • LAD
II (inferior) RCA	• aVL (LV lateral wall) Left Circumflex	• V2 (Septal/LV anterior wall) • LAD	• V5 (LV Lateral wall) • L circumflex
III (Inferior) RCA	• aVF (Inferior) RCA	• V3 (LV anterior wall) • LAD	• V6 (LV Lateral wall) • L circumflex
	• V4R (Right ventricle) • RCA	• V8 (posterior) • L circumflex • Posterior descending branch of RCA	• V9 (posterior) • L circumflex • Posterior descending branch of RCA

TABLE 2: Reciprocal changes

Anatomy/cardiac location	Coronary artery	Leads	Reciprocal change
Posterior LV	RCA/portions of the LAD or circumflex (depending on RCA or left circulation dominance)	V8, V9	V1-V4
Inferior	Right Coronary Artery	II, III, aVF	I, aVL
Anterior	Left anterior descending artery	V3, V4	none
Anteroseptal	Left anterior descending artery	V1-V4	none
Lateral	Left circumflex artery	I, aVL, V5-V6	II, III, aVF
Anterolateral	LAD/L circumflex	I, aVL, V3-V6	II, III, aVF

BOX 1 ST elevation myocardial infarction criteria

- New ST elevation at the J point in two contiguous leads of 2 mm in men or 1.5 mm in women in leads V2-V3
- AND/OR 1 mm of elevation in other contiguous chest leads or limb leads

ST segments, 46 were diagnosed with AMI, with 77% sensitivity and 97% specificity. They concluded that nonconcave ST segments were highly suggestive in adult chest pain patients of acute STEMI.[26]

Current STEMI guidelines state that the physician in the ED should be able to make reperfusion decisions within 10 minutes of obtaining the initial ECG. Additionally, if the initial ECG is nondiagnostic, but the clinical picture is consistent with possible STEMI, serial ECGs at 5- and 10-minute intervals should be subsequently obtained to screen for development of STEMI.[27]

Formal diagnostic criteria on ECG for STEMI defined by the European Society of Cardiology are given in box 1.[1,3,27]

Electrocardiogram ST Segment Elevation Myocardial Infarction Patterns

Inferior Wall Myocardial Infarction

Inferior wall MI is perhaps the most challenging MI pattern for acute management in the ED. It is best seen on the ECG with ST elevations in leads II, III, and aVF. The inferior wall is most often supplied by the right coronary artery (RCA, in about 80%), however, in those with left dominant circulation, the left circumflex can also supply it, and much less frequently, the left anterior descending (LAD) artery.

This distinction is important to note, as inferior wall STEMI can also be suggestive of involvement of other associated vascular territories such as the posterior wall or the right ventricle. Often, the patients presenting with inferior wall MIs can be bradycardic or hypotensive, particularly with proximal lesions of the RCA, due to the proximity of the RCA vascular territory to the major electrical components of the heart. The sinus node is supplied by the RCA in about 60% of cases, and by the left circumflex in the remaining 40%. The atrioventricular (AV) node is supplied by the RCA in 90% of cases, with the left circumflex supplying the remaining 10%, which can subsequently predispose patients with RCA occlusions or left circumflex occlusions to dysrhythmias.[28]

The dominant injured vessel can be indicated by the degree of ST elevation in leads II and III. If there is greater than 1 mm of ST elevation in lead III as compared to lead II, it suggests involvement of the RCA as opposed to the left circumflex due to the direction of the ST segment vector (directed towards the right in lead III).[29-31]

There may also be evidence of ST changes (generally depressions >1 mm) in lead aVL[32] or lead I, which can further implicate the proximal RCA as the occluded vessel. The right ventricle is also supplied by the RCA, and when elevations are noted to be greater in lead III than lead II, the emergency physician should pay close attention to ST changes in lead V1, where elevations combined with an inferior injury pattern can herald proximal RCA occlusion and concomitant RV infarction.[33]

Chia et al. found that ST elevation in lead I was found in 96% of RCA occlusions and therefore concluded that elevation in lead I strongly favors RCA with a sensitivity of 96%, specificity of 85%, positive predictive value of 96%, and negative predictive value of 85%.[34]

Conversely, when the left circumflex is the culprit artery, ST depressions in leads V1 and V2 are more likely. This is because the left circumflex artery produces a stronger vector towards the left (lead II), so there will be more symmetrical elevations in leads II and III and a more isoelectric ST segment in lead I. When combined with a lead II/lead III ratio of 1, these findings better predict left circumflex occlusion/involvement.[34]

This can then be better assessed by placement of lead V4R, which may better demonstrate ST elevations in this setting. V4R should be placed in the same interspace as the left chest leads, in the same location as V4, on the right side of the chest. Elevation greater than or equal to 0.5 mm can indicate RV involvement in the infarct zone.[35]

Right Ventricular Myocardial Infarction

Right ventricular MI occurs most often when there is occlusion proximal to the marginal branches of the RCA, however, can also be seen in left circumflex occlusions or LAD occlusions in those who have left-dominant coronary artery circulation.

Most people have right-dominant circulation, meaning the RCA supplies portions of the right ventricle, the posterior wall of the left ventricle, and the inferior intraventricular septum. In most patients who are RCA dominant, the lateral wall of the right ventricle is supplied by the acute marginal branches, which also support the posterior wall and the posterior intraventricular septum via the posterior descending artery. The anterior wall of the right ventricle is supplied by branches of the LAD.[36,37] A right ventricular myocardial infarction (RVMI) can affect the conduction system of the heart, particularly with proximal RCA lesions due to the vascular territory, which can involve the Bundle of His and the AV node. The most frequent abnormalities found are right bundle branch block (RBBB) and complete heart block.[38]

The presentation in RV infarction can vary from LV infarction, in that you are more likely to appreciate clear lung fields, in conjunction with hypotension (either spontaneously or induced by vasodilator therapy such as nitroglycerin or morphine) and elevated jugular venous pressure (JVP). This triad, although quite specific, only has a sensitivity of 25%.[36,37]

Right ventricular infarction patterns are critical to recognize on ECG. Of note, RV infarctions in one-third of cases are found to accompany inferior wall MI, which is also often caused by occlusion of the RCA. The RVMI is best investigated with lead V4R. In an initial study by Erhardt et al., the researchers demonstrated 70% sensitivity and 100% specificity of lead V4R for right ventricle infarction, as confirmed by autopsy.[39] Additional ECG findings indicative of possible RVMI include ST elevation noted in lead V1 and prominent elevations in lead III in comparison to those in leads II and aVF.

Identifying these RV infarctions is critical, in that once infarctions of the inferior wall and RV are identified, patients should not be given nitroglycerin, or other vasodilator therapy, as they are preload dependent and this can precipitate cardiovascular collapse.

Posterior Wall Myocardial Infarction

A finding of an isolated posterior wall MI is rare, and in isolated posterior MI, the responsible vessel in right-dominant individuals is the posterior LV branch of the RCA, or left circumflex artery in left-dominant patients.[40] The left circumflex artery most often supplies the posterior wall.[41] Portions of the posterior wall can also be supplied by the RCA in some patients. Given this complex blood supply to the posterior left ventricle, it is reasonable to assume that often, in posterior wall MI, there will be other associated ischemic areas such as the inferior lead distribution or lateral wall.

Leads II, III, and aVF may show ST elevations in conjunction with leads V1–V3 showing ST depressions. These ECG findings should be concerning for posterior wall MI, and they can signify a much larger infarct area, thus predisposing the patient to ventricular dysrhythmias, lower ejection fractions, and significantly increased mortality.[41] Therefore, with evidence of either lateral wall or inferior wall ischemia/infarction, posterior left sided leads should be obtained.[42]

Anterior/Lateral Myocardial Infarction

Anterior wall MI is most often due to ischemia stemming from the occlusion of the LAD artery. To identify anterior wall MI on ECG, the septal/anteroseptal leads V1, V2, and V3 should be examined for ST elevations. Anterior-lateral leads are often identified as V3–V6. Reciprocal changes will most frequently be noted in the inferior leads (II, III, aVF), particularly in the occlusive lesions proximal to the take off of S1 (the first septal perforator) or D1 (first diagonal) branch of the LAD.

Additionally, ST elevations in lead aVR may be able to signify proximal occlusion to S1 in the LAD, and is most likely (secondary to the injury current being directed towards the right shoulder) a result of transmural ischemia to the inferior portion of the septum. In a study of 100 patients identified with anterior MI, ST elevations in lead aVR (seen in 43% of patients with proximal lesions to S1 compared to present in 5% distal to S1), complete RBBB (independent indicator for poor prognosis) and ST depressions in lead V5 were all correlated with proximal lesions to S1.[43]

Right bundle branch block is considered a marker of poor prognosis. Typically, mortality/morbidity is not necessarily influenced by the involvement of the conduction system itself, but rather involvement of the conduction system heralds a larger infarct territory. In a study by Ricou et al., 178 patients with anterior MI who had RBBB were found to have higher rates of LV heart failure (72% vs. 52%), increased inhospital (32% vs. 8%) and increased 1-year cardiac mortality rates (17% vs. 7%) when compared to 754 patients who had anterior MI without RBBB.[32]

Anterior MI with occlusions identified proximal to D1 were found to be associated with Q waves in lead aVL (44% in occlusions proximal to D1 compared to 15% Q wave presence in distal lesions). Proximal lesions in the LAD (before the take off of both S1 and D1) were correlated with significant reciprocal depressions greater than 1.0 mm in the inferior leads.[44]

Utility of lead aVR: Lead aVR has been regarded by many as a lead that conveys reciprocal information from the lateral limb and precordial leads, as it does not give a direct view of the ventricles.[45,46] It is an augmented unipolar lead (much like aVL and aVF), in the frontal plane, with aVR having its positive electrode on the right arm, and therefore, offers no direct or specific views of the left ventricle.[46,47] It is geared towards relaying information regarding the upper right portion of the heart including the outflow tract of the right ventricle and basal portion of the intraventricular septum. Until recent years, aVR has been largely ignored in the setting of ECG interpretation in ACS.[48-50]

New studies are showing that ST segment shifts in elevation in aVR can be indicative of many important findings, including multivessel CAD or critical proximal left main coronary artery (LMCA) occlusions. Often, elevations in lead aVR (considered "mirror imaging" of leads V5/V5), with reciprocal ST depression in I, II, and V4-V6 can signify three vessel or LMCA occlusion.[46] This is a profoundly significant finding, in that the LAD artery is crucial for the perfusion of approximately three-fourth of the LV mass. Thus, it would stand to reason that proximal lesions of the trunk can be devastating, with not only profound consequences for the patients ejection fraction, but also can result in arrhythmias for the patient if left undiagnosed.[45-48,50]

Elevations of lead aVR additionally can be of help as predictors of morbidity and mortality in STEMI patients. In a study analyzing 950 patients diagnosed with STEMI, ST elevations were found in 155 (16%) and out of these, 52% of the patients with elevations in aVR were found to have significant LAD occlusions proximal to the S1 branch. Additionally, these patients also experienced higher inhospital mortality rates (19% compared to 5%) as well as lower systolic blood pressures and poorer ejection fractions as well as higher heart rates.[44]

ACUTE CORONARY SYNDROME BIOMARKERS

Early detection of coronary ischemia remains a challenge. In addition to using clinical gestalt and ECG findings, biomarkers and imaging are also critical in assessing the ACS patient. Guideline writing groups have advocated for the diagnosis of AMI based on a rising or falling of cardiac troponin (cTn) in the appropriate clinical situation.[51] When the history and ECG diagnose STEMI, cardiac markers are not required for initial management decisions in the ED.

Markers of Cardiac Injury

Creatinine Phosphokinase

The CK-MB subtype of creatinine phosphokinase (CK) is found in the myocardium. After AMI, CK-MB is detectable in the serum at 3 hours, peaks at 20–24 hours, and becomes normal with 2–4 days after injury.[52,53]

Troponins

Cardiac troponin is the most sensitive and specific biochemical marker used to detect myocardial injury. The European Society for Cardiology (ESC)/World Health Organization (WHO) criteria for the universal definition of AMI is a rising and/or falling pattern of cTn concentrations with at least one value above the 99th percentile limit of the reference value distribution in a patient who has clinical features of myocardial ischemia.[51,54]

Cardiac troponins levels become elevated 2–6 hours from onset of myocardial tissue necrosis. Serum levels peak at 10–24 hours and then again at 72–96 hours due to break down of muscle protein after myocyte death and normalize at 4–14 days.[53,55]

High-sensitivity troponin (hs-cTn) assays can measure cTn in the single digit range of nanograms per liter, therefore providing a more precise calculation of the 99th percentile of cTn concentration in reference subjects.[54,56-58] The Hs-cTns detect troponin release earlier and they detect smaller levels of serum troponin, and therefore, have allowed for the classification of those previously diagnosed as UA to now be diagnosed as having MI.[59-62]

BOX 2 Conditions causing elevated troponin levels in the absence of coronary artery disease

- Heart failure
- Aortic dissection
- Tachyarrhythmias or bradyarrhythmias
- Hypotension
- Hypertensive emergency
- Hypertrophic cardiomyopathy
- Coronary vasculitis
- Coronary endothelial dysfunction
- Myocarditis
- Cardiac incision with surgery
- Peripartum cardiomyopathy
- Frequent defibrillator shocks
- Cardiac contusion
- Cardiotoxic agents
- Severe burns affecting >30% of the body
- Renal failure
- Radiofrequency or cryoablation therapy
- Rhabdomyolysis with cardiac involvement
- Severe pulmonary embolism or pulmonary hypertension
- Apical ballooning syndrome
- Severe acute neurological diseases, e.g. stroke, trauma
- Infiltrative diseases, e.g. amyloidosis, sarcoidosis
- Sepsis
- Acute respiratory failure
- Extreme exertion

Serial enzyme testing of hs-cTn in patients with suspected AMI should be performed on arrival and 3 hours later. The hs-cTn should be measured at 6 hours after admission in patient where there is still a high clinical suspicion for acute MI. Increased baseline hs-cTc without significant dynamic changes is likely a marker of chronic structural heart disease.[54,63]

Box 2 lists possible causes of elevated troponin levels that are not ACS related.[51,54]

Other Cardiac Markers

Cardiac albumin is detectable in serum shortly after transient coronary occlusion. It rises well in advance of myoglobin, CK-MB, and cTn, and has the potential to detect not only infarction, but also early ischemia.[54,64]

Myeloperoxidase is a leukocyte enzyme found in vulnerable coronary plaques that have ruptured. Elevated myeloperoxidase levels are reported to predict short-term risk for adverse cardiac events and death in ED patients with chest pain.[65,52]

N-terminal pro-B-type natriuretic peptide (NT-proBNP) and BNP are widely used as markers for diagnosing congestive heart failure, but they have good predictive value for recurrent ACS events and cardiac-related deaths.[66]

The C-reactive protein (CRP) and highly sensitive CRP (hs-CRP) have long-term prognostic value for cardiac events healthy individuals. C-reactive protein also has potential short-term prognostic implications when combined with other markers such as cTn in patients being evaluated for ACS.[67]

Multiple Marker Strategies

Prior to the implementation of hs-cTn use, using multiple markers seemed to have the potential for improving diagnostic accuracy for the evaluation of ACS. Even at early time points, current laboratory troponins are equivalent if not superior to point-of-care multimarker strategies.[68,69]

With the implementation of hs-cTns, there is no need to test other early markers of acute myocardial necrosis such as myoglobin or CK-MB.[54]

Sabatine used a multimarker approach with a combination of troponin I, CRP, and BNP to assess risk stratification and found that each marker was an independent predictor of the composite of death, MI, or heart failure with the mortality risk nearly doubling as the number of elevated markers increased. Thus, some still advocate for the use of a multimarker approach including troponin and additional markers to enhance risk stratification.[70,71]

Diagnostic Accuracy of Biomarkers for Acute Coronary Syndrome

Presentation Level of Cardiac Enzymes

Standard of care in the evaluation of patients with chest pain includes an ECG, history and physical examination, and laboratory testing which usually includes cardiac biomarkers. Biomarkers have limited utility in patients with ST segment change on the ECG. However, they increase certainty of the diagnosis of ACS in those with ischemic-like changes, nondiagnostic, or normal ECGs. Early positive results of cardiac enzymes can alter the diagnostic course for a patient with a nondiagnostic ECG. Cardiac enzymes are not sensitive for the diagnosis of UA, so the results of a single serum biomarker must be evaluated in context with the history.[72]

The initial cardiac biomarker may not be sufficient to exclude the diagnosis of MI or ACS. A meta-analysis by Goodacre documented the sensitivities and specificities of the troponin at presentation to range from 74 to 82% and 91 to 99% depending on the type of troponin assay utilized. These values are much lower than the sensitivity and specificity obtained from high-sensitivity troponin. Meta-analysis of high-sensitivity troponin assays revealed a sensitivity of 96% and a specificity of 72% for the high-sensitivity troponin T assay while the sensitivity was 83–86% and the specificity was 89–95% for the high-sensitivity troponin I assays.[73] In contrast, a high-sensitivity troponin value below the limit of detection at presentation has a high negative predictive value for excluding the diagnosis of ACS.

Value of Serial Cardiac Enzymes

Serial testing of cardiac enzymes over time increases the sensitivity of the results. The Joint ESC/ACCF/AHA/WHF task force for the universal definition of MI and the National Academy of Clinical Biochemistry recommend a 20% change from an elevated cTn value as an indication of additional myocardial necrosis.[51,74] Studies suggest that an absolute increase of hs-cTnT values is superior to a relative percentage change from the baseline value. Most of this difference is likely due to patients who present late after the onset of symptoms and have higher values at presentation.[75]

The combination of a validated risk stratification tool that identifies patients at low risk for adverse cardiac events and serial negative high-sensitivity troponins can be used to exclude a diagnosis of ACS and identify a very low-risk group for adverse events. The ADAPT trial by Than et al. evaluated an accelerated diagnostic protocol (ADP) that included pretest probability scoring by the Thrombolysis in Myocardial Infarction (TIMI) score, ECG, and 0 + 2 hours values of troponin I. The ADP was found to have a sensitivity of 99.7% and a specificity of 23.4%. Than et al. concluded that a 2-hour ADP could identify a large group of patients who were either suitable for safe early discharge with outpatient follow-up or who could proceed more quickly to further inpatient testing.[69]

Biomarker Summary

Cardiac troponin is the most sensitive and specific biochemical marker of myocardial injury and it is therefore the biomarker of choice for the diagnosis of myocardial necrosis. As troponin assays become more sensitive, excluding the diagnosis of myocardial infarction and identification of groups of patients at lower risk for cardiovascular events can be done using serial less than 3 hours apart in the majority of patients.[54]

CLINICAL DECISION RISK STRATIFICATION TOOLS

Cardiac biomarkers identify patients with MI. In patients with nondiagnostic ECGs, unchanged abnormal ECGs, or normal ECGs, the clinician must decide if emergent additional diagnostic testing needs to be performed to identity patients with UA or high risk for adverse events. The use of validated risk stratification tools for adverse cardiac events or risk of MI can provide the clinician with useful data regarding the likelihood of a cardiac etiology of chest pain. These tools in combination with cardiac biomarkers can assist the clinician with disposition decisions. Clinical decision aids include the TIMI risk score, the HEART score, the Global Registry in Acute Coronary Syndrome (GRACE), the North American Chest Pain Rule (NACPR), the Vancouver Chest Pain Rule, and the pretest consult for ACS. These clinical decision aids were developed using contemporary troponin assays.

Thrombolysis in Myocardial Infarction Risk Score

The TIMI risk score is a risk stratification tool that predicts the risk of adverse events including death and further ischemic events in patients diagnosed with UA/NSTEMI. The TIMI risk score variables are listed in box 3.[76] Adverse event rates increase as the TIMI risk score increases. The TIMI risk scores and the correlating adverse event rates are listed in table 3.

The TIMI risk score is an effective risk stratification tool for ED patients but it should not be used as the sole means for determining patient disposition in the ED because its sensitivity in not adequate to rule out ACS in ED patients.[76-81]

HEART Score

The HEART score was originally developed to help facility decision-making regarding diagnostic and therapeutic strategies for chest pain patients in the ED, in an effort to identify those that may be suitable for discharge without stress testing, etc., as opposed to admission and further inpatient workup, imaging, or provocative studies. It has yet to be adequately validated; however, it does show some promising results for the primary end point goals. Criteria center around the history given by the patient, ECG findings, age, risk factors, and troponin levels obtained during ED stay. Each modifier is given a score based on a point system, with lower HEART scores between 0 and 3 correlating with a 2.5% chance that patients will reach an ultimate poor end point (i.e., ischemic cardiac injury/untoward event) and who are the patients who may be appropriate for discharge and outpatient management. Intermediate HEART scores between 4 and 6 are considered appropriate for admission; with subsequently higher HEART scores correlating with higher risk of acute cardiac event and may ultimately assist in guiding invasive management versus conservative.[82-84]

BOX 3 Thrombolysis in myocardial infarction risk score variables

- Age 65 years or older
- Three or more risk factors for coronary artery disease (HTN, DM, smoking, HDL <40, family history of premature CAD)
- Prior coronary stenosis of 50% or more
- ST segment changes of 0.5 mm or more
- Two or more anginal events in prior 24 hrs
- Use of aspirin in prior 7 days
- Elevated serum cardiac biomarkers

CAD, coronary artery disease; DM, diabetes mellitus; HDL, high density lipoprotein; HTN, hypertension; TIMI, thrombolysis in myocardial infarction.

TABLE 3: Thrombolysis in myocardial infarction (TIMI) risk scores and risk of adverse events[76]

TIMI risk score	Adverse event rate
1	4.7%
2	8.3%
3	13.2%
4	19.9%
5	26.2%
6,7	40.9%

Global Registry in Acute Coronary Syndrome

The GRACE risk model is useful in predicting inhospital and postdischarge mortality or MI. The aggregate of scores is applied to a reference nomogram to determine all-cause mortality from hospital discharge to 6 months. The GRACE risk model can also be used to identify patients who would benefit from an early invasive strategy. The GRACE ACS risk model calculator is available at http://www.outcomes-umassmed.org/grace/. Factors used in the calculation of the GRACE score are listed in table 4.[85-90]

North American Chest Pain Rule

The North American Chest Pain Rule is a risk stratification tool designed to identify ED patients with symptoms suggestive of ACS, but who are at low risk for ACS and thus are safe for early discharge without stress testing or

TABLE 4: GRACE ACS risk model—factors used in calculation[85]

At admission (in-hospital to 6 months)	At discharge (to 6 months)
• Age (years) • HR (BPM) • SBP (mm Hg) • Creatinine (mg/dL) • Congestive heart failure (Killip Class) • Cardiac arrest at admission • ST segment deviation • Elevated cardiac enzymes/markers	• Age (years) • HR (BPM) • SBP (mm Hg) • Creatinine (mg/dL) • Congestive heart failure • In-hospital PCI • In-hospital CABG • Past history of MI • ST segment depression • Elevated cardiac enzymes/markers

ACS, acute coronary syndrome; BPM, beats per minute; CABG, coronary artery bypass graft; GRACE, global registry in acute coronary syndrome; HR, heart rate; MI, myocardial infarction; PCI, percutaneous coronary intervention; SBP, systolic blood pressure.

BOX 4 North American Chest Pain Rule Criteria[90]

High risk criteria

- Age ≥50
- Acute ischemic electrocardiogram changes
- Known coronary artery disease
- Pain typical for acute coronary syndrome
- Troponin >99th percentile

cardiac imaging. The five predictors for outcome are listed in box 4. The NACPR considers patients to be low risk if they do not have any of the high-risk criteria. It has been found to be more than 99% sensitive and 21% specific in evaluating patients as safe for discharge home from the ED but there has not been a prospective clinical trial to further investigate these findings.[52,91]

Vancouver Chest Pain Rule

The Vancouver chest pain rule is also designed to identify patients who are at low risk for ACS and who are safe for early discharge. Criteria include ECG results, historical features, and biomarker measurements. It considers patients younger than 40 years with a normal ECG and no history of ischemic heart disease to be low risk. The CK-MB results are also included. The derivation of the rule documented a 98.8% sensitivity, but recent studies have not validated these results. Replacing the CK-MB with troponin as the biomarker revealed a 91% sensitivity.[65,92] Although the Vancouver chest pain rule has potential, it is not currently recommended since subsequent studies have not validated its results.[53,93]

Pretest Consult for Acute Coronary Syndrome

Kline evaluated an attribute-matching method to generate a pretest probability (PTP) for ACS based on eight clinical variables (attributes) chosen by classification and regression tree analysis of a prospectively collected reference database of 14,796 ED patients evaluated for possible ACS. The eight clinical variables or attributes are listed in box 5. For attribute-matching, a computer program identifies patients within the database who have the exact profile defined by clinician input of the eight attributes. The model only had good utility in patients with very low risk for ACS and cannot be used in patients with ST segment elevation. Using the test threshold approach to diagnostic testing, the authors estimated that patients who have a PTP derived from attribute matching less than 2.5% are unlikely to benefit from further testing for ACS.[94]

BOX 5 Eight clinical variables included in the pretest consult for acute coronary syndrome

- Age
- Gender
- Race
- Diaphoresis
- History of coronary artery disease
- Chest pain worsened with manual palpation
- ST segment depression > –0.5 mm in any two ECG leads
- T-wave inversion > –0.5 mm in any two ECG leads

ECG, electrocardiogram.

Mitchell et al. compared attribute-matching, physician's written unstructured estimate and a logistic regression formula [acute coronary insufficiency-time insensitive predictive instrument (ACI-TIPI)] to determine their diagnostic accuracy in estimating a very low PTP (2%) for ACSs in ED patients evaluated in chest pain units. Unstructured estimate had a sensitivity of 96.1% and a specificity of 27.4%. Attribute-matching had a sensitivity of 98.0% and a specificity of 26.1%. The ACI-TIPI had a sensitivity of 100% and a specificity of 6.1%. They concluded that in a low-risk ED population with symptoms suggestive of ACS, attribute-matching, unstructured estimate, or the ACI-TIPI may identify patients with a PTP less than or equal to 2%, who may not require additional diagnostic testing.[95] This study highlights that the use of clinical decision rules provides the clinician with a standardized mechanism to describe how their decisions are made. However, these decision aids have not been shown to be superior to clinician judgment to identify patients at low risk.

ROLE OF IMAGING IN DIAGNOSIS OF ACUTE CORONARY SYNDROME

In patients who have a nondiagnostic, unchanged, or normal ECG, negative cardiac biomarkers, and the clinician still has concern for an ACS, the AHA/ACC guidelines recommend patients undergo additional diagnostic testing. The goal of coronary imaging in this situation is to find signs of a flow limiting lesions by looking at the coronary vasculature to find evidence of CAD or identifying cardiac tissue findings indicative of epicardial coronary artery flow limitations. Imaging can provide information about the anatomic and dynamic function of the heart, reproduce tissue ischemia, and identify coronary artery lesions.

Echocardiography

Echocardiography is effective in detecting chamber size and shape, wall thickness, regional wall motion abnormalities, and myocardial contractility. Regional wall motion abnormalities on echocardiography can assist in the diagnosis of ACS in patients when the ECG is nondiagnostic and cardiac enzymes are not elevated. Regional wall motion abnormalities documented on echocardiography in a patient without known CAD have a positive predictive value of about 50% for increased likelihood of acute myocardial ischemia. These abnormalities can be visualized within 12–20 seconds after coronary artery occlusion, before the onset of ECG changes or the development of symptoms. The absence of regional wall motion abnormalities has a negative predictive value as high as 98% in cases of suspected MI.[96]

Echocardiography is also essential in diagnosing mechanical complications of MI including cardiac rupture, ventricular septal rupture, acute mitral regurgitation, pericardial effusion, and thrombus formation.[96]

Stress echocardiography obtains images before and after a patient exercises causing graded increases in cardiac workload or after pharmacologic adrenergic stimulating agents, such as dobutamine, or vasodilating agents, such as dipyridamole or adenosine, are given. It has a sensitivity of 61–97% and a specificity of 51–94%. Patients with inducible ischemia identified by stress echocardiography need further evaluation with diagnostic cardiac catheterization.[97] Stress echocardiography is a useful tool to identify patients with flow-limiting lesions during exertion but it is limited by diagnostic difficulties in patients with certain body habitus and requires technician and physician expertise that may not be available at all times.

Myocardial Scintigraphy

Radionuclide myocardial perfusion imaging (rMPI) enables evaluation of cardiac perfusion and function after administration of a radioactive perfusion tracer or radioisotope, commonly technetium-99. Images are usually obtained at rest and after stress. Patients with normal perfusion scans and normal cardiac biomarkers are at low risk for adverse cardiac events. Stress images are obtained after the patient exercises or is given pharmacologic agents or a combination of both. Stress agents used include vasodilators such as adenosine, regadenoson, and dipyridamole and inotropic/chronotropic agents such as dobutamine. Rest and stress images are compared to identify areas of flow-limited obstructive CAD or areas of fixed reduced flow that may result from prior infarction. Stress rMPI detects the presence of CAD by inducing regional ischemia with variable perfusion. Decreased resting perfusion identifies areas of infarction. The sensitivity is 87–93% for detecting coronary stenosis.[98] The radiation exposure is 3-30 mSv.[99]

Cremer et al. reviewed 5,354 patients who had negative troponin tests and subsequent myocardial perfusion images. They noted that patients with TIMI scores less than or equal to 2 had greater than 5% ischemic myocardium in contrast to 19.6% of patients with TIMI scores less than or equal to 3. They concluded that routine provocative testing with myocardial perfusion imaging to detect ischemia prior to ED discharge is low yield in patients with negative troponins and TIMI scores less than or equal to 2 and modest yield in patients with TIMI scores greater than or equal to 3.[100] This study again supports the use of risk stratification tools to help identify patients with sufficiently low risk for adverse cardiac events that additional diagnostic testing is not needed.

Exercise Treadmill Testing

During exercise treadmill testing, 12-lead ECG tracings are obtained as the patient has a graded increase in exercise. Its sensitivity for diagnosing inducible ischemia and obstructive CAD is 68% while the specificity is 77%. The specificity of the test is decreased when ECG abnormalities are present secondary to left ventricular hypertrophy (LVH), electrolyte abnormalities, medications, or artifact. There is also an increase in false-positive results in women.[52,101]

Gibler studied low-risk chest pain patients who underwent exercise testing after serial biomarkers and 9 hours of ECG monitoring. Stress testing had a negative predictive value of 98.7% for the diagnosis of ACS or cardiac event within 30 days.[102] A similar study by Amsterdam et al. looked at immediate exercise testing performed after a single normal cTn level and noted similar sensitivity and specificities with low rates of adverse events.[103]

Absolute contraindications to exercise treadmill testing include recent MI (within 2 days), high-risk UA, uncontrolled cardiac dysrhythmias causing hemodynamic compromise, symptomatic severe aortic stenosis, uncontrolled symptomatic heart failure, acute pulmonary embolus, acute myocarditis or pericarditis, and acute aortic dissection.[104]

Calcium Scoring Coronary Computed Tomography

Calcium scoring coronary computed tomography is a noninvasive means to visualize the wall composition of the coronary arteries. Patients need to have a heart rate less than 65 beats/min to get appropriately gated images, requiring β-blockage for most patients. A calcium score of 0 indicates that there is minimal or no calcified CAD suggesting a lower likelihood of ACS. This scan is usually done as the first phase of the coronary computed tomography angiography (CCTA).[53]

Coronary Computed Tomography Angiography

The best noninvasive method for imaging the coronary arteries is high-resolution CCTA with multidetector or multislice scanners.[105] The diagnostic quality of CCTA is limited if the heart rate is greater 65–70 beats/min, there is an irregular heart rhythm, if the patient is not able to hold their breath for 5 seconds, if there is severe coronary calcification, coronary artery stents are present, or if the segments have a diameter less than 1.5 mm.[106,107] The CCTA can identify CAD in 83–94% of patients. The CCTA delivers 10–15 mSv of radiation, but low-dose radiations protocols are being adopted with radiation dosages ranging from 1 to 8 mSv.[53,108,109] There are, however, logistic challenges to implementation of these protocols.

Cardiac Magnetic Resonance Imaging

Cardiac magnetic resonance (CMR) imaging obtains images during stages of the cardiac cycle and then creates a dynamic clip of myocardial function. The CMR is able to assess cardiac structure and function during a single examination. The T2-weighted images can assess resting wall motion, stress wall motion, resting perfusion, stress perfusion, myocardial edema, and delayed enhancement. The combination of T2 imaging with delayed enhancement helps to differentiate new and old infarcts. The T2 has even identified edema as an early sign of ischemia before troponin elevation. Disadvantages of CMR include exposure to gadolinium-containing contrast agents, prolonged time required for the scan, and lower accuracy compared to CCTA.[53,110,111]

Diagnostic Cardiac Catheterization

Cardiac catheterization with coronary angiography is the gold standard for the diagnosis of CAD. Patients with non-ST segment elevation acute coronary syndrome (NSTEACS) are assigned to one of the three categories depending on their risk assessment—immediate angiography, an invasive approach, or a conservative approach.

Immediate angiography followed by revascularization is performed soon after the diagnosis is made and is indicated for patients assessed to have a poor short or long-term prognosis due to NSTEACS. Immediate angiography is recommended for those with hemodynamic instability, severe LV dysfunction or overt heart failure, recurrent or persistent rest angina despite medical therapy, mechanical complications such as acute mitral regurgitation or ventricular septal defect, sustained ventricular tachycardia, and dynamic ST-T-wave electrocardiographic changes.[112]

The invasive strategy of angiography followed by revascularization is usually performed within 4–48 hours of admission and is aimed at improving long-term prognosis. This approach can limit the extent of MI and improve long-term prognosis. Partial patency of the infarcted artery is noted in 60–85% of these patients.[112,113] A meta-analysis by Bavry et al. concluded that an invasive approach led to better outcomes compared to a conservative approach.[114] Treat angina with aggrastat and determine cost of therapy with invasive or conservative strategy (TACTICS)-TIMI 18 evaluated the relationship between TIMI risk score and benefit from an invasive strategy. There was a significant reduction in death, MI, and rehospitalization for ACS within the 6 month follow-up period with the invasive approach in patients at intermediate TIMI risk with scores of 3–4 and particularly in those with high risk TIMI scores of 5–7.[115,116] Patients at highest risk at presentation have the largest benefit from an early invasive strategy.[117]

If the short-term risk of death or recurrent MI is considered to be low, a conservative approach can be followed where medical therapy is combined with risk stratification with noninvasive testing of LV function and stress testing. Coronary catheterization is indicated for significant ischemia on stress testing, recurrent angina, or reduced LV function.[117,118]

CONCLUSION

Accurate diagnosis of ACS in patients presenting to the ED requires assessment of the history and physical examination, 12-lead ECG, and serum cardiac biomarkers. The history and initial ECG are used to identify STEMI. If STEMI is not identified on the initial ECG, cardiac biomarkers can identify NSTEMI. Troponin is considered the gold standard of the cardiac biomarkers. Cardiac imaging is recommended for patients who are at risk for ACS, but do not have STEMI necessitating need for immediate cardiac catheterization.

REFERENCES

1. Myocardial infarction redefined – a consensus document of The Joint European Society of Cardiology/American College of Cardiology Committee for the redefinition of myocardial infarction. Eur Heart J. 2000;21(18):1502-13.
2. Jacobson C. ECG diagnosis of acute coronary syndrome. AACN Adv Crit Care. 2008;19(1):101-8.
3. Anderson JL, Adams CD, Antman EM, Bridges CR, Califf RM, Casey DE, et al. 2011 ACCF/AHA Focused Update Incorporated Into the ACC/AHA 2007 Guidelines for the Management of Patients With Unstable Angina/Non-ST-Elevation Myocardial Infarction: a report of the American College of Cardiology Foundation/American Heart Association Task Force on Practice Guidelines. Circulation. 2011;123(18):e426-579.
4. Marshall K. Acute coronary syndrome: diagnosis, risk assessment and management. Nurs Stand. 2011;25(23):47-57.
5. Canto JG, Canto EA, Goldberg RJ. Time to standardize and broaden the criteria of acute coronary syndrome symptom presentations in women. Can J Cardiol. 2014;30(7):721-8.
6. Canto JG, Goldberg RJ, Hand MM, Bonow RO, Sopko G, Pepine CJ, et al. Symptom presentation of women with acute coronary syndromes. Arch Intern Med. 2007;167(22):2405-13.
7. Coventry LL, Finn J, Bremner AP. Sex differences in symptom presentation in acute myocardial infarction: a systematic review and meta-analysis. Heart Lung Circ. 2011;20:S6-7.
8. Chen W, Woods SL, Puntillo KA. Gender differences in symptoms associated with acute myocardial infarction: a review of the research. Heart Lung. 2005;34(4):240-7.
9. Shin JY, Martin R, Suls J. Meta-analytic evaluation of gender differences and symptom measurement strategies in acute coronary syndromes. Heart Lung. 2010;39(4):283-95.
10. DeVon HA, Ryan CJ, Ochs AL, Shapiro M. Symptoms across the continuum of acute coronary syndromes: differences between women and men. Am J Crit Care. 2008;17(1):14-25.

11. Aziz F. Coronary artery disease in women: an unsolved dilemma. J Clin Med Res. 2014;6(2):86-90.
12. Bucholz EM, Butala NM, Rathore SS, Dreyer RP, Lansky AJ, Krumholz HM. Sex differences in long-term mortality after myocardial infarction: a systematic review. Circulation. 2014;130(9):757-67.
13. Biava LM, Scacciatella P, Calcagnile C, Dalmasso P, Conrotto F, Fanelli AL, et al. Sex-related differences in patients with ST-elevation myocardial infarction undergoing primary PCI: A long-term mortality study. Cardiovasc Revasc Med. 2015;16(3):135-40.
14. Goodacre S, Locker T, Morris F, Campbell S. How useful are clinical features in the diagnosis of acute, undifferentiated chest pain? Acad Emerg Med. 2002;9(3):203-8.
15. Jneid H. The 2012 ACCF/AHA Focused Update Of The Unstable Angina/Non-ST-Elevation Myocardial Infarction (UA/NSTEMI) Guideline: a critical appraisal. Methodist Debakey Cardiovasc J. 2012;8(3):26-30.
16. Hamm CW, Bassand JP, Agewall S, Bax J, Boersma E, Bueno H, et al. ESC Guidelines for the management of acute coronary syndromes in patients presenting without persistent ST-segment elevation: The Task Force for the management of acute coronary syndromes (ACS) in patients presenting without persistent ST-segment elevation of the European Society of Cardiology (ESC). Eur Heart J. 2011;32(23):2999-3054.
17. Rapezzi C, Biagini E, Branzi A. Guidelines for the diagnosis and treatment of non-ST-segment elevation acute coronary syndromes: the task force for the diagnosis and treatment of non-ST-segment elevation acute coronary syndromes of the European Society of Cardiology. Eur Heart J. 2008;29(2):277-8.
18. Diercks DB, Kirk JD, Lindsell CJ, Pollack CV, Hoekstra JW, Gibler WB, et al. Door-to-ECG time in patients with chest pain presenting to the ED. Am J Emerg Med. 2006;24(1):1-7.
19. Takakuwa KM, Burek GA, Estepa AT, Shofer FS. A method for improving arrival-to-electrocardiogram time in emergency department chest pain patients and the effect on door-to-balloon time for ST-segment elevation myocardial infarction. Acad Emerg Med. 2009;16(10):921-7.
20. Fuchs RM, Achuff SC, Grunwald L, Yin FC, Griffith LS. Electrocardiographic localization of coronary artery narrowings: studies during myocardial ischemia and infarction in patients with one-vessel disease. Circulation. 1982;66(6): 1168-76.
21. Kidambi A, Mather AN, Uddin A, Motwani M, Ripley DP, Herzog BA, et al. Reciprocal ECG change in reperfused ST-elevation myocardial infarction is associated with myocardial salvage and area at risk assessed by cardiovascular magnetic resonance. Heart. 2013;99(22):1658-62.
22. Rautaharju PM, Surawicz B, Gettes LS, Bailey JJ, Childers R, Deal BJ, et al. AHA/ACCF/HRS recommendations for the standardization and interpretation of the electrocardiogram: part IV: the ST segment, T and U waves, and the QT interval: a scientific statement from the American Heart Association Electrocardiography and Arrhythmias Committee, Council on Clinical Cardiology; the American College of Cardiology Foundation; and the Heart Rhythm Society: endorsed by the International Society for Computerized Electrocardiology. Circulation. 2009;119(10):e241-50.
23. Kracoff OH, Adelman AG, Marquis JF, Caspi A, Aldridge HE, Schwartz L. Twelve-lead electrocardiogram recording during percutaneous transluminal coronary angioplasty. Analysis of reciprocal changes. J Electrocardiol. 1990; 23(3):191-8.
24. Ross J. Electorcardiographic ST-segment analysis in the characterization of myocardial ischemia and infarction. Circulation. 1976;53(3):173-81.
25. Falk E. Plaque rupture with severe pre-existing stenosis precipitating coronary thrombosis. Characteristics of coronary atherosclerotic plaques underlying fatal occlusive thrombi. Br Heart J. 1983;50(2):127-34.
26. Nable JV, Brady W. The evolution of electrocardiographic changes in ST-segment elevation myocardial infarction. Am J Emerg Med. 2009;27(6):734-46.
27. American College of Emergency Physicians; Society for Cardiovascular Angiography and Interventions, O'Gara PT, Kushner FG, Ascheim DD, Casey DE, et al. 2013 ACCF/AHA guideline for the management of ST-elevation myocardial infarction: a report of the American College of Cardiology Foundation/American Heart Association Task Force on Practice Guidelines. J Am Coll Cardiol. 2013;61(4):e78-140.
28. Zimetbaum PJ, Josephson ME. Use of the electrocardiogram in acute myocardial infarction. N Engl J Med. 2003;348(10): 933-40.
29. Blanke H, Cohen M, Schlueter GU, Karsch KR, Rentrop KP. Electrocardiographic and coronary arteriographic correlations during acute myocardial infarction. Am J Cardiol. 1984;54(3):249-55.
30. Wong TW, Huang XH, Liu W, Ng K, Ng KS. New electrocardiographic criteria for identifying the culprit artery in inferior wall acute myocardial infarction: usefulness of T-wave amplitude ratio in leads II/III and T-wave polarity in the right V5 lead. Am J Cardiol. 2004;94(9):1168-71.
31. Bayram E, Atalay C. Identification of the culprit artery involved in inferior wall acute myocardial infarction using electrocardiographic criteria. J Int Med Res. 2004;32(1):39-44.
32. Ricou F, Nicod P, Gilpin E, Henning H, Ross J. Influence of right bundle branch block on short- and long-term survival after acute anterior myocardial infarction. J Am Coll Cardiol. 1991;17(4):858-63.
33. Herz I, Assali AR, Adler Y, Solodky A, Sclarovsky S. New electrocardiographic criteria for predicting either the right or left circumflex artery as the culprit coronary artery in inferior wall acute myocardial infarction. Am J Cardiol. 1997;80(10):1343-5.
34. Chia BL, Yip JW, Tan HC, Lim YT. Usefulness of ST elevation II/III ratio and ST deviation in lead I for identifying the culprit artery in inferior wall acute myocardial infarction. Am J Cardiol. 2000;86(3):341-3.
35. Nair R, Glancy DL. ECG discrimination between right and left circumflex coronary arterial occlusion in patients with acute inferior myocardial infarction: value of old criteria and use of lead aVR. Chest. 2002;122(1):134-9.
36. Dell'Italia LJ, Starling MR, O'Rourke RA. Physical examination for exclusion of hemodynamically important right ventricular infarction. Ann Inter Med. 1983;99(5):608-11.
37. Kinch JW, Ryan TJ. Right ventricular infarction. N Engl J Med. 1994;330(17): 1211-17.
38. Bodenhamer J. Electrocardiographic manifestations of right ventricular infarction. Ann Emerg Med. 1989;18(11):1251.
39. Erhardt LR, Sjögren A, Wahlberg I. Single right-sided precordial lead in the diagnosis of right ventricular involvement in inferior myocardial infarction. Am Heart J. 1976;91(5):571-6.
40. Brown DF, Nadel ES. Posterior wall myocardial infarction. J Emerg Med. 2004;27(1):75-8.
41. Brady WJ, Erling B, Pollack M, Chan TC. Electrocardiographic manifestations: acute posterior wall myocardial infarction. J Emerg Med. 2001;20(4):391-401.
42. Aqel RA, Hage FG, Ellipeddi P, Blackmon L, McElderry HT, Kay GN, et al. Usefulness of three posterior chest leads for the detection of posterior wall acute myocardial infarction. Am J Cardiol. 2009;103(2):159-164.
43. Engelen DJ, Gorgels AP, Cheriex EC, De Muinck ED, Ophuis AJ, Dassen WR, et al. Value of the electrocardiogram in localizing the occlusion site in the left anterior descending coronary artery in acute anterior myocardial infarction. J Am Coll Cardiol. 1999;34(2):389-95.
44. Aygul N, Ozdemir K, Tokac M, Aygul MU, Duzenli MA, Abaci A, et al. Value of lead aVR in predicting acute occlusion of proximal left anterior descending coronary artery and in-hospital outcome in ST-elevation myocardial infarction: an electrocardiographic predictor of poor prognosis. J Electrocardiol. 2008;41(4):335-41.
45. Tamura A. Significance of lead aVR in acute coronary syndrome. World J Cardiol. 2014;6(7):630-7.
46. Gorgels AP, Engelen DJ, Wellens HJ. Lead aVR, a mostly ignored but very valuable lead in clinical electrocardiography. J Am Coll Cardiol. 2001;38(5):1355-6.
47. Yamaji H, Iwasaki K, Kusachi S. Prediction of acute left main coronary artery obstruction by 12-lead electrocardiography. ST segment elevation in lead aVR with less ST segment elevation in lead V1. ACC Curr J Rev. 2002;11(2):38-9.
48. Riera AR, Ferreira C, Ferreira Filho C, Dubner S, Barbosa Barros R, Femena F, et al. Clinical Value of Lead aVR. Ann Noninvasive Electrocardiol. 2011; 16(3):295-302.
49. Williamson K, Mattu A, Plautz CU, Binder A, Brady WJ. Electrocardiographic applications of lead aVR. Am J Emerg Med. 2006;24(7):864-74.
50. Rostoff P, Piwowarska W, Konduracka E, Libionka A, Bobrowska-Juszczuk M, Stopyra K, et al. Value of lead aVR in the detection of significant left main coronary artery stenosis in acute coronary syndrome. Kardiol Pol. 2005;62(2):128-35.
51. Thygesen K, Alpert JS, White HD, Joint ESC/ACCF/AHA/WHF Task Force for the Redefinition of Myocardial Infarction. Universal definition of myocardial infarction. Eur Heart J. 2007;28(20):2525-38.
52. Rosen P, Marx J, Hockberger R, Walls R, Adams J. Rosen's Emergency Medicine. Philadelphia, PA: Mosby Elsevier; 2006.
53. Mattu A, Brady W, Bresler M, Stahmer S, Tabas J. Cardiovascular Emergencies. Dallas, TX: American College of Emergency Physicians; 2014.
54. Roffi M, Patrono C, Collet JP, Mueller C, et al. 2015 ESC Guidelines for the management of acute coronary syndromes in patients presenting without

persistent ST-segment elevation: Task Force for the Management of Acute Coronary Syndromes in Patients Presenting without Persistent ST-Segment Elevation of the European Society of Cardiology (ESC). Eur Heart J. 2016;37(3):267-315.

55. Pant S, Deshmukh A, Neupane P, Kumar MPK, Vijayashankar CS. Cardiac biomarkers. In: Lakshmanadoss U (Ed). Novel Strategies in Ischemic Heart Disease. 2012. [online] Available from www.intechopen.com/books/novel-strategies-in-ischemic-heartdisease/biomarkers-in-ischemic-heart-disease. [Accessed February, 2016].
56. Saenger A, Beyrau R, Braun S, Cooray R, Dolci A, Freidank H, et al. Multicenter analytical evaluation of a high-sensitivity troponin T assay. Clin Chim Acta. 2011;412(9-10):748-54.
57. Zaninotto M, Mion M, Novello E, Moretti M, Delprete E, Rocchi MB, et al. Precision performance at low levels and 99th percentile concentration of the Access AccuTnI assay on two different platforms. Clin Chem Lab Med. 2009;47(3):367-71.
58. Todd J, Freese B, Lu A, Held D, Morey J, Livingston R, et al. Ultrasensitive flow-based immunoassays using single-molecule counting. Clin Chem. 2007;53(11):1990-5.
59. Reichlin T, Hochholzer W, Bassetti S, Steuer S, Stelzig C, Hartwiger S, et al. Early diagnosis of myocardial infarction with sensitive cardiac troponin assays. N Eng J Med. 2009;361(9):858-67.
60. Weber M, Bazzino O, Navarro Estrada JL, de Miguel R, Salzberg S, Fuselli JJ, et al. Improved diagnostic and prognostic performance of a new high-sensitive troponin T assay in patients with acute coronary syndrome. Am Heart J. 2011;162(1):81-8.
61. Keller T, Zeller T, Peetz D, Tzikas S, Roth A, Czyz E, et al. Sensitive troponin I assay in early diagnosis of acute myocardial infarction. N Eng J Med. 2009;361(9):868-77.
62. Reichlin T, Irfan A, Twerenbold R, Reiter M, Hochholzer W, Burkhalter H, et al. Utility of absolute and relative changes in cardiac troponin concentrations in the early diagnosis of acute myocardial infarction. Circulation. 2011;124(2):136-45.
63. de Lemos J, Drazner M, Omland T, Ayers C, Khera A, Rohatgi A, et al. Association of troponin T detected with a highly sensitive assay and cardiac structure and mortality risk in the general population. JAMA. 2010;304(22):2503-12.
64. Keating L, Benger JR, Beetham R, Bateman S, Veysey S, Kendall J, et al. The PRIMA study: pre-ischemia-modified albumin in the emergency department. Emerg Med J. 2006;23(10):764-8.
65. Brennan ML, Penn MS, Van Lente F, Nambi V, Shishehbor MH, Aviles RJ, et al: Prognostic value of myeloperoxidase in patients with chest pain. N Engl J Med. 2003;349(17):1595-604.
66. Goetze JP, Christoffersen P, Perko M, Arendrup H, Rehfeld JF, Kastrup J, et al. Increased cardiac BNP expression associated with myocardial ischemia. FASEB J. 2003;17(9):1105 -7.
67. Emerging Risk Factor Collaboration, Kaptoge S, DiAngelantonio E, Lowe G, Pepys MB, Thompson SG, et al. C-reactive protein concentrations and risk of coronary heart disease, stroke and mortality: an individual participant metanalysis. Lancet. 2010;375(9709):132-40.
68. Lee-Lewandrowski E, Januzzi JL, Grisson R, Mohammed AA, Lewandrowski G, Lewandrowski K. Evaluation of first-draw whole blood, point-of-care cardiac markers in the context of the universal definition of myocardial infarction: a comparison of a multimarker panel to troponin alone and to testing in the central laboratory. Arch Pathol Lab Med. 2011;135(4):459-63.
69. Than M, Cullen L, Aldous S, Parsonage WA, Reid CM, Greenslade J, et al. 2-Hour accelerated diagnostic protocol to assess patients with chest pain symptoms using contemporary troponins as the only biomarker: the ADAPT trial. J Am Coll Cardiol. 2012;59(23):2091-8.
70. Sabatine MS, Morrow DA, de Lemos JA, Gibson CM, Murphy SA, Rifai N, et al. Multimarker approach to risk stratification in non-ST elevation acute coronary syndromes: simultaneous assessment of troponin I, C-reactive protein, and B-type natriuretic peptide. Circulation. 2002;105(15):1760-3.
71. Kumar A, Cannon CP. Acute coronary syndromes: diagnosis and management, part I. Mayo Clin Proc. 2009;84(10):917-38.
72. Balk EM, Ioannidis JP, Salem D, Chew PW, Lau J. Accuracy of biomarkers to diagnose acute cardiac ischemia in the emergency department: a meta-analysis. Ann Emerg Med. 2001;37(5):478-94.
73. Goodacre S, Thokala P, Carroll C, Stevens JW, Leaviss J, Al Khalaf M, et al. Systematic review, meta-analysis and economic modelling of diagnostic strategies for suspected acute coronary syndrome. Health Technol Assess. 2013;17(1):v-vi, 1-188.
74. Morrow DA, Cannon CP, Jesse RL, Newby LK, Ravkilde J, Storrow AB, et al. National Academy of Clinical Biochemistry practice guidelines: clinical characteristics and utilization of biomarkers in acute coronary syndromes. Clin Chem. 2007;53(4):552-74.
75. Mueller M, Biener M, Vafaie M, Doerr S, Keller T, Blankenberg S, et al. Absolute and relative kinetic changes of high-sensitivity cardiac troponin T in acute coronary syndrome and in patients with increased troponin in the absence of acute coronary syndrome. Clin Chem. 2012;58(1):209-18.
76. Antman EM, Cohen M, Bernink PJ, McCabe CH, Horacek T, Papuchis G, et al. The TIMI risk score for unstable angina/non-ST Elevation MI: A method for prognostication and therapeutic decision making. JAMA. 2000;284(7):835-42.
77. Hess EP, Agarwal D, Chandra S, Murad MH, Erwin PJ, Hollander JE, et al. Diagnostic accuracy of the TIMI risk score in patients with chest pain in the emergency department: a meta-analysis. CMAJ. 2010;182(10):1039-44.
78. Chase M, Robey JL, Zogby KE, Sease KL, Shofer FS, Hollander JE. Prospective validation of the Thrombolysis in Myocardial Infarction Risk Score in the emergency department chest pain population. Ann Emerg Med. 2006;48(3):252-9.
79. Lyon R, Morris AC, Caesar D, Gray S, Gray A. Chest pain presenting to the Emergency Department—to stratify risk with GRACE or TIMI? Resuscitation. 2007;74(1):90-3.
80. Pollack CV, Sites FD, Shofer FS, Sease KL, Hollander JE. Application of the TIMI risk score for unstable angina and non-ST elevation acute coronary syndrome to an unselected emergency department chest pain population. Acad Emerg Med. 2006;13(1):13-8.
81. Hollander J. Prospective validation of the Thrombolysis in Myocardial Infarction (TIMI) risk score in the emergency department chest pain patient population. Acad Emerg Med. 2005;12(Suppl 1):133.
82. Backus BE, Six AJ, Kelder JC, Mast TP, van den Akker F, Mast EG, et al. Chest pain in the emergency room: a multicenter validation of the HEART Score. Crit Pathw Cardiol. 2010;9(3):164-9.
83. Six AJ, Backus BE, Kelder JC. Chest pain in the emergency room: value of the HEART score. Neth Heart J. 2008;16(6):191-6.
84. Backus BE, Six AJ, Kelder JC, Bosschaert MA, Mast EG, Mosterd A, et al. A prospective validation of the HEART score for chest pain patients at the emergency department. Int J Cardiol. 2013;168(3):2153-8.
85. Granger CB, Goldberg RJ, Dabbous O, Pieper KS, Eagle KA, Cannon CP, et al. Predictors of hospital mortality in the global registry of acute coronary events. Arch Intern Med. 2003;163(19):2345-53.
86. Eagle KA, Lim MJ, Dabbous OH, Pieper KS, Goldberg RJ, Van de Werf F, et al. A validated prediction model for all forms of acute coronary syndrome: estimating the risk of 6-month postdischarge death in an international registry. JAMA. 2004;291(22):2727-33.
87. Abu-Assi E, Ferreira-Gonzalez I, Ribera A, Marsal JR, Cascant P, Heras M, et al. "Do GRACE (Global Registry of Acute Coronary events) risk scores still maintain their performance for predicting mortality in the era of contemporary management of acute coronary syndromes?". Am Heart J. 2010;160(5):826-34.e1-3.
88. Eggers KM, Kempf T, Venge P, Wallentin L, Wollert KC, Lindahl B. Improving long-term risk prediction in patients with acute chest pain: the Global Registry of Acute Coronary Events (GRACE) risk score is enhanced by selected nonnecrosis biomarkers. Am Heart J. 2010;160(1):88-94.
89. Mehta SR, Granger CB, Boden WE, Steg PG, Bassand JP, Faxon DP, et al. Early versus delayed invasive intervention in acute coronary syndromes. N Engl J Med. 2009;360(21):2165-75.
90. Amsterdam EA, Wenger NK, Brindis RG, Casey DE, Ganiats TG, Holmes DR, et al. 2014 AHA/ACC guideline for the management of patients with non-ST-elevation acute coronary syndromes: a report of the American College of Cardiology/American Heart Association Task Force on Practice Guidelines. Circulation. 2014;130(25):e344-426.
91. Mahler SA, Miller CD, Hollander JE, Nagurney JT, Birkhahn R, Singer AJ, et al. Identifying patients for early discharge: performance of decision rules among patients with acute chest pain. Int J Cardiol. 2013;168(2):795-802.
92. Shroeder S, Kopp AF, Kuettner A, Burgstahler C, Herdeg C, Heuschmid M, et al. Influence of heart rate on vessel visibility in noninvasive coronary angiography using new multislice computed tomography: experience in 94 patients. Clin Imaging. 2002; 26(2):106-11.
93. Greenslade JH, Cullen L, Than M, Aldous S, Chu K, Brown AF, et al. Validation of the Vancouver Chest Pain Rule using troponin as the only biomarker: a prospective cohort study. Am J Emerg Med. 2013;31(7):1103-7.

94. Kline JA, Johnson CL, Pollack CV, Diercks DB, Hollander JE, Newgard CD, et al. Pretest probability assessment derived from attribute matching. BMC Med Inform Decis Mak. 2005;5:26.
95. Mitchell AM, Garvey JL, Chandra A, Diercks D, Pollack CV, Kline JA. Prospective multicenter study of quantitative pretest probability assessment to exclude acute coronary syndrome for patients evaluated in emergency department chest pain units. Ann Emerg Med. 2006;47(5):447.
96. Cheitlin M, Armstrong WF, Aurigemma GP, Beller GA, Bierman FZ, Davis JL, et al. ACC/AHA/ASE 2003 guideline update for the clinical application of echocardiography: summary article: a report of the American College of Cardiology/American Heart Association Task Force on Practice Guidelines (ACC/AHA/ASE Committee to Update the 1997 Guidelines for the Clinical Application of Echocardiography). Circulation. 2003;108(9):1146-62.
97. Sabia P, Afrookteh A, Touchstone DA, Keller MW, Esquivel L, Kaul S. Value of regional wall motion abnormality in the emergency room diagnosis of acute myocardial infarction: a prospective study using two-dimensional echocardiography. Circulation. 1991;84 (3 Suppl);185-92.
98. Beller GA. Myocardial perfusion imaging for detection of silent myocardial ischemia. Am J Cardiol. 1988;61(12):22F-28F.
99. Cerqueira MD, Allman KC, Ficaro EP, Hansen CL, Nichols KJ, Thompson RC, et al. Recommendations for reducing radiation exposure in myocardial perfusion imaging. J Nuc Cardiol. 2010;17(4):709-18.
100. Cremer P, Khalaf S, Agarwal S, Mayer-Sabik E, Ellis S, Menon V, et al. Myocardial perfusion imaging in emergency department patients with negative cardiac biomarkers: yield for detecting ischemia, short-term events, and impact of downstream revascularization on mortality. Circ Cardiovasc Imaging. 2014;7(6):912-9.
101. Amsterdam EA, Kirk JD, Diercks DB, Lewis WR, Turnipseed SD. Exercise testing in chest pain units: rationale, implantation, and results. Cardiol Clin. 2005;23(4):503-16, vii.
102. Gibler WB, Runyon JP, Levy RC, Sayre MR, Kacich R, Hattemer CR, et al. A rapid diagnostic and treatment center for patients with chest pain in the emergency department. Ann Emerg Med. 1995;25(1):1-8.
103. Amsterdam EA, Kirk JD, Diercks DB, Lewis WR, Turnipseed SD. Immediate exercise testing to evaluate low-risk patients presenting to the emergency department with chest pain. J Am Coll Cardiol. 2002;40(2):251-6.
104. Gibbons R, Balady GJ, Bricker JT, Chaitman BR, Fletcher GF, Froelicher VF, et al. ACC/AHA 2002 guideline update for exercise testing: summary article: a report of the American College of Cardiology/American Heart Association Task Force on Practice Guidelines (Committee to Update the 1997 Exercise Testing Guidelines). Circulation. 2002;106(14):1883-92.
105. Fox KA, Poole-Wilson P, Clayton TC, Henderson RA, Shaw TR, Wheatley DJ, et al. 5-year outcome of an interventional strategy in non-ST-elevation acute coronary syndrome: the British Heart Foundation RITA 3 randomised trial. Lancet. 2005;366(9489):914-20.
106. Leber AW, Knez A, von Ziegler F, Becker A, Nikolaou K, Paul S, et al. Quantification of obstructive and nonobstructive coronary lesions by 64-slice computed tomography: a comparative study with quantitative coronary angiography and intravascular ultrasound. J Am Coll Cardiol. 2005;46(1):147-54.
107. Raff GL, Gallagher MJ, O'Neill WW, Goldstein JA. Diagnostic accuracy of noninvasive coronary angiography using 64-slice spiral computed tomography. J Am Coll Cardiol. 2005;46(3):552-7.
108. Fine JJ, Hopkins CB, Ruff N, Newton FC. Comparison of accuracy of 64-slice cardiovascular computed tomography with coronary angiography in patients with suspected coronary artery disease. Am J Cardiol. 2006;97(2):173-4.
109. Fazel R, Krumholz HM, Wang Y, Ross JS, Chen J, Ting HH, et al. Exposure to low-dose ionizing radiation from medical imaging procedures. New Engl J Med. 2009;361(9):849-57.
110. Miller CD, Hwang W, Hoekstra JW, Case D, Lefebvre C, Blumstein H, et al. Stress cardiac magnetic resonance imaging with observation unit care reduces cost for patients with emergency chest pain: a randomized trial. Ann Emerg Med. 2010;56(3):209-219.e2.
111. Curry RC, Shash K, Nagurney JT, Rosito G, Shapiro MD, Nomura CH, et al. Cardiac magnetic resonance with T2-weighted imaging improves detection of patients with acute coronary syndrome in the emergency department. Circulation. 2008;118(8):837-44.
112. Liebson PR, Klein LW. The non-Q wave myocardial infarction revisited: 10 years later. Prog Cardivasc Dis. 1997;39(5):399-444.
113. Kerensky RA, Wade M, Deedwania P, Boden WE, Pepine CJ; Veterans Affairs Non-Q-Wave Infarction Stategies in-Hospital (VANQWISH) Trial Investigators. Revisiting the culprit lesion in non-Q wave myocardial infarction. Results from the VANQWISH trial angiographic core laboratory. J Am Coll Cardiol. 2002;39(9):1456-63.
114. Bavry AA, Kumbhani DJ, Rassi AN, Bhatt DL, Askari AT. Benefit of early invasive therapy in acute coronary syndromes: a meta-analysis of contemporary randomized clinical trials. J Am Coll Cardiol. 2006; 48(7):1319-25.
115. Cannon CP, Weintraub WS, Demopoulos LA, Vicari R, Frey MJ, Lakkis N, et al. Comparison of early invasive and conservative strategies in patients with unstable coronary syndromes treated with the glycoprotein IIb/IIIa inhibitor tirofiban. N Engl J Med. 2001;344(25):187987.
116. Sabatine MS, Morrow DA, Giugliano RP, Murphy SA, Demopoulos LA, DiBattiste PM, et al. Implications of upstream glycoprotein IIb/IIIa inhibition and coronary artery stenting in the invasive management of unstable angina/non-ST-elevation myocardial infarction: a comparison of the Thrombolysis In Myocardial Infarction (TIMI) IIIB trial and the Treat angina with Aggrastat and determine Cost of Therapy with Invasive or Conservative Strategy (TACTICS)-TIMI 18 trial. Circulation. 2004;109(7):874-80.
117. Amsterdam EA, Wenger NK, Brindis RG, Casey DE, Ganiats TG, Holmes DR, et al. 2014 AHA/ACC guideline for the management of patients with non-st-elevation acute coronary syndromes: executive summary: a report of the American College of Cardiology/American Heart Association Task Force on Practice Guidelines. J Am Coll Cardiol. 2014; 64(24):2645-87.
118. Authors/Task Force members, Windecker S, Kolh P, Alfonso F, Collet JP, Cremer J, et al. 2014 ESC/EACTS Guidelines on myocardial revascularization: The Task Force on Myocardial Revascularization of the European Society of Cardiology (ESC) and the European Association of Cardio-Thoracic Surgery (EACTS) Developed with the special contribution of the European Association of Percutaneous Cardiovascular Interventions (EAPCI). Eur Heart J. 2014; 35(37):2541-619.

12

CHAPTER

Strategies to Rule-out Acute Myocardial Infarction in the Emergency Department: Who Can Go Home?

Martin Than

INTRODUCTION

Clinicians involved in acute care often worry that patients may come to harm soon after discharge, from the medical complaint that triggered a visit to hospital. Therefore, discharge decisions in emergency medicine are difficult to make and are frequently more challenging than treatment of an immediately life-threatening disease. Patients with symptoms suggestive of acute coronary syndromes (ACSs) contribute approximately 5–10% of annual presentations to emergency departments (EDs) and up to 25% of hospital admissions.[1,2] Accordingly, assessment and safe disposition of these patients is a major challenge. Their safe workup generally requires considerable time and often includes inpatient observation periods, which add to ED and hospital overcrowding. Despite prolonged workup, the actual number of patients finally diagnosed with ACSs can be anything from 20% to much less.[3,4,5] Considerable time and resources are consumed investigating the many patients who do not have an ACS. Consequently, ongoing research explores investigative strategies that identify patient groups who can be discharged early with a low risk of harm from adverse cardiac events.

This chapter will describe the clinical context related to the assessment of patients in the ED with possible acute myocardial infarction (AMI). There will be discussion of the development of clinical decision aids and diagnostic strategies and descriptions of both older and more contemporary tools available to the clinician. All of the approaches subsequently described represent types of diagnostic strategy to investigate patients presenting to the ED with symptoms that are possibly due to acute cardiac ischemia. Some of them can be described as clinical prediction rules, which are methods of identifying and combining the best medical signs and symptoms and other findings in predicting the probability of a specific disease or outcome.[6] In contrast, there is also a purely algorithmic approach based on the numerical values of blood test results. All of these approaches can be described as clinical decisions aids and can form part or all of a diagnostic strategy.

For an emergency physician, the short-term prognosis of a patient is paramount, and therefore, effectively defines the required accuracy (and safety) of an investigative pathway. A recent survey of approximately 1,000 emergency medicine physicians from North America and Australasia found that the most preferred rates of acceptable error were less than or equal to 1 in 100 (1%) or less than or equal 1 in 1,000 (0.1%) in discharging patients from ED with a missed major adverse cardiac event (MACE).[7] These findings suggest that a sensitivity of 99% or higher is the minimum standard that most physicians will accept for a risk scoring system that classifies chest pain patients for early discharge.

In this chapter, where possible, sensitivity will be used as the primary statistic for comparing the safety of different strategies. The prevalence of AMI or ACS in cohorts reported from studies in the ED varies greatly from 1% to greater than 20%. And it is obviously much easier to achieve a high negative predictive value for a rule-out strategy in a very low prevalence population. One approach for assessing the safety impact of a diagnostic strategy at one's own institution is to consider how many patients presenting to the ED each year with possible acute cardiac ischemic symptoms are subsequently found to have a MACE within 30 days and then use the sensitivity to estimate how many of these events might be missed using a particular strategy. For example, for a hospital that sees (a modest) one such event per day, a strategy with a sensitivity of 97% would result in missing approximately 11 patients per year (false negative rate of 3/100 patients in a group of 365 patients per year).

As demonstrated in table 1, the sensitivity is calculated only from disease positive cases, and is thus theoretically independent of the prevalence. In contrast, table 1 demonstrates that negative predictive value is from disease positive and disease negative cases, and is thus, prevalence dependent.

To provide an example from the following literature, consider the following data using the HEART score from Mahler et al. demonstrated in table 2.[8]

TABLE 1: Calculation of sensitivity

		Disease		Sensitivity	a/(a + c)
		+	–	Specificity	d/(d + b)
Test	+	a	b	Positive predictive value	a/(a + b)
	–	c	d	Negative predictive value	c/(c + d)
				Prevalence	(a + b)/(c + d)

TABLE 2: Calculation of sensitivity using the HEART score data from Mahler et al.

		Disease		Sensitivity	58.3
		+	–	Specificity	84.9
HEART score	+	7	159	Positive predictive value	4.2
	–	5	899	Negative predictive value	99.4
				Prevalence	1.1

The disparity between sensitivity and negative predictive value in this data comes from the low prevalence of the study (1.2%). Therefore, when reviewing the data from derivation or validation studies, it is important to review the sensitivity, and consider the negative predictive value in the context of the disease prevalence in the study.

CONTEXT

Traditional Management

Figure 1 demonstrates what currently happens in many hospitals in the developed world, when patients with possible ACS are assessed in the ED.

In this illustration, it has been assumed that the prevalence rate of ACS is approximately 20%. The light bulbs represent decision-making points by the attending clinician in which a decision is made to proceed to another investigation (e.g., exercise stress test or angiography), and/or discharge the patient. One can see that amongst those patients that do have ACS (who really do require admission to hospital and further investigations), a small number of patients may have decisions made at earlier time points such as 2 or 4 hours after arrival at the ED that could lead to essentially unsafe discharge decisions. The proportion of patients (80%) without ACS is noticeably larger, and traditionally, most of these patients remain in hospital (in ED or elsewhere) undergoing prolonged observation and testing either on some sort of chest pain unit or on an inpatient ward.

ACCELERATED DECISION-MAKING FOR RULE-OUT OF ACUTE MYOCARDIAL INFARCTION

Initial research in this area uses the terminology "accelerated diagnostic protocol". This terminology is still used; however, there is some resistance to the concept of using protocols in medicine because it implies a certain rigidity. Subsequently, the expression accelerated diagnostic pathway has also been used and these processes are similar if not identical. Both these phrases are frequently abbreviated to the letters ADP. Perhaps the best phrase of all to use would be "accelerated decision-making pathway", as a scribe below. The objective of an ADP is to facilitate the patient discharge as illustrated in figure 2. In this scenario, strategies to identify those patients at low and intermediate risk of coming to short-term harm have been identified. An ADP facilitates prompter diagnostic decisions through sampling blood at earlier time points for cardiac troponin (cTn). This then

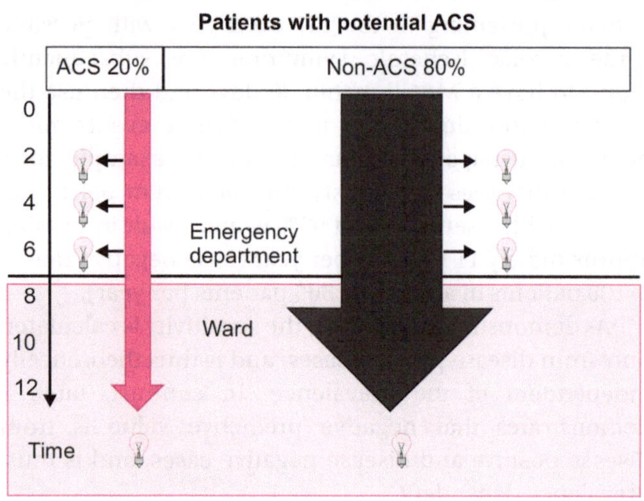

ACS, acute coronary syndrome.

FIG. 1: What has traditionally happened in many hospitals in the developed world when patients with possible acute coronary syndrome are assessed in the emergency department

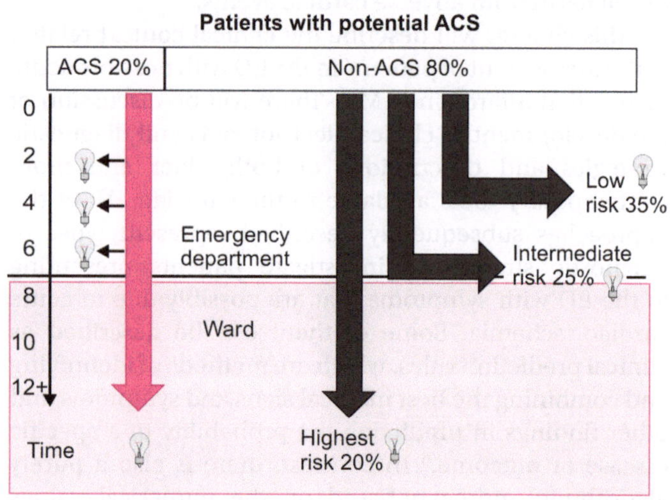

ACS, acute coronary syndrome.

FIG. 2: The objective of an accelerated diagnostic pathway is to facilitate the early patient discharge of low and intermediate risk patients without acute coronary syndrome allows clinicians to rapidly proceed to the same "next step" in clinical management (such as cardiac stress test, imaging, and/or discharge) as would have occurred using a more prolonged serial troponin testing time course to exclude AMI.

OUTCOMES

One challenge in interpreting the medical literature regarding rapid assessment strategies is that different outcomes are used to define key follow-up events. Different definitions for MACEs are used in scientific papers. The principal difference is that some papers define only emergency procedural intervention [percutaneous coronary intervention (PCI) or coronary artery bypass graft (CABG)] as a MACE, whereas others also include procedures that are performed as a result of positive planned follow-up investigations and angiography. The difficulty with the second, more inclusive, approach is that there are wide situational and geographical differences as to which patients get such follow-up procedural interventions. Additionally, it is entirely possible that in some cases, a stenosis seen on cardiac imaging or angiography is an incidental finding and not actually the cause of the patients presenting symptoms. There is no immediate prospect of a unified approach to the reporting of outcomes, and so, clinicians should consider carefully how the outcomes reported match their own patient circumstances.

Clinicians may also have different objectives for an accelerated decision-making pathway. The simplest approach is to apply exactly the same investigations in an accelerated approach as would have been done using a more protracted diagnostic/observational approach. In that case, if a patient with a particular risk profile would normally get an exercise stress test after observation and serial troponin/electrocardiograph (ECG) measurements over a 6-hour period then, in an accelerated decision-making process, the patient would still undergo stress test but the decision to perform this would take place at an earlier time point, and the stress test may potentially take place as an outpatient.

Of course, in an ideal world, a decision-making tool could actually be used to predict who does not need any further testing at all. This has become increasingly possible because traditionally, performing additional investigations such as dynamic stress tests is focused on identifying those patients with unstable angina (UA). As cTns have become increasingly clinically sensitive, more patients who would previously have been diagnosed with UA are now categorized as having a non-ST elevation myocardial infarction (NSTEMI). Certainly, still there are patients who have negative serial troponins who subsequently have positive stress tests and are found to have critical stenoses requiring early intervention (that are thought to have been the cause of the patients presenting chest pain, i.e., the cause of the UA). To a certain extent, the success of a decision-making algorithm in predicting those patients who do not need additional testing depends upon the prevalence of underlying coronary artery disease in the local geographical population.

In the following summaries of existing research on clinical decision aids and ADPs, both AMI and ACS are used as outcomes by the authors.

INVESTIGATIVE STRATEGIES TO FACILITATE EARLY DISCHARGE FROM THE EMERGENCY DEPARTMENT

The ADPs may use "gestalt" clinical judgment or a structured scorer or a combination or both.

Value of Clinical Judgment for "Ruling Out" Acute Coronary Syndromes

Historically, the probability of AMI has been determined using clinical acumen primarily involving historical variables and risk factors learnt at medical school and reinforced during clinical practice. Unfortunately, evidence suggests that neither symptomatic history nor presence of chronic risk factors for coronary artery disease are as predictive as initially thought, when used in the ED context.[9-13] In addition, the experience of the initial-assessing doctors in EDs may vary considerably depending on the hospital setting (i.e., an academic department or a rural hospital). Most existing early rule-out strategies require serial testing for biomarker concentrations, additional biomarkers or the use of a decision rule. In a prospective cohort study, Body et al. evaluated the very simple concept of "ruling out" ACS based on the clinical judgment of the treating physician.[14] The treating clinician's clinical judgment or "gestalt" for the estimated probability of ACS was recorded using a 5-point Likert scale. Based on existing evidence that atypical symptoms do not substantially affect the probability that a patient in the ED has ACS,[12,15,16] it seems unlikely that a clinician's "gestalt" would be sufficient to enable safe "rule out" in the ED. However, the clinical suspicion of the treating physician is an important element of the HEART score.[17]

Among a cohort of 458 patients, the findings of this study confirm that clinical judgment alone cannot be used to either "rule in" or "rule out" ACS. Just over 50% of patients in whom the treating clinician believed that the diagnosis was "definitely ACS" actually developed MACE within 30 days (which included prevalent AMI). On the other hand, just less than 10% of patients in whom the clinician felt that the diagnosis was "definitely not" ACS developed MACE.

However, by combining the clinical judgment of the treating clinician with troponin concentrations measured at the time of presentation and ECG findings, the findings of this study suggest that we may have a promising "rule out" strategy. Ultimately, for patients in whom the clinician believed that the diagnosis was "definitely not" or "probably not" ACS (the first two points on the Likert scale) who also had normal troponin T concentrations (measured with a contemporary, non-high sensitivity assay) in combination with no ECG ischemia, the sensitivity of this strategy was 100% [95% confidence interval (CI) = 95.6–100%] and almost one-quarter of patients could have avoided unnecessary hospital admission. Using the high-sensitivity cTn T (hs-cTnT) assay (Roche Diagnostics Elecsys) would have enabled even patients in whom the clinician felt the diagnosis "could be" ACS to have been discharged while maintaining sensitivity at 100%. This strategy could have enabled more than 40% of patients to be immediately discharged from the ED.[14]

Clearly, these findings must be prospectively validated before clinical implementation is considered as this is the first report and the findings may be overfitted to the cohort in whom they were applied. However, given its simplicity, this rule-out strategy may be particularly desirable in resource-poor environments such as the third world.

Structured Clinical Decision Aids (Scores) for Accelerated Diagnostic Pathways

Methodologies for Developing Structured Clinical Decision Tools

There is no consensus about the best approach to develop risk stratification tools, however, the Transparent Reporting of a Multivariable Prediction Model for Individual Prognosis or Diagnosis (TRIPOD) group has just published consensus guidelines for reporting of such tools.[18] The TRIPOD statement is intended to improve the reporting of prediction modeling studies of all types (development, validation, updating or extending) and in all medical settings (primary, secondary, and tertiary care, and public health), enabling readers to better understand a prediction model study's design, conduct, analysis and interpretation, and to assess the validity, transportability, and application of its results. The TRIPOD was developed through collaboration between prediction research methodologists, medical practitioners, guideline developers, knowledge translation specialists, and journal editors. The TRIPOD contains a 22-item checklist and background document explaining the rationale behind each item, freely available for viewing and downloading on this website.

A large variation of approaches to developing risk scores has been used, ranging from statistical weighting of variables collected in observational studies to clinical judgment, logic, and common sense.

In mathematical models, all relevant clinical variables are collected in their prospective cohort of patients and objective outcomes are determined. Statistical techniques are subsequently employed (most commonly logistic regression analysis or recursive partitioning) to identify those variables which are independent; these are then weighted. There are many variations in techniques on how to develop mathematical models, which are summarized in an excellent textbook by Ewout Steyerberg.[19] Statistically created models tend to be more mathematically sound, but run the risk of being overcomplicated and hard to use.[20] Alternatively, risk scores developed using clinical judgment (such as the HEART score) are more simplistic, and can work well.

An important consideration during development of risk stratification tools is the clinical sensibility of the resulting prediction rule (Table 3). Evaluation of sensibility requires judgment rather than statistical methods.[21] A sensible rule is easy to use, and has content and face validity. This means that it must contain predictors appropriate for the purpose of the rule that are combined in a sensible way, with no obvious items missing (Table 3). Ease of use may be facilitated by presenting a rule developed from logistic regression as a score, where the original predictor weights have been converted to

TABLE 3: Terminology, definitions associated with "sensibility" of clinical prediction rules

Terminology	Meaning
Sensibility	• This refers to whether a prediction rule is both clinically reasonable and easy to use. This is more based on opinion than statistical methodology
Content validity	• For a rule to have content validity, the items included must be sensible, with no obvious omissions, and the way that these variables are organized appears suitable for the objectives of the rule
Face validity	• This is a subjective interpretation of the validity of the rule by the user. The face validity of a rule will depend on the expectations and beliefs of the user, and may not be associated with statistical validity, but is essential for end-user uptake • To maximize face validity and ensure end-user trust, it may be necessary to include variables found to be statistically suboptimal in the final prediction model
User friendliness	• This refers to how easy the rule is to use. This depends on the demands the rule will place on memory, complexity of calculations in the absence of electronic devices, format, and layout of the rule

integers that are easy to add together[20] or as a nomogram, or a risk stratification chart. Though less precise than the original regression formula, such presentations are less complex, easier to apply by memory and usable without electronic assistance. Prediction rules are unlikely to be applied in practice if they are not considered sensible by the end-user, even if they are accurate.[22]

Perhaps the ideal characteristics of a risk stratification system would be:

- It achieves the required diagnostic accuracy (and hence safety) when tested externally and put into clinical practice outside its derivation locations
- It is simple to use
- It is easy to calculate the score, if this needs to be done
- It can be calculated without the aid of a calculator or computer
- It is not too detailed or long (i.e., not too many variables)
- It is easy to implement in different settings
- It is easy to reproduce by different doctors with different experience
- It has good inter-rater agreement
- It can be easily remembered without needing to refer to a secondary source
- It is logical to the user, and results in end-user trust.

While debate about the best method for the development of risk scores may continue, it would seem that if the score works well in clinical practice with appropriate diagnostic accuracy, then how it was created may not matter. It is also likely that whichever scores are adopted by clinicians, there will be an ongoing process of modification and improvement. This is nicely demonstrated by the history of the development and further improvement of scoring systems for the assessment of suspected pulmonary embolism in the ED. The Geneva score[23] has gone through several modifications and simplifications since it was originally published. We are aware of a number of research groups in Australasia, Canada, the United States, the United Kingdom, Germany, and Switzerland that are in the process of developing new, purpose-designed risk scores for patients with possible ACS.

Although sensitivity and negative predictive value are the key parameters of interest when deciding to use a risk assessment score to assist with chest pain rule-out decision-making, it is important to also consider the proportion of patients that will be classified as low risk. Although this is related to the specificity, it is perhaps a better measure of how effective a decision rule will be in changing or impacting upon clinical practice. If the numbers are significantly low, then adopting a risk scoring system in an early rule-out strategy is unlikely to impact upon patient flow and ED overcrowding.

One other consideration is the rapidly changing field of cardiac biomarkers. The risk scoring systems we discuss were designed to be used in conjunction with cardiac biomarkers (and ECG). A new generation of high-sensitivity troponin I assays is almost upon us and high-sensitivity troponin T has been in use in many countries for several years. The inclusion of other supplementary biomarkers, such as heart fatty acid binding protein (H-FABP) and copeptin, may also needs to be investigated in future early rule-out strategies. As such, scoring systems should be flexible to include new technologies.

PRE-EXISTING RISK SCORES

The following descriptions of clinical decision tools are divided into two sections representing older and more contemporary purpose designed scores and algorithms. Some strategies, such as the Thrombolysis in Myocardial Infarction (TIMI) score and Vancouver Chest Pain Rule are mentioned in both sections because advancements have been made.

Many of the earlier risk scores were developed in an era before emergency medicine had a strong academic base. They were usually developed by cardiology research groups and as such focused on identifying patients likely to have ACS, and often some discriminating test results (such as a positive ECG) were present. Differences in reporting styles and populations make it difficult to compare many of the common risk scoring systems. The manner of reporting of diagnostic statistics varies considerably. In many cases, the area under the receiver-operating curve (AUC, or c-statistic—see Box 1) is all that is available.

BOX 1 A brief explanation about receiver operating characteristic curves and c-statistics

- Some of the following decision rules have been analyzed using receiver operator characteristic (ROC) curves. This brief summary is provided to put this in context. The area under the ROC curve (AUC), or c-statistic, is a crude measure for quantifying the diagnostic performance a biomarker. It is sometimes encountered in studies to rule out acute coronary syndrome (ACS). It is not particularly useful in this context as we shall explain. First, to aid understanding, we provide a brief introduction to the AUC and ROC
- The ROC is a plot of sensitivity versus 1-specificity, and the AUC is the area under the curve and therefore is a metric which tells us something about the performance of the biomarker across all sensitivities and specificities. An ideal biomarker would have an AUC of one, meaning 100% sensitivity and 100% specificity. An AUC of 0.5 means the biomarker is no better than a coin toss. Of note, two AUCs may be identical but not have the same ROC. This may be clinically important. For example, one may favor sensitivity over specificity and the other vice versa. For rule-out strategies, it is most important to identify the biomarker that maximizes sensitivity while identifying a clinically meaningful population of low risk patients. What constitutes an acceptable sensitivity (acceptable rate of false negatives) is a judgment call[7]

Goldman

Goldman et al.[24] originally derived the Goldman rule in 1982 from a cohort of 482 patients from a single center using recursive partitioning techniques, and validated the rule in 468 patients from a second center. In 1988, they modified the rule using recursive partitioning on a derivation sample of 1,379 patients, and validated it on a cohort of 4,770 patients.[25] The rule included ECG findings, age, time since symptom onset, prior history of angina or myocardial infarction, and pain characteristics. Notably, the rule did not include biomarker results. The rule achieved 88% sensitivity and 74% specificity in the validation cohort. Grijseels et al.[26] subsequently externally validated the modified Goldman rule in 1995 achieving 74% sensitivity and a 40% specificity. Note that Carlton et al. have now modified and updated the Goldman rule for use in conjunction with high-sensitivity cTn T and this is discussed in the following section.

Acute Cardiac Ischemia Time-insensitive Prediction Instrument

Selker et al. in 1991, published the Acute Cardiac Ischemia Time-insensitive Prediction Instrument (ACI-TIPI) score,[27] which was trialed on a population of 3,453 patients presenting to six hospitals with symptoms suggesting acute cardiac ischemia. The score was derived by means of logistic regression, and included age, sex, chest/arm pain, Q-waves, ST deviation, and T-wave elevation/inversion. The ACI-TIPI uses special software in order to categorize risk and as a result is not easy to use or reproduce. The score was subsequently validated on a new cohort of 2,320 patients, showing a c-statistic of 0.88.[28] The score has since been validated in four other studies, with sensitivity ranging from 84 to 100%, and specificity ranging from 4 to 84%.[29-32]

Thrombolysis in Myocardial Infarction Score

The TIMI risk score for UA/NSTEMI was published by Elliott Antman et al. in 2000.[33] It was validated on 1,957 patients recruited in the multinational, randomized clinical TIMI 11B trial, which compared treatment with unfractionated heparin or enoxaparin. Of note, participants were required to have UA or an NSTEMI in order to be included in the study. Twelve baseline characteristics were screened as candidate predictor variables for developing a risk score and univariate and multivariate analyses were performed to identify seven independent predictive parameters.

The initial results demonstrated that the prevalence of cardiac disease increased as the score increased, from 4.7% for a score of 0–1, to 40.9% with a score of 6–7. The initial score derivation did not involve its use as a rule-out tool, but it has subsequently been validated for this purpose in six other separate studies.[34-39] The sensitivity for these rule-out strategies incorporating the TIMI score ranged from 99.3 to 100%.

It has been common for validators and users of the TIMI score to modify it to accommodate a broader definition of ischemia on the ECG and currently available cardiac biomarkers. For example, Asia-Pacific Evaluation of Chest Pain Trial (ASPECT) and ADAPT studies modified the score to include "any new" ischemia on the ECG, and troponin or multimarker panel testing at 0 and 2 hours after presentation to hospital.[35] This is discussed in the next section.

Platelet Glycoprotein IIb/IIIa in Unstable Angina: Receptor Suppression using Integrilin Therapy

The Platelet Glycoprotein IIb/IIIa in Unstable Angina: Receptor Suppression using Integrilin Therapy (PURSUIT) risk score published in 2000 by Boersma et al. was derived from a population of 9,461 patients enrolled in the PURSUIT randomized controlled trial (comparing glycoprotein IIb/IIIa inhibitor therapy vs. placebo in patients with UA or NSTEMI).[40] The score was derived using multiple regression, which included the parameters: Age, heart rate, systolic blood pressure, ST-segment depression, signs of heart failure, and cardiac enzymes. It yielded a c-statistic of 0.814 for predicting mortality, but only produced a c-statistic of 0.669 for predicting disease. Araujo Goncalves et al.[41] validated the PURSUIT score in 2005 in a cohort of 460 patients admitted to a single center with ACS. They found the score to have a c-statistic of 0.62. The PURSUIT risk score is little used for ED rule-out decision-making because it is not designed for rule-out.

Global Registry of Acute Coronary Events

The Global Registry of Acute Coronary Events (GRACE) score was published by Granger et al. in 2003 and was the product of a multinational collaboration involving 94 hospitals in 14 countries. The score was derived from a cohort of 11,389 patients using multiple regression, and validated in two separate cohorts of 3,972 and 12,142 patients, respectively.[42] Patients needed to have either ECG changes suggesting ACS, serial increase in cardiac enzymes, or documented coronary artery disease to be included, that is, lower risk ED patients were not included. It was found that inclusion of age, Killip class (severity of heart failure),[43] systolic blood pressure, ST-segment deviation, cardiac arrest during presentation, serum creatine, cardiac enzymes, and heart rate accounted for 89.9% of the prognostic information. The final model yielded a c-statistic of 0.83 in the derivation cohort, 0.84

in the smaller validation cohort, and 0.79 in the larger validation cohort. Since its initial publication, the GRACE score has been externally validated in two separate studies, yielding c-statistics of 0.86 and 0.81, respectively.[44,45] It is regarded as a useful tool for predicting those patients that will be at higher risk and as a guide to therapy but not as a rule-out tool.

Marsan (A Clinical Decision Rule for Young Adult Patients with Chest Pain)

In 2005, Marsan et al. modified a rule produced by Walker et al. in 2001.[46] Marsan et al. trialed a population of 1,023 patients and found that chest patients who were younger than 40 years old, with no known cardiac disease, with neither classic cardiac risk factors or an abnormal ECG, and normal biomarkers at presentation were unlikely to suffer an adverse cardiac event within 30 days.[47]

Vancouver Chest Pain Rule

The Vancouver Chest Pain Rule was derived in 2006 by Christenson et al.[48] from a cohort of 769 patients (aged at least 25 years old) presenting to a single center in Vancouver. It is important to note that this decision aid was specifically designed for rule-out purposes. The rule was derived using recursive partitioning, with the result that it is slightly more complex than some of the other risk scoring systems.

In the final model, a patient was considered low-risk if:

- They were younger than 40 years old, with a normal initial ECG, and no prior history of ischemic chest pain; or
- Aging more than or equal to 40 years old with normal ECG results, no previous ischemic chest pain, low risk chest pain characteristics, and either an initial creatine kinase-MB (CK-MB) less than 3 μg/L or an initial CK-MB greater than or equal to 3 μg/L, but without an increase or ECG changes within 2 hours.

This rule proved to be 98.8% sensitive and 32.5% specific in the derivation cohort, with a 28.5% predictive value and 99% negative predictive value. This rule was validated by Jalili et al.[49] who achieved 95.1% sensitivity, 56.3% specificity, 98.6% negative predictive value, and 25.9% positive predictive value in a cohort of 593 consecutive patients aged 25 or older presenting to a single center in Iran.

National Heart Foundation of Australia

In 2006, the Cardiac Society of Australia and New Zealand in collaboration with the National Heart Foundation of Australia published national guidelines for the management of ACSs.[50] The guidelines were formulated by committee consensus using expert opinion and published evidence available at that time. The document included a method for stratifying chest-pain patients at risk of non ST elevation acute coronary syndromes (NSTEACS). The risk score divided patients into low, intermediate, and high risk of NSTEACS using ECG findings, biomarker results, hemodynamic status, syncope, left ventricular ejection fraction, history of PCI, diabetes, heart disease, age, hypertension, family history, smoking, hyperlipidemia, aspirin use, and prior myocardial infarction. The score was later validated by Macdonald et al.[34] in 2011 on a population of 1,758 patients, yielding a c-statistic of 0.82, and Kelly[51] in 2012 in a population of 768 patients yielding a c-statistic of 0.74 (CI = 0.71–0.77) for ACSs, and AMI.

SUMMARY

Of the preexisting risk scores, the TIMI score has probably been most widely used for rule-out of ACS purposes. In contrast, the GRACE score is more commonly used to assist with rule-in management decisions. It is worth noting that of the early scoring systems, only the Vancouver Chest Pain Rule was intentionally developed to facilitate early discharge of patients with possible cardiac chest pain from EDs. This means that there has been plenty of work left to do in the development of purpose-designed risk-assessment tools for the ED.

NEWLY DEVELOPED RISK SCORES

Modified Thrombolysis in Myocardial Infarction Score—Accelerated Diagnostic Protocol Pathway

It has already been mentioned that the TIMI score was not developed for the purpose of facilitating discharge of low risk patients from the ED, and that it was developed from a very high risk group of patients. Despite this, for some years, it was one of the only easy-to-use available risk stratification tools for patients with possible ACS. The ASia-Pacific Evaluation of Chest pain Trial (ASPECT) study involved 3,582 patients from 10 countries in the Asia-Pacific region.[35] It involved using 0- and 2-hour biomarker testing with a point-of-care multimarker panel, ECG, and TIMI. In that study, the ADP identified 9.8% of patients with suspected ACS who could have been discharged early from the ED, with a sensitivity of 99.3% for 30-day MACEs.

The subsequent accelerated diagnostic protocol (ADAPT) study analyzed data from Australasian centers within the ASPECT study and utilized contemporary cTn assays without other biomarkers.[52] In 1,975 patients, the ADAPT-ADP classified 20% of chest pain presentations as low risk with a sensitivity of 99.7%. A modified-ADAPT rule, incorporating results from a highly sensitive assay and patients with a TIMI score of 0 or 1, found

TABLE 4: Modified Thrombolysis In Myocardial Infarction (Modified TIMI) score

Clinical Characteristics: Score **ONE** for every positive response | Score **ZERO** for any negative or 'unknown' response	**Individual scores:**
A. Age ≥65 years = +1	=
B. ≥3 of the following 5 CAD risk factors = +1 , <3 risk factors = 0 ☐ Family history: i.e., at age less than 55 years of age: (1) Angina, (2) MI, (3) Sudden cardiac death without obvious cause ☐ Dislipidemia ☐ Diabetes ☐ Hypertension ☐ Current smoker	=
C. Known CAD (stenosis ≥ 50%): = +1 e.g., a positive investigation or procedure for CAD including: PCI, stent, positive angiogram, positive exercise tolerance test	=
D. ASA (i.e., Acetylsalicylic acid/aspirin) use in past 7 days = +1 Single GP/ambulance dose not included)	=
E. Recent severe angina (e.g. ≥ 2 events in last 24 hours) = +1	=
Total score	=

approximately 40% of patients could be identified as low risk with a sensitivity of 99.2% (Table 4).[35] This was validated in the independent Advantageous Predictors of Acute Coronary Syndromes Evaluation (APACE) cohort with similar accuracy and proportions defined as low risk (sensitivity 99.4% and low risk 39%).[53]

Modified Goldman Risk Score

While originally published by Goldman et al., the Modified Goldman Risk Score was recently incorporated into an ADP by Carlton et al. seeking to identify patients suitable for discharge following a single high-sensitivity troponin (Table 5).[54] The protocol asserted that patients with a Modified Goldman Score less than or equal to 1 (patients get one point for pain at rest, pain similar to previous AMI, pain not relieved by GTN within 15 minutes, pain lasting greater than 60 minutes, pain increasing in frequency, systolic blood pressure less than 100 mm Hg, acute shortness of breath, pain within 6 weeks of AMI or revascularization), as well as a nonischemic ECG and high-sensitivity troponin I less than 14 ng/L.

Carlton et al. validated this ADP in a population of 960 presentations to Poole NHS Foundation Trust district hospital (United Kingdom) with chest pain.[54] In this population, 39.8% were classified as low risk with a 98.8% sensitivity for AMI. Other high-sensitivity troponin T thresholds were investigated, with improved sensitivity (100% at <5 ng/L), at the cost of a smaller low-risk group (29.3% at <5 ng/L). The secondary outcome of MACE within 30 days was also explored, with almost identical results.

Using the modified Goldman risk score as part of an ADP using high-sensitivity troponin T appears to be a safe method of identifying a large low-risk group after

TABLE 5: The Modified Goldman Score and TRUST accelerated diagnostic protocol

Modified Goldman risk score	**1 point for each variable present**
• Typical new-onset chest pain at rest • Pain the same as previous myocardial infarction • Pain not relieved by glyceryl trinitrate • (GTN) spray within 15 min • Pain lasting more than 60 min • Pain occurring with increasing frequency • Hypotension (systolic blood pressure • <100 mm Hg) • Acute shortness of breath • Pain within 6 weeks of a myocardial • Infarction or revascularisation	
Modified Goldman total	
TRUST ADP	
Low risk* (suitable for discharge)	1. Modified Goldman score ≤1 2. Non-ischemic ECG 3. Presentation high-sensitivity troponin T <14 ng/L
Not low risk	1. Modified Goldman score >1 2. Ischemic ECG 3. Presentation high-sensitivity troponin T ≥14 ng/L

*Safety point: Protocol not validated in age ≥80 years.
TRUST, Triage Rule-out Using high-Sensitivity Troponin.

a single biomarker, however, the results of this study require further external validation before they could be implemented.

HEART Score

The HEART score was developed in 2007 by Jacob Six (a cardiologist), Barbra Backus (an emergency medicine physician) et al. first published a study of the HEART score on 120 patients in 2008.[55,56] It achieved a 96.5% sensitivity and a 42.7% specificity. The manner in which the score was developed is interesting. It differs from the other scoring systems in that it is based on a clinical approach rather than a mathematical approach. Jacob Six from Utrecht in The Netherlands was undertaking a teaching ward round with some medical students. In the process of this ward round, he taught students that the key factors to consider when assessing chest pain patients were their history, ECG results, age, risk factors, and their troponin test result. He then realized that these factors actually formed quite a good mnemonic, and work began to see if a score would be useful in clinical practice. It is noticeable that the starting point for the score was clinical knowledge and understanding of the medical scenario and knowledge of the medical literature. This information was used to develop a score that is logical and simple to use. The authors had noted that the Apgar score (a score to assess neonatal well-being immediately after birth),[57] is regarded as very easy to use because of its simplicity. Backus et al. wished simplicity to be a founding principle of the score to help clinicians accept and adopt the risk score system.

As originally described, the score consisted of points given for history, ECG results, age, risk factors, and troponin concentrations.[55,56] For history, two points were given if the history is highly suspicious, one point if it is moderately suspicious, and zero if slightly suspicious. For ECG results, if the ECG was normal then zero points were given. In cases of repolarization abnormalities without significant ST-segment depression, one point was given. Additionally, one point was given for bundle branch block, typical abnormalities indicative of left ventricular hypertrophy, repolarization abnormalities probably due to the use of digoxin, or in case of unchanged known repolarization disturbances. Two points were given for significant ST depression or elevation, when in the absence of a bundle branch block, left ventricular hypertrophy, or the use of digoxin. For age, two points are given for age greater than or equal to 65 years, one point for age 45–65 years and no points for age less than or equal to 45 years. For risk factors, two points are given for greater than or equal to three risk factors or a history of atherosclerotic disease, one point is given for one or two risk factors, and no points are given for no risk factors. For troponin concentrations, two points are given if the troponin level is greater than or equal to two times the threshold for positivity (modified by the authors in validation cohorts[58] to three times the normal limit, one point if the level is greater than 1 to less than three times the normal limit, and no points if the troponin is less than or equal to the normal limit. The original troponin criteria were based on the contemporary nonhigh-sensitivity Beckman Access AccuTroponin I assay with a threshold for positivity of 0.04 µg/L (40 ng/L). The score is summarized in table 6. In subsequent studies, a score of zero to three has become the standard for designating patients as low risk.

Backus et al. tested the score on 880 patients in 2010, yielding a 98.1% sensitivity and 41.6% specificity.[68] Mahler et al. validated the HEART score on a cohort of 1,070 patients.[59] In this population, the score achieved a 58.3% sensitivity, and an 85.0% specificity; however, it must be noted that this population had a very low prevalence of disease (1%) meaning that only a small number of false positive results (five cases) had a large influence on the sensitivity. In 2013, a retrospective validation was published using data from 2,906 patients from the Asia-Pacific ASPECT study in which the prevalence of MACE was 12.9%.[70] In this analysis, the sensitivity was 96.3%. In 2013, there was also a validation published from 10 centers in the Netherlands with a combined prevalence of 17% also resulting in a sensitivity of 96.3%.[63] In this study, the ECG criteria were slightly

TABLE 6: HEART score for chest pain patients

History	Highly suspicious	2
	Moderately suspicious	1
	Slightly suspicious	0
ECG	Significant ST-deviation	2
	Nonspecific repolarisation disturbance/LBTB/PM	1
	Normal	0
Age	≥65 years	2
	>45 and <65 years	1
	≤45 years	0
Risk factors	≥3 risk factors or history of atherosclerotic disease*	2
	1 or 2 risk factors	1
	No risk factors known	0
Troponin	≥3x normal limit	2
	>1 and <3 x normal limit	1
	≤1 x normal limit	0
Total		

*Risk factors for atherosclerotic disease:
Hypercholesterolemia — Cigarette smoking
Hypertension — Positive family history
Diabetes mellitus — Obesity

different with two points also given for negative T-waves. Both latter analyses required retrospective determination of history (H) parameter of the score from other data fields. There has now been a small randomized controlled trial using a modified version of the HEART score that utilizes structured criteria to catergorize "history", excludes patients from being classified as "low risk" if there is a positive troponin result from blood sampling at 0 and 3 hours from arrival at the ED.[62] In this study, the prevalence of MACE was 6% and the sensitivity for MACE for 141 patients randomized to the modified HEART pathway was 100%. Since several adaptations exist for utilization of the HEART score, differences should be considered if undertaking implementation.

North American Chest Pain Rule

The North American chest pain rule was developed by Erik Hess et al. and published in 2012.[63] The initial derivation paper included an internal validation using statistical bootstrapping techniques, and included 2,718 patients from three academic EDs in Ottawa Ontario, Kingston Ontario, and Rochester Minnesota (Box 2). The robust methodology for the study was published in advance in 2008.[64] In this chest-pain rule, patients were classified as low risk if they met the following criteria—older than 50 years of age, atypical chest pain, no history of known coronary disease, nonischemic ECG results, and serial negative troponin test results at least 6 hours from symptom onset. The derived rule was 100% sensitive for a cardiac event within 30 days and categorized 18% of patients as safe for discharge. The model was internally validated using statistical bootstrapping techniques. The authors commented that the rule will differentially affect resource use depending on local practice patterns. They noted that a decrease in resource would be likely in centers where a high proportion of patients undergo prolonged observation. External validation data is awaited.

BOX 2 North American Chest Pain Rule

A patient with chest pain and possible acute coronary syndrome can be safely discharged from the ED without additional diagnostic testing if NONE of the following four criteria are met:

1. New ischemia on initial ECG
2. History of coronary artery disease
3. Pain is typical for acute coronary syndrome
4. Initial cardiac troponin is positive

And

5. Age ≤40 years

Or

Age 41–50 years and repeat troponin at least 6 hours from symptom onset is negative

New Vancouver Chest Pain Diagnostic Algorithm (2012)

Scheuermeyer et al. in Vancouver built on previous work in this area by conducting a single cohort implementation study on 1,116 patients with careful monitoring of patient outcomes.[65] Patients were categorized as low risk if they did not have any high risk features. Patients with perceived high risk features were referred to inpatient cardiology for further assessment and management.
High risk features included:

- History: Pain similar to prior ACS, rest pain for greater than 20 minutes, ongoing pain in the ED, or typical crescendo angina, or a change in angina pattern such as new rest angina;
- Physical findings: Such as a new murmur or clinical heart failure or hemodynamic instability;
- ECG: Results suggestive of ischemia; and
- Cardiac troponin: Elevated.

Patients that were classified as low risk were eligible for early discharge after 2–6 hours. The decision on whether to observe and test for follow-up troponin at 2 or 6 hours was left to the clinician's judgment (gestalt) as to whether the patient was very low risk or not. At the time of discharge, follow-up provocative testing was arranged to take place within 48 hours.

After 30-day follow-up, no patients (0%) had a missed ACS. A "missed" case of ACS was defined as patient that was discharged from the ED with no cardiology referral or outpatient stress testing who proved to have ACS or died at 30 days. At the index visit, 271 patients (24.2%) were referred to cardiology, 579 (51.8%) were discharged home with no follow-up testing and 254 (22.7%) were discharged with follow-up testing. At 30 days, of the 120 patients with ACS, none (0%, 95% CI = 0–2.5%) were missed. However, 21 patients had evidence of reversible ischemia on provocative testing and were readmitted for further investigation without incident. Of the 50 patients who had evidence of reversible ischemia on provocative testing, all were immediately referred for mandatory cardiology consultation; 21 of those patients ultimately proved to have UA. Of the 254 patients referred for stress testing, none represented to the ED prior to their testing, and none had a myocardial infarction. This diagnostic algorithm shows great promise, especially as it was actually implemented in practice.

The Vancouver chest pain diagnostic algorithm was validated on an Australasian population of 1,653 patients by Cullen et al in.[66] Analysis was performed first incorporating a high-sensitivity troponin assay and then separately using a contemporary non-high-sensitivity troponin assay. Utilizing the high-sensitivity assay, 212 patients (13.0%) were eligible for early discharge, with three of these being diagnosed with ACS. The overall prevalence of ACS in this population was high, with 20.4% of the 1,653 patients being diagnosed within 30 days. Using the high-sensitivity assay, the diagnostic sensitivity for ACS was 99.1%, specificity 16.1%. Positive predictive value was 23.3% and negative predictive value 98.6%. Using a contemporary non-high-sensitivity troponin assay, 208 patients (12.6%) were eligible for early discharge with four of these being diagnosed with ACS with a sensitivity of 98.8%.

Manchester Acute Coronary Syndromes Decision Rule

The Manchester Acute Coronary Syndromes (MACS) Decision Rule was derived in a cohort of 698 patients and validated in a further cohort of 463 patients at a separate centre.[67] The rule was derived by logistic regression and incorporates eight variables, of which five relate to a patient's clinical presentation, one relates to the ECG and two are biomarker concentrations (hs-cTnT and H-FABP) measured at the time of presentation to the ED (Box 3).

This decision rule requires the use of a computer to estimate the probability of a MACE occurring within 30 days. Biomarker concentrations are considered as continuous variables, which means that there is no single "cutoff" at which the result is considered to be "positive" but rather a continuum of risk with increasing concentrations. Based on the estimated probability of MACE, patients are stratified into four risk groups, each of which is associated with a suggested destination for the patient following their care in the ED. "Very low risk" patients, who comprise over a quarter of the population, could be immediately discharged from hospital without any further investigation. Patients in the "low risk" group could undergo serial troponin testing in a low dependency environment such as an ED observation ward. "Moderate risk" patients could be investigated further in an acute medical ward. "High risk" patients (approximately 10% of the total) could be considered to have an ACS "ruled in" and would therefore be triaged to a high dependency environment or to specialist care, which could, for example, include a coronary care unit. In the validation study, 1.6% of patients in the "very low risk" group had a MACE within 30 days, although both events were coronary stenoses identified at outpatient angiography without revascularization. In the "high risk" group, over 95% of patients had a MACE.

BOX 3 Variables incorporated in the Manchester Acute Coronary Syndromes Clinical Decision Rule

- High-sensitivity troponin T (Roche Diagnostics Elecsys)
- Heart-type fatty acid binding protein (Randox Laboratories)
- Electrocardiogram sign of ischemia
- Pain in association with vomiting
- Sweating observed in the emergency department
- Hypotension on arrival (systolic blood pressure <100 mm Hg)
- A pattern of worsening angina

The MACS rule requires the use of an additional biomarker, H-FABP, which is not routinely used in clinical practice. In the original studies, the MACS rule was evaluated using a semiautomated assay that requires a large amount of manual input and could not be delivered with the turnaround time that is required for patients attending an ED. However, its use has recently been validated using a fully automated assay that is available on a clinical platform.[68] Before widespread clinical implementation can be considered for the MACS rule, it is important that the findings of the existing studies are prospectively validated in heterogeneous cohorts to ensure that diagnostic performance is maintained. It will also be important to determine whether the inclusion of H-FABP is crucial to maintain the performance of the rule.

Emergency Department Assessment of Chest Pain Score

The Emergency Department Assessment of Chest Pain Score (EDACS score) was derived from a cohort of 1,974 patients from two Australasia centers as a preplanned parallel research to the observational ADAPT study (Table 7). Data were prospectively collected for 37 candidate variables commonly used in clinical care, or reported as having value in predicting AMI among ED patients. Research nurses collected the data using explicit definitions for each candidate variable from a published data dictionary.[69] Clinical symptoms and past medical history were recorded as reported by the patient, without incorporating information from the patient's medical records. Reported rather than previously recorded variables were used, so that the reproducibility of the final prediction rule would not be reliant upon access to the patient's records.

Logistic regression identified age, gender, pain radiating to arms, and diaphoresis as statistical predictors for MACE during initial hospital attendance or within 30 days. Pleuritic pain and pain reproducible on palpation identified as significant negative predictors. Statistical coefficients were converted to whole numbers to create a score. Electrocardiogram and biomarker data were intentionally removed from the derivation process to ensure that the performance would not be dependent on the biomarkers or ECG technology used. This was done to ensure the rule would perform consistently regardless of local assays. Clinician feedback was used to improve the clinical plausibility and the usability of the final score. Following this feedback, points were given to younger patients (<50 years) who had greater than or equal to 3 cardiac risk factors or known ischemic heart disease.

TABLE 7: Emergency Department Assessment of Chest-Pain Score (EDACS)

Clinical characteristics						Individual scores
A. Age	18–45 = +2	51–55 = +6	61–65 = +10	71–75 = +14	81–85 = +18	=
	46–50 = +4	56–60 = +8	66–70 = +12	76–80 = +16	86+ = +20	
B. Risk factors: Age 51+ = 0 **In patients 18–50 only** ☐ Family history premature CAD and age 18-50 = +4 (i.e., Previous AMI, CABG or PCI in men at age <55 years and women at age <65 years) **OR** ≥3 of the following 4 risk factors and age 18–50 = +4						= (maximum=4)
☐ Dislipidemia	☐ Diabetes	☐ Hypertension	☐ Current smoker			
C. Symptoms	Diaphoresis (in association with pain*)			= +3	*Pain that caused presentation to hospital	=
	Pain* occurs or worsened with inspiration (pleuritic)			= −4		=
	Pain * radiates to arm or shoulder			= +5		=
	Pain* reproduced by palpation			= −6		=
D. Gender:	Male = +6	Female = 0				=
					Total score	=

EDACS score*	Risk category	Recommendation
<16	Low risk	Early discharge and outpatient investigation after normal 0 and 2 h TnI and outpatient stress test
≥16	Not low risk	Observation and delayed 2nd TnI: proceed with usual clinical care

*And no new ischemia of ECG; and 0 and 2 h TnI both negative.

The EDACS accelerated diagnostic pathway (EDACS-ADP) categorizes patients with a low EDACS score (<16), as well as normal ECG and troponins at 0 and 2 hours as low risk. Such patients could be discharged early from the ED for outpatient follow-up investigations as long as they had no unstable features (defined as: abnormal vital signs or pain that is ongoing or in a crescendo pattern). This protocol was validated and tested for reproducibility using prospectively collected data from separate cohorts of patients from the same centers. In the derivation (n = 1,974) and validation (n = 608) cohorts, the EDACS-ADP classified 43.2% (sensitivity 99.0%, specificity 51.1%), and 52.8% (sensitivity 100%, specificity 60.7%) as low-risk of MACEs, respectively. The intraclass correlation coefficient for categorization of patients as low-risk was high at 0.87 suggesting good inter-rater agreement.

Subsequently, a retrospective validation of the EDACS-ADP was performed using 763 chest pain patients who presented to St. Paul's Hospital, Vancouver, Canada, between June 2000 and January 2003. Of the 763 patients, 310 (41%) were classified as low risk by the EDACS-ADP. The sensitivity, specificity, negative predictive value, and positive predictive value of the EDACS-ADP for 30-day MACE were 100% (95% CI 94.2–100%), 45.3% (95% CI 41.6–49.1%), 100% (95% CI 98.5–100%), and 17.4% (95% CI 14.1–21.3%), respectively.[70]

The EDACS-ADP is now being used in multiple hospitals in New Zealand and Australia. A single center randomized controlled trial has found the protocol to be both safe and effective at identifying this low-risk group and is in publication.

High-sensitivity Cardiac Troponin T Assay for Rapid Rule Out of Acute Myocardial Infarction

High-sensitivity cardiac troponin T assay for rapid rule out of acute myocardial infarction (TRAPID-AMI) uses a simple algorithm incorporating hs-cTnT baseline values and absolute changes between 0 and 1 hour from ED attendance to allow a safe rule-out as well as an accurate rule-in of AMI. It was developed from 872 patients with acute chest pain to hospitals in Europe.[71] Patients were considered low risk and suitable for rule out of AMI if after blood sampling for troponin on arrival and 1 hour later the hs-cTnT result on arrival is less than 12 ng/L and the dynamic change between the two samples is less than 3 ng/L. Using this approach, 60% of patients could be classified as suitable for rule out with a sensitivity and negative predictive value of 100%. There has since been a multicenter observational validation of this approach involving 1,282 patients from multiple countries. In this validation, 63.4% of patients were categorized as suitable for rule out with a negative predictive value of 99.1%.[73]

One of the attractive aspects of the TRAPID-AMI approach is that it also sets criteria for rule in. These are initial hs-cTnT result of greater than equal to 52 ng/L with a δ at 1 hour of greater than equal to 5 ng/L. The positive predictive value for this approach in the validation study was 77.2% for prediction of AMI as a final adjudicated diagnosis.

CONCLUSION

Clinical decision aids have become popular in emergency medicine to overcome cognitive biases, which affect the clinician's ability to predict an accurate mathematical pretest probability of a patient having a particular pathology. Physicians have difficulty in estimating risks of diseases; frequently erring towards overestimation.[72] Clinical decision aids with or without clinical gestalt have the potential to be important tools in the assessment of patients presenting to the ED with possible AMI, and the accelerated decision-making processes incorporating such aids can be used to facilitate safe early discharge. There is substantial ongoing research in this area. Those clinicians or departments that are thinking of adopting an ADP for local implementation should carefully decide on the outcome of importance (i.e., early rule out of AMI vs. rule out of ACS). Consideration should be given as to whether the setting for the published research for a particular ADP is applicable (and hence transferable) to a local practice setting. This may be particularly important in relation to the disease prevalence since it is relatively easy for an ADP that has been developed and tested in a low prevalence population to categorize a large proportion of patients as being low risk with a high negative predictive value. Considerable caution should be applied in transferring such results into practice setting that has a higher prevalence of AMI and ACS. There may also be differences in the emergency medicine system (e.g., Germany does not have a college of emergency medicine) and in the experience of the training and experience of the staff who are responsible for making assessments and decisions on patients. If changes to a described ADP have occurred over time from the original version described, then clinicians should be clear as to which version they wish to implement and what the evidence for that particular version has been.

REFERENCES

1. Goodacre S, Cross E, Arnold J, Angelini K, Capewell S, Nicholl J. The health care burden of acute chest pain. Heart. Heart. 2005;91(2):229-30.
2. Weinstock MB, Weingart S, Orth F, Van Fossen D, Kaide C, Anderson J, et al. Risk for Clinically Relevant Adverse Cardiac Events in Patients With Chest Pain at Hospital Admission. JAMA Intern Med. 2015;175(7):1207-12.
3. Pollack CV Jr., Sites FD, Shofer FS, Sease KL, Hollander JE. Application of the TIMI risk score for unstable angina and non-ST elevation acute coronary syndrome to an unselected emergency department chest pain population. Acad Emerg Med. [Evaluation Studies]. 2006;13(1):13-8.
4. Chase M, Robey JL, Zogby KE, Sease KL, Shofer FS, Hollander JE. Prospective validation of the Thrombolysis in Myocardial Infarction Risk Score in the emergency department chest pain population. Ann Emerg Med. 2006;48(3):252-9.
5. Hollander JE. The continuing search to identify the very-low-risk chest pain patient. Acad Emerg Med. [Editorial]. 1999;6(10):979-81.
6. McGinn TG, Guyatt GH, Wyer PC, Naylor CD, Stiell IG, Richardson WS. Users' guides to the medical literature: XXII: how to use articles about clinical decision rules. Evidence-Based Medicine Working Group. JAMA. 2000;284(1):79-84.
7. Than M, Herbert M, Flaws D, Cullen L, Hess E, Hollander JE, et al. What is an acceptable risk of major adverse cardiac event in chest pain patients soon after discharge from the Emergency Department: A clinical survey Int J Cardiol 2013;166(3):752-4.
8. Mahler SA, Hiestand BC, Goff DC, Hoekstra JW, Miller CD, et al. Can the HEART Score Safely Reduce Stress Testing and Cardiac Imaging in Patients at Low Risk for Major Adverse Cardiac Events? Crit Pathw Cardiol. 2011;10(3):128-33.
9. Goodacre SW, Angelini K, Arnold SR, Morris F, Revill S, et al. Clinical Predictors of Acute Coronary Syndromes in Patients with Undifferentiated Chest Pain. QJM. 2003;96(12):893-8.
10. Goodacre S, Locker T, Morris F, Campbell S, et al. How Useful are Clinical Features in the Diagnosis of Acute, Undifferentiated Chest Pain? Acad Emerg Med. 2002;9(3):203-8.
11. Body R, McDowell G, Carley S, Mackway-Jones K, et al. Do Risk Factors for Chronic Coronary Heart Disease Help Diagnose Acute Myocardial Infarction in the Emergency Department? Resuscitation. 2008;79(1):41-5.
12. Body R, Carley S, Wibberley C, McDowell G, Ferguson J, Mackway-Jones K. The Value of Symptoms and Signs in the Emergent Diagnosis of Acute Coronary Syndromes. Resuscitation. 2010;81(3):281-6.
13. Han JH, Lindsell CJ, Luber S, Hoekstra KW, Hollander JE, Peacock WF, et al. The Role of Cardiac Risk Factor Burden in Diagnosing Acute Coronary Syndromes in the Emergency Department Setting. Ann Emerg Med. 2007;49(2):145-52.
14. Body R, Cook G, Burrows G, Carley S, Lewis PS, Jarvis J. Can emergency physicians "rule in" and "rule out" acute myocardial infarction with clinical judgement? Emerg Med J. 2014;31(11):872-6.
15. Greenslade JH, Cullen L, Parsonage W, Reid CM, Body R, Richards M, et al. Examining the signs and symptoms experienced by individuals with suspected acute coronary syndrome in the Asia-Pacific region: a prospective observational study. Ann Emerg Med. 2012;60(6):777-785.e3.
16. Carlton EW, Than M, Cullen L, Khattab A, Greaves K, et al. Chest Pain Typicality' in Suspected Acute Coronary Syndromes and the Impact of Clinical Experience. Am J Med. 2015;128(10):1109-1116.e2.
17. Backus B.The HEART score for chest pain patients. Oisterwijk:Uitgeverij BOXPress; 1979.
18. Collins G, Reitsma JB, Altman DG, Moons KGM, et al. Transparent Reporting of a multivariable prediction model for Individual Prognosis or Diagnosis (TRIPOD): the TRIPOD statement. Ann Intern Med. 2015;162(1):55-63.
19. Steyerberg EW. Clinical Prediction Models: A Practical Approach to Development, Validation, and Updating: Springer. 2009.
20. Reilly BM, Evans AT. Translating clinical research into clinical practice: impact of using prediction rules to make decisions. Ann Intern Med. 2006;144(3):201-9.
21. Moons KG, Kengne AP, Woodward M, Royston P, Vergouwe Y, Altman DG, et al. Risk prediction models: I. Development, internal validation, and assessing the incremental value of a new (bio)marker. Heart. 2012;98(9):683-90.
22. Toll DB, Janssen KJ, Vergouwe Y, Moons KG, et al. Validation, updating and impact of clinical prediction rules: a review. J Clin Epidemiol. 2008;61(11):1085-94.
23. Klok FA, Mos IC, Nijkeuter M, Righini M, Perrier A, Le Gal G, et al. Simplification of the revised Geneva score for assessing clinical probability of pulmonary embolism. Arch Intern Med. 2008;168(19):2131-6.
24. Goldman L, Weinberg M, Weisberg M, Olshen R, Cook EF, Sargent RK, et al. A Computer-Derived Protocol to Aid in the Diagnosis of Emergency Room Patients with Acute Chest Pain. N Engl J Med. 1982;307(10):588-96.
25. Goldman L, Cook F, Brand D, Lee TH, Rouan GW, Weisberg MC, et al. A Computer Protocol to Predict Myocardial Infarction in Emergency Department Patients with Chest Pain. N Engl J Med. 1988;318(13):797-803.
26. Grijseels EW, Deckers JW, Hoes AW, Hartman JA, Van der Does E, Van Loenen E, et al. Pre-hospital triage of patients with suspected myocardial infarction. Evaluation of previously developed algorithms and new proposals. Eur Heart J. 1995;16(3):325-32.
27. Selker HP, Griffith MS, Agostino RB. A Tool for Judging Coronary Care Unit Admission Appropriateness, Valid for Both Real-Time and Retrospective Use. Med Care. 1991;29(7):610-27.
28. Selker HP, Beshansky JR, Griffith JL, Audferheide TP, Ballin DS, Bernard SA, et al. Use of the Acute Cardiac Ischemia Time-Insensitive Predictive Instrument (ACI-TIPI) to Assist with Triage of Patients with Chest Pain or other Symptoms Suggestive of Acute Cardiac Ischemia: A Multicenter, Controlled Clinical Trial. Ann Intern Med. 1998;129(11):845-55.
29. Seyal JM, Clark EN, Macfarlane PW. Diagnosis of acute myocardial ischaemia using probabilistic methods. J Cardiovasc Risk 2002;9:115e21.

30. Miller CD, Lindsell CJ, Anantharaman V, Lim SH, Greenway J, Pollack CV, et al. Performance of a population-based cardiac risk stratification tool in Asian patients with chest pain. Acad Emerg Med. 2005;12(5):423-30.
31. Mitchell AM, Garvey JL, Chandra A, Diercks D, Pollack CV, Kline JA. Prospective multicenter study of quantitative pretest probability assessment to exclude acute coronary syndrome for patients evaluated in emergency department chest pain units. Ann Emerg Med. 2006;47(5):447.
32. Kellett J. Early diagnosis of acute myocardial infarction by either electrocardiogram or a logistic regression model: portability of a predictive instrument of acute cardiac ischemia to a small rural coronary care unit. Can J Cardiol 1997;13(11):1033e8.
33. Antman EM, Cohen M, Bernink PJLM, McCabe CH, Horacek T, Papuchis G, et al. The TIMI Risk Score for Unstable Angina/Non-ST Elevation MI. JAMA. 2000;284(7):835-42.
34. Macdonald SPJ, Nagree Y, Fatovich DM, Flavell HL, Loutsky F. Comparison of Two Clinical Scoring Systems for Emergency Department Risk Stratification of Suspected Acute Coronary Syndrome. Emerg Med Australas. 2011;23(6):717-25.
35. Than M, Cullen L, Reid C, Lim SH, Aldous S, Ardagh MW, et al. A 2-h Diagnostic Protocol to Assess Patients with Chest Pain Symptoms in the Asia Pacific Region (ASPECT): a Prospective Observational Validation Study. Lancet. 2011;377(9771):1077-84.
36. Hess EP, Agarwal DT, Chandra S, Murad MH, Erwin PJ, Hollander JE, et al. Diagnostic Accuracy of the TIMI Risk Score in Patients with Chest Pain in the Emergency Department: a Meta-Analysis. CMAJ. 2010 Jul 13;182(10):1039-44.
37. Conway-Morris A, Caesar D, Gray D, Gray A. TIMI Risk Score Accurately Risk Stratifies Patients with Undifferentiated Chest Pain Presenting to an Emergency Department. Heart. 2006 Sep;92(9):1333-4.
38. Tong KL, Kaul S, Wang X, Rinkevich D, Kalvaitis S, Belcik T, et al. Myocardial Contrast Echocardiography Versus Thrombolysis in Myocardial Infarction Score in Patients Presenting to the Emergency Department with Chest Pain and a Nondiagnostic Electrocardiogram. J Am Coll Cardiol. 2005 Sep 6;46(5):920-7.
39. Chase M, Robey JL, Zogby KE, Sease KL, Shofer FS,, Hollander JE. Prospective Validation of the Thrombosis in Myocardial Infarction Risk Score in the Emergency Department Chest Pain Population. . Ann. Emerg. Med. 2006;48(2)252-9.
40. Boersma E, Pieper KS, Steyerberg ES, Wilcox RG, Chang W, Lee KL, et al. Predictors of Outcome in Patients with Acute Coronary Syndromes without Persistant ST-Segment Elevation: Results from an International Trial of 9461 Patients. Circulation. 2000;101(22):2557-67.
41. de Araujo Goncalves P, Ferreira J, Aguiar C, Seabra-Gomes R. TIMI, PURSUIT, and GRACE Risk Scores: Sustained Prognostic Value and Interaction with Revascularisation in NSTE-ACS. Eur. Hear. J. 2005;26:65-872.
42. Granger CB, Goldberg RJ, Dabbous O, Pieper KS, Eagle KA, Cannon CP, et al. Predictors of Hospital Mortality in the Global Registry of Acute Coronary Events. Arch Intern Med. 2003;163(19):2345-53.
43. Killip T, Kimball JT. Treatment of myocardial infarction in a coronary care unit. A two year experience with 250 patients.Am J Cardiol 1967. 20(4):457-64
44. Yusufali, Afzalhussein, Mohammad Zubaid, Ibrahim Al-Zakwani, Alawi A. Alsheikh-Ali, et al. Validation of the GRACE Risk score for hospital mortality in patients with acute coronary syndrome in the Arab Middle East. Angiology. 2011;62(5):390-6.
45. Eggers, Kai M., Kempf T, Venge P, Wallentin L, Wollert KC, et al. Improving long-term risk prediction in patients with acute chest pain: The Global Registry of Acute Coronary Events (GRACE) risk score is enhanced by selected nonnecrosis biomarkers. Am Heart J. 2010;160(1):88-94.
46. Walker NJ, Sites FD, Shofer FS, Hollander JE. Characteristics and outcomes of young adults who present to the emergency department with chest pain. Acad Emerg Med. 2001;8:703-8.
47. Marsan RJ, Shaver KJ, Sease KL, Shofer FS, Sites FD, Hollander JE. Evaluation of a Clinical Decision Rule for Young Adult Patients with Chest Pain. Acad Emerg Med. 2005;12(1):26-31.
48. Christenson J, Innes G, McKnight D, Thompson CR, Wong H, Yu E, et al. A clinical prediction rule for early discharge of patients with chest pain. Ann Emerg Med.2006.47(1):1-10.
49. Jalili M, Hejripour Z, Honarmand AR, Pourtabatabaei N. Validation of the Vancouver Chest Pain Rule: a Prospective Cohort Study. Acad Emerg Med. 2012;19(7):837-42.
50. Acute Coronary Syndrome Guidelines Working Group. Guidelines for the management of acute coronary syndromes 2006. Med J Aust. 2006;184(8):S1-S32.
51. Kelly AM "How useful are the Heart Foundation risk criteria for assessment of emergency department patients with chest pain" Emergency Medicine Australasia. 2012;24(3). pp. 260-5.
52. Than M, Cullen L, Aldous S, Parsonage WA, Reid CM, Greenslade J, et al. 2-Hour accelerated diagnostic protocol to assess patients with chest pain symptoms using contemporary troponins as the only biomarker: the ADAPT trial. J Am Coll Cardiol. 2012;59(23):2091-8.
53. Cullen L, Mueller C, Parsonage WA, Wildi K, Greenslade JH, Twerenbold R, et al. Validation of High-Sensitivity Troponin I in a 2-Hour Diagnostic Strategy to Assess 30-Day Outcomes in Emergency Department Patients With Possible Acute Coronary Syndrome. J Am Coll Cardiol. 2013;62(14):1242-9.
54. Edward W Carlton, Louise Cullen, Martin Than, James Gamble, Ahmed Khattab, Kim Greaves. A novel diagnostic protocol to identify patients suitable for discharge after a single high-sensitivity troponin. Heart. 2015;101(13):1041-6.
55. Six AJ, Backus BE, Kelder JC. Chest Pain in the Emergency Room: Value of the HEART Score. Neth Heart J. 2008;16(6):191-6.
56. Backus B. The HEART score for chest pain patients. Uitgeverij BOXPress, Oisterwijk. 2012; pp. 1-248.
57. APGAR V. A proposal for a new method of evaluation of the newborn infant. Curr Res Anesth Analg. 1953;32(4):260-7.
58. Backus B, Six AJ, Kelder JC, Mast TP, van den Akker F, Mast EG, et al. Chest Pain in the Emergency Room: A Multicentre Validation of the HEART Score. Crit Pathw Cardiol. 2010;9(3):164-9.
59. Mahler SA, Hiestand BC, Goff DC, Hoekstra JW, Miller CD. Can the HEART Score Safely Reduce Stress Testing and Cardiac Imaging in Patients at Low Risk for Major Adverse Cardiac Events? Crit Pathw Cardiol. 2011;10(3):128-33.
60.. Six AJ, Cullen L, Backus BE, Greenslade J, Parsonage W, Aldous S,The HEART Score for the Assessment of Patients With Chest Pain in the Emergency Department. Crit Pathw Cardiol. 2013;12(3):121-6.
61. Backus BE1, Six AJ, Kelder JC, Bosschaert MA, Mast EG, Mosterd A, et al. A prospective validation of the HEART score for chest pain patients at the emergency department. Int J Cardiol. 2013;168(3):2153-8.
62. Mahler SA, Riley RF, Hiestand BC, Russell GB, Hoekstra JW, Lefebvre CW, et al. The HEART Pathway Randomized Trial: Identifying Emergency Department Patients With Acute Chest Pain for Early Discharge. Circ Cardiovasc Qual Outcomes. 2015 Mar;8(2):195-203.
63. Hess EP, Brison RJ, Perry JJ, Calder LJ, Thiruganasambandamoorthy V, Agarwal D, et al. Development of a Clinical Prediction Rule for 30-Day Cardiac Events in Emergency Department Patients with Chest Pain and Possible Acute Coronary Syndrome. Ann Emerg Med. 2012;59(2):115-25.e1.
64. Erik P Hess, George A Wells, Allan Jaffe, Ian G Stiell. A study to derive a clinical decision rule for triage of emergency department patients with chest pain: design and methodology. BMC Emerg Med. 2008;8:3.
65. Scheuermeyer FX, Innes G, Grafstein E, Kiess M, Boychuk B, Yu E, et al. Safety and efficiency of a chest pain diagnostic algorithm with selective outpatient stress testing for emergency department patients with potential ischemic chest pain. Ann Emerg Med. 2012;59(4):256-264.e3.
66. Cullen L1, Greenslade JH2, Than M3, Brown AF4, Hammett CJ5, Lamanna A, et al. The new Vancouver Chest Pain Rule using troponin as the only biomarker: an external validation study. Am J Emerg Med. 2014;32(2):129-34.
67. Body R, Carley S, McDowell G, Pemberton P, Burrows G, Cook G, et al. The Manchester Acute Coronary Syndromes (MACS) decision rule for suspected cardiac chest pain: derivation and external validation. Heart. 2014;100(18):1462-8.
68. Body R, Burrows G, Carley S, Lewis PS, Jarvis J. The Manchester Acute Coronary Syndromes (MACS) decision rule: validation with a new automated assay for heart-type fatty acid binding protein. Emergency Medicine Journal [Internet]. 2014;24:32(10).
69. Cullen L, Than M, Brown AF, Richards M, Parsonage W, Flaws D, et al. Comprehensive standardized data definitions for acute coronary syndrome research in emergency departments in Australasia. Emerg Med Australas. 2010;22(1):35-55.
70. Than M, Flaws D, Sanders S, Doust J, Glasziou P, Kline J, et al. Development and validation of the Emergency Department Assessment of Chest pain Score and 2 h accelerated diagnostic protocol. Emerg Med Australas. 2014;26(1):34-44.
71. Reichlin T, Schindler C, Drexler B, Twerenbold R, Reiter M, Zellweger C, et al.One-hour rule-out and rule-in of acute myocardial infarction using high-sensitivity cardiac troponin T. Arch Intern Med. 2012;172(16):1211-8.
72. Friedmann PD, Brett AS, Mayo-Smith MF. "Differences in generalists' and cardiologists' perceptions of cardiovascular risk and the outcomes of preventive therapy in cardiovascular disease". Ann Intern Med. 1996; 124(4):414-21.
73. Mueller C, Giannitsis E, Christ M, Ordóñez-Llanos J. Multicenter evaluation of a 0-hour/1-hour algorithm in the diagnosis of myocardial infarction with high-sensitivity cardiac troponin T. Ann Emerg Med. 2016;68(1):p76-87.

13 CHAPTER

Acute Coronary Syndrome: Risk Stratification

Lane M Smith, Chadwick D Miller, Simon A Mahler

INTRODUCTION

Acute coronary syndrome (ACS) is a spectrum of diseases ranging from myocardial ischemia to infarction typically due to partial or complete thrombosis of diseased coronary arteries. Acute coronary syndrome is a common condition affecting an estimated 1.4 million Americans each year. The annual cost of ACS in 2010 was $200 billion, and ACS-related expenditures are expected to increase by 200% over the next 20 years.[1] While mortality across the spectrum of ACS has declined over the past 30 years with the increasing use of reperfusion and preventative therapies, there is still significant heterogeneity in ST segment elevation myocardial infarction (STEMI), non-ST segment elevation myocardial infarction (NSTEMI), and unstable angina (UA) outcomes. Current estimates of 30-day mortality for all forms of ACS are between 2 and 3%, but this may be significantly higher if UA is excluded.[2] In addition, ACS prognosis varies based on the presence or absence of comorbid conditions.

The purpose of risk stratifying patients with ACS is two-fold: (i) assist in the development of a reperfusion strategy; and (ii) identify patients at risk for further cardiac events such as sudden cardiac death, recurrent ischemia, heart failure, arrhythmias, and stroke. The process of risk stratification begins immediately upon arrival and continues throughout the hospital course. Due to the variable approach to patients within the ACS spectrum, different risk stratification methods for STEMI and non-ST segment elevation acute coronary syndrome (NSTEACS) are discussed separately.

ST SEGMENT ELEVATION MYOCARDIAL INFARCTION

Recent studies have shown STEMI to carry the worst short-term prognosis compared to other forms of ACS with 30-day mortality between 3 and 10%.[3,4] In addition, early primary reperfusion is the well-defined treatment of choice for STEMI even in patients who are otherwise low risk. Thus, the most useful risk stratifications tools for STEMI are derived from large registries of patients undergoing immediate reperfusion therapy. Since all patients presenting with an STEMI should receive immediate reperfusion, these scores are used to direct downstream patient care after reperfusion or provide triage guidance to higher levels of care for smaller medical centers.

Thrombolysis in Myocardial Infarction Score for ST Segment Elevation Myocardial Infarction

The thrombolysis in myocardial infarction (TIMI) score for STEMI is a widely used method to determine 30-day mortality in patients presenting with STEMI who are eligible for reperfusion.[5] The system was derived from 15,000 patients enrolled in the InTIME II database and identifies nine independent predictors of mortality, which are listed in table 1.

The Killip class is a ranking of heart failure according to the following scheme:[6]

- Killip class I is no clinical signs of heart failure
- Killip class II describes patients with rales, S3 gallop, and elevated jugular venous pressure
- Killip class III are individuals with acute pulmonary edema
- Killip class IV includes patients with cardiogenic shock, hypotension, and peripheral vasoconstriction.

TABLE 1: The nine Thrombolysis in Myocardial Infarction (TIMI) risk factors for mortality and their point values

TIMI risk factors	Point values
Age 65–74 years	2 points
Age >75 years	3 points
History of diabetes, hypertension, or angina	1 point
Systolic blood pressure <100 mm Hg	3 points
Killip class II–IV	2 points
Heart rate >100 beats/min	2 points
Anterior STEMI or left bundle branch block	1 point
Time to reperfusion therapy >4 h	1 point
Weight <67 kg	1 Point

STEMI, ST segment elevation myocardial infarction; TIMI, Thrombolysis in Myocardial Infarction.

TABLE 2: Thrombolysis in Myocardial Infarction risk score mortality for point scores ranging from 0–8

TIMI risk score	Predicted 30-day mortality in STEMI (%)
0	0.8
1	1.6
2	2.2
3	4.4
4	7.3
5	12.4
6	16.1
7	23.4
8	26.8
>8	35.9

STEMI, ST segment elevation myocardial infarction; TIMI, Thrombolysis in Myocardial Infarction.

Mortality at 30 days increases continuously over 0–8 points according to table 2.

This score was further validated among a heterogeneous population of 84,000 STEMI patients in the Third National Registry of Myocardial Infarction database.[7] This included those receiving primary coronary reperfusion, the contemporary therapy of choice, or no acute reperfusion. The TIMI score showed strong prognostic capability for patients receiving some form of acute reperfusion, regardless of the modality. The score underestimated mortality for patients who received no reperfusion. Overall, this score provides an excellent balance of accuracy and ease of use.

Thrombolysis in Myocardial Infarction Risk Index

An even simpler model derived from the same database as the TIMI score uses data obtained at presentation according to the following equation:

$$\text{TIMI risk index} = \frac{\text{Heart rate} \times (\text{Age}/10)^2}{\text{Systolic blood pressure}}$$

A graded relationship between TRI score and inhospital mortality exists for all patients receiving reperfusion therapy according to figure 1.[8] The Thrombolysis In Myocardial Infarction risk index (TRI) has been validated for use outside of the United States as well as in patients undergoing reperfusion by fibrinolysis or cardiac catheterization. Similar to the TIMI score, the TRI underestimates mortality in patients not undergoing reperfusion. The TRI is unique in that no clinical history is required. This makes the score particularly useful for emergency medical service (EMS) providers or in other situations where minimal patient data is available to triage healthcare resources.

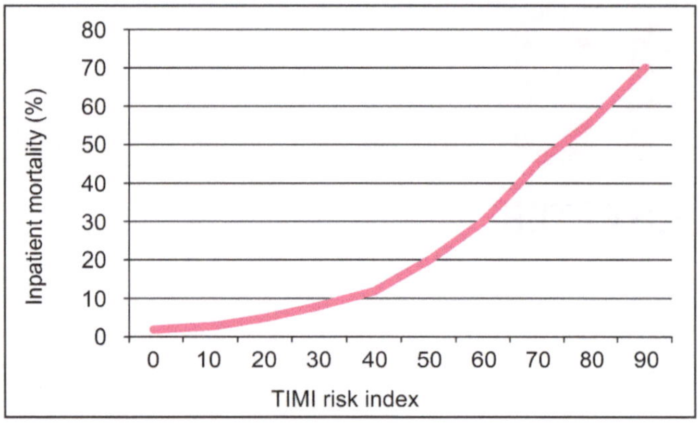

TIMI, Thrombolysis in Myocardial Infarction.

FIG. 1: Inpatient mortality versus Thrombolysis in Myocardial Infarction (TIMI) risk index for ST-segment elevation myocardial infarction patients undergoing reperfusion

Global Registry of Acute Coronary Events Risk Model

The Global Registry of Acute Coronary Events (GRACE) is derived from 100 hospitals that are carefully chosen to be generalizable populations of patients with ACS.[9] It includes both community and tertiary hospitals from 30 countries that represent a diverse spectrum of capabilities within the study regions. More than 11,000 patients were used to develop the original inhospital model of mortality that has been validated using more than 40,000 patients from multiple registries and randomized trials. The original GRACE risk model assigns points to eight risk factors that, when added together, predict inhospital mortality as seen in figure 2.[10] These risk factors and their point values are described in table 3.

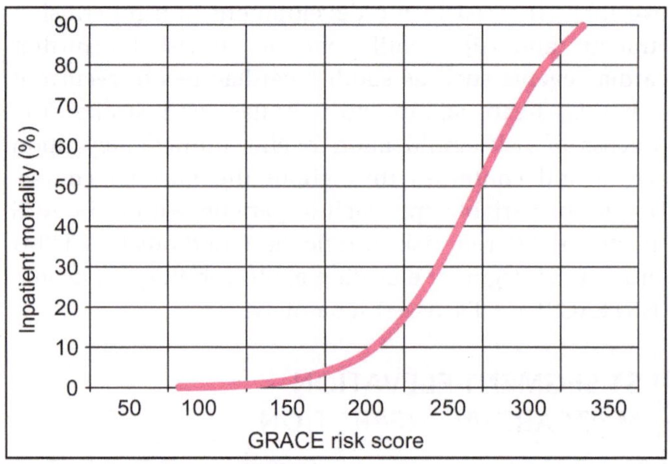

GRACE, Global Registry of Acute Coronary Events.

FIG. 2: Inpatient mortality versus Global Registry of Acute Coronary Events (GRACE) risk score for ST-segment elevation myocardial infarction (STEMI) patients

Source: Nomogram calculated using data from Center for Outcomes Research, University of Massachusetts Medical School; Copyright 1998–2014, *with permission.*

TABLE 3: Global Registry of Acute Coronary Events (GRACE) risk factors

Killip class	Points	SBP (mm Hg)	Points	HR (beats/min)	Points	Age	Points	Creatinine (mg/dL)	Points
I	0	≤80	58	≤50	0	≤30	0	0–0.39	1
II	20	80–99	53	50–69	3	30–39	8	0.49–0.79	4
III	39	100–119	43	70–89	9	40–49	25	0.8–1.19	7
IV	59	120–139	34	90–109	15	50–59	41	1.2–1.59	10
		140–159	24	110–149	24	60–69	58	1.6–1.99	13
		160–199	10	150–199	38	70–79	75	2–3.99	21
		≥200	0	≥200	46	80–89	91	≥4.0	28
						≥90	100		
Other risk factors								**Points**	
Cardiac arrest at admission								39	
ST-segment deviation								28	
Elevation cardiac enzyme levels								14	

SBP, systolic blood pressure; HR, heart rate.

An updated GRACE risk model, Version 2.0, can be used to calculate both inpatient, as seen in figure 2, or 1-year mortality.[11] In addition, a mini-GRACE score is available, which uses a history of renal dysfunction and diuretic use for patients who lack a serum creatinine or Killip classification. More information including a GRACE risk 2.0 calculator and downloadable applications can be found at http://www.outcomes-umassmed.org/grace/.

Alternative Risk Scores and Choosing the Best Scoring Method

Several attempts have been made to improve the predictive value of the TIMI and GRACE risk models. Some have added additional variables, such as hemoglobin concentration, creatinine clearance, and C-reactive protein (CRP) to improve accuracy of the GRACE and TIMI scores.[12,13] Others have used datasets derived from patients receiving only percutaneous coronary intervention (PCI) to better predict mortality in patients receiving the most current reperfusion strategies.[14] A few risk assessment methods have combined scoring methods to improve on the performance of the TIMI and GRACE scores in critically ill patients with STEMI such as the Acute Physiology and Chronic Health Evaluation II (APACHE II) score combined with Killip classification.[15] Each of these alternative scores require data that is not routinely available in the emergency setting and offer no real improvement in accuracy or ease of use when compared to the TIMI or GRACE risk scores.

When it comes to choosing between the TIMI and GRACE risk scores, their prognostic capabilities have been compared with mixed results. Early comparison favored the TIMI score in STEMI patients without cardiogenic shock for determining 30-day and 1-year mortality.[16] However, a subsequent meta-analysis showed that GRACE and TIMI have comparable performance at predicting short- and long-term mortality.[17] Thus, either the TIMI score or GRACE score is a reasonable approach to quantifying early mortality risk after STEMI until more data is collected in the modern era of percutaneous reperfusion.

NON-ST SEGMENT ELEVATION ACUTE CORONARY SYNDROME

Unlike STEMI where emergent revascularization is the standard of care, the early approach to NSTEACS is less clear with fewer than half of patients having an identifiable culprit lesion on cardiac cauterizations.[18] Thus, much of the recent literature has focused on identifying segments of the NSTEACS population that are most likely to benefit from invasive revascularization. A small population of very high-risk patients has been identified as needing emergent intervention prior to further risk stratification.[19,20] Patients presenting with NSTEACS and having the following characteristics should proceed to immediate cardiac catheterization:

- Overt heart failure with cardiogenic shock;
- Ventricular arrhythmias;
- Mechanical complications causing hemodynamic instability [ventricular septal defect, acute mitral regurgitation (MR), critical aortic stenosis, etc.].

For the remaining patients with NSTEACS, two therapeutic approaches have emerged aimed at improving long-term prognosis: Conservative versus early invasive therapy. The conservative approach involves intensive medical therapy followed by a "cooling off" period for several days in patients who become asymptomatic. Provocative testing or noninvasive imaging is often used to determine which patients receiving conservative therapy are most likely to benefit from cardiac catheterization. On the other hand, the early invasive approach focuses on prompt revascularization after medical stabilization.

A number of clinical trials have been performed to determine which approach is superior and the optimal timeframe for an invasive approach. Initial trials were conflicting due to the presence of different primary endpoints, unequal coprimary endpoints, and a wide spectrum of disease severity such as the inclusion of patients having only UA with those having NSTEMI in certain studies.[21-23] However, the general trend of the literature is that moderate- to higher-risk patients and those presenting with significant troponin elevations are most likely to benefit from an early invasive strategy.[24] The 2012 American College of Cardiology/American Heart Association (ACC/AHA) guidelines recommend an early invasive strategy for patients with NSTEACS who are at moderate-to-high risk of adverse events based on objective risk assessment tools such as the TIMI or GRACE model.[25] In addition, the optimal timing of an invasive approach has undergone a paradigm shift in recent years with a 48-hour window being replaced by 24 hours.[26]

Despite guidelines recommending an early invasive strategy in high-risk NSTEACS patients, cardiac catheterization use remains suboptimal.[27] Physician estimations of risk are often inaccurate and as many as 60% of patients deemed to be low risk actually meet criteria for an invasive strategy on subsequent review.[28] Risk stratification tools help clinicians make accurate risk predications and avoid underestimations, which frequently occur when they focus on just one or two factors such as ST deviation or cardiac biomarker elevation.[29] Thus, clinicians should employ one of the risk stratification tools outlined below rather than rely on nonevidence based estimations.

Thrombolysis in Myocardial Infarction Risk Score for Non-ST Segment Elevation Acute Coronary Syndrome

The TIMI risk score for NSTEMI and UA is derived from a cohort of 7,000 patients having NSTEACS.[30] Seven variables are predicative of adverse outcome when present at admission, which included:

- Age ≥ 65 years old
- Presence of three coronary artery disease risk factors
- Known prior coronary stenosis ≥50%
- Presence of ST segment deviation on initial electrocardiogram (ECG)
- At least two episodes of angina in the prior 24 hours
- Elevated cardiac biomarkers
- Use of aspirin in the previous 7 days.

Each variable is assigned one point when present and zero when absent. Of note, aspirin is included in this list due to its association with more significant vascular

TABLE 4: Thrombolysis in Myocardial Infarction (TIMI) risk score for non-ST segment elevation myocardial infarction and unstable angina. Adverse events at 14 days are defined as: All-cause mortality, new or recurrent myocardial infarction, or severe recurrent ischemia requiring revascularization

TIMI risk score	Adverse event rate (%)	Risk assessment
0/1	4.7	Low
2	8.3	
3	13.2	Moderate
4	19.9	
5	26.2	High
6/7	40.9	

TIMI, Thrombolysis in Myocardial Infarction.

disease rather than independently causing a worse outcome. Higher TIMI scores are associated with severe angiographic findings and adverse events at 14 days as seen in table 4.[31]

In addition to predicting outcome, the TIMI score was useful in predicting patient response to treatment. Multiple studies have shown that patients with at least moderate risk TIMI scores (≥3) benefit from an early invasive therapeutic approach.[24,32] Patients with TIMI scores greater than three also derive a greater benefit from anticoagulation and glycoprotein IIb/IIIa inhibitors.[30,33] Additional studies have shown that higher troponin elevations associated with greater degrees of ST segment deviation predict worse outcomes, failed attempts at conservative therapy, and the need for an early invasive strategy.[34]

Thrombolysis in Myocardial Infarction Risk Index for Non-ST Segment Elevation Acute Coronary Syndrome

The TRI uses the same formula and variables collected at presentation that are described for risk assessment in STEMI. As illustrated in figure 3, a graded relationship to in-hospital mortality was seen when this score was applied to more than 300,000 NSTEMI patients in the National Registry of Myocardial Infarction (NRMI) database.[35] Patients with scores less than 30 were deemed to be low risk with mortality rates less than 10%.

Global Registry of Acute Coronary Events Risk Model for Non-ST Segment Elevation Acute Coronary Syndrome

The GRACE risk score can be calculated for NSTEACS using the same variables that were described for patients with STEMI and applied to a nomogram that estimates mortality.[10] This score offers some advantages over the TIMI risk score in that one scoring method can be used for all forms of ACS, estimates for mortality can be made out

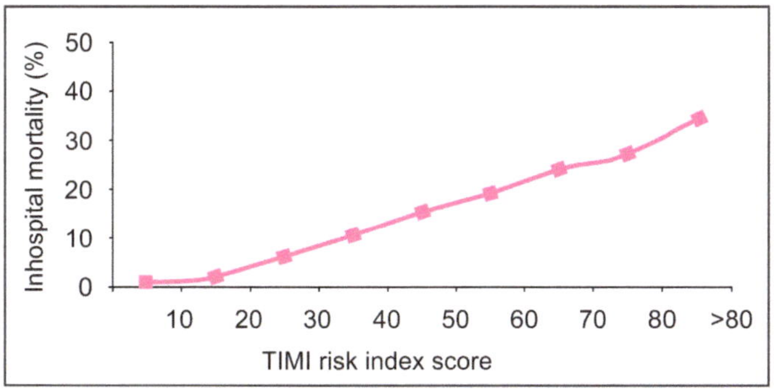

TIMI, Thrombolysis in Myocardial Infarction.

FIG. 3: Inhospital mortality versus Thrombolysis in Myocardial Infarction (TIMI) risk index

to 1 year and the GRACE score does not use a composite endpoint.

Acute Catheterization and Urgent Intervention Triage Strategy-Percutaneous Coronary Intervention Score

The Acute Catheterization and Urgent Intervention Triage Strategy-Percutaneous Coronary Intervention (ACUITY-PCI) score is a risk stratification score for NSTEACS patients undergoing an early invasive treatment option.[36] Unlike the TIMI and GRACE tools that were derived from studies of patients receiving thrombolysis, the ACUITY-PCI score was created from more than 1,600 patients in the angiographic substudy of the ACUITY trial.[37] This score uses a hybrid of clinical, angiographic, and laboratory/electrocardiographic variables to assess the 1-year risk of death or myocardial infarction (MI). These weighted variables include:

- Renal insufficiency (12 points)
- Insulin-treated diabetes (12 points)
- Baseline cardiac biomarkers elevation or ST segment deviation (8 points)
- Bifurcation lesion (4 points)
- Small or diffuse coronary artery disease (2 points)
- Extent of coronary artery disease (1 point per mm of disease).

Adverse events increase across tertiles of the score as seen in table 5. The score has been validated against different cohorts of patients and compared favorably against other risk stratification scores such as the TIMI and GRACE scores.[36]

The ACUITY-PCI score is designed to supplement the TIMI or GRACE scores calculated on admission. Specifically, the score emphasizes the importance of extensive coronary disease or small vessel disease as independent predictors of outcome that are not measured in preangiographic scoring systems. These patterns of disease portrayed a worse prognosis than severe focal lesions and compliment other findings that multiple seemingly minor lesions portend a worse prognosis over prolonged periods of follow-up.[38]

TABLE 5: Acute Catheterization and Urgent Intervention Triage Strategy-Percutaneous Coronary Intervention (ACUITY-PCI) risk score estimates death or myocardial infarction at one year in patients with non-ST segment elevation myocardial infarction acute coronary syndrome undergoing cardiac catheterization

Tertile	ACUITY-PCI score	Death or myocardial infarction (%)
Low	≤12	5
Intermediate	>12 and ≤19	9
High	>19	19

ACUITY-PCI, Acute Catheterization and Urgent Intervention Triage Strategy—Percutaneous Coronary Intervention.

SPECIFIC HIGH-RISK FEATURES

Positive Troponin

Cardiac troponin is the most commonly used biomarker in the assessment of ACS, and elevations are considered indications for an early invasive reprerfusion strategy in NSTEMI ACS. For example, the Thrombolysis And Counterpulsation To Improve Cardiogenic Shock Survival (TACTICS) TIMI-18 trial found that a troponin I threshold of 0.1 ng/mL was able to identify patients likely to benefit from an invasive strategy in the absence of other high-risk features such as congestive heart failure (CHF) or renal insufficiency.[39] Similar results were seen in this study with troponin T values between 0.01 and 0.05 ng/mL. The prognostic significance of troponin T elevation was studied in 7,108 patients who were enrolled in the Global Utilization of Streptokinase and Tissue Plasminogen Activator for Occluded Coronary Arteries (GUSTO) IV ACS trial and did not undergo early revascularization.[40] Patients were grouped according to quartiles of troponin and 30-day mortality increased across the quartiles as seen in table 6.

A similar pattern was seen with the 30-day incidence of recurrent MI as patients with higher troponin T values experienced more frequent reinfarction across the first three quartiles.

Recent advances in troponin sensitivity have improved the ability of this biomarker to detect myocardial damage. This technology draws into question the validity of older diagnostic thresholds for MI as even slight troponin elevations can have prognostic significance. For example, one study found that the implementation of a high sensitivity troponin assay identified more patients as having an NSTEMI and resulted in a 50% reduction in death or recurrent ischemia.[41] This improvement in outcomes was attributed to better comprehensive management of patients who would otherwise not

TABLE 6: Quartiles of troponin T elevation and 30-day mortality increase in patients from the Global Utilization of Streptokinase and Tissue Plasminogen Activator for Occluded Coronary Arteries (GUSTO) IV acute coronary syndrome (ACS) trial

Quartile	Troponin T (ng/mL)	Mortality (%)
First	≤0.01	1.1
Second	0.01–0.12	3.7
Third	0.12–0.47	3.7
Fourth	>0.47	7.4

receive optimal medical and revascularization therapies. Additional studies are forthcoming to best determine an optimal threshold for positive values in the era of high sensitivity assays.

Age and Gender

Advanced age is an important risk factor for poor outcome in patients with ACS. Those older than 75 years of age do worse compared to younger patients and tend to have more severe coronary disease on catherterization.[42] All of the major risk stratification scores, such as the TIMI and GRACE scores, account for this phenomenon with higher points assigned to patients with more advanced age.

Although women have better long-term ACS mortality after adjusting for other comorbid conditions, their 30-day mortality after an MI is historically worse than men's.[43] This is particularly true for women younger than 55 years old, and the differences between the sexes declines with age. However, this gender gap has narrowed in recent years due to better awareness and treatment of ACS in young women.[44] The exact reason for higher early mortality in younger women is not well-understood, but is thought to be due to a higher incidence of atypical symptoms leading to suboptimal early management.

Congestive Heart Failure

Patients presenting with ACS and severe left ventricular (LV) dysfunction are at higher risk of death at 30 days and 1 year compared to those with normal LV function. This was seen in a database of 190,518 patients with STEMI where 19% had Killip class II/III congestive heart failure CHF on admission and suffered a three-fold increase in hospital mortality compared to patients with normal LV function.[45] Patients with CHF were less likely to get standard treatments such as aspirin, β-blockers, and heparin. In addition, patients with a normal ejection fraction (EF) were almost twice as likely to get reperfused by PCI or thrombolytics than those with CHF.

The trend toward worse outcomes was also appreciated in NSTEACS. Using data pooled from seven clinical trials, 46,519 patient with NSTEACS were identified of which 13.5% presented with CHF or developed CHF during their hospitalization.[46] These patients tended to be older, female and suffer four-fold higher mortality at 30 days with an adjusted odds ratio of 1.74 95% confidence interval (CI) = 1.37–2.26. Risk factors for developing CHF during the hospitaliztion included elevated heart rate on admission, diabetes, advanced age, prior MI, or NSTEMI at the time of enrollement. While this study showed no prognostic signifance to the development of CHF during the admission compared to patients presenting with CHF, other studies have shown that patients who develop CHF during their hosptial course have a higher mortality.[47,48] As seen in patients with STEMI, those with NSTEACS and CHF were less likely to undergo revascularization than patients without CHF despite evidence that revascularization improves outcomes in this high-risk patient population.[49]

The impact of CHF on mortality increases across disease severity as measured by Killip class in both STEMI and NSTEACS. Data from the GRACE registry found that hospital mortality across Killip classes I, II, and III was 2.9%, 9.9%, and 20.4%, respectively.[47] Moreover, the presence of Killip class III/IV CHF was prognostically the most significant risk factor for early mortality in a database of 26,000 patients with NSTEACS.[50] Thus, the physical examination in patients with ACS complicated by CHF provides an evidece-based aspect to the assessment of NSTEACS that can be more important than abnormalities in the ECG or cardiac biomarkers.

Ischemic MR has emerged as an important cause of heart failure and increased mortality after ACS. In a cohort of 1,331 geographically defined patients with STEMI or NSTEMI, MR was found in half of the cases.[51] Moderate-to-severe MR was associated with an increased risk of long-term CHF and death that was independent of other risk factors such as age, gender, or Killip class. The degree of MR was often not clinically apparent even in severe cases as the presence of a murmer was inconsistent. In addition, the location of the MI could not predict the development or severity of MR. Echocardiogram was the only accurate means to identify and quantify the degree of MR after myocardial infarction.

Electrocardiogram Abnormalities

Certain electrocardiographic abnormalities in patient presenting with ACS are associated with a worse prognosis. The presence of ST depression in NSTEACS is associated with a two-fold increase in death or MI at 30 days compared to T-wave inversions or a normal ECG.[52] The degree of ST-segement depression and resolution after reperfusion are also significant as patients with greater than or equal to 2 mm of depression and those who fail to resolve their abnormality after reperfusion suffer worse outcomes.[53,54]

Location of the infarct on ECG analysis also carries significant progostic implications in both STEMI and NSTEMI. When compared against patients with inferior wall infarcts, those having anterior infarcts suffer a three-fold increase in inhospital mortality, larger infarct size, lower postinfarct EF, more frequent ventricular arrhythmias, and higher total cardiac mortality.[55] Another study of 4,314 patients presenting with a first-time NSTEMI found that anterior wall infarcts were associated with more frequent cardiac events at 1 year after adjusting for other risk factors.[56]

Arrhythmias

Ventricular and atrial arrhythmias are associated with increased mortality in ACS. Data obtained from 9,211 patient enrolled in The early glycoprotein IIb/IIIa inhibition in non-ST segment elevation acute coronary syndrome (EARLY ACS) trial demonstrated a cumulative incidence of sustained ventricular tachycardia (VT) and ventricular fibrillation (VF) of 1.5% with most cases occuring more than 48 hours after enrollment.[57] Risk factors for VT/VF included prior CHF, EF less than 30%, and three vessel coronary artery disease. Compared to patients without ventricular arrhythmias, those with VT/VF during the first 48 hours of admission had a higher 1-year mortality rate at 13% versus 2.2%. In addition, VT/VF events after the first 48 hours carried an even worse mortality than those occuring early in the admission (hazard ratios 20.7 vs. 7.45).

Atrial fibrillation (AF) is the most common supraventricular arrhytmia in the first 48 hours of ACS and develops in 6–8% of hospitalized patients.[58,59] Both STEMI and NSTEACS patients with AF suffer higher mortality and incidence of ischemic stroke at 30 days and 6 months.[60] This effect on outcome is somewhat attenuated after adjusting for other comorbid conditions such as advanced age, CHF, and ventricular arrhythmias. Other supraventricular arrhythmias, such as supraventricular tachycardia, are rare in ACS and not thought to increase mortality.

Chronic Kidney Disease

Chronic renal failure and end-stage renal disease are independent risk factors for worse outcomes in patients with ACS.[61] The risk of cariovascular death increases with reductions in renal function. Every 10 unit reduction in glomerluar filtration rate (GFR) below 81 mL/min/1.73 m^2 increases the hazard ratio for death and nonfatal cardiovascular outcome by 1.10.[62] Thus, even a small reduction in GFR is considered a significant risk factor for adverse outcome in ACS as reflected in GRACE and ACUITY-PCI risk scoring methods. Patients with poor renal function are less likely to receive revascularization despite being high risk for adverse outcomes.[28] They are also less likely to have appropriate dosing of renally cleared antithrombotic drugs leading to more frequent bleeding complications.[63]

Elevated Non-necrosis Biomarkers

Both CRP and brain natriuretic peptide (BNP) have been studied in a manner similar to troponin T. In the GUSTO IV ACS trial, 30-day mortality increased across quartiles of CRP elevation.[64] In addition, elevation of BNP was associated with higher mortality, recurrent MI and CHF in patients with ACS.[65,66] Other studies have combined biomarkers such as troponin and BNP, and found that patients suspected of ACS with normal values of both had favorable outcomes and were unlikely to benefit from an invasive reprofusion strategy.[67] However, biomarkers other than cardiac troponins are not universally available, have not been incorportated in major risk stratification scores, and are not required to make accurate outcome predictions in ACS.

CONCLUSION

Risk stratification of patients with ACS is an important part of the clinical assessment that begins immediately upon arrival. For patients presenting with STEMI, accurate risk stratification helps guide downstream care after cardiac catherterization. For patients with NSTEACS, risk stratification is an important means to determine which patients would benefit from aggressive reperfusion and medical therapies. A number of evidence-based tools, such as the TIMI risk score and GRACE risk model, have been developed to aid clinicians. These risk scoring methods are shown to be superior to clinicial gestalt and help identify high-risk patients that might otherwise be undertreated. Careful attention should be paid to certain patient populations such as those with CHF and renal dysfunction since they often receive suboptimal medical and reperfusion treatments despite having high-risk features.

REFERENCES

1. Go AS, Mozaffarian D, Roger VL, Benjamin EJ, Berry JD, Blaha MJ, et al. Executive summary: heart disease and stroke statistics—2014 update: A report from the American Heart Association. Circulation. 2014;129:399-410.
2. Roe MT, Messenger JC, Weintraub WS, Cannon CP, Fonarow GC, Dai D, et al. Treatments, trends, and outcomes of acute myocardial infarction and percutaneous coronary intervention. J Am Coll Cardiol. 2010;56:254-63.
3. Jernberg T, Johanson P, Held C, Svennblad B, Lindbäck J, Wallentin L, et al. Association between adoption of evidence-based treatment and survival for patients with ST-elevation myocardial infarction. JAMA. 2011;305:1677-84.
4. Rogers WJ, Frederick PD, Stoehr E, Canto JG, Ornato JP, Gibson CM, et al. Trends in presenting characteristics and hospital mortality among patients with ST elevation and non-ST elevation myocardial infarction in the National Registry of Myocardial Infarction from 1990 to 2006. Am Heart J. 2008;156:1026-34.
5. Morrow DA, Antman EM, Charlesworth A, Cairns R, Murphy SA, de Lemos JA, et al. TIMI risk score for ST-elevation myocardial infarction: A convenient, bedside, clinical score for risk assessment at presentation: An intravenous

nPA for treatment of infracting myocardium early II trial substudy. Circulation. 2000;102:2031-7.
6. Killip T, Kimball JT. Treatment of myocardial infarction in a coronary care unit. A two year experience with 250 patients. Am J Cardiol. 1967;20:457-64.
7. Morrow DA, Antman EM, Parsons L, de Lemos JA, Cannon CP, Giugliano RP, et al. Application of the TIMI risk score for ST-elevation MI in the National Registry of Myocardial Infarct 3. JAMA. 2001;286:1356-9.
8. Wiviott SD, Morrow DA, Frederick PD, Giugliano RP, Gibson CM, McCabe CH, et al. Performance of the thrombolysis in myocardial infarction risk index in the National Registry of Myocardial Infarction-3 and -4: a simple index that predicts mortality in ST-segment elevation myocardial infarction. J Am Coll Cardiol. 2004;44:783-9.
9. GRACE Investigators. Rationale and design of the GRACE (Global Registry of Acute Coronary Events) Project: a multinational registry of patients hospitalized with acute coronary syndromes. Am Heart J. 2001;141:190-9.
10. Granger CB, Goldberg RJ, Dabbous O, Pieper KS, Eagle KA, Cannon CP, et al. Predictors of hospital mortality in the global registry of acute coronary events. Arch Intern Med. 2003;163:2345-53.
11. Fox KA, Fitzgerald G, Puymirat E, Huang W, Carruthers K, Simon T, et al. Should patients with acute coronary disease be stratified for management according to their risk? Derivation, external validation and outcomes using the updated GRACE risk score. BMJ Open. 2014;4:e004425.
12. Giraldez RR, Sabatine MS, Morrow DA, Mohanavelu S, McCabe CH, Antman EM, et al. Baseline hemoglobin concentration and creatinine clearance composite laboratory index improves risk stratification in ST-elevation myocardial infarction. Am Heart J. 2009;157:517-24.
13. Scirica BM, Morrow DA, Cannon CP, de Lemos JA, Murphy S, Sabatine MS, et al. Clinical application of C-reactive protein across the spectrum of acute coronary syndromes. Clin Chem. 2007;53:1800-7.
14. Halkin A, Singh M, Nikolsky E, Grines CL, Tcheng JE, Garcia E, et al. Prediction of mortality after primary percutaneous coronary intervention for acute myocardial infarction: the CADILLAC risk score. J Am Coll Cardiol. 2005;45:1397-405.
15. Mercado-Martínez J, Rivera-Fernández R, Aquilar-Alonso E, García-Alcántara A, Estivill-Torrull A, Aranda-León A, et al. APACHE-II score and Killip class for patients with acute myocardial infarction. Intensive Care Med. 2010;36:1579-86.
16. Lev EL, Kornowski R, Vaknin-Assa H, Porter A, Teplitsky I, Ben-Dor I, et al. Comparison of the predictive value of four different risk scores for outcomes of patients with ST-elevation acute myocardial infarction undergoing percutaneous coronary intervention. Am J Cardiol. 2008;102:6-11.
17. D'Ascenzo F, Biondi-Zoccai G, Moretti C, Bollati M, Omedè P, Sciuto F, et al. TIMI, GRACE and alternative risk scores in Acute Coronary Syndromes: a meta-analysis of 40 derivation studies on 216,552 patients and of 42 validation studies on 31,625 patients. Contemp Clin Trials. 2012;33:507-14.
18. Kerensky RA, Wade M, Deedwania P, Boden WE, Pepine CJ; Veterans Affairs Non-Q-Wave Infarction Stategies in-Hospital (VANQWISH) Trial Investigators. Revisiting the culprit lesion on non-Q-wave myocardial infarction. Results from the VANQWISH trail angiographic core laboratory. J Am Coll Cardiol. 2002;39:1456-63.
19. Hochman JS, Sleeper LA, White HD, Dzavik V, Wong SC, Menon V, et al. One-year survival following early revascularization for cardiogenic shock. JAMA. 2001;285:190-2.
20. O'Connor RE, Brady W, Brooks SC, Diercks D, Egan J, Ghaemmaghami C, et al. Part 10: acute coronary syndromes: 2010 American Heart Association Guidelines for Cardiopulmonary Resuscitation and Emergency Cardiovascular Care. Circulation. 2010;122:S787-817.
21. Effects of tissue plasminogen activator and a comparison of early invasive and conservative strategies in unstable angina and non-Q-wave myocardial infarction. Results of the TIMI IIIB Trial. Thrombolysis in Myocardial Ischemia. Circulation. 1994;89:1545-56.
22. Heggunje PS, Wade MJ, O'Rourke RA, Kleiger RE, Deedwania PC, Lavori PW, et al. Early invasive versus ischemia-guided strategies in the management of non-Q wave myocardial infarction patients with and without prior myocardial infarction; results of Veterans Affairs Non-Q Wave Infarction Strategies in Hospital (VANQWISH) trail. Eur Heart J. 2000;21:2014-25.
23. Fox KA, Poole-Wilson PA, Henderson RA, Clayton TC, Chamberlain DA, Shaw TR, et al. Interventional versus conservative treatment for patients with unstable angina or non-ST-elevation myocardial infarction: the British Heart Foundation RITA3 randomized trial. Randomized Intervention Trial of unstable Angina. Lancet. 2002;360:743-51.
24. Mehta SR, Cannon CP, Fox KA, Wallentin L, Boden WE, Spacek R, et al. Routine vs selective invasive strategies in patients with acute coronary syndromes: a collaborative meta-analysis of randomized trials. JAMA. 2005;293:2908-17.
25. 2012 Writing Committee Members, Jneid H, Anderson JL, Wright RS, Adams CD, Bridges CR, et al. 2012 ACCF/AHA focused update of the guideline for the management of patients with unstable angina/Non-ST-elevation myocardial infarction (updating the 2007 guideline and replacing the 2011 focused update): a report of the American College of Cardiology Foundation/American Heart Association Task Force on practice guidelines. Circulation. 2012;126:875-910.
26. Mehta SR, Granger CB, Boden WE, Steg PG, Bassand JP, Faxon DP, et al. Early versus delayed invasive intervention in acute coronary syndromes. N Engl J Med. 2009;360:2165-75.
27. Graham MM, Ghali WA, Faris PD, Galbraith PD, Tu JV, Norris CM, et al. Population rates of cardiac catheterization and yield of high-risk coronary artery disease. CMAJ. 2005;173:35-9.
28. Lee CH, Tan M, Yan RT, Yan RT, Fitchett D, Grima EA, et al. Use of cardiac catheterization for non-ST-segment elevation acute coronary syndromes according to initial risk: reasons why physicians choose not to refer their patients. Arch Intern Med. 2008;168:291-6.
29. De Abreu M, Mariani JA, Silberstein A, Guridi C, Hecht G, Gagliardi JA, et al. Analysis of the invasive strategy decision in patients with acute coronary syndrome without ST-segment elevation in a real-world setting. Am J Cardiol. 2014;113:1956-61.
30. Antman EM, Cohen M, Bernink PJ, McCabe CH, Horacek T, Papuchis G, et al. The TIMI risk score for unstable angina/non-ST elevation MI: A method for prognostication and therapeutic decision making. JAMA. 2000;284:835-42.
31. Mega JL, Morrow DA, Sabatine MS, Zhao XQ, Snapinn SM, DiBattiste PM, et al. Correlation between the TIMI risk score and high-risk angiographic findings in non-ST-elevation acute coronary syndromes: observations from the Platelet Receptor Inhibition in Ischemic Syndrome Management in Patients Limited by Unstable Signs and Symptoms (PRISM-PLUS) trial. Am Heart J. 2005;149:846-50.
32. Cannon CP, Weintraub, Demopoulos LA, Vicari R, Frey MJ, Lakkis N, et al. Comparison of early invasive and conservative strategies in patients with unstable coronary syndromes treated with the glycoprotein IIb/IIIa inhibitor tirofiban. N Engl J Med. 2001;344:1879-87.
33. Morrow DA, Antman EM, Snappin SM, McCabe CH, Theroux P, Braunwald E. An integrated clinical approach to predicting the benefit of tirofiban in non-ST elevation acute coronary syndromes. Application of the TIMI Risk Score for UA/NSTEMI in PRISM-PLUS. Eur Heart J. 2002;23:223-9.
34. Sabatine MS, Morrow DA, McCabe CH, Antman EM, Gibson CM, Cannon CP. Combination of quantitative ST deviation and troponin elevation provides independent prognostic and therapeutic information in unstable angina and non-ST-elevation myocardial infarction. Am Heart J. 2006;151:25-31.
35. Wiviott SD, Morrow DA, Frederick PD, Antman EM, Braunwald E; National Registry of Myocardial Infarction. Application of the Thrombolysis in Myocardial Infarction risk index in non-ST-segment elevation myocardial infarction: evaluation of patients in the National Registry of Myocardial Infarction. J Am Coll Cardiol. 2006;47:1533-8.
36. Palmerini T, Genereaux P, Caixeta A, Cristea E, Lansky A, Mehran R, et al. A new score for risk stratification of patients with acute coronary syndromes undergoing percutaneous coronary intervention: the ACUITY-PCI (Acute Catheterization and Urgent Intervention Triage Strategy-Percutaneous Coronary Intervention) risk score. JACC Cardiovasc Interv. 2012;5:1108-16.
37. Stone GW, Bertrand M, Colombo A, Dangas G, Farkouh ME, Feit F, et al. Acute Catheterization and Urgent Intervention Triage strategY (ACUITY) trial: study design and rationale. Am Heart J. 2004;148:764-75.
38. Stone GW, Maehara A, Lansky AJ, de Bruyne B, Cristea E, Mintz GS, et al. A prospective natural-history study of coronary atherosclerosis. N Engl J Med. 2011;364:226-35.
39. Morrow DA, Cannon CP, Rifai N, Frey MJ, Vicari R, Lakkis N, et al. Ability of minor elevations of troponins I and T to predict benefit from an early invasive strategy in patients with unstable angina and non-ST elevation myocardial infarction: results from a randomized trial. JAMA. 2001;286:2405-12.
40. James SK, Armstrong P, Barnathan E, Califf R, Lindahl B, Siegbahn A, et al. Troponin and C-reactive protein have different relations to subsequent mortality and myocardial infarction after acute coronary syndrome: a GUSTO-IV substudy. J Am Coll Cardiol. 2003;41:916-24.
41. Mills NL, Churchhouse, AM, Lee KK, Anand A, Gamble D, Shah AS, et al. Implementation of a sensitive troponin I assay and risk of recurrent myocardial

infarction and death in patients with suspected acute coronary syndrome. JAMA. 2011;305:1210-6.

42. Stone PH, Thompson B, Anderson HV, Kronenberg MW, Gibson RS, Rogers WJ, et al. Influence of race, sex, and age on management of unstable angina and non-Q-wave myocardial infarction: The TIMI III registry. JAMA. 1996;275:1104-12.
43. Vaccarino V, Parsons L, Every NR, Barron HV, Krumholz HM. Sex-based differences in early mortality after myocardial infarction. National Registry of Myocardial Infarction 2 Participants. N Engl J Med. 1999;341:217-25.
44. Vaccarino V, Parsons L, Peterson ED, Rogers WJ, Kiefe CI, Canto J. Sex differences in mortality after acute myocardial infarction: changes from 1994 to 2006. Arch Intern Med. 2009;169:1767-74.
45. Wu AH, Parsons L, Every NR, Bates ER; Second National Registry of Myocardial Infarction. Hospital outcomes in patients presenting with congestive heart failure complicating acute myocardial infarction: a report from the Second National Registry of Myocardial Infarction (NRMI-2). J Am Coll Cardiol. 2002;40:1389-94.
46. Bahit MC, Lopes RD, Clare RM, Newby LK, Pieper KS, Van de Werf F, et al. Heart failure complicating non-ST-segment elevation acute coronary syndrome: timing, predictors, and clinical outcomes. JACC Heart Fail. 2013;1:223-9.
47. Steg PG, Dabbous OH, Feldman LJ, Cohen-Solal A, Aumont MC, López-Sendón J, et al. Determinants and prognostic impact of heart failure complicating acute coronary syndromes: observations from the Global Registry of Acute Coronary Events (GRACE). Circulation. 2004;109:494-9.
48. Spencer FA, Meyer TE, Gore, JM, Goldberg RJ. Heterogeneity in the management and outcomes of patients with acute myocardial infarction complicated by heart failure: the National Registry of Myocardial Infarction. Circulation. 2002;105:2605-10.
49. Steg PG, Goldberg RJ, Gore JM, Fox KA, Eagle KA, Flather MD, et al. Baseline characteristics, management practices, and in-hospital outcomes of patients hospitalized with acute coronary syndromes in the Global Registry of Acute Coronary Events (GRACE). Am J Cardiol. 2002;90:358-63.
50. Khot UN, Jia G, Moliterno DJ, Lincoff AM, Khot MB, Harrington RA, et al. Prognostic importance of physical examination for heart failure in non-ST-elevation acute coronary syndromes: the enduring value of Killip classification. JAMA. 2003;290:2174-81.
51. Bursi F, Enriquez-Sarano M, Nkomo VT, Jacobsen SJ, Weston SA, Meverden RA, et al. Heart failure and death after myocardial infarction in the community: the emerging role of mitral regurgitation. Circulation. 2005;111:295-301.
52. Savonitto S, Ardissino D, Granger CB, Morando G, Prando MD, Mafrici A, et al. Prognostic value of the admission electrocardiogram in acute coronary syndromes. JAMA. 1999;281:707-13.
53. Kaul P, Fu Y, Chang WC, Harrington RA, Wagner GS, Goodman SG, et al. Prognostic value of ST segment depression in acute coronary syndromes: insights from PARAGON-A applied to GUSTO-IIb. PARAGON-A and GUSTO IIb Investigators. Platelet IIb/IIIa Antagonism for the Reduction of Acute Global Organization Network. J Am Coll Cardiol. 2001;38:64-71.
54. De Luca G, Maas AC, van 't Hof AW, Ottervanger JP, Hoorntje JC, Gosselink AT, et al. Impact of ST-segment depression resolution on mortality after successful mechanical reperfusion in patients with ST-segment elevation acute myocardial infarction. Am J Cardiol. 2005;95:234-6.
55. Stone PH, Raabe DS, Jaffe AS, Gustafson N, Muller JE, Turi ZG, et al. Prognostic significance of location and type of myocardial infarction: independent adverse outcome associated with anterior location. J Am Coll Cardiol. 1988;11:453-63.
56. Haim H, Hod H, Reisin L, Kornowski R, Reicher-Reiss H, Goldbourt U, et al. Comparison of short- and long-term prognosis in patients with anterior wall versus inferior or lateral wall non-Q-wave acute myocardial infarction. Secondary Prevention Reinfarction Israeli Nifedipine Trial (SPRINT) Study Group. Am J Cardiol. 1997;79:717-21.
57. Piccini JP, White JA, Mehta RH, Lokhnygina Y, Al-Khatib SM, Tricoci P, et al. Sustained ventricular tachycardia and ventricular fibrillation complicating non-ST-segment-elevation acute coronary syndromes. Circulation. 2012;126:41-9.
58. Pizzetti F, Turazza FM, Franzosi MG, Barlera S, Ledda A, Maggioni AP, et al. Incidence and prognostic significance of atrial fibrillation in acute myocardial infarction: the GISSI-3 data. Heart. 2001;86:527-32.
59. Al-Khatib SM, Pieper KS, Lee KL, Mahaffey KW, Hochman JS, Pepine CJ, et al. Atrial fibrillation and mortality among patients with acute coronary syndromes without ST-segment elevation: results from the PURSUIT trial. Am J Cardiol. 2001;88:76-9.
60. Schmitt J, Duray G, Gersh BJ, Hohnloser SH. Atrial fibrillation in acute myocardial infarction: a systematic review of the incidence, clinical features and prognostic implications. Eur Heart J. 2009;30:1038-45.
61. Wright RS, Reeder GS, Herzog CA, Albright RC, Williams BA, Dvorak DL, et al. Acute myocardial infarction and renal dysfunction: a high-risk combination. Ann Intern Med. 2002;137:563-70.
62. Anavekar NS, McMurray JJ, Velazquez EJ, Solomon SD, Kober L, Rouleau JL, et al. Relation between renal dysfunction and cardiovascular outcomes after myocardial infarction. N Engl J Med. 2004;351:1285-95.
63. Melloni C, James SK, White JA, Giugliano RP, Harrington RA, Huber K, et al. Safety and efficacy of adjusted-dose eptifibatide in patients with acute coronary syndromes and reduced renal function. Am Heart J. 2011;162:884-92.
64. James SK, Armstrong P, Barnathan E, Califf R, Lindahl B, Siegbahn A, et al. Troponin and C-reactive protein have different relations to subsequent mortality and myocardial infarction after acute coronary syndrome: a GUSTO-IV substudy. J Am Coll Cardiol. 2003;41:916-24.
65. De Lemos JA, Morrow DA, Bentley JH, Omland T, Sabatine MS, McCabe CH, et al. The prognostic value of B-type natriuretic peptide in patients with acute coronary syndromes. N Engl J Med. 2001;345:1014-21.
66. James SK, Lindahl B, Siegbahn A, Stridsberg M, Venge P, Armstrong P, et al. N-terminal pro-brain natriuretic peptide and other risk markers for the separate prediction of mortality and subsequent myocardial infarction in patients with unstable coronary artery disease: a Global Utilization of Strategies To Open occluded arteries (GUSTO)-IV substudy. Circulation. 2003;108:275-81.
67. James SK Lindbäck J, Tilly J, Siegbahn A, Venge P, Armstrong P, et al. Troponin-T and N-terminal pro-B-type natriuretic peptide predict mortality benefit from coronary revascularization in acute coronary syndromes: a GUSTO-IV substudy. J Am Coll Cardiol. 2006;48:1146-54.

14 CHAPTER

Treatment of Acute Coronary Syndrome in the Emergency Department

Navdeep S Sekhon

INTRODUCTION

Over the past few decades, there have been multiple advances in the treatment of acute coronary syndrome (ACS) that have significantly reduced its morbidity and mortality.[1] In fact, a recent study showed that modern treatment can reduce 1-year mortality by as much as 19%.[2]

The goals of treatments for ACS are multiple. Immediately, it is used to reduce the amount of myocardial necrosis, which helps to preserve left ventricular function and prevent heart failure in patients. In addition, treatments should also help reduce the major adverse cardiac events (MACE) that follow acute myocardial infarction (AMI) which include—cardiovascular death, nonfatal myocardial infarction (MI), and need for urgent revascularization.

The emergency department plays a key role in initiating the care of patients with ACS, and this chapter will discuss the different treatment methodologies for ACS.

USE OF OXYGEN IN ACUTE CORONARY SYNDROME

The application of oxygen to patients with ACS has long been considered the standard of care because oxygen supplementation was thought to increase the delivery of oxygen to at-risk myocardial tissue. In patients who are hypoxic, it is still recommended to correct the hypoxia with supplemental oxygen.[3] However, there have been no randomized controlled trials supporting the routine use of oxygen in ACS in patients who are not hypoxic. Human and animal models have shown that hyperoxemia may have toxic effects that include increased coronary vascular resistance, reduced coronary blood flow, and decreased cardiac index.[4-6] Given these results, it is now recommended by the American Heart Association and the American College of Cardiology to only supply oxygen to patients who have respiratory distress or have an oxygen saturation less than 90%.[3]

ANALGESICS IN ACUTE CORONARY SYNDROME

Use of Narcotic Pain Medications

Morphine has traditionally been the standard of care that all medical students learn as a cornerstone in the treatment of ACS. Morphine is a potent analgesic and anxiolytic, which helps patients symptomatically feel better while they are having their coronary event. Morphine also is a mild venodilator and can reduce heart rate, both of which are beneficial hemodynamically in ACS. However, recent observational studies have suggested that patients receiving narcotic pain medication had worse outcomes compared to those who did not when otherwise matched. The CRUSADE Quality Improvement Initiative showed that patients who had received intravenous morphine had an increased risk of inhospital mortality [odds ratio (OR) = 1.41; 95% confidence interval (CI) = 1.26–1.57].[7] An analysis of the Acute Decompensated Heart Failure National Registry (ADHERE) registry also showed that in nonventilated patients, after risk adjustment, patients who had received IV morphine also had worse outcomes (OR = 4.84; 95% CI = 4.52–5.19; $p < 0.001$).[8] These studies place some doubt on whether morphine should be given routinely in patients with ACS. Given that there are no recent randomized clinical trials and that the aforementioned trials are observational studies which are prone to selection bias, it is reasonable to give morphine if a patient's pain does not respond to nitrates.

Nonsteroidal Anti-inflammatory Drugs in Acute Coronary Syndrome

Multiple studies suggest that the use of nonsteroidal anti-inflammatory drugs (NSAIDs) worsen outcomes.[9,10] The risk of death is worse in patients with non-ST elevation acute coronary syndrome (NSTEACS), prior heart disease, and increases with dose of NSAIDs.[9] This may be a result of the NSAIDs inhibiting cyclooxgenase-2 (COX-2), thereby causing prothrombotic effects. In addition, NSAIDs potentially block the irreversible inhibition of cyclooxygenase-1 (COX-1) by acetylsalicylic acid (ASA), negating its positive effects.[10] Thus, it is reasonable to avoid NSAIDs if possible in ACS.

TREATMENT OF NON-ST SEGMENT ELEVATION MI/UNSTABLE ANGINA

Anti-ischemic Agents in Non-ST Segment Elevation MI/Unstable Angina

Beta-Blockers

Beta-blockers have been a mainstay in the treatment of ACS for decades. Their beneficial effects are thought to be secondary to the decrease in heart rate, blood pressure, and contractility that these drugs induce. These effects reduce myocardial oxygen demand, which can help prevent myocardial necrosis. Early studies showed that the early use of β-blockers in ACS did reduce reinfarction, cardiovascular death, and ventricular dysrhythmias [e.g., International Study of Infarct Survival (ISIS)-1 trial].[11]

This is of particular benefit in unstable angina. The Holland Interuniversity Nifedipine/Metoprolol Trial (HINT) study showed that the early use of β-blockers in unstable angina reduced the progression to infarction[12] and another meta-analysis showed a 13% relative risk reduction in converting to ST elevation myocardial infarctions (STEMI).[13]

However, the use of intravenous β-blockers have been associated with an increase in cardiogenic shock in the ClOpidogrel and Metoprolol in Myocardial Infarction (COMMIT) trial (5.0% vs. 3.9%; $p < 0.0001$), particularly in the high-risk groups of age greater than 70 years, heart rate greater than 110 and systolic blood pressure less than 120 mm Hg.[14] Interestingly, a more recent retrospective review of 72,054 patients showed that patients who received β-blockers within 24 hours had a significant reduction in inhospital mortality (3.9% vs. 6.9%; $p < 0.001$).[15]

Given the results of the COMMIT trial, it is no longer recommended to give intravenous β-blockers in ACS, but rather to give oral β-blockers within the first 24 hours given the known benefits of β-blockade,[3] even though some experts still state that it is appropriate to give intravenous β-blockers in ACS and a recent meta-analysis suggests the same.[16]

Beta-blockers in ACS are contraindicated in patients with active chronic obstructive pulmonary disease (COPD)/asthma exacerbations, signs of congestive heart failure, low-outflow states, second or third degree atrioventricular (AV) blocks without a pacemaker, and earlier-mentioned risk factors for developing heart failure.[3]

Nitrates

Nitrates have a long-standing history in the treatment of ACS. They are endothelium independent vasodilators that cause a decrease in preload and left ventricular end-diastolic volume, which decreases myocardial oxygen consumption. Nitrates can also help dilate atherosclerotic coronary arteries. There is some evidence that nitrates may also prevent platelet aggregation,[17] but may cause a reflex tachycardia as well.

There have not been any randomized clinical trials supporting the use of nitrates, so the basis for its use is mostly from observational studies that demonstrate a reduction in pain, long-term mortality, and resolution of ST-changes.[18]

In ACS, it is beneficial to give sublingual (or buccal) nitroglycerin every 5 minutes until resolution of electrocardiogram (ECG) changes and symptoms for up to a total of three dosages. If this fails, it is reasonable to start intravenous nitroglycerin. Given the short half-life of nitroglycerin, a bolus loading dose will be needed in addition to the continuous infusion. The nitroglycerin should be titrated to resolution of symptoms and/or ECG changes, or until the patient suffers from adverse effects, which are usually hypotension and headache.

Patient on a nitroglycerin drip can rapidly develop tolerance to the drug, so titrating the dosage upwards may become necessary with extended use. In addition, nitroglycerin should not be used in patients with right ventricular infarcts as these patients are preload-dependent and the use of nitroglycerin can cause precipitous drops in blood pressure. These patients are a subset of patients who have inferior STEMIs, and can be identified by doing a right-sided ECG and finding ST elevation in lead V_4R or have the ST elevation greater in lead III than lead II. Patients that have taken phosphodiesterase inhibitors (commonly used to treat erectile dysfunction) should not be given nitrates acutely, as it can cause hypotension and death. In particular, patients who have taken sildenafil or vardenafil within the past 24 hours or tadalafil within the past 48 hours should not receive nitrates.

Calcium Channel Blockers

Calcium channel blockers have been studied in the treatment of ACS. There are three main classes:

- Dihydropyridines (e.g., amlodopine or nifedepine)
- Benzothiazepenes (e.g., diltiazem)
- Phenylethylamines (e.g., verapamil).

The calcium channel blockers have been thought to be beneficial in ACS because they are known to cause coronary vasodilation,[19] and also decrease blood pressure and heart rate to varying degrees. Indeed there have been older studies that suggest that diltiazem and verapamil are equivalent to β-blockers in unstable angina in regards to mortality and progression to infarction.[20,21]

However, with nifedipine, there have been studies[12,22] that showed an increase in mortality with its early use in ACS. In particular, the HINT study had to be stopped early because of an increase in reinfarction.[12] It is thought that this increase in mortality may be secondary to the increased drop in blood pressure associated with the dihydropyridines. Based on these findings, dihydropyridines, such as nifedipine, should be avoided in ACS.

However, the nondihydropyridines (e.g., verapamil or diltiazem) can be used in patients who have contra-indications to β-blockers, such as patients with a concomitant asthma exacerbation, given their benefit in ACS.

Antiplatelet Agents in Non-ST Elevation Acute Coronary Syndrome and Unstable Angina

Antiplatelet agents are helpful in ACS because they inhibit platelet propagation and aggregation, which thereby inhibits thrombus formation. Multiple studies have shown their benefit in ACS. A brief schematic to show the targets of common agents used in ACS is given in flowchart 1.

Acetylsalicylic Acid

Acetylsalicylic acid is a nonreversible COX-1 inhibitor that is a mainstay in the treatment of ACS. Acetylsalicylic acid inhibits platelet activation and aggregation by decreasing the production of thromboxane A2. This causes a downregulation of the glycoprotein (GP) IIb/IIIa receptor on the platelet surface, to which fibrinogen binds to link and activate platelets. Hence, the inhibition of the production of thromboxane A2 reduces thrombus formation and activation.

One of the studies that solidified the role of ASA in ACS was the ISIS-2 trial, which was a randomized, prospective trial of 17,187 patients that compared placebo versus enteric-coated ASA which showed a significant reduction in vascular death at 5 weeks, lowering it from 11.8 to 9.4% (p <0.0001).[23] More recent studies support the benefit of ASA in reducing both short- and long-term mortality, stroke, and reinfarction in patients with ACS.[24,25]

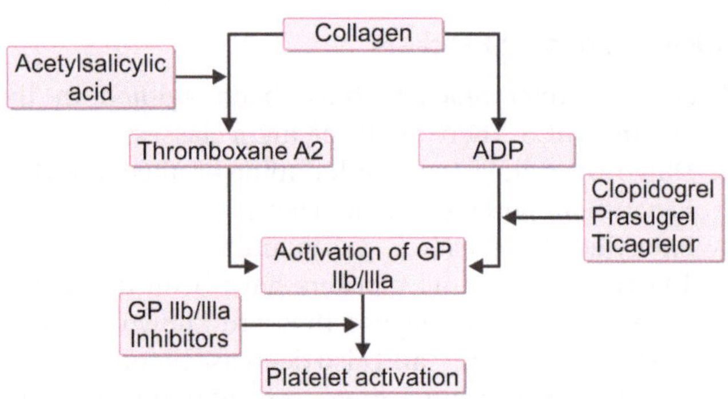

ADP, adenosine diphosphate; GP, glycoprotein.

FLOWCHART 1: Mechanism of action of the antiplatelet agents

Given the evidence, it is recommended that ASA is given to patients with ACS and the American College of Cardiology/American Heart Association (ACC/AHA) recommends an oral dose of 162–325 mg.[3] It is also recommended that patients receive chewable rather than enteric-coated ASA to ensure more rapid and enhanced absorption.[26] If a patient is not able to take medications by mouth, it is reasonable to give it as a suppository or intravenously. However, these routes are not as well studied in ACS. Acetylsalicylic acid also reliably induces inhibition of COX-1, so routine laboratory studies to ensure therapeutic levels are not needed.

Allergic reactions to ASA are rare; the most severe are anaphylaxis, asthma, and rash. If a patient does have a contraindication to ASA, it is reasonable to give clopidogrel in its stead. This recommendation is based on a study of patients with stable ischemic disease where patients who received ASA or clopidogrel had equal outcomes.[27]

Thienopyridines

Thienopyridines are a class of prodrugs that irreversibly block the ability of adenosine diphosphate (ADP) binding the P2Y12 receptor on the cell membrane of platelets. The ADP activates the P2Y12 receptor, which activates platelets and promotes crosslinking with fibrin. Thus, blocking the $P2Y_{12}$ receptor would inhibit platelet aggregation and crosslinking, which is important in the treatment of ACS.[28]

It is important to note that thienopyridines are prodrugs that are metabolized to their active metabolites in the liver by cytochrome P450 (CYP)-dependent enzymes and drugs that affect the function of the CYP system (such as rifampin and ketoconazole) will alter the levels of the active metabolite and alter its efficacy. The two thienopyridines that have been studied the most for the treatment of ACS are clopidogrel and prasugrel.

Clopidogrel

One of the first studies that showed the benefit of clopidogrel when used in combination with ASA in ACS was the Clopidogrel in Unstable Angina to Prevent Recurrent Events (CURE) trial, which was a prospective, randomized trial of 12,562 patients. This trial showed that the use of clopidogrel in addition to ASA decreased the rate of cardiovascular death, nonfatal MI, or stroke at 1 year from 9.3 to 11.4% [relative risk (RR) = 0.80; p <0.001].[29] The use of clopidogrel was associated with an increase in major bleeding (3.7% vs. 2.7%; RR = 1.38; 95% CI = 1.13–1.67; p = 0.001).[29] This reduction in mortality has also been shown for both medically managed and patients who received percutaneous coronary intervention (PCI).[29-31]

The appropriate loading dose of clopidogrel is a matter of some debate. The 600 mg loading dose has been shown to have a more rapid and stronger platelet inhibition compared to the 300 mg dose.[32] The Clopidogrel and Aspirin Optimal Dose Usage to Reduce Recurrent Events–Seventh Organization to Assess Strategies in Ischemic Syndromes (CURRENT OASIS 7) trial also showed a mild reduction in recurrent MI and stent restenosis with the higher dose, at the expense of increased risk of major bleeding with no change in 30-day mortality.[33] Given these findings, the AHA/ACC recommendation is a loading of 300–600 mg orally.[3]

There is also a large variability of response to clopidogrel that results in certain patient attaining inadequate platelet inhibition at standard dosages. This is in part due to the genetic variability in the absorption of clopdiogrel,[34] and the known individual variability in CYP-dependent metabolism.[35] The Gauging Responsiveness With a Verify Now Assay–Impact on Thrombosis and Safety (GRAVITAS) study showed no benefit to poor responders of an increased dose of clopidogrel in patients receiving PCI in terms of death, repeat MI, or stroke. This suggests that a different antiplatelet agent may be preferred in this subgroup of patients.[36]

Prasugrel

Prasugrel is another thienopyridine that has been studied in the treatment of ACS. It is converted to its active metabolite in two steps, first by plasma esterases and second by the CYP enzymes in the liver.[37] Prasugrel has more rapid and consistent platelet inhibition as compared to clopidogrel.[38] However, this increased inhibition is associated with increased risk for major bleeding in the TRial to assess Improvement in Therapeutic Outcomes by optimizing platelet inhibitioN with prasugrel–Thrombolysis In Myocardial Infarction (TRITON-TIMI 38), TaRgeted platelet Inhibition to cLarify the Optimal strateGy to medicallY manage Acute Coronary Syndromes (TRILOGY ACS), and A Comparison of Prasugrel at PCI or Time of Diagnosis of Non-ST Elevation Myocardial Infarction (ACCOAST) trials,[39-41] so it is not recommended for routine upstream use in the emergency department for patients with NSTEACS/unstable angina.

Ticagrelor

Ticagrelor belongs to a novel chemical class called the cyclopentyl-triazolo-pyrimidines, which reversibly binds to the P2Y12 receptor on the platelet surface. This causes the inhibition of platelet aggregation and activation, which is beneficial in ACS. Ticagrelor also has a more rapid and consistent onset of action as compared to clopidogrel. Since it has a half-life of approximately 12 hours, it also has a more rapid offset of action.[42]

The Platelet Inhibition and Patient Outcomes (PLATO) trial was prospective, randomized, multicenter trial of 18,624 patients who presented with ACS and compared the outcomes of patients who received ASA plus ticagrelor versus clopidogrel. This study showed a reduction of death, MI, and stroke in the ticagrelor group [9.8% vs. 11.7%; heart rate (HR) = 0.84; 95% CI = 0.77–0.92; $p < 0.001$], however, at the expense of a small increase in nonprocedure-related major bleeding.[43] Given these findings, it is reasonable to give ticagrelor in addition to patients with ACS in replacement of clopidogrel.

Dyspnea is a common side effect in patients who receive ticagrelor, affecting up to 15% of patients.[43] This dyspnea is usually mild and is not associated with any change in cardiac or pulmonary function tests.[44] Ticagrelor is also associated with ventricular pauses, so it is not recommended in patients who have second or third degree AV blocks unless already treated with a pacemaker.[44]

Glycoprotein IIb/IIIa Inhibitors

The GP IIb/IIIa receptor is an integrin complex and a fibrinogen receptor located on the platelet surface.[45] Glycoprotein IIb/IIIa inhibitors target the final common pathway of platelet aggregation and prevent the cross-linking of platelets by fibrinogen. This inhibits thrombus formation and propagation.

In a meta-analysis of 29,570 patients, Roffi et al. showed that in patients with ACS being managed medically, the use of GP IIb/IIIa inhibitors have no benefit.[46] Furthermore, the Acute Catheterization and Urgent Intervention Triage strategY (ACUITY) Timing trial and the Early Glycoprotein IIb/IIIa Inhibition in Patients With Non-ST Segment Elevation Acute Coronary Syndrome (EARLY-ACS) trial showed that in patients that received PCI, the routine upstream (prior to PCI) use of GP IIb/IIIa was associated with increased major bleeding without a significant reduction in death, MI, or stroke.[47,48]

Thus, the routine upstream use of GP IIb/IIIa inhibitors in ACS is not recommended based on the increased risk of bleeding; however, there is evidence for its use at or during PCI.[49]

Summary of the Role of Antiplatelet Agents in Non-ST Segment Elevation MI/Unstable Angina

The evidence supports the use of aspirin in addition to another antiplatelet agent in patients with NSTEACS/unstable angina. This is commonly called dual antiplatelet therapy (DAPT). The second agent could be either ticagrelor or clopidogrel, with a preference for ticagrelor.[3]

Role of Anticoagulants in Non-ST Segment Elevation MI and Unstable Angina

Anticoagulants have been the standard of care in ACS for decades. The various anticoagulants inhibit thrombus formation by inhibiting thrombin formation and activity. Thrombin is necessary for the formation of fibrinogen, which is used to crosslink platelets and form a thrombus. Thus, inhibiting thrombin formation will retard thrombus formation and propagation. Flowchart 2 demonstrates where in the coagulation cascade the various anticoagulants have their mechanism of action.

Unfractionated Heparin

Unfractionated heparin (UFH) is a heterogeneous mixture of polysaccharide molecules that weigh between 2,000 and 30,000 Da, with most between 15,000 and 18,000 Da. One-third of these molecules have the active polysaccharide sequence that activates antithrombin, causing it to inhibit both thrombin and factor Xa (thromboplastin). It is by this inhibition that UFH gets its anticoagulant effect.[50]

Unfractionated heparin has a narrow therapeutic window, with a therapeutic activated partial thromboplastin time (aPTT) of between 50 and 70 seconds. It is poorly absorbed subcutaneously and has a short half-life, so it has to be given via an intravenous drip with frequent laboratory checks to ensure that dosing is therapeutic. It is also important to note that upon discontinuation of heparin, there often is a transient activation of the coagulation cascade.

The evidence suggests that the use of UFH in ACS causes a reduction of repeat MI in the acute period. A pooled analysis of six trials in the year 2000 compared the use of short-term UFH versus placebo in ACS (NSTEACS). This analysis showed a reduction in MI during the acute phase, but no significant change in mortality and a small increase in major bleeding.[51] A recent Cochrane review came to a similar conclusion.[52] Thus, UFH can be used in ACS to reduce the rate of MI in the acute phase of ACS.

Low Molecular Weight Heparins

Low molecular weight heparins (LMWH), such as enoxaparin, are a class of heparin-derived products that range in molecular weight from 2,000 to 10,000 Da. Their anticoagulant effect comes from their ability to inhibit

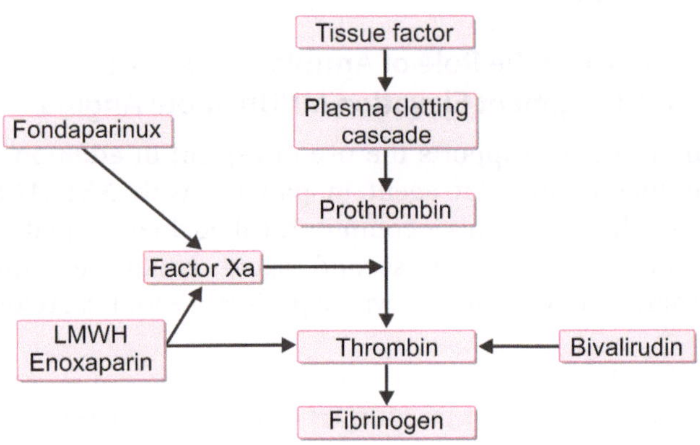

LMWH, Low molecular weight heparins.

FLOWCHART 2: Location of action of different anticoagulants

thrombin and thromboplastin. They are partially excreted by the kidneys, so caution is advised in those with renal impairment.

Low molecular weight heparins do have some advantages over UFH. These advantages include the near complete absorption from subcutaneous injections, which allows for twice daily subcutaneous administration [once daily with enoxaparin with a creatinine clearance (CrCl) <30 mL/min] as opposed to an intravenous drip. Low molecular weight heparins have a predictable dose-effect relationship, ensuring that most patients do not need laboratory testing to monitor treatment.[53] Exceptions are the obese and patients with renal failure, who may require the monitoring of anti-Xa activity to ensure therapeutic action. Another advantage of LMWH is a reduced risk of heparin-induced thrombocytopenia (HIT) compared to UFH.[53]

The outcomes of patients with ACS who receive LMWH are similar to those that receive UFH. A large meta-analysis of 12 trials with 17,157 patients showed similar outcomes.[51] A more recent meta-analysis in 2007 reinforced these results.[54] Thus, it is reasonable to use LMWH as an alternative of UFH in NSTEACS/unstable angina.

Fondaparinux

Fondaparinux is a pentasaccharide that is similar to the antithrombin-binding sequence that is common to all the heparins. It indirectly and reversibly inhibits factor Xa, thereby preventing thrombin generation which inhibits the formation and propagation of thrombus.

Fondaparinux has a half-life of 17 hours and is 100% bioavailable after subcutaneous injection, which allows it to be dosed once daily subcutaneously. It is eliminated through the kidneys, so it should not be used in patients with a CrCl less than 20 mL/min. It is not associated with HIT, and there is no need for laboratory monitoring in these patients. It also does not affect the aPTT, prothrombin time (PT), activated clotting time (ACT), and thrombin time.[50]

The OASIS-5 study randomized 20,078 patients with non-ST segment elevation acute coronary syndromes (NSTEACS) to fondaparinux versus enoxaparin. This study showed that patients who received fondaparinux had a reduced risk of major bleeding at 9 days (2.2% vs. 4.1%; HR = 0.52; 95% CI = 0.44–0.61; p <0.001] while having a similar 9-day primary composite end-point of death, MI, and stroke. However, it was found that patients who received PCI had an increased risk of catheter thrombosis, which disappeared in patients who received a bolus of UFH at time of PCI.[55] This suggests that fondaparinux might be safer to use than LMWH in NSTEACS.

Bivalirudin

Bivalirudin binds directly to thrombin, which inhibits thrombin from inducing the conversion of fibrinogen to fibrin. This helps to prevent the crosslinking of platelets and inhibit thrombus formation and propagation. Its anticoagulation effect can be measured using the ACT.[50]

The ACUITY trial was a large multicenter, open-label, randomized trial with 13,819 patients that suggested that bivalirudin was noninferior to UFH/LMWH. There were no significant differences in the rates of major bleeding, mortality, MI, or stroke.[56] This suggests that bivalirudin can be used as an anticoagulant in NSTEACS.

Thrombolytics in Non-ST Segment Elevation Myocardial Infarction and Unstable Angina

The evidence does not support the routine use of thrombolytics in NSTEACS. The Thrombolysis in Myocardial Infarction (TIMI) IIIB trials showed no change in outcomes, but an increased rate of intracranial hemorrhage.[57] Thus, thrombolytics should not be used routinely in NSTEACS.

COMPLICATIONS OF NON-ST SEGMENT ELEVATION ACUTE CORONARY SYNDROME

Dysrhythmias are a common complication of ACS. The most common dysrhythmias are premature ventricular contractions (PVCs).[58] If the patient develops ventricular tachycardia (which a recent study suggests can occur in up to 6% of patients with ACS),[59] it is reasonable to electrically cardiovert. If this fails, it is reasonable to bolus lidocaine or amiodarone. Care should be given with the use of lidocaine in low cardiac output states as normal dosages can cause toxicity. In these cases, the dosage of lidocaine should be halved.

Conduction disturbances are another complication of NSTEACS, often prompting the need for temporary pacing. With inferior MIs, the conduction blockages are usually secondary to increased vagal tone; however, inferior STEMIs can involve the AV node. Anterior infarctions can also cause high-degree heart block by causing ischemia to the conduction pathways. The patients who would benefit from the implantation of a temporary pacer are listed in box 1.

BOX 1 Indications for placement of temporary pacemaker in patients with acute coronary syndrome[60]

- Sinus node dysfunction not amenable to medical therapy (e.g., atropine)
- Third-degree heart block
- Second-degree heart block with Mobitz type II
- New left bundle branch block
- New right bundle branch with left anterior fascicular block or left posterior fascicular block

MANAGEMENT OF NON-ST SEGMENT ELEVATION MI AND UNSTABLE ANGINA

In summary, there have been many advances in the care of NSTEACS in recent history. The more recent studies suggest that oxygen supplementation should only be used to keep the oxygen saturation greater than 90% and with patients in respiratory distress. The role of nitrates remains to control chest discomfort. The DAPT has become solidified as standard of care, using ASA in addition to either clopidogrel or ticagrelor (which may be superior). In addition to DAPT, patients should also receive anticoagulant therapy. The options for anticoagulants include UFH, LMWH, fondaparinux, and bivalirudin. Thrombolytics and GP IIb/IIIa inhibitors should not routinely be used in the emergency department for the treatment of NSTEACS because of their increased risk of major bleeding. Treatment options for NSTEACS in the emergency department have been provided in box 2.

Disposition

Patients with NSTEACS should be admitted to the hospital under the care of a cardiologist if possible. Moderate- to high-risk patients may require PCI as an inpatient as it improves outcomes,[61-63] so transfer to a hospital with PCI capabilities is reasonable if the presenting hospital does not have those capabilities. In moderate- to high-risk patients, admission to a coronary care unit or intensive care unit is reasonable as it has been shown to improve outcomes. All patients admitted to the hospital should be placed on continuous telemetry monitoring as they are at an increased risk for dysrhythmias.

EMERGENCY DEPARTMENT MANAGEMENT OF ST SEGMENT ELEVATION MI

The ST segment elevation myocardial infarctions are a subset of ACS that causes significant morbidity and mortality. The mortality of STEMI patients at 6 months is as high as 12%.[64] Fortunately, modern medical therapy has reduced mortality at 1 year by up to 5%, which is one of the successes in modern medicine.[65] Most of this benefit is due to the increased focus on early revascularization.

BOX 2 Emergency department management of non-ST segment elevation myocardial infarction and unstable angina[3]

- Oxygen supplementation to keep oxygen saturation >90% and to relieve respiratory distress
- Nitroglycerin to relieve chest discomfort
- Dual antiplatelet therapy: ASA + (clopidogrel or ticagrelor)
- Anticoagulant: UFH, LMWH, fondaparinux, or bivalirudin

ASA, acetylsalicylic acid; LMWH, low molecular weight heparins; NSTEACS, non-ST segment segment elevation acute coronary syndrome; UFH, unfractionated heparin.

Revascularization Techniques for ST Segment Elevation Myocardial Infarctions

Percutaneous Coronary Intervention

Percutaneous coronary intervention has now become the standard of care for patients that have STEMIs. Numerous studies also confirm the superiority of PCI to fibrinolytics.[66-68] Multiple studies also show that the sooner a patient has a PCI after the onset of an STEMI, the better the outcome.[69,70] This has led the medical community to place importance on decreasing the time to PCI to improve patient outcomes. The goal from first medical contact (FMC) to the angioplasty balloon opening the lesion is 90 minutes, 60 minutes in patients with large anterior infarct and earlier presenters.[71]

Early studies showed that most of the benefit from PCI comes in patients who had symptoms for less than 12 hours.[66,72] In addition, in patients who present 12 hours after symptom onset who are still having symptoms or have ECG evidence of ongoing ischemia, an emergent PCI is recommended and been shown to have benefit.[71]

In patients who had symptom onset of the STEMI between 12 and 72 hours ago and are now asymptomatic, the need for emergent PCI is controversial. Two randomized controlled trial of patients who had their STEMI between 12 and 48 hours ago showed a reduction in infarct size and nonsignificant decrease in death, MI, and stroke.[73,74] The Occluded Artery Trial (OAT) showed no significant benefit in asymptomatic patients with STEMI who were greater than 24 hours out.[75] Thus, there is no evidence for emergent PCI in asymptomatic STEMI patients without ECG evidence of ongoing ischemia who are greater than 12 hours from symptom-onset.

If an STEMI patient was to present to a non-PCI facility, these patients should be transferred to a PCI facility if PCI can be arranged within 120 minutes. There were no studies designed to analyze this, but *post hoc* analyses suggest that the benefit of PCI over fibrinolytics persists for door to balloon times up to 120 minutes.[70,76] If a transfer cannot be arranged, it is reasonable to give fibrinolytics.

Antiplatelet Therapy in ST Segment Elevation MI

Acetylsalicylic Acid

The administration of ASA is the standard of care for the treatment of STEMIs. This is based on the ISIS-2 study which showed that in STEMI, the administration of ASA reduced mortality at 1 month by 2.4% compared to placebo.[23] The preferred dose is 324–325 mg administered in a chewable tablet.[71]

Clopidogrel

Clopidogrel has been associated with improved outcomes in patients with STEMI when used in combination with ASA.[77] The suggested dose is 300–600 mg orally, but studies suggest that 600 mg dose is superior with no increase in major bleeding.[33,78] In addition, observational studies suggest that emergency department administration of clopidogrel is associated with improved outcomes compared to catheterization laboratory administration.[79,80] Thus, the use of clopidogrel is recommended in STEMI in combination with ASA in the emergency department.

Prasugrel

Prasugrel is another thienopyridine that is used in the treatment of STEMIs. It is a more potent antiplatelet agent compared to clopidogrel. Studies suggest that prasugrel is superior to clopidogrel in the treatment of STEMI, in particular, the TRITON-TIMI 38 trial which was a double-blind randomized controlled trial of 3,534 patients comparing prasugrel to clopidogrel that showed that prasugrel caused a reduction in repeat MI, in-stent thrombosis, and mortality.[77]

It is important to note that in the elderly (age >75 years) and patients with a prior history of stroke or transient ischemic attack, the use of prasugrel is contraindicated given an increased risk of intracranial bleeding.

Ticagrelor

Ticagrelor is another antiplatelet agent that can be used in an STEMI. The PLATO trial showed that compared to clopidogrel, ticagrelor has decreased mortality, in-stent thrombosis, and recurrent MI but an increased risk for stroke.[81]

Glycoprotein IIb/IIIa Inhibitors

The upstream use of GP IIb/IIIa inhibitors in patients with STEMI is controversial. The Facilitated Intervention with Enhanced Reperfusion Speed to Stop Events (FINESSE) and Bavarian Reperfusion Alternative Evaluation (BRAVE)-3 trials showed no benefit in upstream use of GP IIb/IIIa inhibitors, with a trend towards an increase in major bleeding.[82,83] However, the Ongoing Tirofiban in Myocardial Infarction Evaluation (ON-TIME) 2 trial showed a mild benefit in STEMI. Given the mixed data, it is reasonable to discuss with the cardiologist regarding initiation of GP IIb/IIIa inhibitors in patients with STEMI who will receive PCI.

Anticoagulants Therapy in ST Segment Elevation MI

Unfractionated Heparin

Unfractionated heparin has been used in the treatment of STEMI for a long time. Interestingly enough, there have been no randomized trials comparing its efficacy and safety with placebo. However, it has been used for a long time and considered standard care. The bolus dose should be 70–100 IU/kg intravenous (IV) if there will be no downstream use of GP IIb/IIIa inhibitors, and 50–60 IU/kg if GP IIb/IIIa inhibitors are used.

Low Molecular Weight Heparins

Several nonrandomized trials suggest a benefit with using enoxaparin compared to UFH.[84-86] The STEMI Treated With Primary Angioplasty and Intravenous Lovenox or Unfractionated Heparin (ATOLL) trial was a randomized trial of 910 patients that compared enoxaparin with UFH, which showed a decrease in ischemic complications with the use of enoxaparin.[87] The recommended dose for enoxaparin is 0.5 mg/kg intravenously followed by a 1 mg/kg dose subcutaneously.

Fondaparinux

The OASIS-6 trial showed that in patients receiving PCI, there was no clinical benefit and an increased risk of in-stent stenosis.[88] In light of this, fondaparinux should not be used in STEMIs receiving PCI.

Bivalirudin

The Harmonizing Outcomes with RevasculariZatiON and Stents in Acute Myocardial Infarction (HORIZONS-AMI) trial suggests that the use of bivalirudin is superior to the use of UFH plus GP IIb/IIIa inhibitors.[89] This study caused the ACCP/AHA and the ESC to add bivalirudin as a possible anticoagulant to be used upstream in STEMI (Box 3).

BOX 3 Management of ST segment elevation myocardial infarction that will receive percutaneous coronary intervention[71]

- Dual antiplatelet therapy: ASA 324–325 mg +
  - Ticagrelor 180 mg, prasugrel 60 mg, or clopidogrel 600 mg
- Anticoagulant therapy:
  - UFH 70–100 IU/kg IV bolus or 50–60 IU/kg IV bolus (if using downstream GP IIb/IIIa inhibitor) followed by 12 IU/kg/h infusion

    or
  - Enoxaparin 0.5 mg/kg IV followed by 1.0 mg/kg IV

    or
  - Bivalirudin 0.75 mg/kg IV followed by 1.75 mg/kg/h infusion

PCI, percutaneous coronary intervention; STEMI, ST segment elevation myocardial infarction, UFH, unfractionated heparin; IV, intravenous.

Fibrinolytics

Fibrinolytics are used in STEMI to revascularize the affected coronary arteries. As mentioned above, fibrinolytics should be given to patients who cannot receive a door to balloon time of 120 minutes. The goal for patients is from door to needle (administration of fibrinolytic) of 30 minutes. This necessitates the presence of established protocols to ensure that this occurs on a regular basis. Multiple studies show that patients who receive fibrinolytics have decreased mortality compared to those that do not,[90] but they do have a significant risk of intracranial hemorrhage (0.9-1.0%).[91,92] Patients who are at increased risk for intracranial hemorrhage include patients who have an advanced age, lower weight, female gender, prior stroke, and increased blood pressure upon admission. Interestingly though, it may be in the elderly that fibrinolytics have the greatest benefit.[93] Fibrinolytics should be administered within 12 hours from symptom onset.

Other major bleeding is also a major concern in patients receiving fibrinolytics, some studies suggest that the rate of major bleeding is between 4 and 13%.[91,92,94] It is also important to note that in patients who have received streptokinase in the past, repeat dosages may not be as helpful as the body can produce antibodies to streptokinase.

Given the high rate of potential major bleeding, it is important to adhere to the exclusion criteria (Box 4).

Antithrombotic Agents with the Use of Fibrinolytics

Studies have shown that the addition of ASA and clopidogrel in STEMIs receiving fibrinolytics improve outcomes.[96] The dose of ASA should be from 162 to 325 mg, and the dose clopidogrel should be 300 mg. It is important to note, that in those whose age is greater than 75, it is recommended to given 75 mg of clopidogrel instead to reduce the risk of bleeding. Prasugrel and ticagrelor have not been studied extensively in the use of fibrinolytics, so their use is not recommended.

Anticoagulants with the Use of Fibrinolytics

Unfractionated heparin, enoxaparin, and fondaparinux have been used with fibrinolytics to improve outcomes. The dosages follow:

- Unfractionated heparin: 60 IU/kg IV bolus followed by 12 IU/kg/h infusion
- Enoxaparin: 30 mg IV bolus followed by 1 mg/kg subcutaneous injection. With age older than 75 years, only give 0.75 mg/kg subcutaneous injection, no IV loading dose
- Fondaparinux: 2.5 mg IV bolus.[71]

Timing of Percutaneous Coronary Intervention after Fibrinolytics

If the patient who received fibrinolytics is experiencing cardiogenic shock or severe heart failure, they should be emergently sent to receive a PCI. If there is evidence of repeat vascular occlusion or failure of revascularization, the patients should be sent urgently for PCI. All patients who receive fibrinolytics should have PCI within 24 hours.[71]

Summary of Emergency Department Management of ST Segment Elevation MI Patients Receiving Fibrinolytics

Fibrinolytics should be administered to STEMI patients with a goal door to balloon time of 30 minutes. Adjuvant antithrombotic agents are ASA and clopidogrel. These

BOX 4 Exclusion criteria for the use of fibrinolytics[95]

- Absolute contraindications
  - History of intracranial hemorrhage
  - Known cerebrovascular malformation
  - Known malignant intracranial neoplasm
  - Ischemic stroke within past 3 months
  - Suspected aortic dissection
  - Active bleeding or bleeding diathesis
  - Significant head injury in the past 3 months
  - Intracranial or spinal surgery in the past 2 months
  - Unresponsive, uncontrolled HTN
  - For streptokinase–prior treatment in last 6 months
- Relative contraindications
  - History of poorly controlled, chronic HTN
  - Significant HTN on presentation
  - SBP >180 mm Hg or DBP >110 mm Hg
  - History of cerebrovascular accident >3 months
  - Dementia
  - Known intracranial pathology
  - Traumatic or prolonged (>10 min) CPR
  - Major surgery within 3 weeks
  - Recent internal bleeding (<2–4 weeks)
  - Noncompressible vascular punctures
  - Pregnancy
  - Oral anticoagulant therapy
  - Active peptic ulcer disease

CPR, cardiopulmonary resuscitation; DBP, diastolic blood pressure; HTN, hypertension; SBP, systolic blood pressure.

patients should also receive anticoagulant agents, including UFH, enoxaparin, and fondaparinux. All patients should have a goal for PCI within 24 hours, and patients with evidence of shock of severe heart failure should receive PCI emergently. Patients who fail to revascularize or have repeat occlusion should be sent for PCI urgently.

CONCLUSION

Modern therapy for the treatment of ACS has been shown to improve patient outcomes. All patients who present with ACS should receive dual antiplatelet therapy in addition to anticoagulation. Dual antiplatelet therapy consists of acetylsalicylic acid plus clopidrogel or ticagrelor. For patients that present with an ST elevation myocardial infarction, PCI within 90 minutes from arrival to the emergency department is recommended. If prompt PCI is not possible, thrombolytics should be used within 30 minutes of arrival. For NSTEACS, PCI should be done emergently for hemodynamic instability, signs of heart failure, and refractory angina. For anticoagulation in ACS, heparin, low-molecular weight heparin, or bivalirudin can be used. The evidence only supports the use of fondaparnux in NSTEACS.

REFERENCES

1. Fox KA, Steg PG, Eagle KA, Goodman SG, Anderson FA, Granger CB, et al. Decline in rates of death and heart failure in acute coronary syndromes, 1999-2006. JAMA. 2007;297(17):1892-900.
2. Corbelli JC, Janicke DM, Cziraky MJ, Hoy TA, Corbelli JA. Acute coronary syndrome emergency treatment strategies: Improved treatment and reduced mortality in patients with acute coronary syndrome using guideline-based critical care pathways. Am Heart J. 2009;157(1):61-8.
3. Amsterdam EA, Wenger NK, Brindis RG, Casey DE, Ganiats TG, Holmes DR, et al. 2014 AHA/ACC Guideline for the Management of Patients with Non-ST-Elevation Acute Coronary Syndromes: a report of the American College of Cardiology/American Heart Association Task Force on Practice Guidelines. J Am Coll Cardiol. 2014;64(24):e139-228.
4. Farquhar H, Weatherall M, Wijesinghe M, Perrin K, Ranchord A, Simmonds M, et al. Systematic review of studies of the effect of hyperoxia on coronary blood flow. Am Heart J. 2009;158(3):371-7.
5. Cabello JB, Burls A, Emparanza JI, Bayliss S, Quinn T. Oxygen therapy for acute myocardial infarction. Cochrane Database Syst Rev. 2010;(6):CD007160.
6. Moradkhan R, Sinoway LI. Revisiting the role of oxygen therapy in cardiac patients. J Am Coll Cardiol. 2010;56(13):1013-6.
7. Meine TJ, Roe MT, Chen AY, Patel MR, Washam JB, Ohman EM, et al. Association of intravenous morphine use and outcomes in acute coronary syndromes: results from the CRUSADE Quality Improvement Initiative. Am Heart J. 2005;149(6):1043-9.
8. Peacock WF, Hollander JE, Diercks DB, Lopatin M, Fonarow G, Emerman CL. Morphine and outcomes in acute decompensated heart failure: an ADHERE analysis. Emerg Med J. 2008;25(4):205-9.
9. Bueno H, Bardají A, Patrignani P, Martín-Merino E, García-Rodríguez LA, Spanish Case-Control Study to Assess NSAID-Associated ACS Risk Investigators. Use of non-steroidal antiinflammatory drugs and type-specific risk of acute coronary syndrome. Am J Cardiol. 2010;105(8):1102-6.
10. Gislason GH, Jacobsen S, Rasmussen JN, Rasmussen S, Buch P, Friberg J, et al. Risk of death or reinfarction associated with the use of selective cyclooxygenase-2 inhibitors and nonselective nonsteroidal antiinflammatory drugs after acute myocardial infarction. Circulation. 2006;113(25):2906-13.
11. Randomised trial of intravenous atenolol among 16 027 cases of suspected acute myocardial infarction: ISIS-1. First International Study of Infarct Survival Collaborative Group. Lancet. 1986;2(8498):57-66.
12. Lubsen J, Tijssen JG. Efficacy of nifedipine and metoprolol in the early treatment of unstable angina in the coronary care unit: findings from the Holland Interuniversity Nifedipine/metoprolol Trial (HINT). Am J Cardiol. 1987;60(2):18A-25A.
13. Yusuf S, Wittes J, Friedman L. Overview of results of randomized clinical trials in heart disease. I. Treatments following myocardial infarction. JAMA. 1988;260(14):2088-93.
14. Chen ZM, Pan HC, Chen YP, Peto R, Collins R, Jiang LX, et al. Early intravenous then oral metoprolol in 45,852 patients with acute myocardial infarction: randomised placebo-controlled trial. Lancet. 2005;366(9497):1622-32.
15. Miller CD, Roe MT, Mulgund J, Hoekstra JW, Santos R, Pollack CV, et al. Impact of acute beta-blocker therapy for patients with non-ST-segment elevation myocardial infarction. Am J Med. 2007;120(8):685-92.
16. Chatterjee S, Chaudhuri D, Vedanthan R, Fuster V, Ibanez B, Bangalore S, et al. Early intravenous beta-blockers in patients with acute coronary syndrome--a meta-analysis of randomized trials. Int J Cardiol. 2013;168(2):915-21.
17. Knight CJ, Panesar M, Wilson DJ, Chronos NA, Patel D, Fox K, et al. Different effects of calcium antagonists, nitrates, and beta-blockers on platelet function. Possible importance for the treatment of unstable angina. Circulation. 1997;95(1):125-32.
18. Cotter G, Faibel H, Barash P, Shemesh E, Moshkovitz Y, Metzkor E, et al. High-dose nitrates in the immediate management of unstable angina: optimal dosage, route of administration, and therapeutic goals. Am J Emerg Med. 1998;16(3):219-24.
19. JCS Joint Working Group. Guidelines for diagnosis and treatment of patients with vasospastic angina (coronary spastic angina) (JCS 2008): digest version. Circ J. 2010;74(8):1745-62.
20. Théroux P, Taeymans Y, Morissette D, Bosch X, Pelletier GB, Waters DD. A randomized study comparing propranolol and diltiazem in the treatment of unstable angina. J Am Coll Cardiol. 1985;5(3):717-22.
21. Parodi O, Simonetti I, Michelassi C, Carpeggiani C, Biagini A, L'Abbate A, et al. Comparison of verapamil and propranolol therapy for angina pectoris at rest: a

randomized, multiple-crossover, controlled trial in the coronary care unit. Am J Cardiol. 1986;57(11):899-906.
22. Furberg CD, Psaty BM, Meyer JV. Nifedipine. Dose-related increase in mortality in patients with coronary heart disease. Circulation. 1995;92(5):1326-31.
23. Randomised trial of intravenous streptokinase, oral aspirin, both, or neither among 17,187 cases of suspected acute myocardial infarction: ISIS-2. ISIS-2 (Second International Study of Infarct Survival) Collaborative Group. Lancet. 1988;2(8607):349-60.
24. Antithrombotic Trialists' (ATT) Collaboration, Baigent C, Blackwell L, Collins R, Emberson J, Godwin J, et al. Aspirin in the primary and secondary prevention of vascular disease: collaborative meta-analysis of individual participant data from randomised trials. Lancet. 2009;373(9678):1849-60.
25. Théroux P, Ouimet H, McCans J, Latour JG, Joly P, Lévy G, et al. Aspirin, heparin, or both to treat acute unstable angina. N Engl J Med. 1988;319(17): 1105-11.
26. Grosser T, Fries S, Lawson JA, Kapoor SC, Grant GR, FitzGerald GA. Drug resistance and pseudoresistance: an unintended consequence of enteric coating aspirin. Circulation. 2013;127(3):377-85.
27. CAPRIE Steering Committee. A randomised, blinded, trial of clopidogrel versus aspirin in patients at risk of ischaemic events (CAPRIE). CAPRIE Steering Committee. Lancet. 1996;348(9038):1329-39.
28. Savi P, Nurden P, Nurden AT, Levy-Toledano S, Herbert JM. Clopidogrel: a review of its mechanism of action. Platelets. 1998;9(3-4):251-5.
29. Yusuf S, Zhao F, Mehta SR, Chrolavicius S, Tognoni G, Fox KK, et al. Effects of clopidogrel in addition to aspirin in patients with acute coronary syndromes without ST-segment elevation. N Engl J Med. 2001;345(7):494-502.
30. Solomon MD, Go AS, Shilane D, Boothroyd DB, Leong TK, Kazi DS, et al. Comparative effectiveness of clopidogrel in medically managed patients with unstable angina and non-ST-segment elevation myocardial infarction. J Am Coll Cardiol. 2014;63(21):2249-57.
31. Alexander D, Ou FS, Roe MT, Pollack CV, Ohman EM, Cannon CP, et al. Use of and inhospital outcomes after early clopidogrel therapy in patients not undergoing an early invasive strategy for treatment of non-ST-segment elevation myocardial infarction: results from Can Rapid risk stratification of Unstable angina patients Suppress ADverse outcomes with Early implementation of the American College of Cardiology/American Heart Association guidelines (CRUSADE). Am Heart J. 2008;156(3):606-12.
32. Montalescot G, Sideris G, Meuleman C, Bal-dit-Sollier C, Lellouche N, Steg PG, et al. A randomized comparison of high clopidogrel loading doses in patients with non-ST-segment elevation acute coronary syndromes: the ALBION (Assessment of the Best Loading Dose of Clopidogrel to Blunt Platelet Activation, Inflammation and Ongoing Necrosis) trial. J Am Coll Cardiol. 2006;48(5):931-8.
33. Mehta SR, Tanguay JF, Eikelboom JW, Jolly SS, Joyner CD, Granger CB, et al. Double-dose versus standard-dose clopidogrel and high-dose versus low-dose aspirin in individuals undergoing percutaneous coronary intervention for acute coronary syndromes (CURRENT-OASIS 7): a randomised factorial trial. Lancet. 2010;376(9748):1233-43.
34. von Beckerath N, Taubert D, Pogatsa-Murray G, Schömig E, Kastrati A, Schömig A. Absorption, metabolization, and antiplatelet effects of 300-, 600-, and 900-mg loading doses of clopidogrel: results of the ISAR-CHOICE (Intracoronary Stenting and Antithrombotic Regimen: Choose Between 3 High Oral Doses for Immediate Clopidogrel Effect) Trial. Circulation. 2005;112(19):2946-50.
35. Breet NJ, van Werkum JW, Bouman HJ, Kelder JC, Ruven HJ, Bal ET, et al. Comparison of platelet function tests in predicting clinical outcome in patients undergoing coronary stent implantation. JAMA. 2010;303(8):754-62.
36. Price MJ, Berger PB, Teirstein PS, Tanguay JF, Angiolillo DJ, Spriggs D, et al. Standard- vs high-dose clopidogrel based on platelet function testing after percutaneous coronary intervention: the GRAVITAS randomized trial. JAMA. 2011;305(11):1097-105.
37. Mega JL, Close SL, Wiviott SD, Shen L, Walker JR, Simon T, et al. Genetic variants in ABCB1 and CYP2C19 and cardiovascular outcomes after treatment with clopidogrel and prasugrel in the TRITON-TIMI 38 trial: a pharmacogenetic analysis. Lancet. 2010;376(9749):1312-9.
38. Wiviott SD, Trenk D, Frelinger AL, O'Donoghue M, Neumann FJ, Michelson AD, et al. Prasugrel compared with high loading- and maintenance-dose clopidogrel in patients with planned percutaneous coronary intervention: the Prasugrel in Comparison to Clopidogrel for Inhibition of Platelet Activation and Aggregation-Thrombolysis in Myocardial Infarction 44 trial. Circulation. 2007;116(25):2923-32.
39. Wiviott SD, Braunwald E, McCabe CH, Montalescot G, Ruzyllo W, Gottlieb S, et al. Prasugrel versus clopidogrel in patients with acute coronary syndromes. N Engl J Med. 2007;357(20):2001-15.
40. Roe MT, Armstrong PW, Fox KA, White HD, Prabhakaran D, Goodman SG, et al. Prasugrel versus clopidogrel for acute coronary syndromes without revascularization. N Engl J Med. 2012;367(14):1297-309.
41. Montalescot G, Bolognese L, Dudek D, Goldstein P, Hamm C, Tanguay JF, et al. Pretreatment with prasugrel in non-ST-segment elevation acute coronary syndromes. N Engl J Med. 2013;369(11):999-1010.
42. Gurbel PA, Bliden KP, Butler K, Tantry US, Gesheff T, Wei C, et al. Randomized double-blind assessment of the ONSET and OFFSET of the antiplatelet effects of ticagrelor versus clopidogrel in patients with stable coronary artery disease: the ONSET/OFFSET study. Circulation. 2009;120(25):2577-85.
43. Wallentin L, Becker RC, Budaj A, Cannon CP, Emanuelsson H, Held C, et al. Ticagrelor versus clopidogrel in patients with acute coronary syndromes. N Engl J Med. 2009;361(11):1045-57.
44. Storey RF, Bliden KP, Patil SB, Karunakaran A, Ecob R, Butler K, et al. Incidence of dyspnea and assessment of cardiac and pulmonary function in patients with stable coronary artery disease receiving ticagrelor, clopidogrel, or placebo in the ONSET/OFFSET study. J Am Coll Cardiol. 2010;56(3):185-93.
45. Periayah MH, Halim AS, Yaacob NS, Saad AZ, Hussein AR, Rashid AH, et al. Glycoprotein IIb/IIIa and P2Y12 induction by oligochitosan accelerates platelet aggregation. Biomed Res Int. 2014;2014:653149.
46. Roffi M, Chew DP, Mukherjee D, Bhatt DL, White JA, Moliterno DJ, et al. Platelet glycoprotein IIb/IIIa inhibition in acute coronary syndromes. Gradient of benefit related to the revascularization strategy. Eur Heart J. 2002;23(18):1441-8.
47. Stone GW, Bertrand ME, Moses JW, Ohman EM, Lincoff AM, Ware JH, et al. Routine upstream initiation vs deferred selective use of glycoprotein IIb/IIIa inhibitors in acute coronary syndromes: the ACUITY Timing trial. JAMA. 2007;297(6):591-602.
48. Giugliano RP, White JA, Bode C, Armstrong PW, Montalescot G, Lewis BS, et al. Early versus delayed, provisional eptifibatide in acute coronary syndromes. N Engl J Med. 2009;360(21):2176-90.
49. Kastrati A, Mehilli J, Neumann FJ, Dotzer F, ten Berg J, Bollwein H, et al. Abciximab in patients with acute coronary syndromes undergoing percutaneous coronary intervention after clopidogrel pretreatment: the ISAR-REACT 2 randomized trial. JAMA. 2006;295(13):1531-8.
50. Hamm CW, Bassand JP, Agewall S, Bax J, Boersma E, Bueno H, et al. [ESC guidelines for the management of acute coronary syndromes in patients presenting without persistent ST-segment elevation. The Task Force for the management of acute coronary syndromes (ACS) in patients presenting without persistent ST-segment elevation of the European Society of Cardiology (ESC)]. G Ital Cardiol (Rome). 2012;13(3):171-228.
51. Eikelboom JW, Anand SS, Malmberg K, Weitz JI, Ginsberg JS, Yusuf S. Unfractionated heparin and low-molecular-weight heparin in acute coronary syndrome without ST elevation: a meta-analysis. Lancet. 2000;355(9219):1936-42.
52. Andrade-Castellanos CA, Colunga-Lozano LE, Delgado-Figueroa N, Magee K. Heparin versus placebo for non-ST elevation acute coronary syndromes. Cochrane Database Syst Rev. 2014;6:CD003462.
53. Harrington RA, Becker RC, Cannon CP, Gutterman D, Lincoff AM, Popma JJ, et al. Antithrombotic therapy for non-ST-segment elevation acute coronary syndromes: American College of Chest Physicians Evidence-Based Clinical Practice Guidelines (8th Edition). Chest. 2008;133(6 Suppl):670S-707S.
54. Murphy SA, Gibson CM, Morrow DA, Van de Werf F, Menown IB, Goodman SG, et al. Efficacy and safety of the low-molecular weight heparin enoxaparin compared with unfractionated heparin across the acute coronary syndrome spectrum: a meta-analysis. Eur Heart J. 2007;28(17):2077-86.
55. Fifth Organization to Assess Strategies in Acute Ischemic Syndromes Investigators, Yusuf S, Mehta SR, Chrolavicius S, Afzal R, Pogue J, et al. Comparison of fondaparinux and enoxaparin in acute coronary syndromes. N Engl J Med. 2006;354(14):1464-76.
56. Stone GW, McLaurin BT, Cox DA, Bertrand ME, Lincoff AM, Moses JW, et al. Bivalirudin for patients with acute coronary syndromes. N Engl J Med. 2006;355(21):2203-16.
57. Effects of tissue plasminogen activator and a comparison of early invasive and conservative strategies in unstable angina and non-Q-wave myocardial infarction. Results of the TIMI IIIB Trial. Thrombolysis in Myocardial Ischemia. Circulation. 1994;89(4):1545-56.
58. Julian DG, Valentine PA, Miller GG. Disturbances of rate, rhythm and conduction in acute myocardial infarction: A prospective study of 100 consecutive unselected patients with the aid of electrocardiographic monitoring. Am J Med. 1964;37:915-27.
59. Piccini JP, Schulte PJ, Pieper KS, Mehta RH, White HD, Van de Werf F, et al. Antiarrhythmic drug therapy for sustained ventricular arrhythmias complicating acute myocardial infarction. Crit Care Med. 2011;39(1):78-83.

60. Trappe HJ. Tachyarrhythmias, bradyarrhythmias and acute coronary syndromes. J Emerg Trauma Shock. 2010;3(2):137-42.
61. Mehta SR, Cannon CP, Fox KA, Wallentin L, Boden WE, Spacek R, et al. Routine vs selective invasive strategies in patients with acute coronary syndromes: a collaborative meta-analysis of randomized trials. JAMA. 2005;293(23):2908-17.
62. Bavry AA, Kumbhani DJ, Rassi AN, Bhatt DL, Askari AT. Benefit of early invasive therapy in acute coronary syndromes: a meta-analysis of contemporary randomized clinical trials. J Am Coll Cardiol. 2006;48(7): 1319-25.
63. Fox KA, Clayton TC, Damman P, Pocock SJ, de Winter RJ, Tijssen JG, et al. Long-term outcome of a routine versus selective invasive strategy in patients with non-ST-segment elevation acute coronary syndrome a meta-analysis of individual patient data. J Am Coll Cardiol. 2010;55(22):2435-45.
64. Fox KA, Dabbous OH, Goldberg RJ, Pieper KS, Eagle KA, Van de Werf F, et al. Prediction of risk of death and myocardial infarction in the six months after presentation with acute coronary syndrome: prospective multinational observational study (GRACE). BMJ. 2006;333(7578):1091.
65. Rasoul S, Ottervanger JP, de Boer MJ, Dambrink JH, Hoorntje JC, Gosselink AT, et al. Primary percutaneous coronary intervention for ST-elevation myocardial infarction: from clinical trial to clinical practice. Int J Cardiol. 2009;134(1):104-9.
66. Zijlstra F, Hoorntje JC, de Boer MJ, Reiffers S, Miedema K, Ottervanger JP, et al. Long-term benefit of primary angioplasty as compared with thrombolytic therapy for acute myocardial infarction. N Engl J Med. 1999;341(19):1413-9.
67. Keeley EC, Boura JA, Grines CL. Primary angioplasty versus intravenous thrombolytic therapy for acute myocardial infarction: a quantitative review of 23 randomised trials. Lancet. 2003;361(9351):13-20.
68. Andersen HR, Nielsen TT, Rasmussen K, Thuesen L, Kelbaek H, Thayssen P, et al. A comparison of coronary angioplasty with fibrinolytic therapy in acute myocardial infarction. N Engl J Med. 2003;349(8):733-42.
69. Steg PG, Bonnefoy E, Chabaud S, Lapostolle F, Dubien PY, Cristofini P, et al. Impact of time to treatment on mortality after prehospital fibrinolysis or primary angioplasty: data from the CAPTIM randomized clinical trial. Circulation. 2003;108(23):2851-6.
70. Pinto DS, Kirtane AJ, Nallamothu BK, Murphy SA, Cohen DJ, Laham RJ, et al. Hospital delays in reperfusion for ST-elevation myocardial infarction: implications when selecting a reperfusion strategy. Circulation. 2006;114(19):2019-25.
71. Tamis-Holland JE, O'Gara P. Highlights from the 2013 ACCF/AHA guidelines for the management of ST-elevation myocardial infarction and beyond. Clin Cardiol. 2014;37(4):252-9.
72. A clinical trial comparing primary coronary angioplasty with tissue plasminogen activator for acute myocardial infarction. The Global Use of Strategies to Open Occluded Coronary Arteries in Acute Coronary Syndromes (GUSTO IIb) Angioplasty Substudy Investigators. N Engl J Med. 1997;336(23):1621-8.
73. Schömig A, Mehilli J, Antoniucci D, Ndrepepa G, Markwardt C, Di Pede F, et al. Mechanical reperfusion in patients with acute myocardial infarction presenting more than 12 hours from symptom onset: a randomized controlled trial. JAMA. 2005;293(23):2865-72.
74. Ndrepepa G, Kastrati A, Mehilli J, Antoniucci D, Schömig A. Mechanical reperfusion and long-term mortality in patients with acute myocardial infarction presenting 12 to 48 hours from onset of symptoms. JAMA. 2009;301(5):487-8.
75. Menon V, Pearte CA, Buller CE, Steg PG, Forman SA, White HD, et al. Lack of benefit from percutaneous intervention of persistently occluded infarct arteries after the acute phase of myocardial infarction is time independent: insights from Occluded Artery Trial. Eur Heart J. 2009;30(2):183-91.
76. Boersma E, Primary Coronary Angioplasty vs. Thrombolysis Group. Does time matter? A pooled analysis of randomized clinical trials comparing primary percutaneous coronary intervention and in-hospital fibrinolysis in acute myocardial infarction patients. Eur Heart J. 2006;27(7):779-88.
77. Sabatine MS, Cannon CP, Gibson CM, López-Sendón JL, Montalescot G, Theroux P, et al. Effect of clopidogrel pretreatment before percutaneous coronary intervention in patients with ST-elevation myocardial infarction treated with fibrinolytics: the PCI-CLARITY study. JAMA. 2005;294(10): 1224-32.
78. Patti G, Bárczi G, Orlic D, Mangiacapra F, Colonna G, Pasceri V, et al. Outcome comparison of 600- and 300-mg loading doses of clopidogrel in patients undergoing primary percutaneous coronary intervention for ST-segment elevation myocardial infarction: results from the ARMYDA-6 MI (Antiplatelet therapy for Reduction of MYocardial Damage during Angioplasty-Myocardial Infarction) randomized study. J Am Coll Cardiol. 2011;58(15):1592-9.
79. Koul S, Smith JG, Scherstén F, James S, Lagerqvist B, Erlinge D. Effect of upstream clopidogrel treatment in patients with ST-segment elevation myocardial infarction undergoing primary percutaneous coronary intervention. Eur Heart J. 2011;32(23):2989-97.
80. Dörler J, Edlinger M, Alber HF, Altenberger J, Benzer W, Grimm G, et al. Clopidogrel pre-treatment is associated with reduced in-hospital mortality in primary percutaneous coronary intervention for acute ST-elevation myocardial infarction. Eur Heart J. 2011;32(23):2954-61.
81. Steg PG, James S, Harrington RA, Ardissino D, Becker RC, Cannon CP, et al. Ticagrelor versus clopidogrel in patients with ST-elevation acute coronary syndromes intended for reperfusion with primary percutaneous coronary intervention: A Platelet Inhibition and Patient Outcomes (PLATO) trial subgroup analysis. Circulation. 2010;122(21):2131-41.
82. Ellis SG, Tendera M, de Belder MA, van Boven AJ, Widimsky P, Janssens L, et al. Facilitated PCI in patients with ST-elevation myocardial infarction. N Engl J Med. 2008;358(21):2205-17.
83. Mehilli J, Kastrati A, Schulz S, Früngel S, Nekolla SG, Moshage W, et al. Abciximab in patients with acute ST-segment-elevation myocardial infarction undergoing primary percutaneous coronary intervention after clopidogrel loading: a randomized double-blind trial. Circulation. 2009;119(14):1933-40.
84. Silvain J, Beygui F, Barthélémy O, Pollack C, Cohen M, Zeymer U, et al. Efficacy and safety of enoxaparin versus unfractionated heparin during percutaneous coronary intervention: systematic review and meta-analysis. BMJ. 2012;344:e553.
85. Montalescot G, Ellis SG, de Belder MA, Janssens L, Katz O, Pluta W, et al. Enoxaparin in primary and facilitated percutaneous coronary intervention A formal prospective nonrandomized substudy of the FINESSE trial (Facilitated INtervention with Enhanced Reperfusion Speed to Stop Events). JACC Cardiovasc Interv. 2010;3(2):203-12.
86. Navarese EP, De Luca G, Castriota F, Kozinski M, Gurbel PA, Gibson CM, et al. Low-molecular-weight heparins vs. unfractionated heparin in the setting of percutaneous coronary intervention for ST-elevation myocardial infarction: a meta-analysis. J Thromb Haemost. 2011;9(10):1902-15.
87. Montalescot G, Zeymer U, Silvain J, Boulanger B, Cohen M, Goldstein P, et al. Intravenous enoxaparin or unfractionated heparin in primary percutaneous coronary intervention for ST-elevation myocardial infarction: the international randomised open-label ATOLL trial. Lancet. 2011;378(9792):693-703.
88. Yusuf S, Mehta SR, Chrolavicius S, Afzal R, Pogue J, Granger CB, et al. Effects of fondaparinux on mortality and reinfarction in patients with acute ST-segment elevation myocardial infarction: the OASIS-6 randomized trial. JAMA. 2006;295(13):1519-30.
89. Stone GW, Witzenbichler B, Guagliumi G, Peruga JZ, Brodie BR, Dudek D, et al. Heparin plus a glycoprotein IIb/IIIa inhibitor versus bivalirudin monotherapy and paclitaxel-eluting stents versus bare-metal stents in acute myocardial infarction (HORIZONS-AMI): final 3-year results from a multicentre, randomised controlled trial. Lancet. 2011;377(9784):2193-204.
90. Indications for fibrinolytic therapy in suspected acute myocardial infarction: collaborative overview of early mortality and major morbidity results from all randomised trials of more than 1000 patients. Fibrinolytic Therapy Trialists' (FTT) Collaborative Group. Lancet. 1994;343(8893):311-22.
91. Assessment of the Safety and Efficacy of a New Thrombolytic (ASSENT-2) Investigators, Van De Werf F, Adgey J, Ardissino D, Armstrong PW, Aylward P, et al. Single-bolus tenecteplase compared with front-loaded alteplase in acute myocardial infarction: the ASSENT-2 double-blind randomised trial. Lancet. 1999;354(9180):716-22.
92. A comparison of reteplase with alteplase for acute myocardial infarction. The Global Use of Strategies to Open Occluded Coronary Arteries (GUSTO III) Investigators. N Engl J Med. 1997;337(16):1118-23.
93. White HD. Thrombolytic therapy in the elderly. Lancet. 2000;356(9247):2028-30.
94. Berkowitz SD, Granger CB, Pieper KS, Lee KL, Gore JM, Simoons M, et al. Incidence and predictors of bleeding after contemporary thrombolytic therapy for myocardial infarction. The Global Utilization of Streptokinase and Tissue Plasminogen activator for Occluded coronary arteries (GUSTO) I Investigators. Circulation. 1997;95(11):2508-16.
95. American College of Emergency Physicians; Society for Cardiovascular Angiography and Interventions, O'Gara PT, Kushner FG, Ascheim DD, Casey DE, Chung MK, et al. 2013 ACCF/AHA guideline for the management of ST-elevation myocardial infarction: a report of the American College of Cardiology Foundation/American Heart Association Task Force on Practice Guidelines. J Am Coll Cardiol. 2013;61(4):e78-140.
96. Ferguson JJ. Clopidogrel plus aspirin in patients with acute myocardial infarction treated with fibrinolytic therapy—CLARITY-TIMI 28. Future Cardiol. 2005;1(5):605-10.

15

CHAPTER

Noninvasive Testing

Alexander T Limkakeng, Traci L Thoureen

INTRODUCTION

The evaluation of acute coronary syndrome (ACS) in the emergency department (ED) remains challenging. Each year, over 6 million people present to the ED for evaluation of chest pain or other symptoms concerning for myocardial ischemia.[1] The prevalence of and mortality associated with ischemic heart disease (IHD) is high. Approximately one in three American adults have some form of cardiovascular disease including over 17 million with IHD.[2] Ischemic heart disease is the number one cause of death in both men and women, implicated in approximately one in six deaths.[2]

Clinical evaluation of patients with potential ischemic symptoms should include the history of symptoms, physical exam and resting electrocardiogram (ECG).[3-5] However, history alone is often insufficient to rule out IHD. This is especially true in women, diabetics and the elderly, who tend to present with more atypical symptoms including nausea, vomiting, diaphoresis, and fatigue.[3] A resting ECG obtained within 10 minutes of ED arrival can also aid in risk stratification. However, even in patients without known coronary artery disease (CAD), a nonischemic ECG is associated with a risk of 2%.[6-9] Physical exam can often aid in diagnosing nonischemic causes of symptoms, however, the majority of patients with ACS present with a normal physical exam.[8,10] Biomarkers such as troponin are specific to cardiac muscle, and tend to rise within 3–4 hours of ischemic event.[11,12] However, these tests also have limitations, as 40–60% of patients with ACS present with initial biomarkers below the threshold for clinical decision-making.[13]

For those who do "rule out" by biomarkers, furthermore, there are still significant proportions of patients with IHD that has not yet caused myocardial necrosis.[14] Such patients are at risk for near-term subsequent conversion to myocardial infarction from rupture of an unstable coronary plaque. Additionally, such patients frequently suffer from limiting symptoms that can be ameliorated by percutaneous intervention. Thus, stress testing provides a means to noninvasively assess patients for the entire spectrum of ACS. While it does not definitively rule out the possibility of subsequent adverse cardiac events, it does define patients at very low risk.

WHAT IS A STRESS TEST?

Stress testing is an attempt to briefly induce evidence of regional malperfusion via a stressor or other stimulus and identify that regional malperfusion via medical imaging of the heart. It is comprised of two essential elements: (i) the stressor, which attempts to increase the myocardial oxygen demand and/or differentiate stenosed coronary vessels from healthy ones and (ii) the evaluation component which directly or indirectly evaluates cardiac myocardial perfusion. The goal of this testing is to identify a patient at risk for subsequent adverse cardiac events for whom a cardiac intervention would benefit. Specifically, it attempts to identify malperfusion that is not clinically evident based on resting ECG, cardiac biomarkers, or clinical symptoms alone.

MYOCARDIAL ISCHEMIA PHYSIOLOGY

The observable phenomena of myocardial ischemia have been well described. In their executive summary on stress echocardiography, the European Association of Echocardiography writes: "Myocardial ischaemia results in a typical "cascade" of events in which the various markers are hierarchically ranked in a well-defined time sequence. Flow heterogeneity, especially between the subendocardial and subepicardial perfusion, is the forerunner of ischemia followed by metabolic changes, alteration in regional mechanical function, and only at a later stage by electrocardiographic changes, global left ventricular dysfunction, and pain. The pathophysiological concept of the ischemic cascade is translated clinically into a gradient of sensitivity of different available clinical markers of ischemia, with chest pain being the least and regional malperfusion the most sensitive."[15]

Ischemic myocardium thus can be differentiated from well-perfused segments of the heart by direct imaging, its mechanical (pump) function, electrocardiographic signals, or by clinical symptoms. Stress testing preferentially utilizes the former two means for identifying ischemic myocardium.

INDICATIONS FOR STRESS TESTING

Multiple algorithms and combinations thereof have been developed to risk stratify ED patients with potential IHD and help determine which patients require further testing before discharge.[14,16-19] Patients who are determined to have an intermediate risk probability will benefit most from additional evaluation and testing.[20-22] The American College of Cardiology/American Heart Association (ACC/AHA) recommendations for stress testing are as follows (Boxes 1 and 2).

GENERAL CONTRAINDICATIONS

Stress testing is a noninvasive and generally safe procedure, with adverse events of myocardial infarction (MI) or death occurring in 1 of 2,500 tests.[20] However, certain patients have absolute contraindications to stress testing, and, therefore, cannot safely undergo testing. In patients with relative contraindications, the clinician and the patient should employ shared decision-making in weighing the risk of the test versus the potential benefit derived from the testing results.[24,25] All patients should be informed of the potential risks and benefits of stress testing prior to testing. In general, stress testing is contraindicated in patients with the following conditions (Box 3).

Abdominal aortic aneurysms in the past have been considered a contraindication to stress testing. Best et al.[26] performed a retrospective review which demonstrated a rate of rupture of 0.4%. The risks and benefits of stress testing should be discussed with these patients, but it is considered safe to perform.

STRESSORS

There are several methods to perform cardiac stress testing for a patient. The modality chosen is primarily based on the patient's ability to perform adequate exercise and if

BOX 1 Recommendations for electrocardiogram stress testing

Class I (Evidence or agreement that the test is indicated)

- To diagnose CAD in adult patients with intermediate pretest probability of CAD on the basis of gender, age, and symptoms (specific exceptions noted in class II and III)
- In patients with suspected or known CAD, previously evaluated, who present with significant change in clinical status
- Low-risk unstable angina patients 8–12 hours after presentation who are symptom free and without signs of heart failure
- Intermediate risk unstable angina patients 2–3 days after presentation who are symptom free and without signs of heart failure

Class II (Evidence or consensus is conflicted on whether the test is indicated, class IIa—evidence or agreement leans more towards indicated, class IIb—evidence or agreement is inconclusive)

- Class IIa
  - To diagnose CAD in patients with vasospastic angina
  - Evaluation of intermediate risk unstable angina patients with normal cardiac markers initially and 6–12 hours after onset of symptoms, repeat ECG without significant changes, and no other evidence of ischemia
  - Evaluation of patients with known or suspected exercise-induced arrhythmias
- Class IIb
  - To diagnose CAD in patients with high or low pretest probability based on age, symptoms, gender
  - To diagnose CAD in patients with <1 mm of baseline ST depression and taking digoxin
  - To diagnose CAD in patients with ECG criteria for left ventricular hypertrophy and <1 mm of baseline ST depression
  - To evaluate risk and prognosis in patients with the following ECG abnormalities: WPW syndrome, electronically paced ventricular rhythm, 1 mm or more of resting ST depression, complete LBBB or any interventricular conduction defect with a QRS duration greater than 120 ms

Class III (Evidence or agreement that the test is not indicated)

- To diagnose CAD in patients with the following ECG abnormalities: WPW syndrome, electronically paced ventricular rhythm, >1 mm of resting ST depression, or complete LBBB
- To diagnose CAD in patients with a documented myocardial infarction or prior coronary angiography demonstrating significant disease (however, test can determine ischemia and risk)
- To evaluate risk and prognosis in patients with severe comorbidity likely to limit life expectancy and/or candidacy for revascularization
- To evaluate risk and prognosis in high-risk unstable angina patients
- Routine screening of asymptomatic men or women

CAD, coronary artery disease; ECG, electrocardiogram; LBBB, left bundle branch block; WPW, Wolff-Parkinson-White; PCI, percutaneous coronary intervention; STEMI, ST elevation myocardial infarctions; UFH, unfractionated heparin.

BOX 2 The American College of Cardiology/American Heart Association (ACC/AHA) appropriate use criteria for cardiac radionuclide imaging[22] and stress echocardiogaphy:[23] Criteria with appropriate use score greater than 7 (appropriate)

Detection of CAD/risk assessment: Symptomatic or ischemic equivalent evaluation of ischemic equivalent (nonacute)
- Low pretest probability of CAD
- ECG uninterpretable or unable to exercise
- Intermediate pretest probability of CAD
- ECG interpretable and able to exercise
- Intermediate pretest probability of CAD
- ECG uninterpretable or unable to exercise
- High pretest probability of CAD
- Regardless of ECG interpretability and ability to exercise

Detection of CAD/risk assessment: Symptomatic or ischemic equivalent acute chest pain
- Possible ACS
- ECG: No ischemic changes or with LBBB or electronically paced ventricular rhythm
- Low-risk TIMI score
- Negative troponin levels
- Possible ACS
- ECG: No ischemic changes or with LBBB or electronically paced ventricular rhythm
- Low-risk TIMI score
- Peak troponin: Borderline, equivocal, minimally elevated
- Possible ACS
- ECG: No ischemic changes or with LBBB or electronically paced ventricular rhythm
- High-risk TIMI score
- Negative troponin levels
- Possible ACS
- ECG: No ischemic changes or with LBBB or electronically paced ventricular rhythm
- High-risk TIMI score
- Peak troponin: Borderline, equivocal, minimally elevated
- *Radionuclide imaging only
- Possible ACS
- ECG: No ischemic changes or with LBBB or electronically ventricular paced rhythm
- Initial troponin: Negative
- Recent or ongoing chest pain

Following prior test results, new or worsening symptoms
- Abnormal coronary angiography or abnormal prior stress imaging study

Following prior test results, prior noninvasive evaluation
- Equivocal, borderline, or discordant stress testing where obstructive CAD remains a concern

Following prior coronary angiography (invasive or noninvasive)
- *Radionuclide imaging only
- Coronary stenosis or anatomic abnormality of uncertain significance

Risk assessment: Post-revascularization (PCI or CABG) symptomatic
- Ischemic equivalent

ACS, acute coronary syndrome; CABG, coronary artery bypass graft; CAD, coronary artery disease; ECG, electrocardiogram; LBBB, left bundle branch block; PCI, percutaneous coronary intervention; TIMI, thrombolysis in myocardial infarction.

BOX 3 Stress testing contraindications

- Absolute
  - Acute myocardial infarction within 2 days
  - High-risk unstable angina
  - Uncontrolled cardiac arrhythmia with hemodynamic compromise
  - Uncontrolled arrhythmias causing symptoms or hemodynamic compromise
  - Symptomatic severe aortic stenosis
  - Uncontrolled symptomatic heart failure
  - Acute pulmonary embolism or pulmonary infarction
  - Acute myocarditis or pericarditis
  - Endocarditis
  - Acute aortic dissection
  - Acute noncardiac issue (sepsis, toxicologic)
- Relative
  - Left main coronary artery stenosis
  - Moderate to severe aortic stenosis
  - Electrolyte abnormalities
  - Severe arterial hypertension (>200/110 mm Hg)
  - Tachyarrhythmias or bradyarrhythmias
  - Hypertrophic cardiomyopathy or other forms of outflow tract obstruction
  - Mental or physical impairment leading to inability to exercise adequately
  - High-degree atrioventricular block

there are baseline ECG abnormalities [ST/T changes, left ventricular hypertrophy, left bundle branch block (LBBB), ventricular pre-excitation or paced ventricular rhythm] that would reduce sensitivity of the exercise ECG testing.[27]

Exercise

Patients who have the ability to exercise may undergo treadmill exercise stress testing. The ability to do adequate exercise for the test is defined by ability to have 85% of age-predicted maximum heart rate, more than five metabolic

BOX 4 Patient preparation for exercise stress

- Fast 2–3 hours prior to test
- Hold negative inotropic medications for ideally 24 hours
- Continue to take other medications
- History and exam to assess ability to perform exercise
- Informed consent
- Supine and upright electrocardiogram should be obtained

equivalents workload and exercise for at least 3 minutes to complete stage I of the standard Bruce protocol.[27]

Patients should be coached to perform their best exercise and to advise the provider if they are experiencing symptoms that reproduces their original symptoms (Box 4). Electrocardiogram monitoring leads are attached to the patient in standard configuration. A treadmill machine is usually used. This machine must have variable speed and incline. It should have handrails, but the patient should be discouraged from holding on during testing. The test should be supervised by a physician. Life support equipment should be readily available should a complication arise.

There are several protocols for exercise testing. The most widely used is the Bruce protocol.[28] This protocol is performed measuring exercise capacity in terms of estimated metabolic equivalents of a task, known as METs. One MET estimates the oxygen consumption of a 70 kg, 40-year-old man and equals 3.5 mL/min/kg of body weight.[29] Most activities of daily living require 4–5 METs. If a patient reports difficulties at home with performing daily activities, then modified protocols or pharmacologic stress testing should be considered.[21]

In the standard Bruce protocol, there are three stages separated by 3-minute periods to allow the patient to achieve steady state between the stages. Stage 1 is 1.7 mph at 10% grade (5 METs), stage 2 is 2.5 mph at 12% grade (7 METs), and stage 3 is 3.4 mph at 14% grade (9 METs). For patients who are more limited with their exercise or with older patients, a modified Bruce protocol is used which only has two 3-minute stages. Stage 1 is 1.7 mph without a grade and stage 2 is 1.7 mph with a 5% grade.[21]

There are other protocols that are used less frequently, for example the Naughton, Weber,[30] which start at lower METs and increases by 1–1.5 METs between stages. Other exercise protocols utilize bicycle and arm ergometry.

Although the originator of the Bruce protocol advocated for symptom-limited, not heart rate-limited testing, currently it is common to terminate tests when patients reached 85% of a target heart rate based on age.[31,32] The ACC/AHA guidelines also specify reasons for termination of exercise testing (Table 1).[33]

Pharmacologic Stressors

Patients who are unable to do traditional exercise stress testing because of physical limitations, inability to achieve the exercise end-points, LBBB, or electronically paced rhythms may have testing done with vasodilator agents and/or inotropic agents.[22]

Vasodilators

The vasodilator agents are classified by their action on the adenosine receptor. There are nonselective agents such adenosine and dipyridamole and there are selective agents, namely, binodenoson, regadenoson and apadenoson. There are four types of adenosine receptors, A1, A2A, A2B, and A3. Stimulation of the A2A receptor causes coronary artery dilation, whereas the other receptors cause side effects.[27]

Regadenoson is the only FDA-approved selective adenosine receptor agonist agent at this time. It is the most commonly used vasodilator agent for myocardial perfusion imaging (MPI). In comparison to adenosine, it is less rapidly metabolized, allowing it to be given as a bolus rather than intravenous infusion (Box 5).

TABLE 1: Reasons for termination of a stress test

Absolute indications for termination of testing	Relative indications for termination of testing
• Drop in SBP of more than 10 mm Hg from baseline, despite an increase in workload, when accompanied by other evidence of ischemia • Moderate-to-severe angina • Increasing nervous system symptoms (e.g., ataxia, dizziness, near-syncope) • Signs of poor perfusion (cyanosis or pallor) • Technical difficulties in monitoring ECG tracings or SBP • Subject's desire to stop • Sustained ventricular tachycardia • ST elevation (>1 mm) in leads without diagnostic Q waves (other than V1 or aVR)	• Drop in SBP of 10 mm Hg or more from baseline, despite an increase in workload, in the absence of other evidence of ischemia • ST or QRS changes such as excessive ST depression (horizontal or down-sloping ST-segment depression >2 mm) or marked axis shift • Arrhythmias other than sustained ventricular tachycardia, including multifocal PVCs, triplets of PVCs, supraventricular tachycardia, heart block, or bradyarrhythmias • Fatigue, shortness of breath, wheezing, leg cramps, or claudication • Development of bundle branch block or intraventricular conduction delay that cannot be distinguished from ventricular tachycardia • Increasing chest pain • Hypertensive response (SBP of 250 mm Hg, DBP higher than 115 mm Hg, or both)

DBP, diastolic blood pressure; ECG, electrocardiographic; PVCs, premature ventricular contractions; SBP, systolic blood pressure.

BOX 5 Adenosine/dipyridamole contraindications

- Absolute contraindications
  - Active bronchospasm or current treatment for reactive airway disease
  - Any heart block greater than first degree
  - Systolic blood pressure <90 mm Hg
  - Consumption of methylxanthines or dipyridamole (caffeine or aminophylline)
- Relative contraindications
  - Sick sinus syndrome or bradycardia <40 beats/min
  - History of reactive airway disease not active for a year
- Regadenoson exclusions
  - Second-degree atrioventricular block or sick sinus syndrome
  - Unstable angina

These agents increase myocardial blood flow three- to five-fold in normal coronary arteries independent of myocardial oxygen demand.[34] A perfusion defect is seen when there is a difference between the nondiseased and diseased coronary artery areas that have a limited ability to augment blood flow.

Patients with a history of reactive airway disease or high-grade heart block are not candidates for these agents. Patients must have instructions to withhold caffeine, methylxanthine-containing medications, β-blockers, and nitrates for 24 hours prior to the study. Medications containing dipyridamole and verapamil should be stopped 48 hours prior to the test.[35,36]

Dobutamine

When patients are extremely exercise-limited or have reactive airway disease, the positive inotropic agent, dobutamine, is often used. This drug has a higher side effect profile. If a patient has a contraindication to adenosine (reactive airways disease or significant heart block) or has consumed caffeine in the last 24 hours, however, it may be the stressor of choice (Box 6).[37]

Performance of Pharmacologic Stress Testing

The patient requires a peripheral intravenous line. After recording the height and weight, rest imaging is done for 20 minutes. When this is complete, the patient goes to the treadmill room and electrocardiographic monitoring is started. The patient is positioned supine with adenosine or dobutamine.[37]

With adenosine, the patient receives a weight-based infusion over 4 minutes. Vital signs are recorded each minute of the infusion. The infusion commonly causes flushing, shortness of breath, chest pressure, and leg heaviness but these symptoms are brief and do not usually require modification of the infusion. If the patient has no symptoms of vasodilation after infusion, this may suggest that the adenosine did not reach the patient or that they used caffeine. Bronchospasm and high grade atrioventricular block may occur and requires cessation of the infusion. Bronchospasm may be abated with an aminophylline infusion.[27,38]

If possible, low-level exercise can be done with the adenosine infusion and stopped at the end of the infusion. This exercise can be walking at 1 mph at 0% grade, simple marching, or lifting light weights in the arm contralateral to their peripheral veins.[37] The addition of low-level exercise during pharmacologic stress has been shown to improve the sensitivity of dipyridamole and adenosine stress.[39]

Regadenoson is administered as a single 400 μg bolus (non-weight-based) over 10 seconds followed by a 5 mL saline flush. Twenty seconds after the bolus, the radiotracer is administered. Regadenoson causes a faster and greater increase in heart rate and comparable decrease in blood pressure compared to adenosine.[40]

Dobutamine is also infused with a weight-based dose starting at 10 μg/kg/min and is increased every 3 minutes to a maximum of 40–50 μg/kg/min. The target heart rate is 85% of predicted. If the heart rate does not elevate enough, intravenous atropine may be given. The dobutamine infusion is continued for an additional minute after this occurs. Side effects of dobutamine may include: flushing, palpitations, chest fullness, and nausea. Significant arrhythmia, severe hypertension or marked ischemic ST changes on ECG may require stopping the infusion.[37]

BOX 6 Dobutamine exclusions

- Recent myocardial infarction
- Unstable angina
- Aortic stenosis or obstructive cardiomyopathy
- Atrial tachycardias
- History of ventricular tachycardia
- Uncontrolled hypertension
- Thoracic aortic aneurysm
- Left bundle branch block

ASSESSMENTS

Exercise Parameters and Electrocardiography

One of the reasons for encouraging exercise stress for those who are able is that prognostic information is gained from the patient's ability to exercise and from other parameters.[41] Early studies have demonstrated that an inability to achieve target heart rate is associated with an increased relative risk of death.[42-44]

Electrocardiogram parameters also provide prognostic information. The ECG is monitored in real time during the graded exercise for the same parameters evaluated in a resting ECG for suspicion of ACS (ST segment changes, arrhythmias).[41] In some centers, graded exercise testing is the preferred modality for initial assessment of suspected CAD and it remains a class IA recommendation in patients with intermediate pretest probability, the ability to exercise and interpretable ECGs.[21]

Other parameters have been studied in combination to provide prognosis. One clinically applicable score is the Duke Treadmill Score.[45] It is calculated by the simple formula:

$$\text{Exercise time (minutes)} - [5 \times \text{max ST deviation (mm)}] - (4 \times \text{angina index})$$

The angina index is scored as follows: 0 = no angina during test, 1 = exercise induced angina, 2 = exercise limiting angina. A Duke Treadmill Score greater than 5 is associated with an annual average mortality rate of 0.3% in outpatients and a 0.6% rate in inpatients[46] and a 97% 7-year survival rate.[47]

Clinical Application

Exercise ECG testing has been demonstrated to be safe and effective in triage of ED patients with symptoms of ACS. Multiple studies from the 1990s have demonstrated its safety and high sensitivity and negative predictive value for short-term adverse cardiac events.[48-50] One center published their results using exercise ECG prior to cardiac biomarker rule out and found it safe and effective.[51-54] However, despite these results, most centers have added imaging components to standard stress testing due to the increased diagnostic and prognostic information that is gained.[21]

STRESS ECHOCARDIOGRAPHY

Stress echocardiography is a noninvasive technology that images the heart using ultrasound. In order to diagnose myocardial ischemia from CAD, sonographic images are obtained at baseline and then are compared to those obtained during or immediately after stress. Stress-induced myocardial ischemia is identified by sonographic appearance of worsening wall motion abnormalities or the appearance of new wall motion abnormalities after the stressor.

Physiology

It has been known since as early as 1935 that coronary occlusion results in cardiac wall motion abnormalities.[55] This observation is the fundamental basis for stress echocardiography. By inducing transient myocardial ischemia, wall motion abnormalities that are not present at rest can be visualized with echocardiography. Stress echocardiography utilizes ultrasound to identify these regional wall motion abnormalities to determine myocardial viability.

Indications/Contraindications

In general, there are few contraindications to using echocardiography as the assessment modality for a stress test.[20,21,56] Medical conditions such as chronic obstructive lung disease and obesity can obscure sonographic windows. Most contraindications pertain to the stressor component and relative contraindications mostly relate to optimal test selection. For example, nuclear assessment components are preferred for patients with known single vessel disease due to higher sensitivity or who have had prior nuclear studies for comparison.

Left bundle branch block has historically been considered a relative contraindication to stress echocardiography due to the baseline abnormalities in septal wall motion from left and right ventricular asynchrony. Patients with an underlying LBBB can present diagnostic difficulty in echocardiographic imaging because of the already abnormal conduction of the heart. The ACC/AHA 2007 guidelines recommend pharmacologic stress testing in these patients. Patients with left ventricular hypertrophy can also present increased diagnostic difficulty when undergoing stress echocardiography. However, a systematic review demonstrated that pooled estimates of sensitivity and specificity in this group did not greatly differ from a general population.[57] It is recommended that these patients undergo exercise stress echocardiographic testing when capable.

There is some controversy over the role of gender in stress echocardiography. Some maintain that stress echocardiography may have decreased accuracy in women compared to men due to higher rates of nonobstructive microvascular disease or single vessel disease and differential responses to stressors.[58] However, a systematic review of the question found that although some individual trials showed a difference between men and women in diagnostic accuracy, the pooled data did not show differences in sensitivity and specificity in women and men.[59]

Protocol

As noted earlier, stress echocardiography can be performed using either exercise or pharmacologic agents as the stressor agent. If exercise is used, typically a treadmill is used for ambulatory patients, but bicycle exercise has also been described. If a patient is unable to perform exercise testing, a pharmacologic agent may be utilized instead. Dobutamine is the standard pharmacologic stress agent, with atropine added as needed to achieve the desired heart rate.[60]

Ultrasound technicians as well as personnel trained for management of any dysrhythmias should be at the bedside with standard resuscitation equipment during performance of a stress echocardiogram. Standard ultrasound equipment for echocardiography can be used. The ultrasound machine, a patient stretcher, and the treadmill should all be placed in close proximity to one another so that images can be captured immediately after target heart rate is achieved. Patients should wear a loose fitting gown that can be easily moved to allow for sonographer access to standard echocardiographic windows.

Stressors are administered or applied as noted earlier for stress echocardiography.

A resting echocardiogram is initially obtained to evaluate for ventricular function, chamber sizes, wall thickness, aortic root diameter, pericardial effusion, and valvular structure. These are obtained in standard echocardiographic windows. Parasternal long- and short-axes and apical four- and two-chamber views are acquired. Wall segments examined include anterior, posterior, lateral and inferior walls, anterior and inferior septum, and apex.[15]

Possible adverse effects from stress echocardiography include recurrence of symptoms, rapid large changes in blood pressure and cardiac arrhythmia. However, these adverse effects are rare, occurring in less than 1 in 1,000 exams.[61]

Interpretation

Echocardiography images are typically obtained by certified sonographer technicians and interpreted by board-certified cardiologists. One critique of stress echocardiography is that interpretation is user dependent and necessarily subjective. Nonetheless, when performed properly with standardized techniques, there is high interoperator reproducibility.[15]

The images are then compared to evaluate for wall motion abnormalities in the various regions of the heart (inferior, lateral, septal, anterior, and posterior). As noted before, new or worsening wall motion abnormalities seen on stress echocardiogram can be indicative of obstructive lesions which may be amenable to percutaneous coronary intervention.[15]

Baseline images are classified as either normokinetic or akinetic/dyskinetic. Wall segments that have normal activity at rest and remain normal or become hyperkinetic are considered normal wall segments. Those that become hypokinetic or worse are considered ischemic. Segments that are abnormal at baseline and remain so are necrotic or infarcted. Some segments are abnormal at baseline and show either stunned myocardium or a biphasic response of improving then deteriorating at peak stress. These segments are termed viable.[62]

At least one wall segment that has normal activity at rest and wall motion abnormality with stress is necessary for a stress echocardiogram to be considered abnormal. Generally two adjacent segments are considered necessary to diagnose myocardial ischemia. A Wall Motion Score Index can be calculated. It is merely the sum of the rating on a scale of 1–5 of all 16 wall segments. Higher numbers indicate more severe wall motion abnormalities.[61]

Evidence for Clinical Application

The evidence in support for use of stress echocardiography is extensive. In patients who underwent a normal study, the 3-year cardiac event-free survival was found to be 97%, demonstrating that these patients are risk stratified to a very low risk category.[63] In one study of patients who developed greater than 1 mm ST elevation in two contiguous leads during stress echocardiogram, half of the patients underwent coronary catheterization and all of these patients had greater than 70% stenosis. Multiple vessels were involved in over three-quarters of those patients.[64]

In 2010, the Ontario Health Technology Advisory Committee conducted an extensive systematic review of the literature in support of the use of stress echocardiography. They identified seven systematic reviews summarizing 226 studies comparing stress echocardiography to coronary angiography for the diagnosis of CAD. The pooled estimates of sensitivity and specificity of stress echocardiography from these studies were 80% and 84%, respectively, across stressors, with no significant difference in diagnostic test characteristics between stressors. The diagnostics odds ratio (likelihood ratio +/likelihood ratio –) was 20.64.[61]

In this same review, cost effectiveness was also assessed. Compared to single-photon emission computed tomography (SPECT), three reviews found stress echocardiography to be dominant (lower cost with better outcomes) and three comparisons found stress echocardiography to have incremental cost effectiveness ratios above $50,000/quality adjusted life year. One analysis found that stress echocardiography was associated with lower costs and worse outcomes. Finally, one analysis found stress echocardiography to have higher costs with equivalent outcomes, and thus was considered cost ineffective.[61]

MYOCARDIAL PERFUSION IMAGING

Myocardial perfusion imaging uses radiopharmaceutical tracers to evaluate the changes in myocardial perfusion at rest and following stress. A variety of radioactive nuclides and imaging techniques have been described. For this chapter, we will refer to the most commonly used modality, SPECT with technetium-99m-sestamibi (which has largely replaced thallium as the imaging modality of choice) synonymously with the term MPI although the latter increasingly includes cardiac magnetic resonance imaging (MRI) and traditional CT imaging as well.

Physiology

The normal response to increased oxygen demand is coronary vasodilation and increased perfusion. Healthy coronary vasculature dilates in response to stress, allowing increased perfusion of the myocardium. Diseased stenosed vessels do not responsively dilate in the same way, resulting in a state where there is increased demand but no increase in flow. Ultimately, this leads to symptoms of myocardial ischemia.[22,35]

Indications/Contraindications

Similar to stress echocardiography, there are relatively few contraindications to MPI apart from optimizing patient selection based on pretest probability.[22] Myocardial perfusion imaging does involve exposure to radioactive materials (approximately 12.0 mSv per study), and this should be kept as low as reasonably achievable in keeping with general medical practice.[21,65] Patients who have had recent prior nuclear medicine agents for tests such as ventilation perfusion scans should not receive MPI for at least 24 hours. Similar to echocardiography, obesity and specifically dense breast tissue can lead to artifact and poor visualization. Patients weighing over 400 pounds might require a 2-day protocol in which resting and stress images are obtained separately due to the safe maximum amount of radioactive tracer that can be administered in one dose.[27,66]

Protocol

Various techniques of MPI evaluate this response, aiding in diagnosis, risk stratification, and prognosis of CAD.[36] Some centers have advocated the use of resting MPI alone as a means of ACS evaluation.[67-69] This technique is useful in stable patients with ongoing symptoms. Physical exercise, or dobutamine in patients who are unable to exercise, has traditionally been used to induce increased demand and assess cardiac response to stress.[21] However, direct coronary vasodilators have produced higher quality images, and are now more often used.[36] The two most widely used agents in MPI are dipyridamole or adenosine.[34] Adenosine dilates the coronary vasculature. Dipyridamole inhibits the breakdown of adenosine, leading to the same effect.[70]

In most centers, a technetium-based agent is used to produce images for evaluation. The most commonly used radiopharmaceuticals are sestamibi and tetrofosmin, which are deposited into mitochondria following uptake by cells. Following stress, the radiopharmaceutical of choice is injected intravenously. Myocardial perfusion imaging uses a rest isotope and a stress isotope. At rest, 13.2 mCi of technetium-99m is administered, and 38.8 mCi is used for stress images.[38] The patient has a delay of 45–60 minutes after the isotope is given before images are obtained. The patient is allowed to eat at this point to increase splanchnic blood flow, and the images are obtained about 45–60 minutes after the isotope is injected.[22,37,70]

For scanning, the patient is placed supine with both arms over the head. Multiple rotating heads detect the radiopharmaceuticals to reconstruct an image for evaluation. These protocols are standardized and enable the accurate gathering of information for comparison over time.[70] Images are obtained with ECG gating using a SPECT-90 dual head camera. Analysis of perfusion is aided by software that creates a polar map representing perfusion of three dimensions of myocardium in a two-dimensional plot. In addition, a semiquantitative visual analysis is performed according to standardized methods.[71]

Data indicates that radionuclide testing is safe, with serious complications occurring in less than 0.4% of patients and death in less than 0.05% of patients.[72]

Interpretation

With both exercise and stress perfusion imaging, symptoms, vital sign changes, arrhythmia occurrence, and ECG responses are reported.[37,38] The report will include the type of agent, if used, and if exercise was included.[73] The perfusion images will be examined for the presence of transient ischemic dilation, reversible elevated right ventricular lung tracer uptake, difference in calculated left ventricular ejection fraction between stress and rest (if done), and the patterns of myocardial perfusion. If there is excess extracardiac tracer, it will be described.[73]

In a patient without coronary disease, the images will show homogenous uptake of the tracer throughout the myocardium.[36] Disease is detected when there are differences in the uptake of the tracer at rest versus during stress. A 17-segment division of the image is used to describe location of abnormal uptake using semiquantitative terms.[74] Standardization of this reporting scheme allows physicians to compare disease states over time.[73,75]

Evidence for Clinical Application

Multiple individual studies[76-81] and reviews[21,36,38,82,83] have demonstrated increased prognostic value of MPI over and above clinical and exercise data. For example, the combined annual cardiac death/MI rate was 0.85% in the normal or low-risk MPI versus 5.9% for patients with intermediate to high-risk study.[80] One review found that having greater than or equal to 10% ischemic myocardium on stress nuclear imaging was associated with a median rate of CAD-related death or MI of 4.9%/year.[75] Conversely two reviews found that the annual cardiac event rate for patients with normal or low-risk SPECT studies was 0.6%.[84,85]

In 2010, the Ontario Health Technology Advisory Committee completed a literature review similar to the one performed for stress echocardiography.[36] The pooled estimates of sensitivity and specificity of SPECT for CAD from these studies were 87% and 70% (81% for studies using attenuation correction of images), respectively. The diagnostics odds ratio (likelihood ratio + / likelihood ratio–) was 15.48 (27.01 for studies with attenuation correction). There were no significant differences found between tracer agents or stressor modality.[36]

In studies of direct comparison of SPECT to stress echocardiography, the committee found that SPECT had a modestly higher sensitivity (89% vs. 78%) but lower specificity (70% vs. 88%), respectively. It appears that SPECT is likely less cost-effective than stress echocardiography, with six of eight direct economic comparisons showing that SPECT was either dominated (associated with more cost and worse outcomes) or had incremental cost per quality-adjusted life year of greater than $50,000. In one analysis comparing SPECT to cardiac MRI, however, SPECT dominated.

STRESS TEST SELECTION

Choice of specific modality of stress test should be determined by a number of factors, including patient and institution-specific features. In practice, selection is often driven by local standards, resources and preference. Although institutional resources may limit choices, it is incumbent on clinicians to understand the limitations and strengths of particular modalities in order to optimize decision-making. The following reflects the approach taken by the Duke University Hospital, cardiology, and nuclear cardiology divisions.

When a patient is considered for a stress test, the first question is to discern if the patient can exercise to a satisfactory workload. Often patients who cannot exercise can be identified through common sense and simply asking the patient their own assessment of their ability to exercise. Generally speaking, exercise should be included when possible because of the additional prognostic information provided.[21,86] Additionally, the conditions given in box 7 should be assessed.

BOX 7 History for stress test selection

- Left bundle branch block
- Ventricular pacing
- Ventricular pre-excitation
- Less than 1 mm resting ST-T abnormalities
- Left ventricular hypertrophy
- Taking digoxin
- Prior revascularization
- Ischemia localization

If none of the conditions given in box 7 are present, an exercise ECG may be suitable at some sites. If any are present, stress imaging should be performed. At our institution (Duke University Hospital), the preferred modality, if there are no contraindications, is exercise echocardiography. This is due to technical experience, lack of radiation and evidence of modestly higher specificity.[82,87] If the patient has an LBBB, has known extensive echocardiographic wall motion abnormalities at rest, or is ventricular paced, then a vasodilator stress SPECT can be performed unless they have a contraindication to vasodilator agents (see Table 1). If so, then a dobutamine SPECT or positron emission tomography (PET) can be done. For patients who cannot have stress echocardiogram or SPECT, have prior equivocal stress test results, or have known coronary disease of uncertain significance, cardiac MRI (discussed in another chapter) is also an option.

CONTROVERSIES

Utility of Stress Testing/Overutilization

The utility of stress testing has been called into question. One of the original applications for stress testing was for risk stratification after a myocardial infarction to evaluate patients who would be candidates for coronary artery bypass graft.[88] These patients had known CAD, and underwent stress testing as a means to determine which of those patients had left main disease or diffuse three-vessel disease. The utility has subsequently been applied to patients in whom the burden of CAD is unknown.

Missed myocardial infarction has been cited as the largest source of malpractice payouts for emergency medicine providers, albeit citing pretroponin era data.[89] There is oftentimes an undercurrent of a "can't miss" philosophy to work up of patients presenting with suspicion of ACS.[90] This is due at least in part to overestimation of risk by both physicians and patients.[91] This has led some to argue that there is vast overuse of stress testing.[92,93] In one study, up to 15% to 20% of stress tests that were ordered did not meet appropriate use guidelines.[94] A large review of Medicare beneficiaries found a three-fold increase in the amount of stress testing performed from 1993 to 2001. There was a doubling of coronary angioplasty performed, and a seven fold increase in the use of coronary stenting. In spite of this marked increase in testing and subsequent interventions, the rate of hospitalization from MI did not change over the course of the time period.[95] One study found no change in rates of subsequent admission and 30-day outcomes among patients with prior normal stress testing.[96] Some have argued that the risks of harm from stress testing low-risk chest pain patients actually outweigh any benefits.[93,97-99]

Recent studies suggest limited morbidity or mortality benefit from routine stress testing in low-risk patients. They hypothesize that a cohort of very low-risk patients that can forego or delay stress testing can be identified.[92,97,98,100-102] There have been multiple attempts to derive accelerated diagnostic protocols for direct ED discharge without stress testing with varied success. One of the more widely publicized rules came from the ADAPT trial.[103] This study utilized the TIMI score, the patient's ECG, and two sets of troponins 2 hours apart. Using this workup, the investigators found that the very low-risk cohort had only a 0.25% rate of major adverse cardiac events (death, myocardial infarction, revascularization) at 30 days. Other recent accelerated diagnostic protocols include the Vancouver Chest Pain Rule[18] and North American Rule.[104] Others have likewise found low utility of stress testing patients under the age of 40 years in general.[102,105]

Timing

The optimal timing for performing a stress test is also controversial. The AHA 2010 low-risk chest pain guidelines recommend stress testing be performed within 72 hours of presentation, with 24 hours preferable.[3] In many ED populations, the risk of noncompliance, lack of insurance, or logistical issues dictates that the stress tests be performed during the initial visit. It is safe and reasonable, however, to discharge a low-risk patient with negative biomarkers and a reassuring ECG for outpatient stress test. In a prospective study of 979 patients who met low-risk chest pain criteria and underwent outpatient exercise treadmill testing, there were three (0.3%) nonfatal myocardial infarctions, and no deaths in the follow-up period.[106] Other studies have found similar low rates of adverse events.[107,108]

Nondiagnostic Studies

Another area of uncertainty is the appropriate management of patients with nondiagnostic stress results. Patients may fail to attain adequate target heart rate, or may have artifact, limiting interpretation of imaging. There is a dearth of literature on the subject, although many studies considered nondiagnostic studies in the same category as normal.[36] One abstract found that patients with nondiagnostic stress tests had a significantly higher 30-day risk compared to those with negative tests but in a small sample size (n = 17 patients with indeterminate studies).[109] It is important to recall that inability to attain target heart rate is of itself associated with worse prognosis,[42-44] however, the prognosis for other reasons for nondiagnostic studies is unclear.

Warranty

Many studies have defined the prognostic value of a normal stress test.[72,80,83,85] However, these studies do not directly address the clinical question of how long after a normal stress test a symptomatic patient should be considered low risk. The ACC 2012 guidelines suggest that patients who have "new or worsening symptoms" and prior abnormal stress test, or patients with "equivocal, borderline, or discordant stress testing where obstructive CAD remains a concern" should be retested. It provides an "uncertain" rating of appropriateness for repeat testing after 2 years in patients who have high coronary heart disease (CHD) risk and are asymptomatic or have stable symptoms and prior normal tests.[56] They do not address management of patients with new or worsening symptoms and a prior normal stress test. One study found that in patients with negative stress test within 2 years who presented to the ED with chest pain, only 7% had a 30-day risk for an adverse cardiac event.[110] On the other hand, patients have had ACS in the minutes after a normal stress test.[111]

A large systemic review and meta-analysis performed in 2007 found that in patients who had a normal exercise echocardiogram performed, there was a 1.6% risk of MI or cardiac death in the following 33 months.[112] The same study found that in patients who had a normal exercise nuclear stress test, the risk of myocardial infarction or death from MI at 36 months was 1.2%.[112] In a study evaluating adenosine stress testing, they found an event rate of MI or cardiac death of 1.5% in year one and 1.6% in year two.[113] Thus, a normal stress test in the prior year lowers the pretest probability for ACS, but it does not eliminate the risk entirely.

REFERENCES

1. Bhuiya FA, Pitts SR, McCaig LF. Emergency department visits for chest pain and abdominal pain: United States, 1999-2008. NCHS Data Brief. 2010;(43):1-8.
2. Go AS, Mozaffarian D, Roger VL, Benjamin EJ, Berry JD, Blaha MJ, et al. Executive summary: heart disease and stroke statistics--2014 update: a report from the American Heart Association. Circulation. 2014;129(3):399-410.
3. Amsterdam EA, Kirk JD, Bluemke DA, Diercks D, Farkouh ME, Garvey JL, et al. Testing of low-risk patients presenting to the emergency department with chest pain: a scientific statement from the American Heart Association. Circulation. 2010;122(17):1756-76.
4. Pryor DB, Shaw L, McCants CB, Lee KL, Mark DB, Harrell FE, et al. Value of the history and physical in identifying patients at increased risk for coronary artery disease. Ann Intern Med. 1993;118(2):81-90..
5. Swap CJ, Nagurney JT. Value and limitations of chest pain history in the evaluation of patients with suspected acute coronary syndromes. JAMA. 2005;294(20):2623-9.
6. Zalenski RJ, Cooke D, Rydman R, Sloan EP, Murphy DG. Assessing the diagnostic value of an ECG containing leads V4R, V8, and V9: the 15-lead ECG. Ann Emerg Med. 1993;22(5):786-93.
7. Zalenski RJ, Sloan EP, Chen EH, Hayden RF, Gold IW, Cooke D. The emergency department ECG and immediately life-threatening complications in initially uncomplicated suspected myocardial ischemia. Ann Emerg Med. 1988;17(3):221-6.
8. Lee TH, Goldman L. Evaluation of the patient with acute chest pain. N Engl J Med. 2000;342(16):1187-95.
9. Zalenski RJ, Shamsa F, Pede KJ. Evaluation and risk stratification of patients with chest pain in the emergency department. Predictors of life-threatening events. Emerg Med Clin North Am. 1998;16(3):495-517, vii.

10. Goodacre S, Locker T, Morris F, Campbell S. How useful are clinical features in the diagnosis of acute, undifferentiated chest pain? Acad Emerg Med. 2002;9(3):203-8.
11. Fesmire FM. Improved identification of acute coronary syndromes with delta cardiac serum marker measurements during the emergency department evaluation of chest pain patients. Cardiovasc Toxicol. 2001;1(2):117-23.
12. Hamm CW. Troponin T: a new marker for myocardial cell injury. Ann Med. 1994;26(5):319-20.
13. Morrow DA, Cannon CP, Jesse RL, Newby LK, Ravkilde J, Storrow AB, et al. National Academy of Clinical Biochemistry Laboratory Medicine Practice Guidelines: Clinical characteristics and utilization of biochemical markers in acute coronary syndromes. Circulation. 2007;115(13):e356-75.
14. Limkakeng A, Gibler WB, Pollack C, Hoekstra JW, Sites F, Shofer FS, et al. Combination of Goldman risk and initial cardiac troponin I for emergency department chest pain patient risk stratification. Acad Emerg Med. 2001;8(7): 696-702.
15. Sicari R, Nihoyannopoulos P, Evangelista A, Kasprzak J, Lancellotti P, Poldermans D, et al. Stress Echocardiography Expert Consensus Statement--Executive Summary: European Association of Echocardiography (EAE) (a registered branch of the ESC). Eur Heart J. 2009;30(3):278-89.
16. Wright RS, Anderson JL, Adams CD, Bridges CR, Casey DE, Ettinger SM, et al. 2011 ACCF/AHA focused update incorporated into the ACC/AHA 2007 Guidelines for the Management of Patients with Unstable Angina/Non-ST-Elevation Myocardial Infarction: a report of the American College of Cardiology Foundation/American Heart Association Task Force on Practice Guidelines developed in collaboration with the American Academy of Family Physicians, Society for Cardiovascular Angiography and Interventions, and the Society of Thoracic Surgeons. J Am Coll Cardiol. 2011;57(19):e215-367.
17. Chase M, Robey JL, Zogby KE, Sease KL, Shofer FS, Hollander JE. Prospective Validation of the Thrombolysis in Myocardial Infarction Risk Score in the Emergency Department Chest Pain Population. Ann Emerg Med. 2006; 48(3):252-9.
18. Christenson J, Innes G, McKnight D, Thompson CR, Wong H, Yu E, et al. A clinical prediction rule for early discharge of patients with chest pain. Ann Emerg Med. 2006;47(1):1-10.
19. Fesmire FM. A rapid protocol to identify and exclude acute myocardial infarction: continuous 12-lead ECG monitoring with 2-hour delta CK-MB. Am J Emerg Med. 2000;18(6):698-702.
20. Gibbons RJ, Balady GJ, Bricker JT, Chaitman BR, Fletcher GF, Froelicher VF, et al. ACC/AHA 2002 guideline update for exercise testing: summary article. A report of the American College of Cardiology/American Heart Association Task Force on Practice Guidelines (Committee to Update the 1997 Exercise Testing Guidelines). J Am Coll Cardiol. 2002;40(8):1531-40.
21. Fihn SD, Gardin JM, Abrams J, Berra K, Blankenship JC, Dallas AP, et al. 2012 ACCF/AHA/ACP/AATS/PCNA/SCAI/STS Guideline for the diagnosis and management of patients with stable ischemic heart disease: a report of the American College of Cardiology Foundation/American Heart Association Task Force on Practice Guidelines, and the American College of Physicians, American Association for Thoracic Surgery, Preventive Cardiovascular Nurses Association, Society for Cardiovascular Angiography and Interventions, and Society of Thoracic Surgeons. J Am Coll Cardiol. 2012;60(24):e44-e164.
22. Hendel RC, Berman DS, Di Carli MF, Heidenreich PA, Henkin RE, Pellikka PA, et al. ACCF/ASNC/ACR/AHA/ASE/SCCT/SCMR/SNM 2009 Appropriate Use Criteria for Cardiac Radionuclide Imaging: A Report of the American College of Cardiology Foundation Appropriate Use Criteria Task Force, the American Society of Nuclear Cardiology, the American College of Radiology, the American Heart Association, the American Society of Echocardiography, the Society of Cardiovascular Computed Tomography, the Society for Cardiovascular Magnetic Resonance, and the Society of Nuclear Medicine. J Am Coll Cardiol. 2009;53(23):2201-29.
23. American College of Cardiology Foundation Appropriate Use Criteria Task Force, American Society of Echocardiography, American Heart Association, American Society of Nuclear Cardiology, Heart Failure Society of America, Heart Rhythm Society, et al. ACCF/ASE/AHA/ASNC/HFSA/HRS/SCAI/SCCM/SCCT/SCMR 2011 Appropriate Use Criteria for Echocardiography. A Report of the American College of Cardiology Foundation Appropriate Use Criteria Task Force, American Society of Echocardiography, American Heart Association, American Society of Nuclear Cardiology, Heart Failure Society of America, Heart Rhythm Society, Society for Cardiovascular Angiography and Interventions, Society of Critical Care Medicine, Society of Cardiovascular Computed Tomography, Society for Cardiovascular Magnetic Resonance American College of Chest Physicians. J Am Soc Echocardiogr. 2011;24(3):229-67.
24. Anderson RT, Montori VM, Shah ND, Ting HH, Pencille LJ, Demers M, et al. Effectiveness of the Chest Pain Choice decision aid in emergency department patients with low-risk chest pain: study protocol for a multicenter randomized trial. Trials. 2014;15:166.
25. Hess EP, Coylewright M, Frosch DL, Shah ND. Implementation of shared decision making in cardiovascular care: past, present, and future. Circ Cardiovasc Qual Outcomes. 2014;7(5):797-803.
26. Best PJ, Tajik AJ, Gibbons RJ, Pellikka PA. The safety of treadmill exercise stress testing in patients with abdominal aortic aneurysms. Ann Intern Med. 1998;129(8):628-31.
27. Patel RN, Arteaga RB, Mandawat MK, Thornton JW, Robinson VJ. Pharmacologic stress myocardial perfusion imaging. South Med J. 2007;100(10):1006-14; quiz 1004.
28. Bruce RA, Blackmon JR, Jones JW, Strait G. Exercising testing in adult normal subjects and cardiac patients. Pediatrics. 1963;32:SUPPL 742-56.
29. Akinpelu D, Gonzalez, JM. (2015). Treadmill stress testing technique. [online] Available from: http://emedicine.medscape.com/article/1827089-overview. [Accessed March, 2016].
30. Naughton J, Balke B, Nagle F. Refinements in method of evaluation and physical conditiong before and after myocardial infarction. Am J Cardiol. 1964;14:837-43.
31. Shah BN. On the 50th anniversary of the first description of a multistage exercise treadmill test: re-visiting the birth of the 'Bruce protocol'. Heart. 2013;99(24):1793-4.
32. Tanaka H, Monahan KD, Seals DR. Age-predicted maximal heart rate revisited. J Am Coll Cardiol. 2001;37(1):153-6.
33. Hlatky MA, Pryor DB, Harrell FE, Califf RM, Mark DB, Rosati RA. Factors affecting sensitivity and specificity of exercise electrocardiography. Multivariable analysis. Am J Med. 1984;77(1):64-71.
34. Zoghbi GJ, Iskandrian AE. Selective adenosine agonists and myocardial perfusion imaging. J Nucl Cardiol. 2012;19(1):126-41.
35. Underwood SR, Anagnostopoulos C, Cerqueira M, Ell PJ, Flint EJ, Harbinson M, et al. Myocardial perfusion scintigraphy: the evidence. Eur J Nucl Med Mol Imaging. 2004;31(2):261-91.
36. Health Quality Ontario. Single photon emission computed tomography for the diagnosis of coronary artery disease: an evidence-based analysis. On Health Technol Assess Ser. 2010;10(8):1-64.
37. Miyamoto MI, Vernotico SL, Majmundar H, Thomas GS. Pharmacologic stress myocardial perfusion imaging: a practical approach. J Nucl Cardiol. 2007;14(2):250-5.
38. Ficaro EP. Imaging guidelines for nuclear cardiology procedures. J Nucl Cardiol. 2006;13(6):888.
39. Thomas GS, Prill NV, Majmundar H, Fabrizi RR, Thomas JJ, Hayashida C, et al. Treadmill exercise during adenosine infusion is safe, results in fewer adverse reactions, and improves myocardial perfusion image quality. J Nucl Cardiol. 2000;7(5):439-46.
40. Iskandrian AE, Bateman TM, Belardinelli L, Blackburn B, Cerqueira MD, Hendel RC, et al. Adenosine versus regadenoson comparative evaluation in myocardial perfusion imaging: results of the ADVANCE phase 3 multicenter international trial. J Nucl Cardiol. 2007;14(5):645-58.
41. Chandra A, Rudraiah L, Zalenski RJ. Stress testing for risk stratification of patients with low to moderate probability of acute cardiac ischemia. Emerg Med Clin North Am. 2001;19(1):87-103.
42. Lauer MS, Francis GS, Okin PM, Pashkow FJ, Snader CE, Marwick TH. Impaired chronotropic response to exercise stress testing as a predictor of mortality. JAMA. 1999;281(6):524-9.
43. Lauer MS, Okin PM, Larson MG, Evans JC, Levy D. Impaired heart rate response to graded exercise. Prognostic implications of chronotropic incompetence in the Framingham Heart Study. Circulation. 1996;93(8):1520-6.
44. Wiens RD, Lafia P, Marder CM, Evans RG, Kennedy HL. Chronotropic incompetence in clinical exercise testing. Am J Cardiol. 1984;54(1):74-8.
45. Mark DB. An overview of risk assessment in coronary artery disease. Am J Cardiol. 1994;73(6):19B-25B.
46. Mark DB, Hlatky MA, Harrell FE, Lee KL, Califf RM, Pryor DB. Exercise Treadmill Score for Predicting Prognosis in Coronary Artery Disease. Ann Intern Med. 1987;106(6):793-800.
47. Kwok JM, Miller TD, Christian TF, Hodge DO, Gibbons RJ. Prognostic value of a treadmill exercise score in symptomatic patients with nonspecific ST-T abnormalities on resting ECG. JAMA. 1999;282(11):1047-53.

48. Mikhail MG, Smith FA, Gray M, Britton C, Frederiksen SM. Cost-effectiveness of mandatory stress testing in chest pain center patients. Ann Emerg Med. 1997;29(1):88-98.
49. Polanczyk CA, Johnson PA, Hartley LH, Walls RM, Shaykevich S, Lee TH. Clinical correlates and prognostic significance of early negative exercise tolerance test in patients with acute chest pain seen in the hospital emergency department. Am J Cardiol. 1998;81(3):288-92.
50. Zalenski RJ, McCarren M, Roberts R, Rydman RJ, Jovanovic B, Das K, et al. An evaluation of a chest pain diagnostic protocol to exclude acute cardiac ischemia in the emergency department. Arch Intern Med. 1997;157(10):1085-91.
51. Amsterdam EA, Kirk JD, Diercks DB, Lewis WR, Turnipseed SD. Immediate exercise testing to evaluate low-risk patients presenting to the emergency department with chest pain. J Am Coll Cardiol. 2002;40(2):251-6.
52. Diercks DB, Kirk JD, Turnipseed SD, Amsterdam EA. Utility of immediate exercise treadmill testing in patients taking beta blockers or calcium channel blockers. Am J Cardiol. 2002;90(8):882-5.
53. Kirk JD, Turnipseed S, Lewis WR, Amsterdam EA. Evaluation of chest pain in low-risk patients presenting to the emergency department: the role of immediate exercise testing. Ann Emerg Med. 1998;32(1):1-7.
54. Lewis WR, Amsterdam EA, Turnipseed S, Kirk JD. Immediate exercise testing of low risk patients with known coronary artery disease presenting to the emergency department with chest pain. J Am Coll Cardiol. 1999;33(7):1843-7.
55. Tennant R, Wiggers C. The effects of coronary occlusion on myocardial contraction. Am J Physiol. 1935;112:351-61.
56. Douglas PS, Khandheria B, Stainback RF, Weissman NJ, Peterson ED, Hendel RC, et al. ACCF/ASE/ACEP/AHA/ASNC/SCAI/SCCT/SCMR 2008 appropriateness criteria for stress echocardiography: a report of the American College of Cardiology Foundation Appropriateness Criteria Task Force, American Society of Echocardiography, American College of Emergency Physicians, American Heart Association, American Society of Nuclear Cardiology, Society for Cardiovascular Angiography and Interventions, Society of Cardiovascular Computed Tomography, and Society for Cardiovascular Magnetic Resonance endorsed by the Heart Rhythm Society and the Society of Critical Care Medicine. J Am Coll Cardiol. 2008;51(11):1127-47.
57. Biagini E, Shaw LJ, Poldermans D, Schinkel AF, Rizzello V, Elhendy A, et al. Accuracy of non-invasive techniques for diagnosis of coronary artery disease and prediction of cardiac events in patients with left bundle branch block: a meta-analysis. Eur J Nucl Med Mol Imaging. 2006;33(12):1442-51.
58. Solimene MC. Coronary heart disease in women: a challenge for the 21st century. Clinics (Sao Paulo). 2010;65(1):99-106.
59. Geleijnse ML, Krenning BJ, Soliman OI, Nemes A, Galema TW, ten Cate FJ. Dobutamine stress echocardiography for the detection of coronary artery disease in women. Am J Cardiol. 2007;99(5):714-7.
60. Kamaran M, Teague SM, Finkelhor RS, Dawson N, Bahler RC. Prognostic value of dobutamine stress echocardiography in patients referred because of suspected coronary artery disease. Am J Cardiol. 1995;76(12):887-91.
61. Health Quality Ontario. Stress echocardiography for the diagnosis of coronary artery disease: an evidence-based analysis. Ont Health Technol Assess Ser. 2010;10(9):1-61.
62. Peteiro J, Bouzas-Mosquera A. Exercise echocardiography. World J Cardiol. 2010;2(8):223-32.
63. McCully RB, Roger VL, Mahoney DW, Karon BL, Oh JK, Miller FA, et al. Outcome after normal exercise echocardiography and predictors of subsequent cardiac events: follow-up of 1,325 patients. J Am Coll Cardiol. 1998;31(1):144-9.
64. Arruda AL, Barretto RB, Shub C, Chandrasekaran K, Pellikka PA. Prognostic significance of ST-segment elevation during dobutamine stress echocardiography. Am Heart J. 2006;151(3):744.e1-.e6.
65. Cardiovascular Council Board of Directors. Cardiovascular nuclear imaging: balancing proven clinical value and potential radiation risk. J Nucl Med. 2011;52(7):1162-4.
66. Borges-Neto S, Coleman RE, Jones RH. Perfusion and function at rest and treadmill exercise using technetium-99m-sestamibi: comparison of one- and two-day protocols in normal volunteers. J Nucl Med. 1990;31(7):1128-32.
67. Fesmire FM, Hughes AD, Stout PK, Wojcik JF, Wharton DR. Selective dual nuclear scanning in low-risk patients with chest pain to reliably identify and exclude acute coronary syndromes. Ann Emerg Med. 2001;38(3):207-15.
68. Fesmire FM, Hughes AD, Fody EP, Jackson AP, Fesmire CE, Gilbert MA, et al. The Erlanger chest pain evaluation protocol: a one-year experience with serial 12-lead ECG monitoring, two-hour delta serum marker measurements, and selective nuclear stress testing to identify and exclude acute coronary syndromes. Ann Emerg Med. 2002;40(6):584-94.
69. Barbirato GB, Azevedo JC, Felix RC, Correa PL, Volschan A, Viegas M, et al. Use of resting myocardial scintigraphy during chest pain to exclude diagnosis of acute myocardial infarction. Arq Bras Cardiol. 2009;92(4):269-74.
70. Notghi A, Low CS. Myocardial perfusion scintigraphy: past, present and future. Br J Radiol. 2011;84 Spec No 3:S229-36.
71. Dorbala S, Blankstein R, Skali H, Park MA, Fantony J, Mauceri C, et al. Approaches to reducing radiation dose from radionuclide myocardial perfusion imaging. J Nucl Med. 2015;56(4):592-9..
72. Fraker TD, Fihn SD, 2002 Chronic Stable Angina Writing Committee, American College of Cardiology, American Heart Association, Gibbons RJ, et al. 2007 chronic angina focused update of the ACC/AHA 2002 guidelines for the management of patients with chronic stable angina: a report of the American College of Cardiology/American Heart Association Task Force on Practice Guidelines Writing Group to develop the focused update of the 2002 guidelines for the management of patients with chronic stable angina. J Am Coll Cardiol. 2007;50(23):2264-74.
73. Douglas P, Iskandrian AE, Krumholz HM, Gillam L, Hendel R, Jollis J, et al. Achieving quality in cardiovascular imaging: Proceedings from the American College of Cardiology–Duke University Medical Center Think Tank on Quality in Cardiovascular Imaging. J Am Coll Cardiol. 2006;48(10):2141-51.
74. Salerno M, Elliot L, Shaw LK, Piccini JP, Pagnanelli R, Borges-Neto S. Prognostic validation of an algorithm to convert myocardial perfusion SPECT imaging data from a 12-segment model to a 17-segment model. J Nucl Cardiol. 2009;16(4):605-13.
75. Shaw LJ, Berman DS, Picard MH, Friedrich MG, Kwong RY, Stone GW, et al. Comparative definitions for moderate-severe ischemia in stress nuclear, echocardiography, and magnetic resonance imaging. JACC Cardiovasc Imaging. 2014;7(6):593-604.
76. Borges-Neto S, Shaw LK, Tuttle RH, Alexander JH, Smith WT, Chambless M, et al. Incremental prognostic power of single-photon emission computed tomographic myocardial perfusion imaging in patients with known or suspected coronary artery disease. Am J Cardiol. 2005;95(2):182-8.
77. Liao L, Smith WT, Tuttle RH, Shaw LK, Coleman RE, Borges-Neto S. Prediction of death and nonfatal myocardial infarction in high-risk patients: a comparison between the Duke treadmill score, peak exercise radionuclide angiography, and SPECT perfusion imaging. J Nucl Med. 2005;46(1):5-11.
78. Piccini JP, Horton JR, Shaw LK, Al-Khatib SM, Lee KL, Iskandrian AE, et al. Single-photon emission computed tomography myocardial perfusion defects are associated with an increased risk of all-cause death, cardiovascular death, and sudden cardiac death. Circ Cardiovasc Imaging. 2008;1(3):180-8.
79. Shaw LJ, Berman DS, Hendel RC, Alazraki N, Krawczynska E, Borges-Neto S, et al. Cardiovascular disease risk stratification with stress single-photon emission computed tomography technetium-99m tetrofosmin imaging in patients with the metabolic syndrome and diabetes mellitus. Am J Cardiol. 2006;97(10):1538-44.
80. Shaw LJ, Hendel R, Borges-Neto S, Lauer MS, Alazraki N, Burnette J, et al. Prognostic value of normal exercise and adenosine (99m)Tc-tetrofosmin SPECT imaging: results from the multicenter registry of 4,728 patients. J Nucl Med. 2003;44(2):134-9.
81. Shaw LJ, Hendel RC, Heller GV, Borges-Neto S, Cerqueira M, Berman DS. Prognostic estimation of coronary artery disease risk with resting perfusion abnormalities and stress ischemia on myocardial perfusion SPECT. J Nucl Cardiol. 2008;15(6):762-73.
82. Fleischmann KE, Hunink MG, Kuntz KM, Douglas PS. Exercise echocardiography or exercise SPECT imaging? A meta-analysis of diagnostic test performance. JAMA. 1998;280(10):913-20.
83. Mowatt G, Vale L, Brazzelli M, Hernandez R, Murray A, Scott N, et al. Systematic review of the effectiveness and cost-effectiveness, and economic evaluation, of myocardial perfusion scintigraphy for the diagnosis and management of angina and myocardial infarction. Health Technol Assess. 2004;8(30):iii-iv, 1-207.
84. Iskander S, Iskandrian AE. Risk assessment using single-photon emission computed tomographic technetium-99m sestamibi imaging. J Am Coll Cardiol. 1998;32(1):57-62.
85. Shaw LJ, Iskandrian AE. Prognostic value of gated myocardial perfusion SPECT. J Nucl Cardiol. 2004;11(2):171-85.
86. Myers J, Prakash M, Froelicher V, Do D, Partington S, Atwood JE. Exercise capacity and mortality among men referred for exercise testing. N Engl J Med. 2002;346(11):793-801.

87. Conti A, Sammicheli L, Gallini C, Costanzo EN, Antoniucci D, Barletta G. Assessment of patients with low-risk chest pain in the emergency department: Head-to-head comparison of exercise stress echocardiography and exercise myocardial SPECT. Am Heart J. 2005;149(5):894-901.
88. Fuller CM, Raizner AE, Verani MS, Nahormek PA, Chahine RA, McEntee CW, et al. Early post-myocardial infarction treadmill stress testing. An accurate predictor of multivessel coronary disease and subsequent cardiac events. Ann Intern Med. 1981;94(6):734-9.
89. Rusnak RA, Stair TO, Hansen K, Fastow JS. Litigation against the emergency physician: common features in cases of missed myocardial infarction. Ann Emerg Med. 1989;18(10):1029-34.
90. Pines JM, Isserman JA, Szyld D, Dean AJ, McCusker CM, Hollander JE. The effect of physician risk tolerance and the presence of an observation unit on decision making for ED patients with chest pain. Am J Emerg Med. 2010;28(7):771-9.
91. Newman DH, Ackerman B, Kraushar ML, Lederhandler MH, Masri A, Starikov A, et al. Quantifying Patient-Physician Communication and Perceptions of Risk During Admissions for Possible Acute Coronary Syndromes. Ann Emerg Med. 2015;66(1):13-8, 18.e1.
92. Napoli AM, Arrighi JA, Siket MS, Gibbs FJ. Physician discretion is safe and may lower stress test utilization in emergency department chest pain unit patients. Crit Pathw Cardiol. 2012;11(1):26-31.
93. Prasad V, Cheung M, Cifu A. Chest pain in the emergency department: the case against our current practice of routine noninvasive testing. Arch Intern Med. 2012;172(19):1506-9.
94. Johnson TV, Rose GA, Fenner DJ, Rozario NL. Improving appropriate use of echocardiography and single-photon emission computed tomographic myocardial perfusion imaging: a continuous quality improvement initiative. J Am Soc Echocardiogr. 2014;27(7):749-57.
95. Lucas FL, DeLorenzo MA, Siewers AE, Wennberg DE. Temporal trends in the utilization of diagnostic testing and treatments for cardiovascular disease in the United States, 1993-2001. Circulation. 2006;113(3):374-9.
96. Nerenberg RH, Shofer FS, Robey JL, Brown AM, Hollander JE. Impact of a negative prior stress test on emergency physician disposition decision in ED patients with chest pain syndromes. Am J Emerg Med. 2007;25(1):39-44.
97. Foy AJ, Liu G, Davidson WR, Sciamanna C, Leslie DL. Comparative effectiveness of diagnostic testing strategies in emergency department patients with chest pain: an analysis of downstream testing, interventions, and outcomes. JAMA Intern Med. 2015;175(3):428-36.
98. Hermann LK, Newman DH, Pleasant WA, Rojanasarntikul D, Lakoff D, Goldberg SA, et al. Yield of routine provocative cardiac testing among patients in an emergency department-based chest pain unit. JAMA Intern Med. 2013;173(12):1128-33.
99. Hermann LK, Weingart SD, Duvall WL, Henzlova MJ. The limited utility of routine cardiac stress testing in emergency department chest pain patients younger than 40 years. Ann Emerg Med. 2009;54(1):12-6.
100. Napoli AM. The association between pretest probability of coronary artery disease and stress test utilization and outcomes in a chest pain observation unit. Acad Emerg Med. 2014;21(4):401-7.
101. Napoli AM, Tran S, Wang J. Low-risk chest pain patients younger than 40 years do not benefit from admission and stress testing. Crit Pathw Cardiol. 2013;12(4):201-3.
102. Ely S, Chandra A, Mani G, Drake W, Freeman D, Limkakeng AT. Utility of observation units for young emergency department chest pain patients. J Emerg Med. 2013;44(2):306-12.
103. Than M, Cullen L, Aldous S, Parsonage WA, Reid CM, Greenslade J, et al. 2-Hour accelerated diagnostic protocol to assess patients with chest pain symptoms using contemporary troponins as the only biomarker: the ADAPT trial. J Am Coll Cardiol. 2012;59(23):2091-8.
104. Hess EP, Brison RJ, Perry JJ, Calder LA, Thiruganasambandamoorthy V, Agarwal D, et al. Development of a clinical prediction rule for 30-day cardiac events in emergency department patients with chest pain and possible acute coronary syndrome. Ann Emerg Med. 2012;59(2):115-25.e1.
105. Hermann LK, Weingart SD, Yoon YM, Genes NG, Nelson BP, Shearer PL, et al. Comparison of frequency of inducible myocardial ischemia in patients presenting to emergency department with typical versus atypical or nonanginal chest pain. Am J Cardiol. 2010;105(11):1561-4.
106. Meyer MC, Mooney RP, Sekera AK. A critical pathway for patients with acute chest pain and low risk for short-term adverse cardiac events: role of outpatient stress testing. Ann Emerg Med. 2006;47(5):427-35.
107. Lai C, Noeller TP, Schmidt K, King P, Emerman CL. Short-term risk after initial observation for chest pain. J Emerg Med. 2003;25(4):357-62.
108. Manini AF, Gisondi MA, van der Vlugt TM, Schreiber DH. Adverse cardiac events in emergency department patients with chest pain six months after a negative inpatient evaluation for acute coronary syndrome. Acad Emerg Med. 2002;9(9):896-902.
109. Manini A, McAfee AT, Noble VE, Nualpring S, Bohan JS. Prognostic significance of non-diagnostic stress tests from the chest pain unit. Acad Emerg Med. 2006;13(5 Suppl 1):S186.
110. Engineer RS, Lauer MS, Emerman CL. Chest pain after recent stress test: Is there a warranty? Ann Emerg Med. 2004;44(4):S47.
111. Przybojewski JZ, Thorpe L. Exercise-induced ST-segment elevation possibly caused by coronary artery spasm. A case presentation and review. S Afr Med J. 1985;68(6):419-24.
112. Metz LD, Beattie M, Hom R, Redberg RF, Grady D, Fleischmann KE. The prognostic value of normal exercise myocardial perfusion imaging and exercise echocardiography: a meta-analysis. J Am Coll Cardiol. 2007;49(2): 227-37.
113. Hachamovitch R, Hayes S, Friedman JD, Cohen I, Shaw LJ, Germano G, et al. Determinants of risk and its temporal variation in patients with normal stress myocardial perfusion scans: what is the warranty period of a normal scan? J Am Coll Cardiol. 2003;41(8):1329-40.

SECTION 3

Acute Heart Failure

16

CHAPTER

How to Use Natriuretic Peptides in the Emergency Department?

Boris Arbit, Alan S Maisel

INTRODUCTION

Acute heart failure (AHF) is the leading diagnosis among hospitalized patients in the United States.[1,2] Clinically, heart failure (HF) is a complex syndrome that results from a variety of conditions that prevent the left ventricle from properly filling and ejecting blood. Despite major advances in the therapy of HF, challenges still remain in the timely diagnosis of AHF. The development of biomarkers in AHF stemmed from the need for a fast and reliable test with high sensitivity and specificity to aide the diagnostic workup of patients with acute dyspnea. Differentiating between pulmonary and cardiac causes of acute dyspnea has traditionally been a challenge as the history, physical examination, laboratory, and radiographic findings of the two conditions often overlap. Delayed or erroneous diagnosis for AHF not only causes increased length of hospital stay and healthcare cost, but also leads to increased morbidity and mortality, making the accurate diagnosis imperative. Biomarkers provide objectivity and reproducibility, and over the last 15 years have become an indispensable tool in assisting the diagnostic workup of patients with acute dyspnea.

Among the biomarkers available today, natriuretic peptides (NPs) are the most validated and accepted in the diagnostic evaluation for AHF. The relevant biomarkers in the NP family are B-type natriuretic peptide (BNP), amino N-terminal pro-B-type natriuretic peptide (NT-proBNP), atrial natriuretic peptide (ANP), and mid-region proatrial natriuretic peptide (MR-proANP). Among the four, BNP and NT-proBNP are more validated by clinical trials and more widely used in today's clinical practice (Table 1).

Elevations of NP concentrations correlate well with elevated pulmonary capillary wedge pressure (PCWP) and increased left ventricular wall stress.[1-4] For example, in patients with severe aortic stenosis, BNP concentrations correlated very well with left ventricular wall stress both pre- and postaortic valve replacement. This correlation between NPs and PCWP is also seen in patients with HF.[5,6] This correlation between elevated NP and PCWP and left ventricular wall stress provides

TABLE 1: Characteristics of B-type natriuretic peptide and amino N-terminal prohormone B-type natriuretic peptide

	BNP	NT-proBNP
Components	BNP molecule	NT fragments (1–76) NT-proBNP (1–108)
Molecular weight	4 kDa	8.5 kDa
Genesis	Cleavage from NT-proBNP	Release from ventricular myocytes
Half-life	20 min	120 minutes
Clearance mechanism	Neutral endopeptidase clearance receptors	Renal clearance
Increase with normal aging	+	++++
Correlation with estimated glomerular filtration rate	−0.20	−0.60
Approved cutoff(s) for CHF diagnosis	100 pg/mL	Age <75: 125 pg/mL Age >75: 450 pg/mL
Studies completed	1,370	39
Entry on US market	November, 2000	December, 2002

BNP, B-type natriuretic peptide; NT-proBNP, amino N-terminal prohormone B-type natriuretic peptide; CHF, chronic heart failure.

the physiological basis for using NPs in the diagnostic evaluation of patients with AHF.

B-TYPE NATRIURETIC PEPTIDE

B-type natriuretic peptide was first isolated from the porcine brain leading to its original name "brain natriuretic peptide". It was later found to be a cardiac neurohormone secreted from the cardiac ventricles as a response to ventricular volume expansion and pressure overload.[7] Myocytes release an intracellular 108-amino acid precursor protein, which is cleaved into two fragments—a 32-amino acid protein, BNP and a 76-amino acid N-terminal fragment, NT-proBNP.[8]

The fundamental role of BNP in cardiovascular homeostasis includes increasing glomerular filtration rate (GFR), increasing sodium and water excretion, relaxing arterioles and venules, increasing diastolic relaxation, decreasing myocardial fibrosis, inhibiting cardiac hypertrophy as well as inhibiting renin and aldosterone secretion.

B-type natriuretic peptide levels have been shown to be elevated in patients with left ventricular dysfunction and correlate to New York Heart Association (NYHA) class as well as prognosis.[9,10] Unfortunately, for many years its utility as a diagnostic aid in the urgent-care setting was limited by protracted assay time. As rapid fluorescence immunoassays developed, the biomarker gained wider role in clinical practice. In the year 2000, United States Food and Drug Administration approved BNP as an adjunct to diagnose HF. Current guidelines issued by the American Heart Association/American College of Cardiology (AHA/ACC) for diagnosis of HF endorse Class I A recommendation for use of NP in diagnosis of acutely decompensated HF.[11]

The multicenter Breathing Not Properly trial demonstrated the effectiveness of BNP in the diagnostic workup of patients presenting to the emergency department (ED) with acute dyspnea.[12] In this study, 1,586 patients with acute dyspnea as their chief complaint to the ED were enrolled from seven international sites. The gold standard diagnosis of AHF was made by two cardiologists who were blinded to BNP measurements. There were 883 male and 773 female patients in this study. AHF was diagnosed in 744 patients. In patients with AHF, BNP levels were 675 ± 450 pg/mL, while patients without AHF had BNP levels of 110 ± 225 pg/mL. B-type natriuretic peptide was the single best predictor of AHF with an area under the receiver-operating characteristic curve (AUC) of 0.91 (95% confidence interval: 0.90–0.93, $p < 0.001$). A BNP cutoff of 100 pg/mL had a sensitivity of 90%, specificity of 75% and diagnostic accuracy of 83%. B-type natriuretic peptide levels less than 50 pg/mL were associated with a negative predictive value of 96%. In multiple logistic-regression analysis, BNP above a cutoff of 100 pg/mL was the strongest independent predictor of AHF with an odds ratio of 29.6.

Another pivotal trial that highlighted the role of BNP in the emergency room was the Rapid Emergency Department Heart Failure Outpatient Trial (REDHOT).[13] REDHOT was a 10-center trial in which patients seen in the ED with shortness of breath were consented to have BNP levels drawn on arrival. Entrance criteria included a BNP level more than 100 pg/mL. Physicians were blinded to the actual BNP level and subsequent BNP measurements. Patients were followed up for 90 days after discharge. Of the 464 patients who met the inclusion criteria, 90% were hospitalized. Two-thirds of patients were perceived to be NYHA functional class III or IV. The BNP levels did not differ significantly between patients who were discharged home from the ED and those admitted (976 vs. 766, $p = 0.6$). Using logistic regression analysis, authors found that an ED doctor's intention to admit or discharge a patient had no influence on 90-day outcomes, while the BNP level was a strong predictor of 90-day outcome. Of admitted patients, 11% had BNP levels less than 200 pg/mL (66% of which were perceived NYHA functional class III or IV). The 90-day combined event rate [congestive heart failure (CHF) visits or admissions and mortality] in the group of patients admitted with BNP less than 200 pg/mL and more than 200 pg/mL was 9% and 29%, respectively ($p = 0.006$). The REDHOT showed that perception of severity of CHF among ED physicians did not correlate well with BNP levels; patients sent home from the ED actually showed a trend toward higher BNP levels than did those admitted, yet BNP levels were much stronger predictors of subsequent outcome.

N-TERMINAL PRO-B-TYPE NATRIURETIC PEPTIDE

N-terminal-proBNP is also commonly used in the diagnostic evaluation of patients with AHF. NT-proBNP is a fragment of a prohormone and plays no significant physiologic role. Its clearance is mostly via the kidneys and it has a much longer circulating half-life than BNP, about 60–90 minutes. NT-proBNP concentrations are stable in blood and circulating levels are higher than those of BNP.

The effectiveness of NT-proBNP in the diagnosing patients with AHF was demonstrated by the ProBNP Investigation of Dyspnea in the Emergency Department (PRIDE) study.[14] This study included 599 patients who presented to the ED with acute dyspnea. The study design was very similar to the Breathing Not Properly trial. Among the 599 patients enrolled, 209 had a final diagnosis of AHF. Among patients with AHF, the average NT-proBNP level was 4,054 pg/mL, while the average NT-proBNP level in patients without AHF was 131 pg/mL. The AUC for

NT-proBNP for the diagnosis of AHF was 0.94 (p<0.0001). As NT-proBNP levels varied significantly based on age, different cut points were selected for patients less than 50 years old and over 50 years old. For patients less than 50 years of age, NT-proBNP cutoff of 450 pg/mL had a sensitivity of 93%, specificity of 95%, and diagnostic accuracy of 95% for AHF. For patients over 50 years of age, a NT-proBNP cutoff of 900 pg/mL had a sensitivity of 91%, specificity of 80%, and diagnostic accuracy of 85% for AHF. When the cutoff of 900 pg/mL was applied to the whole patient population, the sensitivity was 90%, specificity was 85% and diagnostic accuracy was 87%. NT-proBNP concentration less than 300 pg/mL had a sensitivity of 99% and negative predictive value of 99%. By multivariate analysis, NT-proBNP was the strongest predictor of AHF with an odds ratio of 44.0 (p <0.0001). N-terminal-proBNP was better than clinician-estimated likelihood for the diagnosis of AHF (AUC = 0.94 vs. AUC = 0.90). Adding NT-proBNP to clinician-estimated likelihood of AHF improved the AUC from 0.90 to 0.96. Among patients with the physician-estimated AHF likelihood of 0–25%, NT-proBNP by optimal cut point had a sensitivity of 96% and specificity of 88% for AHF. Among patients with physician-estimated AHF likelihood of 25–75%, NT-proBNP by optimal cut point had a sensitivity of 93% and specificity of 85% for AHF. In patients with physician-estimated AHF likelihood range of greater than 75%, the sensitivity of NT-proBNP by optimal cut point was 93% and specificity was 84% for AHF.

In a healthcare system where judicious use of resources is a major goal, inclusion of NT-proBNP testing was shown to improve the management of patients presenting to ED with dyspnea through improved diagnosis, cost savings and improvement in selected outcomes.[15] Canadian Multicenter Improved Management of Patients with Congestive Heart Failure (IMPROVE-CHF) Study prospectively compared the clinical and economic impact of a randomized management strategy either guided by NT-proBNP results or without knowledge of NT-proBNP concentrations. Five hundred patients presenting with dyspnea were studied. The median NT-proBNP level among the 230 subjects with a final diagnosis of HF was 3,697 compared with 212 pg/mL in those without HF (p <0.00001). Knowledge of NT-proBNP results reduced the duration of ED visit by 21% (6.3–5.6 h; p = 0.031), the number of patients rehospitalized over 60 days by 35% (51–33; p = 0.046), and direct medical costs of all ED visits, hospitalizations and subsequent outpatient services (US $6,129 to US $5,180 per patient; p = 0.023) over 60 days from enrollment. Adding NT-proBNP to clinical judgment enhanced the accuracy of a diagnosis; the area under the receiver-operating characteristic curve increased from 0.83–0.90 (p <0.0001). The trial was the first prospective randomized analysis to definitively address the question of the additive value of NP testing from both a diagnostic and a cost perspective in a universal healthcare system.

There is no clear superiority of BNP over NT-proBNP for the diagnosis of acute decompensated HF. Indeed, there is a good analytical agreement between BNP and NT-proBNP, but NT-proBNP circulates at higher concentrations than BNP and shows less intra-individual variability. Perhaps the reason NT-proBNP has not been adopted more widely in clinical practice is the earlier availability of BNP assays.

ATRIAL NATRIURETIC PEPTIDE AND MID-REGION PROATRIAL NATRIURETIC PEPTIDE

Atrial natriuretic peptide is a 28-amino acid peptide hormone first isolated from the atrial tissue of rats. Atrial natriuretic peptide is produced in the atria and is a product of the 126-amino acid precursor prohormone ANP (proANP).[16] This prohormone is cleaved into ANP and MR-proANP. The circulating half-life of ANP is 3–5 minutes, while MR-proANP is much more stable and has a considerably longer half-life (up to 50 min).

Although elevations of both BNP and ANP have been associated with AHF, ANP was inferior to BNP in head-to-head studies. For example, in one study by Cowie et al. the AUC of AHF was 0.96 for BNP and 0.93 for ANP. The sensitivity for ANP was 97%, specificity was 72%, and positive predictive value was 55% for AHF. In comparison, the sensitivity of BNP was 97%, specificity was 84%, and positive predictive value was 70% for AHF.[17] The suboptimal result for ANP was due in part to its rapid clearance, which made reliable measurements difficult in typical clinical settings. Recently, biochemical assays targeting the more stable fragment, MR-proANP became available. The diagnostic utility of MR-proANP in AHF was demonstrated in the Biomarker in AHF (BACH) trial, which demonstrated that MR-proANP at cut point of 120 pmol/L was noninferior to BNP at 100 pg/mL for the diagnosis for the AHF. The correlation between MR-proANP and both BNP and NT-proBNP was 0.92. B-type natriuretic peptide at the 100 pg/mL cut point had a sensitivity of 95.6%, specificity of 61.9%, diagnostic accuracy of 73.6%, positive predictive value of 57%, and a negative predictive value of 96.4%. In comparison, MR-proANP with a cut point of 120 pmol/L had a sensitivity of 97%, specificity of 59.9%, diagnostic accuracy of 72.7%, positive predictive value of 56%, and a negative predictive value of 97.4% (Table 2). Furthermore, elevated MR-proANP added significantly to elevated BNP, increasing the C-statistic from 0.787 to 0.816 (p <0.001). Requiring both MR-proANP and BNP to be elevated increased the overall diagnostic accuracy from 73.6% for BNP alone to 76.6% for the combined diagnosis. In patients with intermediate BNP levels and obesity, MR-proANP added

TABLE 2: Mid-region prohormone atrial natriuretic peptide versus B-type natriuretic peptide for diagnosis of acute heart failure (AHF) in the biomarkers in AHF trial[18]

Measure	Sensitivity (%)	Specificity (%)	Accuracy (%)
MR-proANP 120 pmol/L	95.56	59.85	72.64
BNP 100 pg/mL	96.98	61.90	73.50
Difference	1.42	2.05	0.86
Upper 95% limit	2.82	3.84	2.10
Noninferiority p	<0.0001	<0.0001	<0.0001

MR-proANP, mid-region prohormone atrial natriuretic peptide; BNP, B-type natriuretic peptide.

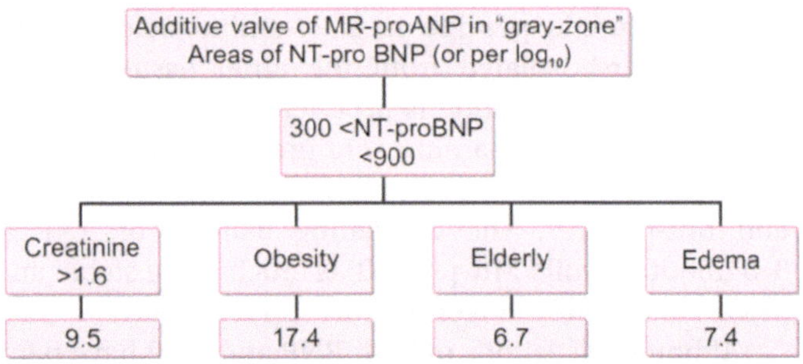

MR-proANP, mid-region prohormone atrial natriuretic peptide; NT-proBNP, N-terminal prohormone B-type natriuretic peptide

FLOWCHART 1: Incremental predictive value of adding mid-region prohormone atrial natriuretic peptide to gray zone amino N-terminal prohormone B-type natriuretic peptide for the diagnosis of acute heart failure

incremental predictive value to BNP for the prediction of AHF. In patients with intermediate NT-proBNP levels, renal insufficiency (creatinine >1.6 mg/dL), obesity, age more than 70 years and edema, MR-proANP also added incremental predictive value to NT-proBNP for the prediction of AHF (Flowchart 1). In the subgroup of patients where the ED physicians were uncertain of the diagnosis, defined as 20–80% probability of AHF on a visual analog scale, the addition of MR-proANP reduced indecision by 29%.[18]

USING NATRIURETIC PEPTIDES IN THE EMERGENCY DEPARTMENT

For patients presenting to the ED with acute dyspnea, the goal of the initial evaluation is timely diagnosis of the etiology of the acute dyspnea, as delays in the initiation of effective therapy are associated with significantly worse outcomes. While acute dyspnea is the most common presenting symptom of AHF, it is certainly not unique to AHF. Other common etiologies of acute dyspnea include pneumonia, viral syndromes, chronic obstructive pulmonary disease, asthma, and pulmonary embolism. While history, physical examination, laboratory, and imaging studies can often provide the clinician with clues, the diagnosis is not always clear during the initial evaluation, which leads to significant delays. This is where NPs come in.

As shown by the evidence outlined above, NPs are excellent independent diagnostic biomarkers for AHF. NPs carry the advantage of widespread availability, high reproducibility, and relative low cost. Natriuretic peptides can be used to diagnose both acute systolic HF and acute diastolic HF. If they are added to the initial panel of laboratory tests when the patient arrives at the ED with acute dyspnea, by the time the clinician completes the history and physical examination, the results may be available. As shown by prior studies, NPs not only have high sensitivity and specificity for AHF, but they also have high discriminatory power in cases where the physician diagnosis of AHF is indeterminant. As the NP assays are fast and reliable, they can lead to significantly reduced ED evaluation time, hospital admission rates, hospital length of stay and overall healthcare cost without increasing mortality or morbidity. In agreement with the recently published recommendations on prehospital and early hospital management of AHF from the Heart Failure Association of the European Society of Cardiology, the European Society of Emergency Medicine and the Society of Academic Emergency Medicine, the authors feel that BNP, NT-proBNP, or MR-proANP should be measured in all patients with acute dyspnea or suspected AHF.[19]

When using NPs in the ED to evaluate patients with acute dyspnea who do not have known HF, the authors propose the following algorithm (Flowchart 2). In patients with acute dyspnea and inconclusive diagnosis by history and physical examination, NP levels should be used to assist the diagnostic evaluation. In patients with BNP levels less than 100 pg/mL or NT-proBNP less than 300 pg/mL, the diagnosis of AHF is very unlikely (<2% likelihood). These patients should be further evaluated for an alternative etiology for their acute dyspnea, such as chronic obstructive pulmonary disease exacerbation, asthma exacerbation, pneumonia, sepsis, pulmonary embolism, cardiac tamponade, constrictive pericarditis, or acute coronary syndrome. In patients with acute dyspnea and BNP levels above 500 pg/mL or NT-proBNP levels above an age-dependent cutoff (>450 pg/mL in patients <50 years old or >900 pg/mL in patients between 50 years and 75 years of age or >1,800 pg/mL in patients >75 years of age), AHF is very highly (>95% likelihood). In these patients, therapy should be initiated for AHF without delay. All patients with AHF should receive diuretics to reduce the intravascular volume and left ventricular preload. In patients without evidence of cardiogenic shock, vasodilators can be added if they are hypertensive. Inotropes can also be considered in these patients if they experience poor tissue perfusion and to aide diuresis. In patients with evidence of cardiogenic shock, inotrope and

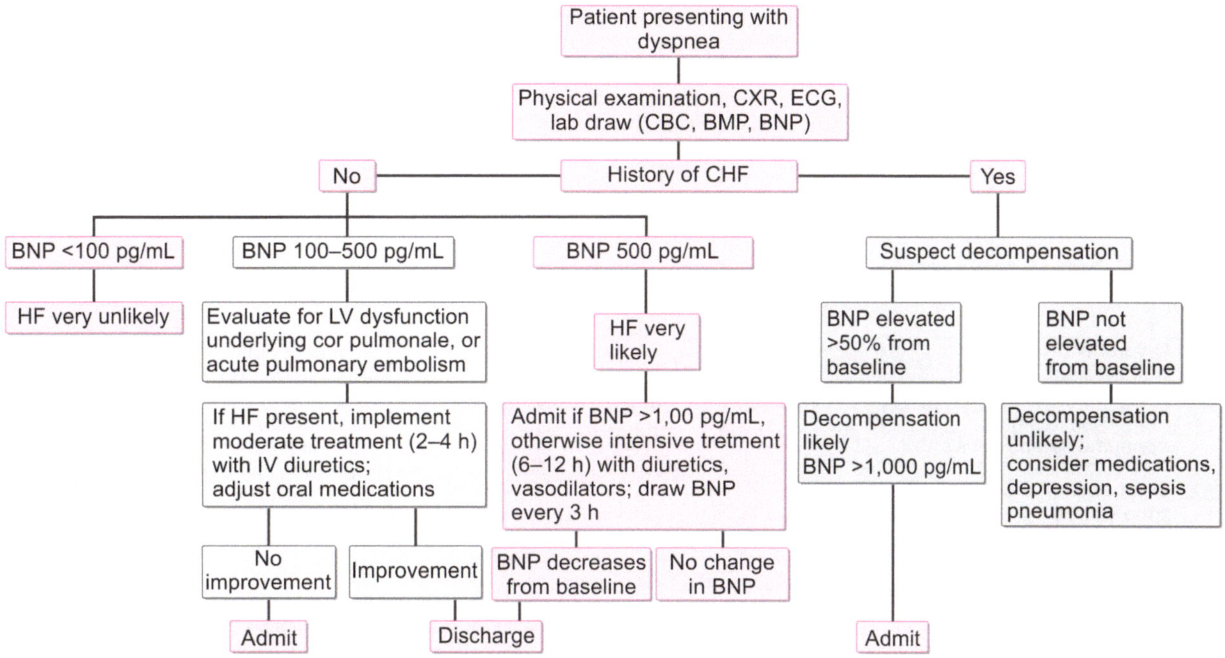

CXR, chest X-ray; ECG, electrocardiogram; CBC, complete blood count; BMP, basic metabolic panel; BNP, B-type natriuretic peptide; CHF, chronic heart failure; HF, heart failure; LV, left ventricular; IV, intravenous.

FLOWCHART 2: Algorithm for the management of heart failure in an emergency department setting

vasodilators may both be necessary in order to improve cardiac output by increasing contractility and decreasing afterload. In patients with NP levels in the gray zone (all ages: BNP between 100 and 500 pg/mL; age <50 years: NT-proBNP between 300 and 450 pg/mL, and age between 50 and 75 years: NT-proBNP between 300 and 900 pg/mL; age >75 years: NT-proBNP between 300 and 1,800 pg/mL), if they had a history of HF or left ventricular dysfunction or strong evidence of AHF, then AHF is highly probable (90% likelihood). These patients should receive empiric treatment for AHF with diuretics and vasodilators as needed and observed closely. If there is no history of HF or strong evidence for AHF or left ventricular dysfunction, then an evaluation for acute coronary syndrome, cor pulmonale or acute pulmonary embolism should be considered. Patients with electrocardiogram and biomarker evidence of acute coronary syndrome should be treated accordingly. Similarly, patients with imaging evidence of acute pulmonary embolism should be initiated on anticoagulation immediately. If there is evidence of existing left ventricular dysfunction or cor pulmonale then the gray zone NP levels are unlikely to represent AHF (<25% likelihood), as these patients tend to have higher NP levels during AHF. These patients should be closely observed and evaluated for an alternative diagnosis. In patients without baseline left ventricular dysfunction, cor pulmonale, acute coronary syndrome, or acute pulmonary embolism, gray zone NP levels may still represent AHF (>75% likelihood). Empiric therapy for AHF should be initiated in these patients and they should be observed closely (Flowchart 3). Although not widely available, MR-proANP can also be used for the diagnostic evaluation of patients with acute dyspnea. Patients with MR-proANP levels below 120 pg/mL are unlikely to have AHF. Patients with MR-proANP levels above 600 pg/mL are very highly to have AHF. The gray zone for MR-proANP is between 120 pg/mL and 600 pg/mL. When available, MR-proANP levels should be checked in patients with BNP or NT-proBNP levels in the diagnostic gray zone to increase the diagnostic accuracy of NPs in patients with obesity (intermediate BNP levels), renal insufficiency (intermediate NT-proBNP levels) and advanced age (intermediate NT-proBNP levels) (Flowchart 1).

In patients with known chronic HF, the diagnosis of AHF with NPs can pose a particular challenge. Patients with existing HF can have significantly elevated NP levels at baseline owing to chronically elevated PCWP due to the severe underlying HF and renal dysfunction that is commonly associated with HF. It is not uncommon to see BNP levels greater than 500 pg/mL and NT-proBNP levels greater than 1,800 pg/mL in patients with existing HF who do not have AHF. In these patients, it would be very helpful to know their "dry" NP levels when they are clinically euvolemic. If their presenting NP levels are elevated more than 50% from baseline, then AHF is likely. Empiric therapy for AHF should be implemented as soon as possible. However, if their presenting NP levels are not elevated more than 50% from baseline, then AHF is unlikely. These patients should be observed (Flowchart 3).

Most of the research has focused on identification of high-risk patients due to the belief that better management of these patients can reduce readmission

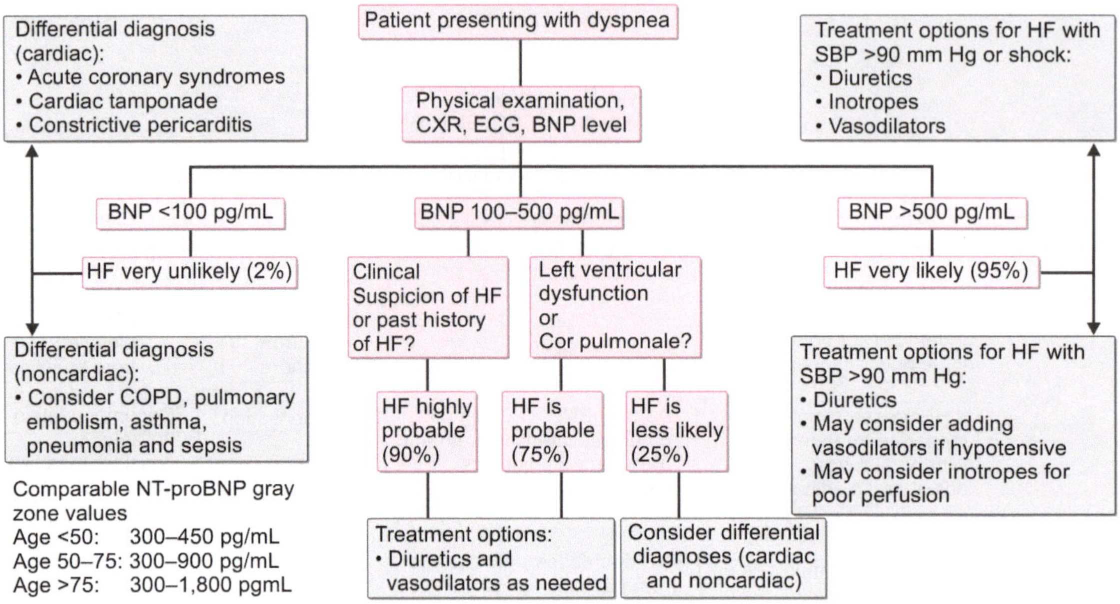

CXR, chest X-ray; HF, heart failure; ECG, electrocardiography; BNP, B-type natriuretic peptide; COPD, chronic obstructive pulmonary disease; NT-proBNP, N-terminal prohormone B-type natriuretic peptide; SBP, systolic blood pressure

FLOWCHART 3: Algorithm on using B-type natriuretic peptide and amino N-terminal prohormone B-type natriuretic peptide levels to rule in and rule out acute heart failure

and mortality rates. Strategies for effective management of low-risk AHF patients in the ED are less clear. Ezekowitz et al. described short- and long-term outcomes in elderly patients (≥65 years) presenting to the ED with AHF. The group showed that patients who were not admitted had a higher rate of repeat ED visits but comparable rates of rehospitalization at 30 days.[20] Approximately 80% of patients with AHF are admitted from the ED,[21] but a group of experts estimated that up to 50% of ED patients with HF could be safely discharged after a brief period of observation, thus avoiding unnecessary admissions and minimizing readmissions.[22]

There may be a role for serial NP monitoring in the ED. As NPs are biomarkers of left ventricular preload and wall stress, a change in NP levels during serial measurement is a reflection of left ventricular preload and wall stress. Thus serial measurements of NP can be used to guide therapy for AHF. While the evidence for NP-guided therapy is not as robust as the evidence for using them in the diagnostic evaluation of AHF, serial NPs measurements should be considered while managing patients with AHF in the ED. The authors propose the following algorithm (Flowchart 2) for NP-guided therapy in AHF patients in the ED. In patients with BNP levels greater than 1,000 pg/mL or NT-proBNP levels greater than 900 pg/mL for age less than 50 years or greater than 1,800 pg/mL for age between 50 and 75 years or greater than 3,600 pg/mL for age greater than 75 years, the AHF is likely severe and these patients would benefit from inpatient therapy. However, if the patient's BNP level is between 500 and 1,000 pg/mL or NT-proBNP level between 300 pg/mL and an age-dependent upper limit (>900 for age <50 years, >1,800 pg/mL for age between 50 and 75 years, and >3,600 pg/mL for age >75 years), an intensive treatment approach with diuretics and vasodilators in the ED can be considered. Natriuretic peptide levels should be checked every 3 hours during this trial of intensive therapy. If the patient experiences improvement in symptoms and a reduction in NP levels, then they can be discharged with close outpatient follow-up. Conversely, if the patient does not experience any improvement in symptoms or if there is no change to NP levels, then the patient should be admitted for further therapy. For patients with known HF who presents with acute dyspnea and natriuretic levels that are 50% higher than baseline, inpatient therapy is often necessary, especially if their presenting BNP level is greater than 1,000 pg/mL or NT-proBNP level is greater than an age-dependent cutoff (>900 pg/mL for age <50 years, >1,800 pg/mL for age between 50 and 75 years and >3,600 pg/mL for age >75 years). Finally, for patients with gray zone NP levels (BNP between 100 and 500 pg/mL, age <50 years; NT-proBNP between 300 and 450 pg/mL, age between 50 years and 75 years' NT-proBNP between 300 pg/mL and 900 pg/mL and age >75 years; NT-proBNP between 300 pg/mL and 1,800 pg/mL) who do not have an alterative explanation for their acute dyspnea, such as acute pulmonary embolism, pneumonia, or chronic obstructive pulmonary disease exacerbation, empiric therapy for AHF should be attempted in the ED. If they experience improvement in their symptoms with empiric AHF therapy, then they can be discharged with close outpatient follow-up and further evaluation for HF. If they do not experience improvement in their symptoms, then they should be admitted for continued observation and evaluation (Flowchart 3).

When using NPs, there are some important caveats that clinicians must keep in mind. First and foremost, NP elevations are not pathognomonic for AHF. Thus, NPs levels should never be used in isolation during the diagnostic evaluation of patients with acute dyspnea. As shown by prior studies, NP levels can increase due to variety of other reasons. As mentioned above, patients with chronic HF can have significantly elevated NP levels even though they are clinically euvolemic. Natriuretic peptide levels can also increase during acute coronary syndrome as left ventricular dysfunction develops during acute myocardial ischemia. Natriuretic peptide levels can also be elevated due to acute and chronic right HF secondary to pulmonary disease, such as chronic pulmonary hypertension and acute pulmonary embolism. Patients in high cardiac output states, such as sepsis, cirrhosis, and hyperthyroidism can also have elevated NP levels without AHF. Other caveats for using NP include advanced age, female gender, obesity, and renal dysfunction. Baseline levels of both BNP and NT-proBNP increase with age. The effect of age on NT-proBNP levels is more profound, thus leading to the age-dependent cutoffs for the diagnostic evaluation of acute dyspnea patients. For unclear reasons, NP levels are higher in women than men. Natriuretic peptide levels can also be elevated in patients with renal dysfunction. As a significant amount of NPs clearance occurs in the kidneys, impaired renal function (GFR $<60\ mL/min/1.7\ m^2$) is associated with inappropriately elevated NP levels. In addition, patients with renal disease are also more likely to have coronary artery disease, left ventricular hypertrophy, and hypertension, which can all cause increases to left ventricular filling pressure and further chronic elevation in NP levels. As NT-proBNP is primarily cleared in the kidneys, the effect of renal impairment is stronger on NT-proBNP than on BNP. Interestingly, obese patients tend to have inappropriately low BNP levels. The exact mechanism of this inverse relationship between obesity and BNP levels is unknown and may be related to increased tissue clearance by membrane-bound NP receptors and decreased production of BNPs in obese patients. As a rule of thumb, BNP levels should be multiplied by a factor of 2–3 in obese patients to account for this inappropriate depression of BNP levels. As NT-proBNP is not cleared by membrane-bound NP receptors, its levels are less affected by obesity. Another aspect of NP levels that the clinician must keep in mind is that although there is a correlation between PCWP and NP levels, NP levels do not change "instantaneously". Only a very small amount of NP is stored in myocytes. In situations of acute increases in left ventricular filling pressure, there is a delay in the rise of NPs as the intracellular production of NPs is ramped up. Thus in patients with clear evidence of flash pulmonary edema, a low NP level cannot be used to rule out AHF. Lastly, not all HF is caused by increases in left ventricular filling pressures. Conditions, such as mitral stenosis and constrictive pericarditis can cause significant HF symptoms without causing elevations of left ventricular filling pressures. Thus the NP levels may be low in these cases.

CONCLUSION

Natriuretic peptides with their low cost, objectivity, reproducibility, and accessibility are excellent adjuncts to physical examination, standard laboratory, and imaging studies in diagnosing AHF in the ED. By providing us with insight into one of the most important pathophysiologic processes in AHF, NPs have revolutionized the evaluation of the patients with acute dyspnea, improving diagnostic accuracy and efficiency of AHF in a variety of clinical settings. They have been widely accepted by clinicians and will continue to play a significant role in the management of patients with acute dyspnea in the ED.

REFERENCES

1. Ikeda T, Matsuda K, Itoh H, Shirakami G, Miyamoto Y, Yoshimasa T, et al. Plasma levels of brain and atrial natriuretic peptides elevate in proportion to left ventricular end-systolic wall stress in patients with aortic stenosis. Am Heart J. 1997;133(3):307-14.
2. Yoshimura M, Yasue H, Okumura K, Ogawa H, Jougasaki M, Mukoyama M, et al. Different secretion patterns of atrial natriuretic peptide and brain natriuretic peptide in patients with congestive heart failure. Circulation. 1993; 87(2):464-9.
3. Lang CC, Choy AM, Turner K, Tobin R, Coutie W, Struthers AD. The effect of intravenous saline loading on plasma levels of brain natriuretic peptide in man. J Hypertens. 1993;11(7):737-41.
4. Haug C, Metzele A, Kochs M, Hombach V, Grunert A. Plasma brain natriuretic peptide and atrial natriuretic peptide concentrations correlate with left ventricular end-diastolic pressure. Clin Cardiol. 1993;16(7):553-7.
5. Massie B, Ports T, Chatterjee K, Parmley W, Ostland J, O'Young J, et al. Long-term vasodilator therapy for heart failure: clinical response and its relationship to hemodynamic measurements. Circulation. 1981;63(2):269-78.
6. Kazanegra R, Cheng V, Garcia A, Krishnaswamy P, Gardetto N, Clopton P, et al. A rapid test for B-type natriuretic peptide correlates with falling wedge pressures in patients treated for decompensated heart failure: a pilot study. J Card Fail. 2001;7(1):21-9.
7. Dickstein K. Natriuretic peptides in detection of heart failure. Lancet. 1998; 351(9095):4.
8. Hunt PJ, Yandle TG, Nicholls MG, Richards AM, Espiner EA. The amino-terminal portion of pro-brain natriuretic peptide (Pro-BNP) circulates in human plasma. Biochem Biophys Res Commun. 1995;214(3):1175-83.
9. Maeda K, Tsutamoto T, Wada A, Hisanaga T, Kinoshita M. Plasma brain natriuretic peptide as a biochemical marker of high left ventricular end-diastolic pressure in patients with symptomatic left ventricular dysfunction. Am Heart J. 1998;135(5):825-32.
10. Clerico A, Iervasi G, Del Chicca M, Emdin M, Maffei S, Nannipieri M, et al. Circulating levels of cardiac natriuretic peptides (ANP and BNP) measured by highly sensitive and specific immunoradiometric assays in normal subjects and in patients with different degrees of heart failure. J Endocrinol Invest. 1998;21(3):170-9.

11. Yancy CW, Jessup M, Bozkurt B, Butler J, Casey DE Jr, Drazner MH, et al. 2013 ACCF/AHA guideline for the management of heart failure: a report of the American College of Cardiology Foundation/American Heart Association Task Force on Practice Guidelines. J Am Coll Cardiol. 2013;62(16):e147-239.
12. Maisel AS, Krishnaswamy P, Nowak RM, McCord J, Hollander JE, Duc P, et al. Rapid measurement of B-type natriuretic peptide in the emergency diagnosis of heart failure. N Engl J Med. 2002;347(3):161-7.
13. Maisel A, Hollander JE, Guss D, McCullough P, Nowak R, Green G, et al. Primary results of the Rapid Emergency Department Heart Failure Outpatient Trial (REDHOT). A multicenter study of B-type natriuretic peptide levels, emergency department decision making, and outcomes in patients presenting with shortness of breath. J Am Coll Cardiol. 2004;44(6):1328-33.
14. Januzzi JL Jr, Camargo CA, Anwaruddin S, Baggish AL, Chen AA, Krauser DG, et al. The N-terminal Pro-BNP investigation of dyspnea in the emergency department (PRIDE) study. Am J Cardiol. 2005;95(8):948-54.
15. Moe GW, Howlett J, Januzzi JL, Zowall H, Investigators CMIMoPWCHFS. N-Terminal Pro–B-Type Natriuretic Peptide Testing Improves the Management of Patients With Suspected Acute Heart Failure Primary Results of the Canadian Prospective Randomized Multicenter IMPROVE-CHF Study. Circulation. 2007; 115(24):3103-10.
16. Xu-Cai YO, Wu Q. Molecular forms of natriuretic peptides in heart failure and their implications. Heart. 2010;96(6):419-24.
17. Cowie MR, Struthers AD, Wood DA, Coats AJ, Thompson SG, Poole-Wilson PA, et al. Value of natriuretic peptides in assessment of patients with possible new heart failure in primary care. Lancet. 1997;350(9088):1349-53.
18. Maisel A, Mueller C, Nowak R, Peacock WF, Landsberg JW, Ponikowski P, et al. Mid-region pro-hormone markers for diagnosis and prognosis in acute dyspnea: results from the BACH (Biomarkers in Acute Heart Failure) trial. J Am Coll Cardiol. 2010;55(19):2062-76.
19. Mebazaa A, Yilmaz MB, Levy P, Ponikowski P, Peacock WF, Laribi S, et al. Recommendations on pre-hospital & early hospital management of acute heart failure: a consensus paper from the Heart Failure Association of the European Society of Cardiology, the European Society of Emergency Medicine and the Society of Academic Emergency Medicine. Eur J Heart Fail. 2015;17(6):544-58.
20. Ezekowitz JA, Bakal JA, Kaul P, Westerhout CM, Armstrong PW. Acute heart failure in the emergency department: Short and long-term outcomes of elderly patients with heart failure. Eur J Heart Fail. 2008;10(3):308-14.
21. Weintraub NL, Collins SP, Pang PS, Levy PD, Anderson AS, Arslanian-Engoren C, et al. Acute heart failure syndromes: emergency department presentation, treatment, and disposition: current approaches and future aims a scientific statement from the American Heart Association. Circulation. 2010;122(19):1975-96.
22. Collins SP, Pang PS, Fonarow GC, Yancy CW, Bonow RO, Gheorghiade M. Is hospital admission for heart failure really necessary?: the role of the emergency department and observation unit in preventing hospitalization and rehospitalization. J Am Coll Cardiol. 2013;61(2):121-6.

17 CHAPTER

Other Biomarkers

Nikola A Kozhuharov, Zaid Sabti, Samyut Shrestha, Christian Müller

INTRODUCTION

Compared to the improved prognosis in chronic heart failure, morbidity and mortality in acute heart failure remain unacceptably high.[1]

This fact may be at least partly due to diagnostic uncertainty in the emergency department and the associated delay in diagnosis and initiation of effective treatment, as well as to incomplete understanding of the pathophysiological mechanisms involved in the different AHF syndromes requiring different management.[2]

The biomarkers introduced in this chapter give the opportunity to overcome these difficulties and to improve the dismal prognosis in AHF.

ROLE OF BIOMARKERS IN ACUTE HEART FAILURE

Acute heart failure is the most common cause of hospitalization for patients over 65 years old, which makes the disease one of the major public health burdens.[3] Mortality following hospitalization for acute heart failure reaches 45% in the first 3 years and up to 15% in the first 6 months following discharge.[4] Improvement of diagnostics and risk assessment in these patients are promising areas for positive change in the situation at hand.

Acute heart failure manifests with symptoms such as difficulty in breathing, weakness, fatigue, and congestion. It is difficult to provide definitive diagnosis based solely on anamnesis and examination. Guidelines issued by cardiology associations recommend measuring the plasma concentrations of B-type natriuretic peptide (BNP) and N-terminal proBNP (NT-proBNP) as a supporting measure. These biomarkers should be viewed as quantitative parameters. The higher the level of natriuretic peptides, the greater the probability of an acute heart failure diagnosis.[1,5,6]

B-type natriuretic peptide and NT-proBNP are the best investigated biomarkers for assessment of prognosis in patients with chronic heart failure and are widely used in the clinical practice. Unfortunately, the prognostic accuracy for death for natriuretic peptides obtained at emergency department presentation is very low. Only measurements of natriuretic peptides performed after 48 h or at hospital discharge have reasonable accuracy for risk prediction.[7] Therefore, other biomarkers have been explored to a low accurate risk stratification already at emergency department presentation.

Notably, the diagnosis of acute heart failure does not describe a uniform disease but a combination of various syndromes.[8] For correct assessment and triaging of the patient, it is necessary to consider the cardiac and noncardiac comorbidities. Therefore, performing tests with other biomarkers in addition to the natriuretic peptides may generate a more complete and precise understanding of the pathophysiology of the disease and facilitate proper triaging and therapy.[9]

CARDIAC TROPONIN I AND CARDIAC TROPONIN T

Cardiac troponin I and troponin T are part of the contractile apparatus of the heart. They are two heart-specific isoforms of the regulatory and structural proteins of the actin filaments in the striated muscles. Their function is related to the conversion of the electrical signals to mechanical contractions.[10]

An increased concentration of cardiac troponin in the blood is associated with myocyte damage. It has not been fully clarified whether this damage has to be irreversible and leading to cell death or reversible and leading to increased permeability of the cell membrane. There are various pathomechanisms for this damage.[8]

The prevalence of increased cardiac troponin levels in patients with acute heart failure is common. With the development of high-sensitivity cardiac troponin assays with low limit of detection, this fact gained additional relevance because the majority of patients with acute heart failure have slightly elevated cardiac troponin levels. Pascual-Figal et al. in a study including 202 patients with acute heart failure showed that the concentration of high-sensitive cardiac troponin T exceeded the 99th percentile in 81% of the patients. The correct interpretation of these findings is a challenge in the routine clinical practice.[11]

There are various causes of cardiac troponin elevation in patients with acute heart failure. Examples of such causes include acute coronary syndrome (ACS), pulmonary embolism, toxins in sepsis, etc.[10]

Indisputably, the ACS is of key importance for rapidly choosing an adequate therapy as well as for the prognosis of patients with acute heart failure.[6] It is a cause of decompensation in up to one-third of the patients.[12] In a cohort from the Finnish Acute Heart Failure Study (FINN-AKVA), an observational clinical trial including 620 patients with acute heart failure, 32% of the enrolled subjects were also diagnosed with ACS. Ischemic heart disease is the most common comorbidity involved in heart decompensation.[13,14]

When clinical signs for cardiac infraction and acute heart failure are present, the diagnostic procedures should be carried out in accordance with the cardiology associations' guidelines on the management of ACS. Alongside clinical assessment and electrocardiogram, cardiac troponin plays a key role in the process. In such cases, biomarkers should be interpreted within the context of the overall clinical diagnostics. If an increase or decrease in cardiac troponin concentration with at least one unit above the 99th percentile of the upper reference limit (URL) is observed, the diagnosis of type 1 myocardial infarction is very likely. This is a condition where one or more coronary arteries become blocked, which results in reduced blood supply to the myocard. In turn, this process leads to cardiac necrosis and the release of troponin in the blood.[15]

Another possible and common cause of troponinemia is the type 2 myocardial infarction. It is defined as myocardial necrosis caused by inadequate oxygen supply to the myocytes, which cannot be solely explained with ischemic heart disease. The causes of type 2 myocardial infarction may be a small-vessel disease, coronary endothelial dysfunction, tachy- or bradyarrhythmias, hypotension, anemia, etc. The therapy of this type of infarction requires elimination of the specific cause for the existing imbalance between the cardiac oxygen demand and supply.[15]

Besides playing a fundamental role in the definition of myocardial infarction, cardiac troponin elevation may also be observed in myocarditis, Takotsubo cardiomyopathy and infiltrative processes, such as amyloidosis, among other conditions. The direct toxic effects of the neurohormones in acute heart failure may also lead to troponinemia.[16]

High concentration of cardiac troponin T and cardiac troponin I in acute heart failure is associated with increase in complications, higher in-hospital mortality, and post-discharge mortality. Cardiac troponin provides this information independently of other factors such as BNP, ejection fraction, etc.[11,17,18]

In analysis of 377 acute heart failure patients from the Basics in Acute Shortness of Breath EvaLuation (BASEL V) study, cardiac troponin concentration exceeded the 99th percentile of the URL in 41% of the patients. A cardiac troponin concentration below that limit was established in 24% of the patients. The high-sensitivity assay did not detect any cardiac troponin in 35% of the patients. The estimated in-hospital mortality rate was least favorable in the group with the most elevated cardiac troponin levels. This correlation could also be observed for the 1-year mortality rate. The odds ratio was 1.03 [95% confidence interval (CI) 1.02–1.05; $p < 0.001$] for each 100 ng elevation in the high-sensitivity cardiac troponin I level.[16] These results are consistent with those reported in the Acute Decompensated Heart Failure National Registry (ADHERE) database. The in-hospital mortality rate was high for patients with cardiac troponin concentrations above the level detectable by the nonhigh-sensitivity cardiac troponin assay. The odds ratio in this case was 2.55 (95% CI = 2.22–2.89; $p < 0.001$).[17]

The data derived from the elevated cardiac troponins during hospitalization for acute heart failure can be supported with serial cardiac troponin measurements during treatment. The increase in this biomarker's concentration during hospitalization helps to identify the patients who are at the highest risk for complications and death.[6] In kidney failure, a common comorbidity, cardiac troponin preserves its predictive value.[16]

Elevated cardiac troponin concentration can be observed in a large number of patients with acute heart failure. Assessed within the context of clinical management, it provides important data on triaging, adequate therapy and patient prognosis. Firstly, cardiac troponin is of fundamental importance for confirming or excluding the ACS as a precipitant of acute heart failure. Secondly, it should be noted that high cardiac troponin levels measured in patients with acute heart failure is an independent predictor for increased in-hospital mortality and long-term mortality.[6] Except in the cases of an ACS, currently there are no direct therapeutic implications from the elevated cardiac troponin levels measured in patients with acute heart failure.

PROCALCITONIN

When a patient experiencing shortness of breath is admitted in the emergency department, it is necessary to formulate a differential diagnosis in order to distinguish between a respiratory tract infection and acute heart failure. These two conditions are the leading causes of emergency admissions in patients over 65 years old, with respectively about 35 and 40%.[19] Bacterial infections precipitate 15–20% of the cases of decompensated heart failure.[20]

Failure to determine the correct diagnosis and the resulting inability to administer adequate and timely treatment increase the risk of complications. A successful outcome may be achieved by the additional use of procalcitonin in the initial diagnostic assessment.

Procalcitonin is a biomarker with a high sensitivity and a high specificity for bacterial infections in emergency department patients with a cut-off level of 0.10 ng/mL.[20] In physiological conditions, it is synthesized by the C-cells of the thyroid gland and is a precursor of the calcitonin hormone. However, procalcitonin can be synthesized at an increased rate by all tissues in response to bacterial infection. This is achieved by two mechanisms. The first mechanism is direct and is due to the effect of lipopolysaccharides and toxins released by bacteria. The second is a response mediated by interleukin 6 (IL-6) and tumor necrosis factor-α. Viral infections reduce the synthesis of procalcitonin through interferon-γ.[21] These properties of the biomarker help to better identify patients with bacterial infections complaining from shortness of breath.

The prospective, international, observational Biomarkers in Acute Heart Failure (BACH) study included 1,641 patients admitted into emergency departments due to shortness of breath. The use of procalcitonin yielded the highest accuracy for diagnosing pneumonia in patients within the overall cohort, with an area under the curve (AUC) in the receiver operating characteristic analysis (ROC analysis) of 0.723 ($p < 0.0001$). For diagnosing pneumonia in patients who also suffered from acute heart failure, the test resulted in an even better AUC of 0.841 ($p < 0.0001$). Elevated levels of procalcitonin indicated a poor prognosis.[22]

Procalcitonin is a valuable biomarker in patients with dyspnea in the emergency department. It brings clarity in a fast manner when differentiating between the two most common diagnoses that lead to these symptoms:

- Acute heart failure
- Bacterial respiratory infections.

The ability of procalcitonin to increase in bacterial infections and to remain the same in case of viral infections facilitates the decision to appoint the antibiotic therapy.

C-REACTIVE PROTEIN

Inflammation plays an important role in heart failure. When infections are present, inflammation may precipitate decompensation. Chronic infection may contribute to the onset and the progression of heart failure.[1]

C-reactive protein (CRP) is one of the most researched biomarkers related to the inflammatory processes. It is synthesized by the hepatocytes in response to IL-6, IL-1, and tumor necrosis factor 4 and 10.[23] C-reactive protein function is related to the ability to activate complement through the classic complement pathway and to modulate the activity of phagocytes. This protein assists in opsonizing bacteria and damaged cells.[23,24]

The role of CRP in acute inflammatory processes makes it a key component in the assessment of emergency department patients with shortness of breath. Pneumonia is the second most common differential diagnosis after acute heart failure in this situation.[19] Considering the levels measured during examination at the emergency department in combination with the dynamic changes in CRP, the specificity of this biomarker for differentiating between both diagnoses reaches 0.927 and its sensitivity 0.960.[25]

One of the biggest disadvantages of CRP is that it does not allow to differentiate between bacterial and viral infection, and chronic inflammatory processes.[19] It is well known that chronic inflammation and in turn the elevated CRP levels lead to complications in the case of an ischemic heart disease. C-reactive protein is a predictor for the development of heart failure.[26] The elevated levels of the biomarker are associated with higher morbidity and mortality in patients with acute heart failure.[27]

In patients with acute heart failure, the elevated CRP levels on admission and their dynamics during therapy provide important data regarding the prognosis. A substudy (n = 794) from the Acute Study of Clinical Effectiveness of Nesiritide in Decompensated Heart Failure (ASCEND-HF) trial, a prospective, interventional trial including overall 7,141 subjects with acute heart failure, showed that high-sensitivity CRP (hsCRP) exceeded the normal levels on emergency admission. Maintaining high levels of hsCRP during therapy was a predictor for prolonged hospitalization. Furthermore, elevated levels 30 days after admission were associated with higher 180-day mortality.[26,28]

The results derived from CRP as a biomarker demonstrated that inflammation plays an important role in acute heart failure. Medications regulating this process, such as valsartan, may improve the prognosis for patients with chronic heart failure.[27] The possible therapeutic benefit of modulating the inflammation in acute heart failure is yet to be understood.

SUPPRESSOR OF TUMORIGENICITY 2

Suppressor of tumorigenicity 2 (ST2) is part of the Toll-like/IL-1-type receptor group. It has a transmembrane (ST2L) and an extracellular soluble isoform (sST2). The ligand for ST2 is IL-33. Interestingly, when the ST2L transmembrane receptor binds to IL-33, the effect of angiotensin, which induces myocardial hypertrophy, is reduced. Similarly, the effect of the fibrosis-inducing nuclear factor-κ B is antagonized. The blood-soluble sST2 isoform competes with ST2L for binding to IL-33, thus reducing the aforementioned effects.[9]

In the presence of endogenous or exogenous stress, the immune system reacts by increasing the synthesis of sST2. Exogenous stress is defined as infections, toxins, etc. Myocardial ischemia, necrosis, and hemodynamic stress are considered endogenous stresses. Furthermore, the sST2 isoform is produced in the lungs and the blood vessels. Bartunek et al. showed that the source of the circulating serum ST2 is extracardial.[29]

The concentration of sST2 in the blood is measured by routine assays, referred to as ST-tests. The concentration of the sST2 isoform is elevated in patients with acute heart failure. The results reported from the N-terminal pro-BNP Investigation of Dyspnea in the Emergency department (PRIDE) study indicated that sST2 helped to identify patients with acute heart failure among emergency department patients with shortness of breath. Notably, in such cases, natriuretic peptides are more commonly used in diagnostics. Soluble suppressor of tumorigenicity 2 provides extremely valuable information for predicting the outcome. It allows to estimate the 1-year mortality rate for patients with shortness of breath in general [hazard ratio (HR) = 5.6; $p < 0.001$) and for patients with acute heart failure (HR = 9.3; $p = 0.03$) in particular. When BNP and sST2 are combined for predicting the mortality for patients with shortness of breath, AUC reaches 0.80 (95% CI = 0.76–0.84, $p < 0.001$).[30]

In a multicenter trial including 346 patients, Rehman et al. reported higher sST2 levels in more severe cases of acute heart failure ($p < 0.001$). On the one hand, there was a correlation between structural and functional changes in the heart, such as left ventricular ejection fraction and remodeling, and sST2. On the other hand, sST2 was not affected by the body mass index (BMI) and the age of the patients.[30,31]

When assessing the sST2 level as a biomarker, it should be kept in mind that sST2 also reflects additional parameters in the pathomechanisms of acute heart failure. The established markers, cardiac troponin and BNP, are useful for looking into necrosis and myocardial stretch, while sST2 provides data on fibrosis. The combination of those three markers may result in better understanding of the disease. Pascual-Figal et al. reported that in a cohort of 107 patients with acute heart failure all patients with normal levels of sST2, BNP and high-sensitivity cardiac troponin survived the 2-year follow-up. The mortality rate for this period among the patients with three positive markers was 53%.[32] The results are illustrated on figure 1.

Data on the dynamics of sST2 in the treatment of patients with acute heart failure is discussed with great interest. Breidthardt et al. studied changes in the sST2 in 207 patients admitted to the emergency department with acute heart failure. Patients have been assigned to receive

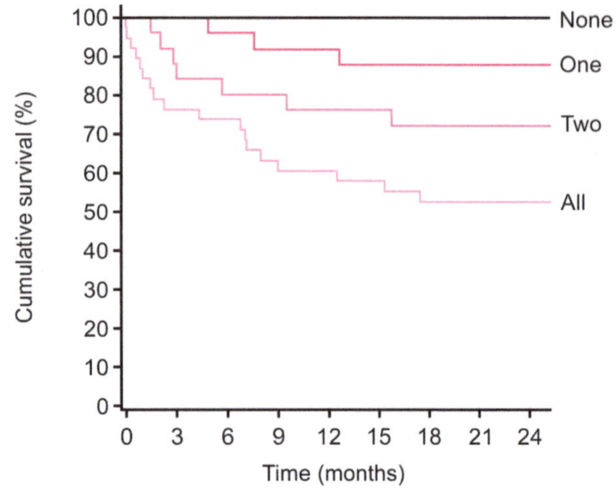

FIG. 1: Complementary role of high-sensitivity troponin T, N-terminal proB-type natriuretic peptide and soluble suppressor of tumorigenicity 2 for the survival of the patients with elevation of one, two, or all three biomarkers

With permission from: Pascual-Figal DA, et al. Soluble ST2, high-sensitivity troponin T- and N-terminal pro-B-type natriuretic peptide: complementary role for risk stratification in acutely decompensated heart failure. Eur J Heart Fail. 2011;13(7):718-25.

diuretic therapy, renin-angiotensin-aldosterone system blockade, and β-blockers according to the individual situation. The authors report a higher 1-year mortality rate in patients whose level of sST2 in the serum was not reduced by more than 25% after 48 hours.[33]

The importance of sST2 in risk assessment was further highlighted by its inclusion in the 2013 Guideline for the Management of Heart Failure issued by The American College of Cardiology Foundation (ACCF)/the American Heart Association (AHA).[3] The reference limit for this marker in case of a heart failure is 35 ng/mL. The higher levels of sST2 help to identify more severe cases which may benefit from intensive therapies and more frequent consultations.[34] In the future, it may also be used to adjust the therapy for prevention of myocardial fibrosis.

GALECTIN 3

The soluble peptide galectin 3 plays an important role in inflammation and myocardial fibrosis. Produced by macrophages during inflammation, this peptide activates the fibroblasts which in turn produce collagen. Therefore, galectin 3 may be viewed as a mediator and a surrogate marker for intensification of the fibrotic processes and the remodeling in the heart.[35] Interestingly, its prognostic value for acute heart failure is higher than that for chronic heart failure.[36]

The PRIDE clinical trial looked into 599 patients with shortness of breath, 209 of whom had acute heart failure. Assessing the data on mortality and rehospitalization derived from patients with cardiac decompensation, van Kimmenade et al. also identified galectin 3 as a factor relevant for the outcome. For the 60-day mortality, the ROC analysis resulted in an AUC of 0.74 (p <0.001) and the multivariate analysis showed an odds ratio of 10.3 (95% CI = 1.6–174.1; p = 0.007) in patients with elevated levels of the biomarker. Furthermore, the odds ratio was 14.3 (95% CI = 5.6–45.1; p <0.001) for the combined 60-day mortality and rehospitalization.[37]

In addition to the short-term prognostic value, galectin 3 also provides data on the long-term prognosis for the patients. This conclusion was drawn by Shah et al. on the basis of 115 emergency department patients experiencing shortness of breath. In patients with acute heart failure, galectin 3 correlated with structural cardiac changes, objectively demonstrated by echocardiography, such as reduced ejection fraction. After a 4-year follow-up, a close correlation between mortality and galectin 3 concentration was reported, with an HR of 14.5 (95% CI = 3.12–67.7; p = 0.001).[38]

Galectin 3 provides valuable data on the prognosis for the subgroup of patients with heart failure with preserved ejection fraction (HFPEF) as well. In a prospective observational study conducted by Carrasco-Sánchez et al., the concentration of galectin 3 in the blood was measured in 419 HFPEF patients and the 1-year mortality rate was assessed. The analysis was adjusted for the covariates age, anemia, NT-proBNP, New York Heart Association (NYHA) classification, and urea. Even following adjustment of the results for the estimated glomerular filtration rate (eGFR), the hazard ratio for patients with galectin 3 concentration exceeding the median of 13.8 ng/mL was 1.46 (95% CI = 1.01–2.11; p <0.001).[39]

Indisputably, the value of a biomarker for assessing the risk of mortality and rehospitalization in patients is of key importance. Providing further insight on the value of galectin 3, an additional analysis from the Coordinating Study Evaluating Outcomes of Advising and Counselling in Heart Failure (COACH) trial indicated that the data collected with this biomarker may help to guide the medicinal therapy. This analysis was performed with the data of 297 patients with acute heart failure who were prescribed spironolactone. Those with higher concentrations of galectin 3 in the blood benefited more from the therapy. The mortality rate in the initial 30 days following discharge was lower.[40]

However, the results from some trials cast doubt on the prognostic value of galectin 3. They discuss the strong dependence of this biomarker on the renal function. Zamora et al. calculated the eGFR using the Chronic Kidney Disease Epidemiology Collaboration (CKD-EPI)-cystatin-C formula in 865 patients with heart failure. They reported a close correlation between galectin 3 and eGFR at r = 0.70 (p <0.001). With this in mind, some authors emphasize the need for further research in order to clarify the prognostic value of galectin 3.[41]

MIDREGIONAL PRO-ADRENOMEDULLIN

Various neurohumoral factors are involved in the development of heart failure. Adrenomedullin is one of the hormones that play an important role in this process. It is a peptide with the properties of a diuretic, a natriuretic and a vasodilator. Adrenomedullin exerts its effect on the circulatory system mainly through the cyclic adenosine monophosphate (cAMP) and the nitric oxide. The widespread distribution of adrenomedullin receptors in the body proves its significance for the pathophysiology of the cardiovascular disease.[42,43]

Adrenomedullin concentration is elevated in patients with acute heart failure and correlates with impaired systolic and diastolic cardiac function.[36] Its measurement in the routine practice is complicated by the instability of this biomarker. Specifically, its plasma half-life is approximately 22 minutes.[44] This issue may be addressed by using midregional pro-adrenomedullin (MR-proADM) assays. Midregional-proADM is a stable fragment of the adrenomedullin hormone precursor and its concentration in the blood matches that of adrenomedullin.[45]

The results from the BACH trial support the role of MR-proADM for predicting the outcome in patients with acute heart failure. It included a total of 1,641 patients admitted with shortness of breath in the emergency departments of 15 centers in various countries. Of these, 568 patients were diagnosed with acute heart failure. For the 90-day mortality rate in this subgroup, after applying MR-proADM the ROC analysis resulted in an AUC of 0.674. This value was better when compared to BNP and NT-proBNP which had an AUC of 0.606 and 0.664, respectively.[7]

The same trial generated interesting data on assessing the short-term risk for the patients. Indeed, this information may clarify the appropriate future treatment and therefore has a key importance for the physician developing a therapy plan for the emergency department patient.

It may justify a decision on a more aggressive medicinal therapy, noninvasive ventilation, or even admission in an intensive care unit. By using MR-proADM in the ROC analysis, it was possible to predict the 7-day mortality rate for the patients, with an AUC of 0.727. Notably, BNP and NT-proBNP did not provide adequate data in this regard, with an AUC of 0.512 and 0.620, respectively.[7] Figure 2 demonstrates the potential of MR-proADM, NT-proBNP and BNP for predicting the 7-day, the 30-day and the 90-day mortality rates. The AUC as per the ROC analysis for the three markers during the initial 90 days are shown.

The data from the PRIDE trial were used in an analysis of the long-term prognostic value of MR-proADM. A total of 560 emergency department patients with shortness of breath, of whom 180 were diagnosed with acute heart failure, were followed up. NT-proBNP had a

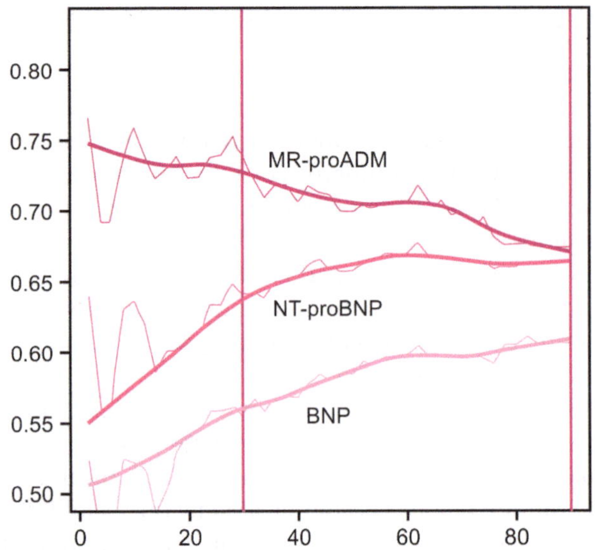

MR-proADM, midregion pro-adrenomedullin; NT-proBNP, N-terminal proB-type natriuretic peptide; BNP, B-type natriuretic peptide.

FIG. 2: Area under the curve for survival to 90 days for mid-region pro-adrenomedullin and N-terminal proB-type natriuretic peptide

With permission from: Maisel A, et al. Mid-region pro-hormone markers for diagnosis and prognosis in acute dyspnea: results from the BACH (Biomarkers in Acute Heart Failure) trial. J Am Coll Cardiol. 2010;55(19):2062-76.

greater prognostic value than the MR-proADM AUC for predicting the 1- or 4-year mortality rate.[46]

Boyer et al. specified that MR-proADM not only provides data on the outcome but also reflects changes in the therapies administered to the patients. Forty-eight patients with heart failure had their MR-proADM concentrations measured at the initiation of therapy and after 24 hours. A reduction of 49% in this biomarker was observed.[47] Further research is necessary to confirm this data and to clarify whether it is possible to use MR-proADM to guide the medicinal therapy.

In conclusion, MR-proADM is a biomarker which may be used as an effective instrument to predict the short-term prognosis after diagnosing a patient with acute heart failure. This prognosis is important when prescribing initial therapy in the emergency department. None of the established natriuretic peptides provides such reliable short-term data and that is where the unique advantage of MR-proADM lies. Further research is necessary to find out whether individualized management of the medicinal therapy in accordance with the MR-proADM levels is possible.

COPEPTIN

Arginine vasopressin (AVP) is a hormone involved in the regulation of the body's individual reaction to endogenous stress. It is also called antidiuretic hormone (ADH), adiuretin or vasopressin. Arginine vasopressin is synthesized in the hypothalamus as a preprohormone. Following its transportation to the pituitary gland, it is released in the blood. Its production may be triggered by various acute conditions such as sepsis, stroke, myocardial infarction, and acute heart failure.[48]

In acute heart failure, AVP exerts its effects trough the V1 and V2 receptors. By binding to the V2 receptor in the blood, AVP reduces the density of the aquaporin 2 channels by activating cAMP. Thus, the natriuresis and the diuresis are reduced. By binding to the V1 receptors, AVP increases the calcium concentration in the cell through activation of phosphatidylinositol. This process leads to arterial vasoconstriction and increased afterload. Thus, a prerequisite for cardiac remodeling is created. Increased inotropy is also observed. The direct activation of the myocyte V1 receptor stimulates cardiac remodeling.[48-50]

The elevation of the vasopressin levels in the blood in acute heart failure has been proven.[51] It is difficult to measure this hormone in the clinical practice due to the short plasma half-life. In such cases, copeptin, which is released during the transformation of preprovasopressin to vasopressin, is a reliable marker. The copeptin concentration in the blood corresponds to that of vasopressin.[49]

Various studies have shown that copeptin has a strong prognostic value in patients with acute heart failure. Potocki et al. compared the prognostic value of copeptin and the natriuretic hormones in 287 emergency department patients with shortness of breath. During the 30-day follow-up period, 29 of the patients died. The ROC analysis had an AUC of 0.83 (95% CI = 0.76–0.90) for predicting the 30-day mortality rate. With BNP and NT-proBNP, the values were 0.76 (95% CI = 0.67–0.84) and 0.63 (95% CI = 0.53–0.74), respectively. After adjustment for the known risk factors, copeptin was the most reliable predictor for the 30-day mortality rate among all patients, with an HR of 3.88 (95% CI = 1.94–7.77; p <0.001), and among the acute heart failure patients, with an HR of 5.99 (95% CI = 2.55–14.07; p <0.001).[52] The ROC curves of the three biomarkers are presented on figure 3.

In the BACH trial including 1,641 emergency department patients with shortness of breath, the 90-day prognostic value of copeptin was assessed. Maisel et al. demonstrated that the quartile with the highest increase in copeptin levels in patients with acute heart failure had the highest mortality rate, with an HR of 3.85 (95% CI = 1.83–8.09; p <0.001).[53] The reduction of copeptin concentration during therapy also had a prognostic value in such patients.[54]

In 2007, Gegenhuber et al. reported a positive correlation between the copeptin levels and the long-term mortality rate. They performed 1-year follow-up in a clinical study of 137 patients with acute heart failure. The ROC analysis showed similar results for copeptin and BNP. The AUC for both markers was 0.69 (95% CI = 0.60–0.76) and 0.72 (95% CI = 0.63–0.79), respectively.[55]

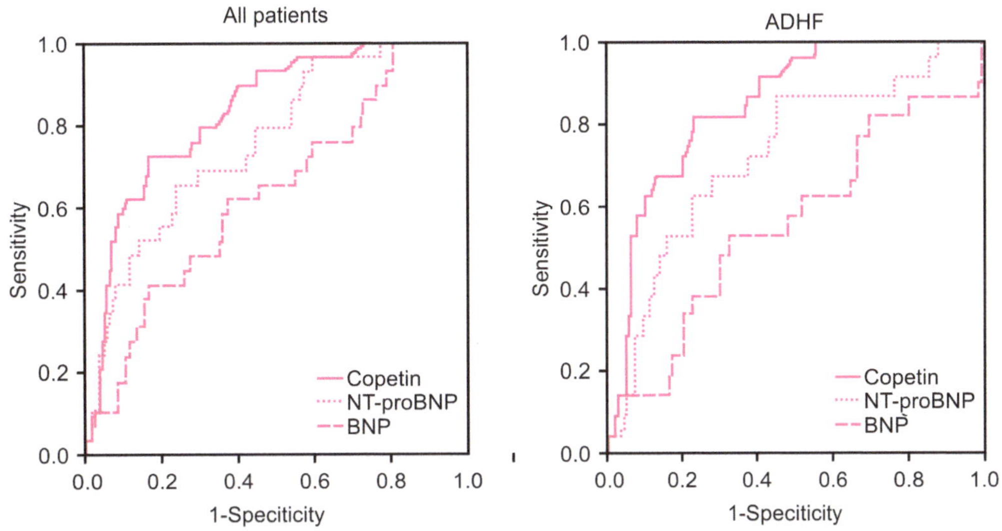

ADHF, acute decompensated heart failure; BNP, B-type natriuretic peptide; NT-proBNP, N-terminal B-type natriuretic peptide.

FIG. 3: Diagnostic accuracy for copeptin, B-type natriuretic peptide and N-terminal proBNP to predict 30-day mortality in patients with dyspnea and in patients with acute decompensated heart failure

Source: Potocki M, Breidthardt T, Mueller A, Reichlin T, Socrates T, Arenja N, et al. Copeptin and risk stratification in patients with acute dyspnea. Crit Care. 2010;14(6):R213.

The evidence available from clinical trials supports the strong short-term and long-term prognostic value of copeptin in patients with acute heart failure. Naturally, the measurements of this biomarker should be interpreted within the clinical context. Its main limitations are related to the broad spectrum of acute diseases which lead to its increase. Furthermore, steroid therapy greatly affects copeptin levels. There is no available data to aid interpretation in such cases.[56]

RENAL BIOMARKERS IN ACUTE HEART FAILURE

Acute kidney injury is one of the most common comorbidities on hospitalization with acute heart failure. It is observed in up to two-thirds of the patients admitted to emergency departments.[57] The coexistence of these two conditions is defined as cardiorenal syndrome. Furthermore, it is irrelevant which organ was affected first.[58]

In such cases, renal function is a strong independent predictor of prognosis. This was demonstrated in ADHERE, where the in-hospital mortality in patients with normal renal function and acute heart failure was under 1.9% compared to 11.2% in patients with severe cardiorenal syndrome.[57]

The biomarker which is most commonly used to evaluate renal function, expressed through the eGFR, is creatinine. This biomarker is a product of the metabolism of creatine in the muscle cells. Creatinine is not only filtered at the glomerulus, but also actively secreted in small quantities in the renal tubule. Different renal factors influence the concentration of creatinine in the blood: the most important being muscle mass, ethnicity, and gender. These parameters are taken into account for the use of formulas that enable the calculation of eGFR through the concentration of creatinine in the serum such as the CKD-EPI equation and the Modification of Diet in Renal Disease (MDRD) study equation.[58]

The use of creatinine in the clinical practice has two main disadvantages. The first one is that its concentration increases only when about 50% of the renal function is lost. This results in inability to recognize milder impairments in renal function. The second one is related to its slow kinetics. The elevation of creatinine levels may only be measured with substantial delay, which makes its use in acute circumstances problematic.[58]

Therefore, in recent years new markers of renal function impairment have been researched. Among them, the most promising one is the neutrophil gelatinase-associated lipocalin (NGAL). It is also known as lipocalin-2 (LCN2) or oncogene 24p3. Neutrophil gelatinase-associated lipocalin was initially discovered in specific granules in the neutrophil granulocytes. In the kidneys, it is synthesized in the epithelial cells of the proximal tubule. The elevated NGAL concentration in the urine is specific for an impairment explained by kidney injury.[5] The increase in NGAL levels in the urine and the blood may be established as early as 2 hours following impairment of the renal function. This is about 2 days sooner compared to creatinine.[58]

These properties of NGAL make it a suitable marker to recognize kidney injury in patients with acute heart failure. Its strong prognostic value in this situation has already been demonstrated in various clinical studies.

Palazzuoli et al. measured BNP, NGAL, and cystatin C on emergency department admission of 231 patients with acute heart failure. Seventy-eight of them developed kidney injury. The mortality and rehospitalization rate was followed up for 6 months. For prediction of acute kidney injury, the use of NGAL with a cut-off point of 134 ng/mL yielded an AUC of 0.81 (95% CI = 0.76–0.88; p <0.001) in an ROC analysis. B-type natriuretic peptide and cystatin C had an AUC of 0.54 (95% CI = 0.45–0.62; p = 0.32) and 0.56 (95% CI = 0.47–0.64; p = 0.15), respectively. When NGAL was used to predict mortality or rehospitalization in patients, the AUC in the ROC analysis was 0.76 (95% CI = 0.70–0.83; p <0.001). B-type natriuretic peptide and cystatin C had an AUC of 0.59 (95% CI = 0.51–0.67; p = 0.01) and 0.67 (95% CI = 0.60–0.75; p = 0.001), respectively.[59] These results demonstrated that NGAL is a reliable and a good tool to predict the development of acute kidney injury in patients with acute heart failure, as well as to predict the 6-month mortality and rehospitalization.

Patients with acute heart failure and renal function impairment are difficult to treat. The complications of the cardiorenal syndrome are associated with longer hospital stay and higher mortality rate. Therefore, close monitoring of renal function in these patients is essential. In the routine clinical practice, it is performed by measuring blood levels of creatinine. The disadvantages of this biomarker may be compensated by introducing new biomarkers such as NGAL, which would facilitate the choice of therapy for these patients and may possibly improve their prognosis.

D-DIMER

Heart failure patients have a high risk of venous thromboembolism (VTE). This may be explained with stasis, inflammatory processes, and endothelial dysfunction, which are also components of Virchow's triad and the pathophysiology in heart failure.[60]

Pulmonary embolism occurs in approximately 5% of emergency department patients with shortness of breath.[7] It is often a precipitant of heart failure decompensation. Various studies have demonstrated that between 6 and 12% of patients with acute heart failure were also diagnosed with pulmonary embolism.[7,61] Darze et al. showed that in patients hospitalized with acute heart failure, the incidence of thromboembolism was increased despite anticoagulant prophylaxis.[62] This data demonstrated the great importance of correctly diagnosing thromboembolic diseases in patients with acute heart failure. Cardiology associations recommend immediate assessment for possible pulmonary embolism when patients present with acute heart failure.[63]

D-dimer has been established as an indispensable part of diagnosing pulmonary embolism. This biomarker allows the rapid exclusion of VTE in the majority of emergency department patients.[64]

The D-dimer molecule is a product of fibrin degradation. The increased concentration of D-dimer in the blood is a sign of simultaneous activation of coagulation and fibrinolysis in the presence of thrombosis. This increase may be measured approximately 2 hours following thrombus development.[65,66]

It should be considered that other causes besides acute thrombosis may also lead to elevated D-dimer levels in the blood. This phenomenon can be explained with the impact of the inflammatory processes on the factors involved in homeostasis.[60] As a result, elevated D-dimer concentrations in the blood may be observed in infections, carcinomas, liver cirrhosis, etc.[67]

When patients present in the emergency department with shortness of breath, it is important to consider the probability of pulmonary embolism as a likely cause for these symptoms. The clinical assessment of the attending physician allows the probability of this disease to be estimated. The results for the D-dimer concentration measured in the blood are interpreted based on this probability.[63,64]

Various scores for establishing the probability of pulmonary embolism are used in clinical practice. The Modified Wells criteria are among the most widely used (Table 1). This score classifies patients into two groups:

- A low-risk group
- A high-risk group.[68]

TABLE 1: Clinical model for predicting the pretest probability of pulmonary embolism

Clinical characteristic	Score
Clinical symptoms of DVT (leg swelling, pain with palpation)	3.0
Other diagnosis less likely than pulmonary embolism	3.0
Heart rate >100	1.5
Immobilization (≥3 days) or surgery in the previous four weeks	1.5
Previous DVT/pulmonary embolism	1.5
Hemoptysis	1.0
Malignancy	1.0
Probalillity	**Score**
Simplified clinical probablility assessment (modified wells criteria)	
High	>4.0
Low	≤4.0

DVT, deep vein thrombosis.

Source: van Belle A, Buller HR, Huisman M V, Huisman PM, Kaasjager K, Kamphuisen PW, et al. Effectiveness of managing suspected pulmonary embolism using an algorithm combining clinical probability, D-dimer testing, and computed tomography. JAMA. American Medical Association. 2006;295(2):172-9.

In the low-risk group, a D-dimer concentration in the blood below 500 ng/mL can rule out the diagnosis of pulmonary embolism. With higher levels of D-dimer concentration in the blood, further diagnostic procedures such as computed tomography or lung scintigraphy are required. High-risk patients with a high pretest probability of pulmonary embolism should undergo diagnostic imaging irrespective of the D-dimer concentration measured in the blood.[64,65] Interestingly, various studies reported 5–50% false-positive results for pulmonary embolism when diagnostic imaging was used in this subgroup. In contrast, in high-risk patients with negative D-dimer, the false-negative results for pulmonary embolism obtained from computed tomography were as low as 1%.[66]

There are cases where additional factors should be considered when using the aforementioned score. In patients over 50 years of age, D-dimer concentration in the blood of 500 ng/mL is known to have a lower specificity for the diagnosis of pulmonary embolism. Douma et al. demonstrated in a prospective study of 5,135 patients over 50 years of age that matching this limit resulted in more precise diagnosing of pulmonary embolism. In their study, they used a D-dimer limit calculated as the product of the patient's age multiplied by 10 ng/mL.[69] The safety of this limit was also confirmed in a large multicenter prospective study.[70]

In patients with infection, carcinoma, liver cirrhosis, or advanced pregnancy, the use of D-dimer concentration in the blood for diagnosing pulmonary embolism is problematic. In such cases, the positive predictive value of the test decreases, while the negative predictive value remains high.[64]

On the one hand, D-dimer has a key role in diagnosing pulmonary embolism, one of the most important differential diagnoses for acute heart failure. On the other hand, its value for assessing the prognosis in patients hospitalized with acute heart failure is of significant interest.

In conclusion, D-dimer is an indispensable biomarker for diagnosing pulmonary embolism in the majority of emergency department patients with shortness of breath. It should be used within the context of the physician's clinical assessment of the probability of pulmonary embolism. This assessment should be based on validated scores such as the Modified Wells score.[68] In patients with a high probability of pulmonary embolism, nonelevated D-dimer is not sufficient to rule out the diagnosis of pulmonary embolism. There are cases where additional factors should be considered when using this biomarker. Matching the reference limits may improve diagnostics in patients over 50 years of age. The use of D-dimer in patients with infections, active malignancy, surgery, injury, cirrhosis, etc. is problematic.[64] The D-dimer value for defining the risk in patients with acute heart failure is a meaningful goal for future research.[71]

CONCLUSION

Assessment of biomarkers, in particular natriuretic peptides, is established as a key step in the process of treating patients with acute heart failure. Within the context of the patient's clinical assessment, their use improves the diagnostic and prognostic estimate of the attending physician.

Acute heart failure is a syndrome which encompasses various pathophysiological processes. The use of other biomarkers in addition to the natriuretic peptides may reflect this complexity more appropriately and in turn provide further guidance for determining the diagnosis, the prognosis and the treatment of the patients.

For initial differentiation between the most common comorbidities accompanying acute heart failure, the biomarkers of necrosis (cardiac troponin I and cardiac troponin T), the biomarkers of systemic inflammation (CRP and procalcitonin) and the biomarkers of renal function (creatinine and NGAL) being some of the most important among these, are of significant importance.

Further to improving diagnostics, the biomarkers described in this chapter, used in addition to the natriuretic peptides, give the opportunity for a more precise identification of patients in high short-term and long-term risk. This in turn may allow for adequate and timely measures in these patients. The next steps may vary from closer monitoring to planning heart transplantation. Furthermore, there are emerging pilot data supporting the use of sST2, copeptin and galectin 3 to guide the specific medicinal therapy in acute heart failure.

It is important to acknowledge that our knowledge on how to best integrate the quantitative biochemical information derived from these measurements into clinical action is still very limited. Derivation and validation of specific changes in patient management are the next step and require extensive further research.

REFERENCES

1. Ponikowski P, Voors AA, Anker SD, et al. 2016 ESC Guidelines for the diagnosis and treatment of acute and chronic heart failure. Eur Heart J. 2016;37(27):2129-200.
2. Mueller C, Christ M, Cowie M, Cullen L, Maisel AS, Masip J, et al. European Society of Cardiology-Acute Cardiovascular Care Association Position paper on acute heart failure: A call for interdisciplinary care. Eur Hear J. Acute Cardiovasc Care. 2017;6(1):81-6.
3. Yancy CW, Jessup M, Bozkurt B, Butler J, Casey DE, Drazner MH, et al. 2013 ACCF/AHA guideline for the management of heart failure: A report of the American College of Cardiology Foundation/American Heart Association Task Force on practice guidelines. Circulation. 2013;128(16):1810-52.
4. Teerlink JR, Cotter G, Davison BA, Felker GM, Filippatos G, Greenberg BH, et al. Serelaxin, recombinant human relaxin-2, for treatment of acute heart failure (RELAX-AHF): a randomised, placebo-controlled trial. Lancet. 2013;381(9860):29-39.

5. Maisel A, Mueller C, Adams K, Anker SD, Aspromonte N, Cleland JG, et al. State of the art: Using natriuretic peptide levels in clinical practice. Eur J Heart Fail. 2008;10(9):824-39.
6. Yancy CW, Jessup M, Bozkurt B, Butler J, Casey DE, Colvin MM, et al. 2017 ACC/AHA/HFSA Focused Update of the 2013 ACCF/AHA Guideline for the Management of Heart Failure: A Report of the American College of Cardiology/American Heart Association Task Force on Clinical Practice Guidelines and the Heart Failure Society of America. J Am Coll Cardiol. 2017;70(6):776-803.
7. Maisel A, Mueller C, Nowak R, Peacock WF, Landsberg JW, Ponikowski P, et al. Mid-region pro-hormone markers for diagnosis and prognosis in acute dyspnea: results from the BACH (Biomarkers in Acute Heart Failure) trial. J Am Coll Cardiol. 2010;55(19):2062-76.
8. Braunwald E. Heart failure. JACC Heart Fail. 2013;1(1):1-20.
9. Maisel AS, Choudhary R. Biomarkers in acute heart failure—state of the art. Nat Rev Cardiol. 2012;9(8):478-90.
10. Omland T, Røsjø H, Giannitsis E, Agewall S. Troponins in heart failure. Clin Chim Acta. 2015;443:78-84.
11. Pascual-Figal DA, Casas T, Ordonez-Llanos J, Manzano-Fernández S, Bonaque JC, Boronat M, et al. Highly sensitive troponin T for risk stratification of acutely destabilized heart failure. Am Heart J. 2012;163(6):1002-10.
12. Tarvasmäki T, Harjola VP, Nieminen MS, Siirilä-Waris K, Tolonen J, Tolppanen H, et al. Acute heart failure with and without concomitant acute coronary syndromes: patient characteristics, management, and survival. J Card Fail. 2014;20(10):723-30.
13. Tarvasmäki T, Harjola VP, Nieminen MS, Siirilä-Waris K, Tolonen J, Tolppanen H, et al. Acute heart failure with and without concomitant acute coronary syndromes: patient characteristics, management, and survival. J Card Fail. 2014;20(10):723-30.
14. Flaherty JD, Bax JJ, De Luca L, Rossi JS, Davidson CJ, Filippatos G, et al. Acute heart failure syndromes in patients with coronary artery disease early assessment and treatment. J Am Coll Cardiol. 2009;53(3):254-63.
15. Roffi M, Patrono C, Collet JP, Mueller C, Valgimigli M, Andreotti F, et al. 2015 ESC Guidelines for the management of acute coronary syndromes in patients presenting without persistent ST-segment elevation: Task Force for the Management of Acute Coronary Syndromes in Patients Presenting without Persistent ST-Segment Elevation of the European Society of Cardiology (ESC). Eur Heart J. 2016;37(3):267-315.
16. Januzzi JL, Filippatos G, Nieminen M, Gheorghiade M. Troponin elevation in patients with heart failure: On behalf of the third Universal Definition of Myocardial Infarction Global Task Force: Heart Failure Section. Eur Heart J. 2012;33(18):2265-71.
17. Peacock WF, De Marco T, Fonarow GC, Diercks D, Wynne J, Apple FS, et al. Cardiac troponin and outcome in acute heart failure. N Engl J Med. 2008;358(20):2117-26.
18. Arenja N, Reichlin T, Drexler B, Oshima S, Denhaerynck K, Haaf P, et al. Sensitive cardiac troponin in the diagnosis and risk stratification of acute heart failure. J Intern Med. 2012;271(6):598-607.
19. Ray P, Birolleau S, Lefort Y, Becquemin MH, Beigelman C, Isnard R, et al. Acute respiratory failure in the elderly: etiology, emergency diagnosis and prognosis. Crit Care. 2006;10(3):R82.
20. Demissei BG, Cleland JG, O'Connor CM, Metra M, Ponikowski P, Teerlink JR, et al. Procalcitonin-based indication of bacterial infection identifies high risk acute heart failure patients. Int J Cardiol. 2015;204:164-71.
21. Davies J. Procalcitonin. J Clin Pathol. 2015;68(9):675-9.
22. Maisel A, Neath SX, Landsberg J, Mueller C, Nowak RM, Peacock WF, et al. Use of procalcitonin for the diagnosis of pneumonia in patients presenting with a chief complaint of dyspnoea: results from the BACH (Biomarkers in Acute Heart Failure) trial. Eur J Heart Fail. 2012;14(3):278-86.
23. Clyne B, Olshaker JS. The C-reactive protein. J Emerg Med. 1999;17(6):1019-25.
24. Pepys MB, Hirschfield GM. C-reactive protein: a critical update. J Clin Invest. 2003;111(12):1805-12.
25. Joffe E, Justo D, Mashav N, Swartzon M, Gur H, Berliner S, et al. C-reactive protein to distinguish pneumonia from acute decompensated heart failure. Clin Biochem. 2009;42(16-17):1628-34.
26. Park JJ, Choi DJ, Yoon CH, Oh IY, Jeon ES, Kim JJ, et al. Prognostic value of C-reactive protein as an inflammatory and N-terminal probrain natriuretic peptide as a neurohumoral marker in acute heart failure (from the Korean Heart Failure registry). Am J Cardiol. 2014;113(3):511-7.
27. Anand IS, Latini R, Florea VG, Kuskowski MA, Rector T, Masson S, et al. C-reactive protein in heart failure: prognostic value and the effect of valsartan. Circulation. 2005;112(10):1428-34.
28. Kalogeropoulos AP, Tang WHW, Hsu A, Felker GM, Hernandez AF, Troughton RW, et al. High-sensitivity C-reactive protein in acute heart failure: insights from the ASCEND-HF trial. J Card Fail. 2014;20(5):319-26.
29. Bartunek J, Delrue L, Van Durme F, Muller O, Casselman F, De Wiest B, et al. Nonmyocardial production of ST2 protein in human hypertrophy and failure is related to diastolic load. J Am Coll Cardiol. 2008;52(25):2166-74.
30. Januzzi JL, Peacock WF, Maisel AS, Chae CU, Jesse RL, Baggish AL, et al. Measurement of the interleukin family member ST2 in patients with acute dyspnea: results from the PRIDE (Pro-Brain Natriuretic Peptide Investigation of Dyspnea in the Emergency Department) study. J Am Coll Cardiol. 2007; 50(7):607-13.
31. Rehman SU, Mueller T, Januzzi JL. Characteristics of the novel interleukin family biomarker ST2 in patients with acute heart failure. J Am Coll Cardiol. 2008;52(18):1458-65.
32. Pascual-Figal DA, Manzano-Fernández S, Boronat M, Casas T, Garrido IP, Bonaque JC, et al. Soluble ST2, high-sensitivity troponin T- and N-terminal pro-B-type natriuretic peptide: complementary role for risk stratification in acutely decompensated heart failure. Eur J Heart Fail. 2011;13(7):718-25.
33. Breidthardt T, Balmelli C, Twerenbold R, Mosimann T, Espinola J, Haaf P, et al. Heart failure therapy-induced early ST2 changes may offer long-term therapy guidance. J Card Fail. 2013;19(12):821-8.
34. Daniels LB, Bayes-Genis A. Using ST2 in cardiovascular patients: a review. Future Cardiol.2014;10(4):525-39.
35. Lala RI, Puschita M, Darabantiu D, Pilat L. Galectin-3 in heart failure pathology – "another brick in the wall"? Acta Cardiol. 2015;70(3):323-31.
36. Mallick A, Januzzi JL. Biomarkers in acute heart failure. Rev Esp Cardiol (Engl Ed). 2015;68(6):514-25.
37. van Kimmenade RR, Januzzi JL, Ellinor PT, Sharma UC, Bakker JA, Low AF, et al. Utility of amino-terminal pro-brain natriuretic peptide, galectin-3, and apelin for the evaluation of patients with acute heart failure. J Am Coll Cardiol. 2006;48(6):1217-24.
38. Shah RV, Chen-Tournoux AA, Picard MH, Van Kimmenade RRJ, Januzzi JL. Galectin-3, cardiac structure and function, and long-term mortality in patients with acutely decompensated heart failure. Eur J Heart Fail. 2010;12(8):826-32.
39. Carrasco-Sánchez FJ, Aramburu-Bodas O, Salamanca-Bautista P, Morales-Rull JL, Galisteo-Almeda L, Páez-Rubio MI, et al. Predictive value of serum galectin-3 levels in patients with acute heart failure with preserved ejection fraction. Int J Cardiol. 2013;169(3):177-82.
40. Maisel A, Xue Y, van Veldhuisen DJ, Voors AA, Jaarsma T, Pang PS, et al. Effect of spironolactone on 30-day death and heart failure rehospitalization (from the COACH Study). Am J Cardiol. 2014;114(5):737-42.
41. Srivatsan V, George M, Shanmugam E. Utility of galectin-3 as a prognostic biomarker in heart failure: where do we stand? Eur J Prev Cardiol. 2015;22(9):1096-110.
42. Peacock WF. Novel biomarkers in acute heart failure: MR-pro-adrenomedullin. Clin Chem Lab Med. 2014;52(10):1433-5.
43. Ishimitsu T, Ono H, Minami J, Matsuoka H. Pathophysiologic and therapeutic implications of adrenomedullin in cardiovascular disorders. Pharmacol Ther. 2006;111(3):909-27.
44. Yuyun MF, Narayan HK, Ng LL. Prognostic significance of adrenomedullin in patients with heart failure and with myocardial infarction. Am J Cardiol. 2015;115(7):986-91.
45. Potocki M, Ziller R, Mueller C. Mid-regional pro-adrenomedullin in acute heart failure: a better biomarker or just another biomarker? Curr Heart Fail Rep. 2012;9(3):244-51.
46. Shah RV, Truong QA, Gaggin HK, Pfannkuche J, Hartmann O, Januzzi JL. Mid-regional pro-atrial natriuretic peptide and pro-adrenomedullin testing for the diagnostic and prognostic evaluation of patients with acute dyspnoea. Eur Heart J. 2012;33(17):2197-205.
47. Boyer B, Hart KW, Sperling MI, Lindsell CJ, Collins SP. Biomarker changes during acute heart failure treatment. Congest Heart Fail. 2012;18(2):91-7.
48. Schrier RW, Abraham WT. Hormones and hemodynamics in heart failure. N Engl J Med. 1999;341(8):577-85.
49. Schurtz G, Lamblin N, Bauters C, Goldstein P, Lemesle G. Copeptin in acute coronary syndromes and heart failure management: State of the art and future directions. Arch Cardiovasc Dis. 2015;108(6-7):398-407.

50. Udelson JE, Smith WB, Hendrix GH, Painchaud CA, Ghazzi M, Thomas I, et al. Acute hemodynamic effects of conivaptan, a dual V1A and V2 vasopressin receptor antagonist, in patients with advanced heart failure. Circulation. 2001;104(20):2417-23.
51. Goldsmith SR, Gheorghiade M. Vasopressin antagonism in heart failure. J Am Coll Cardiol. 2005;46(10):1785-91.
52. Potocki M, Breidthardt T, Mueller A, Reichlin T, Socrates T, Arenja N, et al. Copeptin and risk stratification in patients with acute dyspnea. Crit Care. 2010;14(6):R213.
53. Maisel A, Xue Y, Shah K, Mueller C, Nowak R, Peacock WF, et al. Increased 90-day mortality in patients with acute heart failure with elevated copeptin: secondary results from the Biomarkers in Acute Heart Failure (BACH) study. Circ Heart Fail. 2011;4(5):613-20.
54. Vetrone F, Santarelli S, Russo V, Lalle I, De Berardinis B, Magrini L, et al. Copeptin decrease from admission to discharge has favorable prognostic value for 90-day events in patients admitted with dyspnea. Clin Chem Lab Med. 2014;52(10):1457-64.
55. Gegenhuber A, Struck J, Dieplinger B, Poelz W, Pacher R, Morgenthaler NG, et al. Comparative evaluation of B-type natriuretic peptide, mid-regional pro-A-type natriuretic peptide, mid-regional pro-adrenomedullin, and Copeptin to predict 1-year mortality in patients with acute destabilized heart failure. J Card Fail. 2007;13(1):42-9.
56. Katan M, Christ-Crain M. The stress hormone copeptin: a new prognostic biomarker in acute illness. Swiss Med Wkly. 2010;140:w13101.
57. Heywood JT, Fonarow GC, Costanzo MR, Mathur VS, Wigneswaran JR, Wynne J, et al. High prevalence of renal dysfunction and its impact on outcome in 118,465 patients hospitalized with acute decompensated heart failure: a report from the ADHERE database. J Card Fail. 2007;13(6):422-30.
58. Bouquegneau A, Krzesinski JM, Delanaye P, Cavalier E. Biomarkers and physiopathology in the cardiorenal syndrome. Clin Chim Acta. 2015;443:100-7.
59. Palazzuoli A, Ruocco G, Pellegrini M, De Gori C, Del Castillo G, Franci B, et al. Comparison of Neutrophil Gelatinase-Associated Lipocalin Versus B-Type Natriuretic Peptide and Cystatin C to Predict Early Acute Kidney Injury and Outcome in Patients With Acute Heart Failure. Am J Cardiol. 2015;116(1):104-11.
60. Lip GY, Gibbs CR. Does heart failure confer a hypercoagulable state? Virchow's triad revisited. J Am Coll Cardiol. 1999;33(5):1424-6.
61. Correia LCL, Góes C, Ribeiro H, Cunha M, Paula R de, Esteves JP. Prevalência e preditores de embolia pulmonar em pacientes com insuficiência cardíaca agudamente descompensada. Arq Bras Cardiol. 2012;98(2):120-5.
62. Darze ES, Latado AL, Guimarães AG, Guedes RA, Santos AB, de Moura SS, et al. Incidence and Clinical Predictors of Pulmonary Embolism in Severe Heart Failure Patients Admitted to a Coronary Care Unit. Chest. 2005;128(4):2576-80.
63. Ponikowski P, Voors AA, Anker SD, Bueno H, Cleland JGF, Coats AJS, et al. 2016 ESC Guidelines for the diagnosis and treatment of acute and chronic heart failure. Eur Heart J. 2016;37(27):2129-200.
64. Konstantinides SV, Torbicki A, Agnelli G, Danchin N, Fitzmaurice D, Galiè N, et al. 2014 ESC guidelines on the diagnosis and management of acute pulmonary embolism. Eur Heart J. 2014;35(43):3033-69, 3069a-3069k.
65. Giannitsis E, Mair J, Christersson C, Siegbahn A, Huber K, Jaffe AS, et al. How to use D-dimer in acute cardiovascular care. Eur Heart J Acute Cardiovasc Care. 2015. pii: 2048872615610870. [Epub ahead of print].
66. Mager JJ, Schutgens RE, Haas FJ, Westermann CJ, Biesma DH. The early course of D-dimer concentration following pulmonary artery embolisation. Thromb Haemost. 2001;86(6):1578-9.
67. Zannad F, Stough WG, Regnault V, Gheorghiade M, Deliargyris E, Gibson CM, et al. Is thrombosis a contributor to heart failure pathophysiology? Possible mechanisms, therapeutic opportunities, and clinical investigation challenges. Int J Cardiol; 2013;167(5):1772-82.
68. van Belle A, Büller HR, Huisman M V, Huisman PM, Kaasjager K, Kamphuisen PW, et al. Effectiveness of managing suspected pulmonary embolism using an algorithm combining clinical probability, D-dimer testing, and computed tomography. JAMA. 2006;295(2):172-9.
69. Douma RA, le Gal G, Söhne M, Righini M, Kamphuisen PW, Perrier A, et al. Potential of an age adjusted D-dimer cut-off value to improve the exclusion of pulmonary embolism in older patients: a retrospective analysis of three large cohorts. BMJ. 2010;340:c1475.
70. Righini M, Van Es J, Den Exter PL, Roy PM, Verschuren F, Ghuysen A, et al. Age-adjusted D-dimer cutoff levels to rule out pulmonary embolism: the ADJUST-PE study. JAMA. 2014;311(11):1117-24.
71. Minami Y, Haruki S, Jujo K, Itani R, Shimazaki K, Arashi H, et al. Elevated D-dimer levels predict an adverse outcome in hospitalized patients with acute decompensated heart failure. Int J Cardiol. 2016;204:42-4.

18

CHAPTER

Bioimpedance Vector Analysis in Acute Heart Failure

Salvatore Di Somma, Silvia Navarin

INTRODUCTION

Acute heart failure (AHF) is defined as rapid new-onset or worsening symptoms and signs of heart failure (HF) that results from any structural or functional impairment of the left ventricle.[1] It is a life-threatening condition with a rising prevalence worldwide[2] and requires early diagnosis, risk stratification, and treatment. Despite the improvement in AHF diagnosis and treatment and the consequent reduction in mortality,[3] the rate of rehospitalization for these patients is still very high,[2,4] with a 1-month readmission rate of 25%,[5] congestion being the main reason for it.[6] These patients usually refer to the emergency department (ED), complaining for dyspnea and peripheral edema, both related to fluid overload.[7] However, the presence of signs or symptoms of clinical congestion becomes evident after days or even weeks of so called "hemodynamic congestion".[6] Total body fluid overload is not only a benchmark for AHF diagnosis, but also for its prognosis,[8] since it has already proved the relationship between congestion and patient's poor outcome.[9] However, to the authors' knowledge, although different methods for assessing clinical congestion are available, such as an accurate physical examination, chest X-ray, thorax and inferior vena cava index ultrasound evaluation (Fig. 1), there is still not a standardized algorithm confirmed by guidelines.[6]

Gheorghiade et al. recently proposed an interesting grading congestion score on the basis of the classical method (Table 1).[6] In this complex scenario, the bioimpedance vector analysis (BIVA) found its role showing its additive diagnostic and prognostic value to assess congestion in AHF.[7]

BIOIMPEDANCE VECTOR ANALYSIS

Bioimpedance vector analysis is a noninvasive technique to estimate body composition by bioelectrical impedance measurements.[10,11] All biological structures have a specific resistance, defined as the strength of opposition

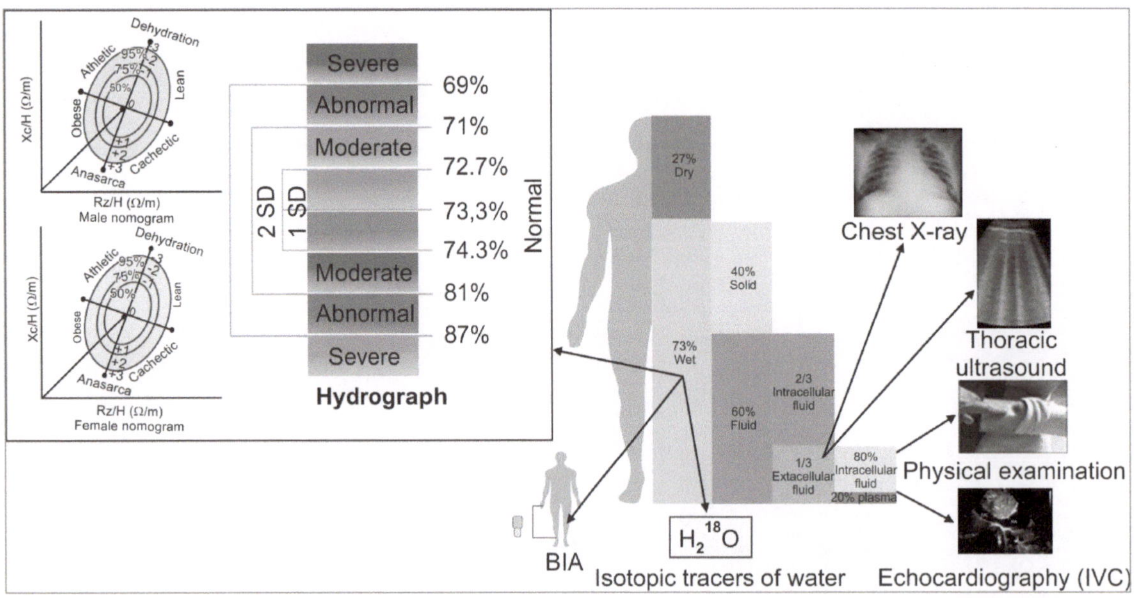

BIA, bioimpedence vector analysis; IVC, inferior vena cava.

FIG. 1: Methods for assessing congestion ***(For color version, see Plate 2)***

TABLE 1: Grading Congestion Score[6]

Variable	Score				
	−1	0	1	2	3
Beside assessment					
Orthopnea*	–	None	Mild	Moderate	Severe/worst
JVP (cm)	<8 and no hepatojugular reflux	–	8–10 or hepatojugular reflux	11–15	>16
Hepatomegly	Absent in the setting of normal JVP	Absent	Liver edge	Moderate pulsatile enlargement	Maddive tender enlargement extending to midline
Edema	–	None	1+	2+	3+/4+
Laboratory					
Natriuretic peptide (one)					
BNP	–	<100	100–299	300–500	>500
NT pro-BNP	–	<400	400–1,500	1,500–3,000	3,000
Dynamic maneuvers					
Orthostatic	Significant decrease in SBP or increase in HR	No change in SBP or HR	–	–	–
–	–	No difficulty	Mild	Moderate	Severe/worst
6 min walk test	>400 m	300–400 m	200–300 m	100–200 m	<100 m
Valsalva maneuver	Normal respinse	–	Absent overshoot pattern	Square wave pattern	–

JVP, jugular venous pressure; BNP, B-type natriuretic peptide; NT pro-BNP, N-terminal proB-type natriuretic peptide; SBP, systolic blood pressure; HR, heart rate.
Congestion grade: <1, none; 1–7, mild; 8–14, moderate; 15–20, severe. Edema, in the absence of other cause of edema.
*Orthopnea: 0, absent; mild (use of one pillow); moderate (use od more than one pillow); severe, sleeps on an armchair on in a seated position.

by a tissue to the electric current flow.[12] The BIVA method measures the opposition of body tissues to the flow of an alternating current of 300 μA, called bioelectrical impedance, administered by four surface electrodes at an operating frequency of 50 kHz.[12] This bioelectrical impedance (Z) consists of two components, resistance (Rz) and reactance (Xc).[13] In order to simplify the measurement, the human body is approximated as a sum of five interconnected cylinders that act as conductors in parallel and while the Rz is inversely related with the amount of total body water, the Xc is considered proportional to body mass.[14,15] Four cutaneous electrodes, two on the wrist and two on the ipsilateral ankle, are applied with an interelectrode distance of at least 5 cm to prevent electrodes interaction. The subject must be supine and avoid skin contacts with the trunk or with the stretcher.[14] Free fluid in thorax and abdomen, as pleural effusion, ascites and urine does not influence BIVA assessment.[13] The results are obtained in 30 seconds and they can be displayed in two ways, as a vector or as a single number expressed in percentage in a scale, called hydrograph (or hydrogram). The first method represents the bivariate vector with its two components (Rz and Xc), adjusted by the patient's height, in a nomogram that is different for men and women.[13] In the same coordinate system, three tolerance ellipses are plotted and they correspond to the 50th, 75th, and 95th vector percentile of the healthy reference population.[1] The major axis of this tolerance ellipses represents hydration status while the minor axis reflects tissue mass. In the second method, the 50th percentile corresponds to the values included in the range between 72.7 and 74.3%.[7] Bioimpedance vector analysis results are very easy and rapid to be interpreted (Fig. 2).

As previously discussed, fluids are good conductors so the length of Z vector, which represents body's impedance, is inversely related to fluid volume. Moreover, several studies have agreed on the delineation of the 75% tolerance ellipse as the boundary of normal tissue hydration.[16] Consequently, vectors outside the upper pole of the 75% ellipse indicate dehydration, whereas vectors outside the lower pole of 75% confidence ellipse represent overhydration (Fig. 2), and shorter the vector, more severe is the condition of fluid overload.[17,18] However, it has been suggested that the window of tolerance for hyper- or dehydration may vary in patients with different diseases.[19] Bioimpedance vector analysis also allows to stratify the severity of both overhydration and dehydration subdividing these two classes into mild, moderate or severe volume abnormalities.[20] Bioimpedance vector analysis device is handy and portable and can be applied in every critical setting, such as the ED, because it does

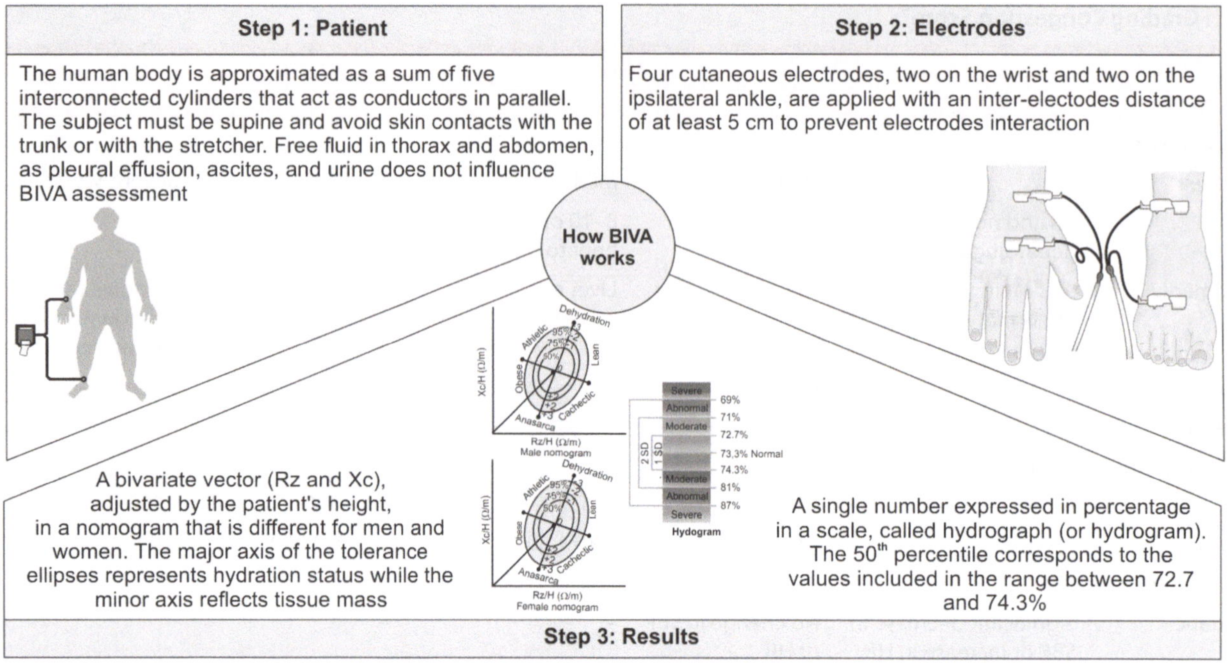

FIG. 2: Bioimpedance vector analysis measurement *(For color version, see Plate 3)*

not require to be plugged and can be easily carried at the patient's bedside (Fig. 2). Furthermore, BIVA technique has shown to be able to detect the change of the amount of body fluid. For example, it has demonstrated the elongation of the vector not only in chronic renal failure patients after hemodyalisis[17] and after peritoneal dialysis[1] ($p < 0.001$ in men, $p = 0.03$ in women), but also in AHF patients after diuretic therapy (Fig. 3).[19,21] Application fields are day by day moving from nephrology to critical care. In intensive care unit patients, the central venous pressure (CVP) was significantly and inversely correlated with individual impedance vector components ($r^2 = 0.28$ and 0.27 with resistance and reactance, respectively), and with both vector components together ($r^2 = 0.31$). Specifically, CVP values greater than 12 mm Hg were associated with shorter impedance vectors, indicating fluid overload. On the other hand, CVP values less than 3 mm Hg were associated with longer impedance vectors, reflecting tissue dehydration. Moreover, the progressive increase of CVP values was associated with shorter and down-sloping impedance vectors on the nomogram.[22]

Bioimpedance Vector Analysis Role in Acute Heart Failure Diagnosis

According to the large number of published studies, the role of BIVA is becoming pivotal for the assessment of total body congestion in AHF.[23] Its appealing characteristics, such as quick and simple use, noninvasiveness, and low cost make this device suitable in a variety of medical settings, such as the ED. Moreover, BIVA technique has already shown to be more accurate and more reliable when compared with other impedance techniques.[7] In AHF patients, BIVA has proved to be strongly related to brain natriuretic peptide (BNP) values,[24] New York Heart Association (NYHA) functional classes[25] and CVP[22] and to allow physicians to detect fluid overload even before the appearance of peripheral edema.[19] Results obtained recently from our group confirmed the additive diagnostic value of BIVA in easily and quickly detecting AHF patients. As summarized in figure 3, patients' vectors were grouped as 95% confidence interval (CI) ellipses of point vectors (Fig. 3). While the white ellipses of the no-AHF cohort demonstrated normal hydration status (inside the 50% tolerance ellipse) in both genders, for congestive patients (grey ellipses) the 95% CI ellipse was displaced along the major axis and between 75 and 95% tolerance ellipses both for females and males, indicating body fluid congestion (Fig. 3). At ED admission, compared with the no-AHF cohort, the hydrogen index (HI) mean value was significantly higher in the AHF group (81.2 ± 6.7% vs. 72.9 ± 3.6%, <0.001), while Xc/H and Rz/H mean values were significantly lower in congestive patients ($p < 0.001$).[26]

It was also demonstrated that combined use of BIVA plus BNP may improve the management of AHF patients in ED, compared to BNP alone. When considered separately, BNP is internationally recognized to represent left ventricle pressure and volume overload, while HI is proportional to total body fluid congestion.[7,27] The combined use of both BNP and BIVA measurements leads to early and accurate AHF diagnosis. However, it is known that a BNP value between 100 and 400 pg/mL is considered to be a "gray zone" with lower diagnostic

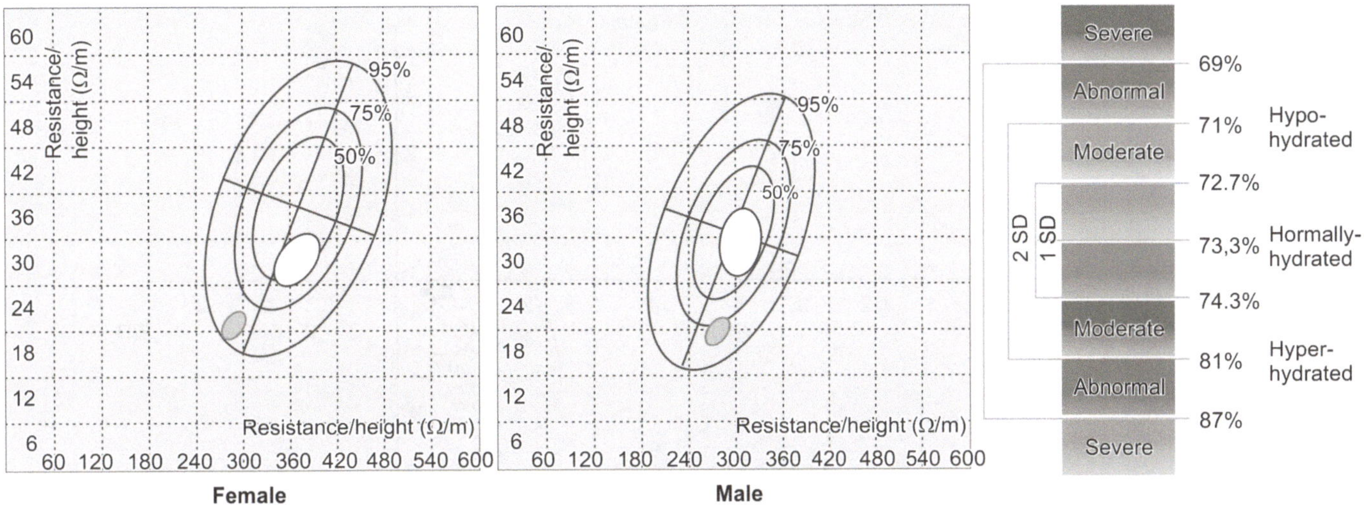

FIG. 3: Vectors' 95% confidence ellipses of congestive patients (gray) and control group (white) for female and for male[26] ***(For color version, see Plate 3)***

accuracy.[28] In this complex scenario, BIVA seems to be helpful for physicians in distinguishing between cardiogenic and noncardiogenic dyspnea.[29] Even if BNP value is between 100 and 400 pg/mL, congestion detected by BIVA with an HI greater than 74.3% proved a strong reclassification power for AHF diagnosis (net reclassification improvement 77%).[26]

The evaluation of total body fluid is fundamental in patients with cardiorenal syndrome too.[30] The results of the study by Ronco et al. suggested the "5B" approach to cardiorenal syndrome patients, that stands for balance of fluids (reflected by body weight), blood pressure, biomarkers, BIVA, and blood volume.[31]

Due to its quick and easy use, BIVA should also be tested in primary care setting for monitoring patients with HF. This innovative application could help primary care physicians in detecting sooner HF decompensation, before it becomes clinically evident, thus preventing HF worsening that may require urgent hospitalization.[7]

Bioimpedance vector analysis alone is probably not the definitive answer to all challenging questions about AHF diagnosis, but it seems to be a useful and promising method for everyday use, especially when coupled with biomarker measurement and with other classical techniques, because it has demonstrated to be accurate, noninvasive, cheap, and easy to use.

Bioimpedance Vector Analysis Role in Acute Heart Failure Prognosis

Available data suggest the prognostic relevance of clinical congestion signs in AHF patients since hospital admission. Retrospective analysis of the studies of left ventricular dysfunction (SOLVD) treatment trial, for example, demonstrated that signs of congestion in patients with HF were associated relative increases in the risk of all cause long-term events, respectively, with 15% of death and with 43% of HF hospitalization within 38 months.[32] Several other studies have also shown that patients with hemodynamic congestion, not yet clinically evident, have poor outcomes.[33]

Due to the unquestionable role of congestion in determining the high rate of rehospitalizations in AHF patients,[6,15] a rapid, cheap, accurate, and bedside device as BIVA for quantifying congestion could be an important prognostic tool to risk stratify these patients, at both hospital admission[26] and hospital discharge.[21] A significant correlation with events (death or rehospitalization) at 3 months was observed in AHF patients with average hydration values greater than 80% at the moment of hospital discharge.[21] The prognostic value of BIVA was also confirmed in a shorter follow-up period (30 days) and with a hydration assessment obtained at the moment of a patient's arrival at ED.[26] An HI value greater than 74.3% was found out to be the predictor of worse 30-day outcome.

Furthermore, the predictive value of BIVA was also investigated in combination with another emerging biomarker: galectin-3 (GAL3), a β-galactoside-binding lectin overexpressed by macrophages during phagocytosis that has been shown to be elevated in patients with AHF as a marker of heart fibrosis.[34] In AHF patients, an early assessment of GAL3 plus BIVA showed to be useful for the risk stratification, detecting patients with higher risk of death and rehospitalization at short and long term, particularly at 30, 60, 90, and 180 days and 12 and 18 months.[35] Moreover, the combination of BIVA + GAL3 showed to increase the prognostic power for death and for rehospitalization, compared to BIVA or GAL3 alone.[35]

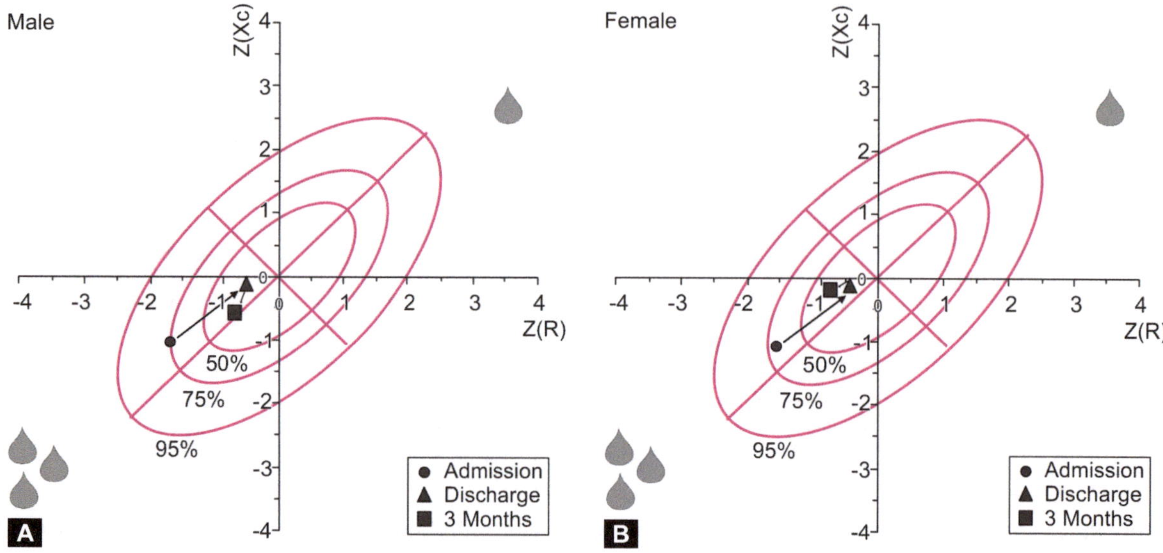

FIG. 4: Bioimpedence vector analysis plots for **A,** males and **B,** females. Graphic representation of mean bioelectrical impedance vector analysis parameters for Acute heart failure population, separated by sex, plotted against the reference population. Means at admission, discharge, and 3 months (clinical stability) are represented by symbols. Arrows denote vector migration

Bioimpedance Vector Analysis Role in Guiding Diuretic Therapy

The main goal of AHF therapy is to remove excess intravascular and extravascular fluid without worsening renal function[6] that occurs in 34% of hospitalized AHF patients and is associated with poor prognosis.[36] Combined with BNP, BIVA showed to be also useful for AHF management, not only for diagnosis and prognosis, since both measures were able to guide physicians' decisions about diuretic therapy, preventing overuse. Valle et al.[19] found that the combined assessment of BNP and BIVA could prevent unnecessary aggressive diuretic therapy, thereby reducing the level of renal complications. Moreover, it was shown that in patients hospitalized for AHF BIVA-BNP- guided management was associated with lower events after discharge, independently of other prognostic variables.[19] Sequential BIVA measurements in AHF patients showed reduction of congestion due to diuretic treatment (Fig. 4). It was proved that the congestion decrease detected by BIVA during hospitalization mirrored the improvement of clinical parameters (dyspnea, weight, and BNP).[37] Thus, BIVA could be considered a dynamic marker of congestion.

However, the use of BIVA in guiding the diuretic treatment has not been adequately studied yet. Further trials with larger patient populations are obviously encouraged to express a definitive consensus on the clinical effectiveness of BIVA. It would be interesting to standardize BIVA employment in AHF patients, in combination with biomarkers, to guide a proper and correct diuretic therapy.

CONCLUSION

Several international trials have already confirmed the accuracy of BIVA in detecting fluid overload in HF patients, even before it becomes clinically evident. These findings suggest the use of BIVA from primary care to ED in order to early recognize AHF patients. A BIVA vector placed outside the lower pole of 75% tolerance ellipse or an HI greater than 74.3% reflects body fluid overload. Moreover, it was proved that AHF patients with shorter BIVA vectors or higher HI have poorer outcome and that BIVA serial measurements reflect patients' answer to diuretic therapy. The combination of BIVA plus biomarkers such as natriuretic peptides, demonstrated to improve the diagnostic and prognostic power in AHF. Its characteristics of accuracy, noninvasiveness, cheapness, velocity, and manageability make BIVA a suitable device for everyday use in every medical setting.

REFERENCES

1. Dickstein K, Cohen-Solal A, Filippatos G, McMurray JJ, Ponikowski P, Poole-Wilson PA, et al. ESC guidelines for the diagnosis and treatment of acute and chronic heart failure 2008: the Task Force for the diagnosis and treatment of acute and chronic heart failure 2008 of the European Society of Cardiology. Developed in collaboration with the Heart Failure Association of the ESC (HFA) and endorsed by the European Society of Intensive Care Medicine (ESICM). Eur J Heart Fail. 2008;10:933-89.
2. Go AS, Mozaffarian D, Roger VL, Benjamin EJ, Berry JD, Borden WB, et al. Heart disease and stroke statistics–2013 update: a report from the American Heart Association. Circulation. 2013;127:e6-e245.
3. Stewart S, MacIntyre K, Hole DJ, Capewell S, McMurray JJ. More 'malignant' than cancer? Five-year survival following a first admission for heart failure. Eur J Heart Fail. 2001;3:315-22.
4. Jhund PS, Macintyre K, Simpson CR, Lewsey JD, Stewart S, Redpath A, et al. Long-term trends in first hospitalization for heart failure and subsequent survival

between 1986 and 2003: a population study of 5.1 million people. Circulation. 2009;119:515-23.
5. Krumholz HM, Merrill AR, Schone EM, Schreiner GC, Chen J, Bradley EH, et al. Patterns of hospital performance in acute myocardial infarction and heart failure 30-day mortality and readmission. Circ Cardiovasc Qual Outcomes. 2009;2:407-13.
6. Gheorghiade M, Follath F, Ponikowski P, Barsuk JH, Blair JE, Cleland JG, et al. Assessing and grading congestion in acute heart failure: a scientific statement from the Acute Heart Failure Committee of the Heart Failure Association of the European Society of Cardiology and endorsed by the European Society of Intensive Care Medicine. Eur J Heart Fail. 2010;12:423-33.
7. Di Somma S, Navarin S, Giordano S, Spadini F, Lippi G, Cervellin G, et al. The emerging role of biomarkers and bio-impedance in evaluating hydration status in patients with acute heart failure. Clin Chem Lab Med. 2012;50:2093-105.
8. Zile MR, Bennett TD, St John Sutton M, Cho YK, Adamson PB, Aaron MF, et al. Transition from chronic compensated to acute decompensated heart failure: pathophysiological insights obtained from continuous monitoring of intracardiac pressures. Circulation. 2008;118:1433-41.
9. Gheorghiade M, Gattis WA, O'Connor CM, Adams KF, Elkayam U, Barbagelata A, et al. Effects of tolvaptan, a vasopressin antagonist, in patients hospitalized with worsening heart failure: a randomized controlled trial. JAMA. 2004;291:1963-71.
10. Piccoli A, Italian CAPD-BIA Study Group. Bioeletric impedance vector distribution in peritoneal dialysis patient with different hydration status. Kidney Int. 2004;65:1050-63.
11. Lukasky HC, Johnson PE, Bolonchuk WW, Lykken GI. Assesment of fat-free mass using bioelectrical impedance measurements of human body. Am J Clin Nutr. 1985;41:810-7.
12. Marino R, Magrini L, Ferri E, Gagliano G, Di Somma S. B-Type natriuretic peptide and non-invasive haemodynamics and hydration assessment in the management of patients with acute heart failure in emergency department. High Blood Press Cardiovasc Prev. 2010;17:219-25.
13. Di Somma S, Lukaski HC, Codognotto M, Peacock WF, Fiorini F, Aspromonte N, et al. Consensus paper on the use of BIVA (Bioelectrical Impedance Vector Analysis) in medicine for the management of body hydration. Emerg Care J. 2011;4:6-14.
14. Peacock FW, Soto MS. Current technique of fluid status assessment. Congest Heart Fail. 2010;16:S45-51.
15. Di Somma S, Gori CS, Grandi T, Risicato MG, Salvatori E. Fluid assessment and management in the emergency department. Contrib Nephrol. 2010;164:227-36.
16. Piccoli A, Italian CAPD-BIA Study Group. Bioelectric impedance vector distribution in peritoneal dialysis patients with different hydration status. Kidney Int. 2004;65:1050-63.
17. Piccoli A. Identification of operational clues to dry weight prescription in hemodialysis using bioimpedance vector analysis. The Italian Hemodialysis-Bioelectrical Impedance Analysis (HD-BIA) Study Group. Kidney Int. 1998;53: 1036-43.
18. Bozzetto S, Piccoli A, Montini G. Bioelectrical impedance vector analysis to evaluate relative hydration status. Pediatr Nephrol. 2010;25:329-34.
19. Valle R, Aspromonte N, Milani L, Peacock FW, Maisel AS, Santini M, et al. Optimizing fluid management in patients with acute decompensated heart failure (ADHF): the emerging role of combined measurement of body hydration status and brain natriuretic peptide (BNP) levels. Heart Fail Rev. 2011;16:519-29.
20. Piccoli A, Rossi B, Pillon L, Bucciante G. A new method for monitoring body fluid variation by bioimpedance analysis: the RXc graph. Kidney Int. 1994;46:534-9.
21. Di Somma S, De Berardinis B, Bongiovanni C, Marino R, Ferri E, Alfei B. Use of BNP and bioimpedance to drive therapy in heart failure patients. Congest Heart Fail. 2010;16:S56-61.
22. Piccoli A, Pittoni G, Facco E, Favaro E, Pillon L. Relationship between central venous pressure and bioimpedance vector analysis in critically ill patients. Crit Care Med. 2000;28:132-7.
23. Tuy T, Peacock F. Noninvasive volume assessment in the emergency department: a look at B-type natriuretic peptide and bioimpedance vector analysis. Contrib Nephrol. 2011;171:187-93.
24. Valle R, Aspromonte A. Use of brain natriuretic peptide and bioimpedance to guide therapy in heart failure patients. Contrib Nephrol. 2010;164:209-16.
25. Castillo Martínez L, Colín Ramírez E, Orea Tejeda A, Asensio Lafuente E, Bernal Rosales LP, Rebollar González V, et al. Bioelectrical impedance and strength measurements in patients with heart failure: comparison with functional class. Nutrition. 2007;23:412-8.
26. Di Somma S, Lalle I, Magrini L, Russo V, Navarin S, Castello L, et al. Additive diagnostic and prognostic value of bioelectrical impedance vector analysis (BIVA) to brain natriuretic peptide 'grey-zone' in patients with acute heart failure in the emergency department. Eur Heart J Acute Cardiovasc Care. 2014;3:167-75.
27. Maisel AS, Krishnaswamy P, Nowak RM, McCord J, Hollander JE, Duc P, et al. Rapid measurement of B-type natriuretic peptide in the emergency diagnosis of heart failure. N Engl J Med. 2002;347:161-7.
28. Maisel A, Mueller C, Adams K, Anker SD, Aspromonte N, Cleland JG, et al. State of the art: using natriuretic peptide levels in clinical practice. Eur J Heart Fail. 2008;10:824-39.
29. Parrinello G, Paterna S, Di Pasquale P, Torres D, Fatta A, Mezzero M, et al. The usefulness of bioelectrical impedance analysis in differentiating dyspnea due to decompensated heart failure. J Card Fail. 2008;14:676-86.
30. Di Somma S, Gori CS, Salvatori E. How to manage cardiorenal syndrome in the emergency room. Contrib Nephrol. 2010;165:93-100.
31. Ronco C, Kaushik M, Valle R, Aspromonte N, Peacock WF. Diagnosis and management of fluid overload in heart failure and cardio-renal syndrome: the "5B" approach. Semin Nephrol. 2012;32:129-41.
32. Drazner MH, Rame JE, Stevenson LW, Dries DL. Prognostic importance of elevated jugular venous pressure and a third heart sound in patients with heart failure. N Engl J Med. 2001;345:574-81.
33. Zile MR, Bennett TD, St John Sutton M, Cho YK, Adamson PB, Aaron MF, et al. Transition from chronic compensated to acute decompensated heart failure: pathophysiological insights obtained from continuous monitoring of intracardiac pressures. Circulation. 2008;118:1433-41.
34. López E, del Pozo V, Miguel T, Sastre B, Seoane C, Civantos E, et al. Inhibition of chronic air way inflammation and remodeling by galectin-3 gene therapy in a murine model. J Immunol. 2006;176:1943-50.
35. De Berardinis B, Magrini L, Zampini G, Zancla B, Salerno G, Cardelli P, et al. Usefulness of combining galectin-3 and BIVA assessments in predicting short- and long-term events in patients admitted for acute heart failure. Biomed Res Int. 2014;2014:983098.
36. Metra M, Nodari S, Parrinello G, Bordonali T, Bugatti S, Danesi R, et al. Worsening renal function in patients hospitalised for acute heart failure: clinical implications and prognostic significance. Eur J Heart Fail. 2008;10:188-95.
37. Alves FD, Souza GC, Aliti GB, Rabelo-Silva ER, Clausell N, Biolo A. Dynamic changes in bioelectrical impedance vector analysis and phase angle in acute decompensated heart failure. Nutrition. 2015;31:84-9.

19

CHAPTER

Echocardiographic Assessment of Acute Heart Failure in the Emergency Department

Jayant K Raikhelkar, Brian D Hoit

INTRODUCTION

Heart failure (HF) is a common cardiovascular disorder that threatens to become a major healthcare epidemic.[1] It is estimated that over 870,000 new cases of HF are diagnosed annually in the United States, with a prevalence of 5.7 million adult Americans and more than 23 million individuals worldwide.[1,2] It is anticipated that the prevalence of HF will increase 46% by 2030 in the United States alone.[2] Heart failure is the leading cause of admission to the hospital for patients aged 65 and older in the United States;[3] it is estimated that annually over 1 million Americans are discharged from the hospital with a diagnosis of HF.[2] The magnitude of this problem makes HF a significant driver of healthcare expenditures. Thus, the total cost related to HF in the United States, approximately 30.7 billion dollars in 2012, is projected to be 69.7 billion dollars by 2030.[2]

Almost all patients with HF will at some point visit the emergency department (ED) with an episode of acute HF.[4] There were 676,000 ED visits for acute HF in 2010 in the United States and approximately 84% of these visits eventually led to hospital admission,[4,5] making the ED a major portal of entry into the hospital for patients with acute HF. In the limited time these patients spend in the ED, correct diagnosis and appropriate stabilizing measures are critical. The ED also serves as the site of decision-making regarding the ultimate disposition of the patient, which may include an ED observation unit, a hospital telemetry unit, an intensive care unit, or discharge home.[4] In this manner, the ED plays critical and comprehensive roles in the management of acute HF in modern medical practice with direct impact on morbidity, mortality, length of stay, and healthcare costs.[6]

Despite its vital role, there is currently limited evidence that ED management can be used to guide the early phase of acute HF care, owing to the lack of large scale clinical trials that specifically recruit patients in the ED setting.[4] Possible contributory factors include ensuring accurate diagnosis of acute HF and long-standing difficulties in establishing a consensus on reasonable end points.[4] The American Heart Association (AHA) issued a scientific statement to describe the state of current management of acute HF in 2010 and it was also addressed in both the 2012 European Society for Cardiology (ESC) as well as the 2013 American College of Cardiology Foundation/American Heart Association (ACC/AHA) guidelines for management of HF.[3,4,7]

DEFINITIONS

Heart failure is defined as a complex clinical syndrome that results from a structural or functional impairment of either ventricular filling or ejection of blood that may be caused by disorders of the pericardium, myocardium, endocardium, heart valves, great vessels, or certain metabolic abnormalities.[3] The hallmarks of HF include the symptoms of dyspnea and fatigue and clinical signs of fluid retention. Acute HF has been defined as the rapid onset or worsening of symptoms and signs of HF.[7] It is a life-threatening condition that requires immediate medical attention and usually leads to urgent admission to the hospital. In contrast, patients with known but compensated HF are classified as having chronic heart failure.[7] Although there are many causes of HF, the majority of cases result from impaired left ventricular function which may be systolic, diastolic or both.[3] The left ventricular ejection fraction (EF), the "lingua franca" and "vox populi" of expressing left ventricular contractile performance, is an important value used to classify HF, prognosticate and assess risk, and select and evaluate the response to medical as well as device therapies. Additionally, clinical trials of HF select patients on the basis of EF; thus, in most studies, HF patients are classified as having HF with either reduced EF (HFrEF, with EF ≤40%) or preserved EF (HFpEF, with EF ≥40%),[3] although partition values as high as 50% have been used.[8]

Although clinical diagnosis by means of history and physical examination plays a central role in the evaluation of the patient with suspected acute HF, these methods lack adequate specificity and sensitivity for definitive diagnosis.[9-11] Cardiovascular imaging, thus plays a crucial adjunctive role in the diagnosis and management of acute HF. Among the imaging modalities available, the 2013 ACCF/ACC guidelines for management of HF state that the most useful diagnostic test in the evaluation of patients with or at risk for HF is a comprehensive two-dimensional echocardiogram with Doppler flow studies.[3] This is explained by its accuracy, portability, safety and well as cost compared to other modalities.[7] Echocardiography has been shown to change therapy in 60–80% of patients in the prehospital setting and lead to improvement in diagnostic accuracy and efficiency in the ED.[11] Although transthoracic echocardiography (TTE) is generally the initial modality employed, transesophageal echocardiography (TEE), contrast echocardiography and lung ultrasonography may be useful. The focused cardiac ultrasound examination and pocket-sized hand-held devices [hand-carried ultrasound (HCU)] are specific protocols and instrumentation, respectively, used in critical care settings such as the ED. In this chapter, we will review the utility of echocardiography in the ED in the setting of acute heart failure.

INSTRUMENTATION

The modern day practice of medicine in the ED mandates balancing the need for accuracy of diagnosis against the need for expeditious decision-making to ensure efficiency in hospital workflow. "Comprehensive echocardiography" is a complete examination of cardiac structure and function using fully equipped high-end platforms performed by a skilled operator and interpreted by an experienced, qualified physician. However, physicians in the ED are required to possess a broad knowledge base in order to manage a multitude of varied medical and surgical emergencies. Although acute HF may be one of the most common diagnoses in the ED, the typical ED physician is unable to dedicate time to acquire echocardiographic skills of those specialized in the field.[12] In addition, the use of traditional scanners in the ED setting is limited by their size, complexity of use and cost.[12] In such circumstances, the use of hand-held cardiac ultrasound (HCU) in the ED is an attractive option. The evolution of echocardiographic technology has led to a number of miniaturized devices suitable for rapid assessment of cardiac structures and function.[12] These devices generally weigh less than 5 kg and cost from $8,000 to $30,000.[13] Current models include Vscan, MobiUS SP1, Acuson P10, and Signos.[12] Cardiac structures and abnormalities that have been accurately detected by HCU include disorders of the left ventricle (enlargement, hypertrophy, systolic function), left atrium (enlargement), right ventricle (enlargement, function) pericardial effusion, and inferior vena cava (IVC) size.[13] The use of HCU has been validated in physicians at various stages of training. For example, a study by Razi et al. showed that internal medicine residents with minimal training with HCU were able to accurately identify patients with acute HF with reduced EF about 22 hours earlier than formal results of a routine complete echocardiogram.[14] Similarly, there was excellent agreement with EF detected by HCU and formal echocardiography in a study of trained cardiologists.[15] While good diagnostic accuracy is reported in the hands of both experienced and inexperienced operators, image quality is reduced compared to high-end platforms, which may result in suboptimal and less reliable studies and the potential for misinterpretation and missed results; accordingly an assessment with these pocket-sized devices should be considered as qualitative and complimentary to the clinical examination. Abnormal studies should be followed up with a comprehensive echocardiographic examination or other studies when this can be done safely. Despite recent improvements in HCU technology, several limitations remain. These include the inability in most cases of HCU to perform several common echocardiographic features including spectral Doppler, tissue Doppler, complex image enhancement, artifact reduction, zoom mode, harmonic imaging, and optimization for cardiac contrast studies.[13] It is expected that this technology will further improve and become less expensive over time.

Comprehensive two-dimensional (2D) echocardiography remains the recommended cardiac ultrasound modality to be used in the diagnosis of acute HF as per the ACC/AHA and the ESC guidelines.[3,7] A complete study with spectral Doppler and tissue Doppler are required to maximize the diagnostic yield. Advanced imaging modalities, including deformation imaging and three-dimensional (3D) echocardiography may be of additional benefit in the acute HF syndrome.[11] However, optimal studies in the setting of acute illness may not be possible and nonstandardized views may be necessary. Other challenges to imaging in the ED may include patient positioning, positive pressure ventilation, the presence of lines and dressings, and the use of inotropic agents and circulatory support.[11]

The use of lung ultrasound may be useful in the patient with dyspnea. The presence of extravascular lung water may be identified by the presence of "B lines" or "ultrasound lung comets (ULC)."[16,17] This sign is due to subpleural interlobular septal thickening caused by edema, which causes reverberation artifacts of the ultrasound beam.[18]

B lines or ULC can be further separated into septal and ground-glass rockets. Septal rockets are due to the thickened interlobular septa, typically distributed about 7 mm apart and are the ultrasound equivalent of Kerley B lines. Ground-glass rockets have been described as confluent with 3 mm intervals, and are thought to be indicative of alveolar flooding. Ultrasound lung comets can be easily visualized using any echocardiographic device by placing the ultrasound probe along the intercostal spaces. Gargani et al. showed that the accuracy of ULC in prediction of cardiac dyspnea approaches that of brain natriuretic peptide [BNP; area under curve (AUC) 0.89 vs. 0.97].[17] Importantly, lung ultrasound detects interstitial edema, but not its underlying cause.

Transesophageal echocardiography is not a first-line imaging modality for HF assessment, but may be needed when TTE is suboptimal or in certain HF scenarios (e.g., acute valvular regurgitation, prosthetic valve dysfunction). Contrast echocardiography using second-generation agents may be used to improve endocardial definition and better assess ventricular function and enhance weak Doppler signals; recent data have confirmed the safety of these agents.[19]

PROTOCOLS

Ultrasound protocols in the ED have been used for over 20 years to facilitate systematic diagnosis and triage, for example, the use of the focused assessment with sonography in trauma (FAST) protocol.[20] Similarly, a point of care problem-oriented focused cardiac ultrasound protocol (FOCUS) has been proposed to streamline care of the patient with suspected cardiac disease, including acute HF (Box 1).[21] It can also be valuable in the patient presenting with dyspnea of unknown etiology. The main difference between standard comprehensive cardiac echocardiography and FOCUS lies in the limited pertinent information obtained. FOCUS provides information required for qualitative gross assessment of cardiac morphology and function usually reported in an absent/present or yes/no fashion.[21] The test can be performed by cardiologists or noncardiologists alike and all types of echocardiographic machines can be used, although HCU is usually the preferred modality. The goals of the FOCUS exam in the ED have been stated in the joint consensus statement of the American Society for Echocardiography (ASE) and American College of Emergency Physicians (ACEP).[20] These include assessments for the following: global cardiac systolic function, marked right and left ventricular enlargement, intravascular volume status, presence of pericardial effusion, guidance for emergent pericardiocentesis, and confirmation of transvenous pacing wire placement. The rapid evaluation of systolic function and intravascular volume status in particular helps to guide the management of acute HF. Although it is not a substitute for a comprehensive echocardiogram, FOCUS in this manner can play an important role in contemporary management of patients with acute HF in the ED.

BOX 1 Use of focused cardiac ultrasound protocol in the emergency department

Structures assessed
- Ventricular size and function
- Pericardial effusion
- Inferior vena cava size

Clinical situations assessed
- Shock
- Cardiac arrest
- Chest pain
- Chest trauma
- Heart failure

Disorders assessed
- Ischemic and nonischemic (e.g., dilated, hypertrophic and restrictive cardiomyopathies, myocarditis) ventricular dysfunction
- Cardiac tamponade
- Pulmonary embolus
- Hypovolemia

TRAINING REQUIREMENTS

The level of competency required for ED cases should be the same for cardiologists and noncardiologists,[22,23] a position endorsed by the European Association of Cardiovascular Imaging.[21] Indeed, special training requirements are suggested for performing and interpreting TTE in patients with acute cardiac conditions.[19] This training includes at least 150 studies in acute/critical care scenarios with an adequate case mix. Additional training is recommended for TEE and advanced techniques such as deformation imaging, 3D echo and myocardial perfusion imaging. Competency may be formally assessed through National Board Certification and by a continuing and committed association with an accredited echocardiography laboratory.

Recommendations for specific training and certification for users of HCU and FOCUS are outlined in a number of society-specific documents.[13,24] A recent expert consensus statement from the American Society of Echocardiography recommends a formal structured training program comprised of didactics, hands-on image acquisition and image interpretation, in an accredited graduate medical education or continuing education program.[13] The ACEP published training guidelines for all emergency ultrasound procedures, including FAST and FOCUS.[24]

Although tools to assess competency in FOCUS and HCU are not currently available, the guiding principles are that the operator performs a significant number of FOCUS studies in the real-life critical-care setting on a representative case mix using the same imaging device (typically HCU). An accredited laboratory is ideally responsible for assistance/consultation, supervision, and quality control.

ECHOCARDIOGRAPHIC DIAGNOSIS OF ACUTE HEART FAILURE

Echocardiography is the main imaging modality to be used along with clinical exam and biomarkers in order to diagnose the acute HF syndrome. Not surprisingly, dyspnea is a class I indication for comprehensive echocardiography; the utility includes classification of the syndrome according to myocardial function, evaluation of the current hemodynamic status of the patient, evaluation of valvular and pericardial disease, and potential identification of ischemia as a cause of the HF syndrome. Accordingly, an echocardiogram should be performed as soon as possible in a patient with suspected acute HF for initiation of appropriate therapies.[25] The goals for a FOCUS examination are to rule out pericardial effusion, identify global left ventricular systolic dysfunction and assess the size of the right ventricle.[20]

Determination of cardiac function in the patient with suspected HF is an essential first step (Fig. 1). Although patients with HF may have reduced (HFrEF) or preserved left ventricular function (HFpEF), those with reduced left ventricular function have been shown to benefit from evidence-based therapies.[3] Indices of left ventricular function include fractional shortening [FS = (LV end diastolic dimension–LV end systolic dimension)/ LV end diastolic dimension], ejection fraction [EF = (LV end diastolic volume –LV end systolic volume)/LV end diastolic volume], mitral annular plane systolic excursion (MAPSE), mitral annular systolic tissue velocity and deformational indices (longitudinal, circumferential, radial strain and strain rates, torsional indices). While fractional shortening can be measured with HCU, the method is only suitable for ventricles with uniform geometry and wall motion.

The recommended method for measurement of EF is the biplane method of disks.[26] The new updated guidelines for chamber quantification by the ASE and the European Association for Cardiovascular Imaging (EACI) state that the normal EF for patients over the age of 20 is

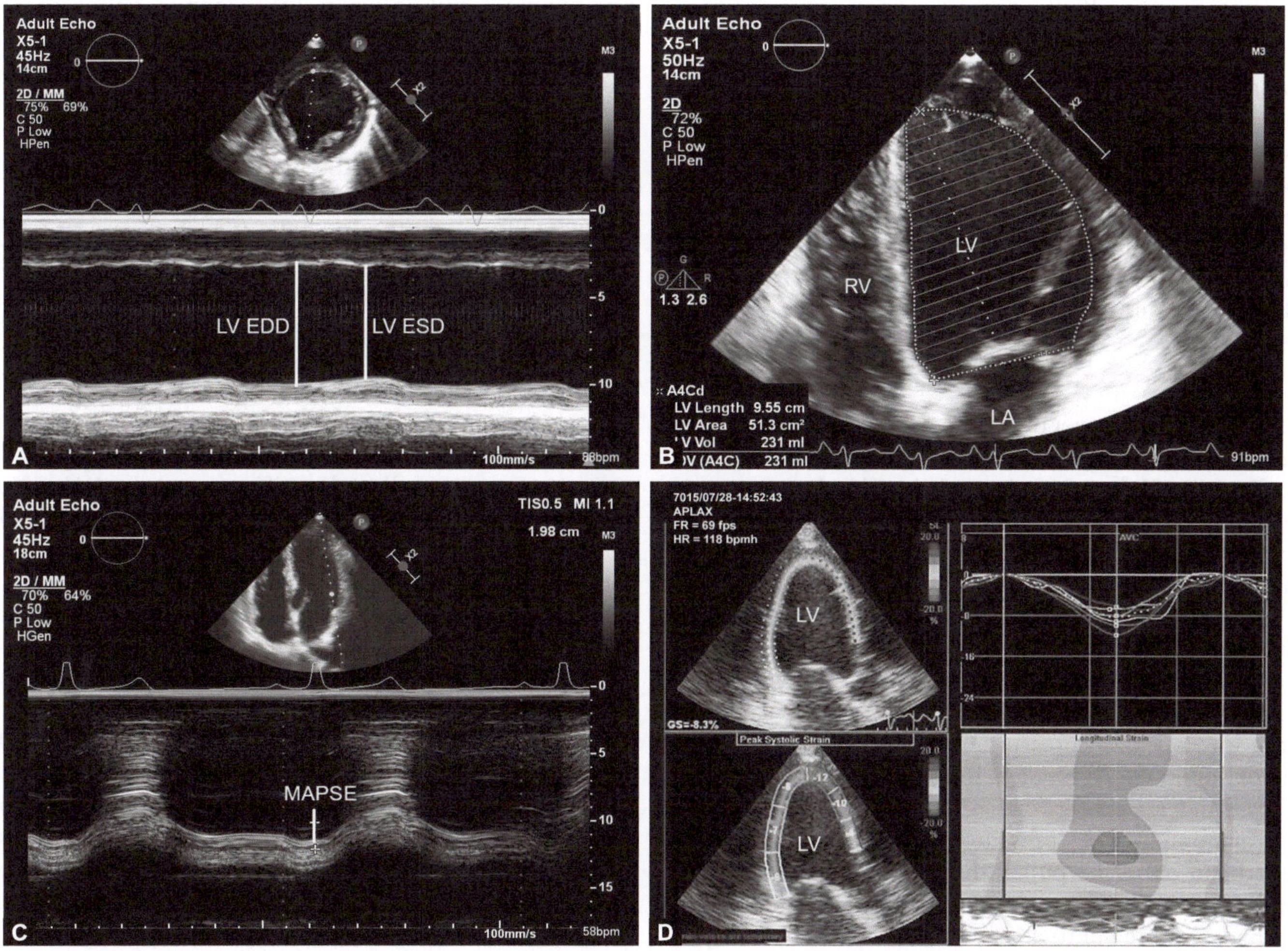

LA, left atrium; RV, right ventricle; LV, left ventricular; EDD, end-diastole; ESD, end-systole; MAPSE; mitral annular plane systolic excursion..

FIG. 1: Left ventricular (LV) function **A,** M-mode of the LV minor axis at end-diastole (LV EDD) and end-systole (LV ESD); **B,** LV end-diastolic volume measured from single plane method of discs. Planimetry of the LV at end-systole is used to calculate ejection fraction; **C,** Mitral annular plane systolic excursion (MAPSE) measured using M-mode echocardiography of the lateral mitral annulus; **D,** LV longitudinal systolic strain measured from two-dimensional speckle tracking echocardiography. Tracking and regional strain values (left), regional strain-time curves (top right), color M-mode of strain *(For color version, see Plate 4)*

53% to 73%.[26] Most studies distinguish HF with reduced EF as less than or equal to 40%.[3] In a study by Logeart et al., the use of echocardiographically determined EF less than 45% showed a sensitivity of 65% and specificity of 85% to predict acute HF.[27] Steg and et al. showed that using a cutoff value of EF 50% had a positive predictive value of 88% in correctly identifying acute HF.[28] Thus, left ventricular function by EF is a useful marker to be used in combination with clinical exam.

Mitral annular plane systolic excursion is a measurement of the mitral ring displacement at systole and is a sensitive parameter to identify early decreases in longitudinal left ventricular dysfunction.[29] The average normal value of MAPSE ranges from 12 to 15 mm and a value less than 8 mm has been shown to be associated with an EF less than 50% with a specificity of 82% and a sensitivity of 98%.[29,30] Similarly, a mitral annular systolic tissue velocity of less than 6.8 cm/s as determined by tissue Doppler imaging was able to detect an EF less than 50% with a sensitivity of 94.1% and specificity of 87%.[31]

Myocardial deformation imaging or strain imaging is a relatively newer imaging modality that is primarily used in early detection of subclinical myocardial dysfunction as seen, for example, in chemotherapy-induced cardiotoxicity.[32] A study by Kraigher-Krainer et al. showed that global longitudinal and circumferential strain are significantly reduced in patients with HFpEF compared to normal patients and patients with hypertensive heart disease without HF.[33]

Diastolic Function

It is estimated that over half of the patients with clinical HF have the syndrome of HF with preserved EF or HFpEF[34] or diastolic HF.[35] Assessment of diastolic dysfunction is thus an important step in evaluation of the patient with acute HF and echocardiography plays a fundamental role in this regard.

Left ventricular performance is dependent upon the ability to alternate from a stiff chamber in systole that ejects stroke volume at arterial pressures to a compliant chamber in diastole that allows the left ventricular to fill from low left atrial pressure.[36] Conceptually, diastole is the period in which blood is transferred from the atria to the ventricles, a process which depends upon the creation and maintenance of a pressure gradient between the two. Blood can either be pulled through the atrioventricular valves by lowered ventricular pressures (suction) or pushed into the ventricles by increased atrial pressures. Abnormalities intrinsic and extrinsic to the myocardium (Box 2) can produce a stiff (or noncompliant) left ventricular during diastole with resultant elevated filling pressures. Determination of elevated filling pressures, either invasively by right heart catheterization (RHC) or noninvasively (by echocardiography) is commonly used to make a diagnosis of the acute HF syndrome. Elevated filling pressures have been defined as a pulmonary capillary wedge pressure (PCWP) greater than 12 mm Hg or an left ventricular end diastolic pressure greater than 16 mm Hg.[36]

BOX 2 Intrinsic and extrinsic factors influencing left ventricular chamber stiffness

Intrinsic to the myocardium	Extrinsic to the myocardium
• LV chamber volume and mass	• RV interaction
• Composition of the LV wall	• Atrial function
• Viscoelasticity	• Pericardial restraint
• Myocardial relaxation	• Pleural and mediastinal pressure
• Coronary turgor	

LV, left ventricular; RV, right ventricular.

Several echocardiographic parameters are used in the assessment of diastolic function and filling pressures. left atrial volume, pulsed-wave (PW) Doppler mitral inflow and tissue Doppler annular velocity play central roles in evaluation of diastolic function.[36] The key measurements of mitral valve inflow include the peak early filling wave (E wave) velocity, the late diastolic filling wave (A wave) velocity, the E/A ratio and the deceleration time (DT) of the E wave (Fig. 2). Normally, early filling predominates over late filling and the E/A ratio (which decreases with age) lies roughly between 1 and 2.[36] In patients with abnormal relaxation (grade 1 diastolic dysfunction), early filling is slowed and filling after atrial systole is increased, leading to an E/A ratio less than 0.8 and a DT greater than 200 m/s.[36] In contrast, with prolonged and severely increased filling pressures, early filling velocities increase (over 1 m/s), DT is abbreviated (<160 ms) owing to increased diastolic stiffness and the E/A ratio is greater than or equal to 2 resulting in a pattern of restrictive filling (grade 3 diastolic dysfunction). An E/A ratio between 0.8 and 1.5 may signify normal diastolic function, or pseudonormal diastolic dysfunction (grade 2 diastolic dysfunction). Tissue Doppler annular velocities (see below) or a Valsalva maneuver (forced expiration against a closed glottis) must be incorporated to make this distinction.[28] A decrease of greater than or equal to 50% of the E/A ratio with Valsalva is highly specific for increased filling pressures in cardiac patients.[37] In patients with dilated cardiomyopathies, Doppler mitral inflow velocities correlate better with cardiac filling pressures (proportional to the grade of dysfunction), functional class and prognosis than does left ventricular EF.[38-40] However, in patients with coronary artery disease (CAD) and preserved EF, mitral variables alone have been shown to correlate poorly with hemodynamics.[41]

Tissue Doppler mitral annular velocities are a vital part of the complete 2D echocardiographic exam (Fig. 3).[36] Measurements include systolic, early diastolic and late

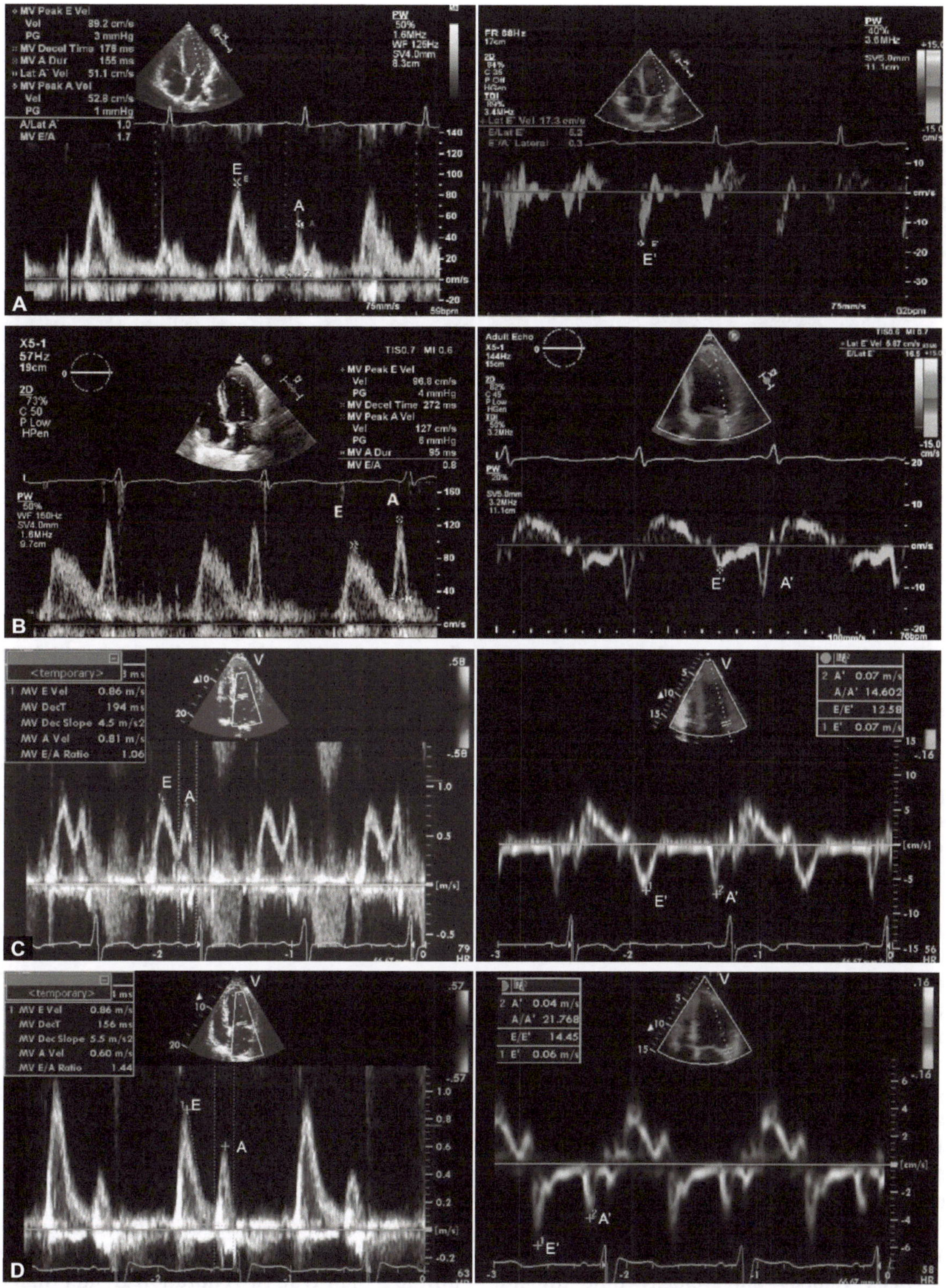

E, early diastolic transmitral flow velocity; A, late diastolic transmitral flow velocity; E′, early diastolic annular velocity; A′, late diastolic annular velocity.

FIG. 2: Transmitral flow (top) and mitral annular tissue velocities (bottom) from patients with **A,** normal diastolic function; **B,** impaired left ventricular (LV) relaxation or grade I diastolic dysfunction (DD); **C,** pseudonormal or grade II DD; and **D,** restrictive filling or grade III DD *(For color version, see Plate 5)*

diastolic annular velocities. The systolic velocities are used to assess systolic function and are similar to the M-mode echo measurement of MAPSE. Late diastolic annular velocity is used as a measure of atrial contractile function. The early diastolic annular velocity (E′ or e′) is directly correlated with the rate of LV relaxation[42] and is,

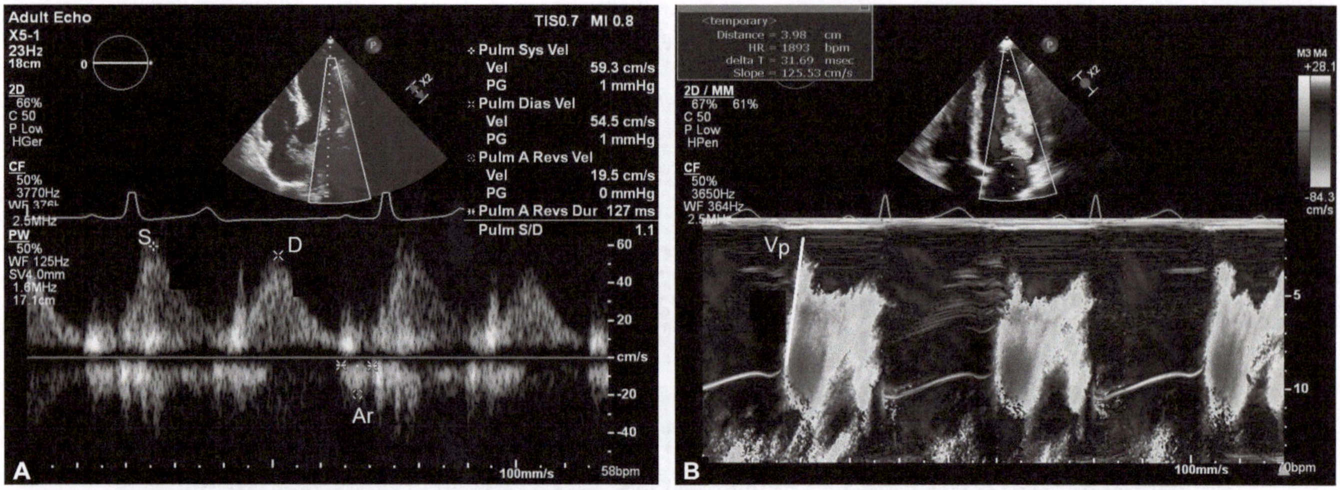

S, systolic PV velocity; D, diastolic PV velocity; Ar, reversed atrial systolic PV velocity.

FIG. 3: Ancillary parameters for grading diastolic dysfunction: **A,** pulmonary venous (PV) Doppler; **B,** flow propagation velocity (Vp) ***(For color version, see Plate 6)***

therefore, particularly useful for measurement of filling pressures and for making the clinically crucial distinction between normal and pseudonormal (grade 2 diastolic dysfunction) filling. It is recommended to measure both the septal e′ as well as the lateral e′ and average the two due to the influence of regional function on these values. The value of e′ is determined not only by left ventricular relaxation, but is also dependent to a certain extent on loading conditions and left ventricular systolic function. Although preload increases the value of e′ in normal individuals,[43] left ventricular filling pressures have been found to have minimal effect on e′ in the setting of impaired relaxation.[44] Thus, in patients with cardiac disease, e′ velocity can be used to correct for the effect of left ventricular relaxation on mitral E velocity. Once mitral inflow velocities have been obtained, the E/e′ ratio is calculated, which is used to estimate left ventricular filling pressures.[36] An E/e′ ratio less than or equal to 8 indicates normal and a ratio greater than or equal to 13 (>15 in patients with reduced EF) indicates elevated left atrial pressure.

Measurements of pulmonary venous flow using PW Doppler and the velocity of early diastolic flow propagation into the left ventricular (V_p) using color M-mode are ancillary methods that may be helpful when transmitral flow and annular tissue Doppler are ambiguous or unavailable (Fig. 3). Common measurements obtained include the peak velocity and velocity time integral (VTI) of systolic (S) and diastolic (D) flow, the S/D ratio and systolic filling fraction, and the duration of reversed flow into the pulmonary veins after atrial contraction (Ar). With increased left ventricular filling pressures and increased left ventricular stiffness, there is a decrease in the S velocity and increase in the D velocity resulting in an S/D ratio less than 1, a systolic filling fraction less than 40% and an increase in the duration of Ar relative to the A wave (Ar-A ≥30 ms).[45-48]

The flow propagation velocity (V_p) is measured as the slope of early diastolic flow on color M-mode from the mitral valve plane to the left ventricular apex. Values of V_p greater than 50 cm/s are considered normal. Slow flow patterns in patients with left ventricular failure are thought to be due to ring vortices that move slowly to the apex.[49] The ratio of peak E velocity to V_p has been shown to be proportional to left atrial pressure;[50] a ratio of greater than 2.5 predicts a PCWP greater than 15 mm Hg with reasonable accuracy in patients with reduced EF.[51]

The main clinical question that arises in management of patients with suspected acute HF is estimation of left ventricular filling pressures, which should be elevated in this state. Parameters that are described above are used in combination to estimate filling pressures. In patients with decreased EF, the first step in evaluation of filling pressures is measurement of the E/A ratio.[36] Patients with a pattern of impaired relaxation with an E/A ratio less than or equal to 1 and E velocity less than or equal to 50 cm/s generally have normal filling pressures. On the other hand, patients with restrictive filling (E/A ≥2 with DT <150 ms) are thought to have elevated filling pressures. In patients with E/A ratios between 1 and 2, additional Doppler parameters must be used to assess filling pressures. A change in E/A ratio with Valsalva maneuver of greater than or equal to 0.5, a systolic peak velocity/diastolic peak velocity ratio in pulmonary venous flow less than 1, an Ar-A duration greater than or equal to 30 ms and E/e′ (using average e′) greater than or equal to 15, are suggestive of elevated filling pressures.[36]

Estimation of filling pressures in patients with preserved EF is more challenging than in those with depressed EF.[36] In these patients, the E/e′ ratio should be calculated first. A ratio less than or equal to 8 identifies patients with normal left ventricular filling pressures, while ratio greater than or equal to 13 is indicative of elevated filling pressures. When the ratio is intermediate, use of other measurements are required. An Ar-A duration greater than or equal to 30 ms, a change in E/A ratio with Valsalva greater than or equal to 0.5 and maximal left atrial volume greater than or equal to 34 mL/m^2 are all indicative of increased left ventricular filling pressures. The presence of two or more of these abnormal parameters increases the confidence of this finding.

A study by Goonewardena et al. showed that determination of the E/e′ ratio by HCU can be used to accurately (AUC of 0.81) estimate elevated left ventricular filling pressures (as determined by PCWP). The greatest accuracy in determination of acute HF with HCU was when it was combined with clinical exam and BNP values (AUC 0.97).[52]

Measurement of Right Heart Pressures

In addition to measurement of left heart volumes and pressures, right heart involvement and estimates of pulmonary artery (PA) and right atrial pressure (RAP) are important in the evaluation, management and prognosis of the patient presenting with acute HF. Right atrial pressure is frequently approximated by IVC diameter and collapsibility during a sniff test (Fig. 4). For an IVC diameter less than 2.1 cm with greater than 50% collapse on inspiration, the RAP is assumed to be 3 mm Hg. For an IVC diameter greater than or equal to 2.1 cm with less than 50% collapse on inspiration, the RAP is assumed to be elevated to 15 mm Hg. If there is an abnormality in only one of the parameters, an intermediate value of 8 mm Hg is used.

The IVC collapse index is used to assess volume status.[6] The size of the IVC decreases with inspiration as more blood exits than fills the vessel, owing to inspiratory negative intrathoracic pressure. The IVC collapse index is defined as the difference in IVC diameter during expiration minus inspiration divided by the IVC diameter during expiration.[6] In patients with intravascular fluid overload, the IVC is dilated with minimal change in the

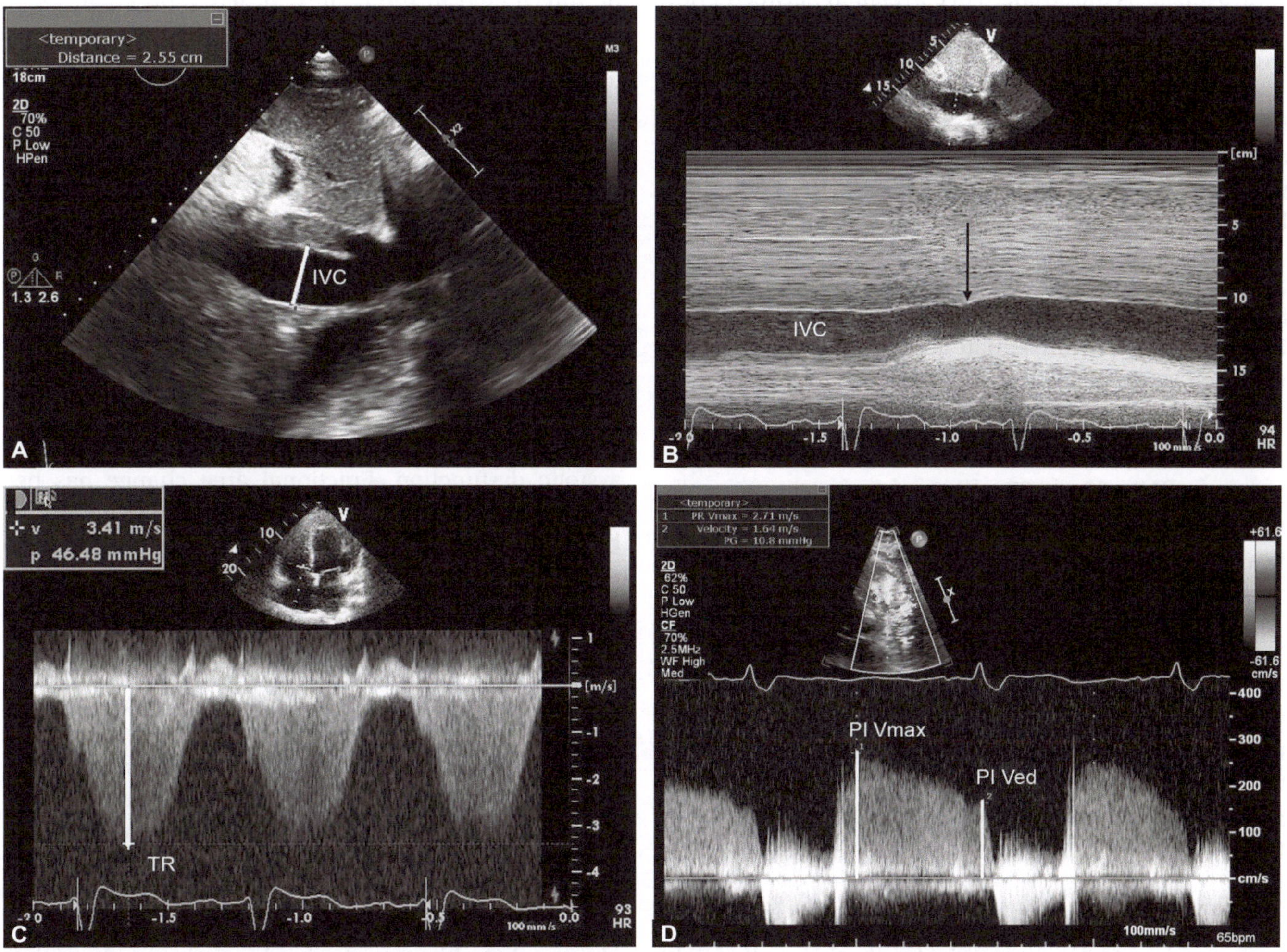

FIG. 4: Doppler-determined right heart pressures: **A,** two-dimensional of the inferior vena cava (IVC); **B,** M-mode of IVC with sniff (arrow); **C,** tricuspid regurgitation (TR) jet used to measure right ventricular (RV) and pulmonary artery (PA) systolic pressure; **D,** pulmonary insufficiency (PI) jet used to measure mean (from PI Vmax, the maximal PI velocity) and end-diastolic PA pressures (from PI Ved, the end-diastolic PI velocity) ***(For color version, see Plate 6)***

respiratory cycle. Thus, the IVC index is closer to 1 in individuals with acute HF compared to those without in whom values are usually between 0.25 and 0.75. A recent study showed the potential use of assessing change in the IVC collapsibility index to monitor the response to therapy in the ED.[53]

Through application of the simplified Bernoulli equation, velocity of the tricuspid regurgitant (TR) jet can be used to calculate right ventricular systolic pressure (RVSP):

$$RVSP = 4v^2 + RAP$$

Where v is the peak velocity in m/s of the TR jet and RAP is estimated from IVC diameter and collapsibility with sniff (Fig. 4). Pulmonary artery systolic pressure (PASP) is equal to RVSP in the absence of pulmonic stenosis or RV outflow obstruction. Tricuspid regurgitant velocity (TRV) greater than or equal to 2.8–2.9 m/s is considered abnormal, but this cutoff may not be accurate in the elderly or the obese.[54] The accuracy of RVSP determination remains controversial as the strength of correlation between PASP and RHC varies widely across the literature and tends to weaken at higher pressures.[55-57]

As with TRV, the velocity of the pulmonary regurgitant jet in early diastole and end-diastole can be applied to estimate mean PA pressure (mPAP) and PA diastolic pressure (PADP), respectively, using the simplified Bernoulli equation and adding an estimate of RAP (Fig. 4).

Pulmonary artery acceleration time is the time from the onset to the peak of the PA flow waveform as measured from pulsed Doppler. Pulmonary artery acceleration time can be used to estimate mPAP with the following validated equations:

$$mPAP = 79 - (0.45 \times \text{PA acceleration time})$$

or

$$mPAP = 90 - (0.62 \times \text{PA acceleration time})$$

If the acceleration time less than 120 ms.[54,58] However, heart rate dependency and sample location dependency and high measurement variability have limited its utility.

A method to assess pulmonary vascular resistance (PVR) employs the ratio of TRV to the time-velocity integral of the right ventricular outflow tract waveform (TVI_{RVOT}). The equation $(TRV/TVI_{RVOT}) \times 10$ was shown to provide a good estimate of PVR, but was inaccurate when very elevated (PVR >6 WU); the ratio TRV^2/TVI_{RVOT} provides a more accurate noninvasive estimate of PVR in the latter instance.[59]

Right Ventricle

In comparison to the left ventricular, the thin-walled right ventricular is highly sensitive to changes in afterload. Thus, the left ventricular can withstand a pressure-overloaded state for a longer period of time than the right ventricular and ventricular enlargement occurs early in the course of pulmonary hypertension relative to systemic hypertension.[60]

The right ventricular is uniquely challenging to image echocardiographically because of its retrosternal position, coarse trabeculations and complex shape that is difficult to model geometrically. As a result, underestimation or overestimation of right ventricular size is a common problem.[54] In addition, measurements are sensitive to probe and patient position and body habitus. Nevertheless, measurement of the linear dimensions of the RV is an integral component of echocardiographic evaluation. Dimensions that should be obtained at end-diastole from a right ventricle-focused apical four-chamber view include the basal, mid-cavity, and longitudinal (Fig. 5). Right ventricular enlargement is diagnosed by diameter greater than 41 mm at the base, 35 mm at mid-cavity, or 83 mm longitudinally.[26] However, these values are not adjusted for age, sex, race, or body size and should therefore be used cautiously. In addition, the right ventricular should be interpreted in the context of left ventricular size, as an enlarged right ventricular may reflect global cardiac dilatation. Enlargement of the proximal and distal RVOT is diagnosed when measurements exceed 35 mm and 27 mm, respectively (Fig. 5).[26]

Measures of right ventricular function include the right ventricular fractional area change (FAC), tricuspid annular plane systolic excursion (TAPSE), the tricuspid annular excursion during systole (RV S′) and the right ventricular index of myocardial performance (RIMP; Fig. 6). Right ventricular FAC is defined as:

$$FAC = \frac{\text{End-diastolic area} - \text{End-systolic area}}{\text{End-diastolic area}} \times 100$$

With FAC less than 35% indicating right ventricular systolic dysfunction. Fractional area change has been shown to correlate with right ventricular EF as determined by magnetic resonance imaging and has also been shown to predict survival.[54] Moreover, it is an independent risk predictor of HF, sudden death, stroke, and/or mortality after myocardial infarction.[61]

Tricuspid annular plane systolic excursion, which represents systolic displacement of the tricuspid annulus toward the right ventricular apex (a measure of longitudinal right ventricular contraction), has been shown to closely correlate with right ventricular EF.[62] It is a simple and highly reproducible measurement, since it does not depend on geometric assumptions or visualization of the endocardial border. Tricuspid annular plane systolic excursion less than 17 mm is considered abnormal,[26] although studies have shown that TAPSE less than 18 mm is associated with significantly reduced survival and TAPSE less than 15 mm is associated with particularly poor outcomes.[26,62] Tricuspid annular plane

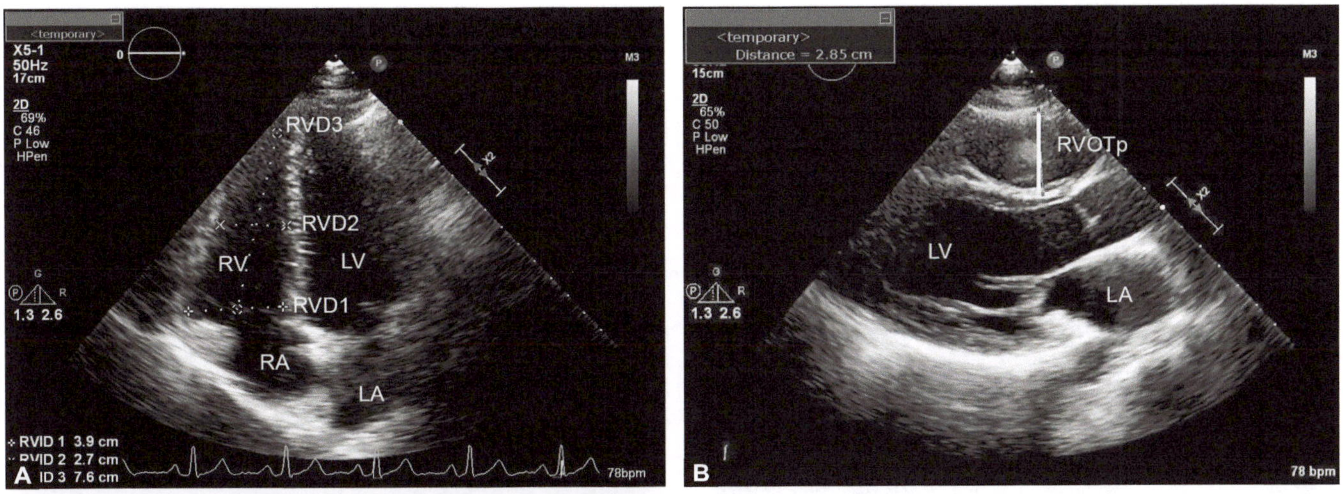

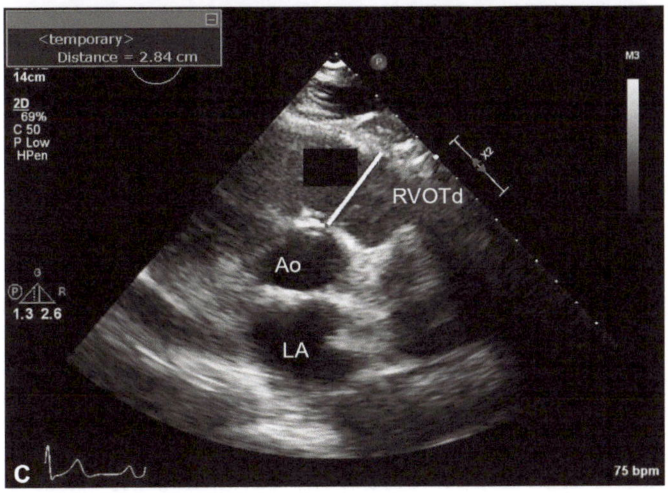

Ao, aorta; RA, right atrium; LA, left atrium.

FIG. 5: Right ventricular (RV) dimensions. **A,** RV dimensions (D1, basal; D2, mid R; and D3, longitudinal) from the RV focused view; **B,** proximal RVOT (RVOTp), from the parasternal long axis; **C,** distal RVOT (RVOTD) from the parasternal short axis

systolic excursion assumes that the systolic motion of the tricuspid annulus represents the function of the entire right ventricular and while this is true in most cases, the relationship deteriorates when wall motion is not uniform throughout the chamber.

Right ventricular S′ can be measured with tissue Doppler and similar to TAPSE, measures longitudinal systolic right ventricular function. Values less than 9.5 cm/s are considered abnormal.[26] S′ is reproducible and correlates well with other measures of RV systolic function. Its principal drawbacks are that uniform wall motion is assumed, and that being a Doppler technique, it is highly dependent on the angle between the ultrasound beam and the direction of tricuspid annular motion.

Right ventricular index of myocardial performance provides an integrated assessment of both systolic and diastolic function. RIMP is calculated as:

$$\text{RIPM} = (\text{IVRT} + \text{IVCT})/\text{RVET}$$

Where IVRT is isovolumic relaxation time, IVCT is isovolumic contraction time and RVET is right ventricular ejection time. These measurements can be obtained with either PW or tissue Doppler, but tissue Doppler minimizes error related to R-R interval variability because only a single scan is necessary; therefore, it is the preferred method.[63] The upper limit of normal is 0.54 for tissue Doppler and 0.43 for PW Doppler. Right ventricular index of myocardial performance requires no geometric assumptions, is reproducible, well-validated, and is an independent predictor of adverse outcomes in patients with pulmonary hypertension.[54,64]

ECHOCARDIOGRAPHY AND B-TYPE NATRIURETIC PEPTIDE

B-type natriuretic peptide (BNP) and N-terminal pro-BNP are secreted by the myocardium in response to increased myocardial wall stress.[65] Use of both of these biomarkers in the diagnosis of acute HF has been validated and is recommended in the European as well as the American HF management guidelines.[3,7] The utility of natriuretic peptides in diagnosis of acute HF has been compared to traditional echocardiographic methods. In a study of 122 patients with suspected acute HF, use of

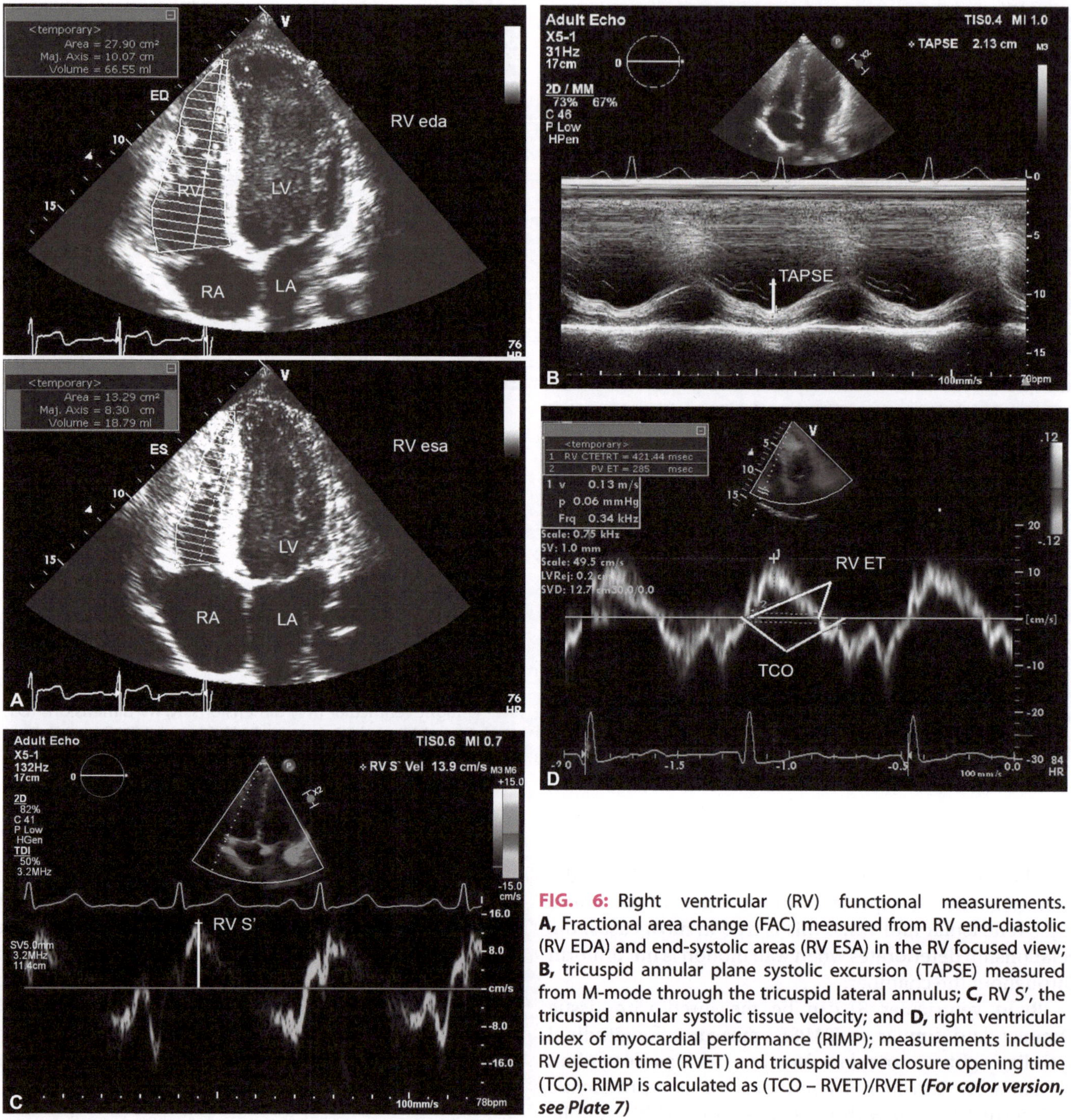

FIG. 6: Right ventricular (RV) functional measurements. **A,** Fractional area change (FAC) measured from RV end-diastolic (RV EDA) and end-systolic areas (RV ESA) in the RV focused view; **B,** tricuspid annular plane systolic excursion (TAPSE) measured from M-mode through the tricuspid lateral annulus; **C,** RV S′, the tricuspid annular systolic tissue velocity; and **D,** right ventricular index of myocardial performance (RIMP); measurements include RV ejection time (RVET) and tricuspid valve closure opening time (TCO). RIMP is calculated as (TCO – RVET)/RVET ***(For color version, see Plate 7)***

comprehensive echo Doppler had a 95% sensitivity and 88% specificity for the diagnosis of acute HF compared to BNP which had a sensitivity of 86% and specificity of 77% at a cutoff value of 250 pg/mL.[66] In this study, an E/e′ value of greater than 15 was found to be as sensitive and specific as BNP in detection of acute HF in patients with both reduced and preserved left ventricular systolic function. In addition, Brenden et al. showed that about 33% of patients admitted with acute HF possess "grey-zone values" of BNP in whom echocardiographic evaluation may be of even greater significance.[67] In a small prospective study of 34 patients with shortness of breath with intermediate levels of BNP and preserved EF, E/e′ greater than 10 was found to be powerful predictor of acute HF with a sensitivity of 100% and specificity of 78.6%.[68] Thus, tissue Doppler plays a useful adjunct role to BNP in the diagnosis of acute HF, especially in cases with indeterminate BNP with preserved left ventricular function.

Acknowledgment

The authors would like to acknowledge Ray Musarra, RCDS, for his assistance with the figures.

REFERENCES

1. Dunlay SM, Roger VL. Understanding the epidemic of heart failure: past, present, and future. Current heart failure reports. Curr Heart Fail Rep. 2014; 11(4):404-15.
2. Mozaffarian D, Benjamin EJ, Go AS, Arnett DK, Blaha MJ, Cushman M, et al. Heart disease and stroke statistics-2015 update: a report from the American Heart Association. Circulation. 2015;131(4):e29-322.
3. Yancy CW, Jessup M, Bozkurt B, Butler J, Casey DE, Drazner MH, et al. 2013 ACCF/AHA guideline for the management of heart failure: a report of the American College of Cardiology Foundation/American Heart Association Task Force on Practice Guidelines. J Am Coll Cardiol. 2013;62(16):e147-239.
4. Weintraub NL, Collins SP, Pang PS, Levy PD, Anderson AS, Arslanian-Engoren C, et al. Acute heart failure syndromes: emergency department presentation, treatment, and disposition: current approaches and future aims: a scientific statement from the American Heart Association. Circulation. 2010;122(19):1975-96.
5. Storrow AB, Jenkins CA, Self WH, Alexander PT, Barrett TW, Han JH, et al. The burden of acute heart failure on U.S. emergency departments. JACC Heart failure. 2014;2(3):269-77.
6. Collins SP, Storrow AB, Levy PD, Albert N, Butler J, Ezekowitz JA, et al. Early management of patients with acute heart failure: state of the art and future directions–a consensus document from the saem/hfsa acute heart failure working group. Acad Emerg Med. 2015;22(1):94-112.
7. McMurray JJ, Adamopoulos S, Anker SD, Auricchio A, Bohm M, Dickstein K, et al. ESC Guidelines for the diagnosis and treatment of acute and chronic heart failure 2012: The Task Force for the Diagnosis and Treatment of Acute and Chronic Heart Failure 2012 of the European Society of Cardiology. Developed in collaboration with the Heart Failure Association (HFA) of the ESC. Eur Heart J. 2012;33(14):1787-847.
8. Vasan RS, Levy D. Defining diastolic heart failure: a call for standardized diagnostic criteria. Circulation. 2000;101(17):2118-21.
9. Dao Q, Krishnaswamy P, Kazanegra R, Harrison A, Amirnovin R, Lenert L, et al. Utility of B-type natriuretic peptide in the diagnosis of congestive heart failure in an urgent-care setting. J Am Coll Cardiol. 2001;37(2):379-85.
10. Davie AP, Francis CM, Caruana L, Sutherland GR, McMurray JJ. Assessing diagnosis in heart failure: which features are any use? QJM. 1997;90(5):335-9.
11. Lancellotti P, Price S, Edvardsen T, Cosyns B, Neskovic AN, Dulgheru R, et al. The use of echocardiography in acute cardiovascular care: recommendations of the European Association of Cardiovascular Imaging and the Acute Cardiovascular Care Association. Eur Heart J Acute Cardiovasc Care. 2014. pii: 2048872614549739.
12. Dalen H, Haugen BO, Graven T. Feasibility and clinical implementation of hand-held echocardiography. Expert Rev Cardiovasc Ther. 2013;11(1):49-54.
13. Spencer KT, Kimura BJ, Korcarz CE, Pellikka PA, Rahko PS, Siegel RJ. Focused cardiac ultrasound: recommendations from the American Society of Echocardiography. J Am Soc Echocardiogr. 2013;26(6):567-81.
14. Razi R, Estrada JR, Doll J, Spencer KT. Bedside hand-carried ultrasound by internal medicine residents versus traditional clinical assessment for the identification of systolic dysfunction in patients admitted with decompensated heart failure. J Am Soc Echocardiogr. 2011;24(12):1319-24.
15. Testuz A, Muller H, Keller PF, Meyer P, Stampfli T, Sekoranja L, et al. Diagnostic accuracy of pocket-size handheld echocardiographs used by cardiologists in the acute care setting. Eur Heart J Cardiovasc Imaging. 2013;14(1):38-42. eng.
16. Gargani L. Lung ultrasound: a new tool for the cardiologist. Cardiovasc Ultrasound. 2011;9:6.
17. Gargani L, Frassi F, Soldati G, Tesorio P, Gheorghiade M, Picano E. Ultrasound lung comets for the differential diagnosis of acute cardiogenic dyspnoea: a comparison with natriuretic peptides. Eur J H Fail. 2008;10(1):70-7.
18. Ricci F, Aquilani R, Radico F, Bianco F, Dipace GG, Miniero E, et al. Role and importance of ultrasound lung comets in acute cardiac care. Eur Heart J Acute Cardiovasc Care. 2015;4(2):103-12.
19. Lancellotti P, Price S, Edvardsen T, Cosyns B, Neskovic AN, Dulgheru R, et al. The use of echocardiography in acute cardiovascular care: recommendations of the European Association of Cardiovascular Imaging and the Acute Cardiovascular Care Association. Eur Heart J Cardiovasc Imaging. 2015;16(2):119-46.
20. Labovitz AJ, Noble VE, Bierig M, Goldstein SA, Jones R, Kort S, et al. Focused cardiac ultrasound in the emergent setting: a consensus statement of the American Society of Echocardiography and American College of Emergency Physicians. J Am Soc Echocardiogr. 2010;23(12):1225-30.
21. Neskovic AN, Edvardsen T, Galderisi M, Garbi M, Gullace G, Jurcut R, et al. Focus cardiac ultrasound: the European Association of Cardiovascular Imaging viewpoint. Eur Heart J Cardiovasc Imaging. 2014;15(9):956-60.
22. Ryan T, Berlacher K, Lindner JR, Mankad SV, Rose GA, Wang A. COCATS 4 Task Force 5: Training in Echocardiography: Endorsed by the American Society of Echocardiography. J Am Soc Echocardiogr. 2015;28(6):615-27.
23. Neskovic AN, Hagendorff A, Lancellotti P, Guarracino F, Varga A, Cosyns B, et al. Emergency echocardiography: the European Association of Cardiovascular Imaging recommendations. Eur Heart J Cardiovasc Imaging. 2013;14(1):1-11.
24. Directors American College of Emergency Physics. (2008). Policy Statement. Emergency Ultrasound Guidelines 2008. [online] Available from: http://www.acep.org/workarea/DownloadAsset.aspx?id=32878. [Accessed March, 2016].
25. Breitkreutz R, Price S, Steiger HV, Seeger FH, Ilper H, Ackermann H, et al. Focused echocardiographic evaluation in life support and peri-resuscitation of emergency patients: a prospective trial. Resuscitation. 2010;81(11):1527-33..
26. Lang RM, Badano LP, Mor-Avi V, Afilalo J, Armstrong A, Ernande L, et al. Recommendations for cardiac chamber quantification by echocardiography in adults: an update from the American Society of Echocardiography and the European Association of Cardiovascular Imaging. J Am Soc Echocardiogr. 2015;28(1):1-39.e14.
27. Logeart D, Saudubray C, Beyne P, Thabut G, Ennezat PV, Chavelas C, et al. Comparative value of Doppler echocardiography and B-type natriuretic peptide assay in the etiologic diagnosis of acute dyspnea. J Am Coll Cardiol. 2002;40(10):1794-800.
28. Steg PG, Joubin L, McCord J, Abraham WT, Hollander JE, Omland T, et al. B-type natriuretic peptide and echocardiographic determination of ejection fraction in the diagnosis of congestive heart failure in patients with acute dyspnea. Chest. 2005;128(1):21-9.
29. Hu K, Liu D, Herrmann S, Niemann M, Gaudron PD, Voelker W, et al. Clinical implication of mitral annular plane systolic excursion for patients with cardiovascular disease. Eur Heart J Cardiovasc Imaging. 2013;14(3):205-12.
30. Simonson JS, Schiller NB. Descent of the base of the left ventricle: an echocardiographic index of left ventricular function. J Am Soc Echocardiogr. 1989;2(1):25-35.
31. Park YS, Park JH, Ahn KT, Jang WI, Park HS, Kim JH, et al. Usefulness of mitral annular systolic velocity in the detection of left ventricular systolic dysfunction: comparison with three dimensional echocardiographic data. J Cardiovasc Ultrasound. 2010;18(1):1-5.
32. Thavendiranathan P, Poulin F, Lim KD, Plana JC, Woo A, Marwick TH. Use of myocardial strain imaging by echocardiography for the early detection of cardiotoxicity in patients during and after cancer chemotherapy: a systematic review. J Am Coll Cardiol. 2014;63(25 Pt A):2751-68.
33. Kraigher-Krainer E, Shah AM, Gupta DK, Santos A, Claggett B, Pieske B, et al. Impaired systolic function by strain imaging in heart failure with preserved ejection fraction. J Am Coll Cardiol. 2014;63(5):447-56.
34. Givertz MM, Slawsky MT, Moraes DL, McIntyre KM, Colucci WS. Noninvasive determination of pulmonary artery wedge pressure in patients with chronic heart failure. Am J Cardiol. 2001;87(10):1213-5; A7.
35. Sharma K, Kass DA. Heart failure with preserved ejection fraction: mechanisms, clinical features, and therapies. Circ Res. 2014;115(1):79-96.
36. Nagueh SF, Appleton CP, Gillebert TC, Marino PN, Oh JK, Smiseth OA, et al. Recommendations for the evaluation of left ventricular diastolic function by echocardiography. J Am Soc Echocardiogr. 2009;22(2):107-33.
37. Hurrell DG, Nishimura RA, Ilstrup DM, Appleton CP. Utility of preload alteration in assessment of left ventricular filling pressure by Doppler echocardiography: a simultaneous catheterization and Doppler echocardiographic study. J Am Coll Cardiol. 1997;30(2):459-67.
38. Pinamonti B, Di Lenarda A, Sinagra G, Camerini F. Restrictive left ventricular filling pattern in dilated cardiomyopathy assessed by Doppler echocardiography: clinical, echocardiographic and hemodynamic correlations and prognostic implications. Heart Muscle Disease Study Group. J Am Coll Cardiol. 1993;22(3):808-15.
39. Vanoverschelde JL, Raphael DA, Robert AR, Cosyns JR. Left ventricular filling in dilated cardiomyopathy: relation to functional class and hemodynamics. J Am Coll Cardiol. 1990;15(6):1288-95.
40. Somaratne JB, Whalley GA, Gamble GD, Doughty RN. Restrictive filling pattern is a powerful predictor of heart failure events postacute myocardial infarction and in established heart failure: a literature-based meta-analysis. J Card Fail. 2007;13(5):346-52.
41. Yamamoto K, Nishimura RA, Chaliki HP, Appleton CP, Holmes DR, Redfield MM. Determination of left ventricular filling pressure by Doppler echocardiography

in patients with coronary artery disease: critical role of left ventricular systolic function. J Am Coll Cardiol. 1997;30(7):1819-26.
42. Ommen SR, Nishimura RA, Appleton CP, Miller FA, Oh JK, Redfield MM, et al. Clinical utility of Doppler echocardiography and tissue Doppler imaging in the estimation of left ventricular filling pressures: A comparative simultaneous Doppler-catheterization study. Circulation. 2000;102(15):1788-94.
43. Hasegawa H, Little WC, Ohno M, Brucks S, Morimoto A, Cheng HJ, et al. Diastolic mitral annular velocity during the development of heart failure. J Am Coll Cardiol. 2003;41(9):1590-7.
44. Nagueh SF, Sun H, Kopelen HA, Middleton KJ, Khoury DS. Hemodynamic determinants of the mitral annulus diastolic velocities by tissue Doppler. J Am Coll Cardiol. 2001;37(1):278-85.
45. Kuecherer HF, Muhiudeen IA, Kusumoto FM, Lee E, Moulinier LE, Cahalan MK, et al. Estimation of mean left atrial pressure from transesophageal pulsed Doppler echocardiography of pulmonary venous flow. Circulation. 1990;82(4):1127-39.
46. Yamamuro A, Yoshida K, Hozumi T, Akasaka T, Takagi T, Kaji S, et al. Noninvasive evaluation of pulmonary capillary wedge pressure in patients with acute myocardial infarction by deceleration time of pulmonary venous flow velocity in diastole. J Am Coll Cardiol. 1999;34(1):90-4.
47. Rossvoll O, Hatle LK. Pulmonary venous flow velocities recorded by transthoracic Doppler ultrasound: relation to left ventricular diastolic pressures. J Am Coll Cardiol. 1993;21(7):1687-96.
48. Appleton CP, Galloway JM, Gonzalez MS, Gaballa M, Basnight MA. Estimation of left ventricular filling pressures using two-dimensional and Doppler echocardiography in adult patients with cardiac disease. Additional value of analyzing left atrial size, left atrial ejection fraction and the difference in duration of pulmonary venous and mitral flow velocity at atrial contraction. J Am Coll Cardiol. 1993;22(7):1972-82.
49. Yotti R, Bermejo J, Antoranz JC, Desco MM, Cortina C, Rojo-Alvarez JL, et al. A noninvasive method for assessing impaired diastolic suction in patients with dilated cardiomyopathy. Circulation. 2005;112(19):2921-9.
50. Garcia MJ, Ares MA, Asher C, Rodriguez L, Vandervoort P, Thomas JD. An index of early left ventricular filling that combined with pulsed Doppler peak E velocity may estimate capillary wedge pressure. J Am Coll Cardiol. 1997; 29(2):448-54.
51. Rivas-Gotz C, Manolios M, Thohan V, Nagueh SF. Impact of left ventricular ejection fraction on estimation of left ventricular filling pressures using tissue Doppler and flow propagation velocity. Am J Cardiol. 2003;91(6):780-4.
52. Goonewardena SN, Blair JE, Manuchehry A, Brennan JM, Keller M, Reeves R, et al. Use of hand carried ultrasound, B-type natriuretic peptide, and clinical assessment in identifying abnormal left ventricular filling pressures in patients referred for right heart catheterization. J Card Fail. 2010;16(1):69-75.
53. Yavaşi Ö, Ünlüer EE, Kayayurt K, Ekinci S, Sağlam C, Surum N, et al. Monitoring the response to treatment of acute heart failure patients by ultrasonographic inferior vena cava collapsibility index. Am J Emerg Med. 2014;32(5):403-7.
54. Karas MG, Kizer JR. Echocardiographic assessment of the right ventricle and associated hemodynamics. Prog Cardiovasc Dis. 2012;55(2):144-60.
55. Farber HW, Foreman AJ, Miller DP, McGoon MD. REVEAL Registry: correlation of right heart catheterization and echocardiography in patients with pulmonary arterial hypertension. Congest Heart Fail. 2011;17(2):56-64.
56. Hinderliter AL, Willis PW, Barst RJ, Rich S, Rubin LJ, Badesch DB, et al. Effects of long-term infusion of prostacyclin (epoprostenol) on echocardiographic measures of right ventricular structure and function in primary pulmonary hypertension. Primary Pulmonary Hypertension Study Group. Circulation. 1997;95(6):1479-86.
57. Fisher MR, Forfia PR, Chamera E, Housten-Harris T, Champion HC, Girgis RE, et al. Accuracy of Doppler echocardiography in the hemodynamic assessment of pulmonary hypertension. Am J Respir Crit Care Med. 2009;179(7):615-21.
58. Dabestani A, Mahan G, Gardin JM, Takenaka K, Burn C, Allfie A, et al. Evaluation of pulmonary artery pressure and resistance by pulsed Doppler echocardiography. Am J Cardiol. 1987;59(6):662-8.
59. Abbas AE, Franey LM, Marwick T, Maeder MT, Kaye DM, Vlahos AP, et al. Noninvasive assessment of pulmonary vascular resistance by Doppler echocardiography. J Am Soc Echocardiogr. 2013;26(10):1170-7.
60. Vonk-Noordegraaf A, Haddad F, Chin KM, Forfia PR, Kawut SM, Lumens J, et al. Right heart adaptation to pulmonary arterial hypertension: physiology and pathobiology. J Am Coll Cardiol. 2013;62(25 Suppl):D22-33.
61. Zornoff LA, Skali H, Pfeffer MA, St John Sutton M, Rouleau JL, Lamas GA, et al. Right ventricular dysfunction and risk of heart failure and mortality after myocardial infarction. J Am Coll Cardiol. 2002;39(9):1450-5.
62. Forfia PR, Fisher MR, Mathai SC, Housten-Harris T, Hemnes AR, Borlaug BA, et al. Tricuspid annular displacement predicts survival in pulmonary hypertension. Am J Respir Crit Care Med. 2006;174(9):1034-41.
63. Rudski LG, Lai WW, Afilalo J, Hua L, Handschumacher MD, Chandrasekaran K, et al. Guidelines for the echocardiographic assessment of the right heart in adults: a report from the American Society of Echocardiography endorsed by the European Association of Echocardiography, a registered branch of the European Society of Cardiology, and the Canadian Society of Echocardiography. J Am Soc Echocardiogr. 2010;23(7):685-713; quiz 86-8.
64. Yeo TC, Dujardin KS, Tei C, Mahoney DW, McGoon MD, Seward JB. Value of a Doppler-derived index combining systolic and diastolic time intervals in predicting outcome in primary pulmonary hypertension. Am J Cardiol. 1998;81(9):1157-61.
65. Oremus M, McKelvie R, Don-Wauchope A, Santaguida PL, Ali U, Balion C, et al. A systematic review of BNP and NT-proBNP in the management of heart failure: overview and methods. Heart Fail Rev. 2014;19(4):413-9.
66. Dokainish H, Zoghbi WA, Lakkis NM, Quinones MA, Nagueh SF. Comparative accuracy of B-type natriuretic peptide and tissue Doppler echocardiography in the diagnosis of congestive heart failure. Am J Cardiol. 2004;93(9):1130-5.
67. Brenden CK, Hollander JE, Guss D, McCullough PA, Nowak R, Green G, et al. Gray zone BNP levels in heart failure patients in the emergency department: results from the Rapid Emergency Department Heart Failure Outpatient Trial (REDHOT) multicenter study. Am Heart J. 2006;151(5): 1006-11.
68. Arques S, Roux E, Sbragia P, Pieri B, Gelisse R, Ambrosi P, et al. Accuracy of tissue Doppler echocardiography in the diagnosis of new-onset congestive heart failure in patients with levels of B-type natriuretic peptide in the midrange and normal left ventricular ejection fraction. Echocardiography. 2006;23(8):627-34.

20 CHAPTER

Emergency Department Acute Heart Failure Treatment

Dick C Kuo, Tyson Pillow

BACKGROUND AND SIGNIFICANCE

Heart failure (HF) affects 23 million worldwide and 5.8 million people in the United States alone and has an increasing prevalence as one ages,[1,2] with prevalence reaching 17.4% in those age 85 or older. The aging population with overall increased survival is further expected to increase HF prevalence[3] by 2030 and the increase in HF prevalence will lead to an estimated 3 million additional cases of HF.[4]

A minimum of 30.7 billion dollars were spent in 2012 in the United States on the care of HF. These costs are projected to more than double by 2030 with approximately 70 million expected annual total costs.[5] In contrast to other cardiovascular diseases, the prevalence and mortality appears to be increasing and prognosis is generally poor[6] HF mortality is high with approximately 50% of patients dying within the first 5 years of diagnosis.[7,8] Mortality at 30 days, 1 year, and 5 years after hospitalization for HF has also been reported at 10.4%, 22%, and 42.3%, respectively.[9]

There are 1 million emergency department (ED) visits and nearly 84% of patients who present to the ED with acute heart failure (AHF) are admitted.[10] Heart failure is the most common cause of acute dyspnea among elderly patients in the ED[11] and among patients presenting to the ED with dyspnea, the most common cause of death.[12] From these statistics, it is obvious that emergency physicians (EPs) play an important role in the care and management of patients with acute or decompensated HF.

DEFINITION

Heart failure is the clinical syndrome that results from left ventricular dysfunction where the heart is unable to pump blood in sufficient quantities to meet metabolic demands. Failure to pump sufficient blood may be the result of either decreased ejection of blood or impairment of ventricular filling. Ejection fraction (EF) is an important concept in HF for classification, treatment and prognosis. The terms preserved EF and reduced EF are now preferred with reduced EF referring to patients with less than or equal to 40% EF, borderline patients with preserved EF of 41–49% and preserved EF with equal to or greater than 50%.[13] Heart failure is also preferred over congestive HF since all patients will not present with volume overload.

RISK FACTORS

Established risk factors for the development of HF include:

- Hypertension
- Previous myocardial infarction (MI) or ischemic heart disease from coronary artery disease
- Diabetes
- Cardiac arrhythmias
- Cardiomyopathies
- High cholesterol
- Smoking and alcohol abuse
- Family history
- Congenital heart disease
- Valvular heart disease
- Obesity and physical inactivity
- Male sex
- African-American race
- Poor socioeconomics
- Micronutrients.

PATHOPHYSIOLOGY

The common pathway to left ventricular dysfunction begins with injury to, or stress on, the myocardium. Left ventricular dysfunction is generally a progressive process with changes in the geometry of the heart known as cardiac remodeling. In cardiac remodeling, the left ventricle becomes dilated and/or hypertrophied and becomes more spherical in it overall shape. These changes to the heart increase the hemodynamic stresses on the walls and decrease its overall performance, which in turn worsen the remodeling process. Cardiac remodeling is a dynamic process and typically precedes the development of symptoms. The remodeling process continues as the disease progresses and ultimately contributes to worsening symptoms.[14]

Recent research has focused on activation of several neurohormones and their role in the progression of HF. Levels of norepinephrine, vasopressin, aldosterone, angiotensin II, endothelin, and cytokines are elevated in HF patients and contribute to the increased hemodynamic stress by causing peripheral vasoconstriction and sodium retention. These neurohormonal factors may also have direct toxicity for cardiac cells and potentiate myocardial fibrosis even further worsening the overall performance of the heart.[14-16]

SIGNS, SYMPTOMS, AND PRESENTATION

The classic symptom is dyspnea. Typically, patients will first become short of breath with exertion. They will note that the degree of activity or intensity of exercise required to become breathless has declined. Orthopnea is also an early symptom. Patients will become dyspneic in the recumbent position, relieved by elevating the head of the bed or elevating the head with pillows. Typically, an increasing number of pillows signals worsening HF. Paroxysmal nocturnal dyspnea (PND) usually occurs at night and is described as the sudden awakening from sleep with the sensation of breathlessness, anxiety, or the feeling of suffocation. Patients frequently remain upright for 30 minutes or longer to obtain relief and may feel the need to open a window. Paroxysmal nocturnal dyspnea may also be associated with bronchospasm that is difficult to distinguish from asthmatic bronchospasm or may coexist in patients with both the diseases. On the extreme edge of presentation is "flash" pulmonary edema, where there is a sudden increase in pulmonary capillary wedge pressure and fulminant left ventricular failure resulting in acute and severe shortness of breath.[17,18] Patients appear in extremis with increased work of breathing, tachypnea and hypoxia. Other symptoms with pulmonary edema include anxiety and diaphoresis. There may be cough and frothy sputum, which on occasion is blood tinged.

Congestive symptoms and signs of volume overload are also common. Peripheral edema is the typical hallmark of volume overload and congestion and frequently precedes or accompanies dyspnea. However, many patients with preserved EF may not exhibit signs or symptoms of volume overload.

Other symptoms include fatigue, chest pain, and palpitations. Renal symptoms include nocturia and oliguria and cerebral symptoms may include headaches, anxiety, memory loss and insomnia. Patients with advanced disease may exhibit confusion and delirium.

CLASSIFICATION AND STAGING

Heart failure is commonly and historically classified according to The New York Heart Association (NYHA) classification for HF in four classes, based on the relationship between symptoms and the amount of effort required to provoke them.[19]

- Class I: No limitation of physical activity
- Class II: Slight limitation of physical activity
- Class III: Marked limitation of physical activity
- Class IV: Symptoms even at rest and are unable to carry on any physical activity without discomfort.

In 2005, the American College of Cardiology/American Heart Association (ACC/AHA) characterized the development of HF in four stages. This staging system recognizes that HF has established risk factors and structural prerequisites, asymptomatic and symptomatic phases, and that specific treatments can be targeted at each stage to reduce morbidity and mortality.[14]

- Stage A: At high risk for HF but without structural heart disease or symptoms of HF
- Stage B: Structural heart disease but without symptoms of HF
- Stage C: Structural heart disease with prior or current symptoms of HF
- Stage D: Refractory HF requiring specialized interventions.

HISTORY AND PHYSICAL EXAMINATION

Initial evaluation of the patient in the ED should always include a quick evaluation of presenting symptoms and vital signs, including respiratory and rate and oxygenation status. In the stable patient, a thorough history and physical should attempt to identify the potential etiology and precipitating factors for decompensation. The ACC/AHA guidelines recommend history to include multiple elements listed in table 1.[14] In addition, emphasis should be placed on chest pain and potential cardiac ischemia, fluid overload, and medication and dietary compliance. History of current or previous atrial fibrillation (AF) or other arrhythmias, any cardiomyopathy and current or past renal failure are also important factors to consider.

Overall early diagnosis is important as delays in diagnosis may lead to delays in treatment, which has been associated with increased mortality.[20] A detailed history and physical is part of every patient's presentation to the ED but should be expedited in unstable patients, and those with severe respiratory distress. History and physical are important steps in confirming the diagnosis as well as excluding other causes of dyspnea; however, history and physical have its limitations

The classic symptoms for HF have poor sensitivity and specificity for the diagnosis of HF, including dyspnea, dyspnea on exertion, and orthopnea. Overall sensitivity and specificity with positive and negative likelihood ratios for common items in the history and physical are shown in table 2. Initial clinical judgment has as specificity of 86% with a positive likelihood ratio of 4.4 and only a

TABLE 1: Important historical factors

History to include	Family history to include
• Hypertension • Diabetes • Dyslipidemia • Valvular heart disease • Coronary or peripheral vascular disease • Myopathy • Rheumatic fever • Mediastinal irradiation • History or symptoms of sleep-disordered breathing • Exposure to cardiotoxic agents • Current and past alcohol consumption • Smoking • Collagen vascular disease • Exposure to sexually transmitted diseases • Thyroid disorder • Pheochromocytoma • Obesity	• Predisposition to atherosclerotic disease (history of myocardial infarction, strokes, and peripheral artery disease) • Sudden cardiac death • Myopathy • Conduction system disease (need for pacemaker) • Tachyarrhythmias • Cardiomyopathy (unexplained heart failure) • Skeletal myopathies

TABLE 2: Accuracy of history and physical findings in emergency department patients[21]

Finding	Sensitivity (%)	Specificity (%)	Positive LR	Negative LR
Initial clinical judgment	61	86	4.4	0.45
History of heart failure	60	90	5.8	0.45
History of MI	40	87	3.1	0.69
History of COPD	34	57	0.81	1.1
PND	41	84	2.6	0.70
Orthopnea	50	77	2.2	0.65
Dyspnea on exertion	84	34	1.3	0.48
Fatigue and weight gain	31	70	1.0	0.99
S3	13	99	11	0.88
Abdomino-jugular reflux	24	96	6.4	0.79
JVD	39	92	5.1	0.66
Rales	60	78	2.8	0.51
Any murmur	27	90	2.6	0.81
Lower extremity edema	50	78	2.3	0.64
S4	5	97	1.6	0.98
Wheezing	22	58	0.52	1.3

COPD, chronic obstructive pulmonary disease; JVD, jugular venous distention; MI, myocardial infarction; PND, paroxysmal nocturnal dyspnea.

few items show better specificity. Dyspnea on exertion (DOE) and orthopnea have overall poor sensitivity and specificity for the diagnosis of HF. Dyspnea on exertion has an 84% sensitivity but has only 34% specificity for the diagnosis of HF. The positive likelihood ratio (LR+) is close to 1 at 1.3 showing that it cannot effectively impact decision-making. Orthopnea only performs marginally better in specificity but loses in sensitivity, with values of 77% and 50%, respectively. The LR+ improving to 2.2 but still well below a likelihood ratio of 5 where values can begin to impact decision-making. Ultimately, a history of prior HF performs singly better than either of these typical presenting symptoms, with a sensitivity of 61%, a specificity of 86% and a LR+ of 5.8.[21]

Typical findings on physical include jugular venous distention (JVD) or distended neck veins, peripheral edema, rales, and possibly an S3 or pulsus alternans. Pulsus alternans may indicate severe left ventricular dysfunction while the S3 on heart examination remains one of the best clinical indicators for HF. Although the sensitivity is low at 13%, its specificity of 99% and LR+ of 11 should confirm a suspected diagnosis of HF in the dyspneic patient. The S3 was also correlated with elevated left ventricular end diastolic pressure (LVEDP), reduced left ventricular ejection fraction (LVEF) and elevated B-type natriuretic peptide (BNP) with a sensitivity of 41%, 52%, and 32%, respectively, and specificities of 92%, 87%, and 92%, respectively.[22]

However, its utility can be limited in a busy and noisy ED where auscultation of a third heart sound if present could be difficult.

Lower extremity edema has a sensitivity and specificity of 50% and 78% and a LR+ of only 2.3. Edema is not limited to the lower extremities and may manifest as scrotal edema, ascites, and hepatomegaly or splenomegaly. Rales on auscultation of the lung fields have a sensitivity of 60% and specificity of 78% with an only slightly better LR+ of 2.8. Abdominojugular reflux and JVD are the only other parameters with LR+ greater than 5. Abdominojugular reflux involves manual compression of the right upper quadrant to elevate jugular venous pressure. This sign has a LR+ of 6.4 with sensitivity and specificity of 24% and 96%, respectively, while JVD itself has a LR+ of 5.1 and a sensitivity and specificity of 39% and 92%, respectively. The high specificity of a gallop and JVD was also reported in an earlier study in 1997 by Davie et al. This study also found the displaced apical impulse to have a sensitivity of 66% and a specificity of 96% with the best overall positive and negative predictive values of 75% and 94%, respectively.[23]

The majority of HF signs and symptoms have low sensitivity overall but higher specificity with the exception of DOE and will perform better as tests for ruling in the diagnosis of HF as opposed to ruling it out.

DIFFERENTIAL DIAGNOSIS

Many of the symptoms for HF are nonspecific and the differential can be fairly broad. In patients that initially present with dyspnea, decreased exercise tolerance and fatigue, the differential includes myocardial ischemia, pulmonary disease, deconditioning and sleep apnea among many others. Efforts should focus on exclusion of other causes of dyspnea and their major treatment branch points, while continuing to consider AHF.

Acute severe exacerbations of asthma and chronic obstructive pulmonary disease often mimic AHF, and may occur simultaneously. Chronic obstructive pulmonary disease especially has a high prevalence and a similar presentation and it may be difficult to distinguish between the two disease processes and may represent the most troublesome competing diagnosis. Table 3 gives an overview of the differential for dyspnea and AHF. Other mimics to consider include large pulmonary embolus and severe pneumonia as well as the multiple causes of noncardiogenic pulmonary edema such as, the Acute Respiratory Distress Syndrome (ARDS), toxins, high altitude and opiate overdose. Acute coronary syndrome (ACS) with dyspnea as an anginal equivalent is also an important consideration in the differential.

In patients with fluid retention and peripheral edema, the differential includes renal disease, medication side effects, venous insufficiency or thrombosis, and cirrhosis.

Chest X-Ray and Imaging

Obtaining a chest X-ray (CXR) is common in patients that are short of breath and the evaluation of the HF patient is no different. Unstable patients may have portable CXRs performed as tolerated. Findings associated with HF include cardiomegaly, increased size of the vascular pedicle, and redistribution of pulmonary blood flow to the upper lobes seen as increased vascular markings in the upper lobes commonly referred to as cephalization. As HF progresses to interstitial edema, Kerly B lines become visible as well as peribronchial cuffing and increased size of the fissures. With alveolar edema there is consolidation that begins in the perihilar region and air bronchograms. The entire lung may take on a cottonwool appearance that is typically associated with pulmonary edema. The CXR may demonstrate findings that support the diagnosis of HF but is frequently nondiagnostic.

TABLE 3: Differential for dyspnea and acute heart failure

Cardiac	Pulmonary	Other
• Myocardial ischemia • Atrial fibrillation • Arrhythmia • Pericardial effusion	• Chronic obstructive pulmonary disease • Asthma • Pneumonia • Pleural effusion • Pulmonary embolus • Pneumothorax • Pulmonary infarcts • Aspiration • Foreign body • Pulmonary hypertension • Cancer	• Noncardiogenic pulmonary edema • Metabolic acidosis • Anaphylaxis • Mediastinitis • Pneumo-mediastinum • Toxins • Medication effects • Renal failure or disease • Anemia • Cirrhosis • Panic attack

Similar to many of our findings on history and physical, a normal CXR does not exclude HF as the presenting diagnosis.[24] Chest X-ray also has the potential to identify other causes of dyspnea such as pneumonia, pneumothorax, pleural effusion, or findings consistent with chronic obstructive pulmonary disease.

Bedside ultrasound is an emerging technique in the evaluation of potential HF patients. The utility of bedside ultrasound for the diagnosis of HF was studied by Anderson et al. who compared three different ultrasound modalities. This study evaluated the combination of cardiac ultrasound for left ventricular EF, inferior vena cava collapsibility, and pulmonary interstitial edema (i.e., B lines) to establish a HF diagnosis. The combination of all three modalities resulted in a specificity of 100% (95% confidence interval = 95 - 100) but showed poor sensitivity (36%). In addition, any combination of two of the modalities had a specificity of 93% or greater.[25] Similar to previous discussed findings, ultrasound has a high specificity but a low sensitivity once again making it a reasonable test to confirm the presence of HF, but a poor choice to rule out the disease process.

In another study by Al Deeb et al., a systematic review looked at seven total studies (two in the ED, two in the intensive care unit, two in inpatient, and one in prehospital setting) evaluating the use of B lines to diagnose acute cardiogenic pulmonary edema (ACPE).[26] The sensitivity of ultrasound using B lines to diagnosis ACPE is 94.1% and the specificity is 92.4%. This study suggests that a ultrasound showing B lines can be used to further substantiate an EP's working diagnosis of ACPE. In the setting of initial low pretest probability for ACPE, lack of B lines on ultrasound can almost exclude the diagnosis of ACPE.

Bedside ultrasound is rapidly expanding in its use by EPs as more and more EPs are trained and become adept with its use. Although its use in the acutely dyspneic patient may be limited due to availability and discomfort associated with performing all of the above measurements in a supine position, if available may provide a more expeditious radiologic study than CXR.

Electrocardiogram

An electrocardiogram (ECG) should be performed on all dyspneic patients and those with a suspicion of HF.

This test should be performed as soon as possible after presentation to the ED. Electrocardiogram testing can quickly identify arrhythmias and signs of current or past myocardial ischemia or even ST segment elevation in acute myocardial infarction (STEMI). Other findings that may require prompt treatment include AF with rapid ventricular response (RVR), primary ventricular arrhythmias or any other tachy or brady dysrhythmia. Electrocardiogram testing can create multiple branch points in patient management and accurate interpretation is an essential skill for every EP. Although it may not typically contribute directly to the diagnosis of HF, the ECG in patients with HF from systolic dysfunction is frequently significantly abnormal and patients with a normal ECG rarely have abnormal systolic function.[27]

Laboratory

Basic laboratory testing is recommended for potential HF patients.[13] This includes a complete blood count (CBC) and serum electrolytes with blood urea nitrogen (BUN) and creatinine. The CBC can at a minimum identify anemia as a concomitant or exacerbating factor. Liver function tests may be abnormal indicating hepatic congestion, and thyroid stimulating hormone (TSH) levels can help determine if hypothyroidism or hyperthyroidism is contributing to the disease process.

Blood urea nitrogen and creatinine as measurements of renal function are important laboratory tests in acute decompensated HF patients as renal function is a major predictor of mortality and severity of disease. A decreased glomerular filtration rate (GFR) is one of the strongest predictors of short-term mortality. There is an approximate 7% increase risk in mortality for every 10 mL/min decrease in GRF.[28,29] At least one in four patients admitted to the hospital for HF has a GFR less than 60 mL/min/1.73 m^2, and patients who experience worsening renal function have increased short- and long-term mortality and are associated with longer hospital stays.[30]

Cardiorenal syndrome is the bidirectional interaction between HF and worsening renal function. Patients admitted with HF frequently have impaired renal function. In data from the Acute Decompensated Heart Failure National Registry (ADHERE) of patients admitted for HF, approximately 30% of patients had a creatinine greater than 2.0 mg/dL and only 9% of patients had a normal estimated GFR.[31] As preciously described mortality is increased in patients with worsening GFR and patients with chronic kidney disease have an increased risk for HF. It is also believed that the decrease in renal function limits the ability to relieve congestive symptoms. Decreased GFR is believed to be due to the decrease in renal blood flow but this is not the only likely explanation as cardiorenal syndrome occurs in a variety of clinical settings.[32]

Troponin is recommended in addition to other typical lab tests. Troponin appears to be a major marker for increased mortality. Hospitalized patients with an elevated troponin have a significantly higher acute mortality as compared to those with a troponin below the local cut point[33] and should be considered as potential candidates for more aggressive therapy. Furthermore, when a higher sensitivity troponin assay is available (Verisens RUO Human cTnI Assay, patients with a persistently elevated or rising troponin had a much higher 90-day mortality and a higher HF-related readmission rate.[34]

B-type Natriuretic Peptide

Given the degree of clinical uncertainty, clinicians and researchers have long searched for a rapid test that could easily confirm or exclude the diagnosis of HF.

B-type natriuretic peptide is released by the ventricles in response to increased wall tension. In 2002, Maisel et al.[35] showed that a BNP greater than 100 pg/mL was a better predictor of HF than clinical judgment, with a sensitivity of 90% and a specificity of 76% and an overall accuracy of 83%. Lower values were associated with higher negative predictive values. A value of less than 50 pg/mL had a negative predictive value of 96%. B-type natriuretic peptide may prove especially useful when the diagnosis is uncertain.

The use of BNP testing has become an important ED diagnostic adjunct. Levels less than 100 pg/mL reliably exclude the diagnosis of HF while levels above 400–500 pg/mL are consistent with the diagnosis of HF. This ultimately leaves a gray zone from 100 to 400 pg/mL that requires additional testing to determine an accurate diagnosis.[36,37] N-terminal pro-BNP (NT-proBNP) is a metabolic byproduct of BNP synthesis that performs in a similar fashion diagnostically to BNP. Levels of NT-proBNP below 300 pg/mL exclude a diagnosis of HF, and levels above 900 pg/mL are highly suggestive, with a 300–900 pg/mL gray zone requiring additional confirmatory testing.[38,39] Measurement of BNP or NT-proBNP can be useful for establishing prognosis or disease severity in acutely decompensated HF[40-42] but is less established in its use to guide therapy.[43]

As patients age, their NT-proBNP also rises and requires adjustment for age. In patients older than 75 years, the recommended cut point is 1,800 pg/mL. Both BNP and NT-proBNP testing can also be confounded in the presence of obesity.[44] There is an inverse association with body mass index (BMI) and increasing BMI is associated with lower than expected levels of BNP and NT-proBNP in both healthy volunteers and patients with HF. Natriuretic peptides are also positively confounded by the presence of renal failure[45] and patients with decreased GFR have increased circulating levels of BNP and NT-proBNP. To adjust for these potential confounders, it has

TABLE 4: Differential for elevated natriuretic peptide levels

Cardiac	Noncardiac
• Heart failure • Acute coronary syndrome • Valvular disease • Heart muscle disease • Myocarditis • Left ventricular hypertrophy • Pericardial disease • Atrial fibrillation • Cardiac surgery • Cardioversion	• Advancing age • Anemia • Renal failure • Obstructive sleep apnea • Pulmonary embolus • Severe pneumonia • Pulmonary hypertension • Sepsis • Severe burns • Toxic metabolic insults • Cancer chemotherapy • Envenomation

been recommended that in patients with a BMI in excess of 35, the measured BNP levels should be doubled, and halved in the presence of renal failure[46] (defined as an estimated GFR below 60 mL/min). Table 4 gives a list of potential causes for elevated natriuretic peptides.

The newer biomarkers, galectin-3 (GAL3) and sST2 are two promising biomarkers that have been recently developed[47] but their clinical utility has yet to be defined in the setting of the ED.

TREATMENT

Once the diagnosis of HF is established, treatment should be initiated rapidly. The newest therapy in the maintenance treatment of HF patients is the combination of an angiotensin-receptor blocker with the newer neprilysin inhibitor.[48] Long-term outcomes for HF patients continue to improve and evolve from the discovery of the beneficial effect of β-blockers in HF patients.[49] Although chronic treatments to reduce long-term mortality of HF are not always indicated in the early treatment of ADHF, however, continuation of guideline-directed medical therapy (GDMT) is indicated as long as there is no contraindication to their administration.[13]

Initial Evaluation and Stabilization in Patients with Acute Severe Symptoms

All patients are initially triaged in the ED and the sickest patients are typically seen and treated expeditiously. Treatment in the ED always starts with the airway, breathing, and circulation (ABC) and the initial evaluation of the patient with suspected ADHF seeks to identify those with potential respiratory failure and severe respiratory distress, as well as those patients with significantly elevated blood pressure that is contributing to their symptoms. Primary goals in the patient with acute severe symptoms include support of oxygenation, ventilation and hemodynamic stabilization. Every EP evaluating a patient with acute dyspnea will assess the airway and evaluate the need for immediate intubation. The patient will be assessed for potential difficulties in intubation as well and measures will be initiated to support oxygenation and ventilation.

Blood pressure is an important consideration in the treatment of patients with acute decompensated HF who present to an ED. The Society of Academic Emergency Medicine (SAEM) and the Heart Failure Society of America (HFSA) recently published a consensus document on the early management of AHF which suggested that treatment of AHF be divided into three categories with regards to blood pressure: (i) hypertensive patients with SBP greater than 140 mm Hg, (ii) normotensive patients with SBP 140–110 mm Hg, and (iii) hypotensive patients with SBP less than 110 mm Hg.[50]

Flash Pulmonary Edema

Severe respiratory distress in ADHF is usually a result of flash pulmonary edema (FPE) and may result in complete respiratory failure. Flash pulmonary edema has been clinically associated with renal artery stenosis, coronary artery disease, particular blood pressure profiles, obstructive sleep apnea, diastolic dysfunction, valvular heart disease, and Takotsubo cardiomyopathy,[17] and occurs with acute increases in left ventricular end diastolic filling pressure (LVEDP). Elevated LVEDP leads to an increase in interstitial edema and ultimately increased alveolar fluid and pulmonary edema. Although FPE is considered a form of cardiogenic pulmonary edema, it is also associated with neurohormonal changes involving the renin angiotensin system, increased endothelin-1 and catecholamines, and decreased nitric oxide synthesis that leads to increased permeability of the pulmonary capillary endothelium.[17,18]

Treatment for Flash Pulmonary Edema and Severe Respiratory Distress

A quick decision point is necessary on the initial evaluation of the patient. Patients with FPE are always potential candidates for intubation. Patients that are speaking in one word sentences may be placed on a trial of noninvasive ventilation (NIV). Patients whose respiratory function does not allow even one word sentences, who are confused or obtunded require intubation. However, hypoxic patents in severe respiratory distress will sometimes be unable to cooperate or tolerate the mask associated with NIV. Patients unable to cooperate should be considered candidates for endotracheal intubation.

The two kinds of NIV that are commonly used consist of continuous positive airway pressure (CPAP) and bilevel positive airway pressure (BiPAP). Continuous positive airway pressure will treat type I respiratory failure (oxygenation) while BiPAP will treat both type I and type II (ventilation) respiratory failure, but the physiologic differences between the two types of NIV have little bearing on the treatment of FPE. Importantly, NIV should not be considered as solo therapy. The use of NIV may temporize the need for intubation, and buy time for the implementation of other therapies.

Continuous positive airway pressure was first described as a treatment for pulmonary edema in 1935.[51] In 1991, Bersten et al. found that CPAP decreased the need for intubation and mechanical ventilation when compared to oxygen alone. However, there was no significant difference found for in-hospital mortality or length of stay.[52] Since then there have been multiple clinical trials based in the ED[53,54] and multiple meta-analysis and systemic reviews[55-57] investigating the role of CPAP and NIV in acute pulmonary edema. In addition, Cochrane reviews[58,59] eventually established NIV as a beneficial treatment for acute pulmonary edema. Noninvasive ventilation significantly reduces inhospital mortality and the need for intubation with a number needed to treat (NNT) of 13 and 8, respectively.

Patients that do not require intubation or NIV will likely benefit from the administration of oxygen. Oxygen should be administered to maintain an oxygen saturation of greater than 90% but is not required or recommended if the patient is not hypoxic or tachypneic.

Diuretics and vasodilators are the most common medical therapies that are given in acute decompensated HF. In FPE, most patients are hypertensive on presentation with SBP greater than 140 mm Hg and vasodilator therapy is the key component in their care. In these patients with elevated blood pressure redistribution is more predominant than volume overload[60] and hypertensive patients require immediate afterload reduction with vasodilator therapy.

Nitrates are the vasodilator of choice and the nitrate of choice in the ED is nitroglycerin. Nitroglycerin can be initially administered sublingual until intravenous therapy can be established. Intravenous nitroglycerin works rapidly and is easily titratable to reach a goal blood pressure. Nitroglycerin provides rapid reduction in left ventricular filling pressures and at higher doses decreases systemic afterload. Congestive symptoms are improved and stroke volume and cardiac output are increased. Although IV nitroglycerin is recommended and commonly used there have been no large studies examining its efficacy in the ED setting or in its use in FPE. A recent Cochrane review found no difference between nitrates and alternate therapies for multiple end points but only four studies, three of which were ultimately excluded from their analysis, leaving only one study to base their overall conclusions. The authors did finally conclude that there is a lack of data to draw any firm conclusions regarding the use of nitrates and current evidence is based on a few low-quality studies.[61]

Intravenous nitroglycerin in patients with chest pain is typically started at an initial dose of 10 µg/min and titrated upward as tolerated. For comparison purposes, sublingual nitroglycerin, typically 0.4 mg or 400 µg, is given every 5 minutes for chest pain equating to a dose of 80 µg/min. This strategy will not be effective in the hypertensive HF patient and intravenous nitroglycerin should be started at considerably higher doses. Doses of 120 µg/min are typically required to significantly decrease pulmonary capillary wedge pressure.[62] Levy et al. used doses of as much as 2,000 µg every 3 minutes in 29 patients in an open label nonrandomized study and compared their results to 45 patients not given high dose nitroglycerin. The median dose of nitroglycerin was 6.5 mg and the nitroglycerin group had lower intubation rates, intensive care unit admissions, and a trend to lower mortality.[63] If waiting for the intravenous nitroglycerin preparation, 0.4 mg sublingual nitroglycerin can be given routinely every 60 seconds until there is a blood pressure response or the patient's dyspnea improves.

Nitrates or other vasodilators should not be used when the patient presents initially with hypotension and nitrates are specifically contraindicated when there has been recent use of phosphodiesterase-5 inhibitors such as sildenafil. Concomitant use may precipitate severe hypotension. Hypotension may also result with the use of vasodilators in the setting of isolated right HF and right-sided myocardial infarction where patients are extremely preload dependent. The alternatives to nitroglycerin include other vasodilators such as sodium nitroprusside and nesiritide. Sodium nitroprusside has also been shown to be effective in the treatment of HF from systolic dysfunction.[64,65] It is rapidly titratable and can quickly bring down blood pressure. Sodium nitroprusside has the adverse effect of accumulation of cyanide derivatives so that prolonged therapy is not recommended. Nesiritide is another alternative and has also been shown to be not worse than other vasodilators.[66,67] Of note, nesiritide has a longer half-life than either nitroglycerin or nitroprusside and side effects such as induced hypotension may persist longer.

Other considerations include the timing of vasoactives. Vasoactives are defined as IV medications that are used to alter the patient's hemodynamic status (e.g., nitroglycerin, nitroprusside, nesiritide, dopamine, dobutamine, etc.). Outcomes appear improved in patients with shorter times to receive their vasoactive medication. Delayed administration of vasoactive medications is associated with increased mortality, especially in patients with high BNP.[68]

Of note, there are no published HF guidelines that directly address the treatment of acute or FPE and the closest mention is the administration of intravenous medications for the treatment of acute decompensated HF. Nitrates and other vasodilators are recommended as adjunct to diuretic therapy but this is not specific for FPE, and NIV has no specific recommendation at all.[13]

Patients without Flash Pulmonary Edema

In patients that are normotensive (SBP 110–140 mm Hg) with congestion as their primary complaint, diuretics remain the mainstay of treatment. The most recent ACCF/AHA (American College of Cardiology Foundation/American Heart Association) 2013 guidelines on the evaluation and treatment of HF state that diuretics are an essential component of treatment in patients with evidence of significant fluid overload.[13] In 2011, the Diuretic Strategies in Patients with Acute Decompensated Heart Failure or DOSE trial investigated the optimum dosing strategies for diuretics in hospitalized HF patients. The study found that there was no difference between administration by either bolus or continuous infusion and no differences between high or low doses of diuretic. This prospective, double blind, randomized multicenter trial enrolled 308 patients in an investigation that evaluated patients' global assessment of symptoms and also the change in serum creatinine from baseline. There was a nonstatistically significant trend toward greater improvement in the high dose furosemide group, as well as greater diuresis. However, these effects were associated with a transient worsening of renal function.[69] Diuretics should be administered in an intravenous dose equal to 1–2.5 times the patient's usual daily PO regimen. In patients that have not previously received diuretic therapy, typical dosing would be to start furosemide at 40 mg intravenous or bumetanide at 1 mg intravenous for the hospitalized patient. Subsequent dosing can then be adjusted according to urine output. The addition of a second diuretic, low-dose dopamine or ultrafiltration should be considered if diuresis is not effective.[13]

While there is historical precedent that morphine may be of value, no reasonable data exists to support its use. European society guidelines suggest opiates such as morphine may be useful to reduce anxiety and relieve the distress associated with dyspnea.[70] However, there is data to suggest morphine should not be used in acute decompensated HF. In fact, data from over 60,000 patients in the ADHERE registry found an associated increase in intensive care unit admissions and mortality associated with morphine use,[71] and there are no specific recommendations from the ACCF/AHA guidelines.

Patients Presenting with Hypotension

Patients that present with acute decompensated HF and hypotension (SBP <110 mm Hg) are critically ill and are caught in a treatment dilemma. Hypotension is an extremely poor prognostic sign in AHF and mortality is high. Even though the patient has HF a small fluid bolus can be initiated and the response measured. If unresponsive and blood pressure remains low, inotropes should be considered. Although inotropes may raise blood pressure, they are highly arrhythmogenic. Overall, inotropes have not been shown to decrease mortality in patients that present with ADHF and hypotension unless it is as a bridge to mechanical therapy (e.g., left ventricular assist device).[72-74]

Despite the disheartening data, patients with cardiogenic shock should receive temporary intravenous inotropic support to maintain systemic perfusion and to prevent end-organ damage until other definitive therapy (revascularization, heart transplantation, left ventricular assist device) is available or until symptoms resolve.[13] The lowest possible dose needed to achieve an increase in blood pressure should be used to limit potential arrhythmogenic effects. Inotropic support may also be recommended as bridge therapy for patients who are candidates for mechanical circulatory support or cardiac transplantation.[75-77] Of the common inotrope choices available in the United States (dopamine, dobutamine, and milrinone), none have proven any superiority over another.

Inotropic agents should not be used in the absence of specific indications in patients without documented severe systolic dysfunction, low blood pressure, impaired perfusion, and evidence of significantly decreased cardiac output. Recent ACCF/AHA guidelines give a class III (harm) warning.[13]

ACUTE CORONARY SYNDROME AND HEART FAILURE

Acute coronary syndrome is a significant cause of de novo HF and a common precipitant of worsening HF. In patients presenting with ACS and HF, those patients with hyperglycemia have been reported to have worse outcomes.[78] Acute coronary syndrome is a spectrum of diseases that includes acute myocardial infarction and non-ST elevation myocardial infarction (NSTEMI) and guidelines have been developed to help treat these situations when complicated by HF.[79,80] Patients presenting with STEMI and signs of congestive HF or cardiogenic shock require emergent percutaneous coronary intervention (PCI) and revascularization.[79,81] These patients may also require mechanical circulatory support.

Patients with NSTEMI and HF on presentation are classified as high-risk patients and an invasive strategy (typically involving PCI) is recommended in their care.[80] In addition, in patients with angina and suitable coronary anatomy, especially significant left main or equivalent stenosis, PCI and/or coronary artery bypass grafting (CABG) is also indicated. In patients with mild to moderate systolic dysfunction, CABG is reasonable to improve survival when there is significant multivessel or left anterior descending coronary artery stenosis when viable myocardium remains.[13]

ATRIAL FIBRILLATION AND HEART FAILURE

Atrial fibrillation is also a common coexisting condition with HF and the two have a bidirectional relationship. Patients with HF are more likely than the general population to develop AF, and AF is a strong independent risk factor for the development of HF.[82] The prevalence of AF increases as NYHA classification increases where 40% of patients with class IV HF will have AF.[83] This bidirectional relationship between AF and HF can worsen and perpetuate each other. Heart failure can promote RVR in AF and AF can easily worsen symptoms in HF patients.

Patients that present to the ED with AHF and AF with RVR require immediate electrical cardioversion if unstable (severe decompensated HF, hypotension, associated cardiac ischemia or signs of decreased tissue perfusion).[84] Patients that are stable require rapid rate control. In patients without pre-excitation, intravenous β-blockers or a nondihydropyridine calcium channel blocker can slow ventricular heart rate in the acute setting in the ED.[85-88] Amiodarone might also be useful for rate control in patients without pre-excitation and should be considered if other medications are unsuccessful.[89-91] With pre-excitation and AF, any nodal blocking agents (digoxin, nondihydropyridine calcium channel antagonists, or amiodarone) should not be administered. Of note, 2014 ACC/AHA AF guidelines gave a class III (harm) warning for nondihydropyridine calcium channel blockers and state that they should not be used in decompensated HF. However, this recommendation is only supported by level C evidence (expert opinion).[84]

DISCHARGE VERSUS ADMISSION

The overall goals of therapy are to improve symptoms and restore normal oxygenation while optimizing the patient's volume status. Risk of rehospitalization is high in patients who did not receive adequate diuresis or during their initial hospitalization.[92] Identifying the etiology of de novo HF and any precipitating factors that have contributed to decompensation and hospitalization are also important considerations so that they may be addressed to minimize their effects on potential future episodes of AHF and readmissions.

Overall, EPs have a low threshold for admitting patients with HF and a low-risk tolerance for discharge decisions. Over 80% of patients presenting to the ED for HF are admitted[10] and EPs define low-risk patients as those with a less than 1% chance of 30-day mortality, hospital death or serious complication. Additionally, EPs considered 0.5% risk for 30-day mortality or other major complication as the discharge threshold.[93] Missing from current guidelines are decision rules or recommendations directed at ED disposition decision-making.[13,50] While high risk appears easy to define, in comparison, low-risk patients that meet the EPs discharge threshold appear much more elusive, and there have been many past and current attempts to define this group without measurable success.[50]

The recent SAEM/HFSA consensus document[50] recommends of those patients that present to the ED with AHF, patients can be placed in high-risk groups if they have hypotension, hypoxia, renal insufficiency, or cardiac ischemia or infarction, and moderate-risk groups if they have significant active comorbidities, or significant self-care barriers or poor response to ED treatment. Low-risk patients are those that exhibit none of these factors. Low-risk patients that respond to initial ED care and do not require further treatment can be discharged home.[50] Patients discharged from the ED should have early physician follow-up and a collaborative care plan since these concepts have been shown to lower readmission rates and improve outcomes.[94,95]

Patients require admission in the high-risk group and intensive care unit care is necessary for invasive monitoring, diagnostics or treatment or if patients require intravenous vasodilators or inotropic support. The intermediate-risk group can be considered for inpatient versus observation unit. Observation unit patients are patients without high-risk features whose active comorbidities and self-care barriers can be adequately addressed in less than 24 hours and who are expected to respond to continued treatment in less than 24 hours.[50] Patients admitted to an ED observation unit have demonstrated readmission rates not higher than admitted patients with fewer bed days amongst discharged patients.[96]

There is ongoing work evaluating decision-making in the disposition of patients with new novel approaches being suggested.[50] One of the newer innovations uses an implantable pressure sensor to measure LVEDP. When therapy was guided by LVEDP readmission rates, up to 1 year were reduced when compared to patients that were managed by clinical assessment alone.[97]

CONCLUSION

Emergency physicians continue to play a significant role in the early management of AHF patients. The definitive diagnosis of HF can be elusive given the poor historical performance of many signs and symptoms but focus on specific findings and advances in biomarkers has improved overall diagnostic ability. Although there are no ED-specific treatment guidelines, therapies for AHF have been expanded to include NIV and vasodilators. There are numerous published guidelines available and the recent SAEM/HFSA consensus document has suggested a new framework for the treatment of AHF based upon blood pressure. The same document has also created a new algorithm for the risk stratification and disposition of AHF patients although more data is needed to validate disposition models in addition to treatment in the ED setting.

Conflict of interest: The authors have no conflict of interest to report.

REFERENCES

1. Roger VL, Go AS, Lloyd-Jones DM, Benjamin EJ, Berry JD, Borden WB, et al. Executive summary: heart disease and stroke statistics–2012 update: a report from the American Heart Association. Circulation. 2012;125(1):188-97.
2. Bleumink GS, Knetsch AM, Sturkenboom MC, Straus SM, Hofman A, Deckers JW, et al. Quantifying the heart failure epidemic: prevalence, incidence rate, lifetime risk and prognosis of heart failure. The Rotterdam Study. Eur Heart J. 2004;25(18):1614-19.
3. Go AS, Mozaffarian D, Roger VL, Benjamin EJ, Berry JD, Blaha MJ, et al. Heart disease and stroke statistics–2014 update: A report from the American Heart Association. Circulation. 2014;129(3):e28-e292.
4. Heidenreich PA, Trogdon JG, Khavjou OA, Butler J, Dracup K, Ezekowitz MD, et al. Forecasting the future of cardiovascular disease in the United States: a policy statement from the American Heart Association. Circulation. 2011;123(8):933-44.
5. Heidenreich PA, Albert NM, Allen LA, Bluemke DA, Butler J, Fonarow GC, et al. Forecasting the impact of heart failure in the United States: a policy statement from the American Heart Association. Circ Heart Fail. 2013;6(3):606-19.
6. Liu L. Changes in cardiovascular hospitalization and comorbidity of heart failure in the United States: findings from the National Hospital Discharge Surveys 1980–2006. Int J Cardiol. 2011;149(1):39-45.
7. Levy D, Kenchaiah S, Larson MG, Benjamin EJ, Kupka MJ, Ho KK, et al. Long-term trends in the incidence of and survival with heart failure. N Engl J Med. 2002;347(18):1397-402.
8. Roger VL, Go AS, Lloyd-Jones DM, Adams RJ, Berry JD, Brown TM, et al. Heart disease and stroke statistics–2011 update: a report from the American Heart Association. Circulation. 2011;123(4):e18-e209.
9. Loehr LR, Rosamond WD, Chang PP, Folsom AR, Chambless LE. Heart failure incidence and survival (from the Atherosclerosis Risk in Communities study). Am J Cardiol. 2008;101(7):1016-22.
10. Storrow AB, Jenkins CA, Self WH, Alexander PT, Barrett TW, Han JH, et al. The burden of acute heart failure on U.S. emergency departments. JACC Heart Fail. 2014;2(3):269-77.
11. Ray P, Birolleau S, Lefort Y, Becquemin MH, Beigelman C, Isnard R, et al. Acute respiratory failure in the elderly: etiology, emergency diagnosis and prognosis. Crit Care. 2006;10(3):R82.
12. Bordin P, Da Col PG, Peruzzo P, Stanta G, Guralnik JM, Cattin L. Causes of death and clinical diagnostic errors in extreme aged hospitalized people: a retrospective clinical-necropsy survey. J Gerontol A Biol Sci Med Sci. 1999;54(11):M554-9.
13. Writing Committee Members, Yancy C, Jessup M, Bozkurt B, Butler J, Casey DE, et al. 2013 ACCF/AHA guideline for the management of heart failure: a report of the American College of Cardiology Foundation/American Heart Association Task Force on Practice Guidelines. Circulation. 2013;128(16):e240-327.
14. Hunt SA, Abraham WT, Chin MH, Feldman AM, Francis GS, Ganiats TG, et al. ACC/AHA 2005 Guideline Update for the Diagnosis and Management of Chronic Heart Failure in the Adult: a report of the American College of Cardiology/American Heart Association Task Force on Practice Guidelines (Writing Committee to Update the 2001 Guidelines for the Evaluation and Management of Heart Failure): developed in collaboration with the American College of Chest Physicians and the International Society for Heart and Lung Transplantation: endorsed by the Heart Rhythm Society. Circulation. 2005;112(12):e154-235.
15. Johnson FL. Pathophysiology and etiology of heart failure. Cardiol Clin. 2014;32(1):9-19.
16. Schrier RW, Abraham WT. Hormones and hemodynamics in heart failure. N Engl J Med. 1999;341(8):577-85.
17. Rimoldi SF, Yuzefpolskaya M, Allemann Y, Messerli F. Flash pulmonary edema. Prog Cardiovasc Dis. 2009;52(3):249-59.
18. Ware LB, Matthay MA. Clinical practice. Acute pulmonary edema. N Engl J Med. 2005;353:2788-96.
19. American Heart Association. (2015). Classes of Heart Failure. [online] Available from: http://www.heart.org/HEARTORG/Conditions/HeartFailure/AboutHeartFailure/Classes-of-Heart-Failure_UCM_306328_Article.jsp. [Accessed March, 2016].
20. Peacock WF, Fonarow GC, Emerman CL, Mills RM, Wynne J, ADHERE Scientific Advisory Committee and Investigators, et al. Impact of early initiation of intravenous therapy for acute decompensated heart failure on outcomes in ADHERE. Cardiology. 2007;107(1):44-51.
21. Wang CS, FitzGerald JM, Schulzer M, Mak E, Ayas NT. Does this dyspneic patient in the emergency department have congestive heart failure? JAMA. 2005;294(15):1944-56.
22. Marcus GM, Gerber IL, McKeown BH, Vessey JC, Jordan MV, Huddleston M, et al. Association between phonocardiographic third and fourth heart sounds and objective measures of left ventricular function. JAMA. 2005;293(18):2238-44.
23. Davie AP, Francis CM, Caruana L, Sutherland GR, McMurray JJ. Assessing diagnosis in heart failure: which features are any use? QJM. 1997;90(5):335-9.
24. Collins SP, Lindsell CJ, Storrow AB, Abraham WT, ADHERE Scientific Advisory Committee, Investigators and Study Group. Prevalence of negative chest radiography results in the emergency department patient with decompensated heart failure. Ann Emerg Med. 2006;47(1):13-8.
25. Anderson KL, Jenq KY, Fields JM, Panebianco NL, Dean AJ. Diagnosing heart failure among acutely dyspneic patients with cardiac, inferior vena cava, and lung ultrasonography. Am J Emerg Med. 2013;31(8):1208-14.
26. Al Deeb M, Barbic S, Featherstone R, Dankoff J, Barbic D. Point-of-care ultrasonography for the diagnosis of acute cardiogenic pulmonary edema in patients presenting with acute dyspnea: a systematic review and meta-analysis. Acad Emerg Med. 2014;21(8):843-52.
27. Davie AP, Francis CM, Love MP, Caruana L, Starkey IR, Shaw TR, et al. Value of the electrocardiogram in identifying heart failure due to left ventricular systolic dysfunction. BMJ. 1996;312(7052):222.
28. Smith GL, Lichtman JH, Bracken MB, Shlipak MG, Phillips CO, DiCapua P, et al. Renal impairment and outcomes in heart failure: systematic review and meta-analysis. J Am Coll Cardiol. 2006;47(10):1987-96.
29. Hillege HL, Nitsch D, Pfeffer MA, Swedberg K, McMurray JJ, Yusuf S, et al. Renal function as a predictor of outcome in a broad spectrum of patients with heart failure. Circulation. 2006;113(5):671-8.
30. Fonarow GC, Adams KF, Abraham WT, Yancy CW, Boscardin WJ; ADHERE Scientific Advisory Committee, Study Group, and Investigators. Risk stratification for in-hospital mortality in acutely decompensated heart failure: classification and regression tree analysis. JAMA. 2005;293(5):572-80.
31. Heywood JT, Fonarow GC, Costanzo MR, Mathur VS, Wigneswaran JR, Wynne J, et al. High prevalence of renal dysfunction and its impact on outcome in 118,465 patients hospitalized with acute decompensated heart failure: a report from the ADHERE database. J Card Fail. 2007;13(6):422-30.
32. Bock JS, Gottlieb SS. Cardiorenal syndrome: new perspectives. Circulation. 2010;121(23):2592-600.
33. Peacock WF, De Marco T, Fonarow GC, Diercks D, Wynne J, Apple FS, et al. Cardiac troponin and outcome in acute heart failure. N Engl J Med. 2008;358(20):2117-26.
34. Xue Y, Clopton P, Peacock WF, Maisel AS. Serial changes in high-sensitive troponin I predict outcome in patients with decompensated heart failure. Eur J Heart Fail. 2011;13(1):37-42.
35. Maisel AS, Krishnaswamy P, Nowak RM, McCord J, Hollander JE, Duc P, et al. Rapid measurement of B-type natriuretic peptide in the emergency diagnosis of heart failure. N Engl J Med. 2002;347(3):161-7.
36. Mayo DD, Colletti JE, Kuo DC. Brain natriuretic peptide (BNP) testing in the emergency department. J Emerg Med. 2006;31(2):201-10.
37. Mueller C, Scholer A, Laule-Kilian K, Martina B, Schindler C, Buser P, et al. Use of B-type natriuretic peptide in the evaluation and management of acute dyspnea. N Engl J Med. 2004;350(7):647-54.
38. Van Kimmenade RR, Pinto YM, Bayes-Genis A, Lainchbury JG, Richards AM, Januzzi JL. Usefulness of intermediate amino-terminal pro-brain natriuretic peptide concentrations for diagnosis and prognosis of acute heart failure. Am J Cardiol. 2006;98(3):386-90.

39. Moe GW, Howlett J, Januzzi JL, Zowall H; Canadian Multicenter Improved Management of Patients With Congestive Heart Failure (IMPROVE-CHF) Study Investigators. N-terminal pro-B-type natriuretic peptide testing improves the management of patients with suspected acute heart failure: primary results of the Canadian prospective randomized multicenter IMPROVE-CHF study. Circulation. 2007;115(24):3103-10.
40. Bettencourt P, Azevedo A, Pimenta J, Friões F, Ferreira S, Ferreira A. N-terminal-pro-brain natriuretic peptide predicts outcome after hospital discharge in heart failure patients. Circulation. 2004;110(15):2168-74.
41. Fonarow GC, Peacock WF, Horwich TB, Phillips CO, Givertz MM, Lopatin M, et al. Usefulness of B-type natriuretic peptide and cardiac troponin levels to predict in-hospital mortality from ADHERE. Am J Cardiol. 2008;101(2):231-7.
42. Maisel A, Hollander JE, Guss D, McCullough P, Nowak R, Green G, et al. Primary results of the Rapid Emergency Department Heart Failure Outpatient Trial (REDHOT): a multicenter study of B-type natriuretic peptide levels, emergency department decision making, and outcomes in patients presenting with shortness of breath. J Am Coll Cardiol. 2004;44(6):1328-33.
43. Dhaliwal AS, Deswal A, Pritchett A, Aguilar D, Kar B, Souchek J, et al. Reduction in BNP levels with treatment of decompensated heart failure and future clinical events. J Card Fail. 2009;15(4):293-9.
44. Krauser DG, Lloyd-Jones DM, Chae CU, Cameron R, Anwaruddin S, Baggish AL, et al. Effect of body mass index on natriuretic peptide levels in patients with acute congestive heart failure: a ProBNP Investigation of Dyspnea in the Emergency Department (PRIDE) substudy. Am Heart J. 2005;149(4):744-50.
45. McCullough PA, Duc P, Omland T, McCord J, Nowak RM, Hollander JE, et al. B-type natriuretic peptide and renal function in the diagnosis of heart failure: an analysis from the Breathing Not Properly Multinational Study. Am J Kidney Dis. 2003;41(3):571-9.
46. Anwaruddin S, Lloyd-Jones DM, Baggish A, Chen A, Krauser D, Tung R, et al. Renal function, congestive heart failure, and amino-terminal pro-brain natriuretic peptide measurement: results from the ProBNP Investigation of Dyspnea in the Emergency Department (PRIDE) Study. J Am Coll Cardiol. 2006;47(1):91-7.
47. Karayannis G, Triposkiadis F, Skoularigis J, Georgoulias P, Butler J, Giamouzis G. The emerging role of Galectin-3 and ST2 in heart failure: practical considerations and pitfalls using novel biomarkers. Curr Heart Fail Rep. 2013;10(4):441-9.
48. McMurray JJ, Packer M, Desai AS, Gong J, Lefkowitz MP, Rizkala AR, et al. Angiotensin-neprilysin inhibition versus enalapril in heart failure. N Engl J Med. 2014;371(11):993-1004.
49. Sacks CA, Jarcho JA, Curfman GD. Paradigm shifts in heart-failure therapy: a timeline. N Engl J Med. 2014;371(11):989-91.
50. Collins SP, Storrow AB, Levy PD, Albert N, Butler J, Ezekowitz JA, et al. Early management of patients with acute heart failure: state of the art and future directions--a consensus document from the SAEM/HFSA acute heart failure working group. Acad Emerg Med. 2015;22(1):94-112.
51. Poulton EP. Left-sided heart failure with pulmonary edema: its treatment with the "pulmonary plus pressure machine". Lancet. 1936;228:981-3.
52. Bersten AD, Holt AW, Vedig AE, Skowronski GA, Baggoley CJ. Treatment of severe cardiogenic pulmonary edema with continuous positive airway pressure delivered by face mask. N Engl J Med. 1991;325(26):1825-30.
53. Moritz F, Brousse B, Gellee B, Chajara A, L'Her E, Hellot MF, et al. Continuous positive airway pressure versus bilevel noninvasive ventilation in acute cardiogenic pulmonary edema: a randomized multicenter trial. Ann Emerg Med. 2007;50(6):666-75, 675.e1.
54. Liesching T, Nelson DL, Cormier KL, Sucov A, Short K, Warburton R, et al. Randomized trial of bilevel versus continuous positive airway pressure for acute pulmonary edema. J Emerg Med. 2014;46(1):130-40.
55. Pang D, Keenan SP, Cook DJ, Sibbald WJ. The effect of positive pressure airway support on mortality and the need for intubation in cardiogenic pulmonary edema: a systematic review. Chest. 1998;114(4):1185-92.
56. Peter JV, Moran JL, Phillips-Hughes J, Graham P, Bersten AD. Effect of non-invasive positive pressure ventilation (NIPPV) on mortality in patients with acute cardiogenic pulmonary oedema: a meta-analysis. Lancet. 2006;367(9517):1155-63.
57. Weng CL, Zhao YT, Liu QH, Fu CJ, Sun F, Ma YL, et al. Meta-analysis: non-invasive ventilation in acute cardiogenic pulmonary edema. Ann Intern Med. 2010;152(8):590-600.
58. Vital FM, Saconato H, Ladeira MT, Sen A, Hawkes CA, Soares B, et al. Non-invasive positive pressure ventilation (CPAP or bilevel NPPV) for cardiogenic pulmonary edema. Cochrane Database Syst Rev. 2008;(3):CD005351.
59. Vital FM, Ladeira MT, Atallah AN. Non-invasive positive pressure ventilation (CPAP or bilevel NPPV) for cardiogenic pulmonary oedema. Cochrane Database Syst Rev. 2013;5:CD005351.
60. Cotter G, Felker GM, Adams KF, Milo-Cotter O, O'Connor CM. The pathophysiology of acute heart failure–is it all about fluid accumulation? Am Heart J. 2008;155(1):9-18.
61. Wakai A1, McCabe A, Kidney R, Brooks SC, Seupaul RA, Diercks DB, et al. Nitrates for acute heart failure syndromes. Cochrane Database Syst Rev. 2013;8:CD005151.
62. Elkayam U, Akhter MW, Singh H, Khan S, Usman A. Comparison of effects on left ventricular filling pressure of intravenous nesiritide and high-dose nitroglycerin in patients with decompensated heart failure. Am J Cardiol. 2004;93(2):237-40.
63. Levy P, Compton S, Welch R, Delgado G, Jennett A, Penugonda N, et al. Treatment of severe decompensated heart failure with high-dose intravenous nitroglycerin: a feasibility and outcome analysis. Ann Emerg Med. 2007;50(2):144-52.
64. Cioffi G, Stefenelli C, Tarantini L, Opasich C. Hemodynamic response to intensive unloading therapy (furosemide and nitroprusside) in patients >70 years of age with left ventricular systolic dysfunction and decompensated chronic heart failure. Am J Cardiol. 2003;92(9):1050-6.
65. Mullens W, Abrahams Z, Francis GS, Skouri HN, Starling RC, Young JB, et al. Sodium nitroprusside for advanced low-output heart failure. J Am Coll Cardiol. 2008;52(3):200-7.
66. Colucci WS, Elkayam U, Horton DP, Abraham WT, Bourge RC, Johnson AD, et al. Intravenous nesiritide, a natriuretic peptide, in the treatment of decompensated congestive heart failure. Nesiritide Study Group. N Engl J Med. 2000;343(4): 246-53.
67. O'Connor CM, Starling RC, Hernandez AF, Armstrong PW, Dickstein K, Hasselblad V, et al. Effect of nesiritide in patients with acute decompensated heart failure. N Engl J Med. 2011;365(1):32-43.
68. Maisel AS, Peacock WF, McMullin N, Jessie R, Fonarow GC, Wynne J, et al. Timing of immunoreactive B-type natriuretic peptide levels and treatment delay in acute decom- pensated heart failure: an ADHERE (Acute Decompensated Heart Failure National Registry) analysis. J Am Coll Cardiol. 2008;52(7):534-40.
69. Felker GM, Lee KL, Bull DA, Redfield MM, Stevenson LW, Goldsmith SR, et al. Diuretic strategies in patients with acute decompensated heart failure. N Engl J Med. 2011;364(9):797-805.
70. McMurray JJ, Adamopoulos S, Anker SD, Auricchio A, Bohm M, Dickstein K, et al. ESC Guidelines for the diagnosis and treatment of acute and chronic heart failure 2012: The Task Force for the Diagnosis and Treatment of Acute and Chronic Heart Failure 2012 of the European Society of Cardiology. Developed in collaboration with the Heart Failure Association (HFA) of the ESC. Eur J Heart Fail. 2012;14(8):803-69.
71. Peacock WF, Hollander JE, Diercks DB, Lopatin M, Fonarow G, Emerman CL. Morphine and outcomes in acute decompensated heart failure: an ADHERE analysis. Emerg Med J. 2008;25(4):205-9.
72. Cuffe MS, Califf RM, Adams KF, Benza R, Bourge R, Colucci WS, et al. Short-term intravenous milrinone for acute exacerbation of chronic heart failure: a randomized controlled trial. JAMA. 2002;287(12):1541-7.
73. Elkayam U, Tasissa G, Binanay C, Stevenson LW, Gheorghiade M, Warnica JW, et al. Use and impact of inotropes and vasodilator therapy in hospitalized patients with severe heart failure. Am Heart J. 2007;153(1): 98-104.
74. Abraham WT, Adams KF, Fonarow GC, Costanzo MR, Berkowitz RL, LeJemtel TH, et al. In-hospital mortality in patients with acute decompensated heart failure requiring intravenous vasoactive medications: an analysis from the Acute Decompensated Heart Failure National Registry (ADHERE). J Am Coll Cardiol. 2005;46(1):57-64.
75. O'Connor CM, Gattis WA, Uretsky BF, Adams KF, McNulty SE, Grossman SH, et al. Continuous intravenous dobutamine is associated with an increased risk of death in patients with advanced heart failure: insights from the Flolan International Randomized Survival Trial (FIRST). Am Heart J. 1999;138(1 Pt 1):78-86.
76. Hershberger RE, Nauman D, Walker TL, Dutton D, Burgess D. Care processes and clinical outcomes of continuous outpatient support with inotropes (COSI) in patients with refractory endstage heart failure. J Card Fail. 2003;9(3):180-7.
77. Gorodeski EZ, Chu EC, Reese JR, Shishehbor MH, Hsich E, Starling RC. Prognosis on chronic dobutamine or milrinone infusions for stage D heart failure. Circ Heart Fail. 2009;2(4):320-4.
78. Lazzeri C, Valente S, Chiostri M, D'Alfonso MG, Spini V, Angelotti P, et al. Admission Glycaemia and Acute Insulin Resistance in Heart Failure Complicating Acute Coronary Syndrome. Heart Lung Circ. 2015;24(11):1074-80.

79. O'Gara PT, Kushner FG, Ascheim DD, Casey DE, Chung MK, de Lemos JA, et al. 2013 ACCF/AHA guideline for the management of ST-elevation myocardial infarction: executive summary: a report of the American College of Cardiology Foundation/American Heart Association Task Force on Practice Guidelines. Circulation. 2013;127(4):529-55.
80. Anderson JL, Adams CD, Antman EM, Bridges CR, Califf RM, Casey DE, et al. 2012 ACCF/AHA focused update incorporated into the ACCF/AHA 2007 guidelines for the management of patients with unstable angina/non-ST-elevation myocardial infarction: a report of the American College of Cardiology Foundation/American Heart Association Task Force on Practice Guidelines. J Am Coll Cardiol. 2013;61(23):e179-347.
81. Wu AH, Parsons L, Every NR, Bates ER, Second National Registry of Myocardial Infarction. Hospital outcomes in patients presenting with congestive heart failure complicating acute myocardial infarction: a report from the Second National Registry of Myocardial Infarction (NRMI-2). J Am Coll Cardiol. 2002;40(8):1389-94.
82. Wang TJ, Larson MG, Levy D, Vasan RS, Leip EP, Wolf PA, et al. Temporal relations of atrial fibrillation and congestive heart failure and their joint influence on mortality: the Framingham Heart Study. Circulation. 2003; 107(23):2920-5.
83. Maisel WH, Stevenson LW. Atrial fibrillation in heart failure: epidemiology, pathophysiology, and rationale for therapy. Am J Cardiol. 2003;91(6A): 2D-8D.
84. January CT, Wann LS, Alpert JS, Calkins H, Cigarroa JE, Cleveland JC, et al. 2014 AHA/ACC/HRS guideline for the management of patients with atrial fibrillation: executive summary: a report of the American College of Cardiology/ American Heart Association Task Force on practice guidelines and the Heart Rhythm Society. Circulation. 2014;130(23):2071-104.
85. Abrams J, Allen J, Allin D, Anderson J, Anderson S, Blanski L, et al. Efficacy and safety of esmolol vs propranolol in the treatment of supraventricular tachyarrhythmias: a multicenter double-blind clinical trial. Am Heart J. 1985; 110(5):913-22.
86. Ellenbogen KA, Dias VC, Plumb VJ, Heywood JT, Mirvis DM. A placebo-controlled trial of continuous intravenous diltiazem infusion for 24-hour heart rate control during atrial fibrillation and atrial flutter: a multicenter study. J Am Coll Cardiol. 1991;18(4):891-7.
87. Siu CW, Lau CP, Lee WL, Lam KF, Tse HF. Intravenous diltiazem is superior to intravenous amiodarone or digoxin for achieving ventricular rate control in patients with acute uncomplicated atrial fibrillation. Crit Care Med. 2009;37(7):2174-9.
88. Platia EV, Michelson EL, Porterfield JK, Das G. Esmolol versus verapamil in the acute treatment of atrial fibrillation or atrial flutter. Am J Cardiol. 1989;63(13):925-9.
89. Delle Karth G, Geppert A, Neunteufl T, Priglinger U, Haumer M, Gschwandtner M, et al. Amiodarone versus diltiazem for rate control in critically ill patients with atrial tachyarrhythmias. Crit Care Med. 2001;29(6):1149-53.
90. Hou ZY, Chang MS, Chen CY, Tu MS, Lin SL, Chiang HT, et al. Acute treatment of recent-onset atrial fibrillation and flutter with a tailored dosing regimen of intravenous amiodarone. A randomized, digoxin-controlled study. Eur Heart J. 1995;16(4):521-8.
91. Clemo HF, Wood MA, Gilligan DM, Ellenbogen KA. Intravenous amiodarone for acute heart rate control in the critically ill patient with atrial tachyarrhythmias. Am J Cardiol. 1998;81(5):594-8.
92. Konstam MA. Relating quality of care to clinical outcomes in heart failure: in search of the missing link. J Card Fail 2001;7(4):299-301.
93. McCausland JB, Machi MS, Yealy DM. Emergency physicians' risk attitudes in acute decompensated heart failure patients. Acad Emerg Med. 2010;17(1):108-10.
94. Hernandez AF, Greiner MA, Fonarow GC, Hammill BG, Heidenreich PA, Yancy CW, et al. Relationship between early physician follow-up and 30-day readmission among Medicare beneficiaries hospitalized for heart failure. JAMA. 2010;303(17):1716-22.
95. Lee DS, Stukel TA, Austin PC, Alter DA, Schull MJ, You JJ, et al. Improved outcomes with early collaborative care of ambulatory heart failure patients discharged from the emergency department. Circulation. 2010;122(18):1806-14.
96. Schrager J, Wheatley M, Georgiopoulou V, Osborne A, Kalogeropoulos A, Hung O, et al. Favorable bed utilization and readmission rates for emergency department observation unit heart failure patients. Acad Emerg Med. 2013;20(6):554-61.
97. Sharma GV, Woods PA, Lindsey N, O'Connell C, Connolly L, Joseph J, et al. Noninvasive monitoring of left ventricular end-diastolic pressure reduces rehospitalization rates in patients hospitalized for heart failure: a randomized controlled trial. J Card Fail. 2011;17(9):718-25.

21 CHAPTER

The Role of Observation Units in Acute Heart Failure

Edgardo Ordonez

INTRODUCTION

Based on recent estimations in 2010, there were approximately 676,000 emergency department (ED) visits for acute heart failure (AHF).[1] In addition, heart failure (HF) costs the nation an estimated 32 billion a year and this number is projected to increase to around 43 billion by the year 2020.[2] As ED visits for AHF continue to increase, the emergency provider must have options for the disposition of these patients. Previous experience shows that most ED AHF visits result in hospitalization, with four out of five patients being admitted.[3-5] It has been recently estimated that approximately 50% of patients who present to the ED with AHF could be discharged after a brief period of observation.[6]

The observation unit (OU) can serve as both a safe and cost-effective option to provide care for patients with AHF.[3,4,7-11] The OU can also be helpful to further risk stratify patients and initiate treatment in the outpatient setting and allow for a period in which the need for inpatient admission can further be determined. Other elements that are essential to the management of AHF in the OU would be to optimize pharmacotherapy, patient education on diet, smoking cessation and medication adherence, consultation with a cardiologist or heart failure specialists as needed, and arrangement of postdischarge follow-up.[4]

RISK STRATIFICATION AND PATIENT SELECTION FOR THE OBSERVATION UNIT

Determining the appropriate AHF patient for the OU is not as straightforward as other diagnoses given that many patients with AHF have comorbidities that can make their disposition decision more difficult. Several decision rules and risk calculators help ED providers delineate low-risk patients that are appropriate for outpatient or OU evaluation and management of other disease processes such as the CURB-65 score for pneumonia, Pulmonary Embolism Severity Index (PESI), thrombolysis in myocardial infarction (TIMI) score for unstable angina/non ST-segment elevation myocardial infarction (UA/NSTEMI), and the San Francisco Syncope Rule. In patients with AHF, there are criteria that aid in determining high-risk patients, such as hypotension, hyponatremia, renal dysfunction, elevated troponin levels, and elevated natriuretic peptides, but unfortunately, absence of those criteria does not necessarily deem patients to be low-risk.[12-18] Additionally, these patients are generally too medically complex for the OU setting.

The Society for Cardiovascular Patient Care (SCPC) has previously published recommendations for the management of the AHF patient in the OU.[19] Included in those recommendations are risk stratification criteria used to appropriately select patients for OU disposition based on the available evidence.[19] Below is a brief discussion of each variable along with the most recent recommendations by the SCPC if applicable. Boxes 1 and 2 show sample transfer and exclusion criteria, respectively.

Hemodynamic Status

Systolic hypertension is common in patients hospitalized with AHF and is an independent predictor of morbidity and mortality. Georghiade et al. published data using a cohort from the OPTIMIZE-HF (Organized Program to Initiate Lifesaving Treatment In Hospitalized Patients

BOX 1 Sample transfer criteria

Sample transfer criteria

- Patient ≥18 years of age, with diagnosis and planned treatment for acute heart failure requiring further management beyond initial ED treatment
- Patients with the following findings:
  - Dyspnea at rest or minimal exertion per the patient
  - Evidence of extracellular volume expansion by at least one of the following: JVD, rales, ascites, edema or positive chest X-ray defined as cardiomegaly, pulmonary vascular congestion, Kerley B-lines, pulmonary edema, and/or pleural effusion
  - Elevated BNP level >100

BNP, B-type natriuretic peptides; ED, emergency department; JVD, jugular venous distention.

BOX 2 Sample exclusion criteria

- Unstable vital signs (BP >220/120 or SBP <90, HR >130, RR ≥32, 02 sat <90%)
- Temperature >38.5
- On renal replacement therapy or creatinine ≥3
- Blood urea nitrogen ≥40
- Sodium <135
- Troponin level >99th percentile
- EKG with findings suggestive of acute ischemia
- Treatment with intravenous infusion vasoactive drugs in the hour prior to enrollment
- Heart failure due to atrial fibrillation with rapid ventricular response
- Other comorbidities acutely exacerbated
- Patients requiring noninvasive positive pressure ventilation

BP, blood pressure; ECG, electrocardiogram; HR, heart rate; SBP, systolic blood pressure.

With Heart Failure) registry, which showed that patients with lower systolic blood pressure (SBP) at admission had higher hospital and postdischarge mortality rates. Higher SBP at admission was associated with lower in-hospital mortality rates: 7.2% (<120 mm Hg), 3.6% (120–139 mm Hg), 2.5% (140–161 mm Hg), and 1.7% (>161 mm Hg; p <0.001).[12] Another study by Fonarow also looked at SBP as a variable of predicting inpatient mortality, and used this as a way to develop a risk stratification tool. Patients were considered low, intermediate, or high risk, with an SBP of less than 115 mm Hg considered a high predictor of mortality.[17]

Notes: The Society for Cardiovascular Patient Care recommends systolic blood pressure greater than or equal to 100 mm Hg on presentation; consider systolic blood pressure greater than 120 mm Hg.

Serum Sodium Concentration

Hyponatremia is defined as a serum sodium concentration of less than 135 mmol/L and can be associated with hypervolemic, hypovolemic, and euvolemic states. The majority of patients with AHF will have a dilutional hyponatremia secondary to hypervolemia. It is commonly found in patients hospitalized with AHF, and rates of hyponatremia of about 20–21% have been noted in several studies.[13,18,20-23] It has been shown that hospitalized patients with hyponatremia at the time of AHF presentation have poorer prognosis, longer hospital stays, and overall increased morbidity and mortality than those patients with normal serum sodium concentrations.[13,18,20-23]

Notes: The Society for Cardiovascular Patient Care recommends serum sodium concentration greater than or equal to 135 mmol/L on presentation.

Renal Function

Renal function can be assessed by evaluating serum blood urea nitrogen (BUN), serum creatinine, or glomerular filtration rate. Patients with AHF and concomitant renal disease is now increasing in incidence, and having both organ dysfunctions provides higher morbidity and mortality than each individual disease entity alone.[24] Several studies have showed that a higher baseline BUN was a powerful predictor of mortality, even in the absence of severe renal failure in patients with AHF.[14,25,26] A study by Formiga et al. also concluded that patients with an elevated creatinine had increased in-hospital mortality.[27] Having renal disease can make for more difficult OU treatment due to the delicate balance of the need of aggressive diuresis with monitoring of renal function.

Notes: The Society for Cardiovascular Patient Care recommends blood urea nitrogen less than 40 mg/dL.

The Society for Cardiovascular Patient Care recommends creatinine less than 3 mg/dL.

Cardiac Ischemia

A study published by Chin et al. found that ischemic electrocardiographic changes, among the other variables previously discussed, were associated with major complication or death in the hospital.[28] Additionally, Peacock et al. analyzed the Acute Decompensated Heart Failure National Registry for patients hospitalized with AHF and an elevated troponin. In this study, patients who had a positive troponin had a lower SBP on admission, a lower ejection fraction (EF), and higher inhospital mortality, independent of other predictive variables, than those who did not have an elevated troponin.[15] Similar findings of adverse outcomes have previously been published by Kuwabara et al.[29] and have recently been found in a study by Braga et al.[30] In general, a troponin level below the 99th percentile, as established by the each individual hospitals laboratory, would be appropriate for an OU stay.

Notes: The Society for Cardiovascular Patient Care recommends absence of new ischemic ECG changes and/or elevated troponin levels.

Natriuretic Peptides

The B-type natriuretic peptides (BNP) can be a useful tool for ED providers in diagnosing congestive HF as the cause of a patient's dyspnea.[31] As an example, it may aid in differentiating congestive HF from chronic obstructive pulmonary disease in patients with both conditions, and guide appropriate treatment and disposition. This biomarker is a neurohormone that is increased as a response to volume expansion and pressure overload occurring in the ventricles.[32] The use of this biomarker allows for more diagnostic certainty along with other signs of AHF to determine appropriateness for an OU stay. Currently, there are no clear cutoffs as to what BNP levels would be appropriate for an OU stay, although it is known that increasing BNP levels correlate with disease severity.

Notes: The Society for Cardiovascular Patient Care recommends B-type natriuretic peptides less than 1,000 pg/mL or N-terminal pro (NT)-BNP less than 5,000 pg/mL.

Other Risk Stratification Factors

Several other factors should be considered when determining if a patient is appropriate for an OU admission. As previously stated, the most recent SCPC recommendations have provided some criteria as guidelines. Patients who have not previously been diagnosed with HF may be better suited for an inpatient admission. It is important to consider the patient's respiratory status, and whether there is an increased respiratory rate, or if the patient is requiring noninvasive ventilation at the time of OU entry. Those who are receiving an intravenous infusion, that is being actively titrated, would also not be ideal candidates. It would be beneficial if the patient has had at least a partial response to the therapy that has been initiated in the ED. Additionally, and at times equally important, is that each patient have access to adequate social support and follow-up.[19] If patients do not meet the criteria as above, the patient may better be served in an inpatient setting, as the hospitalization is likely to span more than an 8–24 hour stay.

TREATMENT IN THE OBSERVATION UNIT

Oxygen Therapy and Respiratory Support

The immediate treatment of AHF, given its transient nature, encompasses both respiratory support and pharmacologic therapy. It is generally accepted that noninvasive ventilation such as continuous positive airway pressure or bilevel positive airway pressure is an adjunct in the treatment of AHF that helps prevent the need for intubation.[33] While such interventions would not be appropriately carried out in the OU setting, patients may be appropriate for the OU if they initially required them in the emergency setting, as these patients may rapidly improve with concurrent pharmacologic treatments. Patients in the OU may still require some form of respiratory support, such as nasal cannula or oxygen via facemask, and would be appropriate to manage in this setting to determine the ability to titrate the patient off this treatment during the observation period.

Diuretics

Patients with AHF are generally volume overloaded. Diuretics are considered one of the first-line agents for the treatment of AHF patients with evidence of volume overload, as they can relieve symptoms and improve oxygenation.[34] Given that these patients usually present to the outpatient or emergency setting severely symptomatic, it is recommended that intravenous treatment over oral therapy be initiated, given its greater and more consistent bioavailability. In the emergency setting, patients are generally given an initial bolus of intravenous diuretic that may be equal to or up to two and a half time greater than their usual home dose of oral diuretic. Diuretic naïve patients may receive less.

Common loop diuretics used currently are furosemide and bumetanide. They can be given as both a bolus dose or as a continuous infusion. Felker et al. recently published that there were no significant differences in patient's global assessment of symptoms or in the change in renal function when loop diuretic therapy in the form of furosemide was administered by bolus, as compared to intravenous infusion or at a high dose as compared with a low dose.[35] This information is pertinent to patients who may be appropriate for an OU stay, as continuous infusions may be burdensome for some units to manage with their nursing staffing models. Peak diuresis tends to occur within the first 30–60 minutes after administration in the ED, and the OU would allow for continued diuretic dosing, monitoring of intake and output, weights, hemodynamics, and oxygenation. Additionally, continued assessment of renal function and electrolytes, which can be negatively affected by the use of diuretics, can be evaluated.

Clinicians need to take into account that diuretic therapy, especially in moderate to high doses, does not go without risks. As previously discussed in risk stratification, due to the increasing incidence of patients with AHF and renal disease, diuretic therapy can potentially worsen this and lead to increased morbidity and mortality.

Vasodilators

In addition to diuretic therapy, pharmacologic treatment for AHF may consist of vasodilators such as nitrates, nitroprusside, and nesiritide. These agents are frequently used in patients with congestive symptoms along with normal to elevated blood pressures.[36] One of the earliest trials to show the benefits of nitrates was published by Cotter et al. using isosorbide dinitrate.[37] Nitroglycerin is the most commonly used vasodilator and can be given in sublingual, transdermal, or intravenous forms. It has a significantly shorter half-life than isosorbide dinitrate and thus a more desirable safety profile for intravenous use. Nitroglycerin is known to reduce left ventricular pressures and lowers afterload while increasing stroke volume and cardiac output. Its dosing ranges from 5 µg/min to a max of 200 µg/min, but general starting doses in hypertensive AHF patients will be 50 µg/min or greater. The need for titration and frequent hemodynamic monitoring due to its use is integral in the initial emergency setting but would not be appropriate for the OU.

In some cases, nitroglycerin is not effective in blood pressure and symptom control in AHF, and a more potent vasodilator, such as nitroprusside is indicated. Nitroprusside produces significant reduction in pulmonary capillary wedge pressure and an increase in cardiac output. It is generally started at a dose of 5–10 µg/min and titrated upwards.[38] However, there are limitations to its use due to the potential accumulation of cyanide. Patients requiring a nitroprusside infusion would most likely need and intensive care unit setting and would not be suitable candidates for the OU.

Nesiritide is a natriuretic peptide identical to BNP and has been used in the treatment of AHF. Initial trials had shown that nesiritide decreased pulmonary capillary wedge pressures and also dyspnea in patients with AHF.[39,40] A multicenter trial showed that a nesiritide treatment group in the ED of OU setting was shown to have decreased rates of hospitalization compared to the standard treatment group, although the findings were not statistically significant. However, rates of hospital rehospitalization were statistically significantly lower in the nesiritide treatment group.[41] More recently, a large randomized controlled trial by O'Connor et al. found that nesiritide was not associated with an increase or a decrease in the rate of death and rehospitalization, and had a small nonsignificant effect on dyspnea when used in combination with other therapies. It also was noted to have increased rates of hypotension.[42] While there is still debate as to whether or not nesiritide will become more standard in the treatment of AHF, its ability to be a nontitratable infusion makes it an attractive option for potential OU protocols.

Angiotensin-converting Enzyme Inhibitors

The majority of patient with HF and a reduced EF will benefit from angiotensin-converting enzyme (ACE) inhibitors. Current guidelines by several expert panels endorse its use as standard therapy for HF and as an appropriate medication to initiate in OU setting unless there is a contraindication.[19,34,36] Several randomized trials have shown the benefits of ACE inhibitors in symptom improvement, reduction in hospitalization, and a reduction in mortality in patients with HF, and systolic dysfunction.[43,44]

Angiotensin converting enzyme inhibitors are avoided in patients with previous exposures leading to severe life-threatening reactions (e.g., angioedema). It is also contraindicated in patients who are pregnant or who plan to become pregnant. Caution must be taken in prescribing ACE inhibitors to patients with very low systemic blood pressures or severely increased serum creatinine levels of less than 3 mg/dL. Additional caution must be taken with patients who have an elevated serum potassium level less than 5 mEq/L, as initiation of an ACE inhibitor can potentiate the hyperkalemia.

There are many options of ACE inhibitors to choose from and it is up to the clinician to make the decision on which ACE inhibitor to use. It is advisable to start at the lowest available dose and titrate upwards as tolerated. Monitoring of serum creatinine and potassium levels can be done at 1–2 weeks after initiation of therapy and possibly after dose adjustments if indicated. If patients cannot tolerate ACE inhibitors, angiotensin receptor blockers (ARBs) are a suitable replacement.

Beta-blockers

As with ACE inhibitors, β-blockers are a mainstay in the treatment of patient with HF and a reduced EF, and are also supported by guidelines of several expert panels.[19,34,36] Studies have shown symptom improvement, decreased hospitalizations, and survival benefits in patients with HF and a reduced EF who are on β-blocker therapy.[45-48] Ideally, β-blockers should not be started on patients who have decompensated HF as this can worsen their outcome. As with ACE inhibitors, β-blockers should be initiated at a low dose and can be instituted after or in conjunction with ACE inhibitor therapy. The most commonly used β-blockers for HF are carvedilol, sustained release metoprolol succinate, and bisoprolol. Patients previously on β-blocker therapy can be continued on this therapy in the OU, while those not previously on therapy can have it initiated in this setting.

Aldosterone Antagonists

Aldosterone receptor antagonists are recommended in patients with New York Heart Association (NYHA) class II–IV HF and who have an EF of 35% or less, unless contraindicated, to reduce morbidity and mortality.[34,49] The Randomized Aldactone Evaluation Study (RALES) trial showed a significant reduction in all-cause mortality and decreased hospitalization in patients with HF and reduced EF.[50] Similar results were seen with the aldosterone antagonist eplerenone in a separate trial.[51] Patients should have a serum creatinine less than 2.5 mg/dL in males and 2 mg/dL in females, with serum potassium less than 5 mEq/L. Monitoring of renal function and potassium levels will be indicated after initiation of therapy. As with other chronic therapy above, this medication can be continued in the OU or initiated, if the patient had not previously been on treatment, at the lowest starting dose.

Hydralazine and Isosorbide Dinitrate

Hydralazine plus nitrate therapy, when compared to placebo, has been shown to have a favorable effect on left ventricular function and mortality on patients with chronic HF who were on digoxin and a diuretic, with a greater mortality benefit noted in African-Americans.[52,53] Follow-up studies have further evaluated the combination of hydralazine and isosorbide dinitrate. In one comparison to the efficacy of ACE inhibitors, there was a trend towards reduction in mortality in the ACE inhibitor group, but posthoc analyses showed the mortality benefit with ACE inhibitors was seen only in white patients with hypertension.[53,54]

Additional studies evaluated the efficacy of the combination of hydralazine and isosorbide dinitrate on African-American patients who were already on some standard HF treatment regimen. Results showed significantly lower rates of mortality in the combination group versus placebo.[55,56] Subsequent studies have further solidified that combination therapy with hydralazine and isosorbide dinitrate was associated with a substantial reduction in HF hospitalizations, echocardiographic parameters, morbidity, and mortality.[57,58]

The American College of Cardiology and American Heart Association (ACC/AHA) guidelines state that, the combination of hydralazine and isosorbide dinitrate is recommended for self-described African-American patients with NYHA class III–IV HF with a reduced EF receiving optimal therapy with ACE inhibitors and β-blockers, unless contraindicated.[34] It also recommends the combination in all patients with current or prior symptomatic HF with a reduced EF who cannot be given and ACE inhibitor or ARB due to drug intolerance, hypotension, or renal insufficiency.[34]

Digoxin

Digoxin has long been used in patients with HF due to systolic dysfunction. While it is known that digoxin does not decrease mortality in patients with HF, it has previously been published to show benefits in improving symptoms of HF while also decreasing hospitalizations.[59-61] Digoxin is not generally used for the treatment of AHF, but it may be initiated after stabilization. Patients with chronic HF who are on first line therapy can be considered for its use, as it is supported by current guidelines to help decrease hospitalizations for HF.[34]

DIAGNOSTIC EVALUATION

Laboratory Studies

Given that patients with AHF in the OU are on aggressive diuretic therapy up to 2.5 times their normal home dosing, and will ideally have increased urine output, it is imperative to monitor electrolytes during periods of diuresis. This is especially true for potassium and magnesium, as depletion of these electrolytes can cause conduction disturbances and cardiac rhythms that can potentially be fatal. The potassium level should be kept between 4 and 5 mEq/L. Magnesium levels should be supplemented if there is a deficiency. The OU also allows for evaluation of serial cardiac biomarkers as indicated to evaluate for ischemia as the cause of AHF. A troponin greater than 99th percentile should exclude patients from OU admission, or if found later, transition them to the inpatient setting.

Electrocardiogram and Continuous Cardiac Monitoring

Cardiac monitoring is an essential diagnostic tool used in the OU setting for AHF patients and goes hand in hand with laboratory evaluation. If there are conduction disturbances, abnormal rhythms, or evidence of ischemia on electrocardiography or cardiac monitoring, this can prompt rapid evaluation of electrolytes or cardiac biomarkers and subsequent appropriate treatment.

Respiratory Monitoring

Given that patients with AHF are mainly symptomatic with dyspnea, respiratory support in the form of nasal cannula or facemask is appropriate in the OU setting. Continuous pulse oximetry allows the clinician frequent assessments of the patients response to therapy. The goal would be to have the patient return to their baseline oxygenation requirement.

Hemodynamic Monitoring

A significant number of patients with AHF in the OU will initially have presented to the ED with elevated SBP, with some of them requiring intravenous vasoactive medications to improve blood pressure and symptoms. While those patients on titratable medications are not OU appropriate, due to the need of increased hemodynamic monitoring, there is still a need for frequent assessment of hemodynamics due to the potential increased urine output causing a drop in blood pressure.

Echocardiography

Echocardiography provides valuable information for the clinician such as atrial, ventricular, and valvular structure and function. It is essential that all patients with new onset HF have echocardiography performed. For patients with chronic HF the ACC/AHA performance measures suggest that adult patients have left ventricular ejection fraction (LVEF) assessment documented within a 12-month period in the outpatient setting. For those that are inpatient, LVEF assessment is to be performed either before arrival or during hospitalization, or have documentation to show that it is planned after discharge.[62] This noninvasive test is appropriate to be done in the OU setting, if indicated.

CONSULTATIONS IN THE OBSERVATION UNIT

The OU setting provides a good time frame to obtain important consultations that may help improve the patient's outpatient treatment plan and follow-up. These can include, but are not limited to, cardiologists/HF specialists, advanced practice providers, nurses, health educators, dietitians, pharmacists, and social workers/case managers.

PATIENT EDUCATION IN THE OBSERVATION UNIT

Educating patients with HF on several topics related to their disease process is essential in reducing hospital admissions and readmissions, while also decreasing healthcare costs. Unfortunately, patients who present to the ED with AHF tend to have comorbid conditions, are on multiple medications, and have poor adherence to their regimens. The management of patients with HF is multifactorial and must encompass not only medication adherence, but also lifestyle modification, dietary restrictions, frequent follow-up, and continued education. It is important for the clinician and support staff to understand any barriers the patient may have, be they financial, social support, time constraints, or transportation issues in order to offer and provide optimal care for the patient.

Medication Adherence

Medication nonadherence is common in patients with HF, and plays a major role in preventable rehospitalizations. A recent meta-analysis of the literature showed that medication adherence ranged from 10 to 93%, with most investigators publishing rates between 40% and 60%.[63] Several factors are important when considering medication adherence in patients and the World Health Organization (WHO) developed a report on adherence to long-term therapies to describe this framework.[64] The five dimensions of this framework are: (i) socioeconomic factors, (ii) healthcare system-related factors, (iii) condition-related factors, (iv) treatment-related factors and (v) patient-related factors (Fig. 1).

The OU setting can provide time to do in-depth medication reconciliation with the patient. Each facility will have its own method of performing this, but in order to ensure that the most up-to-date information is obtained, it can be requested that patients' families or caregivers bring any medications from home to compare to what is documented in the patient chart and to correct any discrepancies prior to discharge. It is also important to obtain information on herbal supplements, vitamins, minerals, or any other over-the-counter medications used. This will help reduce any dosing errors, duplicates, and omissions, while also reviewing any potential drug interactions.

Dietary Adherence

A sodium-restricted diet is reasonable for patients with HF to reduce congestive symptoms and is supported by current guidelines.[19,34,36] Several studies have noted the relationship between sodium and hypertension, left

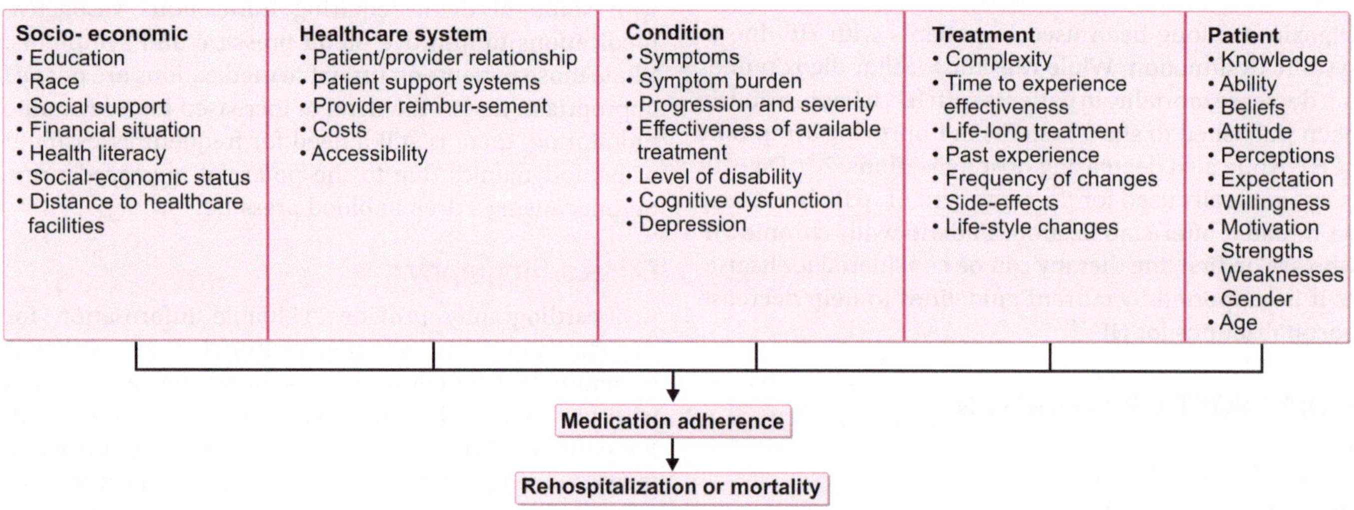

FIG. 1: World Health Organization's multidimensional adherence model and rehospitalization

ventricular hypertrophy and cardiovascular disease.[65-68] The exact cutoff for sodium restriction is unclear because of confounding data suggesting that some patients with HF with a reduced EF have worse outcomes with sodium restriction.[69-71]

Counseling on sodium restriction should involve not only the patient, but also family members and caregivers, as they may be involved in the daily food planning. Patients may benefit from completing a food diary over a specific time frame to assess what average food consumption is and where improvements can be made. It would also be helpful to encourage them to read food labels, make alternative food choices when possible, and substitute salt with other herbs and spices to improve the flavor of foods. Printed materials, web-based education materials, or referral to a dietitian can also help provide the patient with helpful resources to adhere to a strict diet.

Smoking Cessation

Smoking is a known independent risk factor of mortality in patients with HF.[72] Several guidelines recommend smoking cessation as part of patient education.[19,34,36] This can be done in the OU setting, given the ample time for patient interaction. Other options include referrals to smoking cessation classes. In addition, depending on the patient motivation to change behavior at the time of OU treatment, it may be plausible to start the patient on pharmacologic treatment to reduce the cravings of nicotine.

Alcohol Consumption

As with the general public, patients with HF should limit their alcohol intake. The Heart Failure Society of America (HFSA) and SCPC's recommend limiting alcohol to less than 2 drinks/day for men and less than 1 drink/day for women.[19,36] Those with alcohol-related cardiomyopathy should abstain from alcohol altogether.

Symptom Monitoring

Patients with HF need to be educated on monitoring their symptoms at home to help prevent ED visits, hospitalizations, and rehospitalizations. A few factors that the patient must be aware of and monitor are daily weights, increased dyspnea, increased edema, or worsening fatigue. A multicenter randomized trial utilizing a technology-based daily weight and symptom-monitoring system for patients with advanced HF was shown to significantly reduce mortality, although there was no difference in rehospitalization rates.[73] Unfortunately, adherence to daily weight monitoring in published trials ranges from 20 to 80%.[74] Symptom monitoring continues to be poorly performed by HF patients.[75] This is an area that must continue to be reinforced and would be beneficial to implement as part of the OU educational program.

Below are the SCPC's published recommendations on patient education elements in the OU setting:[19]

- Medication adherence
  - Instructions regarding importance of taking medication as prescribed including its purpose, recommend schedule and what to do if a dose is missed
  - Identify those patients at high risk for non-adherence who may benefit from referral to a comprehensive disease management program.
- Dietary adherence
  - A dietary intake of 2,000–3,000 mg of sodium per day is strongly recommended
  - Identify those patients at high risk for non-adherence
  - Review sources of high sodium, including hidden sources. Include family members in instruction since they can unknowingly become contributors to a patient's decompensation
  - Review recent dietary intake to identify possible sodium indiscretion contributing to current decompensation.
- Smoking cessation
  - All current smokers should receive information and reinforcement on smoking cessation
  - Refer to smoking cessation program
  - Consider prescribing oral or topical agents for nicotine cravings.
- Alcohol consumption
  - Limit alcohol consumption (<2 drinks/day for men, <1 drink/day for women)
  - Refer to abstinence program as needed.
- Symptom monitoring
  - Daily weights should be encouraged, using the same scale, wearing similar clothing, at same time per day.
  - Notification of clinician with change in weight and/or symptoms; i.e., weight gain of 3 or more pounds overnight or 5 pounds over 3 days, increased dyspnea, increase fatigue, dizziness, etc.

DISPOSITION AND DISCHARGE CRITERIA FROM THE OBSERVATION UNIT

The disposition of the patient from the OU is either to admit as an inpatient due to worsening or lack of improvement of the clinical condition, or to discharge the patient home to further continue outpatient management in a nonhospitalized setting. The decision can be based on several factors including the patient's subjective feeling of improvement, objective parameters and clinician judgment.

Clinical Congestion

Both objective and subjective criteria for clinical congestion can be used to assess a patient's improvement in the OU setting. Evaluation of jugular venous pressure (JVP), rales on lung examination, edema, urine output, and weight can provide objective criteria by which clinicians can base disposition decisions. Patients may also express decreased dyspnea and orthopnea. It would be beneficial to ambulate patients prior to discharge to determine if exertional dyspnea or dyspnea greater than baseline remains. A 3-minute walk test has previously been proposed as a way to assess patients for discharge decisions in the ED who presented with cardiopulmonary conditions.[76] Also, due to increased urine output from excessive diuresis, patients may become orthostatic and experience symptoms of dizziness, which would alert the clinician that the patient might warrant further observation.

Vital Signs

As with most OU protocols, patients would be discharged when they are in stable condition, and those who are not would be admitted to an inpatient bed. Vital signs provide more objective criteria by which to evaluate a patient's clinical condition and improvement. It is important to look at both blood pressure and heart rate as objective parameters for readiness for OU discharge as they are known to be significant independent predictors of mortality in patients with AHF.[17] It has been recommended that patients with AHF have a blood pressure less than 160 mm Hg at the time of discharge.[77] Oxygen saturation is another criterion used for discharge and previous recommendations have used 90% oxygen saturation as a suitable number, although there is no clear evidence behind that recommendation.[10]

Renal Function

As previously noted in the risk stratification section, both BUN and creatinine have been shown to be predictors of mortality in patients with AHF at the time of presentation. Furthermore, it has been shown that worsening of renal function during treatment is also a predictor of inhospital mortality.[77-79] A worsening of the serum creatinine by more than 0.3 mg/dL from hospital admission correlated with worse patient outcomes and would suggest that these patients, if in the OU setting, warrant further treatment until the creatinine improves or stabilizes, or inpatient admission. Equally important is to evaluate serum sodium levels to ensure that the patient has not developed hyponatremia, as this has also been shown to be a predictor of mortality as previously detailed.[13,18,20,22,23,80]

Support System

It must be noted that the management of the patient with HF requires a multidisciplinary team approach. Emergency physicians, OU physicians, advanced practice providers, nurses, pharmacists, dietitians, and socials workers/case managers all play an integral role in diagnosing, treating, planning, and implementing the total care of the HF patient. Issues that caused the patient to present to the ED acutely decompensated must be addressed, whether they be due to medication nonadherence, dietary nonadherence, depression, financial constraints, transportation issues, or inadequate follow-up arrangements. Family members should be engaged and encouraged to be involved as much as possible. A follow-up appointment and/or in home health nurse visit would ideally be scheduled prior to discharge from the OU. Documentation to meet all Joint Commission Accreditation Health Care Organizations (JCAHO) core measures should be in the chart.

The SCPC has published recommendations on optimal discharge criteria for patients with AHF from the OU.[19] These criteria were further validated in a clinical trial by Collins et al.[81] The parameters below have been adapted from their recommendations as criteria for discharge from the OU.

- Improvement in clinical congestion
  - Decrease in jugular venous pressure
  - Resolution of rales
  - Resolution of orthopnea
  - Improvement of edema
  - Improvement of dyspnea
  - Ability to ambulate without dyspnea above baseline or orthostasis
  - Decrease in weight
  - Adequate urine output.
- Stable vital signs
  - Blood pressure
  - Heart rate without tachycardia or bradycardia
  - Oxygen saturation greater than 90% on room air or from baseline oxygen source.
- Evaluation of renal function
  - No significant alterations in serum creatinine
  - No significant alterations in serum electrolytes, in particular (Na, K, Mg).
- Support system
  - Reasons for decompensation have been addressed and/or reversed
  - Patient and family education completed
  - Follow-up visit within 7–10 days after OU stay
  - Completion of JCAHO core measures.

CONCLUSION

The role of OUs in the management of AHF will continue to play an increasing role in reducing hospital admissions, readmissions and healthcare costs. As outlined in this chapter, essential elements in successful OUs include utilizing evidence-based protocols for diagnosing, risk-stratifying, and managing patients with specific endpoints that can determine the need for admission. Due to the medical complexity of many patients with AHF, the OU affords the optimal setting to give patients sufficient time to be stabilized, treated aggressively, given education and have barriers addressed prior to a disposition. With new and emerging diagnostic and treatment modalities on the horizon, the OU may also play a critical role in their implementation. Boxes 3 and 4 outline a sample OU treatment protocol and order set for reference.

BOX 3 Sample observation unit treatment protocol for heart failure

Essential elements

- Monitoring
  - Cardiac monitoring
  - Pulse oximetry
  - Daily weights
  - Intake and output
- Diagnostic testing
  - Electrocardiograms
  - Cardiac biomarkers
  - Serum electrolytes
  - Echocardiogram
- Treatment algorithm
  - Diuretics
  - Vasodilators (if indicated)
  - Oxygen therapy
  - Electrolyte replacement
- Dietary
  - Low sodium diet
  - Fluid restriction
- Patient education
  - Educational videos, handouts on HF
  - Bedside teaching
  - Smoking cessation counseling
  - Dietitic consultation
- Discharge planning
  - Social work/case management
  - Cardiology/HF specialist

HF, heart failure.

BOX 4 Sample order set

- Vital signs: Q 4 hours
  - Optimize systolic blood pressure: notify MD if too high or low
    - Optimum systolic BP = lowest pressure that supports renal function (Urine output >0.5 cc/kg/h with reasonable BUN/creatinine) and CNS activity (mentation) without significant or long suffering orthostatic symptoms

Continued

Continued

- Respiratory
  - Continuous pulse oximetry
  - Oxygen via nasal cannula, keep O_2 saturation >92%
- Intake and output: Q 4 hours (insert Foley catheter PRN, especially if heavy diuresis interrupts sleep)
  - Fluid restriction: 1,800 cc per 24 hours fluid restriction
- Laboratory Studies
  - BMP and CBC 14 hours after admission or 2 hours before discharge (if planned discharge is before 14 hours)
  - Follow potassium (Table 1) and magnesium (Table 2) nomograms for hypokalemia
  - Troponin level at 0, 3, and 6 hours to assess for ischemia
- Diagnostic studies
  - If ejection fraction has never been measured or was measured over 1 year ago and was normal, order 2D-echocardiography
  - Continuous ECG monitoring and 12 lead ECG if indicated
- Interventions
  - Smoking cessation counseling
  - Heart failure medication education
  - ACE-inhibitor/ARB trial
  - Arrange for outpatient follow-up appointment within 1 week
- Medications
  - Initiate intravenous furosemide protocol as follows:
    - Give IV furosemide dose equivalent to prior outpatient total daily dose up to 180 mg maximum (single dose) or → 40 mg IV (if never taken furosemide before)
- Guidelines
  - If normal renal function: expect 500 cc urine in 2 h/onset of action: 5 min
  - If renal insufficiency: expect >250 cc urine in 2 h/peak concentration in HF 2–4 h
  - After 3 h, if furosemide is effective but diuresis target has not been reached or if Furosemide has been ineffective in delivering expected 2 h urine output, double dose of Furosemide and administer IV
  - After 6 h if no diuretic given and/or total OU urine output is <1,000 cc, notify MD
  - If patient has a very pronounced diuresis response (>2 L) from diuretics and/or vasodilator therapy, obtain a K^+ level
  - If resting heart rate <60 or >120 and/or NEW rhythm or conduction disturbances: STAT metabolic panel, basic, and Mg^{++} level

ACE, angiotensin-converting enzyme; ARB, angiotensin receptor blocker; IV, intravenous; BP, blood pressure; BMP, basic metabolic profile; BUN, blood urea nitrogen; CBC, complete blood count; CNS, central nervous system; ECG, electrocardiogram; 2D, two-dimmential; HF, heart failure; MD, medical doctor.

TABLE 1: Potassium (give intravenous or per oral dose unless specifically stated)

Level	IV dose	PO dose	Recheck K^+
3.7–3.9 mEq/dL	20 mEq*	40 mEq*	12 h or in the morning
3.4–3.6 mEq/dL	20 mEq × 2 doses*	40 mEq × 2 doses*	6 h or in the morning
3.0–3.3 mEq/dL	20 mEq × 4 doses	40 mEq × 3 doses*	4 h after last dose
<3.0 mEq/dL	20 mEq × 6 doses*	Give IV only	1 h after last infusion

* Before giving dose, assess last serum creatinine level. If serum creatinine level is above 2.5 mg/dL (reflecting renal insufficiency), decrease dose by 50%.
IV, intravenous; PO, per oral.

TABLE 2: Magnesium (give intravenous or per oral dose unless specifically stated)

Level	IV dose	PO dose	Recheck K^+
1.9 mg/dL	Give PO only	Magnesium oxide (uromag) 140 mg	In the morning
1.3–1.8 mg/dL	1 g $MgSO_4$ for every* 0.1 mg/dL below 1.9 mg/dL	Give IV only	In the morning
1.2 mg/dL or below	8 g $MgSO_4$**	Give IV only	6 h after last infusion or in the morning

*Mix 1 to 2 g $MgSO_4$ in 50 mL of D5W or NaCL 0.9% and infuse over 1-h period.
Mix 3–6 g $MgSO_4$ in 150 mL of D5W or NaCL 0.9%; rate should not exceed 2 g per hour.
**Mix 2 g $MgSO_4$ in 50 mL of D5W or NaCL 0.9% and infuse over 30 min period.
Repeat three more times to achieve adequate level.
IV, intravenous; PO, per oral; D5W, 5% dextrose in water.

REFERENCES

1. Centers for Disease Control and Prevention, N.C.F.H.S. (2010). National Ambulatory Medical Care Survey and 2010 National Hospital Ambulatory Medical Care Survey. Ambulatory health care data: questionnaires, datasets, and related documentation. For methodology, see National Center for Health Statistics, Public Use Data File Documentation: 2010 National Ambulatory Medical Care Survey and Public Use Data File Documentation: 2010 National Hospital Ambulatory Medical Care Survey. [online] Available from: http://www.cdc.gov/nchs/ahcd/ahcd_questionnaires.htm. [Accessed March, 2016].
2. Go AS, Mozaffarian D, Roger VL, Benjamin EJ, Berry JD, Blaha MJ, et al. Heart disease and stroke statistics--2014 update: a report from the American Heart Association. Circulation. 2014;129(3): p. e28-e292.
3. Collins SP, Schauer DP, Gupta A, Brunner H, Storrow AB, Eckman MH. Cost-effectiveness analysis of ED decision making in patients with non-high-risk heart failure. Am J Emerg Med. 2009;27(3):293-302.
4. Peacock WF, Remer EE, Aponte J, Moffa DA, Emerman CE, Albert NM. Effective observation unit treatment of decompensated heart failure. Congest Heart Fail. 2002;8:68-73.
5. Blecker S, Ladapo JA, Doran KM, Goldfeld KS, Katz S. Emergency department visits for heart failure and subsequent hospitalization or observation unit admission. Am Heart J. 2014;168(6):901-8.e1.
6. Collins SP, Pang PS, Fonarow GC, Yancy CW, Bonow RO, Gheorghiade M. Is hospital admission for heart failure really necessary?: the role of the emergency department and observation unit in preventing hospitalization and rehospitalization. J Am Coll Cardiol. 2013;61(2):121-6.
7. Diercks DB, Peacock WF, Kirk JD, Weber JE. ED patients with heart failure: identification of an observational unit-appropriate cohort. Am J Emerg Med. 2006;24(3):319-24.
8. Peacock WF. Emergency department observation unit management of heart failure. Crit Pathw Cardiol. 2003;2(4):207-20.
9. Peacock WF. Heart failure management in the emergency department observation unit. Prog Cardiovasc Dis. 2004;46(5): 465-85.
10. Peacock WF. Using the emergency department clinical decision unit for acute decompensated heart failure. Cardiol Clin. 2005;23(4):569-88, viii.
11. Peacock WF, Young J, Collins S, Diercks D, Emerman C. Heart failure observation units: optimizing care. Ann Emerg Med. 2006;47(1):22-33.
12. Georghiade M, Abraham WT, Albert NM, Greenberg BH, O'Connor CM, She L, et al. Systolic blood pressure at admission, clinical characteristics, and outcomes in patients hospitalized with acute heart failure. JAMA. 2006;296(18):2217-26.
13. Gheorghiade M, Rossi JS, Cotts W, Shin DD, Hellkamp AS, Piña IL, et al. Characterization and prognostic value of persistent hyponatremia in patients with severe heart failure in the ESCAPE Trial. Arch Intern Med. 2007;167(18):1998-2005.
14. Filippatos G, Rossi J, Lloyd-Jones DM, Stough WG, Ouyang J, Shin DD, et al. Prognostic value of BUN in patients hospitalized with worsening heart failure: insights from the Acute and Chronic Therapeutic Impact of a Vasopressin Antagonist in Chronic Heart Failure (ACTIV in CHF) study. J Card Fail. 2007;13(5):360-4.
15. Peacock WF, De Marco T, Fonarow GC, Diercks D, Wynne J, Apple FS, et al. Cardiac troponin and outcome in heart failure. N Engl J Med. 2008;358(20):2117-26.
16. Januzzi JL, Camargo CA, Anwaruddin S, Baggish AL, Chen AA, Krauser DG, et al. The N-terminal Pro-BNP investigation of dyspnea in the emergency department (PRIDE) study. Am J Cardiol. 2005;95(8):948-54.
17. Fonarow GC, Adams KF, Abraham WT, Yancy CW, Boscardin WJ, ADHERE Scientific Advisory Committee, Study Group, and Investigators. Risk stratification for in-hospital mortality in acutely decompensated heart failure classification and regression tree analysis. JAMA. 2005;293(5):572-80.
18. Gheorghiade M, Abraham WT, Albert NM, Gattis Stough W, Greenberg BH, O'Connor CM, et al. Relationship between admission serum sodium concentration and clinical outcomes in patients hospitalized for heart failure: an analysis from the OPTIMIZE-HF registry. Eur Heart J. 2007;28(8): 980-8.
19. Peacock WF, Fonarow GC, Ander DS, Collins SP, Gheorghiade M, Kirk JD, et al. Society of Chest Pain Centers recommendations for the evaluation and management of the observation stay acute heart failure patient-parts 1-6. Acute Card Care. 2009;11(1)3-42.
20. Konstam MA, Gheorghiade M, Burnett JC, Grinfeld L, Maggioni AP, Swedberg K, et al. Effects of oral tolvaptan in patients hospitalized for worsening heart failure: the EVEREST Outcome Trial. JAMA. 2007;297(12):1319-31.
21. Budnitz DS, Lovegrove MC, Crosby AE. Emergency department visits for overdoses of acetaminophen-containing products. Am J Prev Med. 2011;40(6):585-92.

22. Klein L, O'Connor CM, Leimberger JD, Gattis-Stough W, Piña IL, Felker GM, et al. Lower serum sodium is associated with increased short-term mortality in hospitalized patients with worsening heart failure: results from the Outcomes of a Prospective Trial of Intravenous Milrinone for Exacerbations of Chronic Heart Failure (OPTIME-CHF) study. Circulation. 2005;111(19):2454-60.
23. Oren RM. Hyponatremia in congestive heart failure. Am J Cardiol. 2005;95(9A):2B-7B.
24. Bongartz LG, Cramer MJ, Doevendans PA, Joles JA, Braam B. The severe cardiorenal syndrome: 'Guyton revisited'. Eur Heart J. 2005; 26(1):11-7.
25. Aronson D, Mittleman MA, Burger AJ. Elevated blood urea nitrogen level as a predictor of mortality in patients admitted for decompensated heart failure. Am J Med. 2004;116(7):466-73.
26. Felker GM, Leimberger JD, Califf RM, Cuffe MS, Massie BM, Adams KF, et al. Risk stratification after hospitalization for decompensated heart failure. J Card Fail. 2004;10(6):460-6.
27. Formiga F, Chivite D, Manito N, Casas S, Riera A, Pujol R. Predictors of in-hospital mortality present at admission among patients hospitalised because of decompensated heart failure. Cardiology. 2007;108(2):73-8.
28. Chin MH, Goldman L. Correlates of major complications or death in patients admitted to the hospital with congestive heart failure. Arch Intern Med. 1996;156:1814-20.
29. Kuwabara Y, Sato Y, Miyamoto T, Taniguchi R, Matsuoka T, Isoda K, et al. Persistently increased serum concentrations of cardiac troponin in patients with acutely decompensated heart failure are predictive of adverse outcomes. Circ J. 2007;71:1047-51.
30. Braga JR, Tu JV, Austin PC, Chong A, You JJ, Farkouh ME, et al. Outcomes and care of patients with acute heart failure syndromes and cardiac troponin elevation. Circ Heart Fail. 2013;6(2):193-202.
31. McCullough PA, Nowak RM, McCord J, Hollander JE, Herrmann HC, Steg PG, et al. B-type natriuretic peptide and clinical judgment in emergency diagnosis of heart failure: analysis from breathing not properly (BNP) multinational study. Circulation. 2002;106(4):416-22.
32. Chen HH, Burnett JC. Natriuretic peptides in the pathophysiology of congestive heart failure. Curr Cardiol Rep. 2000;2(3):198-205.
33. Collins SP, Mielniczuk LM, Whittingham HA, Boseley ME, Schramm DR, Storrow AB. The use of noninvasive ventilation in emergency department patients with acute cardiogenic pulmonary edema: a systematic review. Ann Emerg Med. 2006;48(3):260-9, 269.e1-4.
34. Yancy CW, Jessup M, Bozkurt B, Butler J, Casey DE, Drazner MH, et al. 2013 ACCF/AHA guideline for the management of heart failure: a report of the American College of Cardiology Foundation/American Heart Association Task Force on practice guidelines. Circulation. 2013;128(16):1810-52.
35. Felker GM, Lee KL, Bull DA, Redfield MM, Stevenson LW, Goldsmith SR, et al. Diuretic strategies in patients with acute decompensated heart failure. N Engl J Med. 2011;364(9):797-805.
36. Heart Failure Society of America, Lindenfeld J, Albert NM, Boehmer JP, Collins SP, Ezekowitz JA, et al. HFSA 2010 Comprehensive Heart Failure Practice Guideline. J Card Fail. 2010;16(6):475-539.
37. Cotter G, Metzkor E, Kaluski E, Faigenberg Z, Miller R, Simovitz A, et al. Randomised trial of high-dose isosorbide dinitrate plus low-dose furosemide versus high-dose furosemide plus low-dose isosorbide dinitrate in severe pulmonary oedema. Lancet. 1998;351(9100):389-393.
38. Palmer RF, Lasseter KC. Drug therapy. Sodium nitroprusside. N Engl J Med. 1975;292(6):294-7.
39. Colucci WS, Elkayam U, Horton DP, Abraham WT, Bourge RC, Johnson AD, et al. Intravenous nesiritide, a natriuretic peptide, in the treatment of decompensated congestive heart failure. N Engl J Med. 2000;343(4):246-53.
40. Publication Committee for the VMAC Investigators (Vasodilatation in the Management of Acute CHF). Intravenous nesiritide vs nitroglycerin for treatment of decompensated congestive heart failure: a randomized controlled trial. JAMA. 2002;287(12):1531-40.
41. Peacock WF, Holland R, Gyarmathy R, Dunbar L, Klapholz M, Horton DP, et al. Observation unit treatment of heart failure with nesiritide: results from the proaction trial. J Emerg Med. 2005;29(3):243-52.
42. Phelan HA, Richter AA, Scott WW, Pruitt JH, Madden CJ, Rickert KL, et al. Does isolated traumatic subarachnoid hemorrhage merit a lower intensity level of observation than other TBI? J Neurotrauma. 2014;31(20):1733-6.
43. Effect of enalapril on survival in patients with reduced left ventricular ejection fractions and congestive heart failure. The SOLVD Investigators. N Engl J Med. 1991;325(5):293-302.
44. Effect of enalapril on mortality and the development of heart failure in asymptomatic patients with reduced left ventricular ejection fractions. The SOLVD Investigattors. N Engl J Med. 1992;327(10):685-91.
45. Colucci WS, Packer M, Bristow MR, Gilbert EM, Cohn JN, Fowler MB, et al. Carvedilol inhibits clinical progression in patients with mild symptoms of heart failure. Circulation. 1996;94:2800-6.
46. A randomized controlled trial of beta blockade in heart failure: The Cardiac Insufficiency Bisoprolol Study (CIBIS). CIBIS Investigators and Committees. Circulation. 1994;90(4):1765-73.
47. The Cardiac Insufficiency Bisoprolol Study II (CIBIS-II): a randomised trial. Lancet. 1999;353(9146):9-13.
48. Bristow MR, Gilbert EM, Abraham WT, Adams KF, Fowler MB, Hershberger RE, et al. Carvedilol produces dose-related improvements in left ventricular function and survival in subjects with chronic heart failure. MOCHA Investigators. Circulation. 1996;94(11):2807-16.
49. Butler J, Ezekowitz JA, Collins SP, Givertz MM, Teerlink JR, Walsh MN, et al. Update on aldosterone antagonists use in heart failure with reduced left ventricular ejection fraction. Heart Failure Society of America Guidelines Committee. J Card Fail. 2012;18(4):265-81.
50. Pitt B, Zannad F, Remme WJ, Cody R, Castaigne A, Perez A, et al. The effect of spironolactone on morbidity and mortality in patients with severe heart failure. N Engl J Med. 1999;341(10):709-17.
51. Zannad F, McMurray JJ, Krum H, van Veldhuisen DJ, Swedberg K, Shi H, et al. Eplerenone in patients with systolic heart failure and mild symptoms. N Engl J Med. 2011;364(1):11-21.
52. Cohn JN, Archibald DG, Ziesche S, Franciosa JA, Harston WE, Tristani FE, et al. Effect of vasodilator therapy on mortality in chronic congestive heart failure. Results of a Veterans Administration Cooperative Study. N Engl J Med. 1986;314(24):1547-52.
53. Carson PE, Ziesche S, Johnson G, Cohn JN. Racial differences in response to therapy for heart failure: analysis of the vasodilator-heart failure trials. Vasodilator-Heart Failure Trial Study Group. J Card Fail. 1999;5(3):178-87.
54. Cohn JN, Johnson G, Ziesche S, Cobb F, Francis G, Tristani F, et al. A comparison of enalapril with hydralazine-isosorbide dinitrate in the treatment of chronic congestive heart failure. N Engl J Med. 1991;325(5):303-10.
55. Taylor AL, Ziesche S, Yancy C, Carson P, D'Agostino R, Ferdinand K, et al. Combination of isosorbide dinitrate and hydralazine in blacks with heart failure. N Engl J Med. 2004;351(20):2049-57.
56. Taylor AL, Ziesche S, Yancy CW, Carson P, Ferdinand K, Taylor M, et al. Early and sustained benefit on event-free survival and heart failure hospitalization from fixed-dose combination of isosorbide dinitrate/hydralazine: consistency across subgroups in the African-American Heart Failure Trial. Circulation. 2007;115(13):1747-53.
57. Anand IS, Win S, Rector TS, Cohn JN, Taylor AL. Effect of fixed-dose combination of isosorbide dinitrate and hydralazine on all hospitalizations and on 30-day readmission rates in patients with heart failure: results from the African-American Heart Failure Trial. Circ Heart Fail. 2014;7(5):759-65.
58. Ferdinand KC, Elkayam U, Mancini D, Ofili E, Piña I, Anand I, et al. Use of isosorbide dinitrate and hydralazine in African-Americans with heart failure 9 years after the African-American Heart Failure Trial. Am J Cardiol. 2014;114(1):151-9.
59. Eichhorn EJ, Gheorghiade M. Digoxin. Prog Cardiovasc Dis. 2002;44(4): 251-66.
60. Uretsky BF, Young JB, Shahidi FE, Yellen LG, Harrison MC, Jolly MK. Randomized study assessing the effect of digoxin withdrawal in patients with mild to moderate chronic congestive heart failure: results of the PROVED trial. PROVED Investigative Group. J Am Coll Cardiol. 1993;22(4):955-62.
61. Packer M, Gheorghiade M, Young JB, Costantini PJ, Adams KF, Cody RJ, et al. Withdrawal of digoxin from patients with chronic heart failure treated with angiotensin-converting-enzyme inhibitors. RADIANCE Study. N Engl J Med. 1993;329(1):1-7.
62. American College of Cardiology/American Heart Association Task Force on Performance Measures, Bonow RO, Masoudi FA, Rumsfeld JS, Delong E, Estes NA, et al. ACC/AHA classification of care metrics: performance measures and quality metrics: a report of the American College of Cardiology/American Heart Association Task Force on Performance Measures. Circulation. 2008;118(24):2662-6.
63. Wu JR, Moser DK, Lennie TA, Burkhart PV. Medication adherence in patients who have heart failure: a review of the literature. Nurs Clin North Am. 2008;43(1):133-53; vii-viii.

64. De Geest S, Sabate E. Adherence to long-term therapies: evidence for action. Eur J Cardiovasc Nurs. 2003;2(4):323.
65. He FJ, Li J, Macgregor GA. Effect of longer term modest salt reduction on blood pressure: Cochrane systematic review and meta-analysis of randomised trials. BMJ. 2013;346:f1325.
66. Effects of weight loss and sodium reduction intervention on blood pressure and hypertension incidence in overweight people with high-normal blood pressure. The Trials of Hypertension Prevention, phase II. The Trials of Hypertension Prevention Collaborative Research Group. Arch Intern Med. 1997;157(6):657-67.
67. Jula AM, Karanko HM. Effects on left ventricular hypertrophy of long-term nonpharmacological treatment with sodium restriction in mild-to moderate essential hypertension. Circulation. 1994;89(3):1023-31.
68. Cook NR, Cutler JA, Obarzanek E, Buring JE, Rexrode KM, Kumanyika SK, et al. Long term effects of dietary sodium reduction on cardiovascular disease outcomes: observational follow-up of the trials of hypertension prevention (TOHP). BMJ. 2007;334(7599):885-8.
69. Paterna S, Parrinello G, Cannizzaro S, Fasullo S, Torres D, Sarullo FM, et al. Medium term effects of different dosage of diuretic, sodium, and fluid administration on neurohormonal and clinical outcome in patients with recently compensated heart failure. Am J Cardiol. 2009;103(1):93-102.
70. Paterna S, Gaspare P, Fasullo S, Sarullo FM, Di Pasquale P. Normal-sodium diet compared with low-sodium diet in compensated congestive heart failure: is sodium an old enemy or a new friend? Clin Sci (Lond). 2008;114(3):221-30.
71. Parrinello G, Di Pasquale P, Licata G, Torres D, Giammanco M, Fasullo S, et al. Long-term effects of dietary sodium intake on cytokines and neurohormonal activation in patients with recently compensated congestive heart failure. J Card Fail. 2009;15(10):864-73.
72. Pocock SJ, Wang D, Pfeffer MA, Yusuf S, McMurray JJ, Swedberg KB, et al. Predictors of mortality and morbidity in patients with chronic heart failure. Eur Heart J. 2006;27(1):65-75.
73. Goldberg LR, Piette JD, Walsh MN, Frank TA, Jaski BE, Smith AL, et al. Randomized trial of a daily electronic home monitoring system in patients with advanced heart failure: the Weight Monitoring in Heart Failure (WHARF) trial. Am Heart J. 2003;146(4):705-12.
74. Evangelista LS, Shinnick MA. What do we know about adherence and self-care. J Cardiovasc Nurs. 2008;23(3):250-7.
75. Moser DK, Doering LV, Chung ML. Vulnerabilities of patients recovering from an exacerbation of chronic heart failure. Am Heart J. 2005;150(5):984.
76. Pan AM, Stiell IG, Clement CM, Acheson J, Aaron SD. Feasibility of a structured 3-minute walk test as a clinical decision tool for patients presenting to the emergency department with acute dyspnoea. Emerg Med J. 2009;26(4): 278-82.
77. Forman DE, Butler J, Wang Y, Abraham WT, O'Connor CM, Gottlieb SS, et al. Incidence, predictors at admission, and impact of worsening renal function among patients hospitalized with heart failure. J Am Coll Cardiol. 2004;43(1): 61-7.
78. Chittineni H, Miyawaki N, Gulipelli S, Fishbane S. Risk for acute renal failure in patients hospitalized for decompensated congestive heart failure. Am J Nephrol. 2007;27(1):55-62.
79. Gotsman I, Zwas D, Planer D, Admon D, Lotan C, Keren A. The significance of serum urea and renal function in patients with heart failure. Medicine (Baltimore). 2010;89(4):197-203.
80. Gheorghiade M, Gattis WA, O'Connor CM, Adams KF, Elkayam U, Barbagelata A. Effects of tolvaptan, a vasopressin antagonist, in patients hospitalized with worsening heart failure a randomized controlled trial. JAMA. 2004;291(16): 1963-71.
81. Collins SP, Lindsell CJ, Naftilan AJ, Peacock WF, Diercks D, Hiestand B, et al. Low-risk acute heart failure patients: external validation of the Society of Chest Pain Center's recommendations. Crit Pathw Cardiol. 2009;8(3):99-103.

22 CHAPTER

Cardiogenic Shock

W Barton Campbell

INTRODUCTION

Shock is a frequently encountered, often fatal, emergency. Shock occurs as a consequence of insufficient tissue perfusion resulting in vital organ ischemic malfunction. Early shock is often reversible; more prolonged shock may cause irreversible ischemic damage of vital organs. Prompt recognition of shock and its proximate cause is essential. Shock results from diverse causes and varies in severity. It may develop quickly or insidiously. Shock pathogenesis is broadly grouped into distributive (62% from sepsis, 4% from nonsepsis), hypovolemic (16%), cardiogenic (16%), and obstructive (2%) causes.[1] It is often, in varying degree, due to a combination of causes mentioned in table 1.

Cardiogenic shock was described in 1942 by Dr Eugene Stead Jr and Dr Richard Ebert.[2] It has been variably defined in the literature but is commonly recognized in the appropriate clinical setting by evidence of impaired organ function and hypotension with systolic blood pressures less than 80–90 mm Hg over at least 30 minutes duration. As Stead and Ebert noted, some combination of pallor, cold extremities, diaphoresis, weak arterial pulses, elevated jugular venous pressures, dyspnea, tachypnea, confusion, diminished urine output, and lactic acidosis is variably present.

INCIDENCE AND PATHOGENESIS

Cardiogenic shock most commonly presents in the setting of acute myocardial infarction (AMI). Occurring in 5–10% of all myocardial infarction cases, shock is more common in anteroseptal ST elevation AMI (STEMI) than STEMI in other locations or non-STEMI.[3] Shock is the leading cause of death in AMI. Cardiogenic shock mortality rates are historically near 50%.[4] Of the 41,000 patients with STEMI in GUSTO-1 (Global Utilization of Streptokinase and Tissue Plasminogen Activator for Occluded Coronary Arteries), 7.2% had cardiogenic shock. Of these, 11% had shock on admission while 89% developed shock during hospitalization. The STEMI mortality was 55% in those with cardiogenic shock and 3% in those without. Patients given thrombolytic therapy and those who underwent angioplasty of the culprit vessel had reduced mortality.[5]

The incidence of STEMI-induced cardiogenic shock has been increasing since 2003, apparently related to increased numbers of patients with prior myocardial damage. Mortality rates over this period, however, have been decreasing concomitant with increased early revascularization and mechanical circulatory support (vide infra).[6] Cardiogenic shock less commonly occurs in a variety of other cardiovascular problems for which little demographic data is available. Prompt recognition of cardiogenic shock and its underlying pathogenesis is essential in reducing the likelihood of mortality.

A markedly impaired left ventricular ejection fraction (LVEF) with reduced cardiac output (CO) is the usual cause of cardiogenic shock in STEMI. Coronary artery occlusion causes prompt loss of contraction in the ischemic myocardium. Stroke volume falls causing hypotension, which activates baroreceptors resulting in increased sympathetic tone and catecholamine release. The catecholamine surge causes peripheral vasoconstriction increasing left ventricular (LV) afterload. The resultant increased LV wall stress and myocardial oxygen demand extend the zone of myocardial ischemic damage. Left ventricular diastolic compliance deteriorates causing an increase in LV diastolic pressures. Left atrial and pulmonary venous pressures rise accordingly, causing increased lung stiffness or pulmonary edema. An inflammatory response to the ischemic myocardial insult causes release of cytokines such as interleukin-6 and interleukin-8. Cytokine release can further depress myocardial contractility and activate neutrophils.[7] Cytokines are known to activate nitric oxide synthase causing production of nitric oxide. Such changes cause impaired vasoregulation. Decreasing systemic vascular resistance with diminished coronary artery perfusion pressure may be the result of this concomitant inflammatory process.[8]

Inferior myocardial infarction (MI) is usually due to occlusion of the right coronary artery (RCA) which supplies the inferior LV septum in 90% of people and

TABLE 1: A generalized categorization of circulatory shock and some common causes

Types of shock	Distributive (66%)	Hypovolemic (16%)	Obstructive (2%)	Cardiogenic (16%)
Cardiac output	Normal to slight increase	Decreased	Decreased	Decreased
Pulmonary wedge pressure	Little change	Decreased	Usually increased	Increased
Systemic vascular resistance	Usually decreased	Compensatory increase	Compensatory increase	Compensatory increase
Right atrial (jugular venous) pressure	Little change	Decreased	Increased	Usually increased
Common causes	Infection: • Multiple organisms (62%)	Hemorrhage: • Gastrointestinal bleed • Operative bleed • Aneurysmal rupture • Retroperitoneal bleed	• Pulmonary embolus • Tamponade • Tension • Pneumothorax • Valvular or arterial obstruction	Impaired myocardial contractility due to ischemic or nonischemic causes.
Less common causes	• Systemic inflammatory response syndrome • Neurologic • Endocrinologic • Toxic shock • Venomization	• Diarrhea • Burns • Vomiting • Pancreatitis • Diuresis • Crush injury	–	• Acute valvular incompetence • Impaired ventricular compliance

has a smaller LV myocardial distribution. When RCA occlusion is proximal to the RCA acute marginal branch to the right ventricular (RV) free wall, dysfunction (often mislabeled "right ventricular infarction") impairs RV stroke volume. The diminished RV output drops LV filling pressure (preload), reducing LV stroke volume. The dysfunctional RV free wall also expands into the closed pericardial space resulting in increased intrapericardial pressures. Due to this tethering effect, the free wall of the right ventricle cannot further expand to accommodate venous return to the right heart. The increased inspiratory RV volume is therefore accommodated by a shift of the septum into the left ventricle. This further diminishes the LV stroke volume. Right atrial (RA) and jugular venous pressures are elevated, usually exceeding pulmonary arterial wedge (PAW) pressures. Right ventricular free wall dysfunction, as it is not due to infarcted but only ischemic myocardium, invariably recovers with time.[9] Right ventricular free wall involvement in the presence of inferior MI has been shown to increase the likelihood of cardiogenic shock.[10]

Mitral regurgitation (MR), if present, will further impair CO and exacerbate shock. Mitral regurgitation is not uncommon with inferior MI and is caused by inferior medial papillary muscle dysfunction or rupture. The posterior descending branch of the RCA supplies the inferior myocardial wall and is the sole blood supply to the inferior medial papillary muscle. Inferior medial papillary muscle dysfunction may resolve if ischemia improves. Necrotic rupture of the papillary muscle body, or even a papillary muscle tip, invariably causes severe, often life-threatening regurgitation, usually with shock, and requires rapid mitral surgical repair or valve replacement of the resulting "flail" mitral leaflet. Severe MR with a flail leaflet is less frequently due to a ruptured chordae tendineae which can occur spontaneously with or without an MI. Commonly, MR results from dysfunctional LV enlargement which laterally displaces the papillary muscles and causes mitral annular dilatation.

Rupture of a necrotic interventricular septum, an "infarct ventricular septal defect (VSD)", reduces effective LV CO in direct proportion to the degree of the ensuing left to right shunt. This complication may occur on the first infarct day or several days later. It is more frequent in inferior than anteroseptal MI. Mortality is approximately 50–60%. If the shunt is severe, urgent (even though high risk) surgical repair must be considered.[11] Rupture of the LV free wall usually results in sudden cardiac death characterized by pulseless electrical activity. Rarely, the rupture may have a relatively slow leak leading to cardiac tamponade. If recognized promptly, these patients may occasionally be salvaged by rapid surgical repair. Pericardiocentesis should be avoided as decompression of the pericardial space will increase bleeding through the necrotic ventricular wall defect.

Cardiac tamponade is a common cause of cardiogenic shock. Tamponade can result from any condition that allows fluid to accumulate in the pericardial space in a volume sufficient to cause increased intrapericardial pressures. It may occur with pericarditis, aortic dissection rupture, or from cardiac procedures, including balloon angioplasty or ablation procedures, with bleeding or effusion into the pericardial space. When increased intrapericardial pressure squeezes the heart to the point that it impairs cardiac venous return, tamponade results causing reduced stroke volume and arterial pressure. An inspiratory leftward septal shift into the LV occurs as the increased intrapericardial pressure does not allow RV free wall expansion to accommodate the increased venous return during inspiration. This septal shift with diminished LV volume causes hypotension with an inspiratory drop in systolic blood pressure (and narrowed pulse pressure) called "pulsus paradoxicus". Pulsus paradoxicus can be readily recognized while manually taking the blood pressure. The cuff is slowly deflated to the point where Korotkoff sounds are first heard during expiration. After noting this systolic value, further deflation continues to a point where Korotkoff sounds are heard throughout a normal respiratory cycle (deep breathing is avoided as it causes increased drop in intrapleural pressures). A difference of over 8 mm Hg (torr) between expiratory systolic blood pressure and the appearance of inspiratory systolic blood pressure is considered significant. Tachycardia results from increased baroreceptor activity in the setting of hypotension. The increased RV diastolic pressure approximates RA pressure, as both the right atrium and the free wall of the RV are compressed by the increased pressure in the pericardial space. Normally, with opening of the tricuspid valve, blood flows from the right atrium into the lower pressure right ventricle in early diastole. The resulting fall in RA pressure creates the Y descent from the intra-atrial V wave. With opening of the tricuspid valve in tamponade, little transvalve flow results and there is no significant Y descent. This is recognized in the jugular venous pulse as an absent V wave. A significant V wave excludes the diagnosis of tamponade. Hypotension, tachycardia, pulsus paradoxicus, elevated jugular venous pressures, and loss of the V wave (due to the absent Y descent) are pathognomonic of tamponade. The diagnosis of tamponade may be confirmed by an echocardiogram, if readily available. The echocardiogram is useful for the demonstration of pericardial fluid or clot with an associated inspiratory diminution in LV volume due to the septal shift. The presence of RA collapse and RV free wall early diastolic collapse are confirmatory findings. Rapid bedside recognition of tamponade and prompt pericardiocentesis to decompress the pericardial space is often essential for survival. If tamponade or impending tamponade is suspected, diuretics should be avoided and volume should be given as needed to maintain an adequately high venous filling pressure needed to counteract the high intrapericardial pressures.

Myocarditis, especially of the "fulminant" variety, may cause cardiogenic shock if inflamed myocardium decreases LV contractility to the point of significantly impaired CO. Myocarditis, often with accompanying pericarditis, usually causes persistent chest discomfort. "Fulminant" myocarditis, frequently accompanied by fever, is rapidly severe, often presenting with cardiogenic shock occurring within 24–48 hours of onset. If these patients can be kept alive, they commonly improve and may recover normal LV function. Mechanical circulatory assist devices are commonly required for survival (vide infra). One recent study suggested a 93% 5-year survival rate without transplant compared to a 45% survivorship in those with nonfulminant myocarditis.[12] Chronic indolent myocarditis may slowly progress to cariogenic shock and carries a much worse prognosis.

Stress-induced ("takotsubo") cardiomyopathy is frequently associated with profound LV and occasionally RV hypokinesis. It is most commonly (~82% of patients) apical in distribution and has been referred to as "apical ballooning cardiomyopathy". Its presentation is quite similar to AMI, including EKG repolarization changes and elevated biomarkers (troponins and creatine kinase-myocardial band). This presentation requires urgent coronary angiography to exclude AMI due to coronary occlusion. Takotsubo cardiomyopathy is recognized by the absence of hemodynamically significant coronary artery stenoses. Takotsubo dyskinesia is not localized to the territory of one coronary artery. In a recent evaluation of 1,750 patients with takotsubo cardiomyopathy, 90% were female and nearly 30% had psychogenic etiologies. Stress-induced cardiomyopathy is associated with cardiogenic shock in approximately 10% of the patients who survived to reach the hospital. Patients with stress-induced cardiomyopathy frequently recover completely within a week or two.[13] Shock may occur in some of these patients in the absence of profound impairment of ejection fraction.[14] In a recent report on 32 patients with takotsubo cardiomyopathy (identified out of a cohort of 3,272 patients who presented with apparent troponin positive acute coronary syndrome), six (20%) were shown to have left ventricular outflow tract (LVOT) obstruction. These six patients were older and had more hemodynamic instability. Their echocardiograms disclosed septal bulging into the LVOT accompanied by systolic anterior motion of the mitral valve with resultant MR similar to the changes seen in hypertrophic obstructive cardiomyopathy. This subset of patients was managed with volume and β-blockers as opposed to inotropic medications which could worsen the dynamic outflow tract obstruction. The authors suggest that echocardiography be done promptly on admission to identify and allow the proper hemodynamic approach to these atypical takotsubo variants.[15]

Peripartum cardiomyopathy is an uncommon condition occurring in approximately 1 per 4,000 live births in the United States. It is more commonly seen in Africa and Caribbean countries where the incidence may be as high as 1:300 births. The frequency is greater in older women (>30 years) who are multiparous, who have hypertension, or are of African descent.[16] Peripartum cardiomyopathy usually occurs in the month prior to or within 2 months following parturition. Arrhythmias and thromboembolic disease are prevalent and the incidence of cardiogenic shock is reported at 15–25%. The pathogenesis of peripartum cardiomyopathy remains cryptic.[17]

Acute aortic valvular regurgitation, usually from abrupt rupture of a cusp, commonly presents as cardiogenic shock. Frequent causes are aortic valve endocarditis and Stanford A (ascending aorta) aortic dissection. Unlike patients with chronic aortic insufficiency, these patients do not have a wide pulse pressure and the LV chamber is not dilated. On auscultation, the S1 is soft and the diastolic murmur is commonly a low frequency apical (Austin Flint) murmur due to the aortic insufficiency jet forcing the anterior leaflet of the mitral valve into a nearly closed position in diastole.[18] The murmur is characteristically very soft or undetectable. When suspected, aortic valvular incompetence can be easily detected with echocardiography. Rapid surgical intervention is usually required for survival.

Less common causes of cardiogenic shock include various types of vascular mechanical obstruction which often require prompt surgical intervention. A left atrial "ball valve" myxoma may intermittently occlude the mitral valve orifice. Rarely, other tumors can occlude the LVOT. Massive pulmonary embolus is a cause of mechanical syncope or cardiogenic shock due to pulmonary artery occlusion and impaired left heart filling. Surgical embolectomy or thrombolytic therapy may be required. Following chest trauma, localized bleeding into the aortic wall can create an acquired profound coarctation near the ligamentum arteriosum. The resulting severe increase in LV afterload may result in cardiogenic shock with absent lower extremity pulses. Transesophageal echocardiography may be required to identify the intramural bleed/coarctation as the genesis of global LV hypokinesis. Rapid surgical intervention is required (personal observation). A tension pneumothorax occurs when a communication between the lung parenchyma and the pleural space acts as a one-way valve causing increased intrapleural pressure. This can occur following blunt chest trauma, surgical trauma, or as a complication of mechanical ventilation. The increased intrapleural pressure can impair venous return to the heart resulting in a mechanical cariogenic shock. Hypotension, elevated jugular venous pressures, and distant breath sounds are present. Needle aspiration or surgical (chest tube) decompression of the pleural space is lifesaving and usually must be immediate.

Arrhythmias, either bradycardia or tachycardia, may further compromise CO in patients with any type of cardiogenic shock and must be treated accordingly. Tachycardia of any etiology may cause a cardiomyopathy. Tachycardia-induced cardiomyopathies may cause heart failure, but quite rarely cause cardiogenic shock.[19]

Cardiac transplantation currently has an 85% 1-year survival. Approximately 2.5% of heart transplant patients develop cardiogenic shock. Causes of severe cardiac failure and shock in these patients include graft failure, multiple organ failure, and infection. Some common post-transplant infections such as "cytomegalovirus and toxoplasma gondii" may be amenable to treatment if diagnosed.[20] Transplant patients who have recurrent heart failure or shock requiring retransplantation have a 46% 1-year survival.[21]

Toxic cardiomyopathies are a quite rare cause of cardiogenic shock. Excessive use of ethanol, especially over a long period of time, may cause severe dilative cardiomyopathy.[22] Cocaine and its derivatives cause ischemic cardiomyopathies including MI.

Cocaine also has a direct toxic effect on heart muscle. Sudden cardiac death is not uncommon but cardiogenic shock occurs infrequently.[23] Levamisole, a common cocaine adulterant, known to cause agranulocytosis and vasculitis has a cardiotoxic and vasoconstrictor effect via its amphetamine-like metabolite, aminorex.[24]

Noncompaction cardiomyopathy is an uncommon condition characterized by deep LV trabeculation exceeding 50% of LV wall thickness. It is usually recognized echocardiographically. It may be found at any age and often presents with heart failure requiring usual therapy. The incidence of cardiogenic shock and end-stage heart failure is estimated at 5–12%.[25]

Postcardiotomy cardiogenic shock is estimated to occur in approximately 1% of cardiothoracic surgical cases. It may develop intraoperatively, resulting in inability to wean from the bypass pump, or it may develop up to 48 hours following the surgical procedure. The pathogenesis is variable, often related to the surgical complexity and operative time, intraoperative myocardial ischemia, age, and premorbid conditions. A surgically precipitated systemic inflammatory response can compromise recovery. In-hospital mortality rates from this variety of cardiogenic shock are reported to be 60–70%.[26]

DIAGNOSIS

Circulatory shock can be diagnosed if evidence of multisystem organ hypoperfusion is recognized. Cardiogenic (as opposed to distributive or hypovolemic) circulatory shock is usually differentiated by the clinical setting and by the presence of elevated right and left heart filling pressures. It occurs most frequently in AMI and less commonly in one of the other problems discussed above. Shock may be present abruptly or insidiously and occurs in variable degrees. Patients with cardiogenic shock have a variable combination of hypotension (with systolic pressures usually below 80–90 mm Hg and mean blood pressures below 65 mm Hg), tachycardia, abnormal mentation, peripheral vasoconstriction with moist, cool, pale, or cyanotic extremities, elevated jugular venous pressures with a positive hepatic jugular reflux, dyspnea, tachypnea, and oliguria. Central arterial pulses usually have a "thready" quality due to impaired stroke volume and narrowed pulse pressure. A murmur or gallop may be present. Rales (crackles) may reflect increased left heart pressures.

Laboratory data show a widened anion gap due to metabolic acidosis. Lactate levels (normally <2.5 mmol/L) are elevated due to anaerobic metabolism. Serial monitoring of lactate levels help guide therapy. A decreasing lactate level is associated with improved survival.[27] Bicarbonate and pCO_2 are commonly low in compensation for the lactic acidosis. Increased troponin levels suggest myocardial damage and the brain natriuretic peptide (BNP) or its precursor, the N-terminal pro-BNP level is usually elevated. If acute tubular necrosis (ATN) is not present, fractional excretion of urinary Na^+ (FENa) levels will be low (often $<1\%$) due to diminished glomerular perfusion. "Muddy brown" urinary casts and a FENa above 3% are indicative of ATN, but elevated FENa levels may also be seen with diuretic therapy.

The EKG is helpful in diagnosing and localizing STEMI. Left bundle branch block may be due to STEMI or other types of myocardial injury. Evidence of LV enlargement or nonspecific ST-T changes is often present. Right-sided chest leads are routine in the setting of inferior infarctions, as J point elevation in V3r and V4r strongly suggest an accompanying RV free wall ischemic injury. PR-segment depression suggests pericarditis. Electrical alternans with diminished voltage is suggestive of pericardial effusion which may cause tamponade. Pulmonary embolus may be associated with tachycardia, T inversion in right precordial leads, a rightward and anterior rotation in late QRS forces, or none of these findings.

The echocardiogram usually shows a reduced ejection fraction and/or severe valvular incompetence. In the SHOCK trial of patients with cardiogenic shock due to AMI, the average LVEF was 30% and a lower LVEF was associated with an increased 1-year mortality.[28] A normal RV or LV ejection fraction does not exclude the diagnosis of cardiogenic shock but certainly confers a better prognosis. Echocardiographic moderate to severe MR compared to mild or no regurgitation also carried a worse prognosis in the SHOCK trial.[28]

The echocardiogram may be diagnostic in tamponade or valvular heart problems and assist in the diagnosis of many of the cardiac problems listed above. An echocardiogram can provide an estimate of the RV peak systolic pressures, LV end diastolic pressures, and RA pressures.

Although no randomized trials exist, bedside hemodynamic monitoring assists in the recognition of cardiogenic versus noncardiogenic (distributive or hypovolemic) shock, and has been routinely performed in the critical care unit for over 45 years. It is essential in measuring response to therapeutic maneuvers.[29] Cardiogenic shock is characterized by an elevated pulmonary wedge (PAW) pressure, often exceeding 18 torr. Thermodilution or Fick cardiac index is characteristically less than 2 L/min/m^2. When CO falls, tissue extraction of nutrients and O_2 must increase resulting in a fall in mixed venous O_2 (MVO_2) content [Content is calculated by hemoglobin × 1.34 (which estimates the O_2 carrying capacity) × saturation]. Changes in MVO_2 saturations, obtained from the pulmonary artery, reflect changing CO. Cardiac output equals O_2 consumption over the A-V O_2 difference (arterial O_2 content minus MVO_2 content). Therefore, as arterial VO_2 and O_2 consumption are usually little changed, a falling MVO_2 widens the denominator and implies a falling CO.[30] Normally, MVO_2 at rest (although quite variable) is approximately 75%. In a resting patient, an MVO_2 of 65% or less suggests diminished CO in the absence of increased O_2 consumption. High MVO_2 saturations in patients with clinical cardiogenic shock suggest a possible left to right intracardiac shunt. In such a patient with a new murmur and recent MI, an infarct VSD is likely present. This can be confirmed by demonstrating a "step up" in O_2 saturation between the right atrium and pulmonary artery. The magnitude of the step up will be proportional to the degree of the left to right shunt. Hemodynamic monitoring helps guide therapy. Measurement of right heart and PAW pressures enables the attainment of optimal filling pressures. Relatively low wedge pressures (12 torr or less) indicate a component of hypovolemia, perhaps due to occult bleeding or aggressive diuresis, requiring volume resuscitation. Optimal PAW pressure (which reflects left heart filling pressure) maintains optimal LV stroke volume via the Starling effect. Optimal PAW pressures vary but are usually found at approximately 15–16 torr and are confirmed by following MVO_2 saturation changes with varying filling (PAW) pressures. Excessively high PAW pressures contribute to increased lung stiffness and possible pulmonary edema. Large V waves (>10 torr above mean PAW pressure) are suggestive, but not pathognomonic, of acute severe MR.[31] An intra-arterial catheter allows ongoing direct pressure measurement and provides a more reliable guide to appropriate use of vasopressors.

Intravascular resistance is directly related to mean pressure and inversely related to stroke volume. It is a calculated variable (Resistance = mean pressure/CO).

Resistances should be calculated when obtaining the thermodilution or Fick CO. High vascular resistance in cardiogenic shock implies maintenance of blood pressure at the expense of CO. Some patients with cardiogenic shock due to STEMI develop relatively low vascular resistances and may be resistant to vasopressor therapy. This resembles the Systemic Inflammatory Response Syndrome resulting from a chemokine-mediated degree of distributive shock (vide supra). In the SHOCK trial, 18% of STEMI cardiogenic shock patients had fever and/or leukocytosis and a significant percentage of these later developed a positive blood culture. These patients had a worsened prognosis.[32]

TREATMENT

Treatment of cardiogenic shock must be individualized with a therapeutic approach appropriate to the underlying pathogenesis. The ST segment elevation myocardial infarction, which is most common cause of cardiogenic shock, accrues from acute coronary arterial thrombotic occlusion, caused by atherosclerotic plaque cap rupture and release of core thromboplastic material causing *in situ* platelet aggregation and intra-arterial thrombosis. Rapid re-establishment of adequate flow in the occluded coronary artery clearly reduces the mortality risk and severity of cardiogenic shock. Urgent coronary angiography to identify the occluded "culprit" artery with balloon angioplasty and stenting [percutaneous coronary intervention (PCI)] to re-establish a good arterial lumen and adequate coronary flow is the preferred approach. Time is of the essence. Time from arrival in the emergency room to inflation of the intervention balloon should be less than 90 minutes.[33] Early, as opposed to delayed, reopening of the occluded artery clearly improves outcome as does the adequacy of restoration of coronary flow. In a German registry study of 1,333 patients with AMI and cardiogenic shock, patients with restoration of normal [thrombolysis in myocardial infarction (TIMI) = 3] coronary flow had a lower in-hospital mortality (37%) than those with poor (TIMI = 0–1) postprocedural flow (78%). Age was also a factor. Inpatient mortality in patients younger than 55 years was 30% while in those older than 75 years, mortality was 63%.[34] Multivessel severe coronary stenoses (defined as at least one additional vessel with a diameter of 2.5 mm or greater and a >70% stenosis, or a left main occlusion) are more common (65–75%) than single vessel disease in patients with AMI-induced cardiogenic shock. Compared to those with single vessel disease, patients with multivessel or left main coronary disease have an adverse 6 month mortality. Nonrevascularized AMI patients who develop late cardiogenic shock (4 or more days after admission) have an in-hospital mortality of greater than 80%.[35] Survival is improved if initial multivessel PCI is performed as opposed to opening the presumed culprit vessel only. In a study of 266 patients with cardiogenic shock following AMI and cardiac arrest, patients with single artery occlusion had a 6 months survivorship of 42.3% while those with multivessel disease had a 29.6% survivorship. Among multivessel patients who had PCI of the culprit artery only, the 6 months survivorship was 20.4% while those with initial multivessel PCI had a 43.9% survival.[36] The survival advantage of primary PCI over fibrinolytic reperfusion declines rapidly with time. This has prompted community and regional networking for rapid transport to tertiary care centers and rapid mobilization of PCI capable cardiac catheterization laboratories. Associated strategies facilitating early intervention include performing and transmitting prehospital EKGs, bypassing the emergency room thus allowing direct door to catheterization laboratory access and prehospital mobilization of the catheterization laboratory with 24-hour rapid availability of the team.[37]

Patients without access within 2 hours to a tertiary care catheterization laboratory facility should be given prompt intravenous thrombolytic therapy and then transferred to the appropriate tertiary care facility for follow-up.[38] Tenecteplase, a tissue plasminogen activator, is our thrombolytic agent of choice. It is given as a single intravenous bolus over 10 seconds. Dosage (see package insert) is weight based and is 40 mg for a 70–80 kg person. The incidence of intracranial hemorrhage is 0.9%.[39] Persistent ST elevation usually suggests failure of thrombolytic therapy. Coronary angiography should be performed in such patients to delineate thrombolytic failure. Successful PCI of a persistent occlusion following intravenous fibrinolytic therapy improves event free survival in the setting of thrombolytic failure. In the REACT trial of 427 STEMI patients with failed fibrinolysis, PCI, carried out on average nearly 7 hours after onset of symptoms, resulted in an event free survival rate of 85% compared to 70% in a conservative treatment group. Repeat intravenous fibrinolytic administration was of no benefit with a trend toward an adverse outcome.[40]

Coronary artery bypass grafting (CABG) is a third option for re-establishment of coronary flow in a patient with AMI (STEMI) and cardiogenic shock. Coronary artery bypass grafting has the disadvantage of requiring more time for re-establishment of coronary flow. It may be appropriate for some patients with multivessel or left main coronary disease. It is often the best option if concomitant surgical repair of an infarct VSD or MR is required. Although, some studies of CABG for AMI complicated by cardiogenic shock show an in-hospital mortality of approximately 40%, this relatively good result may be due to selection bias. It is unclear that coronary arterial bypass surgery is as effective as PCI or thrombolytic therapy for AMI-induced cardiogenic shock. In the United States, immediate CABG for AMI with cardiogenic shock is performed in approximately 3% of patients.[41]

Platelet aggregation is fundamental in initiating coronary thrombosis. Inhibition of platelet aggregation with aspirin, 160 mg, chewed (for rapid effect) and swallowed, is now routine initial therapy in STEMI. The efficacy of immediate aspirin was documented in the International Study of Infarct Survival-2 (ISIS-2) trial in 1988. Over 17,000 patients with suspected acute (within the prior 24 hours) MI were randomized to oral aspirin, intravenous streptokinase, neither or both. The 5 week mortality was 9.1% in the aspirin alone group and 11.8 % in the placebo group. Aspirin plus thrombolytic therapy (streptokinase, which is no longer available in this country) further reduced mortality to 8.0% versus 13.2% in the control group. Aspirin should be continued at a daily dose of 81 mg.[42]

Further inhibition of platelet aggregation in STEMI patients results from routine initial administration of thienopyridine drugs such as clopidogrel (Plavix). Plavix is given in an oral loading dose of 300 mg followed by 75 mg daily. If cardiothoracic surgery is a consideration, clopidogrel is usually held due to the increased surgical bleeding risk. Several studies have shown a small but real reduction in mortality with the early addition of thienopyridines to aspirin in the setting of AMI.[43,44]

In STEMI, clot formation is a dynamic process with ongoing fibrin deposition and lysis. All thrombolytic agents increase platelet aggregation even as they activate plasmin production and promote fibrinolysis. Thrombin inhibitors, given concomitantly with thrombolytic agents, improve the incidence of late coronary patency.[45] Low molecular weight heparins, which interfere with the clot formation cascade by inhibiting factor 10a, are effective but in the absence of available factor 10a measurements, we prefer unfractionated heparin in patients going to the catheterization laboratory (or possibly to surgery) due to the availability of monitoring parameters and its reversibility. In patients who are receiving thrombolytic therapy an initial heparin bolus of 70 units/kg (4,000 units maximum) is given followed by an infusion of 20 units/kg/h (1,000 units/h maximum). The activated partial thromboplastin time (aPTT) is monitored and should be kept at 50–70 seconds. Patients going directly for PCI receive a similar bolus. The activated clotting time is targeted at approximately 250 seconds. Bivalirudin has not been evaluated in this setting. Inhibition of platelet IIb-IIIa receptors has not been well studied and remains controversial in STEMI with cariogenic shock. Data from the PURSUIT (Platelet Glycoprotein IIb/IIIa in Unstable Angina: Receptor Suppression Using Integrilin Therapy) showed a similar incidence of cardiogenic shock in non-STEMI patients who had received the IIb-IIIa receptor blocker, eptifibatide, compared to those who had not.[46]

As discussed earlier, a right heart catheter facilitates diagnosis and is essential for monitoring changes in hemodynamic status. Some patients with apparent cardiogenic shock may be hypovolemic, especially if they have occult bleeding, vomiting, or excessive diuresis. These patients will be recognized by PAW or pulmonary artery diastolic pressures that are inappropriately low for the clinical picture (<15 torr) and with cardiac indices usually less than 2 L/min/m^2. They require volume resuscitation with IV crystalloid. A rapidly infused 250 cc bolus of isotonic sodium chloride, followed by more as needed, should be given with a target PAW pressure of 15–17 torr and followed with serial MVO_2 saturations (vide supra). Right heart pressures are used to diagnose RV dysfunction, especially in the setting of inferior MI where RA pressures will equal or exceed the PAW pressure. An inappropriately high right heart CO or high MVO_2 in a setting of apparent cardiogenic shock usually implies a left to right shunt which can be confirmed by demonstrating a significant "step-up" in O_2 saturation between the superior vena cava and pulmonary artery.

Profound hypotension which persists following an appropriate volume challenge and optimization of PAW pressures, usually requires intravenous inotropic and/or vasopressor agents in an attempt to improve organ perfusion and attenuate lactic acidosis. β-blockers and nondihydropyridine (diltiazem and verapamil) calcium-channel blockers should be avoided because of their negative inotropic effect. Inotropic agents increase myocardial O_2 requirements and may worsen MI—especially in the nonrevascularized patient. They are also arrhythmogenic. For these reasons, they should always be given at the lowest possible effective dosage. Due to endogenous sympathetic activation and catecholamine release, patients with cardiogenic shock usually present with elevated systemic vascular resistances and inotropic agents may be minimally effective in this setting. Intravenous norepinephrine (Levophed), which stimulates α and β-1 adrenergic receptors, is an inotrope and a vasopressor drug. In the setting of persistent hypotension with cardiogenic shock, norepinephrine is the preferred initial pressor choice. It is started at a dose of 0.1 mcg/kg/min and infused through a central venus catheter. It is titrated upward with dose adjustments every 2–3 minutes until an adequate response is obtained. The half-life is approximately 1 minute but can be prolonged with renal insufficiency. Continuous intra-arterial pressure monitoring is helpful and a pulmonary artery (Swan-Ganz) catheter is needed to monitor MVO_2 content and calculate pulmonary artery and systemic vascular resistance response to the infusion. This is the only means of knowing whether COs are decreasing with inotropic therapy if arterial blood pressures are unchanged (due to increasing systemic vascular resistances). Lactate levels are helpful in monitoring adequate vital organ perfusion (vide supra) and blood samples can be pulled from these catheters. The most effective systemic pressures vary from patient to patient and must be individualized. In the vast majority, a mean blood pressure of 65 torr will be adequate.[47] A recent randomized comparison evaluating dopamine versus norepinephrine as the pressor of choice in circulatory shock included 280 patients with cardiogenic shock. In the cardiogenic shock group, 28-day mortality was 52.5% in the dopamine group and 48.5% in the norepinephrine group. Arrhythmias (most commonly atrial fibrillation) occurred in 24% of dopamine infusion patients and 12% of norepinephrine patients.[48] When norepinephrine is ineffective at high dose, dobutamine, a β-1 agonist with predominate inotropic (and relatively little vasopressor) activity, is often added at an initial IV dose of 2 mcg/kg/min and titrated upward to a maximum of 40 mcg/kg/min.

Vasopressin, a relatively pure vasoconstrictor, is rarely used in cardiogenic shock. Phenylephrine is a pure α agonist with no notable inotropic activity and is given as a pure vasopressor (not commonly appropriate in cardiogenic shock).

Intubation, sedation and ventilation are usually required to decrease work of breathing and to improve O_2 delivery in acidemic, tachypneic, circulatory shock patients. In the randomized SHOCK trial, 88% of the early revascularization group was on mechanical ventilation.[49] Arterial blood gas monitoring is used to monitor adequate oxygen content and pH. The pCO_2 (reflecting alveolar ventilation) should be reduced to a level adequate to provide respiratory compensation for the metabolic acidosis.

Mechanical devices designed to augment CO are increasingly used for refractory cardiogenic shock. Intra-aortic balloon counter pulsation (IABP) has been in use for nearly 50 years.[50] A flexible catheter around which the deflated balloon is wrapped is inserted through a sheath into the femoral artery and advanced into the descending thoracic aorta just distal to the left subclavian artery. A lumen attached to the control console and running into the balloon allows rapid early diastolic intra-aortic balloon inflation and presystolic deflation with low-viscosity helium. The control console triggers the inflation of the balloon just at the dicrotic notch in early diastole with balloon deflation just prior to systole (triggered to the R wave on the EKG). This results in increased diastolic intra-aortic pressures due to the sudden increased intra-aortic volume, and decreased systemic aortic resistances, due to the abrupt volume removal from the aorta just prior to systole. Myocardial wall stress (and therefore the myocardial oxygen requirement) is reduced. The augmented diastolic perfusion pressure improves diastolic coronary flow. Although this device has been used for many years in patients with cardiogenic shock, no appropriate studies have documented its efficacy in cardiogenic shock. In 1985, a small randomized trial was unable to show a mortality difference in patients randomized to IABP with intravenous nitroglycerin versus a control group.[51] In the landmark SHOCK trial, 85% of patients in both groups were on IABP and some studies suggest reduced mortality with IABP in conjunction with thrombolysis.[49] A multicenter trial from Germany randomized 600 patients with cardiogenic shock complicating AMI to use of IABP or a control group. All patients had revascularization with early PCI. At 12 months, mortality was 52% in the IABP group and 51% in the control group.[52] Intraaortic balloon counter pulsation is of value in cardiogenic shock accompanying infarct VSD or severe mitral insufficiency as both are improved by decreasing after load. It may be of value in patients given thrombolytic therapy who lack early access to PCI. Advantages of IABP are that it can be put in place percutaneously at the bedside (and checked for appropriate position with a chest X-ray). It is the cheapest mechanical circulatory assist device. It obviously cannot be used in patients with aortic insufficiency. Significant complications include mechanical ischemia of the leg, the renal, or the mesenteric circulation, dissection, cholesterol emboli, thrombus and thrombotic embolus, bleeding, and infection. Care must be taken to position the tip at least a centimeter inferior to the left subclavian artery to decrease the probability of stroke. If the device must be left in for over a week, an axillary, as opposed to the usual femoral arterial insertion site, may reduce the likelihood of infection. Unlike other mechanical circulatory assist devices, IABP does not directly pump blood from the venous circuit or left ventricle into the arterial circulation.

Newer percutaneous ventricular assist devices (VADs) which are hemodynamically more effective than IABP are now frequently selected for treating cardiogenic shock. An effective VAD will decrease pulmonary artery wedge (left ventricular end-diastolic pressure) pressures, decrease myocardial oxygen requirements and directly increase CO and arterial blood pressure. Two popular percutaneous devices, approved for use in the USA, are the TandemHeart™ (made by Cardiac Assist Inc.) and the Impella® (made by Abiomed Inc.). Patients placed on these devices are given intravenous heparin with a targeted aPTT of 55–65 seconds.

The TandemHeart has a venous catheter which is percutaneously placed through the femoral or jugular vein into the right atrium and then across the atrial septum into the left atrium via a transseptal puncture. The arterial catheter is advanced via a femoral arterial puncture into the iliac artery. The left atrial to arterial blood goes through a console with a centrifugal impeller pump providing continuous flow of oxygenated left atrial blood to the iliac artery at flows of up to 4.5 L/min (limited by cannula size). An early randomized comparison of the TandemHeart to IABP, in 41 patients with AMI and cardiogenic shock, was carried out by the Leipzig group. TandemHeart patients had significant improvement in CO, blood pressure, and serum lactate when compared to IABP patients. Both groups were sent to early coronary revascularization; however, both groups had a 30-day mortality of 45%. The TandemHeart group had significantly more major bleeds and limb ischemia even though this device was removed slightly earlier (average of 3.5 days vs. 4 days) than the IABP device.[53]

The Impella device is frequently utilized for cardiogenic shock or in support of high-risk coronary angioplasty in our institution. The percutaneous placement of the Impella is more facile than with the TandemHeart. It provides continuous flow via a microaxial rotary inclined plane around a central 9 Fr catheter which is placed across the aortic valve—usually via femoral arterial access. The tip has a pig-tail configuration to facilitate crossing the aortic valve. Impella devices come as a 2.5 L/min model with a 12 Fr diameter, and a recently introduced 14 Fr 3.5 L/min model. The largest size, a 5 L/min pump, is 22 Fr and requires a surgical cut-down for arterial access. The Impella device impels blood from the LV chamber across the aortic valve to the aortic root. A RV Impella (right ventricle to pulmonary artery) is also available. In a European registry of 120 patients with acute cardiogenic shock, the Impella 2.5 device was easily percutaneously placed in 95% of the cases. It was left in place for an average of 2 days. The blood lactate level was significantly reduced from 5.8 to 2.5 mmol/L following Impella placement. However, the 30-day mortality was 64%. The authors suggested that this high mortality reflected inappropriately late use of the Impella in these very ill registry patients. Twenty-three percent of the patients had significant bleeding and 8% of patients had evidence of hemolysis.[54] A more recent review of 47 cardiogenic shock patients from a single institution was published by a cardiothoracic surgical group. Postcardiotomy cardiogenic shock was present in 68%. The Impella 5.0 device was utilized in 80% with 20% receiving the Impella 2.5 L/min device. The 30-day mortality rate was 30%. The 5.0 devices were surgically implanted and the 2.5 Impellas were placed percutaneously. Device malfunction occurred in five patients. The average duration of Impella support was 5.4 days. Weaning from the device was started after inotropic support had been stopped and was accomplished by decreasing pump support in decrements of two levels while assessing patient response every 2 hours. The low mortality in this small series is noteworthy.[55] The Impella device had FDA approval for 6 hours of use in cardiogenic shock. A case report of a 61-year-old man with AMI complicated by severe cardiogenic shock, who survived following 35 days of support with the Impella 5.0, demonstrates that much longer time may be required for survival.[56] The Impella 5.0 may be an efficacious bridge to cardiac transplantation or implantation of a durable LV assist device. A report from Baylor University described 40 patients with cardiogenic shock who were supported with the Impella 5.0 until heart transplant or left ventricular assist device, which occurred on average over 7 days later (range of 1–22 days). The cardiac index improved from 1.8 L/min/m^2 to 2.9 L/min/m^2 and pulmonary artery diastolic pressure fell from a mean of 34–24 torr post-Impella insertion. Thirty patients (75%) survived to their next therapy.[57] Complications include a high risk of bleeding, which usually occurred when removing the Impella device. This problem can and should be minimized in higher risk patients with vascular surgical removal. Hemolysis, limb ischemia, clotting, aortic valve injury, and arterial dissection or perforation are recognized risks of the Impella device. Randomized prospective trials, although difficult due to the multiple variables encountered in cardiogenic shock, are needed to place this expensive, important technology in proper clinical perspective.

Extracorporeal membrane oxygenation (V-A ECMO) with veno-arterial bypass is another frequently employed option for mechanical circulatory support in cardiogenic shock. A mechanical heart and lung apparatus was first developed by Gibbon in 1954.[58] Modern ECMO devices pass venous blood through a membrane oxygenator (which also removes CO_2) and a warmer with a rotary pump returning blood to the arterial circulation. Extracorporeal membrane oxygenation devices have been used over the last 50 years for life support in a variety of clinical situations. Extracorporeal membrane oxygenation is frequently employed for postcardiotomy cardiogenic shock and inability to wean from the bypass pump in the operative suite. A perfusion technologist should be in constant attendance in the intensive care suite during employment of ECMO. A review of 123 patients with cardiogenic shock of various etiologies at Beth Israel Deaconess Medical Center in Boston showed an in-hospital mortality of 61% in ECMO treated patients.[59] A smaller consecutive series of 18 patients with cardiogenic shock due to AMI reported a 33% in-hospital mortality. The average ECMO duration was 3.2 days. Ninety four percent required transfusion.[60] A meta-analysis of 1,866 adult patients with cardiogenic shock treated with V-A ECMO reported in-hospital survivals ranging from 21 to 65% suggesting a large variability in *pre-hoc* severity of illness. There was a high reported frequency of severe complications including acute kidney injury in 56% and major bleeding in 41%. Neurologic complications occurred in 13% with stroke in 6%. Other problems included lower extremity ischemia (17%) resulting in compartment syndrome in 10%. Significant infection was reported in 30%. Intrathoracic bleeding or tamponade was seen in 42%.[61] Extracorporeal membrane oxygenation increases after load due to the intra-arterial infusion of blood during systole. Concomitant use of IABP with ECMO can theoretically reduce the after load and provide better decompression of the left ventricle. This approach has not been adequately studied.[62] Platelet consumption and an induced consumptive coagulopathy are associated with ECMO.[63] Patients successfully weaned from ECMO may have good long-term survival rates. An Australian report of 104 ECMO survivors in adult patients with cardiogenic shock reported a 79% 1 year survivorship.[64]

In the changing field of mechanical circulatory support technology, the use of percutaneous devices is estimated to have increased over 1,500% compared with a negligible increase in nonpercutaneous devices from 2007 to 2011. Over this time, rates of in-hospital mortality from cardiogenic shock appear to have decreased. There is also apparent decrease in hospital costs associated with shorter hospital stays.[65] Effective therapy of shock must be implemented quickly before the late stage shock with multiorgan failure becomes irreversible. Pharmaceutical approaches to cardiogenic shock have had little apparent success. In AMI complicated by cardiogenic shock, rapid restoration of intracoronary blood flow has been shown to reduce mortality.[49] Mechanical circulatory assist devices are expensive and carry significant risks. Their increasing use is associated with an apparent decrease in mortality that may or may not be causal.[64]

Cardiogenic shock varies in severity, etiology, and presentation making registry outcomes difficult to interpret. Large, randomized, prospective trials, expensive, and difficult to effectively implement, are needed to place the use (and timing) of circulatory assist devices in appropriate perspective in the therapy of diverse types of cardiogenic shock. Available resources and skills vary significantly among institutions. The expense of these devices appropriately raises ethical concerns about the ability to pay and over or under utilization of facilities.[66] Although, cardiogenic shock has many causes and therapy must be directed at the underlying pathogenetic process, AMI remains the overwhelming most frequent problem. A tertiary care hospital cardiogenic shock team should be constantly available to facilitate rapid, state of the art intervention including revascularization and early deployment of mechanical devices in appropriately selected patients. Systemic approaches facilitating rapid recognition and transport to adequately equipped and staffed tertiary care hospitals in a designated area are becoming more plentiful. As technology evolves and new data are acquired, we can be optimistic about the likelihood of further mortality reduction in cardiogenic shock.

REFERENCES

1. Vincent JL, De Backer D. Circulatory shock. N Engl J Med. 2013; 369(18):1726-34.
2. Stead E, Ebert R. Shock syndrome produced by failure of the heart. Arch Intern Med. 1942;69(3):369.
3. Fox KA, Anderson FA, Dabbous OH, Steg PG, López-Sendón J, Van de Werf F, et al. Intervention in acute coronary syndromes: do patients undergo intervention on the basis of the risk characteristics? The Global Registry of Acute Coronary Events (GRACE). Heart. 2007;93(2):177-82.
4. Fox KA, Steg PG, Eagle KA, Goodman SG, Anderson FA, Granger CB, et al. Decline in rates of death and heart failure in acute coronary syndromes, 1999-2006. JAMA. 2007;297(17):1892-900.
5. Holmes D, Bates ER, Kleiman NS, Sadowski Z, Horgan JH, Morris DC, et al. Contemporary reperfusion therapy for cardiogenic shock: the GUSTO-I trial experience. The GUSTO-I Investigators. Global Utilization of Streptokinase and Tissue Plasminogen Activator for Occluded Coronary Arteries. J Am Coll Cardiol. 1995;26(3):668-74.
6. Kolte D, Khera S, Aronow WS, Mujib M, Palaniswamy C, Sule S, et al. Trends in incidence, management, and outcomes of cardiogenic shock complicating ST-elevation myocardial infarction in the United States. J Am Heart Assoc. 2014;3(1):e000590.
7. Frangogiannis NG, Smith CW, Entman ML. The inflammatory response in myocardial infarction. Cardiovasc Res. 2002;53(1):31-47.
8. Wildhirt SM, Dudek RR, Suzuki H, Bing RJ. Involvement of inducible nitric oxide synthase in the inflammatory process of myocardial infarction. Int J Cardiol. 1995;50(3):253-61.
9. Goldstein JA. Pathophysiology and management of right heart ischemia. J Am Coll Cardiol. 2002;40(5):841-53.
10. Mehta SR, Eikelboom JW, Natarajan MK, Diaz R, Yi C, Gibbons RJ, et al. Impact of right ventricular involvement on mortality and morbidity in patients with inferior myocardial infarction. J Am Coll Cardiol. 2001;37(1):37-43.
11. Moore CA, Nygaard TW, Kaiser DL, Cooper AA, Gibson RS. Postinfarction ventricular septal rupture: the importance of location of infarction and right ventricular function in determining survival. Circulation. 1986;74(1):45-55.
12. McCarthy RE, Boehmer JP, Hruban RH, Hutchins GM, Kasper EK, Hare JM, et al. Long-term outcome of fulminant myocarditis as compared to acute (non-fulminant) myocarditis. N Engl J Med. 2003;342(10):690-5.
13. Templin C, Ghadri JR, Diekmann J, Napp LC, Bataiosu DR, Jaguszewski M, et al. Clinical features and outcomes of takotsubo (stress) cardiomyopathy. N Engl J Med. 2015;373(10):929-38.
14. Singh K, Neil CJ, Nguyen TH, Stansborough J, Chong CR, Dawson D, et al. Dissociation of early shock in takotsubo cardiomyopathy from either right or left ventricular systolic dysfunction. Heart Lung Circ. 2014; 23(12):1141-8.
15. De Baker O, Debonnaire P, Gevaert S, Missault L, Gheeraert P, Muyldermans L. Prevalence, associated factors and management implications of left ventricular outflow tract obstruction in takotsubo cardiomyopathy: a two-year two-center experience. BMC Cardiovasc Disord. 2114;14:147.
16. Sliwa K, Bohm M. Incidence and prevalence of pregnancy related heart disease. Cardiovasc Res. 2014;101(4):554-60.
17. Goland S, Modi K, Bitar F, Janmohamed M, Mirocha JM, Czer LS, et al. Cinical profile and predictors of complications in peripartum cardiomyopathy. J Card Fail. 2009;15(8): 645-50.
18. Stout KK, Verner ED. Acute valvular regurgitation. Circulation. 2009;119(25): 3232.
19. Gopinathannair R, Etheridge SP, Marchlinski FE, Spinale FG, Lakkireddy D, Olshansky B. Arrhythmia-Induced Cardiomyopathies: Mechanisms, Recognition, and Management. J Am Coll Cardiol. 2015;66(15):1714-28.
20. Lund LH, Edwards LB, Kucheryavaya AY, Benden C, Dipchand AI, Goldfarb S, et al. The Registry of the International Society for Heart and Lung Transplantation: 32nd Official Adult Heart Transplant Report--2015; Focus theme: Early Graft Failure. J Heart Lung Transplant. 2015;34(10):1244-54.
21. Lund LH, Edwards LB, Kucheryavaya AY, Benden C, Christie JD, Dipchand AI, et al. The Registry of the International Society for Heart and Lung Transplantation: 31st Official Adult Heart Transplant Report--2014; Focus theme: Retransplantation. J Heart Lung Transplant. 2014;33(10):996-1008.
22. Faucher L, Babuty D, Poret P, Casset-Senon D, Autret ML, Cosnay P, et al. Comparison of long-term outcome of alcoholic and idiopathic dilated cardiomyopathy. Eur Heart J. 2000;21(4): 306-14.
23. Lange RA, Hillis D. Cardiovascular complications of cocaine use. N Engl J Med. 2001;345(5):351-8.
24. Karch SB, Mari F, Bartolini V, Bertol E. Aminorex poisoning in cocaine abusers. Int J Cardiol. 2012;158(3):344-6.
25. Bhatia NL, Tajik AJ, Wilansky S, Steidley DE, Mookadam F. Isolated noncompaction of the left ventricular myocardium in adults: a systematic overview. J Card Fail. 2011;17(9):771-8.

26. Fukuhara S, Takeda K, Garan AR, Kurlansky P, Hastie J, Naka Y, et al. Contemporary mechanical circulatory support for postcardiotomy shock. Gen Thorac Cardiovasc Surg. 2016;64(4):183-91.
27. Jansen TC, van Bommel J, Schoonderbeek FJ, Sleeswijk Visser SJ, van der Klooster JM, Lima AP, et al. Early lactate-guided therapy in intensive care unit patients: A multi-center open label randomized controlled trial. Am J Resp Crit Care Med. 2010;182(6):752-61.
28. Picard MH, Davidoff R, Sleeper LA, Mendes LA, Thompson CR, Dzavik V, et al. Echocardiographic predictors of survival and response to early revascularization in cardiogenic shock. Circulation. 2003;107(2):279-84.
29. Carabello B, Cohn PF, Alpert JS. Hemodynamic monitoring in patients with hypotension after myocardial infarction. The role of the medical center in relation to the community hospital. Chest. 1978;74(1):5-9.
30. Fick A. Uber die Messing des Blutquantums in den Herzventrikeln. Sitz der Physic-Med get Wurtzberg. 1870, p. 16.
31. Richard AD, Kay R, Smith H, Rentrop P, Holt J, Gorlin R. Large V waves in the pulmonary wedge pressure tracing in the absence of mitral regurgitation. Am J Cardiol. 1982;50(5):1044-50.
32. Kohsaka S, Menon V, Lowe AM, Lange M, Dzavik V, Sleeper LA, et al. Systemic inflammatory response syndrome after acute myocardial infarction complicated by cardiogenic shock. Arch Intern Med. 2005;165(14):1643-50.
33. O'Gara PT, Kushner FG, Ascheim DD, Casey DE, Chung MK, de Lemos JA, et al. 2013 ACCF/AHA Guideline for the management of ST-elevation myocardial infarction: executive summary: a report of the American College of Cardiology Foundation/American Heart Association Task Force on Practice Guidelines. Circulation. 2013;127(4) :529-55.
34. Zeymer U, Vogt A, Zahn R, Weber MA, Tebbe U, Gottwik M, et al. Predictors of in-hospital mortality in 1333 patients with acute myocardial infarction complicated by cardiogenic shock treated with primary percutaneous coronary intervention (PCI); Results of the primary PCI registry of the Arbeitsgemeinschaft Leitende Kardiologische Krankenhausärzte (ALKK). Eur Heart J. 2004;25(4);322-8.
35. Lindholm MG, Køber L, Boesgaard S, Torp-Pedersen C, Aldershvile J, Trandolapril Cardiac Evaluation study group. Cardiogenic shock complicating acute myocardial infarction; prognostic impact of early and late shock development. Eur Heart J. 2003;24(3):258-65.
36. Mylotte D, Morice MC, Eltchaninoff H, Garot J, Louvard Y, Lefèvre T, et al. Primary percutaneous coronary intervention in patients with acute myocardial infarction, resuscitated cardiac arrest and cardiogenic shock: the role of primary multivessel revascularization. JACC Cardiolvasc Interv. 2013;6(2):115-25.
37. Bagai A, Dangas GD, Stone GW, Granger CB. Reperfusion strategies in acute coronary syndromes. Circ Res. 2014;114(12):1918-28.
38. Pinto DS, Frederick PD, Chakrabarti AK, Kirtane AJ, Ullman E, Dejam A, et al. Benefit of transferring ST-segment-elevation myocardial infarction patients for percutaneous coronary intervention compared with administration of onsite fibrinolytic declines as delays increase. Circulation. 2011;124(23):2512-21.
39. Assessment of the Safety and Efficacy of a New Thrombolytic (ASSENT-2) Investigators, Van de Werf F, Adgey J, Ardissino D, Armstrong PW, Aylward P, et al. Single-bolus tenecteplase compared with front-loaded alteplase in acute myocardial infarction: the ASSENT-2 double-blind randomized trial. Lancet. 1999;354(9180):716-22.
40. Gershlick AH, Stephens-Lloyd A, Hughes S, Abrams KR, Stevens SE, Uren NG, et al. Rescue angioplasty after failed thrombolytic therapy for acute myocardial infarction. N Engl J Med. 2005;353(26):2758-68.
41. Babaev A, Frederick PD, Pasta DJ, Every N, Sichrovsky T, Hochman JS, et al. Trends in management and outcomes of patients with acute myocardial infarction complicated by cardiogenic shock. JAMA. 2005;294(4):448-54.
42. Randomized trial of intravenous streptokinase, oral aspirin, both or neither among 17,187 cases of suspected acute myocardial infarction: ISIS-2. ISIS-2 (Second International Study of Infarct Survival) Collaborative Group. Lancet. 1988;2(8607):349-60.
43. Chen ZM, Jiang LX, Chen YP, Xie JX, Pan HC, Peto R, et al. Addition of clopidogrel to aspirin in 45,852 patients with acute myocardial infarction: randomized placebo-controlled trial. Lancet. 2005;366(9497):1607-21.
44. Sabatini MS, Cannon CP, Gibson CM, López-Sendón JL, Montalescot G, Theroux P, et al. Addition of clopidogrel to aspirin and fibrinolytic therapy for myocardial infarction with ST elevation. N Engl J Med. 2005;352(12):1179-89.
45. White HD, Braunwald E, Murphy SA, Jacob AJ, Gotcheva N, Polonetsky L, et al. Enoxaparin vs, unfractionated heparin with fibrinolysis for ST elevation myocardial infarction in elderly and younger patients: results from the ExTRA CT-TIMI 25. Eur Heart J. 2007;28(9):1066-71.
46. Hasdai D, Harrington RA, Hochman JS, Califf RM, Battler A, Box JW, et al. Platelet glycoprotein IIb-IIIa blockade and outcome of cardiogenic shock complicating acute coronary syndromes without persistent ST-segment elevation. J Am Coll Cardiol. 2000;36(3):685-92.
47. Cecconi M, De Backer D, Antonelli M, Beale R, Bakker J, Hofer C, et al. Consensus on circulatory shock and hemodynamic monitoring. Task Force of the European Society of Intensive Care Medicine. Intensive Care Med. 2014;40(12):1795-815.
48. De Baker D, Biston P, Devriendt J, Madl C, Chochrad D, Aldecoa C, et al. Comparison of dopamine and norepinephrine in the treatment of shock. N Engl J Med. 2010;362(9):779-89.
49. Hochman JS, Sleeper LA, Webb JG, Sanborn TA, White HD, Talley JD, et al. Early revascularization in acute myocardial infarction complicated by cardiogenic shock. SHOCK Investigators. Should We Emergently Revascularize Occluded Coronaries for Cardiogenic Shock. N Engl J Med. 1999;341(9):625-34.
50. Kantrowitz A, Krakauer JS, Rosenbaum A, Butner AN, Freed PS, Jaron D. Phase-shift balloon pumping in medically refractory cardiogenic shock. Results in 27 patients. Arch Surg. 1969;99(6):739-43.
51. Flaherty JT, Becker LC, Weiss JL, Brinker JA, Bulkley BH, Gerstenblith G, et al. Results of a randomized prospective trial of intraaortic balloon counterpulsation and intravenous nitroglycerin in patients with acute myocardial infarction. J Am Coll Cardiol. 1985;6(2):434-46.
52. Thiele H, Zeymer U, Neumann FJ, Ferenc M, Olbrich HG, Hausleiter J, et al. Intra-aortic balloon counterpulsation in acute myocardial infarction complicated by cardiogenic shock (IABP-SHOCK II): final 12 month results of a randomized, open-label trial. Lancet. 2013;382(9905):1638-45.
53. Thiele H, Sick P, Boudriot E, Diederich KW, Hambrecht R, Niebauer J, et al. Randomized comparison of intra-aortic balloon support with a percutaneous left ventricular assist device in patients with a revascularized acute myocardial infarction complicated by cardiogenic shock. Eur Heart J. 2005;26(13):1276-83.
54. Lauten A, Engström AE, Jung C, Empen K, Erne P, Cook S, et al. Percutaneous left-ventricular support with the Impella-2.5-assist device in acute cardiogenic shock: results of the Impella-EUROSHOCK-Registry. Circ Heart Fail. 2013;6(1):23-30.
55. Lemaire A, Anderson MB, Lee LY, Scholz P, Prendergast T, Goodman A, et al. The Impella device for acute mechanical circulatory support in patients with cardiogenic shock. Ann Thorac Surg. 2014;97(1):133-8.
56. Castillo-Sang MA, Prasad SM, Singh J, Ewald GA, Silvestry SC. Thirty-five day Impella 5.0 support via right axillary side graft cannulation for acute cardiogenic shock. Innovations (Phila). 2013;8(4):307-9.
57. Lima B, Kale P, Gonzalez-Stawinski GV, Kuiper JJ, Carey S, Hall SA. Effectiveness and Safety of the Impella 5.0 as a Bridge to Cardiac Transplantation or Durable Left Ventricular Assist Device. Am J Cardiol. 2016;117(10):1622-8.
58. Gibbon JH. Application of a mechanical heart and lung apparatus to cardiac surgery. Minn Med. 1954;37(3):171-85; passim.
59. Carroll BJ, Shah RV, Murthy V, McCullough SA, Reza N, Thomas SS, et al. Clinical features and outcomes in adults with cardiogenic shock supported by extracorporeal membrane oxygenation. Am J Cardiol. 2015; 116(10):1624-30.
60. Esper SA, Bermudez C, Dueweke EJ, Kormos R, Subramaniam K, Mulukutla S, et al. Extracorporeal membrane oxygenation support in acute coronary syndromes complicated by cardiogenic shock. Catheter Cardiovasc Interv. 2015;86(Suppl 1):S45-50.
61. Cheng R, Hachamovitch R, Kittleson M, Patel J, Arabia F, Moriguchi J, et al. Complications of extracorporeal membrane oxygenation for treatment of cardiogenic shock and cardiac arrest: a meta-analysis of 1,866 adult patients. Ann Thorac Surg. 2014;97(2):610-6.
62. Ma P, Zhang Z, Song T, Yang Y, Meng G, Zhao J, et al Combining ECMO with IABP for the treatment of critically ill adult heart failure patients. Heart Lung Circ. 2014;23(4):363-6.
63. Tanaka KA, Esper S, Bolliger D. Perioperative factor concentrate therapy. Br J Anaesth. 2013;111(Suppl 1):i35-49.
64. Burrell AJ, Pellegrino VA, Wolfe R, Wong WK, Cooper DJ, Kaye DM, et al. Long-term survival of adults with cardiogenic shock after venoarterial extracorporeal membrane oxygenation. J Crit Care. 2015;30(5):949-56.
65. Stretch R, Sauer CM, Yuh DD, Bonde P. National trends in the utilization of short-term mechanical circulatory support: incidence, outcomes, and cost analysis. J Am Coll Cardiol. 2014;64(14):1407-15.
66. Rajagopalan N, Guglin M, Million K, Yanagida R, Hoopes CW. Success of left ventricular assist device therapy in uninsured patients. Int J Cardiol. 2014; 177(3):1087-8.

23 CHAPTER

Acute Pericarditis

Jacqueline J Denysiak, Daniel C Walters, Lori B Daniels

INTRODUCTION

The simplest definition of acute pericarditis is inflammation of the pericardial sac. To understand acute pericarditis, it helps to review anatomy of the heart. The heart wall is composed of several layers: from inside to outside, there is endocardium, myocardium, and finally epicardium. Then, there is a double-layered sac known as the pericardium that encases the heart.[1] The pericardium is fibroelastic, fluid-containing, and has two components: an outer fibrous layer made of connective tissue, and an inner serous layer which is a closed sac composed of two layers itself. The inner layer or visceral pericardium lines the epicardial tissue, while the tougher, thickened, membranous outer layer known as the parietal pericardium lines the fibrous pericardium. Normally, there is less than 25–50 mL of serous fluid in the space between the visceral and parietal pericardium.[2] However, in the setting of inflammation as well as other disease processes, the potential space can become filled with up to several liters of a transudative, exudative, or sanguineous fluid, depending on the etiology. This is a common occurrence with the inflammation of pericarditis.[2,3]

An understanding of pericardial structure assists in comprehending its purposes. These include limiting the distention of cardiac chambers, decreasing torsion and friction of the heart against other contents of the mediastinum by providing lubrication within the pericardial space, and also preventing the spread of infection or neoplastic processes by providing an immunologic barrier.[4] The focus of this chapter will be on acute pericarditis, the causes, clinical findings, treatments, and prognosis of which will be discussed further.

CAUSES

A simple classification of acute pericarditis involves subdividing the disease into fibrinous, serous, hemorrhagic, and suppurative or purulent categories. Fibrinous pericarditis is most commonly presumed to be idiopathic or postviral infection, often preceded by a flu-like, upper respiratory tract or gastrointestinal illness. Some of the most common viruses implicated in acute pericarditis include coxsackie viruses A and B, echovirus, cytomegalovirus, human immunodeficiency virus and hepatitis A and B.[5] Serous acute pericarditis can occur in the immediate post-acute myocardial infarction (AMI) time period or several weeks after AMI, and is also known as Dressler's syndrome. It can also be seen in the setting of uremia, collagen vascular disease, autoimmune disease, and in patients with neoplasms. Hodgkin's lymphoma, breast and lung cancers are some of the neoplasms most commonly associated with pericarditis.[6]

Less common but notable causes of serous acute pericarditis include drug-induced lupus syndrome, post-pericardiectomy, amyloidosis, postradiation therapy and post-trauma.[7] Suppurative or purulent acute pericarditis is usually caused by *pneumococcus* or *Streptococcus* but is relatively rare in recent times thanks to the widespread use of antibiotics.[8]

Hemorrhagic pericarditis is typically seen in a traumatic or iatrogenic (e.g., postpacemaker, postcardiopulmonary resuscitation) setting when acute blood loss into the pericardial space triggers an inflammatory response. However, causes of hemorrhagic pericarditis are not limited to trauma. For instance, depending on the anatomic location, invasive thoracic tumors may cause bleeding into the pericardial sac as well.[9,10] In practice, the etiology of acute pericarditis is often unknown and gets categorized as "idiopathic" or "viral" without a specific virus implicated; roughly 80–85% of patients diagnosed with acute pericarditis will be labeled as such (Table 1).[11-14]

TABLE 1: Pericarditis[11-14]

Etiology	Incidence
Idiopathic or viral	~85%
Autoimmune or connective tissue disease or pericardial injury	~5–10%
Neoplastic	~5%
Bacterial	~1–5%
Postmyocardial infarction	1–5%

CLINICAL FINDINGS

Symptoms

A classic presentation of acute pericarditis is a patient presenting with chest pain that is described as "pleuritic", meaning pain that is sharp and worse with deep inspiration. The pain is also typically affected by the position of the patient, classically alleviated when leaning forward or sitting upright and exacerbated by lying flat. This presentation is in contrast to the classic pain of ischemic heart disease, known as angina, which is characteristically described as a dull, heavy chest discomfort, often episodic, without positional change, and possibly radiating to the patient's jaw, neck, arms, or back. The pain of pericarditis typically does not change with exertion and is often persistent, lasting hours to days from onset prior to treatment being sought.[15]

Physical Examination

On physical examination, a pericardial friction rub is a particularly specific, but not sensitive, finding for acute pericarditis.[16] Described as a scratching, high-pitched sound with three components, a friction rub is caused by the increased inflammation and contact between the visceral and parietal pericardium. Though not essential for diagnosis, auscultation of a pericardial friction rub is pathognomonic for acute pericarditis. The friction rub can be intermittently present and can vary in intensity throughout the disease course.

Should the inflammation seen in acute pericarditis result in more significant fluid accumulation within the pericardial space (known as a pericardial effusion), a pericardial friction rub may be less common, as the accumulated fluid prevents direct approximation and rubbing of the inflamed layers of the pericardium against each other. On the other hand, there are additional physical examination findings of note which may occur. These findings tend to be particularly notable if the effusion is large enough to cause cardiac tamponade, a state in which the elevated pressures within the pericardial space impedes filling of the cardiac chambers to result in hemodynamic compromise. Notable findings on physical examination associated with larger pericardial effusions and with cardiac tamponade include jugular venous distention, hypotension, and distant or muffled heart sounds; taken together, this triad of findings is known as Beck's triad. Pulsus paradoxus has a sensitivity of 82% for cardiac tamponade, while findings of tachycardia and elevated jugular venous pressure have sensitivities of 77% and 76%, respectively.[17,18]

DIFFERENTIAL DIAGNOSIS

The differential diagnosis for a patient with an acute onset of chest pain is broad. Potential lethal diagnoses that must be considered include aortic dissection, AMI, tension pneumothorax, and pulmonary embolism. It is critical to rule these out before continuing with the diagnostic workup for acute pericarditis. Other items on the differential diagnosis include but are not limited to pneumonia, gastroesophageal reflux, acute pancreatitis, costochondritis, and anxiety/somatization disorder.

LABORATORY EVALUATION

Complete blood count with differential diagnosis, coagulation profile, blood urea nitrogen test, and creatinine levels; the inflammatory markers erythrocyte sedimentation rate and/or C-reactive protein, and cardiac biomarkers including cardiac troponin with or without a natriuretic peptide, should be ordered in the workup of acute pericarditis. Leukocytosis may be present in the event of infectious, autoimmune, or neoplastic causes of acute pericarditis, and elevation of inflammatory markers is typically seen regardless of etiology. Blood cultures are often ordered for early infectious evaluation. Cardiac troponin is ordered to assess for possible acute coronary syndrome or myocarditis. A D-dimer may also be considered for assessment of pulmonary embolism and/or aortic dissection in those patients who are considered low risk. In the appropriate clinical scenario, thyroid function could also be checked.[19]

DIAGNOSTIC PROCEDURES

Electrocardiogram

Electrocardiogram (ECG) is critical in the workup of possible pericarditis to assess for potentially lethal myocardial ischemia and/or infarction. It can also be diagnostic of pericarditis. There are a number of classic ECG findings in acute pericarditis, which progress through a series of stages (Figs 1 to 3). These include diffuse ST-segment elevation, typically concave up, often with reciprocal ST depression in lead aVR. In addition, there may be widespread PR depressions, most notably in leads V5 and V6, along with PR elevation in lead aVR, both of which are very specific findings. As the disease course progresses over the ensuing week or so, the ECG will evolve and show diffuse T-wave inversions after a brief period of ST and PR segment normalization. In most patients, the T waves subsequently normalize as well. In a patient with a large pericardial effusion, low-voltage QRS complexes and electrical alternans may be also observed. Low-voltage ECGs are caused by a dampening of the recorded electrical impulses as they pass through the expanded and fluid-filled pericardial effusion. Electrical alternans is a beat-to-beat variation in the electrical impulses noted on the ECG. This is due to

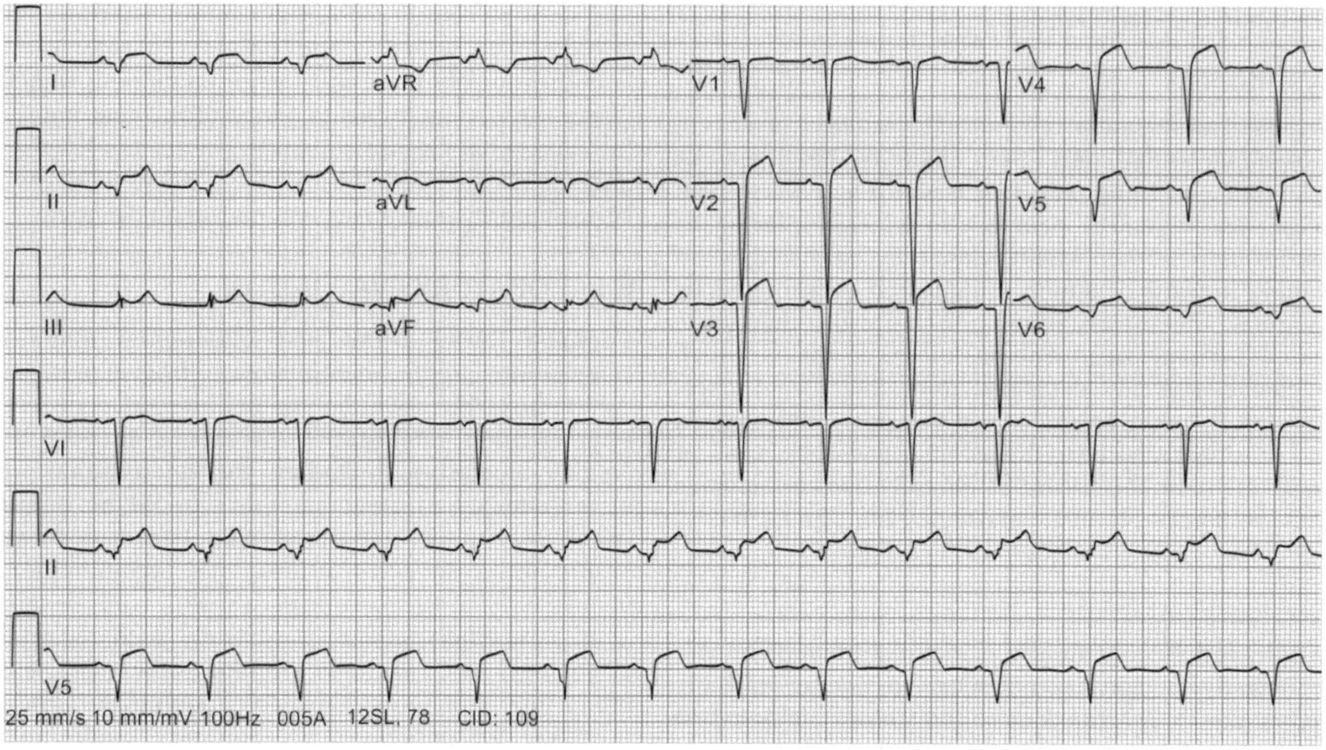

FIG. 1: Electrocardiogram of a patient with acute pericarditis, demonstrating diffuse ST elevation

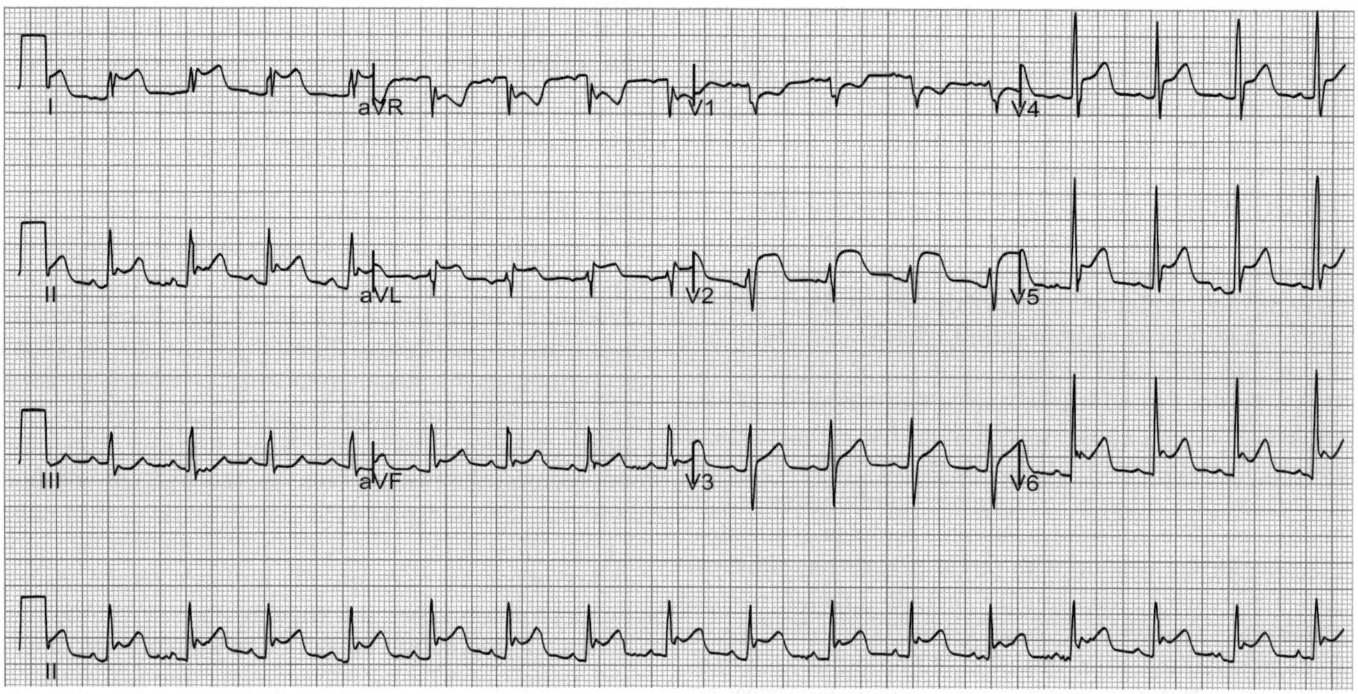

FIG. 2: Electrocardiogram notable for diffuse concave-up ST elevation in most leads. Leads V4-V6 demonstrate Spodick's sign, characterized by downward TP segment. There is also PR elevation in lead aVR, and PR depression in several other leads

swinging movement of the entire heart to and from and is reflected in the alternating heights of larger and smaller QRS complexes; in more extreme cases, there can also be beat-to-beat changes in QRS axis.[4]

Chest X-ray

Most commonly, patients with acute pericarditis have normal chest X-rays. However, if a large pericardial effusion is present there may be an enlarged cardiac

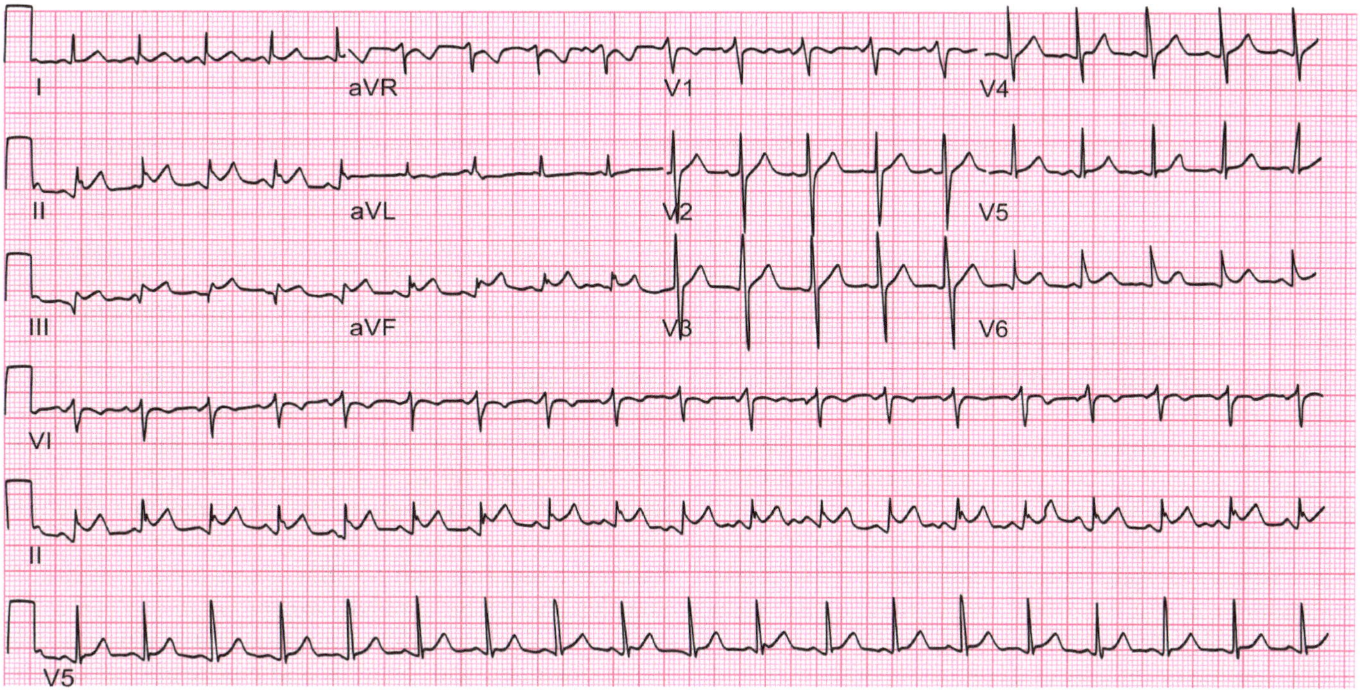

FIG. 3: Typical electrocardiogram of patient with acute pericarditis

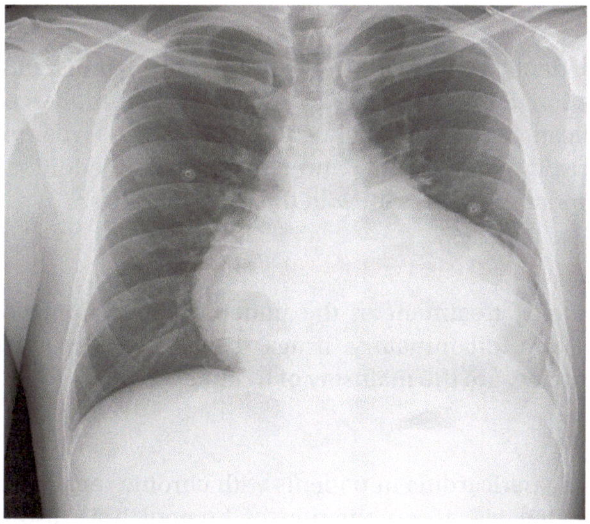

FIG. 4: Chest X-ray of a patient with large pericardial effusion demonstrating characteristic "water bottle" heart secondary to effusion from pericarditis

Courtesy: Dr Daniel G Blanchard.

silhouette. Some have described the associated globular shape as a "water bottle" heart (Fig. 4).[15] Rate of accumulation of pericardial fluid is often determined by etiology, and may determine if and when enlargement of the cardiac silhouette is seen. For instance, a patient with rapid accumulation of fluid due to trauma will have radiographic evidence sooner than someone with uremic pericarditis, which may slowly accumulate over days or weeks.[20] Although seeing an enlarged cardiac silhouette may support the diagnosis of acute pericarditis with a pericardial effusion, it is not considered the gold standard.[21]

Echocardiogram

Transthoracic echocardiogram is routinely performed in patients with suspected acute pericarditis, though frequently is normal. The echocardiogram serves multiple purposes, including assessing for the presence of pericardial effusion with potential for subsequent cardiac tamponade, and for any wall motion abnormalities that may be suggestive of ischemic chest pain as opposed to acute pericarditis.[22]

Magnetic Resonance Imaging

Cardiac magnetic resonance imaging is sometimes performed to assist with the diagnosis of acute pericarditis via detection of pericardial inflammation, especially when the diagnosis is suspected but the ECG and echocardiogram are unrevealing.[23] Intravenous gadolinium, which causes pericardial enhancement, is suggestive of inflammation. If there is concomitant myocardial inflammation (myopericarditis), this can often be visualized as well.

Invasive Testing

Pericardiocentesis, a procedure in which a needle is used to remove fluid from within the pericardial sac, is a diagnostic and potentially therapeutic procedure for patients with acute pericarditis and resultant pericardial effusion. Most patients with acute pericarditis do not require pericardiocentesis; however, it may be indicated for diagnostic purposes in those patients in whom an infectious or neoplastic etiology is of concern. It is also indicated for therapeutic purposes in those with pericardial effusions resulting in hemodynamic compromise (i.e., cardiac tamponade).[24] When fluid is aspirated from the pericardial space, the gross appearance of the fluid is evaluated to be sanguineous, serosanguineous, serous, or purulent. The fluid is then sent to the laboratory to obtain cell counts and white blood cell differential, though these are not generally helpful in differentiating a transudative from an exudative process in this setting. Cytology of the fluid should routinely be performed to assess for other cells within the fluid, including assessment for any possible malignant etiology.[6]

If tuberculosis is a consideration, acid-fast bacillus stain, mycobacterial culture, adenosine deaminase level, interferon-γ or lysozyme, and/or polymerase chain reaction testing for tuberculosis could be obtained.[25] Finally, routine Gram stain and culture of pericardial fluid is typically recommended to assess for any other potential infectious etiology. The pericardiocentesis procedure is not, however, without risk. Dysrhythmias, cardiac wall puncture, hemothorax, and pneumothorax are serious complications that may occur.[7]

Pericardial Biopsy

Pericardial biopsy is not performed as commonly as the other procedures and imaging discussed above, but may be indicated after prior pericardiocentesis when there is moderate or severe pericardial effusion with or without tamponade that has either not resolved after appropriate treatment, that has resolved and then recurred, or if there is suspicion of primary or secondary neoplastic disease that has gone undiagnosed. This is performed by cardiothoracic surgeons in a controlled operating room setting, often in the setting of concomitant therapeutic surgical pericardial drainage (a pericardial "window").

TREATMENT

Patients with acute pericarditis should be advised to avoid strenuous activity until their symptoms resolve, as strenuous physical activity can cause a recurrence of symptoms. Further treatment of acute pericarditis depends on the underlying cause.[26]

Viral, Traumatic, Connective Tissue Disorder-associated Causes, and Idiopathic Pericarditis

A majority of patients diagnosed will fall into the idiopathic or viral etiology. Medical treatment for these subtypes includes a combination of nonsteroidal anti-inflammatory drugs (NSAIDs) and colchicine. The COPE (COlchicine for Acute PEricarditis) trial demonstrated a decrease in the recurrence rate of pericarditis with the coadministration of colchicine in combination with conventional NSAID-based therapy, in patients diagnosed with idiopathic, viral, traumatic, or connective-tissue disorder-associated acute pericarditis.[27] This combination has become the *de facto* standard of care in patients able to tolerate both therapies. Typical doses of colchicine are 0.5–1.0 mg daily for 3 months. An NSAID, such as ibuprofen 600–800 mg 3 times per day, or indomethacin 50 mg three times per day, can be given for 2–3 weeks or until symptoms reside, and then tapered off. For patients in whom a secondary indication for aspirin use is present, such as AMI, high-dose aspirin therapy may be substituted for NSAID use (i.e., 650–1,000 mg three times per day). For patients with recurrence of disease, this same regimen is often employed with a longer duration of colchicine treatment for up to 6 months, with NSAIDs as well if symptomatic.[28] Steroids should be avoided, except when indicated for treatment of an underlying connective tissue disease, or when treatment with NSAIDs and colchicine has clearly failed (and an infectious etiology has been excluded), as they can increase the likelihood of recurrent pericarditis.[21]

Tubercular

In patients with acute pericarditis due to tuberculosis infection, the treatment plan is focused on antitubercular medications, specifically RIPE therapy (rifampin, isoniazid, pyrazinamide and ethambutol), in addition to symptomatic treatment with the use of NSAIDs.[29]

Other Infectious Etiology

Generally, treatment of the underlying infection along with anti-inflammatory drugs, such as NSAIDs and colchicine, are the mainstay of treatment.

Uremic

Uremic pericarditis in patients with chronic renal failure is treated via a combination of hemodialysis, aspirin, and colchicine.[27] Rarely, steroids can be useful in this subgroup as well.[30]

Cardiac Tamponade

This is addressed in a subsequent chapter, however if acute pericarditis is complicated by cardiac tamponade, emergent treatment with pericardiocentesis is indicated. This is a true medical emergency.

Indications for Hospitalization

Risk factors for poor prognosis in acute pericarditis have been identified as a fever more than 38°C (especially if accompanied by leukocytosis), subacute course, a large pericardial effusion and/or cardiac tamponade, and failure to respond to aspirin/NSAID therapy within 1 week.[11] Unlike acute coronary syndromes, elevated cardiac troponin (suggestive of myocardial involvement, or myopericarditis) may not be a negative prognostic marker.[14] For those patients presenting with predictors concerning for poor prognosis, it is reasonable to hospitalize and complete a thorough diagnostic or etiologic evaluation while initiating therapy.[13] For those patients who do not meet high-risk criteria, outpatient management is a reasonable choice, though close follow-up is required.[31]

PROGNOSIS

Morbidity and Mortality

Mortality associated with acute pericarditis is low at roughly 1%, and is independently associated with age and concurrent sepsis or co-infection.[32] Characteristic morbidity associated with acute pericarditis is caused by cardiac tamponade, transformation to a hemorrhagic process (often iatrogenic from anticoagulant medications), evolution of disease to pericardial constriction, and recurrence of the primary disease. Morbidity has been shown to be associated with a specific etiologic cause as opposed to an idiopathic or viral diagnosis. Approximately 1–2% of patients with a first episode of acute pericarditis will go on to develop pericardial constriction, though constriction occurs in less than 1% after idiopathic or viral pericarditis, compared to about 8% after a nonviral or nonidiopathic etiology and is especially common after purulent pericarditis (~33%).[33] Acute cardiac tamponade occurs in about 1% of patients with idiopathic or viral disease versus about 20% of those with a specific etiologic cause identified.[33,34]

Recurrence

Recurrence of disease is very common, and varies depending on the etiology of the disease, as well as with differing treatment regimens. Difficulties in precise etiologic diagnosis have limited the ability to precisely characterize the rate of recurrence by disease subtype. In the absence of colchicine therapy, overall rate of recurrence has been as high as 30% in patients with idiopathic acute pericarditis treated with aspirin or NSAIDs.[35] In contrast, combination treatment with colchicine and NSAIDs results in a recurrence rate of approximately 10%.[27] Those patients diagnosed with idiopathic or viral disease have a lower rate of recurrence (16.5%) than those diagnosed with a specific cause (27.6%).[11] In hospitalized patients, prior diagnosis of the disease is noted in 22% of patients, including 18.5% and 28.2% of men and women, respectively.[33] Some studies suggest that recurrence may reflect an autoimmune process,[36] as evidenced by elevation of inflammatory markers identified locally within the pericardial fluid yet absent systemically.[37] Further support is lent by the typical improvement seen with anti-inflammatory and immunosuppressant treatment. Colchicine in combination with aspirin or NSAIDs remains the standard therapy for recurrent pericarditis with data from multiple randomized, controlled trials demonstrating reduction in the frequency of recurrence and more rapid symptom alleviation compared to aspirin or NSAIDs alone.[21,35] Refractory cases may be treated with systemic glucocorticoids, advanced immunosuppressive therapies, and rarely pericardiectomy.

CONCLUSION

Acute pericarditis is a complex disease that can be triggered by many different inflammatory processes. The key to diagnosis involves careful history taking, astute physical examination skills, ECG and imaging interpretation, and the use of laboratory findings to assess for evidence of inflammation. Although the exact etiology may never be identified, sampling of the pericardial effusion, if present, may help in identifying the cause, and is of particular importance in cases where an infection or malignancy is suspected or possible. The treatment of acute pericarditis is rooted in identifying the etiology and treating the underlying condition, along with anti-inflammatory medications. For the most common cases of idiopathic and viral causes, NSAIDs for 2–3 weeks (or until symptoms abate) along with colchicine for 3 months has become the mainstay of treatment. Patients identified as high risk should be hospitalized for initial stages of treatment to allow for close monitoring and assessment of response to treatment. Mortality from acute pericarditis remains low, however, if pericarditis is associated with a large or growing effusion and subsequent tamponade, emergent management and fluid drainage is indicated.

REFERENCES

1. Spodick DH. The Pericardium: A Comprehensive Textbook. New York, NY, USA: Marcel Dekker; 1997.
2. Braunwald E. Pericardial disease. In: Longo DL, Fauci AS, Kasper DL, Hauser SL, Jameson JL, Loscalzo J, editors. Harrison's Principles of Internal Medicine, 19th edition. New York, NY, USA: The McGraw-Hill Education; 2015. pp. 1571-7.
3. Lange RA, Hillis LD. Clinical practice. Acute pericarditis. N Engl J Med. 2004;351(21):2195-202.
4. Troughton RW, Asher CR, Klein AL. Pericarditis. Lancet. 2004;363(9410): 717-27.
5. Campbell PT, Li JS, Wall TC, O'Connor CM, Van Trigt P, Kenney RT, et al. Cytomegalovirus pericarditis: a case series and review of the literature. Am J Med Sci. 1995;309(4):229-34.
6. Maisch B, Ristic A, Pankuweit S. Evaluation and management of pericardial effusion in patients with neoplastic disease. Prog Cardiovasc Dis. 2010;53(2): 157-63.
7. Cho BC, Kang SM, Kim DH, Ko YG, Choi D, Ha JW, et al. Clinical and echocardiographic characteristics of pericardial effusion in patients who underwent echocardiographically guided pericardiocentesis: Yonsei Cardiovascular Center experience, 1993-2003. Yonsei Med J. 2004;45(3):462-8.

8. Rubin RH, Moellering RC. Clinical, microbiologic and therapeutic aspects of purulent pericarditis. Am J Med. 1975;59(1):68-78.
9. Maisch B, Ristic AD. Practical aspects of the management of pericardial disease. Heart. 2003;89(9):1096-103.
10. Atar S, Chiu J, Forrester JS, Siegel RJ. Bloody pericardial effusion in patients with cardiac tamponade: is the cause cancerous, tuberculous, or iatrogenic in the 1990s? Chest. 1999;116(6):1564-9.
11. Imazio M, Cecchi E, Demichelis B, Ierna S, Demarie D, Ghisio A, et al. Indicators of poor prognosis of acute pericarditis. Circulation. 2007;115(21):2739-44.
12. Zayas R, Anguita M, Torres F, Gimenez D, Bergillos F, Ruiz M, et al. Incidence of specific etiology and role of methods for specific etiologic diagnosis of primary acute pericarditis. Am J Cardiol. 1995;75(5):378-82.
13. Imazio M, Brucato A, Ferrazzi P, Rovere ME, Gandino A, Cemin R, et al. Colchicine reduces postoperative atrial fibrillation: results of the Colchicine for the Prevention of the Postpericardiotomy Syndrome (COPPS) atrial fibrillation substudy. Circulation. 2011;124(21):2290-5.
14. Imazio M, Brucato A, Barbieri A, Ferroni F, Maestroni S, Ligabue G, et al. Good prognosis for pericarditis with and without myocardial involvement: results from a multicenter, prospective cohort study. Circulation. 2013;128(1):42-9.
15. Agabegi SS, Agabegi ED, Ring AC. Step-up to Medicine, 4th edition. Philadelphia, PA, USA: Wolters Kluwer Health; 2012.
16. Spodick DH. Pericardial rub. Prospective, Multiple observer investigation of pericardial friction in 100 patients. Am J Cardiol. 1975;35(3):357-62.
17. Curtiss EI, Reddy PS, Uretsky BF, Cecchetti AA. Pulsus paradoxus: definition and relation to the severity of cardiac tamponade. Am Heart J. 1988;115(2):391-8.
18. Guberman BA, Fowler NO, Engel PJ, Gueron M, Allen JM. Cardiac tamponade in medical patients. Circulation. 1981;64(3):633-40.
19. Kabadi UM, Kumar SP. Pericardial effusion in primary hypothyroidism. Am Heart J. 1990;120(6 Pt 1):1393-5.
20. Gunukula SR, Spodick DH. Pericardial disease in renal patients. Semin Nephrol. 2001;21(1):52-6.
21. Imazio M, Bobbio M, Cecchi E, Demarie D, Pomari F, Moratti M, et al. Colchicine as first-choice therapy for recurrent pericarditis: results of the CORE (COlchicine for REcurrent pericarditis) trial. Arch Intern Med. 2005;165(17):1987-91.
22. Klein AL, Abbara S, Agler DA, Appleton CP, Asher CR, Hoit B, et al. American Society of Echocardiography clinical recommendations for multimodality cardiovascular imaging of patients with pericardial disease: endorsed by the Society for Cardiovascular Magnetic Resonance and Society of Cardiovascular Computed Tomography. J Am Soc Echocardiogr. 2013;26(9):965-1012.
23. Rajiah P. Cardiac MRI: Part 2, pericardial diseases. AJR Am J Roentgenol. 2011;197(4):W621-34.
24. Mercé J, Sagristà-Sauleda J, Permanyer-Miralda G, Soler-Soler J. Should pericardial drainage be performed routinely in patients who have a large pericardial effusion without tamponade? Am J Med. 1998;105(2):106-9.
25. Fowler NO. Tuberculous pericarditis. JAMA. 1991;266(1):99-103.
26. Imazio M, Gaita F. Diagnosis and treatment of pericarditis. Heart. 2015;101(14):1159-68.
27. Imazio M, Bobbio M, Cecchi E, Demarie D, Demichelis B, Pomari F, et al. Colchicine in addition to conventional therapy for acute pericarditis: results of the COlchicine for acute PEricarditis (COPE) trial. Circulation. 2005;112(13):2012-6.
28. Imazio M, Gaita F, LeWinter M. Evaluation and Treatment of Pericarditis: A Systematic Review. JAMA. 2015;314(14):1498-506.
29. Cohn DL, Catlin BJ, Peterson KL, Judson FN, Sbarbaro JA. A 62-dose, 6-month therapy for pulmonary and extrapulmonary tuberculosis. A twice-weekly, directly observed, and cost-effective regimen. Ann Intern Med. 1990;112(6):407-15.
30. Iyoda M, Ajiro Y, Sato K, Kuroki A, Shibata T, Kitazawa K, et al. A case of refractory uremic pleuropericarditis--successful corticosteroid treatment. Clin Nephrol. 2006;65(4):290-3.
31. Imazio M, Demichelis B, Parrini I, Giuggia M, Cecchi E, Gaschino G, et al. Day-hospital treatment of acute pericarditis: a management program for outpatient therapy. J Am Coll Cardiol. 2004;43(6):1042-6.
32. Kyto V, Sipila J, Rautava P. Clinical profile and influences on outcomes in patients hospitalized for acute pericarditis. Circulation. 2014;130(18):1601-6.
33. Imazio M, Brucato A, Maestroni S, Cumetti D, Belli R, Trinchero R, et al. Risk of constrictive pericarditis after acute pericarditis. Circulation. 2011;124(11):1270-5.
34. Adler Y, Charron P, Imazio M, Badano L, Baron-Esquivias G, Bogaert J, et al. 2015 ESC Guidelines for the diagnosis and management of pericardial diseases: The Task Force for the Diagnosis and Management of Pericardial Diseases of the European Society of Cardiology (ESC) Endorsed by: The European Association for Cardio-Thoracic Surgery (EACTS). Eur Heart J. 2015;36(42):2921-64.
35. Imazio M, Brucato A, Cemin R, Ferrua S, Belli R, Maestroni S, et al. Colchicine for recurrent pericarditis (CORP): a randomized trial. Ann Intern Med. 2011;155(7):409-14.
36. Brucato A, Brambilla G, Moreo A, Alberti A, Munforti C, Ghirardello A, et al. Long-term outcomes in difficult-to-treat patients with recurrent pericarditis. Am J Cardiol. 2006;98(2):267-71.
37. Pankuweit S, Wadlich A, Meyer E, Portig I, Hufnagel G, Maisch B. Cytokine activation in pericardial fluids in different forms of pericarditis. Herz. 2000;25(8):748-54.

24 CHAPTER

Cardiac Tamponade

Nicholas W Wettersten, Denise D Barnard

INTRODUCTION

Cardiac tamponade is a life-threatening cardiovascular emergency, which requires prompt diagnosis and treatment to avert death. The state can develop rapidly or insidiously. Clinicians should retain a high degree of clinical suspicion for tamponade in patients with shock or refractory hypotension and tachycardia. The pathophysiology stems from external compression of the heart by pericardial fluid restricting filling and, therefore, preload, stroke volume, and cardiac output. Removal of the fluid results in a prompt reversal of physiology and can dramatically improve a patient's condition. This chapter covers the pathophysiology, keys to diagnosis, and treatment of cardiac tamponade.

PATHOPHYSIOLOGY

Pericardial Anatomy and Physiology

The pericardium envelops the heart and consists of two layers, the visceral and parietal pericardium.[1] The visceral pericardium is a monolayer of cells adherent to the heart and extending to the great vessels before reflecting upon itself as the parietal pericardium. The parietal pericardium is a thin fibrous relatively inelastic tissue consisting mainly of collagen and elastin. The monolayer of cells of the visceral pericardium and reflected layer on the parietal pericardium is called the serosa, while the fibrous portion of the parietal pericardium is called the fibrosa.

The pericardium is highly innervated primarily by the phrenic nerve with partial innervation from the vagus nerve.[1] The anterior and posterior parietal pericardium contain lymphatics.[2] Damage to these lymphatics, such as by inflammation, may contribute to the accumulation of fluid and development of tamponade.[3]

Though unnecessary for normal cardiac function, as congenital absence or surgical removal of the pericardium leads to no detriment in cardiac function, its presence does influence normal cardiac physiology.[1,3] The pericardium helps to maintain the position of the heart in the chest by adhering to the great vessels, sternum, anterior mediastinum, and diaphragm.[2] It serves as a protective barrier for the heart from extracardiac inflammation and infection.[2] The intrapericardial fluid reduces the friction of heart movement.[2] The pericardium's most important physiologic function, with implications in tamponade, is its biomechanical interaction with the heart.

Under normal conditions, the pericardium and surrounding tissues variably restrict cardiac dimensions, dilation, and output.[2,4-6] This pressure-volume relationship between the heart and pericardium follows a J-shaped curve (Fig. 1). At low cardiac volumes, the pericardium is relatively compliant and the heart can fill with minimal pericardial restriction.[7] However, after a certain volume, the pericardium quickly becomes noncompliant and can no longer distend without significant increases in pressure. At this upper limit, further cardiac filling is severely restricted. This function protects the heart from

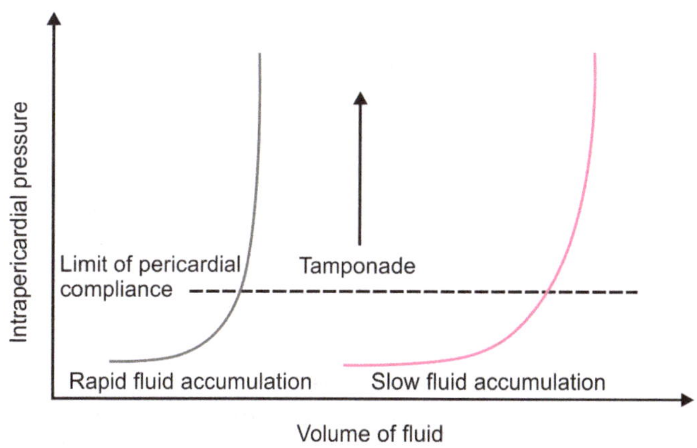

FIG. 1: The J-shaped pressure-volume relationship between the heart and pericardium with increasing intrapericardial fluid. The left curve represents the effects of rapid fluid accumulation. When fluid accumulates faster than the pericardium can stretch and comply, the limit of pericardial compliance is reached quickly and intrapericardial pressure changes rapidly with small changes in fluid. With slow fluid accumulation, the pericardium can comply and stretch to accommodate a much greater volume until limits of compliance are finally met and tamponade develops as represented with the curve on the right

acute increases in loading conditions with acute cardiac dilatation.[7,8]

The volume the pericardium can distend before becoming noncompliant and restrictive to cardiac filling, is called the pericardial reserve volume. A normal pericardium contains less than 50 mL of fluid and can only tolerate 100–200 mL.[9] The pericardium can adapt and distend over time from either chronic cardiac dilatation or a gradually expanding pericardial effusion.[9-12] This shifts the pressure-volume J curve to the right and liters of fluid can fill the pericardial space or intracardiac cavity before the pericardium restricts further filling (Fig. 1). This has implications for the acuity in which a pericardial effusion develops tamponade.

The pressure-volume relationship can be directly measured as the transmural filling pressure, the difference between the intracardiac pressure and the intrapericardial pressure. At the flat portion of the J curve, the intracardiac pressure is positive from venous return. Because the pericardium lies within the thoracic cavity, the intrapericardial pressure reflects intrathoracic pressure and is either zero or negative. Combined, the intracardiac and intrapericardial pressures create a positive pressure gradient for filling the right-sided cardiac chambers. As the heart fills and approaches the reserve volume, the intrapericardial pressure becomes increasingly positive and the transmural filling pressure approaches zero, restricting further cardiac filling. This transmural filling pressure is not uniform around the heart and has regional variation.[13] A key factor affecting the transmural filling pressure is respiration.

The cardiac chambers, pericardial space, pericardium and pulmonary veins lie within the thoracic cavity and are subject to the effects of the respiratory cycle on intrathoracic pressure. The superior vena cava (SVC) and inferior vena cava (IVC) are only partially in the thoracic cavity and are less subject to the changes in intrathoracic pressure. This latter point is key to why intrathoracic pressure significantly affects right-sided filling but not left-sided. With inspiration, intrathoracic pressure decreases, thereby decreasing intrapericardial and intracardiac pressures while venous return remains positive and not significantly changed by the negative intrathoracic pressure. Overall, this leads to a larger transmural filling pressure and augmented filling of the right-sided cardiac chambers. For the left-sided cardiac chambers, the decrease in intrathoracic pressure equally decreases pressure in the pulmonary veins and left-sided chambers, therefore, leading to no change in the filling gradient.[14] In sum, inspiration augments filling of the right-sided chambers with no change in left-sided filling. Expiration has the reverse effect with decreased filling of right-sided chambers but again no change in left-sided filling. This respiratory variation in conjunction with ventricular interdependence explains pulsus paradoxus.

As cardiac filling reaches the pericardial reserve volume, the pericardium exerts ventricular interdependence and diastolic interaction.[2] At the steep portion of the J-curve, the pericardium transmits the intracavitary filling pressures between ventricles through shifting of the interventricular septum. The bowing of the septum into the opposite ventricle affects the loading conditions and diastolic pressure of the opposing ventricle. With inspiration increasing right-sided filling compared to the left, the interventricular septum is displaced into the left ventricle. This increases left ventricular diastolic pressure, reducing preload and, therefore, reducing stroke volume and cardiac output. The end result is a lower systolic blood pressure during inspiration. With expiration, systolic blood pressure rises as the right ventricular filling gradient decreases and the interventricular septum does not bow into the left ventricle. This normal respiratory variation in systolic blood pressure, the normal pulsus paradoxus, is less than 10 mm Hg.

Pathophysiology of Tamponade

Cardiac tamponade occurs over a continuum of hemodynamic changes.[12] When a pericardial effusion forms, it reduces the pericardial reserve volume and shifts the starting point of the pressure-volume relationship further up the J curve. Subsequently the amount of blood, and therefore preload, that can enter the heart before the pericardium restricts filling is diminished. A pericardial effusion increases intrapericardial pressure thereby decreasing the transmural filling pressure. Since the pericardium can accommodate large volumes if developing over a prolonged time course, the progression to tamponade is highly variable.

To counterbalance a decreasing transmural filling pressure, neurohormonal activation results in multiple compensatory mechanisms. Venous constriction increases venous return, thereby increasing intracavitary pressure and the transmural filling pressure. Because of decreasing preload, stroke volume is maintained by decreasing end-systolic volume and increasing contractility. As stroke volume falls further, heart rate must increase to maintain cardiac output. Eventually, the pericardial reserve volume and transmural filling pressure approach zero and the noncompliant portion of the pressure-volume relationship is reached, compensatory mechanisms are overcome and severe tamponade ensues with circulatory collapse and imminent death without relief.

This progression occurs over a spectrum from mild to severe tamponade based on the difference between intrapericardial pressure and intracardiac pressure with predominant effects on the right ventricle.[9,12,15] In mild tamponade, intrapericardial pressure is less than both right atrial and wedge pressure. With moderate tamponade, intrapericardial pressure is greater than right atrial pressure but still less than wedge. Severe tamponade is the classical description of significant elevation and equalization of intracardiac pressures (right atrial and wedge), often greater than 10 mm Hg above baseline, with equalization to intrapericardial pressure.[9]

This last state occurs with a normal myocardium; however, a diseased myocardium can have severe tamponade without equalization of pressures. With chronic left ventricular systolic dysfunction, left ventricular end-diastolic pressure will remain elevated and not equalize though severe tamponade is present.[16] Conversely, with right ventricular hypertrophy and elevated right heart pressures, severe tamponade can be present without the intrapericardial pressure equaling right ventricular diastolic pressure and no apparent hemodynamic effect on the right ventricle.[17,18] Therefore, caution should be exercised to prematurely discount tamponade if hemodynamic or echocardiographic parameters do not appear conclusive.[9]

As a state of severe tamponade is approached, respiratory variation in cardiac filling, ventricular interdependence, and diastolic interaction become more prominent.[2] This leads to an exaggerated pulsus paradoxus. As explained above, it is normal to have a respiratory variation in systolic blood pressure with inspiration resulting in a drop of less than 10 mm Hg because of increased right ventricular filling and bowing of the interventricular septum into the left ventricle. However in tamponade, the increased venous return cannot expand the right ventricular free wall against a noncompliant pericardium and effusion. As a result, the interventricular septum is displaced further into the left ventricle decreasing left ventricular preload and subsequently blood pressure. This results in a greater than 10 mm Hg respiratory variation in peak systolic blood pressure and an abnormal pulsus paradoxus.

ETIOLOGY

Large population-based studies on the etiologies of pericardial effusions and tamponade are lacking.[19] The causes of pericarditis are often the causes of effusions and tamponade (Table 1). Current data comes from case series often in which investigators performed extensive evaluations to determine the etiology.[20-24] Etiologies for pericardial effusions include idiopathic, neoplastic, infectious, iatrogenic, autoimmune/collagen vascular diseases, heart failure, hypothyroidism, uremia, trauma, radiation induced, postmyocardial infarction, and post-operative, mainly cardiac surgery and heart transplant.

Infectious causes can be from any type of organism including viral, bacterial, fungal, mycobacterial and protozoal. With extensive testing, Levy et al. were able to determine many unique infections causing effusions,

TABLE 1: The percentages that different etiologies were found to cause pericardial effusions, with and without tamponade, from case series.[20-24] For each case series, the total number of cases evaluated and the percentage that an etiology was found to cause the effusion is reported. Cases presenting as moderate-to-large effusions without tamponade are presented separately from those presenting with cardiac tamponade

Case series	Pericardial effusions			Pericardial tamponade		
	Corey et al.	Sagrista-Sauleda et al.	Levy et al.	Sagrista-Sauleda et al.	Ben-Horin	Kabukcu
Number of cases	57	203	204	119	169	50
Etiology						
Idiopathic	7	30	37	29	26	20
Neoplasm	23	8	15	22	34	30
Infectious	27	2	22	8	4	14
Autoimmune/CVD	12	7	14	0	4	12
Uremia	12	7	2	3	6	22
Heart failure	–	8	–	0	0.5	–
Hypothyroidism	–	–	10	–	–	–
Iatrogenic	–	14	–	18	–	–
Radiation induced	14	–	–	–	2	–
Postinfarction	–	8	–	8	–	–
Postpericardiotomy	–	–	–	–	5	–
Trauma	–	–	–	–	12	–
Other	9	14	–	12	7	–

CVD, collagen vascular disease.

such as *Bartonella, Coxiella burnetii, Mycoplasma pneumoniae*, and *Toxoplasma*.[22] Tuberculosis is now a rare cause of a pericardial effusion; however, it used to be considered a common cause of a bloody effusion. In a series of 64 patients with bloody effusions, only one patient had tuberculosis while the most common causes were iatrogenic (31%), malignancy (26%), coronary artery disease (11%), or idiopathic (10%).[25] In general, though infectious etiologies other than viral are uncommon.

With the rise of advanced invasive cardiac procedures, iatrogenic effusions and tamponade have risen. Any cardiac procedure has a risk of causing an effusion and tamponade; however, those considered higher risk are listed in box 1.[26] With percutaneous coronary interventions, one institution found an event rate of 0.12%.[27] Cases were twice as common in patients treated with atheroablative devices. Despite the low event rate, mortality was high at 42%.

Pericardial effusions following cardiac surgery are common, but infrequently cause significant cardiac tamponade. In a series of 122 patients, 103 (84%) had effusions postoperatively with 66 (64%) completely resolving by 50 days postoperatively.[28] A separate series found an incidence of 64% in 780 patients.[29] Most of these effusions were small-to-moderate in size. Large effusions with tamponade are uncommon occurring in 1–2% of postcardiac surgery patients.[29,30] Effusions are more common after coronary artery bypass grafting, but tamponade more frequently occurs after valve surgery.[29,30] Anticoagulation was found to increase the risk of tamponade.[30]

Table 1 displays the etiologies, which caused either a moderate-to-large effusion with tamponade or without tamponade in different case series. There are notable differences in the prevalence that an etiology causes an effusion versus tamponade. Effusions are most often idiopathic, but are not the leading cause of tamponade. Infections are also common causes of effusion, but unlikely causes of tamponade. Effusions from malignancies are infrequent but are the leading cause of tamponade. Tamponade of unknown etiology can often later be attributed to an undiagnosed malignancy.[24] Iatrogenic effusions commonly lead to tamponade. Taking these differences into consideration is important when assessing a patient's risk for tamponade. Given the frequency with which malignancies cause tamponade, it should be in the differential for unexplained dyspnea or tachycardia in a cancer patient.

BOX 1 **Percutaneous cardiac procedures associated with an increased risk of iatrogenic cardiac tamponade[26]**

- Coronary intervention
- Valve repair and replacement
- Mitral valvuloplasty
- Patent foramen ovale closure
- Transseptal puncture
- Atrial fibrillation ablation
- Pacemaker implantation
- Left atrial appendage closure

Often, the clinical scenario directs the clinician to the cause of an effusion and tamponade (postcardiac procedure, pericarditis symptoms, metastatic cancer).[23] When the cause is not clear, there may be some helpful clinical indicators for cause. One study found patients with inflammatory signs were more likely to have acute idiopathic pericarditis, those with large effusions without inflammatory signs or tamponade were likely to have chronic idiopathic pericarditis, and those with tamponade but no inflammatory signs to have malignancy.[21] A later study confirmed that patients presenting with tamponade more often had malignancy; however, it did not confirm the association with inflammatory signs.[24] Extensive testing for infectious etiologies may be indicated given the large variety of infections found to cause effusions.[20,22] Testing should take into consideration local infectious risk factors and patient population risk factors.[22]

When an effusion is drained for tamponade or performed electively for diagnosis, fluid qualities and testing may be helpful. Bloody effusions are more likely malignant and cytology may confirm or diagnose malignancy.[24] Light's criteria are used to differentiate transudative and exudative pleural effusions, and are often applied to pericardial fluid. However, a study of pericardial fluid found the normal composition to contain a lactate dehydrogenase (LDH) 2.4 times the serum level, a pericardial to serum protein content ratio of 0.6, and a predominance of lymphocytes suggesting that Light's criteria cannot be applied to pericardial fluid with any accuracy.[31] Malignant effusions have been found to have higher levels of tumor markers, hemoglobin, white blood cells, and LDH compared to nonmalignant effusions; however, the tumor marker CA 72-4 in a bloody effusion had a high diagnostic accuracy for distinguishing a malignant effusion from a benign effusion.[32] Potential novel markers for diagnosis are osteoprotegerin and TNF-related apoptosis-inducing ligand with high ratios of pericardial to serum levels for both suggestive of a malignant effusion.[33] Lastly, pericardial biopsy is sometimes helpful with diagnosis. When performed, pericardioscopy with extensive biopsying (18–20 samples) has been shown to have the highest yield.[34]

DIAGNOSIS

Tamponade can be categorized as "surgical" or "medical". Surgical tamponade classically is the result of a catastrophic event with hemorrhage into the pericardium that requires immediate surgical intervention (type A aortic dissection, coronary perforation in catheterization laboratory). Medical tamponade is a slower process likely stemming from inflammation. These two present differently and develop over different time courses with surgical tamponade developing hemodynamic compromise in minutes-to-hours and medical tamponade developing over days-to-weeks.[35]

Symptoms and Signs

The presenting symptoms and signs of tamponade are varied and nonspecific. Patients may complain of dyspnea, orthopnea, fullness, chest tightness, abdominal pain, dysphagia, or nausea.[19,35] In addition, if the provoking condition is an infection or malignancy, the patient's primary symptoms may be fever, weakness, lethargy, cough, or nonspecific pain. Alternatively, patients may present with end-organ complications of tamponade, such as renal failure, ascites or mesenteric ischemia.[35] In a review of the literature, dyspnea had the highest sensitivity at 87–88%.[19] Chest pain, cough, lethargy, fever, and palpitations were present in 25% or less of patients.[19] Overall, history is highly limited.

As with history, the majority of physical examination findings are nonspecific. Patients often have tachycardia and tachypnea.[19] Heart sounds may be muffled and a pericardial friction rub may be appreciated.[19,35,36] Jugular venous pressure (JVP) is often elevated with a preserved *x* descent but a lost or diminished *y* descent.[19,37] Though hypotension and cardiovascular collapse is the terminal end-point of untreated tamponade, 27–43% of patients presenting with subacute tamponade are hypertensive.[38,39] Hypertension is believed to be from profound sympathetic activation and often resolves with drainage of the effusion.[38] Hypertension should be cautiously treated, if at all, in patients with tamponade. The classical finding of Beck's triad with hypotension, elevated JVP, and distant heart sounds was described in surgical tamponade and is not a common finding of medical tamponade.[19]

One key physical examination finding for diagnosis is pulsus paradoxus. Pulsus paradoxus is a normal physiologic event where systolic blood pressure decreases with inspiration because of the respiratory variation of intrathoracic pressure and ventricular interdependence. As ventricular interdependence is exaggerated in tamponade, so is pulsus paradoxus. It is assessed while the patient is performing normal respirations, not exaggerated inspiratory or expiratory effort. A sphygmomanometer is inflated above the systolic blood pressure and slowly deflated while listening for when the first Korotkoff sound is heard intermittently with respiratory variation. The cuff is deflated further until the first Korotkoff sound is heard continuously. The difference between the pressure, when the first Korotkoff sound is heard intermittently and when it is heard continuously, is the pulsus paradoxus.[19]

BOX 2 Causes other than cardiac tamponade for an exaggerated pulsus paradoxus

- Severe obstructive pulmomary disease
- Congestive heart failure
- Mitral stenosis
- Massive pulmonary embolus
- Severe hypovolemic shock
- Obesity
- Tense ascites
- Right ventricular infarction
- Constrictive pericarditis
- Restrictive cardiomyopathy
- Pneumothorax

A normal pulsus paradoxus has a pressure difference of less than 10 mm Hg. A pressure difference greater than 10 mm Hg is considered abnormal and in the right context concerning for tamponade. In one study assessing pulsus paradoxus, a difference of greater than 10 mm Hg had a positive likelihood ratio of 3.3 and negative likelihood ratio of 0.03, while a difference greater than 12 mm Hg had a positive likelihood ratio of 5.9 and negative likelihood ratio of 0.03.[19,40] These findings highlight that a normal pulsus paradoxus strongly suggests a patient does not have tamponade while a pulsus paradoxus greater than 10 mm Hg increases the likelihood of tamponade, a likelihood that increases as the difference in pressures increases. It is important to recognize though that many other conditions can cause an exaggerated pulsus paradoxus (Box 2).[19,41] Also, left ventricular dysfunction may result in an absent pulsus paradoxus.[16]

Electrocardiography and Chest Radiography

Electrocardiographic findings include low voltage, electrical alternans, atrial arrhythmias, bundle branch blocks, ST segment elevation, and PR depression.[19,35] Electrical alternans is the beat-to-beat variation in the amplitude of the P, QRS, or ST-T-waves from the heart moving in the effusion (Fig. 2). Electrocardiographic findings lack sensitivity for tamponade, yet some findings are specific.[19] Low voltage has been found to be specific for a pericardial effusion and tamponade.[42,43] In addition, PR segment depression and electrical alternans were specific in one study, though only PR segment depression was associated with tamponade.[43]

Chest radiography may be normal or show an enlarged globular heart or "water bottle" heart (Fig. 3).[19,35] On lateral X-ray, an epicardial fat stripe, "double lucency" sign or "epicardial halo" sign may be seen. Cardiomegaly on chest radiography is a sensitive sign, but not specific.[19]

Echocardiography

One of the most important diagnostic modalities for assessing the hemodynamic significance of a pericardial effusion and the presence of cardiac tamponade is echocardiography. Echocardiographic findings and diagnostic criteria for tamponade are listed in box 3.[35,44,45] Right

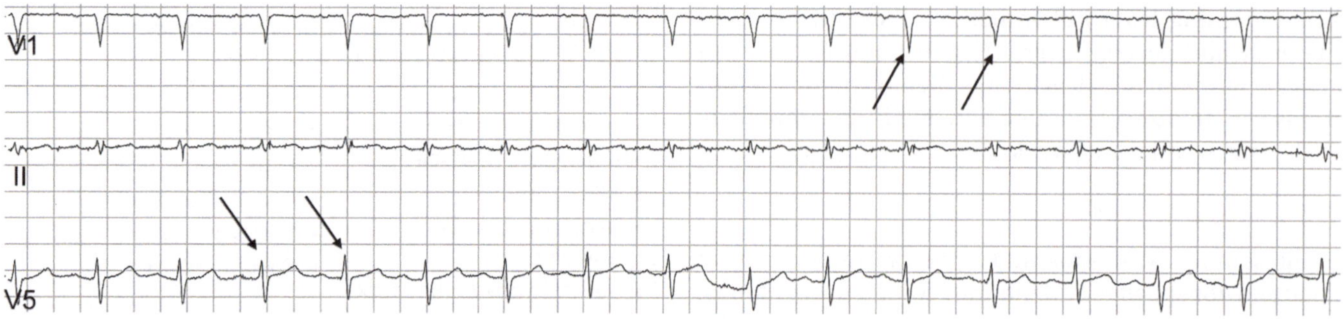

FIG. 2: Electrical alternans. Note the beat-to-beat change in S wave height in V1 and R wave height in V5 (highlighted with arrows)

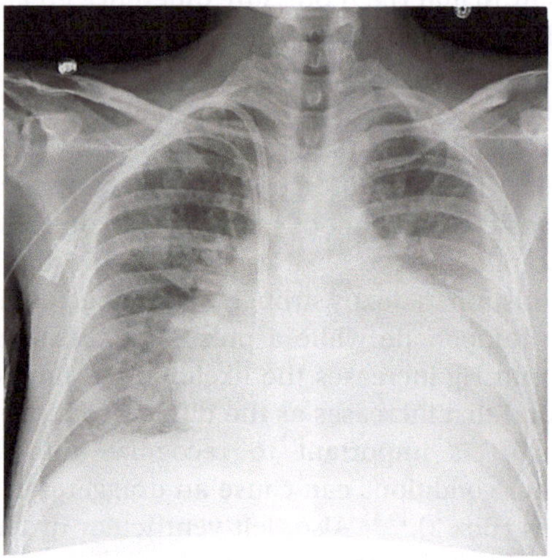

FIG. 3: Example of a water bottle heart. The enlarged cardiac silhouette almost fills the thorax. This patient had a large pericardial effusion with tamponade believed to be from uremia (note tunneled dialysis catheter). Cardiac silhouettes can be even more dramatic filling the entire thorax

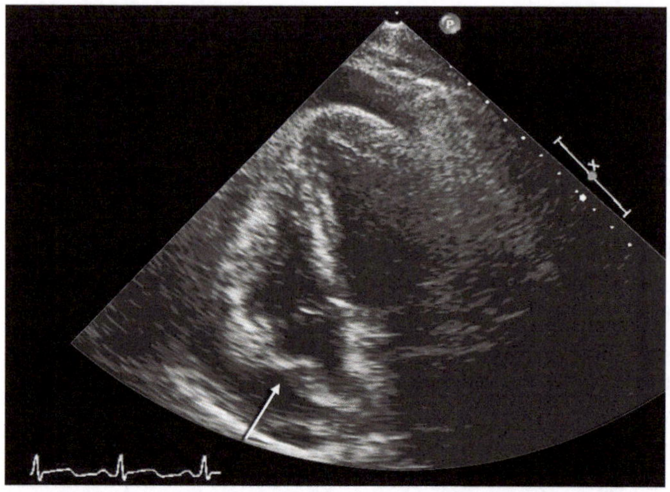

FIG. 4: Right atrial collapse on an echocardiogram from the apical four chamber view. A large effusion is seen and the right atrium is buckling inward as highlighted by white arrow

BOX 3 Potential echocardiographic findings suggestive of cardiac tamponade (see text for discussion of sensitivities and specificities)

- Right atrial collapse >1/3 of cardiac cycle
- Late diastolic collapse of right atrium
- Left atrial collapse
- Early right ventricular diastolic collapse
- Respiratory variation in right ventricular and left ventricular chamber size (septal shifting)
- Respiratory variation in right ventricular and left ventricular filling >25%
- Plethoric inferior vena cava without inspiratory collapse
- Respiratory variation in hepatic vein flow

atrial collapse is an early finding for a hemodynamically significant effusion, but does not necessarily indicate tamponade is present (Fig. 4). Reported sensitivity and specificity for this finding range from 60 to 100%.[46,47] This variability likely results from different criteria used to define right atrial collapse. The longer the right atrium is inverted during a cardiac cycle, the more sensitive and specific this finding is for tamponade. With a criterion that inversion persists for at least one-third the cardiac cycle, sensitivity is 94% and specificity is 100%.[48]

Right ventricular diastolic collapse is slightly less sensitive but more specific than right atrial collapse with reported sensitivity of 60–90% and specificity of 80–100% (Fig. 5).[46,47] The lower sensitivity and higher specificity stems from the higher intracardiac pressures of the right ventricle compared to the right atrium; therefore, the pressure in the intrapericardial space is often greater and more hemodynamically significant to cause right ventricular diastolic collapse.[17,18,49] The sensitivity and specificity for any chamber collapse are 90% and 65%, respectively.[47] The presence of simultaneous chamber collapse is 45% sensitive and 92% specific.[47]

A large respiratory variation in mitral and tricuspid inflow can be indicative of tamponade.[50] With inspiration, the right-sided filling gradient is augmented while the left-sided filling gradient is unchanged resulting in increased right ventricular filling, decreased left ventricular filling and bowing of interventricular septum into the left

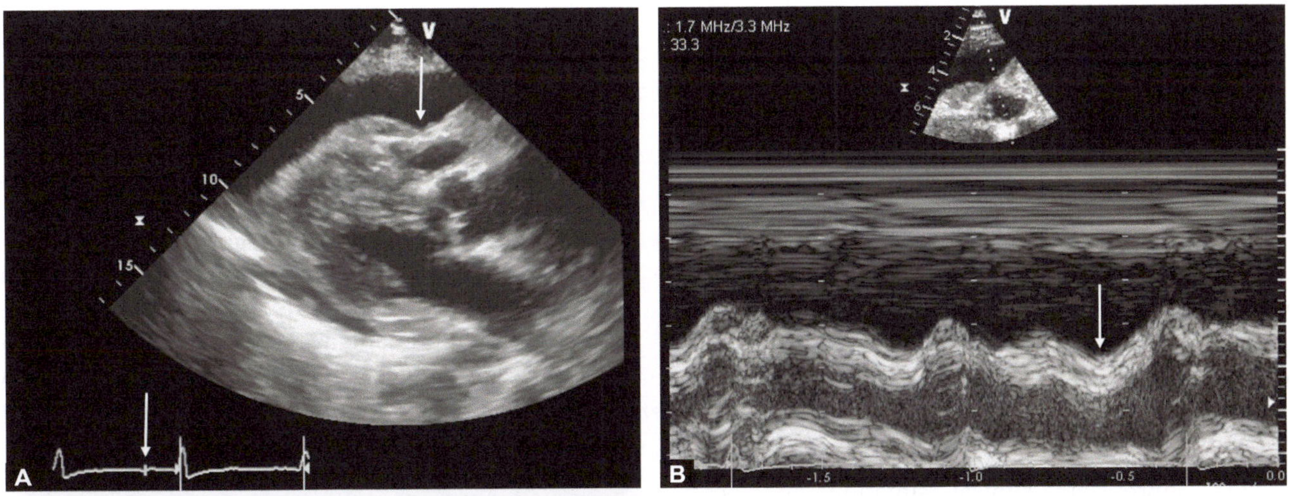

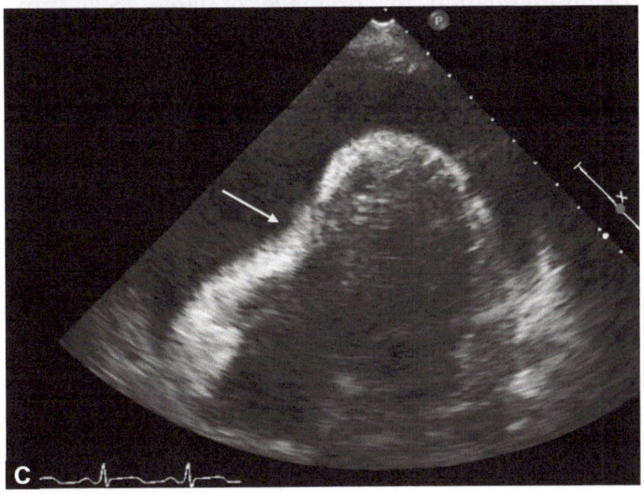

FIG. 5: **A,** Right ventricular diastolic collapse on echocardiogram from the parasternal long view. The white arrows demonstrate the right ventricle collapsing inward with the electrocardiography lead highlighting diastole; **B,** This is better appreciated on M-mode where the right ventricular free wall is seen moving into the right ventricle during diastole (white arrow); **C,** Right ventricular diastolic collapse from the apical four chamber view, collapse highlighted by white arrow

ventricle (see the pathophysiology section for further details). As a result, tricuspid inflow is accentuated with inspiration and attenuated with expiration. The reverse is found for mitral inflow with inflow attenuated with inspiration but accentuated with expiration. A respiratory variation of 25% or more in transvalvular flow is strongly suggestive of tamponade (Fig. 6).[44] The difference in respiratory variation increases as the hemodynamic influence of an effusion increases.[14]

An analogous respiratory variation can be seen in the hepatic veins and the SVC. Findings suggestive of tamponade include a marked predominance of the systolic component over the diastolic component, expiratory accentuation of this variance and expiratory inversion of the diastolic component.[47] These findings have a sensitivity of 75% and specificity of 91%.[47]

A dilated IVC with minimal inspiratory collapse (plethoric) is a very sensitive marker (97%) for tamponade, but not specific (40%).[51] Uncommon echocardiographic findings include left atrial collapse and left ventricular collapse.[46] These usually arise in unique situations or following cardiac surgery.[52]

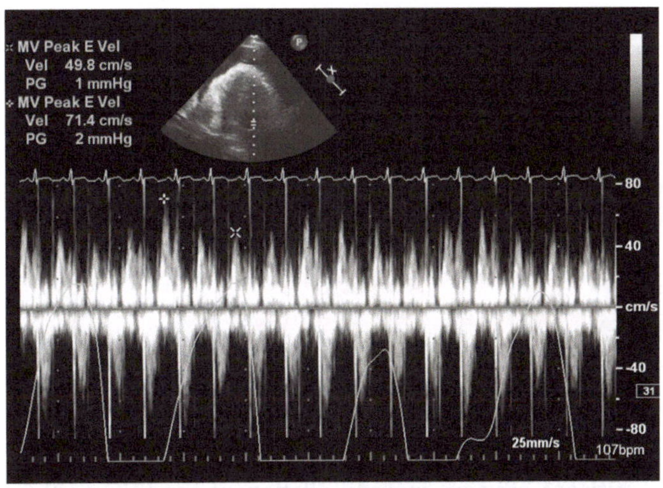

FIG. 6: Respiratory variation in mitral inflow in tamponade with pulse-wave Doppler. At end expiration, mitral inflow is greatest measured at 71.4 cm/s and at end inspiration, it is the smallest measured at 49.8 cm/s. The difference is 21.6 cm/s for over a 30% variation consistent with tamponade

Echocardiographic findings of tamponade must be placed in clinical context and the presence or absence of these findings alone should not determine the treatment course. In one study, 34% of patients with effusions but not tamponade showed collapse of one or more chambers.[47] Alternatively, echocardiographic findings can be absent in numerous conditions. Specifically patients with right ventricular hypertrophy or chronic right ventricular volume overload can lack any echocardiographic findings and develop tamponade.[37,41,46] Echocardiographic findings have been shown repeatedly to be unreliable with right ventricular overload.[17,18] Concomitant left ventricular dysfunction may also present with tamponade with small effusions and variable clinical findings.

Right Heart Catheterization

With the appropriate clinical situation and echocardiographic findings, right heart catheterization is unnecessary for the diagnosis of tamponade, but its findings can be definitive for tamponade. Tamponade occurs along a hemodynamic spectrum, which can be appreciated during right heart catheterization.[17] As an effusion grows and intrapericardial pressure increases, the hemodynamic influence is translated onto the heart. Early hemodynamic influence is appreciated first on echocardiography as right atrial collapse. On right heart catheterization, this correlates with an increase in right atrial pressure with loss of the *y* descent and a more pronounced *a* wave. Further hemodynamic progression leads to right ventricular diastolic collapse on echocardiography. At this point, right heart catheterization shows elevation and equalization of the mean right atrial pressure, right ventricular diastolic pressure, pulmonary diastolic pressure, and wedge pressure with these pressures equaling the intrapericardial pressure. In addition, as tamponade progresses over this hemodynamic spectrum, heart rate increases while stroke volume and cardiac output drop. With removal of the effusion, the hemodynamic and echocardiographic findings revert to normal in a reverse pattern in which they developed.[17]

Computed Tomography and Magnetic Resonance Imaging

Cardiac computed tomography (CT) and cardiac magnetic resonance imaging (MRI) are rarely indicated for the diagnosis of a pericardial effusion or tamponade. Cardiac CT findings suggestive of a hemodynamically significant effusion include dilation of the SVC or IVC, flattening of interventricular septum or compression of the coronary sinus.[53] Cardiac CT or MRI may be helpful for evaluation of a posterior loculated effusion, though transesophageal echocardiogram can often adequately visualize the posterior pericardium. Cardiac CT or MRI may be helpful in better defining the nature of an effusion or a potential mass in the pericardium.

TREATMENT

As tamponade occurs along a spectrum and no single noninvasive test definitively diagnoses tamponade, the management of a large pericardial effusion is not always clear. In a series of 71 patients with large effusions without tamponade, 26 underwent pericardiocentesis.[54] Pericardiocentesis only had a diagnostic yield of 7% and, at a median follow-up of 10 months, 61 of the effusions had resolved and no patients developed tamponade.[54] In a series of 28 patients with large chronic (>3 months duration) idiopathic pericardial effusions, 8 patients (29%) developed tamponade unexpectedly while pericardiocentesis led to resolution of the effusion in 8 of 19 patients (42%).[55] This latter series has led to the recommendation for drainage of large (>20 mm on echocardiography) asymptomatic pericardial effusions, though this should likely only be performed if the effusion persists over 3 months.[35]

Acute Medical Management

The role of medical therapy in the management of cardiac tamponade is limited. Often rapid intravenous fluids are given to increase the transmural pressure in favor of right ventricular filling; however, a fluid responsiveness is only seen in approximately 50% of patients.[56] A study in dogs showed volume resuscitation only improved conditions when the dogs were hypovolemic with minimal impact when the subjects were normovolemic or hypervolemic.[57] This benefit was only seen when the right atrial pressure was less than 12 mm Hg.[57] A small trial in human subjects with tamponade showed a systolic blood pressure less than 100 mm Hg predictive of a favorable response to fluids.[56] Excessive volume resuscitation may also be detrimental as it has been reported to induce tamponade.[58]

Vasodilator therapy with nitroprusside in conjunction with volume resuscitation had previously been advocated based on animal studies.[59] However, in a small cohort study with human subjects in tamponade, no benefit was seen from nitroprusside or volume resuscitation.[60] In addition, vasopressor and inodilator therapy has shown no benefit.[61] Definitive management of tamponade requires procedural drainage of the effusion.

Procedural Drainage

Definitive management of tamponade requires drainage of the effusion. This is most often performed percutaneously with pericardiocentesis; however, surgical drainage is sometimes indicated. Surgical drainage is advocated for acute traumatic hemopericardium, purulent pericarditis, and loculated effusions not safely amenable to percutaneous drainage.[35] Potential surgical procedures include subxiphoid pericardiotomy, pleuropericardial window, peritoneal-pericardial window, partial pericardiectomy, or wide anterior pericardiectomy. The choice of surgical procedure will depend on the clinical status of the patient, the nature of effusion and local practice patterns. Surgical drainage is associated with a high 30-day mortality of 19.4% with malignant effusions and 5.5% with benign effusions in one series.[62]

Given the mortality associated with surgical drainage, pericardiocentesis is the preferred method for drainage. Pericardiocentesis should rarely be performed "blind" but done with fluoroscopic or preferably echocardiographic guidance. It is often performed in the cardiac catheterization laboratory. Traditionally, pericardial effusions were accessed from a subcostal location using landmark guidance. However, with the use of echocardiography, the interventionalist can find the largest portion of the pericardial effusion closest to the skin for safest access.[63] In the largest reported series of echocardiographic-guided pericardiocentesis involving 1,127 pericardiocenteses, the success rate was 97% with a complication rate of only 4.7% (1.2% major and 3.5% minor).[64] In this series, the para-apical site was the most common site of access (63%) followed by subcostal then other nontraditional sites including left axillary, left parasternal, right parasternal, and posterolateral.[64]

Pericardiocentesis Procedure

The optimal site to access a pericardial effusion will vary based on echocardiographic findings and procedural technique may change based on access site. If echocardiography is not used, the procedure is often performed in the cardiac catheterization laboratory with fluoroscopy used for guidance. However, if a patient is in a critical condition, where the acuity does not allow for imaging, a subcostal/paraxiphoid landmark-based approach is preferred and will be described initially.[37] Subsequently, the modifications and variations for echocardiographic and fluoroscopically guided pericardiocentesis will be discussed. Of note, for any pericardiocentesis, the use of electrocardiographic guidance is no longer advised.[35,37]

Pericardiocentesis was considered an absolute contraindication with type A aortic dissection.[35] However, a case series showed that controlled pericardial drainage in hemodynamically compromised patients prior to the operating room was safe and effective.[65] Relative contraindications include uncorrected coagulopathy, anticoagulation, thrombocytopenia with platelets of less than 50,000, and a small posterior loculated effusion.[35] Major complications of the procedure include death, laceration and/or perforation of the myocardium, laceration of a coronary, pericardial or internal mammary arteries, injury to abdominal viscera, pneumothorax, ventricular tachycardia, air embolism, and potential for infection.[35,64] Minor complications include vasovagal bradycardia, nonsustained supraventricular tachycardia, and pleuropericardial fistula.[64]

For the subcostal/paraxiphoid approach, the patient is positioned supine.[35,37] A long 16-gauge or 18-gauge needle, often with a polytetrafluoroethylene sheath, is inserted at a 15–30° angle to the skin between the xiphoid process and left costal margin. The needle is advanced to bypass the costal margin and toward the left shoulder. This path should remain outside of the pleural space and avoid coronary, pericardial and internal mammary arteries. As the needle is advanced, negative pressure is applied to aspirate for fluid or if the needle has a stylet, this is intermittently removed to assess for flow. Once access is obtained, if the needle has a sheath it is advanced into the space and the needle withdrawn; otherwise, the needle is left in place.

At this time, the operator may choose to remove all of the pericardial effusion (using the sheath) and withdraw from the pericardial space; however, prolonged pericardial drainage significantly reduces the risk of recurrence of the effusion and is highly recommended.[66,67] In addition, no more than 1 L of fluid removal is advised to prevent acute right ventricular dilation.[68] For prolonged drainage, a soft J-tipped guidewire is introduced, the sheath removed, dilation is performed, and then a multiholed pigtail catheter is placed. Alternatively, a 5–8 French sheath is introduced and the multiholed pigtail catheter is introduced through the sheath.[63] One advantage of the latter method is if the pigtail catheter clogs and cannot be cleared, it is relatively simple to replace the catheter through the sheath.

The catheter should be left in place until drainage falls to less than 25 mL a day.[35] While the catheter is in place, fluid should be aspirated/drained intermittently every 4–6 hours. Between aspirations, saline or heparinized saline (approximately 100 units per mL) should be left to dwell in the drain to prevent blockage.[63] Alternatively, the drain may be connected to a drainage bag and left to gravity. In this situation, flushing should occur more frequently (every 2–4 h) to prevent clogging of the drain. While the drain is in place, serial echocardiograms should be performed to ensure adequate drainage.

With fluoroscopic guidance, the subcostal/paraxiphoid approach is the preferred access site, though a tangential approach using the epicardial halo sign has been described.[35] Fluoroscopy allows visualization of the appropriate positioning of the needle and guidewire. Before dilating and placing the drain, a few milliliters of contrast solution can be injected after access is obtained and should layer inferiorly indicating appropriate positioning.[35]

With echocardiographic guidance, a thorough examination should be performed to find the ideal access site avoiding major organs.[63] Once the optimal site is obtained, the angle of the echocardiogram's transducer should be noted for angulation of the needle. As the site will vary based on echocardiographic findings, the patient may be positioned supine or in a modified left lateral decubitus position. To confirm appropriate needle position with echocardiography, the needle may be directly visualized in the pericardial space. Once access is obtained, agitated bacteriostatic saline can be injected into the pericardial space and visualized with echocardiography with an appearance similar to a bubble study.

OUTCOMES

Whether a pericardial effusion fully resolves or recurs depends on the nature of the effusion.[69] Viral and idiopathic effusions tend to have good outcomes without recurrence. Purulent effusions depend on the nature of the infection, response to treatment, and initial drainage therapy. Malignant effusions have poor outcomes in general and increased likelihood of recurrence. Factors found to predict recurrence of an effusion and tamponade include lack of extended drainage, incomplete drainage, loculated effusion, and malignancy.[66]

Should a pericardial effusion recur, a second drainage may be attempted or a more permanent drainage procedure performed.[55] This can be done with a surgical pericardial window or percutaneous balloon pericardiotomy. The latter has been found to be safe and effective especially in patients with malignant effusions who may have a poor functional status.[70,71] Complications include fever, pneumothorax, left pleural effusion, and bleeding.[69] In addition, double-balloon pericardiotomy has also been used and the timing of balloon pericardiotomy does not affect outcome.[72] Should these percutaneous approaches fail, surgical management may be indicated.

SPECIAL CASES

Postcardiac Procedures

With the rise of cardiac procedures, both percutaneous and surgical, iatrogenic tamponade has risen and in fact became the most common reason for pericardiocentesis in one series.[64] As discussed earlier (etiology section), multiple different percutaneous procedures can lead to effusions and tamponade at a low incidence but high mortality.[26,27] Pericardial effusions occur in approximately two-thirds of patients postcardiac surgery, but only 1–2% develops tamponade with anticoagulation therapy increasing risk of tamponade.[28-30] Signs and symptoms are nonspecific and include malaise, dyspnea, chest pain, tachycardia, fever, elevated jugular venous distension, and hypotension, all of which could be expected findings in a postoperative setting.[73] Pulsus paradoxus was found in only 17% of patients.[73] Classic echocardiographic findings are less reliable but can still be seen.[29,73,74] Additionally, effusions are more often to be loculated and potentially causing localized compression and transesophageal echocardiography may be necessary for evaluation.[52,73] Pericardiocentesis has a high success rate treating tamponade both postsurgery (97%) and percutaneous procedures (99%).[73,75]

Low-pressure Tamponade

Low-pressure tamponade is an under-recognized form of tamponade where low intrapericardial pressures result in tamponade physiology because of low cardiac filling pressures.[76] Patients with low-pressure are less likely to have clinical signs of tamponade, but do demonstrate common symptoms and echocardiographic findings of tamponade. Right heart catheterization is the key in diagnosis and shows similar findings to classic tamponade with equalization of intrapericardial pressure and right atrial pressure, but at lower intracardiac pressures than classic tamponade. Pericardiocentesis in these patients improves cardiac output and clinical status.[76] A patient presenting with symptoms and echocardiographic findings of tamponade, but without clinical signs should prompt the provider to consider low-pressure tamponade.

Effusive-constrictive Pericarditis

Effusive-constrictive pericarditis is a hemodynamic state in which the visceral pericardium exerts constrictive physiology on the heart and a pericardial effusion exerts hemodynamic influence but not necessarily tamponade.[77,78] It is an uncommon condition but the exact incidence is unknown.[79] Etiologies are similar to causes of pericarditis and pericardial effusions, though tuberculosis causes a higher incidence of effusive-constrictive disease.[79] It may be suspected prior to pericardiocentesis based on echocardiographic findings consistent with constriction; however, these findings are insensitive.[77,79] Definitive diagnosis is made with right heart catheterization during pericardiocentesis. With drainage of the effusion, intrapericardial pressure will drop, but right atrial pressure will remain elevated and there is a classic constrictive dip-plateau of diastolic filling. Most patients improve clinically with pericardiocentesis because the hemodynamic influences of the effusion are removed; however, patients deteriorate later from the constrictive physiology.[79] As constrictive physiology can occasionally spontaneously resolve, a trial of medical therapy with anti-inflammatory medications or steroids and observation is recommended.[77,79] However, if constriction does not resolve or the patient deteriorates then definitive therapy with surgical pericardiectomy is necessary but carries a high mortality.[79]

CONCLUSION

Cardiac tamponade is a life-threatening condition that requires prompt diagnosis and treatment. Symptoms and signs are nonspecific except for pulsus paradoxus. Echocardiography is the most important diagnostic tool; however, it does have limitations and positive or negative findings do not definitively rule-in or rule-out tamponade. Medical therapy has a limited role in management and definitive management is with drainage of the effusion, most often by echocardiographic-guided pericardiocentesis. It is critical to remember that tamponade occurs along a hemodynamic spectrum and therapy is instituted early prior to patient deterioration.

REFERENCES

1. Spodick DH. Macrophysiology, microphysiology, and anatomy of the pericardium: a synopsis. Am Heart J. 1992;124(4):1046-51.
2. Shabetai R. The pericardium: an essay on some recent developments. Am J Cardiol. 1978;42(6):1036-43.
3. Spodick DH. The normal and diseased pericardium: current concepts of pericardial physiology, diagnosis and treatment. J Am Coll Cardiol. 1983;1(1): 240-51.
4. Hammond HK, White FC, Bhargava V, Shabetai R. Heart size and maximal cardiac output are limited by the pericardium. Am J Physiol. 1992;263(6 Pt 2):H1675-81.
5. Freeman GL, Little WC. Comparison of in situ and in vitro studies of pericardial pressure-volume relation in dogs. Am J Physiol. 1986;251(2 Pt 2):H421-7.
6. Freeman GL, LeWinter MM. Determinants of intrapericardial pressure in dogs. J App Physiol. 1986;60(3):758-64.
7. Applegate RJ, Johnston WE, Vinten-Johansen J, Klopfenstein HS, Little WC. Restraining effect of intact pericardium during acute volume loading. Am J Physiol. 1992;262(6 Pt 2):H1725-33.
8. Spodick DH. Threshold of pericardial constraint: the pericardial reserve volume and auxiliary pericardial functions. J Am Coll Cardiol. 1985;6(2): 296-7.
9. Shabetai R. Pericardial effusion: haemodynamic spectrum. Heart. 2004;90(3): 255-6.
10. Freeman GL, LeWinter MM. Pericardial adaptations during chronic cardiac dilation in dogs. Circ Res. 1984;54(3):294-300.
11. Reddy PS, Curtiss EI, O'Toole JD, Shaver JA. Cardiac tamponade: hemodynamic observations in man. Circulation. 1978;58(2):265-72.
12. Reddy PS, Curtiss EI, Uretsky BF. Spectrum of hemodynamic changes in cardiac tamponade. Am J Cardiol. 1990;66(20):1487-91.
13. Hoit BD, Lew WY, LeWinter M. Regional variation in pericardial contact pressure in the canine ventricle. Am J Physiol. 1988;255(6 Pt 2):H1370-7.
14. Gonzalez MS, Basnight MA, Appleton CP. Experimental pericardial effusion: relation of abnormal respiratory variation in mitral flow velocity to hemodynamics and diastolic right heart collapse. J Am Coll Cardiol. 1991;17(1):239-48.
15. Ditchey R, Engler R, LeWinter M, Pavelec R, Bhargava V, Covell J, et al. The role of the right heart in acute cardiac tamponade in dogs. Circ Res. 1981;48(5):701-10.
16. Hoit BD, Gabel M, Fowler NO. Cardiac tamponade in left ventricular dysfunction. Circulation. 1990;82(4):1370-6.
17. Singh S, Wann LS, Schuchard GH, Klopfenstein HS, Leimgruber PP, Keelan MH, Jr, et al. Right ventricular and right atrial collapse in patients with cardiac tamponade--a combined echocardiographic and hemodynamic study. Circulation. 1984;70(6):966-71.
18. Leimgruber PP, Klopfenstein HS, Wann LS, Brooks HL. The hemodynamic derangement associated with right ventricular diastolic collapse in cardiac tamponade: an experimental echocardiographic study. Circulation. 1983;68(3): 612-20.
19. Roy CL, Minor MA, Brookhart MA, Choudhry NK. Does this patient with a pericardial effusion have cardiac tamponade? JAMA. 2007;297(16):1810-8.
20. Corey GR, Campbell PT, Van Trigt P, Kenney RT, O'Connor CM, Sheikh KH, et al. Etiology of large pericardial effusions. Am J Med. 1993;95(2):209-13.
21. Sagrista-Sauleda J, Merce J, Permanyer-Miralda G, Soler-Soler J. Clinical clues to the causes of large pericardial effusions. Am J Med. 2000;109(2): 95-101.
22. Levy PY, Corey R, Berger P, Habib G, Bonnet JL, Levy S, et al. Etiologic diagnosis of 204 pericardial effusions. Medicine. 2003;82(6):385-91.
23. Kabukcu M, Demircioglu F, Yanik E, Basarici I, Ersel F. Pericardial tamponade and large pericardial effusions: causal factors and efficacy of percutaneous catheter drainage in 50 patients. Tex Heart Inst J. 2004;31(4):398-403.
24. Ben-Horin S, Bank I, Guetta V, Livneh A. Large symptomatic pericardial effusion as the presentation of unrecognized cancer: a study in 173 consecutive patients undergoing pericardiocentesis. Medicine. 2006;85(1):49-53.
25. Atar S, Chiu J, Forrester JS, Siegel RJ. Bloody pericardial effusion in patients with cardiac tamponade: is the cause cancerous, tuberculous, or iatrogenic in the 1990s? Chest. 1999;116(6):1564-9.
26. Holmes DR Jr, Nishimura R, Fountain R, Turi ZG. Iatrogenic pericardial effusion and tamponade in the percutaneous intracardiac intervention era. JACC Cardiovasc Interv. 2009;2(8):705-17.
27. Fejka M, Dixon SR, Safian RD, O'Neill WW, Grines CL, Finta B, et al. Diagnosis, management, and clinical outcome of cardiac tamponade complicating percutaneous coronary intervention. Am J Cardiol. 2002;90(11):1183-6.
28. Weitzman LB, Tinker WP, Kronzon I, Cohen ML, Glassman E, Spencer FC. The incidence and natural history of pericardial effusion after cardiac surgery—an echocardiographic study. Circulation. 1984;69(3):506-11.
29. Pepi M, Muratori M, Barbier P, Doria E, Arena V, Berti M, et al. Pericardial effusion after cardiac surgery: incidence, site, size, and haemodynamic consequences. Br Heart J. 1994;72(4):327-31.
30. Kuvin JT, Harati NA, Pandian NG, Bojar RM, Khabbaz KR. Postoperative cardiac tamponade in the modern surgical era. Ann Thorac Surg. 2002;74(4):1148-53.
31. Ben-Horin S, Shinfeld A, Kachel E, Chetrit A, Livneh A. The composition of normal pericardial fluid and its implications for diagnosing pericardial effusions. Am J Med. 2005;118(6):636-40.
32. Karatolios K, Pankuweit S, Maisch B. Diagnostic value of biochemical biomarkers in malignant and non-malignant pericardial effusion. Heart Fail Rev. 2013;18(3):337-44.
33. Karatolios K, Pankuweit S, Goettsch C, Hofbauer LC, Timmesfeld N, Al-Fakhri N, et al. Osteoprotegerin (OPG) and TNF-related apoptosis-inducing ligand (TRAIL) levels in malignant and benign pericardial effusions. Clin Biochem. 2012;45(3):237-42.
34. Seferovic PM, Ristic AD, Maksimovic R, Tatic V, Ostojic M, Kanjuh V. Diagnostic value of pericardial biopsy: improvement with extensive sampling enabled by pericardioscopy. Circulation. 2003;107(7):978-83.
35. Maisch B, Seferovic PM, Ristic AD, Erbel R, Rienmuller R, Adler Y, et al. Guidelines on the diagnosis and management of pericardial diseases executive summary; The Task force on the diagnosis and management of pericardial diseases of the European society of cardiology. Eur Heart J. 2004;25(7):587-610.
36. Spodick DH. Pericardial rub. Prospective, Multiple observer investigation of pericardial friction in 100 patients. Am J Cardiol. 1975;35(3):357-62.
37. Spodick DH. Acute cardiac tamponade. N Engl J Med. 2003;349(7):684-90.
38. Argulian E, Herzog E, Halpern DG, Messerli FH. Paradoxical hypertension with cardiac tamponade. Am J Cardiol. 2012;110(7):1066-9.
39. Brown AL, Brown J Jr, Stephens MR. Elevated blood pressure among Harlem residents. Nurse Pract. 1982;7(3):26-9, 33-5, 58.
40. Curtiss EI, Reddy PS, Uretsky BF, Cecchetti AA. Pulsus paradoxus: definition and relation to the severity of cardiac tamponade. Am Heart J. 1988;115(2):391-8.
41. Argulian E, Messerli F. Misconceptions and facts about pericardial effusion and tamponade. Am J Med. 2013;126(10):858-61.
42. Bruch C, Schmermund A, Dagres N, Bartel T, Caspari G, Sack S, et al. Changes in QRS voltage in cardiac tamponade and pericardial effusion: reversibility after pericardiocentesis and after anti-inflammatory drug treatment. J Am Coll Cardiol. 2001;38(1):219-26.
43. Eisenberg MJ, de Romeral LM, Heidenreich PA, Schiller NB, Evans GT Jr. The diagnosis of pericardial effusion and cardiac tamponade by 12-lead ECG. A technology assessment. Chest. 1996;110(2):318-24.
44. Otto CM. (2013). Textbook of clinical echocardiography. [online] Available from http://proxy.lib.umich.edu/login?url=https://www.clinicalkey.com/dura/browse/bookChapter/3-s2.0-C20110057484. [Accessed July, 2016].
45. Oh JK, Seward JB, Tajik AJ. The Echo Manual. 3rd ed. Philadelphia: Lippincott Williams & Wilkins; 2006. p. 431.
46. Reydel B, Spodick DH. Frequency and significance of chamber collapses during cardiac tamponade. Am Heart J. 1990;119(5):1160-3.

47. Merce J, Sagrista-Sauleda J, Permanyer-Miralda G, Evangelista A, Soler-Soler J. Correlation between clinical and Doppler echocardiographic findings in patients with moderate and large pericardial effusion: implications for the diagnosis of cardiac tamponade. Am Heart J. 1999;138(4 Pt 1):759-64.
48. Gillam LD, Guyer DE, Gibson TC, King ME, Marshall JE, Weyman AE. Hydrodynamic compression of the right atrium: a new echocardiographic sign of cardiac tamponade. Circulation. 1983;68(2):294-301.
49. Klopfenstein HS, Schuchard GH, Wann LS, Palmer TE, Hartz AJ, Gross CM, et al. The relative merits of pulsus paradoxus and right ventricular diastolic collapse in the early detection of cardiac tamponade: an experimental echocardiographic study. Circulation. 1985;71(4):829-33.
50. Appleton CP, Hatle LK, Popp RL. Cardiac tamponade and pericardial effusion: respiratory variation in transvalvular flow velocities studied by Doppler echocardiography. J Am Coll Cardiol. 1988;11(5):1020-30.
51. Himelman RB, Kircher B, Rockey DC, Schiller NB. Inferior vena cava plethora with blunted respiratory response: a sensitive echocardiographic sign of cardiac tamponade. J Am Coll Cardiol. 1988;12(6):1470-7.
52. Fusman B, Schwinger ME, Charney R, Ausubel K, Cohen MV. Isolated collapse of left-sided heart chambers in cardiac tamponade: demonstration by two-dimensional echocardiography. Am Heart J. 1991;121(2 Pt 1):613-6.
53. Restrepo CS, Lemos DF, Lemos JA, Velasquez E, Diethelm L, Ovella TA, et al. Imaging findings in cardiac tamponade with emphasis on CT. Radiographics. 2007;27(6):1595-610.
54. Merce J, Sagrista-Sauleda J, Permanyer-Miralda G, Soler-Soler J. Should pericardial drainage be performed routinely in patients who have a large pericardial effusion without tamponade? Am J Med. 1998;105(2):106-9.
55. Sagrista-Sauleda J, Angel J, Permanyer-Miralda G, Soler-Soler J. Long-term follow-up of idiopathic chronic pericardial effusion. N Engl J Med. 1999; 341(27):2054-9.
56. Sagrista-Sauleda J, Angel J, Sambola A, Permanyer-Miralda G. Hemodynamic effects of volume expansion in patients with cardiac tamponade. Circulation. 2008;117(12):1545-9.
57. Grose R, Greenberg MA, Yipintsoi T, Cohen MV. Cardiac tamponade in dogs with normal coronary arteries. I. Effect of changing intravascular volume on hemodynamics and myocardial blood flow. Basic Res Cardiol. 1984;79(5):531-41.
58. Hashim R, Frankel H, Tandon M, Rabinovici R. Fluid resuscitation-induced cardiac tamponade. J Trauma. 2002;53(6):1183-4.
59. Gascho JA, Martins JB, Marcus ML, Kerber RE. Effects of volume expansion and vasodilators in acute pericardial tamponade. Am J Physiol. 1981;240(1):H49-53.
60. Kerber RE, Gascho JA, Litchfield R, Wolfson P, Ott D, Pandian NG. Hemodynamic effects of volume expansion and nitroprusside compared with pericardiocentesis in patients with acute cardiac tamponade. N Engl J Med. 1982;307(15):929-31.
61. Martins JB, Manuel WJ, Marcus ML, Kerber RE. Comparative effects of catecholamines in cardiac tamponade: experimental and clinical studies.Am J Cardiol. 1980;46(1):59-66.
62. Piehler JM, Pluth JR, Schaff HV, Danielson GK, Orszulak TA, Puga FJ. Surgical management of effusive pericardial disease. Influence of extent of pericardial resection on clinical course. J Thorac Cardiovasc Surg. 1985;90(4):506-16.
63. Callahan JA, Seward JB. Pericardiocentesis guided by two-dimensional echocardiography. Echocardiography. 1997;14(5):497-504.
64. Tsang TS, Enriquez-Sarano M, Freeman WK, Barnes ME, Sinak LJ, Gersh BJ, et al. Consecutive 1127 therapeutic echocardiographically guided pericardiocenteses: clinical profile, practice patterns, and outcomes spanning 21 years. Mayo Clin Proc. 2002;77(5):429-36.
65. Hayashi T, Tsukube T, Yamashita T, Haraguchi T, Matsukawa R, Kozawa S, et al. Impact of controlled pericardial drainage on critical cardiac tamponade with acute type A aortic dissection. Circulation. 2012;126(11 Suppl 1):S97-S101.
66. Rafique AM, Patel N, Biner S, Eshaghian S, Mendoza F, Cercek B, et al. Frequency of recurrence of pericardial tamponade in patients with extended versus nonextended pericardial catheter drainage. Am J Cardiol. 2011; 108(12):1820-5.
67. Tsang TS, Barnes ME, Gersh BJ, Bailey KR, Seward JB. Outcomes of clinically significant idiopathic pericardial effusion requiring intervention. Am J Cardiol. 2003;91(6):704-7.
68. Armstrong WF, Feigenbaum H, Dillon JC. Acute right ventricular dilation and echocardiographic volume overload following pericardiocentesis for relief of cardiac tamponade. Am Heart J. 1984;107(6):1266-70.
69. Sagrista-Sauleda J, Merce AS, Soler-Soler J. Diagnosis and management of pericardial effusion. World J Cardiol. 2011;3(5):135-43.
70. Ziskind AA, Pearce AC, Lemmon CC, Burstein S, Gimple LW, Herrmann HC, et al. Percutaneous balloon pericardiotomy for the treatment of cardiac tamponade and large pericardial effusions: description of technique and report of the first 50 cases. J Am Coll Cardiol. 1993;21(1):1-5.
71. Swanson N, Mirza I, Wijesinghe N, Devlin G. Primary percutaneous balloon pericardiotomy for malignant pericardial effusion. Catheter Cardiovasc Interv. 2008;71(4):504-7.
72. Wang HJ, Hsu KL, Chiang FT, Tseng CD, Tseng YZ, Liau CS. Technical and prognostic outcomes of double-balloon pericardiotomy for large malignancy-related pericardial effusions. Chest. 2002;122(3):893-9.
73. Tsang TS, Barnes ME, Hayes SN, Freeman WK, Dearani JA, Butler SL, et al. Clinical and echocardiographic characteristics of significant pericardial effusions following cardiothoracic surgery and outcomes of echo-guided pericardiocentesis for management: Mayo Clinic experience, 1979-1998. Chest. 1999;116(2):322-31.
74. Bommer WJ, Follette D, Pollock M, Arena F, Bognar M, Berkoff H. Tamponade in patients undergoing cardiac surgery: a clinical-echocardiographic diagnosis. Am Heart J. 1995;130(6):1216-23.
75. Tsang TS, Freeman WK, Barnes ME, Reeder GS, Packer DL, Seward JB. Rescue echocardiographically guided pericardiocentesis for cardiac perforation complicating catheter-based procedures. The Mayo Clinic experience. J Am Coll Cardiol. 1998;32(5):1345-50.
76. Sagrista-Sauleda J, Angel J, Sambola A, Alguersuari J, Permanyer-Miralda G, Soler-Soler J. Low-pressure cardiac tamponade: clinical and hemodynamic profile. Circulation. 2006;114(9):945-52.
77. Sagrista-Sauleda J, Angel J, Sanchez A, Permanyer-Miralda G, Soler-Soler J. Effusive-constrictive pericarditis. N Engl J Med. 2004;350(5):469-75.
78. Hancock EW. Subacute effusive-constrictive pericarditis. Circulation. 1971; 43(2):183-92.
79. Syed FF, Ntsekhe M, Mayosi BM, Oh JK. Effusive-constrictive pericarditis. Heart Fail Rev. 2013;18(3):277-87.

25 CHAPTER

Hypertensive Emergencies

Phillip D Levy, Aaron M Brody

INTRODUCTION

Hypertension is the most common cardiovascular condition encountered in clinical practice. It affects 31% of Americans and approximately 1 billion people worldwide.[1,2] Hypertension is the also the primary risk factor for severe cardiovascular disease, such as stroke, myocardial infarction, heart failure, and kidney failure. The risk of developing these complications increases with the degree of blood pressure (BP) elevation, doubling for each rise of 20 mm Hg systolic blood pressure (SBP), and 10 mm Hg diastolic blood pressure (DBP) above 115/75 mm Hg.[3] Conversely, effective BP control can lower the risk for myocardial infarction, stroke, and heart failure by 25%, 40%, and 50%, respectively.[4]

Hypertension is primarily a chronic disease, and its symptoms tend to be nonspecific and mild. However, up to 1 in 100 patients with hypertension will sustain a true life-threatening hypertensive emergency during the course of their disease, [5] which warrants immediate treatment. While from an epidemiological perspective, hypertensive emergencies remain relatively rare, accounting for between 0.5 and 1.1% of hospital admissions,[6,7] marked BP elevation (defined as SBP >180 mm Hg) complicates up to 13% of all hospital admissions.[8] Hospital mortality rates for patients with hypertensive emergencies range from 3 to 10% in various studies,[9,10] and are associated directly with the degree of SBP elevation (from 6.9 to 19.7% for 180–189 mm Hg and >220 mm Hg, respectively).[8]

An essential element of treating hypertensive emergencies is distinguishing these episodes from marked yet asymptomatic BP elevations. Even at profound levels, the BP itself, in absence of acute end-organ damage, does not pose a risk for immediate morbidity or mortality, and does not require urgent reduction. In fact, treating has not been shown to improve outcomes or to decrease repeat emergency department (ED) visits.[11] The American College of Emergency Physicians specifically advocates against this practice in published clinical policies.[12,13] These patients require prompt referral to primary care, and, for select patients, initiation or titration of long-term antihypertensive therapy at discharge from the ED.[13,14] Conversely, when end-organ damage is identified, prompt reduction of BP can significantly reduce severe adverse outcomes.

The prompt reduction of BP in hypertensive emergencies, typically utilizing parenteral agents is recommended in order to reduce morbidity and mortality. This practice is based on clinical experience and evidence from observational studies[15-18] despite a lack of clear-cut clinical trial evidence showing a mortality benefit.[19,20] Even for specific disease processes, such as acute stroke or heart failure, in which higher level evidence is available, there is often no definitive evidence-based consensus regarding the single best agent or even BP target, leading to confusion among clinicians and heterogeneity in practice.[10] Perhaps, most important to remember is that treatment should be tailored to the specific diagnosis, and that each manifestation of a hypertensive emergency has different BP targets with differing goals for rate of reduction and agents of choice. This said, several principles of management are relevant across the range of hypertensive emergencies:

- Proactive diagnostic measures should be taken to identify end-organ damage when history or physical examination suggests it may be present
- Treatment should be initiated and monitored in accordance with the organ system involved, rather than focusing on the BP value in isolation
- Blood pressure should be closely monitored for the duration of therapy, in order to assess effectiveness of treatment, and to identify clinically significant hypotension
- Treatment does not end in hospital, and all patients require close primary care follow-up after discharge to ensure long-term BP control.

DEFINITION

Hypertensive emergency is defined as acute BP elevation, accompanied by life-threatening end-organ damage. Although there is no consensus regarding a BP threshold, typically, such damage does not occur with BPs lower than 180/110 mm Hg, and this value is often used as a cutoff in epidemiological studies.[9] Historically, terms such as "hypertensive crisis", "hypertensive urgency", and "accelerated" or "malignant" hypertension have been used to describe such patients. Unfortunately, these terms are ill defined, and often used interchangeably. A more consistent and evidence-based approach focuses on the presence (or absence) of signs or symptoms attributable to acute end-organ damage within the context of established or potentially new-onset hypertension, thus identifying those patients who will benefit from rapid reduction of BP. Use of the singular term "hypertensive emergency" best encompasses this and classic presentations of such acute end-organ damage include cardiogenic pulmonary edema, aortic dissection, myocardial ischemia, acute kidney injury (AKI), hemorrhagic and ischemic stroke, and hypertensive encephalopathy.

PATHOPHYSIOLOGY

Increased BP is a physiological consequence of aging, but the onset of hypertension in young and middle-aged individuals represents a complex interplay of multiple pathways including neurohormonal dysregulation [involving the sympathetic nervous system (SNS) and renin–angiotensin–aldosterone systems (RAAS) primarily), vascular modulation, sodium intake, psychosocial stress and obesity. Cardiac and renal functions also play a crucial role, by both contributing to elevated BP and as long-term consequences of hypertension. Despite an advanced pathophysiological understanding, the definitive cause of hypertension remains unknown in more than 90% of patients. These individuals are labeled as having primary or essential hypertension and the cause is considered idiopathic. In the subset of patients with an identifiable, discrete cause of their elevated BP, the term secondary hypertension applies. While immediate treatment for most will not differ, relevance of this distinction for hypertensive emergencies lies in the need for more comprehensive diagnostic work-up, as well as disease-specific management for some conditions such as renal artery stenosis.

When BP is uncontrolled in chronic hypertension, persistent vasoconstriction leads to a number of adverse consequences that eventually manifest as damage to "end" organs, most importantly the heart, brain, and kidneys. In the macrocirculation, the heart and large blood vessels are most affected, through the mechanisms of increased afterload and shear forces on the vessel walls. Continued elevations in systemic vascular resistance (SVR) cause significant augmentation of the pressure wave reflected from the periphery back to the central circulation (termed the augmentation index) during diastole,[21] thus driving up left ventricular (LV) afterload. The resulting increase in aortic wall stiffness manifests with a rise in the central aortic pressure and increase in the pressure amplitude of the waveform.[22,23] This impedes forward flow from the heart, which leads to increased demand for contractile force from the left ventricle to maintain aortic valve opening and the duration of ventricular ejection.[24] This in turn increases intraventricular wall tension, which, together with ongoing stimulation from the SNS and RAAS, promotes cardiomyocyte hypertrophy and myocardial fibrosis.[25] Initially, this process is adaptive to physiological requirements, and leads to an increase in LV mass, which enhances the ventricle's function against excessive afterload. However, the resulting cardiac remodeling eventually leads to stiffening and impaired diastolic function with elevated filling pressure and resistance to inflow from the left atrium.[26] When a sudden increase in afterload occurs as in the setting of a hypertensive emergency, an abrupt decrease in stroke volume follows. This precipitates backflow of blood into the pulmonary arteries leading to capillary leak and rapid onset of "flash pulmonary edema".[27] In patients with more gradual increases in afterload, a slower rise in LV end-diastolic pressure may cause excess wall tension with compression of the subendocardial microvasculature and myocardial ischemia.[28] Over time, this contributes to LV wall thinning, chamber dilation, and, eventually, systolic dysfunction.

Changes in the microcirculation affect diverse organ systems, causing the clinical symptoms of noncardiac end-organ damage.[29,30] The initial, compensatory effect of vascular remodeling with arteriolar intimal hypertrophy eventually becomes a pathological response, and manifests as critical luminal narrowing and the potential for regional ischemia from occlusion or loss of vessel wall integrity.[31] Autoregulation, which is the intrinsic capacity of resistance vessels to rapidly dilate or constrict in response to dynamic perfusion pressure changes, works to maintain relatively constant blood flow to end organs. This process is protective within a narrow range, but eventually fails to modulate the persistent pressure elevations of chronic, uncontrolled hypertension. Small-vessel ischemic episodes, many of which are clinically silent are the primary cause of chronic end-organ damage. The accumulation of these insults over time leads to clinically significant disease, including progressive white matter (i.e., multi-infarct) disease in the brain[32] and hypertensive nephropathy.[33] Cerebral microbleeds, which are identified by imaging of hemosiderin deposits on brain magnetic resonance imaging (MRI), are a relatively new class of subclinical brain injury associated with chronic hypertension and portend more rapid cognitive decline in older adults.[34]

Distinct from the pathogenesis of end-organ damage that occurs with poorly controlled hypertension over time, a hypertensive emergency results from acute endothelial injury caused by a dramatic rise in vascular pressure that overwhelms autoregulatory mechanisms. A subsequent decrease in nitric oxide (NO)-mediated vascular smooth muscle relaxation and excess release of endothelin, a vasoconstrictor cytokine, further increase SVR.[35] The mechanical effect of this process is uncontrolled vessel wall tension, leading to dilatation and, eventually, rupture of terminal arterioles. The endothelial cells respond through a variety of inflammatory and procoaguable pathways, causing fibrin deposits and tissue ischemia.[36-38]

An important, though difficult, distinction should be made between severely elevated BP as a cause of acute end-organ damage and as a result. In many hypertensive emergencies, the severely elevated BP is both, and in some cases, such as stroke, it may even serve a protective function working to drive perfusion to areas of ischemia. Blood pressure can be elevated as a result of the stress and anxiety associated with critical illness, through activation of the SNS. As evidence of this, BP often decreases spontaneously on repeat measurement, even in the absence of specific antihypertensive therapy. However, this effect is inconsistent,[39] and acute stress or anxiety should not be anticipated as the major contributor to BP elevation in the setting of a hypertensive emergency.

CLINICAL FEATURES

As noted, there is no absolute level of BP that defines a hypertensive emergency, but acute end-organ damage does not occur in the absence of severe elevations (i.e., ≥180/110 mm Hg). However, absent signs or symptoms suggestive of acute end-organ damage, excessively high BP alone (regardless of the level) does not herald imminent onset of a hypertensive emergency. Moreover, the majority of hypertensive emergencies occur in patients with chronic hypertension,[7,9] many of who have some degree of underlying, chronic end-organ damage. This is especially true for African-Americans, who are more likely to have poorly controlled chronic hypertension and associated pressure mediated consequences than Whites.[9,40]

Generally, the heart, brain, or kidneys are the organ systems most likely to be involved in patients with a hypertensive emergency. The pattern of presentation points to the organ system involved—focal neurologic deficit or altered mentation suggest brain injury, whereas chest pain or shortness of breath are indicative of cardiac involvement. Milder symptoms, such as headache,[41] dizziness, and epistaxis,[42] are frequently associated with elevated BP, but do not indicate in and of themselves hypertensive emergencies. Absent evidence of acute end-organ damage, ED treatment should focus on symptomatic relief, and reinforcement of adherence to long-term chronic antihypertensive therapy rather than acute BP reduction.

Hypertensive encephalopathy is perhaps the best example of a true hypertensive emergency, where acutely elevated BP is the primary factor precipitating acute onset of symptomatic end-organ damage. Through selective vasodilation and constriction, the brain has autoregulatory mechanisms to ensure consistent cerebral blood flow. This is effective over a wide range of systemic BPs. When these mechanisms fail, often as a result of the vascular changes associated with uncontrolled hypertension, acutely elevated intracranial pressure ensues causing diffuse cerebral edema. This leads to vasospasm, ischemia, increased vascular permeability, punctate hemorrhages, and interstitial edema. The hallmarks of the clinical presentation are severe headache, vomiting, and altered mental status. In severe cases, these may progress to seizures or coma. Retinal involvement may cause a range of symptoms from blurred vision to complete blindness. The physical examination findings are also neurological in nature. Typically, patients present with delirium and generalized depressed mental status. Focal deficits, when found, do not follow a singular anatomic pattern and may occur bilaterally, consistent with diffuse cerebral dysfunction rather than an anatomically localized stroke syndrome or space-occupying lesions. Papilledema, although difficult to recognize, is often present, along with significant hypertensive retinopathy. Computed tomography (CT) may not show acute hemorrhage or other acute pathology; however, diffuse or regional cerebral edema and small hemorrhages have been reported in case series. The clinical presentation of diffuse cerebral dysfunction, an absence of hemorrhage, acute ischemia, or space occupying lesion on CT scan, along with markedly elevated systemic BP, is sufficient to make a presumptive diagnosis of hypertensive encephalopathy. This condition is fully reversible with early, aggressive BP reduction, and this therapeutic response also serves to confirm the diagnosis. Recently published data from the Nationwide Inpatient Sample suggest that the overall inhospital mortality rate is less than1%.[43]

Posterior reversible encephalopathy syndrome (PRES) is a recently defined neurological presentation caused by increased vascular permeability secondary to endothelial damage with vasogenic edema. While it is associated with various medical conditions, such as kidney disease, malignancies, cytotoxic therapy, and autoimmune diseases, severe BP elevation is the most common cause, and accounts for approximately half of the reported cases in the literature.[44] The clinical presentation is similar to that of hypertensive encephalopathy, albeit with less global and more region specific features.[45] The PRES is characterized by a constellation of symptoms related to posterior cerebral impairment, including visual changes, headache, altered mental status, and seizures. This condition is diagnosed by the visualization of bilateral hyperintensities on T2 and fluid attenuated inversion recovery (FLAIR) MRI. As the name suggests, PRES is reversible by treating the underlying cause, and mortality

TABLE 1: Hypertension in the context of systemic illness

Medical condition	Mechanism of Blood pressure elevation	Blood pressure treatment
Thyrotoxicosis[46]	Excess thyroid hormone leads to vasodilation, and the compensatory activation of the RAAS increases intravascular volume, leading to increased preload	Propranolol 1 mg/min IV, may repeat q2–5 min to a maximum dose of 5 mg
Pheochromocytoma[47]	α-adrenergic effects of catecholamines causes vasospasm	Phentolamine 2.5–5 mg IV, repeat as needed
Neuroleptic malignant syndrome[48]	Unknown; may relate to loss of tonic inhibition of the SNS	No specific treatment beyond discontinuation of antipsychotic medications. Benzodiazepines (Lorazepam 1–2 mg IV) may be beneficial
Serotonin syndrome[49]	Excess activation of peripheral serotonin receptors (5-HT2A)	Mild: Diazepam 5 mg IV/PO Severe: Esmolol 500 µg/kg IV bolus, followed by 50 µg/kg/min maintenance

RAAS, renin angiotension aldosterone systems; SNS, sympathetic nervous system; IV, intravenous.

is rare, although many patients have persistent minor neurological deficits.[44]

Altered mental status or seizures may also be present with acute intracranial hemorrhage (ICH), or in the setting or pregnancy, eclampsia. As mentioned, focal neurological deficits typically point to a stroke syndrome, which may be ischemic or hemorrhagic. Other clinical features such as chest pain, shortness of breath, or peripheral edema reflect cardiovascular or renal involvement, perhaps from acute coronary syndrome (ACS), aortic dissection, acute heart failure (AHF), or AKI. The latter may be difficult to distinguish from underlying chronic kidney disease (CKD) in a patient with long-standing uncontrolled hypertension and poor healthcare access, but when associated with acute symptoms, the safest course of action is to presume it represents a hypertensive emergency and work back from there.

Acute medical conditions (thyroid storm and pheochromocytoma) and adverse drug reactions (neuroleptic malignant syndrome and serotonin syndrome), which cause hypermetabolic states, can acutely elevate BP, through impairment of electrolyte homeostasis, and activation of the SNS and RAAS pathways. A distinction between the BP elevations associated with these conditions, and a true hypertensive emergency, is the contributory role of the BP itself to the pathological process. In the conditions listed above, the BP elevation is a result of the underlying pathology. While it may exacerbate symptoms, and be associated with acute end-organ damage in select circumstances, the BP does not have a direct role in the etiology of the disease. Treatment of the underlying disorder will often resolve the BP elevation, although BP reduction may play a role in supportive management. Although a complete discussion of each of these conditions is outside the scope of this chapter, table 1 summarizes the pathophysiological processes leading to BP elevation, and addresses appropriate management of hypertension in the context of these conditions.

Patients often present to the ED with an incidental finding of severely elevated BP, from use of home monitors, measurements in quasi-medical settings such as pharmacies and health fairs, and routine vital signs in outpatient clinics. Many will have a history of poorly controlled hypertension, but for those who do not, these incidental measurements may hint at a diagnosis of hypertension. However, the overwhelming majority of these patients do not have a hypertensive emergency. In order to differentiate these patients from those with elevated BP and acute end-organ damage, the term "asymptomatic" hypertension is often applied. However, this term can be misleading, as many of these patients have symptoms which may or may not relate to their BP elevation, such as low grade headache, dizziness, atypical chest pain, generalized or focal weakness and paresthesia, visual disturbances, or mild dyspnea. With the exception of dyspnea, the occurrence of such symptoms appears to be unrelated to the degree of BP elevation.[50] When present, such symptoms should prompt the clinician to carefully evaluate for signs of end-organ damage, and obtain ancillary studies as appropriate. Of note, despite widespread belief among the lay community and some physicians that acute, severe hypertension contributes to epistaxis, there is no evidence to support a causal relationship.[42,51]

EVALUATION

In isolation, no diagnostic test can reliably differentiate between elevated BP with and without end-organ damage, and it is important to incorporate clinical judgment based upon patient history and physical examination findings to determine when further evaluation is warranted. When indicated, ancillary testing should be guided by the suspected end-organ injury pattern. Laboratory testing to look for acute or worsening renal dysfunction (i.e., basic metabolic panel and urinalysis) and microangiopathic hemolytic anemia (i.e., complete blood count with manual differential and peripheral smear) should be considered in the vast majority of cases. When AHF, or ACS are suspected, electrocardiogram (ECG), cardiac biomarkers (i.e., high-sensitivity troponin and brain natriuretic peptide), and a chest radiograph are essential. However, in the absence of such symptoms, routine ECG for evaluation of LV hypertrophy or other indicators of hypertensive heart disease is not recommended as this test has limited sensitivity and specificity for such a diagnosis.[52] Advanced cardiovascular imaging by CT, transesophageal echocardiogram, or MRI should be considered if there is clinical suspicion for aortic dissection. Brain imaging by CT or MRI should be considered when neurologic findings are present. Beyond this, other laboratory tests should be utilized to exclude toxic, metabolic, and infectious processes.

Fundoscopy can play a critical role in the evaluation of patients with severely elevated BP and vague symptoms. Hypertensive retinopathy provides evidence of underlying end-organ damage, and is strongly associated with an enhanced risk of stroke in patients with hypertension.[53] Lesions of acute retinopathy are distinct from more chronic changes, which include arterial narrowing, "copper" or "silver" wiring of the arterioles, arteriovenous nicking, and retinal hemorrhages. Findings including focal intraretinal periarteriolar transudates (whitish ovoid lesions deep in the retina), focal retinal pigment epithelial lesions (evidence of choroidal injury), macular and optic disc edema, and cotton-wool spots (fluffy white lesions that consist of swollen, ischemic axons caused by small-vessel occlusion), all should increase the suspicion of an acute rather than a chronic problem.[54] Hard exudates, which consist of lipid deposits located deep in the retina, are also a common but late occurrence. While specific, these abnormalities are not sensitive for the diagnosis of hypertensive emergency and may be absent in up to 30% of patients.[55] Utility of fundoscopy is limited by technical challenges including the need to dilate pupils for accurate assessment and a lack of experience among ED providers. Nonmydriatic digital fundus photography is a modality which may help overcome these barriers, and has shown promise in detection of findings associated with both chronic and acute hypertensive retinopathy in ED settings.[56]

Bedside ultrasound is gaining acceptance as an important diagnostic tool in many academic EDs. Cardiac dysfunction,[57,58] pulmonary edema,[59] and aortic dissection[60] can all be diagnosed using this modality, with varying degrees of accuracy. Additionally, bedside ultrasound is useful for evaluation symptoms that may accompany elevated BP, such as undifferentiated dyspnea,[61] pneumonia,[62] pneumothorax,[63] pulmonary embolism,[64] and cardiac tamponade,[65] can all be visualized by experienced operators. This test has the advantage of performance at the patients' bedside, and thus does not necessitate moving unstable patients. It can be also immediately interpreted, and thus uniquely meets the needs of critically ill patients.

Invasive blood pressure (IBP) monitoring via an arterial catheter provides a continuous, precise measure of BP, and is recommended for use in certain critically ill patients and those undergoing major cardiovascular surgeries. Significant differences have been found between IBP and noninvasive measurements.[66,67] This finding has been replicated for patients with acute ischemic stroke (AIS), and the differences are more pronounced at the higher range of BPs (SBP >180 mm Hg).[68] This discrepancy could have major therapeutic implications, such as the decision to utilize thrombolysis, which is contraindicated when BP is greater than 185/110 mm Hg, as well as initiation and titration of antihypertensive therapy. Despite these theoretical advantages, a retrospective database study found no mortality benefit associated with the use of IBP monitoring.[69] Conversely, arterial cannulation is associated with severe complications such as limb ischemia[70] and catheter-associated blood stream infections.[71] Newer continuous noninvasive BP monitoring systems utilizing arterial tonometry may provide the benefits of IBP without the associated risks, but these devices are not yet considered equivalent in accuracy to intra-arterial monitoring.[72]

MANAGEMENT

Acute Blood Pressure Control

Antihypertensive Therapy

All hypertensive emergencies will require BP reduction to preserve organ function, and prevent patient deterioration. While the agent and BP goals differ for each specific presentation, the objective is always to safely and effectively lower BP in a relatively rapid fashion while maintaining peripheral perfusion. In the past, oral (i.e., clonidine) and sublingual (i.e., captopril, nifedipine, nitroglycerin) preparations have been used, but most patients who truly require acute BP reduction will benefit from the predictable, controlled effects of a parenteral agent, either by repeated intravenous boluses or by titratable infusion.

Mean arterial pressure (MAP) is the area under the curve of the arterial pressure wave during one cardiac cycle.

It represents the sum of the circulatory forces that impact BP and the relationship between cardiac function and vascular effects is defined by the equation

$$MAP = (CO \times SVR) + CVP$$

where SVR is the systemic vascular resistance, which is comprised of the sum of the resistance of the entire arterial system. The arterioles are the primary site of BP regulation, and have much higher resistance than larger vessels. Thus, the vasogenic tone of the arterioles vessels is the primary driver of SVR. The SVR is also known as afterload. CO is cardiac output and reflects the contractile force of the left ventricle. Central venous pressure (CVP) represents intravascular volume, and is the effective hydrostatic force of the circulatory system. This parameter is the preload on the heart. In clinical practice, a close estimation of MAP can be calculated using the equation

$$MAP = DBP + 1/3\ (SBP - DBP)$$

However, this approximation is only correct at normal resting heart rates. When the heart rate increases, the fraction of the cardiac cycle the heart spends in diastole decreases, and the MAP is closer to a simple arithmetic mean of the SBP and DBP.

Each antihypertensive medication or class of medications has specific interactions with each part of this equation, and thus, the hemodynamic response varies substantially, as shown in table 2. Some intravenous antihypertensive agents exert their effect directly through receptors on the endothelial and smooth muscle cells of the blood vessels, while others work indirectly through an increase in production or release of endogenous vasodilators. The clinical effect is dependent on the mechanism of action, and thus, agents must be chosen carefully, to address the appropriate element of the BP elevation—preload, cardiac output, or afterload.[73]

A multicenter prospective registry identified labetalol and nitroglycerin as the most commonly used intravenous antihypertensive medications,[50,74] but a systematic review did not demonstrate clear superiority of any single agent.[19] While studies such as CLUE (Evaluation of intravenous niCardipine and Labetalol Use in the Emergency department),[42,51,75] suggest more favorable effects on BP reduction with nicardipine, a dihydropyridine calcium channel blocker, comparative outcome trials are lacking. A general guide to the pharmacodynamic profiles of the various intravenous antihypertensive agents is provided in table 3. Depending on the desired hemodynamic response profile, certain agents may be more appealing than others for a specific indication, as illustrated in table 4.

TABLE 2: Hemodynamic effect profile of common intravenous antihypertensive agents

Class	Agents	CO	SVR	CVP
Adrenergic inhibitors				
α1-blockers	Phentolamine, urapidil*	+	–	–
β1-blockers	Esmolol, metoprolol	–	+/–	+/–
Mixed α1/β-blockers	Labetalol	–	–	+/–
Angiotensin converting enzyme inhibitors	Enalaprilat	+/–	–	+/–
Calcium channel blockers				
Dihydropyridine	Clevidipine, nicardipine	+	–	+/–
Nondihydro-pyridine	Diltiazem, verapamil	–	–	+/–
Direct-acting vasodilators	Hydralazine	+	–	+/–
Dopamine-1 receptor agonists	Fenoldopam	+/–	–	+/–
Loop diuretics	Furosemide, bumetanide, torsemide	+/–	–	–
Nitric oxide donors	Sodium nitroprusside, nitroglycerin, isosorbide dinitrate	+	–	–

*Also has 5-HT1A agonist properties.

CO, cardiac output; CVP, central venous pressure; SVR, systemic vascular resistance.

With permission from: Levy P. Hypertensive emergencies: On the cutting edge. Advancing the standard of care: Cardiovascular and neurovascular emergencies. EMCREG-International Symposia Monograph; February 2011. pp. 19-26 (www.emcreg.org).

Blood Pressure Goals

The goal in treating hypertensive emergencies is not reduction of BP per se; rather, it is resolution of acute organ injury. Despite lack of clinical trial data[20] to support specific BP goals, the JNC 7 in 2003 recommended targeting a maximal reduction in MAP of 20–25% within the first hour and a goal BP of 160/100 mm Hg by 2–6 hours, followed by gradual normalization (>140/90 mm Hg) over the next 48 hours.[17] The European Society of Hypertension and the European Society of Cardiology (ESH/ESC) published guidelines in 2013, in which they advised reducing BP by 25% in the "first hours", followed by a subsequent cautious reduction. These recommendations are based on expert opinion, and arise from an understanding of the cerebral autoregulation curve. Under normal circumstances, cerebral blood flow is maintained within a wide range of pressures (MAP 60–160 mm Hg). This curve shifts to the right in patients with chronic hypertension and tends to settle at a point approximately 25% below baseline MAP (Fig. 1). Because most patients with a hypertensive emergency have underlying chronic hypertension, reducing MAP rapidly below 100 mm Hg could lead to a decrease in cerebral blood flow.[76] However, BP during a hypertensive emergency is often markedly elevated beyond baseline and well above the lower limit of an individual's autoregulation curve.[9] Consequently, a margin of safety exists, and antihypertensive therapy often serves to bring BP down to the perfusion plateau from the ascending portion of the autoregulation curve, rather than along this plateau and down the descending limb, where hypoperfusion can ensue.

TABLE 3: User's guide to intravenous antihypertensive therapy

Medication by class	Bolus or loading dose	Infusion rate	Time to onset	Duration of action
Adrenergic inhibitors				
Phentolamine	5–15 mg q5 min	0.2–0.5 mg/min	1–2 min	10–30 min
Urapidil	12.5–50 mg q5 min	9–30 mg/h	1–2 min	2.5 h
Esmolol	0.5–1 mg/kg × 1	50–300 µg/kg/min	1–2 min	20 min
Metoprolol	5 mg q5 min	None	10–30 min	5–8 h
Labetalol	20–80 mg q10 min	1–2 mg/min	2–5 min	3–6 h
ACE inhibitor				
Enalaprilat	0.625–1.25 mg q15 min up to 5 mg max	1–2 mg/h	15–30 min	6–12 h
Calcium channel blockers				
Clevidipine	None	2–32 µg/h	1–2 min	1–5 min
Nicardipine	None	5–15 mg/h	5–15 min	4–6 h
Diltiazem	0.25–0.35 mg/kg q15 min	5–15 mg/h	5–15 min	6 h
Verapamil	2.5–5 mg IV q15 min	None	5–15 min	6 h
Direct-acting vasodilator				
Hydralazine	5–20 mg q30 min	1.5–5 µg/kg/min	10–20 min	2–4 h
Dopamine antagonist				
Fenoldopam	None	0.1–0.3 µg/kg/min; titrate by 0.1 µg/kg	<5 min	30 min
Loop diuretics				
Furosemide	40–240 mg q12 h	10–40 mg/h	30–60 min	2–4 h
Bumetanide	0.5–4 mg q12 h	None	30–60 min	2–4 h
Torsemide	10–20 mg q12 h	None	30–60 min	2–4 h
Nitric oxide donors				
Sodium nitroprusside	None	0.25–10 µg/kg/min	Immediate	1–2 min
Nitroglycerin	1–2 mg q5 min	5–400 µg/min	2–5 min	5–10 min
Isosorbide dinitrate	3–4 mg q5 min	1–10 mg/h	2–5 min	5–10 min

ACE, angiotensin converting enzyme; FDA, Food and Drug Administration; IV, intravenously.

TABLE 4: Indication-specific approach to management of hypertensive emergencies

Indication	Goals of treatment	Primary agents	Secondary agents	Caveats
Acute coronary syndromes	Diminish cardiac workload and improve coronary artery perfusion	Nitroglycerin	Esmolol, labetalol, metoprolol, nicardipine	Routine use of intravenous β-blocker therapy is controversial
Acute heart failure syndromes	Reduce impedance to forward flow and diminish cardiac workload	Nitroglycerin, furosemide	Clevidipine, enalaprilat, nicardipine, sodium nitroprusside	Intubation or noninvasive ventilatory support decreases preload and may drop BP. Enalaprilat may cause sustained hypotension
Aortic dissection	Reduce shear force and dP/dt	Esmolol plus sodium nitroprusside	Esmolol plus dihydropyridine calcium channel blocker (clevidipine or nicardipine), labetalol as monotherapy	Avoid β-blockers if aortic regurgitation is present
Acute ischemic stroke*	Reduce hemorrhagic conversion and edema while avoiding regional hypoperfusion	Nicardipine or labetalol	Clevidipine, esmolol	Acute BP reduction is indicated only with planned fibrinolytic administration or when secondary target-organ dysfunction is involved

Continued

Continued

Indication	Goals of treatment	Primary agents	Secondary agents	Caveats
Acute intracerebral hemorrhage*	Reduce hematoma expansion and perihematomal edema	Nicardipine or labetalol	Clevidipine, esmolol	BP may decrease with pain management alone
Hypertensive encephalopathy*	Decrease brain edema, reduce intracranial pressure, and improve autoregulatory control	Nicardipine or labetalol	Clevidipine, esmolol, enalaprilat	Other causes of altered mental status should be considered in the workup
Acute kidney injury	Decrease pressure in renal parenchyma and glomerular apparatus	Fenoldopam, clevidipine, nicardipine	Labetalol, sodium nitroprusside	Angiotensin converting enzyme inhibitors and diuretics should be avoided
Preeclampsia and eclampsia	Decrease intracranial pressure while maintaining placental perfusion	Hydralazine	Labetalol, nicardipine	Intravenous magnesium (6 g initially) is indicated in all cases. Emergent cesarean section is definitive treatment
Sympathetic crisis	Reduce α1-adrenergic receptor-mediated vasoconstriction	Phentolamine, nitroglycerin	Clevidipine, nicardipine, sodium nitroprusside	Benzodiazepines are first-line therapy when sympathetic crisis is caused by cocaine or amphetamines. β-blocker monotherapy (including labetalol) is contraindicated

*Nitric oxide donors and hydralazine should be avoided with these indications.

BP, blood pressure; dP/dt, change in pressure/change in time; FDA, Food and Drug Administration.

With permission from: Levy P. Hypertensive emergencies: On the cutting edge. Advancing the standard of care: Cardiovascular and neurovascular emergencies. EMCREG-International Symposia Monograph; February 2011. pp. 19-26 (www.emcreg.org).

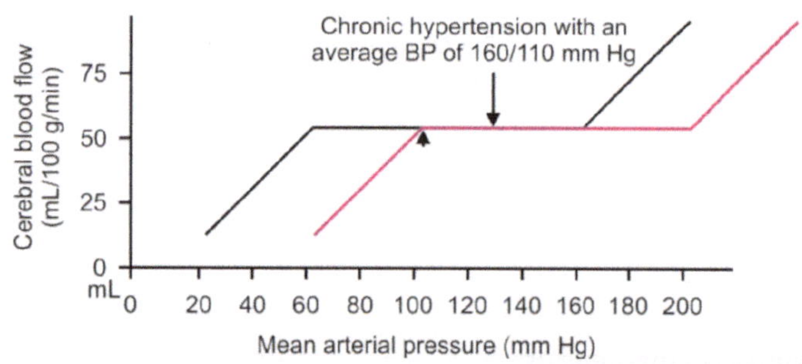

FIG. 1: The cerebral blood pressure autoregulation curve (black line) and its right-shift response to chronic hypertension (red line). Data shown are for a hypothetical patient with chronic hypertension and poor blood pressure control at baseline (average mean arterial pressure indicated by black arrow). As indicated by the black arrowhead, the lower limit of the shifted autoregulation curve in this scenario sits at a point approximately 25% below the "average" baseline mean arterial pressure

Use of a single BP goal for all hypertensive emergencies, in all patients, fails to account for this variability and may prevent effective interruption of the pathophysiology causing acute end-organ damage. Clinicians must base therapy goals on their best understanding of where a patient is currently on their individual autoregulation curve, and therapy should be directed at achieving a BP range where the body's homeostatic mechanisms can effectively re-establish autoregulation. Therefore, the best approach is to focus on condition-specific targets and to tailor these to the patient, considering the effects of chronic hypertension. In general, BP reduction has a large role in symptom resolution in cardiac injury patterns, such as AHF and ACS, while the effect in hypertensive emergencies involving the central nervous system (other than hypertensive encephalopathy) may be less apparent. An overview of respective treatment goals and relevant caveats for differing indications can be found in table 4.

Acute Coronary Syndrome and Acute Heart Failure

In hypertensive emergencies that involve the heart, such as ACS and AHF, afterload reduction is the most critical element of BP control. The physiological goals in ACS are to decrease cardiac oxygen demand and increase coronary perfusion. Both of these are achieved by afterload reduction, and when this goal is met, anginal symptoms typically resolve, especially once coronary referpusion therapy is administered. An acute rise in SVR and, more specifically, the augmentation index contributes greatly to the symptoms of AHF. Thus, interventions targeting afterload reduction can offset these forces, and enable more effective ventricular contractions. Administration of NO donors (medications that exert their effect by providing an exogenous source of NO) such as nitroglycerin, despite small reductions in preload, have the effect of increasing CO through this mechanism. The NO donors are effective for both ACS and AHF, as they produce small vessel dilation, decreasing SVR, and diminish the intensity of the retrograde pressure wave reflection. This leads to improvements in systolic ejection time, and improves coronary artery filling.[77-79]

Acute BP reduction using boluses of high-dose isosorbide dinitrate and nitroglycerin are associated with rapid symptom resolution, and decreased incidence of mechanical ventilation and myocardial infarction among patients with severe, hypertensive AHF.[80] At higher doses (e.g., nitroglycerin given by 1–2 mg by boluses or infused at rates >250 μg/min), these agents reduction afterload profoundly, yet are generally well-tolerated, even with MAP reductions of 30–40%. High-dose nitroglycerin has distinct advantages over alternatives such as sodium nitroprusside, obviating the need for arterial line monitoring and the risk of cyanide poisoning. An important caveat is that NO donors should not be used in patients who have taken a phosphodiesterase-5 (PDE5) inhibitor such as sildenafil (Viagra) or tadalafil (Cialis), typically prescribed for erectile dysfunction within the preceding 48 hours as this can result in profound and persistent hypotension.[81]

Short-acting angiotensin converting enzyme inhibitors (ACEI) are another class of drugs that are well-tolerated and are effective in rapid symptom resolution in patients with hypertensive AHF. A rapid-acting sublingual preparation, captopril, is available, and is effective for this indication;[82] however, enalaprilat, which can be administered by intravenous bolus or infusion is the preferred ACEI in the setting of AHF. Cautious dosages (0.625–1.25 mg/dose up to a maximum of 2.5 mg over 30 min) are recommended as the drug is relatively long-acting and can precipitate a sustained drop in BP.[83] Third- and fourth-generation intravenous dihydropyridine calcium channel blockers (i.e., nicardipine and clevidipine) are emerging as potential alternatives, with small trials suggesting that this class can safely and effectively reduce BP while improving dyspnea more rapidly than standard therapy in hypertensive AHF.[84,85] These agents have the advantage of a short half-life, and thus facilitate more precise titration. Beta-adrenergic antagonists play a major role in the chronic management of both HF and IHD. However, labetalol and other intravenous agents, such as metoprolol, should be avoided in the first hours of treatment, as they produce a decrease in CO, and in ACS, may increase the risk of developing cardiogenic shock.[9,74]

The rate of BP reduction, and eventual BP targets for patients with hypertensive ACS and AHF should be titrated to patients' symptoms, specifically dyspnea. When BP is rapidly normalized (i.e., decreased to ≤120/80 mm Hg), adverse events are more likely to occur, particularly in the setting of compromised cardiac function.[56] Persistent BP elevations can be tolerated in clinically improving patients during the acute phase. Normalization of BP can be achieved with reinitiation, or uptitration of oral antihypertensive medications over several days.

Aortic Dissection

Aortic dissection is unique among hypertensive emergencies in regards to BP goals. The BP reduction to a specific target (SBP <110 mm Hg), along with reduction of the heart rate (to <60 beats/min) is essential, as it decreases propagation of the dissection injury and reduces the likelihood of perioperative and inhospital death.[17,86] The immediate goal is to reduce intimal shear forces by driving down the pressure that results from LV ejection with each cardiac cycle (termed dP/dt). This goal is achieved by first decreasing heart rate and stroke volume through administration of a rapid-acting β-blocker. Beta-adrenergic blockade should be achieved prior to direct reduction of BP, as vasodilation can lead to reflex tachycardia, thus paradoxically worsening dP/dT. Esmolol, which has a rapid onset of action, is the drug of choice for initial therapy. Once heart rate of less than 60 beats/min is achieved, vasodilatory agents, such as sodium nitroprusside, nicardipine, or clevidipine, should be administered with a goal of rapidly reducing SBP below 120 mm Hg. Labetalol has both α- and β-blocker properties, and is an acceptable alternative as monotherapy, particularly if used as a continuous infusion. A caveat to the use of β-adrenergic agents is their propensity to decrease CO in patients with compromised cardiac function. Another contraindication is severe aortic regurgitation, as β-blockade can precipitate pulmonary edema in these patients.[87] Diltiazem and verapamil, which are both mixed calcium channel blockers (i.e., agents with both cardiac and vascular effects), may also be used, though neither is ideal as monotherapy. Eventually, most patients with aortic dissection will require multiple medications to control their BP, both during the initial course and after discharge. In addition to antihypertensive therapy, aggressive pain management using hydromorphone or morphine should be considered, recognizing that these agents have potential added effects on BP control.

Acute Ischemic Stroke

The role of acutely elevated BP is extremely variable in AIS. Understanding the nuances of this association is critical to achieve optimal outcomes. A U-shaped relationship exists between mortality and BP, with worse outcomes at the high and low extremes.[88] The optimal range is wide, and appears to lie between 120–200 mm Hg systolic and 81–110 mm Hg diastolic pressures. Despite several large-scale prospective clinical trials, results and interpretation of these data are inconclusive. Hence, consensus on a specific target or threshold for treatment does not exist. Current American Heart Association/American Stroke Association (AHA/ASA) guidelines call for a BP reduction to below 185/110 mm Hg only when systemic thrombolysis is planned, and maintenance of BP at less than 180/110 mm Hg in these cases.[89] In patients with other contraindication to thrombolysis, antihypertensive therapy is not indicated unless BP is greater than 220/120 mm Hg, and even in such cases, the goal is to decrease by approximately 15% gradually, over the first 24 hours after symptom onset. The AHA/ASA guidelines are based on a metaregression of BP control trials in stroke that suggest—(i) an association between large rises or falls in BP and worse outcome; and (ii) a decrease in death and/or dependency with more modest BP reduction at immediate- and intermediate-term follow-up.[90] However, these associations were not statistically significant, and large confidence intervals surround the odds ratios. Of note, the antihypertensive interventions included in this analysis targeted BP reduction within 1 week after ictus, and thus, may not be relevant to acute phase management.

Since publication of these recommendations, two large randomized studies have been completed [the Scandinavian Candesartan Acute Stroke Trial (SCAST; n = 2,029)[91] and the China Antihypertensive Trial in Acute Ischemic Stroke (CATIS; n = 4,071)[92]]. Results from these trials confirm that there is no specific benefit with BP reduction over the first 24 hours. The SCAST trial actually showed a trend towards higher risk of poor functional outcome in treated patients. Thus, there appears to be a limited role for acute antihypertensive therapy in patients with AIS who are not candidates for thrombolysis. That said, a subanalysis of SCAST also showed a nonsignificant trend towards reduced vascular events (but not functional outcomes) among those treated within 6 hours of symptom onset. While this suggests that patients may have an increased susceptibility towards BP elevation very early in the clinical course of the disease, such a hypothesis will require further validation before its clinical relevance can be understood.

For selected patients where immediate BP reduction is indicated, labetalol and nicardipine are the agents of choice. These drugs maintain adequate cerebral perfusion while producing reductions in SVR.[93] Nicardipine may have some advantages over labetalol as it results in a more rapid and sustained achievement of BP goals with reduced BP variability—a potentially important determinant of patient outcome.[94,95] The NO donors (i.e., nitroglycerin and sodium nitroprusside) are highly effective antihypertensive options, but they should be avoided, as there is a risk of increased intracranial pressure[96] secondary to cerebral vasodilation.

Spontaneous Intracranial Hemorrhage

Chronic hypertension is a major risk factor for spontaneous ICH, and up to 90% of patients with ICH present with elevated BP.[97] Persistently elevated BP contributes to hematoma expansion, vasogenic edema, and increases the probability of rebleeding. Similar to AIS, a U-shaped curve relationship exists between admission BP and mortality, with poorer outcomes at both extremes.[88] The optimal BP appears to be 141-160 mm Hg/101-110 mm Hg, with a large systematic review,[98] as well as several multicenter trials show improved functional outcomes with SBP reductions to 140-150 mm Hg.[99,100] In contrast to ischemic stroke, there is very little evidence to suggest adverse outcomes from profound, treatment-related BP reductions in ICH. According to the most recent AHA/ASA guidelines, rapid reduction is recommended when SBP exceeds 200 mm Hg or MAP exceeds 150 mm Hg, with a goal of reducing SBP to 140 mm Hg.[101] With less severe BP elevations (SBP >180 mm Hg or MAP >130 mm Hg), more permissive targets are indicated (BP 160/90 mm Hg or MAP 110 mm Hg).

These guidelines reflect the best evidence available at time of publication, but they lack the efficacy data needed to recommend an ideal time frame within to achieve BP goals. In the recently published Second Intensive Blood Pressure Reduction in Acute Cerebral Hemorrhage Trial (INTERACT2; n = 2,829) further results are available which enhance the AHA/ASA guidelines. These data show an association between intensive antihypertensive therapy targeting a SBP of 140 mm Hg within the first hour, and improved functional outcome at 90 days for patients with a wide range of systolic BPs (150–220 mm Hg), though no difference in mortality or major disability was demonstrated.[102] A post hoc analysis of patients in this study (n = 1,092) found that patients who achieved a reduction in SBP greater than or equal to 20 mm Hg within the first hour of treatment demonstrated a 35% reduction in the risk for poor neurological outcome.[103] This finding suggests that acute BP reduction has a role in optimizing outcomes in ICH. The ongoing, large, prospective Antihypertensive Treatment of Cerebral Hemorrhage (ATACH-II) study (NCT01176565), which will enroll 1,280 patients includes an intervention-arm target SBP of less than 140 mm Hg within 4.5 hours of ICH onset.[104] When complete, this study will provide critical guidance into the timing and intensity of antihypertensive therapy in patients with ICH.

Consistent with therapeutic recommendations for AIS, labetalol and nicardipine are first-line agents for acute BP reduction. However, clinical trial evidence to preference these medications is lacking, as subjects enrolled in INTERACT2 received antihypertensive medications at physician discretion. Urapidil, an α-adrenergic antagonist (which is not FDA approved), was the most commonly used agent (32.5%) in the intensive treatment arm, followed by nitroglycerin or nitroprusside (27.0%), nicardipine (16.2%) and labetalol (14.4%). Analysis of an association between therapeutic agents and outcomes has not been published. Thus, ATACH-II will provide further insight into this question, as nicardipine will be used exclusively in the intervention[103] arm of this pending trial. Nimodipine, an oral dihydropyridine calcium channel blocker, is indicated for treatment of subarachnoid hemorrhage, but its effects are likely due to prevention of vasospasm, rather than reduction of systemic hypertension.

Hypertensive Encephalopathy and Posterior Reversible Encephalopathy Syndrome

As opposed to acute stroke syndromes, where BP elevations may be partially reactive and compensatory, the relationship between BP elevation and the severity of neurologic injury is direct in hypertensive encephalopathy. As this is a diagnosis of exclusion, other possible etiologies should be ruled out prior to initiation of aggressive BP reduction. However, when indicated, and appropriately administered, antihypertensive therapy will reverse the symptoms, and confirm the diagnosis of hypertensive encephalopathy. The physiological rationale is to re-establish autoregulatory control over cerebral blood flow, and this is achieved by bringing cerebral blood flow back down to the pressure curve plateau. Once this goal is achieved, intracerebral edema will decrease, and symptoms will resolve. Reductions of MAP by 30–40% may be needed, but BP treatment should be titrated to clinical improvement, rather than an absolute numerical target.[105]

Hypertensive encephalopathy is an extremely rare condition, and no high level data exists to promote specific therapeutic regimens. Based on expert opinion, the agents of choice are labetalol and nicardipine, as they produce a level decrease in resistance across cerebral and systemic arterioles.[106] In contrast, NO donors (nitroglycerin and nitroprusside), though widely used for this indication, can actually lead to patient deterioration as these agents can increase intracranial pressure through preferential cerebral (vs. peripheral) vasodilation with resultant brain edema.[107] Several case reports have described neurological deterioration with administration of nitroglycerin in PRES, a subtype of hypertensive encephalopathy, supporting this as an actual rather than theoretical concern.[96] Hydralazine, a direct-acting vasodilator that inhibits calcium release from the sarcoplasmic reticulum, may cause similar differential circulatory effects. These agents should be reserved for cases where BP is refractory to other therapies.

Acute Kidney Injury

Acute kidney injury is the clinical endpoint of many diseases that cause rapid worsening of renal function. It is defined by an increase in serum creatinine of either greater than or equal to 0.3 mg/dL in 48 hours, greater than or equal to 1.5 times baseline in 7 days, or urine output of less than 0.5 mL/kg/h over 6 hours.[108] Chronic poor BP control can lead to gradual but insidious decreases in kidney function, to the point of necessitating chronic renal replacement therapy, and this progress is more common in African-American populations. Against this background, it is sometimes difficult to distinguish AKI from CKD especially in patients with limited access to care, for whom baseline renal function may not be known. Specifically, deterioration of kidney function may be directly related to severe hypertension through prerenal causes, extrinsic alterations in glomerular filtration rate (GFR) or intrinsic nephron destruction caused by acute pressure overload. The first two etiologies may also be secondary to antihypertensive therapies; diuretics causing volume depletion, and GFR alterations triggered by drug-mediated afferent arteriolar vasoconstriction from ACE inhibitors. Additionally, inappropriate rapid reduction of BP may lead to renal hypoperfusion and AKI. Consequently, a grasp of the etiology is critical to proper management of these patients, as therapies are widely divergent. Some patients require fluid administration to augment volume and increase perfusion, while others need intravenous antihypertensive therapy to mitigate acute hypertensive nephron damage. Vascular causes of renal injury, such as renal artery occlusion, are also prevalent in hypertensive patients, and these pathologies are suggested by hematuria and appropriate findings on sonographic or CT imaging. Simple laboratory testing is useful to differentiate between prerenal and intrinsic renal causes of AKI, and will guide therapeutic interventions. A blood urea nitrogen (BUN)/creatinine ratio over 20 and a fractional excretion of sodium [FENa; calculated as (urine sodium/serum sodium ÷ urine creatinine/serum creatinine) × 100] below 1%—or for those on chronic diuretic therapy, a fractional excretion of urea [FEurea; calculated as (urine urea/serum urea ÷ urine creatinine/serum creatinine) × 100] below 35%—suggest a prerenal cause. When intrinsic renal function is intact, the kidney will reabsorb as much sodium as possible, and the FENa will be low. However, when intrinsic renal function is impaired, the kidney will not concentrate urine to maintain adequate sodium homeostasis.

In cases of intrinsic, pressure-related nephron injury, acute BP reduction is indicated. Fenoldopam, a potent dopamine 1A receptor agonist, has historically been preferred as it leads to improved perfusion of the corticomedullary region and has been associated with a reduction in need for subsequent dialysis and rate of inhospital death.[109] ACEIs, such as enalaprilat, should be avoided as they create greater vasodilation in efferent than afferent arterioles, which increases the risk of further deterioration in GFR. Rapid-acting, dihydropyridine calcium channel blockers, such as clevidipine and nicardipine, have no adverse effect on glomerular autoregulation and are acceptable alternatives to fenoldopam. Other agents, including labetalol and sodium nitroprusside, may also be used, although less data are available to support use of these medications.

Preeclampsia and Eclampsia

Until definitive management by delivery of the fetus can be achieved, BP control is an essential element of managing women with severe preeclampsia and eclampsia. These conditions represent an overwhelming of cerebral autoregulation, and rapid BP reduction is essential to reduce cerebral edema and maintain blood flow to the brain.[110] Patients with preeclampsia and eclampsia are typically young, healthy and without a history of chronically elevated BP. Thus, attempts to therapeutically manipulate the autoregulation curve will be different than in other hypertensive emergencies. There is generally not a resetting of the autoregulation curve in these patients, and adverse consequences can develop at seemingly "low" BPs, compared to other pathologies discussed in this chapter. Accordingly, the threshold for intervention is much lower than the standard mentioned previously (i.e., SBP exceeding 160 mm Hg).[111]

Magnesium sulfate is the first-line therapy for all women with preeclampsia and eclampsia. It has several beneficial effects for these patients as it: (i) relaxes smooth muscle (partly through calcium antagonism), which leads to some decrease in peripheral and cerebral vascular resistance; (ii) limits cerebral edema formation by protecting the blood-brain barrier; and (iii) has central anticonvulsant activity.[112] However, its effects on SVR are minor, and additional agents should be used to reduce BP. Hydralazine and labetalol by intravenous bolus are the classic treatments for acute hypertensive complications in pregnancy. Both are effective for this indication, and are uniquely appropriate for this population since they do not significantly impact placental blood flow.[113] Nicardipine, though less frequently utilized, is a reasonable alternative and may produce a greater decrease in BP than labetalol.[114]

Sympathetic Crises

The acute BP elevations associated with hyperadrenergic states may arise from either endogenous (i.e., pheochromocytoma) or exogenous sources of catecholamine excess. In most clinical settings, the latter are more common that the former. Sympathomimetic toxicity is caused by intake (through various routes) of substances that interfere with norepinephrine metabolism or directly activate α-adrenergic receptors. Substances that are commonly encountered include cocaine, amphetamines, and tyramine containing foods in patients taking monoaminase inhibitor antidepressants. The net result is a cardiostimulatory and vasopressor response that manifests clinically as tachycardia and marked hypertension. Although the vasopressor response has been demonstrated in animal models, in humans, the central cardiostimulatory effect is predominant.[115] In patients manifesting psychiatric symptoms of sympathomimetic toxicity, such cardiac and vascular stimulation is compounded by central sympathetic activation. In these cases, hemodynamic derangements can often be improved by administration of benzodiazepines and other sedative medications, without direct antihypertensive therapy.[116]

When BP is persistently elevated, acute end-organ damage with cardiac or cerebral ischemia, cardiac arrest can ensue. To prevent these outcomes, acute BP reduction is essential. Phentolamine, a reversible pure α-blocker, is considered first-line therapy, producing a reliable decrease in peripheral and coronary vasoconstriction with little adverse effect.[117,118] Nitroglycerin can also be used and is specifically indicated for patients with associated chest pain and suspected coronary artery vasospasm.[119] Dexmedetomidine, a centrally acting α-2 agonist has been suggested, based on physiologic studies, as a potential drug for this indication,[120] and it has the additional benefit of generalized sedation when patients are severely agitated. Heart rate control may also be needed (especially in patients with pheochromocytoma, in whom adrenal release of epinephrine may be particularly high), and a short-acting β-blocker, such as esmolol, is ideal for this purpose. However, to avoid precipitation of unopposed α-receptor activity and a worsening of hypertension, β-blocker therapy should be paired with a vasodilator. Although labetalol has combined α- and β-blocker properties, β-receptor effects strongly predominate when the drug is administered in intravenous form (α to β ratio of 1:7). Consequently, intravenous labetalol is susceptible to a similar differential response and should be used with caution in the setting of catecholamine excess. For patients who present with apparent catecholaminergic excess due withdrawal effects of noncompliance with chronic clonidine therapy, an α-2 agonist that acts at the presynaptic receptors to decrease norepinephrine release, treatment with oral clonidine may be sufficient, provided acute end-organ damage is absent.

DISPOSITION

Individuals without evidence of acute end-organ damage can be discharged home, but hypertensive emergency patients warrant admission, most often to an intensive care unit. Clinical features, such as chest pain, dyspnea on exertion, or worsening renal function, may confuse the picture, and short-term management in an observation unit can be useful to determine whether the acute presentation represents a true emergency.

Outcomes associated with a given hypertensive emergency are largely a function of the underlying acute end-organ injury pattern. However, data from STAT suggest that severe hypertension (at least in the subset of patients in whom intravenous antihypertensives are administered) is a high-risk condition with inhospital and 30-day mortality rates of 6.9% and 11%, respectively, and a 90-day readmission rate of nearly 40%.[9,121] When associated with AKI, mortality is even greater, with an odds ratio of 1.05 ($p = 0.03$) per 10 mL/min estimated glomerular filtration rate decline.[122] Although risk for short-term deterioration is minimal in patients with elevated BP who lack evidence of acute end-organ damage, the long-term risk of cardiovascular, cerebrovascular, and renovascular disease is relatively high,[98] underscoring the need for development of effective, patient-centric models of chronic hypertension care at the system level.[99,100,123,124]

CONCLUSION

Hypertensive emergencies are true, life-threatening conditions that warrant immediate intervention. Differentiating such emergencies from more benign presentations with BP elevation but no evidence of acute end-organ damage is critical for initiation of appropriate management. Aggressive, intravenous antihypertensive therapy and admission to the hospital is the general rule for virtually all hypertensive emergencies, though specific intervention should be guided by the pattern of organ injury, not the BP itself. In the absence of acute end-organ damage, management should focus on chronic oral antihypertensive therapy and assurance of outpatient follow-up, rather than treatment aimed at short-term BP control.

REFERENCES

1. Go AS, Mozaffarian D, Roger VL, Benjamin EJ, Berry JD, Blaha MJ, et al. Heart disease and stroke statistics--2014 update: a report from the American Heart Association. Circulation. 2014;129(3):e28-292.
2. Lackland DT, Weber MA. Global burden of cardiovascular disease and stroke: hypertension at the core. Can J Cardiol. 2015;31(5):569-71.
3. Lewington S, Clarke R, Qizilbash N, Peto R, Collins R, Prospective Studies Collaboration. Age-specific relevance of usual blood pressure to vascular mortality: a meta-analysis of individual data for one million adults in 61 prospective studies. Lancet. 2002;360(9349):1903-13.
4. Law MR, Morris JK, Wald NJ. Use of blood pressure lowering drugs in the prevention of cardiovascular disease: meta-analysis of 147 randomised trials in the context of expectations from prospective epidemiological studies. BMJ. 2009;338:b1665.
5. Deshmukh A, Kumar G, Kumar N, Nanchal R, Gobal F, Sakhuja A, et al. Effect of Joint National Committee VII report on hospitalizations for hypertensive emergencies in the United States. Am J Cardiol. 2011;108(9):1277-82.
6. Papadopoulos DP, Sanidas EA, Viniou NA, Gennimata V, Chantziara V, Barbetseas I, et al. Cardiovascular hypertensive emergencies. Curr Hypertens Rep. 2015;17(2):5.
7. Pinna G, Pascale C, Fornengo P, Arras S, Piras C, Panzarasa P, et al. Hospital admissions for hypertensive crisis in the emergency departments: a large multicenter Italian study. PloS One. 2014;9(4):e93542.
8. Shorr AF, Zilberberg MD, Sun X, Johannes RS, Gupta V, Tabak YP. Severe acute hypertension among inpatients admitted from the emergency department. J Hosp Med. 2012;7(3):203-10.
9. Katz JN, Gore JM, Amin A, Anderson FA, Dasta JF, Ferguson JJ, et al. Practice patterns, outcomes, and end-organ dysfunction for patients with acute severe hypertension: the Studying the Treatment of Acute hyperTension (STAT) registry. Am Heart J. 2009;158(4):599-606.e1.
10. Devlin JW, Dasta JF, Kleinschmidt K, Roberts RJ, Lapointe M, Varon J, et al. Patterns of antihypertensive treatment in patients with acute severe hypertension from a nonneurologic cause: Studying the Treatment of Acute Hypertension (STAT) registry. Pharmacotherapy. 2010;30(11): 1087-96.
11. Levy PD, Mahn JJ, Miller J, Shelby A, Brody A, Davidson R, et al. Blood pressure treatment and outcomes in hypertensive patients without acute target organ damage: a retrospective cohort. Am J Emerg Med. 2015;33(9):1219-24.
12. Decker WW, Godwin SA, Hess EP, Lenamond CC, Jagoda AS, American College of Emergency Physicians Clinical Policies Subcommittee (Writing Committee) on Asymptomatic Hypertension in the ED. Clinical Policy: critical issues in the evaluation and management of adult patients with asymptomatic hypertension in the emergency department. Ann Emerg Med. 2006;47(3):237-49.
13. Wolf SJ, Lo B, Shih RD, Smith MD, Fesmire FM, American College of Emergency Physicians Clinical Policies Committee. Clinical policy: critical issues in the evaluation and management of adult patients in the emergency department with asymptomatic elevated blood pressure. Ann Emerg Med. 2013;62(1):59-68.
14. Levy PD, Cline D. Asymptomatic hypertension in the emergency department: a matter of critical public health importance. Acad Emerg Med. 2009;16(11): 1251-7.
15. Marik PE, Rivera R. Hypertensive emergencies: an update. Curr Opin Crit Care. 2011;17(6):569-80.
16. Muiesan ML, Salvetti M, Amadoro V, di Somma S, Perlini S, Semplicini A, et al. An update on hypertensive emergencies and urgencies. J Cardiovasc Med (Hagerstown). 2015;16(5):372-82.
17. Chobanian AV, Bakris GL, Black HR, Cushman WC, Green LA, Izzo JL, et al. The Seventh Report of the Joint National Committee on Prevention, Detection, Evaluation, and Treatment of High Blood Pressure: the JNC 7 report. JAMA. 2003;289(19):2560-72.
18. Mancia G, Fagard R, Narkiewicz K, Redon J, Zanchetti A, Böhm M, et al. 2013 ESH/ESC guidelines for the management of arterial hypertension: the Task Force for the Management of Arterial Hypertension of the European Society Of Hypertension (ESH) and of the European Society Of Cardiology (ESC). Eur Heart J. 2013;34(28):2159-219.
19. Perez MI, Musini VM. Pharmacological interventions for hypertensive emergencies: a Cochrane systematic review. J Hum Hypertens. 2008; 22(9):596-607.
20. Vadera R. Does antihypertensive drug therapy decrease morbidity or mortality in patients with a hypertensive emergency? Ann Emerg Med. 2011;57(1):64-5.
21. Nürnberger J, Keflioglu-Scheiber A, Opazo Saez AM, Wenzel RR, Philipp T, Schäfers RF. Augmentation index is associated with cardiovascular risk. J Hypertens. 2002;20(12):2407-14.
22. Munir S, Guilcher A, Kamalesh T, Clapp B, Redwood S, Marber M, et al. Peripheral augmentation index defines the relationship between central and peripheral pulse pressure. Hypertension. 2008;51(1):112-8.
23. Ooi H, Chung W, Biolo A. Arterial stiffness and vascular load in heart failure. Congest Heart Fail. 2008;14(1):31-6.
24. Chirinos JA, Segers P. Noninvasive evaluation of left ventricular afterload: part 2: arterial pressure-flow and pressure-volume relations in humans. Hypertension. 2010;56(4):563-70.
25. Sharma K, Kass DA. Heart failure with preserved ejection fraction: mechanisms, clinical features, and therapies. Circ Res. 2014;115(1):79-96.
26. Santos M, Shah AM. Alterations in cardiac structure and function in hypertension. Curr Hypertens Rep. 2014;16(5):428.
27. Rimoldi SF, Yuzefpolskaya M, Allemann Y, Messerli F. Flash pulmonary edema. Prog Cardiovasc Dis. 2009;52(3):249-59.
28. Mundhenke M, Schwartzkopff B, Strauer BE. Structural analysis of arteriolar and myocardial remodelling in the subendocardial region of patients with hypertensive heart disease and hypertrophic cardiomyopathy. Virchows Arch. 1997;431(4):265-73.
29. Bidani AK, Polichnowski AJ, Loutzenhiser R, Griffin KA. Renal microvascular dysfunction, hypertension and CKD progression. Curr Opin Nephrol Hypertens. 2013;22(1):1-9.
30. Scuteri A, Nilsson PM, Tzourio C, Redon J, Laurent S. Microvascular brain damage with aging and hypertension: pathophysiological consideration and clinical implications. J Hypertens. 2011;29(8):1469-77.
31. Mulvany MJ. Small artery remodelling in hypertension. Basic Clin Pharmacol Toxicol. 2012;110(1):49-55.

32. Staals J, Makin SD, Doubal FN, Dennis MS, Wardlaw JM. Stroke subtype, vascular risk factors, and total MRI brain small-vessel disease burden. Neurology. 2014;83(14):1228-34.
33. Wang XC, Liu CH, Chen YJ, Wu Y, Yang LS, Liu HM, et al. Clinical and pathological analysis of the kidney in patients with hypertensive nephropathy. Exp Ther Med. 2013;6(5):1243-6.
34. Wu R, Feng C, Zhao Y, Jin AP, Fang M, Liu X. A meta-analysis of association between cerebral microbleeds and cognitive impairment. Med Sci Monit. 2014;20:2189-98.
35. Ault MJ, Ellrodt AG. Pathophysiological events leading to the end-organ effects of acute hypertension. Am J Emerg Med. 1985;3(6 Suppl):10-5.
36. Schiffrin EL. Vascular remodeling in hypertension: mechanisms and treatment. Hypertension. 2012;59(2):367-74.
37. Mayet J, Hughes A. Cardiac and vascular pathophysiology in hypertension. Heart. 2003;89(9):1104-9.
38. van den Born BJ, Löwenberg EC, van der Hoeven NV, de Laat B, Meijers JC, Levi M, et al. Endothelial dysfunction, platelet activation, thrombogenesis and fibrinolysis in patients with hypertensive crisis. J Hypertens. 2011;29(5):922-7.
39. Tanabe P, Persell SD, Adams JG, Mccormick JC, Martinovich Z, Baker DW. Increased blood pressure in the emergency department: pain, anxiety, or undiagnosed hypertension? Ann Emerg Med. 2008;51(3):221-9.
40. Flack JM, Okwuosa T, Sudhakar R, Ference B, Levy P. Should African Americans have a lower blood pressure goal than other ethnic groups to prevent organ damage? Curr Cardiol Rep. 2012;14(6):660-6.
41. Friedman BW, Mistry B, West JR, Wollowitz A. The association between headache and elevated blood pressure among patients presenting to an ED. Am J Emerg Med. 2014;32(9):976-81.
42. Theodosis P, Mouktaroudi M, Papadogiannis D, Ladas S, Papaspyrou S. Epistaxis of patients admitted in the emergency department is not indicative of underlying arterial hypertension. Rhinology. 2009;47(3):260-3.
43. Polgreen LA, Suneja M, Tang F, Carter BL, Polgreen PM. Increasing trend in admissions for malignant hypertension and hypertensive encephalopathy in the United States. Hypertension. 2015;65(5):1002-7.
44. Thompson RJ, Sharp B, Pothof J, Hamedani A. Posterior reversible encephalopathy syndrome in the emergency department: case series and literature review. West J Emerg Med. 2015;16(1):5-10.
45. Hinchey J, Chaves C, Appignani B, Breen J, Pao L, Wang A, et al. A reversible posterior leukoencephalopathy syndrome. N Engl J Med. 1996;334(8):494-500.
46. Karras DJ, Ufberg JW, Harrigan RA, Wald DA, Botros MS, Mcnamara RM. Lack of relationship between hypertension-associated symptoms and blood pressure in hypertensive ED patients. Am J Emerg Med. 2005;23(2):106-10.
47. Kikidis D, Tsioufis K, Papanikolaou V, Zerva K, Hantzakos A. Is epistaxis associated with arterial hypertension? A systematic review of the literature. Eur Arch Otorhinolaryngol. 2014;271(2):237-43.
48. Mahn JJ, Dubey E, Brody A, Welch R, Zalenski R, Flack JM, et al. Test characteristics of electrocardiography for detection of left ventricular hypertrophy in asymptomatic emergency department patients with hypertension. Acad Emerg Med. 2014;21(9):996-1002.
49. Ong YT, Wong TY, Klein R, Klein BE, Mitchell P, Sharrett AR, et al. Hypertensive retinopathy and risk of stroke. Hypertension. 2013;62(4): 706-11.
50. Hayreh SS. Classification of hypertensive fundus changes and their order of appearance. Ophthalmologica. 1989;198(4):247-60.
51. Amraoui F, van Montfrans GA, van den Born BJ. Value of retinal examination in hypertensive encephalopathy. J Hum Hypertens. 2010;24(4):274-9.
52. Bruce BB, Thulasi P, Fraser CL, Keadey MT, Ward A, Heilpern KL, et al. Diagnostic accuracy and use of nonmydriatic ocular fundus photography by emergency physicians: phase II of the FOTO-ED study. Ann Emerg Med. 2013;62(1):28-33.e1.
53. Sobczyk D, Nycz K, Andruszkiewicz P. Validity of a 5-minute focused echocardiography with A-F mnemonic performed by non-echocardiographers in the management of patients with acute chest pain. Cardiovasc Ultrasound. 2015;13:16.
54. Holst JM, Kilker BA, Wright S, Hoffmann B. Heart failure with preserved ejection fraction: echocardiographic valve protocol for emergency physicians. Eur J Emerg Med. 2014;21(6):394-402.
55. Eicken JJ, Billington M, Noble VE. Pulmonary ultrasound examination for edema, effusion, and thromboembolism. Glob Heart. 2013;8(4):313-21.
56. Tsung AH, Nickels LC, De Portu G, Flach EF, Stead LG. Aortic dissection and thrombosis diagnosed by emergency ultrasound in a patient with leg pain and paralysis. Case Rep Vasc Med. 2013;2013:490126.
57. Cibinel GA, Casoli G, Elia F, Padoan M, Pivetta E, Lupia E, et al. Diagnostic accuracy and reproducibility of pleural and lung ultrasound in discriminating cardiogenic causes of acute dyspnea in the emergency department. Intern Emerg Med. 2012;7(1):65-70.
58. Liu XL, Lian R, Tao YK, Gu CD, Zhang GQ. Lung ultrasonography: an effective way to diagnose community-acquired pneumonia. Emerg Med J. 2015;32(6):433-8.
59. Unluer EE, Karagoz A. Bedside ultrasonographic diagnosis of pneumothorax. Interv Med Appl Sci. 2014;6(3):133-6.
60. Borloz MP, Frohna WJ, Phillips CA, Antonis MS. Emergency department focused bedside echocardiography in massive pulmonary embolism. J Emerg Med. 2011;41(6):658-60.
61. Goodman A, Perera P, Mailhot T, Mandavia D. The role of bedside ultrasound in the diagnosis of pericardial effusion and cardiac tamponade. J Emerg Trauma Shock. 2012;5(1):72-5.
62. Ribezzo S, Spina E, Di Bartolomeo S, Sanson G. Noninvasive techniques for blood pressure measurement are not a reliable alternative to direct measurement: a randomized crossover trial in ICU. ScientificWorldJournal. 2014;2014:353628.
63. Romagnoli S, Ricci Z, Quattrone D, Tofani L, Tujjar O, Villa G, et al. Accuracy of invasive arterial pressure monitoring in cardiovascular patients: an observational study. Crit Care. 2014;18(6):644.
64. Manios E, Vemmos K, Tsivgoulis G, Barlas G, Koroboki E, Spengos K, et al. Comparison of noninvasive oscillometric and intra-arterial blood pressure measurements in hyperacute stroke. Blood Press Monit. 2007;12(3): 149-56.
65. Gershengorn HB, Wunsch H, Scales DC, Zarychanski R, Rubenfeld G, Garland A. Association between arterial catheter use and hospital mortality in intensive care units. JAMA Intern Med. 2014;174(11):1746-54.
66. Valentine RJ, Modrall JG, Clagett GP. Hand ischemia after radial artery cannulation. J Am Coll Surg. 2005;201(1):18-22.
67. Gowardman JR, Lipman J, Rickard CM. Assessment of peripheral arterial catheters as a source of sepsis in the critically ill: a narrative review. J Hosp Infect. 2010;75(1):12-8.
68. Kim SH, Lilot M, Sidhu KS, Rinehart J, Yu Z, Canales C, et al. Accuracy and precision of continuous noninvasive arterial pressure monitoring compared with invasive arterial pressure: a systematic review and meta-analysis. Anesthesiology. 2014;120(5):1080-97.
69. Levy D, Larson MG, Vasan RS, Kannel WB, Ho KK. The progression from hypertension to congestive heart failure. JAMA. 1996;275(20):1557-62.
70. Karras DJ, Kruus LK, Cienki JJ, Wald MM, Chiang WK, Shayne P, et al. Evaluation and treatment of patients with severely elevated blood pressure in academic emergency departments: a multicenter study. Ann Emerg Med. 2006;47(3):230-6.
71. Fuchs FD, Moreira LB, Pires CP, Torres FS, Furtado MV, Moraes RS, et al. Absence of association between hypertension and epistaxis: a population-based study. Blood Press. 2003;12(3):145-8.
72. Shayne PH, Pitts SR. Severely increased blood pressure in the emergency department. Ann Emerg Med. 2003;41(4):513-29.
73. Levy P, Compton S, Welch R, Delgado G, Jennett A, Penugonda N, et al. Treatment of severe decompensated heart failure with high-dose intravenous nitroglycerin: a feasibility and outcome analysis. Ann Emerg Med. 2007;50(2):144-52.
74. Den Uil CA, Caliskan K, Lagrand WK, van der Ent M, Jewbali Ls, van Kuijk JP, et al. Dose-dependent benefit of nitroglycerin on microcirculation of patients with severe heart failure. Intensive Care Med. 2009;35(11):1893-9.
75. Soma J, Angelsen BA, Techn D, Aakhus S, Skjaerpe T. Sublingual nitroglycerin delays arterial wave reflections despite increased aortic "stiffness" in patients with hypertension: a Doppler echocardiography study. J Am Soc Echocardiogr. 2000;13(12):1100-8.
76. Cotter G, Metzkor E, Kaluski E, Faigenberg Z, Miller R, Simovitz A, et al. Randomised trial of high-dose isosorbide dinitrate plus low-dose furosemide versus high-dose furosemide plus low-dose isosorbide dinitrate in severe pulmonary oedema. Lancet. 1998;351(9100):389-93.
77. Kloner RA, Hutter AM, Emmick JT, Mitchell MI, Denne J, Jackson G. Time course of the interaction between tadalafil and nitrates. J Am Coll Cardiol. 2003;42(10):1855-60.
78. Hamilton RJ, Carter WA, Gallagher EJ. Rapid improvement of acute pulmonary edema with sublingual captopril. Acad Emerg Med. 1996; 3(3):205-12.
79. Rhoney D, Peacock WF. Intravenous therapy for hypertensive emergencies, part 1. Am J Health Syst Pharm. 2009;66(15):1343-52.
80. Peacock WF, Chandra A, Char D, Collins S, Der Sahakian G, Ding L, et al. Clevidipine in acute heart failure: results of the a study of blood pressure control in acute heart failure-a pilot study (PRONTO). Am Heart J. 2014;167(4):529-36.

81. Peacock F, Varon J, Ebrahimi R, Dunbar L, Pollack CV. Clevidipine for severe hypertension in acute heart failure: a velocity trial analysis. Congest Heart Fail. 2010;16(2):55-9.
82. Cheung AT, Hobson RW. Hypertension in vascular surgery: aortic dissection and carotid revascularization. Ann Emerg Med. 2008;51(3 Suppl):S28-33.
83. American College of Cardiology/American Heart Association Task Force on Practice Guidelines, Society of Cardiovascular Anesthesiologists, Society for Cardiovascular Angiography and Interventions, Society of Thoracic Surgeons, Bonow RO, Carabello BA, et al. ACC/AHA 2006 guidelines for the management of patients with valvular heart disease: a report of the American College Of Cardiology/American Heart Association Task Force On Practice Guidelines (writing committee to revise the 1998 Guidelines for the Management of Patients With Valvular Heart Disease): developed in collaboration with the Society Of Cardiovascular Anesthesiologists: endorsed by the Society for Cardiovascular Angiography and Interventions and the Society Of Thoracic Surgeons. Circulation. 2006;114(5):e84-231.
84. Vemmos KN, Tsivgoulis G, Spengos K, Zakopoulos N, Synetos A, Manios E, et al. U-shaped relationship between mortality and admission blood pressure in patients with acute stroke. J Intern Med. 2004;255(2):257-65.
85. Jauch EC, Saver JL, Adams HP, Bruno A, Connors JJ, Demaerschalk BM, et al. Guidelines for the early management of patients with acute ischemic stroke: a guideline for healthcare professionals from the American Heart Association/American Stroke Association. Stroke. 2013;44(3):870-947.
86. Geeganage CM, Bath PM. Relationship between therapeutic changes in blood pressure and outcomes in acute stroke: a metaregression. Hypertension. 2009;54(4):775-81.
87. Sandset EC, Bath PM, Boysen G, Jatuzis D, Korv J, Luders S, et al. The angiotensin-receptor blocker candesartan for treatment of acute stroke (SCAST): a randomised, placebo-controlled, double-blind trial. Lancet. 2011; 377(9767):741-50.
88. He J, Zhang Y, Xu T, Zhao Q, Wang D, Chen CS, et al. Effects of immediate blood pressure reduction on death and major disability in patients with acute ischemic stroke: the CATIS randomized clinical trial. JAMA. 2014;311(5):479-89.
89. Liu-Deryke X, Janisse J, Coplin WM, Parker D, Norris G, Rhoney DH. A comparison of nicardipine and labetalol for acute hypertension management following stroke. Neurocrit Care. 2008;9(2):167-76.
90. Narotam PK, Puri V, Roberts JM, Taylon C, Vora Y, Nathoo N. Management of hypertensive emergencies in acute brain disease: evaluation of the treatment effects of intravenous nicardipine on cerebral oxygenation. J Neurosurg. 2008;109(6):1065-74.
91. Liu-Deryke X, Levy PD, Parker D, Coplin W, Rhoney DH. A prospective evaluation of labetalol versus nicardipine for blood pressure management in patients with acute stroke. Neurocrit Care. 2013;19(1):41-7.
92. Sheta MA, Paladugu M, Mendelson J, Holland NR. When should nitroglycerine be avoided in hypertensive encephalopathy? Hypertension. 2011;58(5):e187-8.
93. Asdaghi N, Manawadu D, Butcher K. Therapeutic management of acute intracerebral haemorrhage. Expert Opin Pharmacother. 2007;8(18): 3097-116.
94. Tsivgoulis G, Katsanos AH, Butcher KS, Boviatsis E, Triantafyllou N, Rizos I, et al. Intensive blood pressure reduction in acute intracerebral hemorrhage: a meta-analysis. Neurology. 2014;83(17):1523-9.
95. Anderson CS, Huang Y, Arima H, Heeley E, Skulina C, Parsons MW, et al. Effects of early intensive blood pressure-lowering treatment on the growth of hematoma and perihematomal edema in acute intracerebral hemorrhage: the Intensive Blood Pressure Reduction in Acute Cerebral Haemorrhage Trial (INTERACT). Stroke. 2010;41(2):307-12.
96. Qureshi AI, Palesch YY, Martin R, Novitzke J, Cruz-Flores S, Ehtisham A, et al. Effect of systolic blood pressure reduction on hematoma expansion, perihematomal edema, and 3-month outcome among patients with intracerebral hemorrhage: results from the antihypertensive treatment of acute cerebral hemorrhage study. Arch Neurol. 2010;67(5):570-6.
97. Morgenstern LB, Hemphill JC, Anderson C, Becker K, Broderick JP, Connolly ES, et al. Guidelines for the management of spontaneous intracerebral hemorrhage: a guideline for healthcare professionals from the American Heart Association/American Stroke Association. Stroke. 2010;41(9):2108-29.
98. Anderson CS, Heeley E, Huang Y, Wang J, Stapf C, Delcourt C, et al. Rapid blood-pressure lowering in patients with acute intracerebral hemorrhage. N Engl J Med. 2013;368(25):2355-65.
99. Wang X, Arima H, Heeley E, Delcourt C, Huang Y, Wang J, et al. Magnitude of blood pressure reduction and clinical outcomes in acute intracerebral hemorrhage: intensive blood pressure reduction in acute cerebral hemorrhage trial study. Hypertension. 2015;65(5):1026-32.
100. Qureshi AI, Palesch YY. Antihypertensive Treatment of Acute Cerebral Hemorrhage (ATACH) II: design, methods, and rationale. Neurocrit Care. 2011;15(3):559-76.
101. Williams O, Brust JC. Hypertensive Encephalopathy. Curr Treat Options Cardiovasc Med. 2004;6(3):209-16.
102. Pancioli AM. Hypertension management in neurologic emergencies. Ann Emerg Med. 2008;51(3 Suppl):S24-7.
103. Immink RV, van den Born BJ, van Montfrans GA, Kim YS, Hollmann MW, van Lieshout JJ. Cerebral hemodynamics during treatment with sodium nitroprusside versus labetalol in malignant hypertension. Hypertension. 2008; 52(2):236-40.
104. Khwaja A. KDIGO clinical practice guidelines for acute kidney injury. Nephron Clin Pract. 2012;120(4):c179-84.
105. Landoni G, Biondi-Zoccai GG, Tumlin JA, Bove T, De Luca M, Calabrò MG, et al. Beneficial impact of fenoldopam in critically ill patients with or at risk for acute renal failure: a meta-analysis of randomized clinical trials. Am J Kidney Dis. 2007;49(1):56-68.
106. Euser AG, Cipolla MJ. Cerebral blood flow autoregulation and edema formation during pregnancy in anesthetized rats. Hypertension. 2007; 49(2):334-40.
107. ACOG Committee on Practice Bulletins--Obstetrics. ACOG practice bulletin. Diagnosis and management of preeclampsia and eclampsia. Number 33, January 2002. Obstet Gynecol. 2002;99(1):159-67.
108. Euser AG, Cipolla MJ. Magnesium sulfate for the treatment of eclampsia: a brief review. Stroke. 2009;40(4):1169-75.
109. Vigil-De Gracia P, Lasso M, Ruiz E, Vega-Malek JC, de Mena FT, López JC, et al. Severe hypertension in pregnancy: hydralazine or labetalol. A randomized clinical trial. Eur J Obstet Gynecol Reprod Biol. 2006;128(1-2):157-62.
110. Elatrous S, Nouira S, Ouanes Besbes L, Marghli S, Boussarssar M, Sakkouhi M, et al. Short-term treatment of severe hypertension of pregnancy: prospective comparison of nicardipine and labetalol. Intensive Care Med. 2002;28(9):1281-6.
111. Tuncel M, Wang Z, Arbique D, Fadel PJ, Victor RG, Vongpatanasin W. Mechanism of the blood pressure--raising effect of cocaine in humans. Circulation. 2002;105(9):1054-9.
112. Baumann BM, Perrone J, Hornig SE, Shofer FS, Hollander JE. Randomized, double-blind, placebo-controlled trial of diazepam, nitroglycerin, or both for treatment of patients with potential cocaine-associated acute coronary syndromes. Acad Emerg Med. 2000;7(8):878-85.
113. Chan GM, Sharma R, Price D, Hoffman RS, Nelson LS. Phentolamine therapy for cocaine-association acute coronary syndrome (CAACS). J Med Toxicol. 2006;2(3):108-11.
114. Hollander JE, Carter WA, Hoffman RS. Use of phentolamine for cocaine-induced myocardial ischemia. N Engl J Med. 1992;327(5):361.
115. Hollander JE, Hoffman RS, Gennis P, Fairweather P, Disano MJ, Schumb DA, et al. Nitroglycerin in the treatment of cocaine associated chest pain--clinical safety and efficacy. J Toxicol Clin Toxicol. 1994;32(3):243-56.
116. Kontak AC, Victor RG, Vongpatanasin W. Dexmedetomidine as a novel countermeasure for cocaine-induced central sympathoexcitation in cocaine-addicted humans. Hypertension. 2013;61(2):388-94.
117. Gore JM, Peterson E, Amin A, Anderson FA, Dasta JF, Levy PD, et al. Predictors of 90-day readmission among patients with acute severe hypertension. The cross-sectional observational Studying the Treatment of Acute hyperTension (STAT) Study. Am Heart J. 2010;160(3):521-7.e1.
118. Szczech LA, Granger CB, Dasta JF, Amin A, Peacock WF, Mccullough PA, et al. Acute kidney injury and cardiovascular outcomes in acute severe hypertension. Circulation. 2010;121(20):2183-91.
119. Nishikawa T, Ueba T, Kajiwara M, Iwata R, Miyamatsu N, Yamashita K. Preventive effect of aggressive blood pressure lowering on hematoma enlargement in patients with ultra-acute intracerebral hemorrhage. Neurol Med Chir (Tokyo). 2010;50(11):966-71.
120. Arima H, Anderson CS, Wang JG, Huang Y, Heeley E, Neal B, et al. Lower treatment blood pressure is associated with greatest reduction in hematoma growth after acute intracerebral hemorrhage. Hypertension. 2010;56(5):852-8.
121. Devereaux D, Tewelde SZ. Hyperthyroidism and thyrotoxicosis. Emerg Med Clin North Am. 2014;32(2):277-92.
122. Pappachan JM, Raskauskiene D, Sriraman R, Edavalath M, Hanna FW. Diagnosis and management of pheochromocytoma: a practical guide to clinicians. Curr Hypertens Rep. 2014;16(7):442.
123. Langan J, Martin D, Shajahan P, Smith DJ. Antipsychotic dose escalation as a trigger for neuroleptic malignant syndrome (NMS): literature review and case series report. BMC Psychiatry. 2012;12:214.
124. Volpi-Abadie J, Kaye AM, Kaye AD. Serotonin syndrome. Ochsner J. 2013; 13(4):533-40.

26 CHAPTER

Aortic Dissection

D Mark Courtney

INTRODUCTION

The emergency care of patients with suspected aortic dissection hinges on considering the diagnosis in the right cohort of patients, utilizing appropriate diagnostic testing in a timely manner, and when diagnosed, utilizing a multidisciplinary team-based approach to care. In many ways, this is no different from other cardiovascular emergencies presented in this textbook. However, the challenges are significant. Chest pain is an exceedingly common symptom among emergency doctors and a chief complaint for more than 5 million emergency department visits annually in the United States. Aortic dissection may also present without chest pain, but with back pain, neck pain, arm pain, abdominal pain, neurologic deficit, and even syncope, shock, and cardiac arrest. Compared with acute myocardial infarction (MI) and pulmonary embolism (PE), two of the more common diagnoses among patients with chest complaints, aortic dissection is comparatively less common. There are estimates of hospitalization in the United States in 2010 of 493,000 for MI, 146,000 for PE, but only 8,000 for acute aortic dissection. The timely identification of this less common but equally or more time critical diagnosis is a challenge for clinicians.

Aortic dissection typically results from a defect in the intima of the aorta that allows high-pressure blood to dissect into the media layer and propagate in a linear manner creating a false lumen. This typically starts either in (i) the ascending aorta between the aortic valve and brachiocephalic artery, (ii) the arch, or (iii) the descending aorta, distal to the left subclavian artery take off. This intimal defect allows arterial high-pressure blood to propagate through the potential space between the intima and the media. This creates a false lumen, as this blood can extend distally down the descending aorta, and can also extend retrograde and into the pericardium.

Pathology exists when this dissection prevents normal blood flow to critical vessels: carotid artery-stroke, spinal artery-paralysis, mesenteric arteries: mesenteric ischemia, renal artery: renal failure, limb arteries: limb ischemia. Other pathophysiologic consequences are important to consider. Retrograde dissection may: (i) fill the pericardium leading to tamponade, (ii) result in acute severe aortic valve insufficiency, or (iii) obstruct flow through the coronary ostia leading to acute MI. The dissection may also rupture through the adventitia leading to hemothorax, which is often rapidly fatal. Clearly, this is a time-dependent critical emergency diagnosis (Table 1).

Categorization of aortic dissection is important and will be commented on further in the management section of this chapter, but essentially aortic dissection is categorized based on where the medial defect is located. The most commonly used current classification is the Stanford system, which categorizes type A dissections as those with a medial defect involving the ascending aorta (portion between the aortic valve and the brachiocephalic artery), or type B dissections as those with a medial defect that does not involve the ascending aorta (hence, this is distal to the brachiocephalic artery).[1] It is interesting that with this definition, a dissection involving the arch that is at, or distal to, the brachiocephalic artery and does not involve the ascending aorta, is considered type B. An older classification system by DeBakey is also

TABLE 1: Pathophysiology and clinical syndromes of aortic dissection

Anatomic abnormality	Clinical consequence
Retrograde propagation	
Into pericardium	Tamponade, shock
Disrupting aortic annulus	Aortic insufficiency
Obstructing coronary arteries	Acute myocardial infarction
Forward propagation	
Obstruction of cerebral blood flow	Transient ischemic attack or stroke symptoms
Obstruction of spinal blood flow	Spinal ischemia with deficit level of weakness/paralysis
Obstruction of mesenteric arteries	Mesenteric ischemia
Obstruction of renal arteries	Renal failure
Disruption through adventitia (free rupture)	Hemothorax, shock, often fatal

used and describes: type I dissections (originate in the ascending aorta and propagate distally), type II (originate in ascending aorta and is confined there), and type III dissections (originate and are confined to the descending aorta).

This chapter will focus on what cognitive tools exist to guide clinicians in considering this diagnosis in the right cohort of patients, at the right time. We will then present evidence-based guidance on test interpretation. Finally, we will comment on team-based strategies of management.

CONSIDERING THE DIAGNOSIS

As indicated, aortic dissection can be considered in a wide range of symptoms. However, it is not practical to test every patient with chest pain, back pain, arm pain, abdominal pain, or syncope for this disease. When considering the undifferentiated patient, the clinician formulates a "pretest probability of disease".[2] This is typically done unconsciously, as the clinician considers what the likelihood is, or is not, for this individual patient in front of them to have that disease. For some patients this is easy. The substernal chest pain smoker with diaphoresis who reports pain exactly like a prior MI has very high pretest probability for MI. For many patients, it is challenging when presentation is more vague. For some conditions, validated pretest probability scoring instruments exist that can be used to aid in estimating a pretest probability of disease, such as the Wells score for PE. Unfortunately, for aortic dissection there is no broadly used, prospectively validated pretest probability prediction rule to use as a decision aid. The clinician must, therefore, rely on the history and examination in formulating a pretest probability for a given patient and then must decide if that probability is sufficient to warrant testing. If the probability that a patient has aortic dissection is very low, perhaps less than 1% to 2%, the clinician may determine that adverse aspects of testing [intravenous contrast, radiation, time, cost to healthcare system, charge to patient] do not warrant testing. Increasingly, patients are participating in some of the decision-making regarding testing or not testing for cardiac disease in a process that has been termed "shared decision-making".[3]

CLUES FROM THE HISTORY AND EXAMINATION IN FORMULATING A PRETEST PROBABILITY FOR ACUTE AORTIC DISSECTION

Nature of Pain

Pain is a hallmark feature of aortic dissection. It is possible to have acute aortic dissection without pain, but this is uncommon. Even the nature of the way patients describe pain is important in considering who to test further. Classic teaching and understanding of the pathophysiological process of aortic dissection suggests that its nature as an acute vascular event is associated with abrupt onset and severe nature of pain. Indeed when Michael DeBakey, one of the pioneers of vascular surgery and the leader in early surgical treatment of aortic dissection, experienced this at age 97, he described it as "sharp ... intolerable". His vivid description of this, as well as the amazing story of becoming among the oldest survivors of the surgery he pioneered is fascinating.[4]

This nature of aortic pain described in the emergency setting as abrupt in onset and with a "ripping" or "tearing" severe quality goes back at least 40 years.[5] Most contemporary data on the presentation and outcome of aortic dissection comes from the International Registry of Acute Aortic Dissections (IRAD), which in 2000 first published description of pooled data from 464 confirmed aortic dissection patients from 12 international centers.[6] Since then, IRAD has grown to include 30 centers in 11 countries contributing data on over 3,800 confirmed acute aortic dissection patients.[7] However, it is important to understand that registry data that include only patients with the confirmed disease tell us significant information about those who have the disease, but "do not tell us much about the large number of patients tested for aortic dissection who did not". Initial IRAD data reported that among the 464 confirmed cased of dissection, 95% reported some pain, 85% reported abrupt onset, 90% reported it as severe, and 50% reported it as ripping or tearing. Often, patients described pain that migrates or radiates from the chest to the neck, back, arm, flank, or abdomen. Though migrating pain is classically taught as unique for dissection it is by no means universal. It can be seen variably from between 12 and 55% of cases.[1] Regardless, the quality and nature of pain can be an important initial clue to suspect aortic dissection.

Nonpain Symptoms

Not all patients present with pain. It is possible for dissection to simply present with collapse and shock. This can be due to retrograde propagation into the pericardium with tamponade. In the right clinical context, bedside ultrasound available and evaluation of possible tamponade should be done in anyone with unexplained syncope and shock or persistent hypotension. It is also possible that patients may present with focal neurological signs such as stroke. This can occur with obstruction of cerebral blood flow due to dissection involving arch vessels. Finally, nontraumatic abrupt weakness consistent with a spinal level deficit can be the presentation of dissection resulting in spinal ischemia.

BOX 1 Past medical history suggestive of risk factors for aortic dissection

Increased aortic wall stress
- Hypertension
- Pheochromocytoma
- Cocaine or other stimulant use
- Coarctation of the aorta

Abnormality of aortic media
- Genetic
  - Marfan syndrome
  - Ehlers–Danlos syndrome
  - Turner syndrome
  - Bicuspid aortic valve
- Vasuclitis
  - Takayasu arteritis
  - Giant cell arteritis
  - Behçet arteritis
- Other
  - Pregnancy (particularly 3rd trimester)
  - Polycystic kidney disease
  - Infection: From bacteremia or local source

TABLE 2: Sensitivity of history and examination elements for acute aortic dissection[10]

	Sensitivity	95% Confidence interval
History		
History of hypertension	64%	54–72%
Any pain	90%	85–94%
Chest pain	67%	56–77%
Back pain	32%	19–47%
Sudden onset of pain	84%	80–89%
Severe pain	90%	88–92%
Ripping or tearing pain	39%	14–69%
Migrating pain	31%	12–55%
Syncope	9%	8–12%
Examination		
Elevated blood pressure	49%	41–57%
Pulse deficit	31%	24–39%
Focal neurological deficit	17%	12–23%
Shock	19%	15–26%

Past Medical History

Patients with hypertension represent the largest group with the most common risk factor for aortic dissection. Other disease states that put increased wall tension on the aorta are summarized in box 1. In addition to these, there are several disease states both genetic and acquired that result in abnormality of the aortic media, which should also be considered.

EXAMINATION ELEMENTS

Examination that reveals neurological deficits, new aortic murmur, or elements of tamponade should result in consideration of aortic dissection. Blood pressure is important to consider and follow serially, but it can be misleading as patients may present with hypertension, normotension, or shock. Blood pressure differences in limbs and pulse deficits can be a clue to dissection. Certainly, absence of a pulse in one limb relative to the other can be an obvious abnormality, but this is not common. Though, there is not absolute agreement on what level of difference constitutes a "positive" finding when checking for a blood pressure differential between arms, one publication suggests a difference of at least 20 mm Hg may be a reasonable cutoff.[8] However, blood pressure difference is a nonspecific finding with up to 19% of normal patients having a blood pressure differential of greater than 20 mm Hg.[9]

One study that nicely summarized elements from the history and examination in a meta-analysis was published in 2002.[10] Klompas et al. reviewed 21 studies including a total of 1,848 patients, and produced pooled data on the sensitivity—how well characteristics can "rule out" the presence of dissection. The most important findings are summarized in table 2. Collectively, this work demonstrates that none of the elements from the history or examination alone are powerful enough to rule out the presence of dissection. They are clues that should prompt consideration of the diagnosis, but like many entities in emergency medicine, confirmation depends on an index of suspicion in the right patient and confirmatory imaging.

Chest Radiography and Aortic Dissection

The chest radiograph is not sufficiently sensitive to be used alone to exclude the diagnosis. Along with an electrocardiogram, it should be one of the earliest things ordered in the evaluation of a patient for possible dissection, and if abnormal, it may identify alternative diagnoses or it may have findings that could represent dissection. One publication suggested that a mediastinum to thoracic ratio of greater than 30% could be used as a cutoff to identify abnormal examinations.[11] This can be measured as the ratio of width of the mediastinum at the level of the aortic knob divided by the width of the thorax from one costophrenic angle to the other. However, published sensitivity of this finding is only 76%, again pointing out the need for more definitive imaging to exclude the diagnosis.

Chest radiograph in combination with other features may be useful. Van Kodolitsch described a triad of: "Aortic pain" (sudden or ripping or tearing) + pulse or blood pressure differential + mediastinal widening on chest X-ray.[8] When zero of the findings were present, the likelihood was significantly lower that dissection was present. However, 4% of those who did not have any components of the triad still had dissection, which was largely a function of this study being done in a sample with very high prevalence of disease, to begin with. Still, this is one way of integrating features from the history, examination and chest radiograph. If done in a lower prevalence of disease sample, it is possible this approach would provide more reassuring negative predictive value.

Is There a Pretest Probability Score for Aortic Dissection?

The short answer at this time is no. However, work in 2010, as part of a consensus effort, described the aortic disease detection (ADD) score.[12] If zero of the factors were present, a patient could be considered very low risk for aortic disease. It is summarized in table 3. A problem with this approach is that it may apply to an extremely small subset of patients—those who clinicians are not considering for aortic dissection any way. The summary of it can be simplified that patients with a normal examination, no predisposing conditions, nonabrupt onset, nonsevere pain, and nonripping-tearing quality are low risk.

Use of D-dimer

As of the date of this writing, there has not been a prospective management study investigating use of D-dimer to exclude aortic dissection in the emergency or acute care setting. Nazerian in 2014 published a study with retrospective analysis of D-dimer performance when coupled with the ADD risk score, and showed that of the patients who had none of the ADD score elements and a negative D-dimer, none had dissection.[13] Again, this is retrospective analysis of the ADD score and application of the D-dimer. None of the patients had management decisions done in real time based on the D-dimer.

The American College of Emergency Physicians in late 2014 released Current guidelines on pretest probability and testing for aortic dissection based on consensus from an expert panel.[14] This clinical policy statement cited a lack of class I or II evidence, and recommended that the ADD score alone should not be used to exclude dissection and the D-dimer alone should not be used for exclusion. Future prospective research evaluating both pretest probability assessment and D-dimer use was recommended.

TABLE 3: Aortic Disease Detection score[12]

Predisposing conditions	Pain features	Physical examination elements
Marfan or other connective tissue disease	Abrupt onset	Pulse asymmetry or blood pressure differential >20 mm Hg
Family history of aortic disease	Severe intensity (7 or greater out of 10 or documented as severe, or requiring >2 analgesic doses)	Focal neurological deficit
Patient history of aortic valve disease	Ripping or tearing	New murmur of aortic insufficiency
Recent aortic manipulation	–	Shock or hypotension (<90 mm Hg)
Known thoracic aortic aneurysm	–	–

DIAGNOSTIC APPROACHES FOR CONFIRMATION

The diagnostic gold standard currently is CT angiography (CTA). In most cases, this is the most rapid way to visualize an intimal flap, false lumen, and assess the location and clinical significance. Current multidetector CT machines with post-image acquisition formatting can result in high resolution visualization in a variety of planes. However, standard vascular imaging requires iodinated contrast, which can be problematic in renal insufficiency. Approach varies by hospital, but typically patients with a glomerular filtration rate (GFR) 45–60 mL/min can be imaged with a reduced osmolar agent and a reduced volume of contrast. For GFR 30–44 mL/min, a similar approach can be used if discussion between radiology and the clinician results in decision to proceed. Additionally, reduction in tube current can be done for vascular studies to optimize visualization in these lower contrast settings. For GFR less than 30 mL/min, iodinated contrast is typically contraindicated. Options in this case are: attempt echocardiographic diagnosis, which typically is done as a transesophageal echocardiography (TEE) approach to maximize diagnostic accuracy, transthoracic echocardiography (less sensitive), or magnetic resonance imaging (MRI) studies. All of these are significantly more time-consuming, require expertise to conduct and interpret study results, and are typically not first-line approaches to diagnostic confirmation when CTA is available. One meta-analysis pooled findings from other studies and compared CTA, TEE, and MRI with respect to diagnostic performance. Authors reported sensitivity for CTA of 100% (95% CI = 96–100) and specificity of 98% (95% CI = 87–99). Transesophageal echocardiography had slightly lower sensitivity (98%) and specificity (95%). Magnetic resonance imaging was similar with sensitivity of 98% and specificity of 98%.[15]

TEAM-BASED MANAGEMENT APPROACHES

Historically, the approach to acute aortic dissection, once confirmed, is to minimize further propagation of the medial defect. It has been suggested that minimizing shearing forces through blood pressure reduction as well as the frequency of these shearing forces through heart rate reduction is the optimal pharmacological approach. Some form of medical management can and should be done while simultaneously determining the need for and timing of operative intervention. Classically, type A dissection is managed surgically while type B dissection often can be managed nonoperatively. However, it is possible in the context of complicated type B dissections or those with ischemia that an operative treatment may be considered. Therefore, consultation with cardiothoracic or cardiovascular surgery is important for any acute aortic dissection.

Other members of a team-based approach include critical care physicians from either medical ICU, surgical ICU, or cardiac ICU setting who will continue care for the patient. Having their input in risk stratification, interpretation of diagnostic tests, evaluation for ischemic, and other complications outlined above is critical. Furthermore, team-based decisions about what pharmacological approach to be taken is important to smooth transitions of care as much as possible.

Pharmacological Approach

Beta blockade to lower blood pressure and heart rate with an agent such as intravenous esmolol, which is rapidly acting but short in duration when stopped, is often used initially. Intravenous labetalol may also be used emergently and may have benefits over esmolol in providing more dual reduction in blood pressure as well as heart rate. In patients with clear contraindications to beta blockade, calcium blockade with diltiazem is a reasonable alternative. However, caution is needed in patients with significant aortic insufficiency as these drugs may reduce the reflex tachycardia that is important in acute aortic insufficiency. After β-blockade, if blood pressure is still unacceptably high, addition of a vasodilator can be used. Historically, this has most often been nitroprusside, but intravenous nitroglycerin is efficacious in this setting as well.

What Blood Pressure or Heart Rate Goals Should be Targeted?

Many specialty societies[1] have suggested targeting a rate of 60 beats/min or less and a systolic blood pressure of 120 mm Hg or less, but there is no direct human data to suggest that these targets are critical or that there is independent reduction in morbidity or mortality based on independent effects of blood pressure and pulse control. It is done largely out of consensus and historical precedence.

Analgesia

In addition to lowering pulse and blood pressure with cardiovascular acting agents, treatment of pain can be an important adjunct. Opiates such as intravenous morphine or dilaudid are often needed.

Hypotension

Hypotension in aortic dissection is ominous. Verification of blood pressure in multiple limbs and perhaps with an intravascular arterial pressure transducer (which should be strongly considered in all acute aortic dissection patients) can be initial management steps. Transient low blood pressure can be treated with volume resuscitation initially and, if refractory, with vasopressor agents. However, this is at best temporizing as hypotension is typically secondary to vascular catastrophe; either tamponade, free wall rupture into the thorax or abdomen, or occasionally complete obstruction of the true lumen with the false lumen. Again, the importance of a team-based evaluation is critical. Adequate treatment of nearly all causes of hypotension in aortic dissection is operative, and team-based decision-making requires presence and dialog between all parties—emergency care, surgical, intensive care, patient, and family.

REFERENCES

1. Hiratzka LF, Bakris GL, Beckman JA, Bersin RM, Carr VF, Casey DE, et al. 2010 ACCF/AHA/AATS/ACR/ASA/SCA/SCAI/SIR/STS/SVM guidelines for the diagnosis and management of patients with Thoracic Aortic Disease: a report of the American College of Cardiology Foundation/American Heart Association Task Force on Practice Guidelines, American Association for Thoracic Surgery, American College of Radiology, American Stroke Association, Society of Cardiovascular Anesthesiologists, Society for Cardiovascular Angiography and Interventions, Society of Interventional Radiology, Society of Thoracic Surgeons, and Society for Vascular Medicine. Circulation. 2010;121(13):e266-369.
2. Gallagher EJ. Clinical utility of likelihood ratios. Ann Emerg Med. 1998; 31(3):391-7.
3. Hess EP, Grudzen CR, Thomson R, Raja AS, Carpenter CR. Shared Decision-making in the Emergency Department: Respecting Patient Autonomy When Seconds Count. Acad Emerg Med. 2015;22(7):856-64.
4. Altman LK. (2006). The man on the table devised the surgery. The New York Times. [online] Available from: http://www.nytimes.com/2006/12/25/health/25surgeon.html?page&_r=0. [Accessed April, 2016].
5. Kleiger RE. Chest pain in patients seen in emergency clinics. JAMA. 1976; 236(6):595-7.
6. Hagan PG, Nienaber CA, Isselbacher EM, Bruckman D, Karavite DJ, Russman PL, et al. The International Registry of Acute Aortic Dissection (IRAD): new insights into an old disease. JAMA. 2000;283(7):897-903.
7. International Registry of Acute Aortic Dissections (IRAD). Aortic Dissection. [online] Available from: http://www.iradonline.org/irad.html. [Accessed April, 2016].
8. von Kodolitsch Y, Schwartz AG, Nienaber CA. Clinical prediction of acute aortic dissection. Arch Intern Med. 2000;160(19):2977-82.
9. Singer AJ, Hollander JE. Blood pressure. Assessment of interarm differences. Arch Intern Med. 1996;156(17):2005-8.

10. Klompas M. Does this patient have an acute thoracic aortic dissection? JAMA. 2002;287(17):2262-72.
11. Shirakabe A, Hata N, Yokoyama S, Shinada T, Suzuki Y, Kobayashi N, et al. Diagnostic score to differentiate acute aortic dissection in the emergency room. Circ J. 2008;72(6):986-90.
12. Rogers AM, Hermann LK, Booher AM, Nienaber CA, Williams DM, Kazerooni EA, et al. Sensitivity of the aortic dissection detection risk score, a novel guideline-based tool for identification of acute aortic dissection at initial presentation: results from the international registry of acute aortic dissection. Circulation. 2011;123(20):2213-8.
13. Nazerian P, Morello F, Vanni S, Bono A, Castelli M, Forno D, et al. Combined use of aortic dissection detection risk score and D-dimer in the diagnostic workup of suspected acute aortic dissection. Int J Cardiol. 2014;175(1):78-82.
14. American College of Emergency Physicians Clinical Policies Subcommittee (Writing Committee) on Thoracic Aortic Dissection, Diercks DB, Promes SB, Schuur JD, Shah K, Valente JH, et al. Clinical policy: critical issues in the evaluation and management of adult patients with suspected acute nontraumatic thoracic aortic dissection. Ann Emerg Med. 2015;65(1):32-42.e12.
15. Shiga T, Wajima Z, Apfel CC, Inoue T, Ohe Y. Diagnostic accuracy of transesophageal echocardiography, helical computed tomography, and magnetic resonance imaging for suspected thoracic aortic dissection: systematic review and meta-analysis. Arch Intern Med. 2006;166(13):1350-6.

27 CHAPTER

Cardiac Trauma

Michael Jaung, Zubaid R Rafique

INTRODUCTION

Traumatic injuries are the leading cause of death for persons less than age 40 in the United States.[1] Although the prevalence of cardiac injury in blunt and penetrating trauma varies widely in the literature, it is a significant cause of mortality and morbidity both in the prehospital and hospital settings.

Described as early as the 17th century, cardiac trauma has long challenged physicians. Today, there are multiple programs, guidelines, and protocols that instruct providers on the diagnosis and management of blunt and penetrating cardiac injuries in the setting of polytrauma; however, there continues to be gaps in our knowledge and more research is needed.

This chapter will cover the clinical manifestations, pathophysiology, diagnosis, and emergency management of cardiac trauma. Emphasis is placed on nonlethal pathologies since such patients are likely to survive and arrive at a trauma center, and thus, benefit from emergency evaluation and intervention.

BLUNT CARDIAC INJURY

Blunt cardiac injury (BCI) is a broad amalgamation of pathologies that occur to the heart and great vessels. Although falls cause the highest incidence of overall trauma in the United States, motor vehicle collisions (MVCs), pedestrians struck by motor vehicles, and motorcycle crashes are the most common cause of BCI.[2] Other causes are falls, assault, and occupational and sport-related injuries.

Injuries to the heart and great vessels are thought to be caused by the increased intrathoracic pressure due to direct blunt injury to the chest. Some describe the phenomenon as an "osseous pinch," where the intrathoracic organs are caught in between the sternum and the thoracic spine. Others explain that the shear forces from acceleration and deceleration of visceral organs are the real culprit.[3] In either case, blunt trauma to the chest can cause both structural and electrical defect and sometimes both can occur simultaneously.

Clinical Manifestations

Clinical symptoms and signs specific for cardiac injury are not well-studied. Patients with BCI usually have a history of high-risk trauma, including high-speed MVC with extrication, motorcycle crash, and falls greater than 6 feet. The most common presenting symptoms are chest pain and dyspnea (Table 1). Patients suffering severe BCI often present with signs of hemorrhagic or cardiogenic shock, hypotension, altered mental status, tachypnea, and arrhythmias. Other physical signs include thoracic wall abrasions, thoracic crepitus, sternal step-off, and distended jugular veins. The most common signs and symptoms for aortic rupture are nonspecific and present in less than half of cases—dyspnea, back pain, and disparate extremity blood pressures.

Early identification and management of shock is a cornerstone of the advanced trauma life support (ATLS) program. The clinical signs of shock and BCI should be identified in an algorithmic manner during the primary and secondary surveys. This is especially important as patients with BCI commonly have concomitant intrathoracic, intracranial and abdominal injuries that confound the physical signs and symptoms, and thus, make diagnosis and management difficult.

Pathophysiology

Structural

Lethal Injuries

Lethal injuries often result in immediate death due to catastrophic hemorrhage. Autopsy studies have shown

TABLE 1: Symptoms and signs of blunt cardiac injury

Symptoms	Signs	
Chest pain	Abrasions	Pulmonary edema
Dyspnea	Lacerations	Muffled heart sounds
Back pain	Hematomas	Heart murmur
Dizziness	Crepitus	Persistent tachycardia
Palpitations	Venous distension	Arrhythmia
Syncope	Hypotension, without signs of exsanguination	

that transmural rupture of the cardiac wall is the most common cause of lethal injury, followed by venous-atrial tear and coronary artery dissection or tear.[4] Since the right side of the heart is closer to the anterior chest wall, cardiac injuries disproportionately affect the right ventricle and right atrium. Other injures include tears of the venous-atrial confluence at the inferior vena cava and pulmonary veins and dissection or tear of the left anterior descending coronary artery.

Cardiac Contusion and Cardiac Concussion

There is a spectrum of cardiac wall abnormalities spanning from cardiac contusion to concussion. Although contusions lead to myocyte injury and necrosis similar to myocardial infarction, the pattern of injury is different. Instead of ischemic watershed injuries following a vascular distribution, traumatic contusions have distinct boundaries and are usually confined only to traumatized myocytes.[5] On the other hand, there is no myocyte necrosis or injury in cardiac concussions. However, they can manifest as wall-motion abnormalities exhibiting "myocardial stunning" and usually resolve spontaneously.

Intramural Hematoma

Intramural hematomas develop from shearing of smaller vessels within the myocardium. In trauma, they most commonly occur in the right ventricle. Large hematomas can cause arrhythmias including bundle branch blocks and premature ventricular contractions. The sequelae of these hematomas are well-studied in patients following cardiac percutaneous procedures. Usually hematomas are managed conservatively as they resolve without intervention.

Valvular Injury

Injury to cardiac valves can be caused by papillary muscle rupture, chordae injury, and direct injury to valve leaflets. These injuries can lead to acute valvular regurgitation and heart failure. Tricuspid valve injury has also been shown to lead varying degrees of atrioventricular block.

Ventricular Septal Rupture

Acute ventricular septal ruptures are rare in BCI. The membranous portion of the septum is more commonly affected, and a defect may be asymptomatic depending on its severity.

Coronary Artery Injury

Nonlethal injuries to coronary arteries are rare and include dissections and tears. Pericardial effusions and tamponade can develop from these injuries as well as acute myocardial infarction. They occur more commonly in the left anterior descending artery and left main system.

Aortic Isthmus Tear

Although large aortic ruptures are usually lethal, there is a subset of aortic injuries that have been described in BCI. The majority of patients who arrive at the hospital with aortic injury have a tear at the isthmus. It is thought that the periadventitial tissue may prevent larger ruptures. If untreated, these aortic tears can lead to pseudoaneurysms.

Electrical

Ventricular Fibrillation and Tachycardia

The prevalence of ventricular fibrillation and tachycardia in adults with BCI is unknown as patients with these dysrhythmias usually die prior to arrival at the hospital. Although limited information is available on this cohort, the mechanism of dysrhythmia is presumed to be similar to commotio cordis as observed in children and adolescents.

Commotio Cordis

The phenomenon of commotio cordis is sudden cardiac arrest in a child or adolescent after a BCI without structural cardiac injury. It has been documented and studied in the United States with a national registry, and the vast majority of cases occur in competitive and recreational sports after a blunt blow to the chest by a ball, kick, or other object. Animal studies and anecdotal evidence suggest that these cases are often nonresponsive to cardiopulmonary resuscitation. Commotio cordis is thought to be caused by a combination of blunt injury during cardiac repolarization leading to refractory ventricular fibrillation as well as coronary vasospasm or changes in myocardial contractility.[4] Mortality rates were initially high even with prompt resuscitation and defibrillation; however, recently improvement has been noted with preventative measures and increased access to automatic external defibrillators.

Atrial Fibrillation

Atrial fibrillation is the second most common arrhythmia seen in BCI after sinus tachycardia. The mechanism is unknown, but there are likely systemic factors as atrial fibrillation is also commonly seen after significant intracranial and abdominal trauma without BCI.

Supraventricular Tachycardia

Rarely, paroxysmal supraventricular tachycardia can develop after BCI. These patients are at higher risk of decompensation compared to patients with supra-ventricular tachycardias from a medical cause.

Conduction Abnormalities

As described earlier, atrioventricular blocks can develop in the setting of intramural hematomas. Bundle branch blocks have been observed in patients with BCI with no structural injury, and the most common abnormality is the right bundle branch block.

Late Complications

There have been rare reports of delayed complications due to BCI in patients who later presented to the hospital after initial evaluation. These include cases of delayed cardiac rupture or fistula causing pericardial effusion and tamponade. Patients with structural BCI can continue to have cardiac wall abnormalities months after discharge from the hospital, which can lead to congestive heart failure. Those with electrical abnormalities can develop atrioventricular block and other arrhythmias.

Diagnosis

In patients where BCI is suspected either by mechanism or clinical manifestations identified on the primary and secondary surveys, further diagnostic evaluation is warranted in tandem with and after completion of the initial patient assessment. Figure 1 outlines the algorithm for evaluation of BCI, and table 2 shows the grading of blunt cardiac injuries.

Electrocardiogram

Electrocardiograms (ECGs) can help reveal both structural and electrical injury in patient with suspected BCI. Cardiac monitoring should be initiated as part of the primary survey. Unstable arrhythmias need to be investigated with an ECG in tandem with the secondary survey and stabilized according to the ATLS protocol. For stable patients, ECGs should be performed on all patients with suspected BCI, including patients who may be admitted for other injuries. It is recommended that patients with a new abnormality on ECG, which includes arrhythmias, ST changes, ischemia, or heart

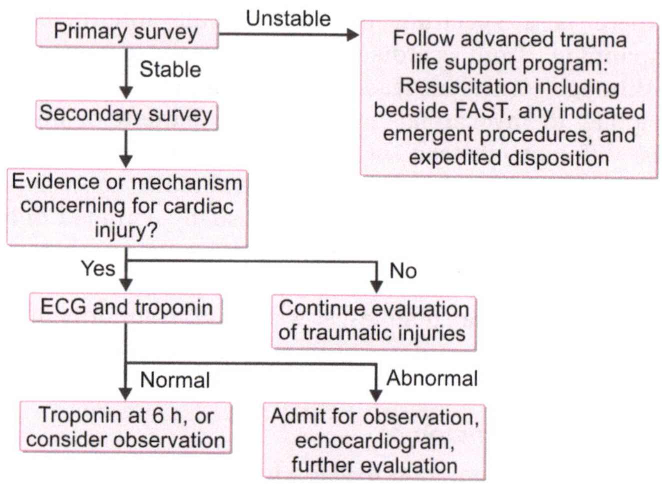

FAST, focused assessment with sonography for trauma; ECG, electrocardiogram.

FIG. 1: Evaluation of blunt cardiac injury

TABLE 2: Grading of cardiac injury

Grade*	Injury description
I	• Blunt cardiac injury with minor electrocardiogram abnormality (nonspecific ST or T-wave changes, premature atrial, or ventricular contraction or persistent sinus tachycardia) • Blunt or penetrating pericardial wound without cardiac injury, cardiac tamponade, or cardiac herniation
II	• Blunt cardiac injury with heart block (right or left bundle branch, left anterior fascicular, or atrioventricular) or ischemic changes (ST depression or T-wave inversion) without cardiac failure • Penetrating tangential myocardial wound up to, but not extending through endocardium, without tamponade
III	• Blunt cardiac injury with sustained (≥5 beats/min) or multifocal ventricular contractions • Blunt or penetrating cardiac injury with septal rupture, pulmonary or tricuspid valvular incompetence, papillary muscle dysfunction, or distal coronary arterial occlusion without cardiac failure • Blunt pericardial laceration with cardiac herniation • Blunt cardiac injury with cardiac failure • Penetrating tangential myocardial wound up to, but not extending through, endocardium, with tamponade
IV	• Blunt or penetrating cardiac injury with septal rupture, pulmonary or tricuspid valvular incompetence, papillary muscle dysfunction or distal coronary arterial occlusion producing cardiac failure • Blunt or penetrating cardiac injury with aortic or mitral valve incompetence • Blunt or penetrating cardiac injury of the right ventricle, right atrium, or left atrium
V	• Blunt or penetrating cardiac injury with proximal coronary arterial occlusion • Blunt or penetrating left ventricular perforation • Stellate wound with <50% tissue loss of the right ventricle, right atrium or left atrium
VI	• Blunt avulsion of the heart; penetrating wound producing >50% tissue loss of a chamber

*Advance one grade for multiple penetrating wounds to a single chamber or multiple chamber involvement.

block should be admitted with continuous telemetry and further evaluation.[6] It should be noted that a normal ECG without any abnormalities does not exclude BCI.

Cardiac Enzymes

The use of cardiac enzymes in identification of BCI has been extensively studied. Less specific cardiac enzyme studies including creatine kinase (CK) and CK-myocardial band (MB) were shown to not be able to distinguish between patients with and without BCI diagnosed on echocardiogram. Multiple studies have found varying evidence to support the use of cardiac troponin I and T in screening for BCI. In a study by Rajan el al.,[7] a troponin I of less than 1.05 μg/L at 6 hours ruled out BCI. Other studies suggest that a normal EKG and a negative troponin essentially rule out BCI with almost a 100% negative predictive value. Thus, the Eastern Association for the Surgery of Trauma practice management guideline recommends both an ECG and a cardiac troponin to evaluate BCI.[6]

Plain Radiographs

Chest radiographs are not sensitive in detecting BCI; however, they are routinely indicated to rapidly diagnose intrathoracic trauma not already identified in the primary and secondary surveys. There are multiple findings on chest radiograph that can indicate BCI including widened mediastinum, enlarged cardiac silhouette and pneumopericardium. Traditionally, sternal fractures were associated with BCI, but recent studies have found that sternal fractures alone do not warrant further investigation if there are no ECG changes.

Echocardiogram

Bedside ultrasound using the focused assessment with sonography for trauma (FAST) examination is an essential part of the primary and secondary surveys in hypotensive patients after blunt trauma. With an experienced operator, the sensitivity for detecting a pericardial effusion approaches 100% (Fig. 2).[8] A significant limitation is when there are poorly visualized transthoracic windows due to concurrent pneumothorax or hemothorax. In these situations, it is recommended to perform serial ultrasound exams after placement of a thoracostomy tube. Bedside ultrasound for evaluation of other structural injuries to the heart in the setting of trauma has not been evaluated.

Transthoracic and transesophageal echocardiograms are not recommended as screening tools for BCI in stable patients without ECG abnormalities or elevated cardiac enzymes. For patients who are persistently hypotensive or have other evidence of BCI, echocardiogram is the best modality for identifying most cardiac injuries. Although an echocardiogram may be a poor modality for evaluating aortic injuries because of its limited visualization of the distal ascending aorta and proximal aortic arch, it may be the only modality for an unstable patient.

Computed Tomography

In the stable patient with suspected BCI, CT is a valuable tool to further evaluate intrathoracic injuries. A constellation of findings can indicate tamponade: pericardial effusion, distension of the inferior vena cava and renal veins, and periportal congestion.[9] Computed tomography can also identify the cause of a pericardial effusion including ventricular rupture, aortic root injury and coronary artery injury. It is the preferred tool to evaluate for thoracic aortic injury and can identify extravasation, para-aortic hematoma, filling defects, intimal flaps, and thrombi.

Other Modalities

Angiography, nuclear medicine, and magnetic resonance imaging are not recommended in the screening of patients for BCI.

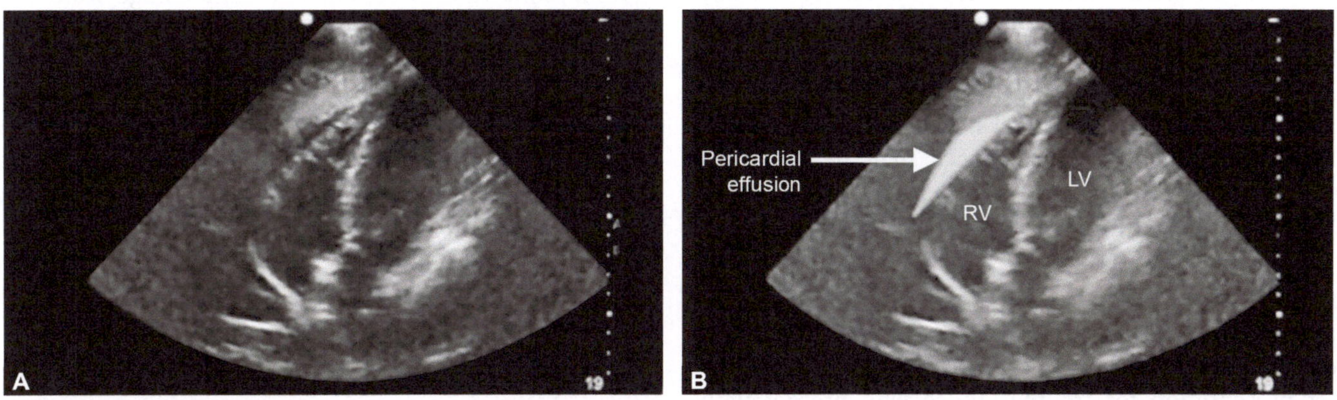

LV, left ventricle; RV, right ventricle.

FIG. 2: Bedside ultrasound showing pericardial effusion. The top and bottom are the same views of the heart showing pericardial effusion

MANAGEMENT

Hemodynamically, unstable BCI should be managed according to the ATLS program in close conjunction with consultants. Interventions may include airway protection, volume resuscitation with blood products, vasopressors, invasive monitoring and central venous access, thoracostomy, and pericardiocentesis. Early identification and stabilization should be prioritized so that definitive treatment for the patient is not delayed.

Hemodynamically stable patients with BCI who require other immediate management for intracranial, thoracic, or abdominal injury will often undergo those interventions prior to further management of BCI.

Structural

Many structural injuries in stable patients are managed conservatively. These include isolated sternal fractures, cardiac contusions, and intramural hematomas. Patients should be on continuous telemetry while hospitalized and serial ECGs and cardiac enzymes are warranted.

Other structural injuries such as valvular injury, coronary artery injury, ventricular septal defects, and aortic injuries will require operative repair even if the patient is stable. In limited situations, these injuries are also managed conservatively. For aortic tears, aggressive blood pressure control is indicated to prevent further injury and complications.

Electrical

There are very limited indications for invasive interventions if a patient with BCI undergoes a cardiac arrest. The use of emergent thoracotomy is highly dependent on available trauma surgeons for immediate definitive management and is described further in the procedures section. With the exception of commotio cordis, cardiac arrest in BCI is usually due to catastrophic hemorrhage causing exsanguination into the thoracic cavity or pericardial space.

Other electrical abnormalities should be closely managed emergently to prevent decompensation. In atrial fibrillation and supraventricular tachycardia, rhythm control is warranted. Pacing should be considered for unstable atrioventricular blocks. Other atrioventricular blocks and bundle branch blocks may be managed conservatively, and all patients should be admitted for further observation and evaluation.

Late Complications

Patients with delayed presentation of cardiac rupture or pericardial effusion should be managed as if it is their first presentation for trauma. Those who present with new onset congestive heart failure from cardiomyopathy or pericarditis should be managed medically.

PENETRATING CARDIAC INJURY

Epidemiology

Penetrating cardiac injury (PCI) is one of the most lethal traumatic injuries. Similar to BCI, the common causes of death are from catastrophic hemorrhage or cardiac tamponade, leading to high mortality rates in prehospital and hospital settings. Case series studies have found that patients with stab wounds have lower mortality rates than those with gunshot wounds.[10]

Clinical Manifestation

Traditionally, PCI was suspected with any injury within the "cardiac box", which is the area from the level of the suprasternal notch to xiphoid process inferiorly and bilateral nipple lines laterally. In reality, the trajectory of any penetrating wound to the neck, abdomen, back, or flank can lead to cardiac injury. Anterior structures of the heart are more commonly affected—the right ventricle followed by the left ventricle. The specific chamber has not been shown to be predictive of survival. Hemorrhage into the pericardium and thoracic cavity can lead to hypovolemic or obstructive shock. In rare cases, injury to the coronary arteries can cause myocardial ischemia.

Diagnosis

Unlike BCI, ECGs and cardiac enzymes are usually not helpful in evaluating PCI. An EKG can be consistent with tamponade and evaluate for ischemic injury and arrhythmias, but neither a negative EKG nor cardiac enzyme rule out PCI.

The FAST bedside examination is also commonly applied to PCI, and it may be the only modality available to evaluate for pericardial effusion in the unstable patient. These echocardiograms are also limited by the operator experience and inadequate windows when there is significant pneumothorax or hemothorax. There have been rare reports of missed pericardial effusion even after placement of a thoracostomy tube and serial FAST examinations due to concurrent hemorrhage from the pericardium into the thoracic cavity.[11]

Less than 50% of patients with PCI will have changes on a plain chest radiograph indicating injury. In stable patients, CT and transthoracic echocardiogram can be used to further characterize injury, but nearly all patients with PCI will require definitive treatment in the operating room. Previous invasive diagnostic procedures included pericardiocentesis, subxiphoid pericardial window, and measuring central venous pressures are no longer used in the initial evaluation of PCI.

Management

The initial evaluation and management in PCI should follow the ATLS program with focus on early identification and stabilization of shock. For patients who present in cardiac arrest after having signs of life in prehospital setting, an emergency thoracotomy is indicated if trauma surgical care is immediately available for further management. For patients with cardiac tamponade, a pericardiocentesis should be considered.

Stable patients with PCI require close monitoring while emergency evaluation is completed and they await procedures. These patients are at high risk of decompensation from hemorrhage, hypothermia, acidosis, and coagulopathy.

There have been rare cases of delayed acute myocardial infarction following PCI as well as the development of pseudoaneurysms of the heart and aorta and complications from retained missiles.[12] These patients usually develop these complications postoperatively prior to discharge.

PROCEDURES

The resuscitation of cardiac injury patients can require multiple interventions as outlined above for airway protection and evacuation of concomitant hemothorax or pneumothorax. In this section, two emergency procedures specific to cardiac trauma—thoracotomy and pericardiocentesis—has been discussed.

Emergency Thoracotomy

There are very limited indications for an emergency department (ED) resuscitative thoracotomy. In penetrating injury, thoracotomy is indicated for a patient in cardiac arrest with initial signs of cardiac activity and the arrest witnessed in prehospital or hospital setting within 15 minutes of thoracotomy.[13] In blunt injury, there are varying recommendations for thoracotomy. Previously, it was indicated only in patients with cardiac arrest witnessed after arrival in the hospital. A recent review of thoracotomy outcomes in BCI recommend considering thoracotomy within 15 minutes of cardiac arrest.[14] In both PCI and BCI, a general surgeon must be immediately available for definitive treatment if patient is resuscitated.

An emergency thoracotomy allows for evaluation of hemopericardium, direct control of intrathoracic exsanguination and open cardiac massage. Cross-clamping of the descending aorta slows abdominal blood loss, and it increases perfusion to the brain and heart.

Pericardiocentesis

Emergency pericardiocentesis is indicated for patients in shock with pericardial effusion identified on ultrasound and operative thoracostomy is not immediately available.[15] It should be performed with ultrasound guidance, and as much pericardial fluid should be evacuated as possible. A temporary catheter can be left in place for periodic drainage until definitive operative treatment is available.

CONCLUSION

Cardiac injury is a significant cause of mortality in trauma patients, and its diagnosis and treatment are challenging for physicians. The primary goal in evaluation of traumatic cardiac injury is early identification and management. Hemodynamically unstable patients are most commonly in hypovolemic or obstructive shock. They require immediate resuscitation, evaluation with bedside ultrasound and prompt consultation for definitive surgical care.

The spectrum of BCI is wide, and is summarized in table 3. In stable patients, structural and electrical injuries from BCI can be screened in the ED with an ECG and cardiac troponin. Any abnormalities warrant admission and further evaluation and monitoring; however, most pathologies are managed conservatively.

Penetrating injuries from gunshot wounds lead to higher rates of mortality compared to stab wounds. When identified in the ED, PCI warrants admission and nearly all cases require operative management. Emergency thoracotomy and pericardiocentesis both have limited indications but can be life-saving in critically injured patients with BCI or PCI.

TABLE 3: Types of blunt cardiac and great vessel injury

Blunt cardiac injury	Diagnosis	Treatment
Cardiac contusion, intramural hematomas	Electrocardiogram, echocardiogram, troponin	Conservative management
Valvular injury, septal rupture	Murmur, echocardiogram	Surgical depending on clinical scenario
Coronary artery injury	Electrocardiogram, troponin	Surgical or percutaneous evaluation
Aortic tear	Echocardiogram, computed tomography	Surgical depending on clinical scenario
Commotio cordis	Electrocardiogram	Early resuscitation and defibrillation
Supraventricular tachycardias	Electrocardiogram	Cardioversion
Conduction abnormalities	Electrocardiogram	Conservative management, placement of pacemaker depending on scenario

The literature on the evaluation and management of BCI and PCI continues to evolve. More research and education is needed to address the high mortality rate in the prehospital, ED and hospital settings.

REFERENCES

1. Nance ML. National Trauma Data Bank 2013 Annual Report. Chicago, IL: American College of Surgeons; 2014.
2. Teixeria PG, Ceorgiou C, Inaha K, Dubose J, Plurad D, Chan L, et al. Blunt cardiac trauma: lessons learned from the medical examiner. J Trauma. 2009;67(6):1259-64.
3. Navid F, Gleason TG. Great vessel and cardiac trauma: diagnostic and management strategies. Semin Thorac Cardiovasc Surg. 2008;20(1):31-8.
4. Yousef R, Carr JA. Blunt cardiac trauma: a review of the current knowledge and management. Ann Thorac Surg. 2014;98(3):1134-40.
5. El-Chami MF, Nicholson W, Helmy T. Blunt cardiac trauma. J Emerg Med. 2008;35(2):127-33.
6. Clancy K, Velopulos C, Bilaniuk JW, Collier B, Crowley W, Kurek S, et al. Screening for blunt cardiac injury: an Eastern Association for the Surgery of Trauma practice management guideline. J Trauma Acute Care Surg. 2012;73 (5 Suppl 4):S301-6.
7. Rajan G, Zellweger R. Cardiac troponin I as a predictor of arrhythmia and ventricular dysfunction in trauma patients with myocardial contusion. J Trauma. 2004;57(4):801-8.
8. Mandavia D, Joseph A. Bedside echocardiography in chest trauma. Emerg Med Clin North Am. 2004;22(3):601-19.
9. Restrepo CS, Gutierrez FR, Marmol-Velez JA, Ocazionez D, Martinez-Jimenez S. Imaging patients with cardiac trauma. Radiographics. 2012; 32(3):633-49.
10. Pereira BM, Nogueira VB, Calderan TR, Villaca MP, Pertrucci O, Fraga GP. Penetrating cardiac trauma: 20-y experience from a university teaching hospital. J Surg Res. 2013;183(2):792-7.
11. Ball CG, Williams BH, Wyrzykowski AD, Nicholas JM, Rozycki GS, Felciano DV. A caveat to the performance of pericardial ultrasound in patients with penetrating cardiac wounds. J Trauma. 2009;67(5):1123-4.
12. Talving P, Demetriades D. Cardiac trauma during teenage years. Pediatr Clin North Am. 2014;61(1):111-30.
13. Fairfax LM, Hsee L, Civil ID. Resuscitative thoracotomy in penetrating trauma. World J Surg. 2015;39(6):1343-51.
14. Slessor D, Huntor S. To be blunt: are we wasting our time? Emergency department thoracotomy following blunt trauma: a systematic review and meta-analysis. Ann Emerg Med. 2015;65(3):297-307.
15. Lee TH, Ouellet JF, Cook M, Schreiber MA, Kortbeek JB. Pericardiocentesis in trauma: a systematic review. J Trauma Acute Care Surg. 2013;75(4): 543-9.

SECTION 4

Arrhythmias

28 CHAPTER

Atrial Fibrillation and Atrial Flutter

David E Krummen, Amir A Schricker

INTRODUCTION

Atrial fibrillation (AF) and atrial flutter (AFL) are frequently encountered in clinical practice, resulting in approximately 600,000 emergency department (ED) visits in North America annually.[1] Symptoms from AF vary widely, from debilitating palpitations, chest pain, and shortness of breath to asymptomatic patients who present with stroke as the first manifestation of AF or AFL. Because of the high frequency of these arrhythmias in patients seeking medical attention, a comprehensive understanding of their management strategies is essential for healthcare providers.

The purpose of this chapter is to review the epidemiology, presentation, diagnosis, and management of AF and AFL according to current guidelines.[2,3] Additionally, the special situations of AF in heart failure and AF in patients with accessory pathways are discussed. In general, care of the patient with AF is governed by the following three principles: (i) prevention of thromboembolism; (ii) appropriate heart rate control; and (iii) maintenance of sinus rhythm if significant symptoms are still present after achieving adequate rate control. Importantly, improvements in atrial arrhythmia care have demonstrated significant reductions in morbidity and mortality over time,[4] and significant improvements in quality of life[5] for affected patients.

EPIDEMIOLOGY

Atrial fibrillation is the most common sustained arrhythmia,[6] occurring in approximately 1% of the population and increasing steadily with age.[7] The risk of AF reaches almost 10% in patients over the age of 80 years. Atrial fibrillation is uncommon in childhood but increases to approximately 6% in those older than 65 years. Atrial flutter occurs somewhat less frequently,[8] and may occur separately or in conjunction with AF. The true prevalence of AF and AFL, however, is unknown as they are often asymptomatic;[9,10] recent work using implantable loop recorders (ILRs) in patients with cryptogenic stroke and no prior diagnosis of atrial arrhythmias reveals AF in approximately 12% at 1 year.[11] In addition to stroke, AF and AFL are associated with increased risks of heart failure, hospitalization, dementia,[12] and mortality.[13,14]

Risk factors for AF include transient reversible causes, chronic medical conditions, and underlying heart disease. Transient causes include thyrotoxicosis,[15] excessive alcohol ingestion,[16] acute myocardial infarction (MI), recent cardiac surgery, pericarditis, and pulmonary disease. Specifically, during acute MI, AF and AFL may occur in up to 10% of patients,[17] and in postcardiac surgery patients up to 50%. Chronic medical conditions, such as advanced age, hypertension, and obesity are well-established risk factors for AF. Increasingly, obstructive sleep apnea is also recognized as an independent risk factor.[5] Underlying heart disease conditions such as ischemic heart disease, congestive heart failure (CHF),[18] and valvular disease are also significant contributors to arrhythmia development.

Atrial flutter risk factors are similar to those for AF with the exception that patients recently undergoing left atrial AF ablation[19] or surgery are at greater risk for AFL.

Several groups have attempted to develop risk scores to predict an individual's risk of developing AF. A recent study incorporates age, sex, blood pressure, treatment for hypertension, PR interval, cardiac murmur, body mass index, and heart failure.[20] Further work integrates serum biomarkers including B-type natriuretic peptide (BNP) and C-reactive protein (CRP) to improve upon clinical characteristics.[21] Still others have found correlations between biomarkers of atrial fibrosis such as galectin-3[22] or biomarker assessment of the extracellular matrix [tissue inhibitor of matrix metalloproteinase (TIMP)][23] and AF incidence. However, such markers are not routinely used clinically due to suboptimal sensitivity and specificity.

CLASSIFICATION OF ATRIAL FLUTTER AND ATRIAL FIBRILLATION

Current guidelines propose the following classification scheme for AF:[2]

- Paroxysmal AF: Recurrent AF episodes that terminate spontaneously or with intervention within 7 days

- Persistent AF: Characterized as AF with episodes that last longer than 7 days
- Long-standing persistent AF: Refers to AF that has lasted for more than 12 months
- Permanent AF: Used to describe AF when a joint decision is made by the patient and physician to cease further attempts to restore and/or maintain sinus rhythm
- Nonvalvular AF: Refers to AF in the absence of rheumatic mitral stenosis, a mechanical or bioprosthetic heart valve, or mitral valve repair.

This classification scheme applies to recurrent episodes of AF lasting more than 30 seconds that are unrelated to reversible causes.

Atrial flutter is classified by the anatomic location of the macroreentrant circuit:[3]

- Typical AFL: A reentrant circuit in the right atrium that passes through (and is dependent upon) the cavotricuspid isthmus (CTI), usually in a counterclockwise direction; clockwise rotation is also seen ("reverse typical AFL"). Classically, typical flutter activity manifests on the electrocardiogram (ECG) as sawtooth waves in the inferior leads (i.e., lead II, III, and aVF) and/or V1 (Fig. 1)
- Atypical AFL: A reentrant circuit that does not depend upon the CTI and can occur in either atrium; a sawtooth pattern in the inferior leads is usually not observed in atypical AFL.

CLINICAL PRESENTATION

Up to 90% of paroxysmal atrial tachyarrhythmia episodes may be asymptomatic, even with rapid heart rates. A significant proportion of patients with asymptomatic arrhythmia may present with stroke as their first symptom.[11] Symptoms due to AF and AFL vary and are often due to the degree of heart rate elevation. Common symptoms include palpitations, tachycardia, shortness of breath, weakness and fatigue. Less commonly patients may present with chest pain or syncope. Sometimes the only symptom may be heart rate irregularity, detected by a home blood pressure machine[24] or by consumer devices.[25]

CLINICAL EVALUATION

History and Physical Examination

A complete history and physical examination is an essential part of the workup of patients with AF and AFL. Important aspects of the patient's history include the timeline of symptoms, frequency duration and severity of episodes, and precipitating factors. Additionally, a detailed history of the patient's past medical problems, including CHF, hypertension, diabetes, history of stroke, and presence of ischemic cardiac or peripheral vascular disease are important for decisions regarding anticoagulation.[2]

A comprehensive physical examination, including a detailed cardiac examination, should be performed in all patients. First, vital signs should be assessed to determine hemodynamic stability. Cardiac examination during AF will often reveal an irregular ventricular rate; however, in patients with pacemakers and atrioventricular (AV) block, the heart rate can be regular.[26] Conversely, AFL is more commonly regular, but may be irregular due to variable AV nodal block.[27] Specific aspects to consider include findings associated with hyperthyroidism[15] and the presence of valvular disease. Additionally, evidence for CHF, such as distended neck veins or pulmonary edema, should be evaluated during physical examination to guide potential diuresis.

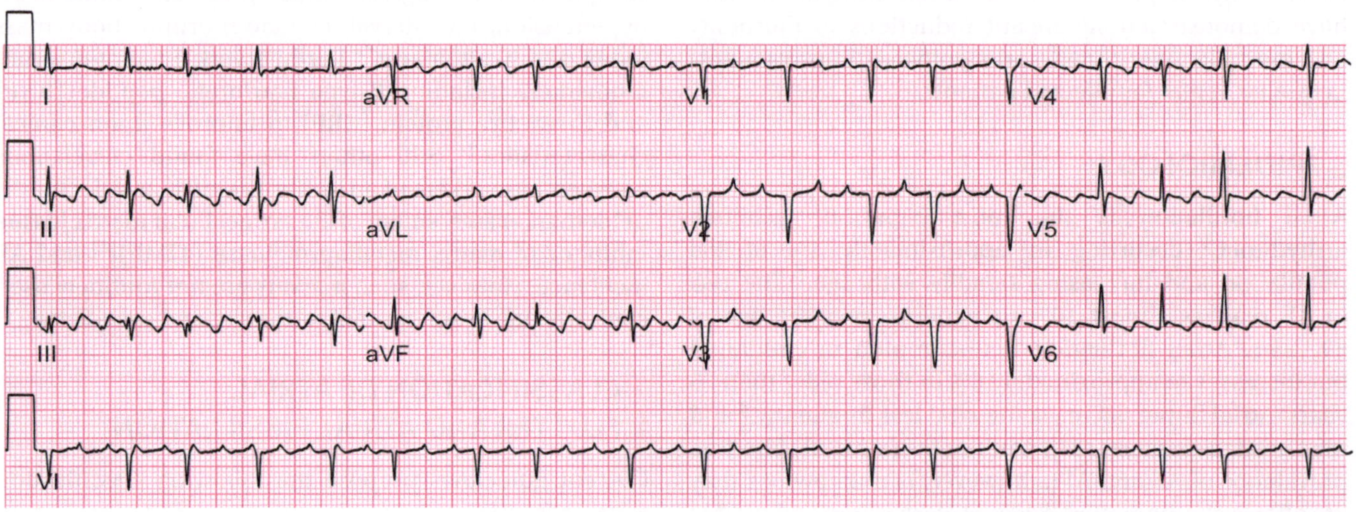

FIG. 1: Electrocardiogram (ECG) of typical atrial flutter. The ECG shows sawtooth flutter waves in leads II, III, and aVF. Note the presence of variable atrioventricular nodal block

Laboratory Tests

Laboratory testing should be performed to assess for electrolyte abnormalities, renal dysfunction, thyroid abnormalities, and other potentially reversible causes. Tests should include a chemistry panel with renal function, complete blood count, thyroid function panel, and cardiac markers if chest pain is present.

Electrocardiogram

Atrial Fibrillation

The ECG is an essential tool in the diagnosis and management of AF, which is characterized by an absence of clear P waves, a coarse and undulating baseline and an irregularly irregular RR interval. An example ECG showing AF is shown in figure 2. Atrial fibrillation needs to be distinguished from sinus rhythm with frequent premature atrial complexes, multifocal atrial tachycardia, and AFL with variable AV block.

Other important electrocardiographic information includes evidence of current or prior MI, left ventricular hypertrophy, ventricular preexcitation over an accessory pathway [Wolff-Parkinson-White (WPW) syndrome, see later], conduction system disease, electrolyte abnormalities, and evidence for pericarditis.

Atrial Flutter

Typical AFL typically features an organized atrial rate approximately 300 beats/min (range 240–350 beats/min), with a usual ventricular response of 150 beats/min (i.e., during 2:1 AV block) or 75 beats/min (i.e., 4:1 AV block). Occasionally, AFL presents with a varying degree of AV block resulting in an irregularly irregular rhythm, which may be confused with AF.[27] Typical flutter classically manifests on the ECG with sawtooth waves in the inferior leads (i.e., lead II, III, and aVF; Fig. 1). However, this is not universal. In contrast, atypical AFL typically does not exhibit classic sawtooth waves and may require alternative methods, such as invasive electrophysiology study, for definitive diagnosis.[26]

Echocardiogram

A transthoracic echocardiogram is routinely performed to assess for structural disease such as scar from prior MI or significant left ventricular hypertrophy as these are contraindications to class I[28,29] and class III[2] anti-arrhythmics, respectively. Additionally, a transesophageal echocardiogram (TEE) may be necessary to assess for a left atrial appendage thrombus if cardioversion is considered.

TREATMENT: ATRIAL FIBRILLATION

The treatment of a hemodynamically unstable patient is immediate direct-current (DC) cardioversion. For others, the central goals of AF and AFL management are the initiation of appropriate anticoagulation for prevention of systemic embolization, control of ventricular heart rate and restoring sinus rhythm, if symptoms are present once rate control has been achieved.

Anticoagulation

All patients, regardless of management strategy, require protection from systemic embolization. Current guidelines[2,3] recommend the use of the CHA_2DS_2-VASc scoring system in patients with AF or AFL to assess the risk of systemic embolization (Table 1).

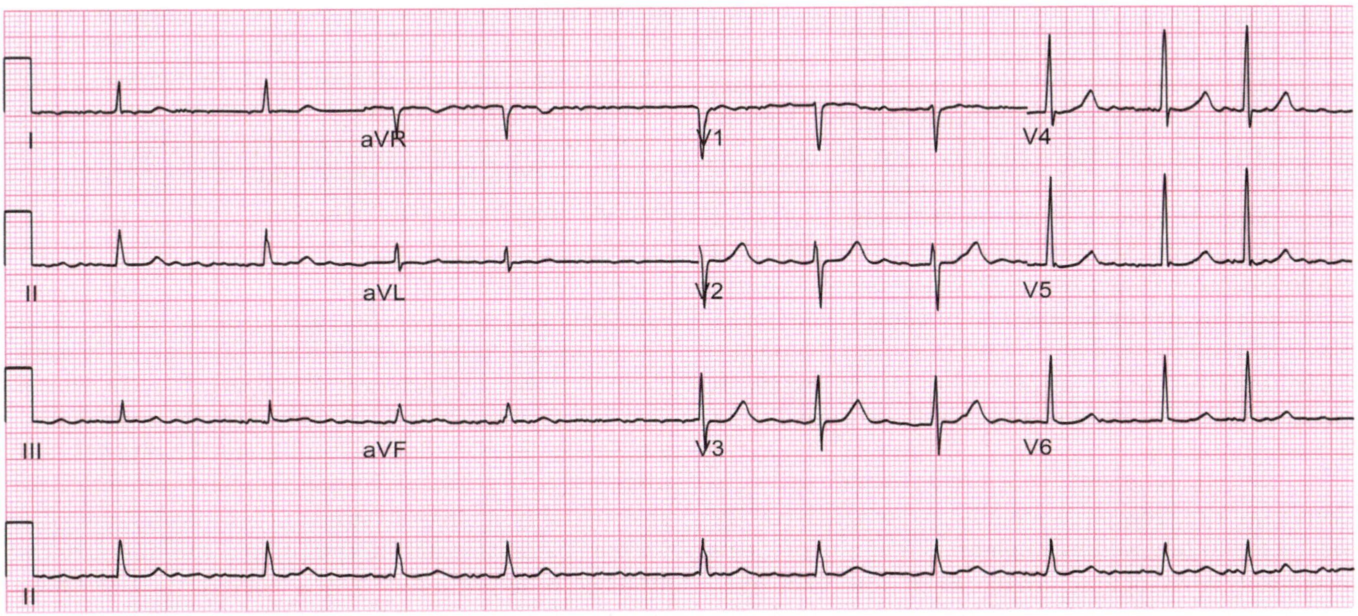

FIG. 2: 12-lead electrocardiogram with rhythm strip of atrial fibrillation. Note the lack of P-waves and irregularly irregular rhythm

TABLE 1: Components of the CHA_2DS_2-VASc scoring system[2]

	Condition	Points
C	Congestive heart failure (or left ventricular systolic dysfunction)	1
H	Hypertension, or treated hypertension on medications	1
A_2	Age ≥75 years	2
D	Diabetes mellitus	1
S_2	Prior stroke or TIA	2
V	Vascular disease (e.g., peripheral artery disease)	1
A	Age 65–74 years	1
Sc	Sex category (i.e., female gender)	1

TIA; transient ischemic attack.

Patients whose CHA_2DS_2-VASc score is 2 or more require long-term oral anticoagulation. Traditionally, oral anticoagulation consisted of treatment with the vitamin K antagonist warfarin [with a goal international normalized ratio (INR) of 2.0–3.0]. More recently, newer agents have been introduced and include direct thrombin inhibitors, such as dabigatran,[30] and factor Xa inhibitors, such as rivaroxaban,[31] apixaban,[32] and edoxaban.[33] Alternatively, left atrial appendage closure devices are now approved for patients who are at high risk of stroke but cannot tolerate oral anticoagulation.[34]

Patients with a score of 0 may be managed with aspirin therapy alone. Patients whose score is 1 may be treated with either aspirin or oral anticoagulation therapy.

Ventricular Rate Control

Prior work has shown that prolonged tachycardia can result in tachycardia-induced cardiomyopathy.[35,36] The second cornerstone of AF and AFL management is to control the heart rate, which has been shown to improve the ejection fraction (EF).[37,38] This may be accomplished with AV nodal blocking agents such as β-blockers or calcium-channel blockers. Digoxin may be used in combination with these agents for additional rate control. Table 2 summarizes rate-control medications.

Results from the Rate Control Versus Electrical Cardioversion II (RACE) II trial[39] have established the initial target heart rate as less than or equal to 110 beats/min. If palpitations and other symptoms from AF or AFL persist, however, more aggressive heart rate control is required; typically targeting a heart rate between 70 and 80 beats/min at rest.

For symptomatic and refractory AF where adequate ventricular rate control is unable to be achieved, AV node ablation followed by implantation of a permanent pacemaker is an option.[2] If the EF is less than 50%, such patients should be considered for a biventricular pacemaker.[40]

TABLE 2: Medications to achieve ventricular rate control in atrial fibrillation[2,38]

	Intravenous doses	Oral maintenance doses
β-blockers		
Metoprolol	2.5–5 mg bolus every 5 min, up to 3 doses	25–100 mg BD (metoprolol succinate ER: 50–200 mg daily)
Esmolol	Bolus: 500 μg/kg Continuous: 50–200 μg/kg/min	N/A
Carvedilol	N/A	3.125–25 mg BD (up to 50 mg BD if >85 kg)
Calcium-channel blockers		
Diltiazem	Bolus: 0.25 mg/kg (average 20 mg) every 5 min Continuous: 5–15 mg/h	120–480 mg daily
Verapamil	0.075–0.15 mg/kg	120–480 mg daily (slow-release available)
Digitalis		
Digoxin	Load: 500 μg, followed every 6 h by 250 μg twice	0.125–0.375 μg daily
Other		
Amiodarone	150 mg over 10 min, then 0.5–1 mg/min	200 mg daily

Restoring and Maintaining Sinus Rhythm

In patients with nonparoxysmal AF, typically at least one attempt to restore sinus rhythm is made.[2] This may be accomplished by achieving therapeutic anticoagulation for 3 weeks and then performing cardioversion. Alternatively, if cardioversion cannot be delayed, a TEE may be performed to rule out a left atrial appendage thrombus, and if a thrombus is not present cardioversion may be performed. Flowchart 1 provides an overview of the cardioversion decision process.

Long-term Management

An important step in the management of AF is to decide upon a long-term treatment strategy. In general, there are two management strategies: (i) rate control and (ii) rhythm control. Notably, several large studies compared the rate and rhythm control strategies, and there was no significant difference in long-arm morbidity and mortality[41,42] between them.

For patients without symptoms, the rate control strategy is appropriate. When significant arrhythmia symptoms are present, a rhythm control strategy improves quality of life.[5] In this strategy, the patient is

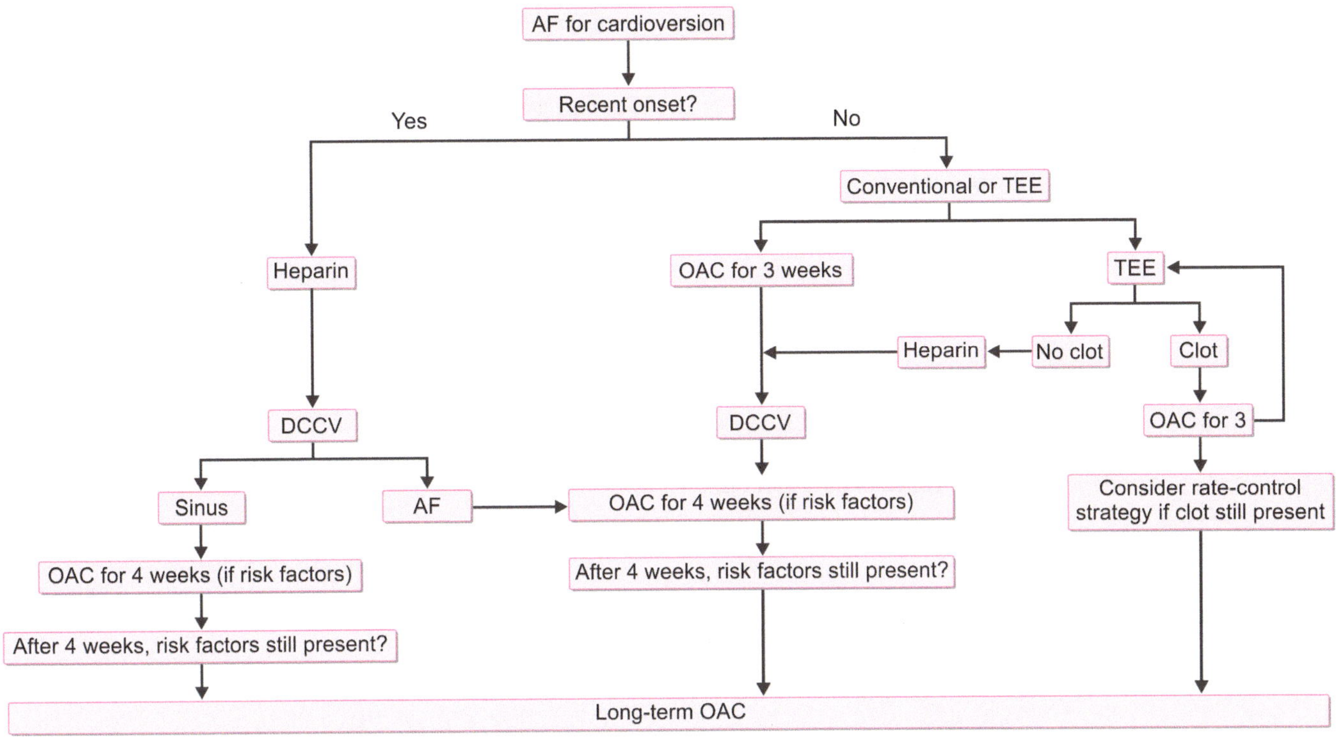

AF, atrial fibrillation; DCCV, direct current cardioversion; OAC, oral anticoagulation; TEE, transesophageal echocardiogram.

FLOWCHART 1: Flowchart to guide cardioversion of hemodynamically stable atrial fibrillation (AF). Recent onset refers to AF of duration less than 48 hours

placed on appropriate anticoagulation and attempts are made to restore and maintain sinus rhythm, either via cardioversion (pharmacologic or direct current) or ablation. Although several older studies have shown no benefit to the rhythm control strategy,[41] more recent studies have shown benefit in younger, healthier patients with significant symptoms.[43] Recent trials have also shown benefits for the rhythm control strategy with ablation in patients with heart failure.[44,45] Rhythm control may involve the following modalities, alone or in combination.

Direct Current Cardioversion

Direct current cardioversion is effective greater than 75% of the time, with increased chances of success depending on the duration of AF and the size of the left atrium. The success rate is approximately 90% when AF duration is less than 1 year, compared to 50% when AF has been present for more than 5 years. As noted earlier, a common strategy involves achieving adequate anticoagulation for 3 weeks prior to cardioversion. An alternative is to perform a TEE prior to cardioversion to verify the absence of left atrial appendage thrombus.

Antiarrhythmic Medications

Antiarrhythmic medications are typically administered by a cardiologist or electrophysiologist, as the side effects and safety profile require close supervision.[46] Some options are described as follows:

- Class IC antiarrhythmic drugs: Therapy with class IC antiarrhythmic agents is associated with increased mortality in patients with underlying cardiovascular disease, as shown in the Cardiac Arrhythmia Suppression Trial (CAST).[47] However, in patients without structural or ischemic heart disease, these agents may be safely used to prevent AF.[2] Most commonly used examples from this antiarrhythmic class include flecainide and propafenone
- Class III antiarrhythmic drugs: The major action of these drugs is to prolong refractoriness in cardiac tissue. Dofetilide may be safely used in patients with ischemic heart disease or CHF; sotalol can be used in patients with coronary artery disease. Significant left ventricular hypertrophy is a contraindication for these antiarrhythmics. During initiation of these medications, patients must be closely monitored, and dofetilide must be administered in hospital for the first six doses to observe for QTc prolongation. Amiodarone is the most effective antiarrhythmic drug and may also be used in patients with ischemic heart disease or heart failure, but also has significant long-term side effects, some of which are irreversible. Dronedarone is the newest of the class III agents; unlike amiodarone and dofetilide, dronedarone is contraindicated in patients with CHF.

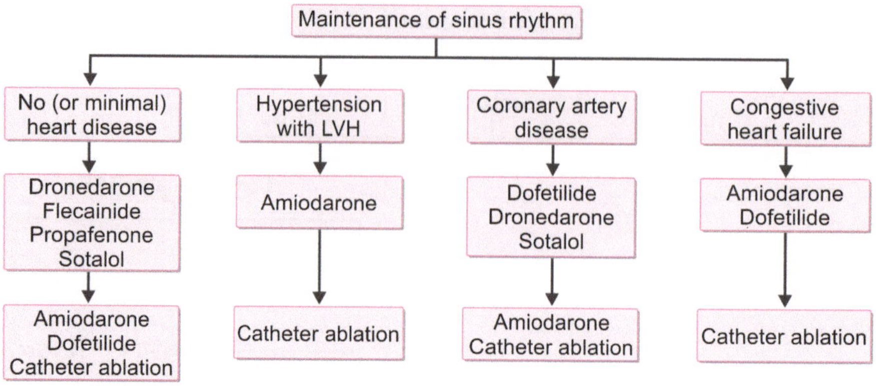

LVH, left ventricular hypertrophy.

FLOWCHART 2: Rhythm control flowchart. Note that antiarrhythmic choice is highly dependent upon concomitant heart disease

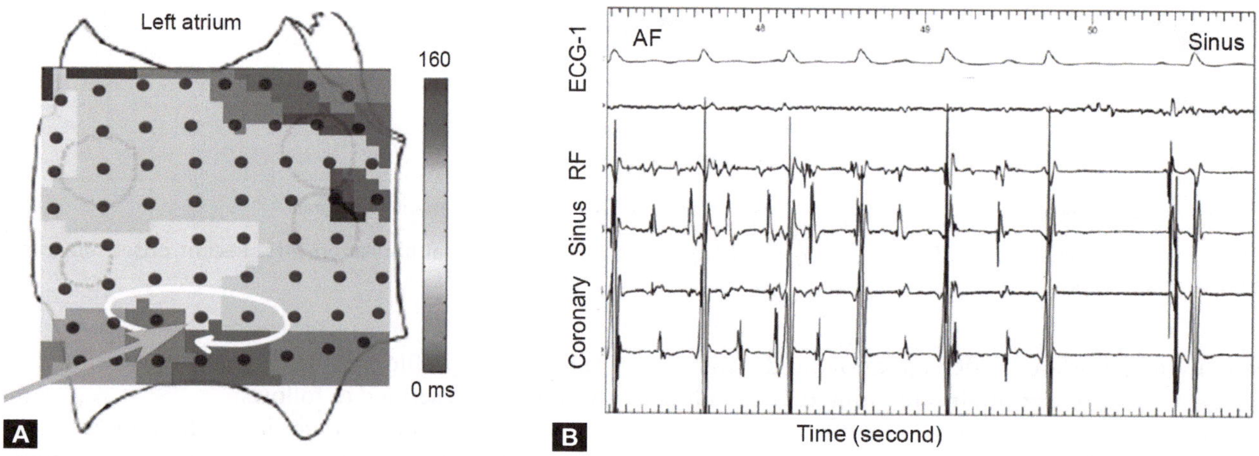

AF, atrial fibrillation; RF, radio frequency; ECG, electrocardiogram.

FIG. 3: Mapping and ablation of localized sources of atrial fibrillation (AF). **A,** Isochronal representation of left atrial electrical activation during AF shows a clockwise rotor (white circular arrow). **B,** Focal ablation at the site indicated by the green arrow terminated AF to sinus rhythm ***(For color version, see Plate 8)***

Although effective, amiodarone is typically avoided for long-term therapy in younger patients when possible due to the risk of irreversible side effects such as pulmonary fibrosis. Instead, class IC and the class III agents dofetilide, sotalol, and dronedarone are used as indicated in flowchart 2.

Catheter Ablation

Ablation is indicated for symptomatic patients who have failed, are not candidates for, or desire to avoid antiarrhythmic drugs. Ablation is most commonly performed by an electrophysiologist, but also may be performed by a cardiothoracic surgeon during concomitant open-heart surgery, such as valve replacement or coronary artery bypass grafting.

The goals of the ablation procedure are to electrically isolate the pulmonary veins, as the pulmonary veins have been identified as the source of AF-triggering ectopy. Additional ablation strategies for patients with recurrent AF include additional linear ablation[48] and complex fractionated atrial activity.[49] Unfortunately, improved outcomes with these approaches were not seen in recent randomized clinical trials.[50,51]

An emerging body of data suggests that localized sources, such as electrical rotors (Fig. 3) and focal drivers, sustain AF and may be successfully targeted to improve ablation success.[52-54] Other groups have shown efficacy with extensive ablation including pulmonary vein isolation, left atrial posterior wall, and additional trigger elimination in patients with nonparoxysmal AF.[55] Additional trials are required to further define the optimal approach to AF ablation.

TREATMENT: ATRIAL FLUTTER

While overall the clinical management of AFL is similar to AF with respect to anticoagulation,[3] differences exist

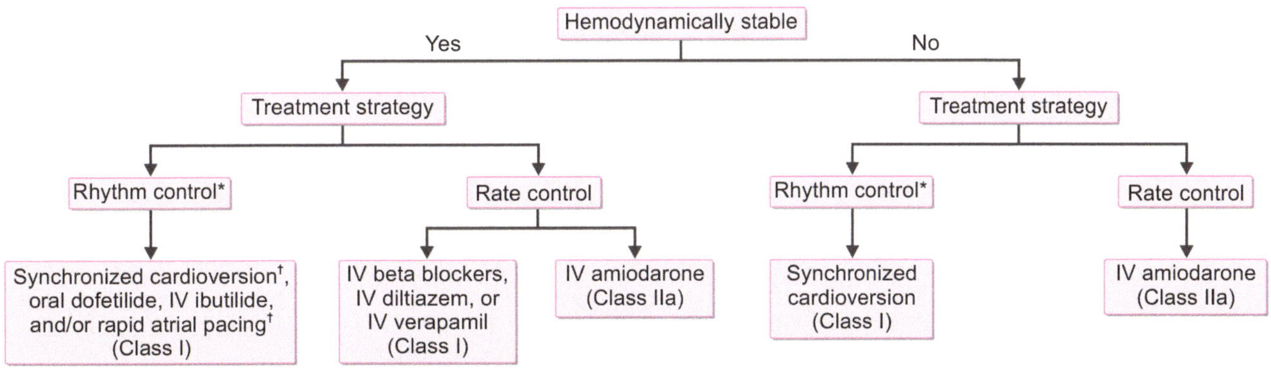

IV, intravenous

*Anticoagulation as per guideline is required.

†For rhythms that break or recur spontaneously, synchronized cardioversion or rapid atrial pacing is not appropriate.

FLOWCHART 3: Acute management of atrial flutter

With permission from: Page RL, Joglar JA, Caldwell MA, Calkins H, Conti JB, Deal BJ, et al. 2015 ACC/AHA/HRS Guideline for the Management of Adult Patients With Supraventricular Tachycardia: A Report of the American College of Cardiology/American Heart Association Task Force on Clinical Practice Guidelines and the Heart Rhythm Society. J Am Coll Cardiol. 2016;67(13):e27-115.

with respect to rate control and rhythm control options both in the acute setting and for long-term management. The acute management of AFL is shown in flowchart 3.

As with AF, unstable patients should be considered for synchronized cardioversion. Alternatively, if the risk of stroke is felt to be excessive (e.g., AFL has been present for >48 hours without anticoagulation), intravenous amiodarone is recommended for acute rate control.

Stable patients with AFL should also be stratified into those who are candidates for rhythm control or rate control. For patients with AFL less than 48 hours without anticoagulation (or any duration of AFL with >3 weeks of oral anticoagulation), rhythm control may be considered. In addition to synchronized cardioversion, therapy with oral dofetilide, intravenous ibutilide or atrial pacing (such as when a pacemaker is present) are first-line therapies for the acute management of AFL.[3] For rate control patients, intravenous β-blockers, diltiazem, or verapamil are the primary options.

For the long-term management of AFL, an important difference for patients with AFL versus AF is that catheter ablation is the first-line therapy for patients in whom rhythm control is desired; antiarrhythmic therapy is second line. This is because trials have shown an excellent success rate and low risk of complications with catheter ablation of typical AFL[56] and atypical AFL[57] using available technologies.

ATRIAL FIBRILLATION, ATRIAL FLUTTER AND HEART FAILURE

Overall, patients with CHF should receive similar care for AF and AFL as patients without CHF.[58] However, there are important stipulations to keep in mind.

- Typically, β-blockers are recommended as first line for rate control, as patients with heart failure require this medication for long-term management. Digoxin should be considered if a second agent is needed
- Antiarrhythmic therapy for CHF patients is predominantly limited to dofetilide[59] and amiodarone. Dofetilide requires inpatient administration, but has a low long-term side effect profile. Amiodarone is effective, but cumulative toxicity and recent reports showing increased hazard with amiodarone therapy[60] limit the long-term appeal of this medication
- Patients who fail medical rate control may be candidates for AV node ablation and biventricular pacing[40]
- Although ablation therapy is less likely to be effective in patients with heart failure, successful ablation may help to improve quality of life and left ventricular function.[44,45]

SPECIAL SITUATION: ATRIAL FIBRILLATION OR ATRIAL FLUTTER AND WOLFF–PARKINSON-WHITE SYNDROME

Occasionally, AF or AFL occurs in conjunction with the WPW syndrome, in which there is an accessory pathway connecting the atria to the ventricles. This condition, also discussed in chapter 32, presents an increased risk of sudden death due to AF rapidly conducting to the ventricles via the accessory pathway leading to a very rapid ventricular rate (Fig. 4).

In summary, unstable patients should receive urgent cardioversion.[3] More stable patients should receive therapy with an antiarrhythmic drug such as intravenous ibutilide[61] or intravenous procainamide, rather than a

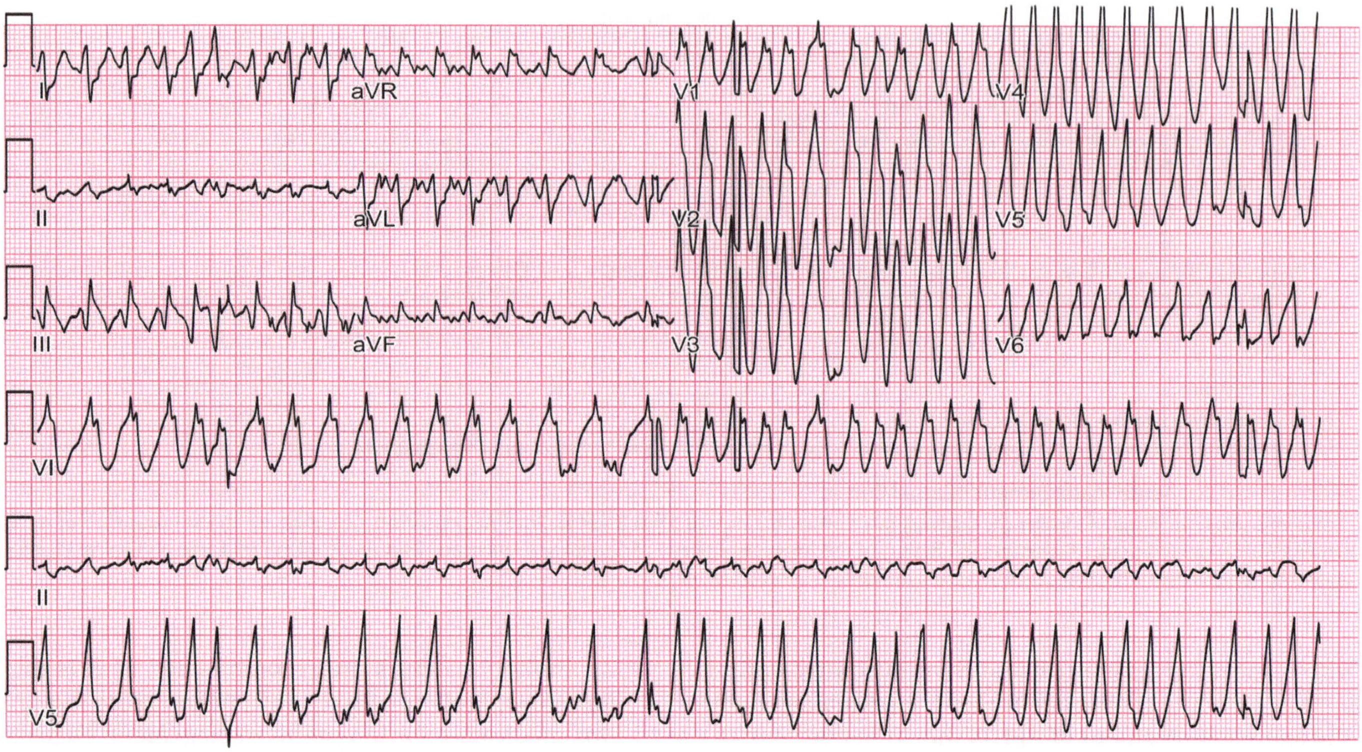

FIG. 4: Atrial fibrillation (AF) with an accessory pathway. The electrocardiogram shows rapid, irregular, and variable excitation of the ventricles during AF with an anterograde-conducting accessory pathway. Following acute management with urgent cardioversion, the patient was referred for successful ablation of a left lateral accessory pathway

pure AV nodal blocking agent, which may paradoxically increase the ventricular rate and lead to ventricular fibrillation. Thereafter, patients should be referred for catheter ablation of the accessory pathway. In patients who are not candidates for ablation, class IC agents may be used in the absence of structural heart disease. Sotalol, dofetilide, or amiodarone may be considered in patients with structural heart disease.[3]

PROGNOSIS

Patient with AF and AFL are at a significantly increased risk of stroke, CHF, and mortality. However, improving AF therapies have decreased morbidity and mortality from these arrhythmias over time.[4] Furthermore, restoration of sinus rhythm improves quality of life in patients with significant symptoms despite adequate rate control.[5] Despite these advances, additional work is required to prevent arrhythmia-related strokes and bleeding complications, to achieve better control heart rate in select patients refractory to standard AV nodal blocking medications, and to improve AF and AFL ablation success rates.

CONCLUSION

In this chapter, an overview of AF and AFL management, focusing on acute management has been presented. A comprehensive discussion of all aspects of current guidelines is beyond the scope of this chapter; for issues not addressed in this work, readers are advised to consult the excellent guidelines by January et al.[2] and Page et al.[3]

REFERENCES

1. Atzema CL, Austin PC, Miller E, Chong AS, Yun L, Dorian P. A population-based description of atrial fibrillation in the emergency department, 2002 to 2010. Ann Emerg Med. 2013;62(6):570-7. e7.
2. January CT, Wann LS, Alpert JS, Calkins H, Cigarroa JE, Cleveland JC, et al. 2014 AHA/ACC/HRS guideline for the management of patients with atrial fibrillation: a report of the American College of Cardiology/American Heart Association Task Force on Practice Guidelines and the Heart Rhythm Society. J Am Coll Cardiol. 2014;64(21):e1-76.
3. Page RL, Joglar JA, Caldwell MA, Calkins H, Conti JB, Deal BJ, et al. 2015 ACC/AHA/HRS Guideline for the Management of Adult Patients With Supraventricular Tachycardia: A Report of the American College of Cardiology/American Heart Association Task Force on Clinical Practice Guidelines and the Heart Rhythm Society. J Am Coll Cardiol. 2016;67(13):e27-115.
4. Schnabel RB, Yin X, Gona P, Larson MG, Beiser AS, McManus DD, et al. 50 year trends in atrial fibrillation prevalence, incidence, risk factors, and mortality in the Framingham Heart Study: a cohort study. Lancet. 2015;386(9989):154-62.
5. Hagens VE, Ranchor AV, Van Sonderen E, Bosker HA, Kamp O, Tijssen JG, et al. Effect of rate or rhythm control on quality of life in persistent atrial fibrillation. Results from the Rate Control Versus Electrical Cardioversion (RACE) Study. J Am Coll Cardiol. 2004;43(2):241-7.
6. Chugh SS, Blackshear JL, Shen WK, Hammill SC, Gersh BJ. Epidemiology and natural history of atrial fibrillation: clinical implications. J Am Coll Cardiol. 2001;37(2):371-8.
7. Go AS, Hylek EM, Phillips KA, Chang Y, Henault LE, Selby JV, et al. Prevalence of diagnosed atrial fibrillation in adults: national implications for rhythm

management and stroke prevention: the AnTicoagulation and Risk Factors in Atrial Fibrillation (ATRIA) Study. JAMA. 2001;285(18):2370-5.
8. Granada J, Uribe W, Chyou PH, Maassen K, Vierkant R, Smith PN, et al. Incidence and predictors of atrial flutter in the general population. J Am Coll Cardiol. 2000;36(7):2242-6.
9. Lim HS, Lip GY. Asymptomatic atrial fibrillation on device interrogation. J Cardiovasc Electrophysiol. 2008;19(8):891-3.
10. Brambatti M, Connolly SJ, Gold MR, Morillo CA, Capucci A, Muto C, et al. Temporal relationship between subclinical atrial fibrillation and embolic events. Circulation. 2014;129(21):2094-9.
11. Sanna T, Diener HC, Passman RS, Di Lazzaro V, Bernstein RA, Morillo CA, et al. Cryptogenic stroke and underlying atrial fibrillation. N Engl J Med. 2014;370(26):2478-86.
12. Miyasaka Y, Barnes ME, Gersh BJ, Cha SS, Bailey KR, Abhayaratna WP, et al. Secular trends in incidence of atrial fibrillation in Olmsted County, Minnesota, 1980 to 2000, and implications on the projections for future prevalence. Circulation. 2006;114(2):119-25.
13. Crandall MA, Horne BD, Day JD, Anderson JL, Muhlestein JB, Crandall BG, et al. Atrial fibrillation significantly increases total mortality and stroke risk beyond that conveyed by the CHADS2 risk factors. Pacing Clin Electrophysiol. 2009;32(8):981-6.
14. Mamas MA, Caldwell JC, Chacko S, Garratt CJ, Fath-Ordoubadi F, Neyses L. A meta-analysis of the prognostic significance of atrial fibrillation in chronic heart failure. Eur J Heart Fail. 2009;11(7):676-83.
15. Forfar JC, Miller HC, Toft AD. Occult thyrotoxicosis: a correctable cause of "idiopathic" atrial fibrillation. Am J Cardiol. 1979;44(1):9-12.
16. Ettinger PO, Wu CF, De La Cruz C, Weisse AB, Ahmed SS, Regan TJ. Arrhythmias and the "Holiday Heart": alcohol-associated cardiac rhythm disorders. Am Heart J. 1978;95(5):555-62.
17. Liberthson RR, Salisbury KW, Hutter AM, DeSanctis RW. Atrial tachyarrhythmias in acute myocardial infarction. Am J Med. 1976;60(7):956-60.
18. Wang TJ, Larson MG, Levy D, Vasan RS, Leip EP, Wolf PA, et al. Temporal relations of atrial fibrillation and congestive heart failure and their joint influence on mortality: the Framingham Heart Study. Circulation. 2003;107(23):2920-5.
19. Gerstenfeld EP, Callans DJ, Sauer W, Jacobson J, Marchlinski FE. Reentrant and nonreentrant focal left atrial tachycardias occur after pulmonary vein isolation. Heart Rhythm. 2005;2(11):1195-202.
20. Schnabel RB, Sullivan LM, Levy D, Pencina MJ, Massaro JM, D'Agostino RB, et al. Development of a risk score for atrial fibrillation (Framingham Heart Study): a community-based cohort study. Lancet. 2009;373(9665):739-45.
21. Schnabel RB, Larson MG, Yamamoto JF, Sullivan LM, Pencina MJ, Meigs JB, et al. Relations of biomarkers of distinct pathophysiological pathways and atrial fibrillation incidence in the community. Circulation. 2010;121(2):200-7.
22. Ho JE, Yin X, Levy D, Vasan RS, Magnani JW, Ellinor PT, et al. Galectin 3 and incident atrial fibrillation in the community. Am Heart J. 2014;167(5):729-34.e1.
23. Kalogeropoulos AS, Tsiodras S, Rigopoulos AG, Sakadakis EA, Triantafyllis A, Kremastinos DT, et al. Novel association patterns of cardiac remodeling markers in patients with essential hypertension and atrial fibrillation. BMC Cardiovasc Disord. 2011;11:77.
24. Wiesel J, Fitzig L, Herschman Y, Messineo FC. Detection of atrial fibrillation using a modified microlife blood pressure monitor. Am J Hypertens. 2009;22(8): 848-52.
25. McManus DD, Lee J, Maitas O, Esa N, Pidikiti R, Carlucci A, et al. A novel application for the detection of an irregular pulse using an iPhone 4S in patients with atrial fibrillation. Heart Rhythm. 2013;10(3):315-9.
26. Krummen DE, Patel M, Nguyen H, Ho G, Kazi DS, Clopton P, et al. Accurate ECG diagnosis of atrial tachyarrhythmias using quantitative analysis: A prospective diagnostic and cost-effectiveness study. J Cardiovasc Electrophysiol. 2010; 21(11):1251-9.
27. Krummen DE, Feld GK, Narayan SM. Diagnostic accuracy of irregularly irregular RR intervals in separating atrial fibrillation from atrial flutter. Am J Cardiol. 2006;98(9):209-14.
28. Echt DS, Liebson PR, Mitchell LB, Peters RW, Obias-Manno D, Barker AH, et al. Mortality and morbidity in patients receiving encainide, flecainide, or placebo. The Cardiac Arrhythmia Suppression Trial. N Engl J Med. 1991;324(12):781-8.
29. Anderson JL, Platia EV, Hallstrom A, Henthorn RW, Buckingham TA, Carlson MD, et al. Interaction of baseline characteristics with the hazard of encainide, flecainide, and moricizine therapy in patients with myocardial infarction. A possible explanation for increased mortality in the Cardiac Arrhythmia Suppression Trial (CAST). Circulation. 1994;90(6): 2843-52.
30. Connolly SJ, Ezekowitz MD, Yusuf S, Eikelboom J, Oldgren J, Parekh A, et al. Dabigatran versus warfarin in patients with atrial fibrillation. N Engl J Med. 2009;361(12):1139-51.
31. Patel MR, Mahaffey KW, Garg J, Pan G, Singer DE, Hacke W, et al. Rivaroxaban versus warfarin in nonvalvular atrial fibrillation. N Engl J Med. 2011;365(10):883-91.
32. Granger CB, Alexander JH, McMurray JJ, Lopes RD, Hylek EM, Hanna M, et al. Apixaban versus warfarin in patients with atrial fibrillation. N Engl J Med. 2011;365(11):981-92.
33. Giugliano RP, Ruff CT, Braunwald E, Murphy SA, Wiviott SD, Halperin JL, et al. Edoxaban versus warfarin in patients with atrial fibrillation. N Engl J Med. 2013;369(22):2093-104.
34. Reddy VY, Sievert H, Halperin J, Doshi SK, Buchbinder M, Neuzil P, et al. Percutaneous left atrial appendage closure vs warfarin for atrial fibrillation: a randomized clinical trial. JAMA. 2014;312(19):1988-98.
35. Luchsinger JA, Steinberg JS. Resolution of cardiomyopathy after ablation of atrial flutter. J Am Coll Cardiol. 1998;32(1):205-10.
36. Redfield MM, Kay GN, Jenkins LS, Mianulli M, Jensen DN, Ellenbogen KA. Tachycardia-related cardiomyopathy: a common cause of ventricular dysfunction in patients with atrial fibrillation referred for atrioventricular ablation. Mayo Clin Proc. 2000;75(8):790-5.
37. Joglar JA, Acusta AP, Shusterman NH, Ramaswamy K, Kowal RC, Barbera SJ, et al. Effect of carvedilol on survival and hemodynamics in patients with atrial fibrillation and left ventricular dysfunction: retrospective analysis of the US Carvedilol Heart Failure Trials Program. Am Heart J. 2001;142(3):498-501.
38. Camm AJ, Kirchhof P, Lip GY, Schotten U, Savelieva I, Ernst S, et al. Guidelines for the management of atrial fibrillation: the Task Force for the Management of Atrial Fibrillation of the European Society of Cardiology (ESC). Eur Heart J. 2010;31(19):2369-429.
39. Van Gelder IC, Groenveld HF, Crijns HJ, Tuininga YS, Tijssen JG, Alings AM, et al. Lenient versus strict rate control in patients with atrial fibrillation. N Engl J Med. 2010;362(15):1363-73.
40. Curtis AB, Worley SJ, Adamson PB, Chung ES, Niazi I, Sherfesee L, et al. Biventricular pacing for atrioventricular block and systolic dysfunction. N Engl J Med. 2013;368(17):1585-93.
41. Wyse DG, Waldo AL, DiMarco JP, Domanski MJ, Rosenberg Y, Schron EB, et al. A comparison of rate control and rhythm control in patients with atrial fibrillation. N Engl J Med. 2002;347(23):1825-33.
42. Van Gelder IC, Hagens VE, Bosker HA, Kingma JH, Kamp O, Kingma T, et al. A comparison of rate control and rhythm control in patients with recurrent persistent atrial fibrillation. N Engl J Med. 2002;347(23):1834-40.
43. Ogawa S, Yamashita T, Yamazaki T, Aizawa Y, Atarashi H, Inoue H, et al. Optimal treatment strategy for patients with paroxysmal atrial fibrillation: J-RHYTHM Study. Circ J. 2009;73(2):242-8.
44. Jones DG, Haldar SK, Hussain W, Sharma R, Francis DP, Rahman-Haley SL, et al. A randomized trial to assess catheter ablation versus rate control in the management of persistent atrial fibrillation in heart failure. J Am Coll Cardiol. 2013;61(18):1894-903.
45. Hunter RJ, Berriman TJ, Diab I, Kamdar R, Richmond L, Baker V, et al. A randomized controlled trial of catheter ablation versus medical treatment of atrial fibrillation in heart failure (the CAMTAF trial). Circ Arrhythm Electrophysiol. 2014;7(1):31-8.
46. Goodman LS, Brunton LL, Chabner B, Knollmann BC. Goodman & Gilman's Pharmacological Basis of Therapeutics, 12th edition. New York: McGraw-Hill; 2011.
47. Pratt CM, Moye LA. The cardiac arrhythmia suppression trial. Casting suppression in a different light. Circulation. 1995;91(1):245-7.
48. Pappone C, Rosanio S, Oreto G, Tocchi M, Gugliotta F, Vicedomini G, et al. Circumferential radiofrequency ablation of pulmonary vein ostia: A new anatomic approach for curing atrial fibrillation. Circulation. 2000;102(21): 2619-28.
49. Nademanee K, McKenzie J, Kosar E, Schwab M, Sunsaneewitayakul B, Vasavakul T, et al. A new approach for catheter ablation of atrial fibrillation: mapping of the electrophysiologic substrate. J Am Coll Cardiol. 2004;43(11):2044-53.
50. Verma A, Jiang CY, Betts TR, Chen J, Deisenhofer I, Mantovan R, et al. Approaches to catheter ablation for persistent atrial fibrillation. N Engl J Med. 2015;372(19):1812-22.

51. Wong KC, Paisey JR, Sopher M, Balasubramaniam R, Jones M, Qureshi N, et al. No Benefit of Complex Fractionated Atrial Electrogram Ablation in Addition to Circumferential Pulmonary Vein Ablation and Linear Ablation: Benefit of Complex Ablation Study. Circ Arrhythm Electrophysiol. 2015;8(6): 1316-24.
52. Narayan SM, Krummen DE, Shivkumar K, Clopton P, Rappel WJ, Miller JM. Treatment of Atrial Fibrillation by the Ablation of Localized Sources: CONFIRM (Conventional Ablation for Atrial Fibrillation With or Without Focal Impulse and Rotor Modulation) Trial. J Am Coll Cardiol. 2012;60(7):628-36.
53. Miller JM, Kowal RC, Swarup V, Daubert JP, Daoud EG, Day JD, et al. Initial independent outcomes from focal impulse and rotor modulation ablation for atrial fibrillation: multicenter FIRM registry. J Cardiovasc Electrophysiol. 2014;25(9):921-9.
54. Tomassoni G, Duggal S, Muir M, Hutchins L, Turner K, McLoney AM, et al. Long-term Follow-up of FIRM-guided Ablation of Atrial Fibrillation: A Single-center Experience. J Innov Card Rhythm Manag. 2015;6:2145-51.
55. Pump A, Di Biase L, Price J, Mohanty P, Bai R, Santangeli P, et al. Efficacy of catheter ablation in nonparoxysmal atrial fibrillation patients with severe enlarged left atrium and its impact on left atrial structural remodeling. J Cardiovas Electrophysiol. 2013;24(11):1224-31.
56. Feld G, Wharton M, Plumb V, Daoud E, Friehling T, Epstein L. Radiofrequency catheter ablation of type 1 atrial flutter using large-tip 8- or 10-mm electrode catheters and a high-output radiofrequency energy generator: results of a multicenter safety and efficacy study. J Am Coll Cardiol. 2004;43(8):1466-72.
57. Bai R, Fahmy TS, Patel D, Di Biase L, Riedlbauchova L, Wazni OM, et al. Radiofrequency ablation of atypical atrial flutter after cardiac surgery or atrial fibrillation ablation: a randomized comparison of open-irrigation-tip and 8-mm-tip catheters. Heart Rhythm. 2007;4(12):1489-96.
58. Roy D, Talajic M, Nattel S, Wyse DG, Dorian P, Lee KL, et al. Rhythm control versus rate control for atrial fibrillation and heart failure. N Engl J Med. 2008;358(25):2667-77.
59. Torp-Pedersen C, Moller M, Bloch-Thomsen PE, Køber L, Sandøe E, Egstrup K, et al. Dofetilide in patients with congestive heart failure and left ventricular dysfunction. Danish Investigations of Arrhythmia and Mortality on Dofetilide Study Group. N Engl J Med. 1999;341(12):857-65.
60. Saksena S, Slee A, Waldo AL, Freemantle N, Reynolds M, Rosenberg Y, et al. Cardiovascular outcomes in the AFFIRM Trial (Atrial Fibrillation Follow-Up Investigation of Rhythm Management). An assessment of individual antiarrhythmic drug therapies compared with rate control with propensity score-matched analyses. J Am Coll Cardiol. 2011;58(19):1975-85.
61. Glatter KA, Dorostkar PC, Yang Y, Lee RJ, Van Hare GF, Keung E, et al. Electrophysiological effects of ibutilide in patients with accessory pathways. Circulation. 2001;104(16):1933-9.

29 CHAPTER

Ventricular Tachycardia and Ventricular Fibrillation

David E Krummen, Gautam G Lalan, Amir A Schricker

INTRODUCTION

Ventricular tachycardia (VT) and ventricular fibrillation (VF) are common life-threatening ventricular arrhythmias accounting for approximately 4.25 million deaths worldwide annually.[1] Patients with ventricular arrhythmias are commonly unstable with a high risk of severe morbidity and mortality; rapid identification and intervention are important to their management. Therefore, a comprehensive understanding of the evaluation and management of these arrhythmias is essential for practitioners in the acute care setting. The purpose of this chapter is to review the diagnosis, evaluation, initial treatment, and long-term management of patients with ventricular arrhythmias according to recent studies and society guidelines.[1-3]

EPIDEMIOLOGY

Several factors have been identified which significantly increase an individual's risk of ventricular arrhythmias. Demographic characteristics include male sex and advanced age; for males the incidence of sudden cardiac death (SCD) is 6.88 per 1,00,000 patient-years compared with 1.40 per 100,000 patient-years in females.[4] Increasing age is also associated with SCD, predominantly due to greater incidence of coronary heart disease (CHD) and heart failure. Although generally low, recent work has found that the rate of cardiac arrest for patients under age 35 is higher than previously estimated at 2.28 per 100,000 patients-years.[5]

In older patients, ventricular arrhythmias are predominantly seen in association with CHD,[6,7] congestive heart failure,[8] and infiltrative diseases such as sarcoidosis. In younger populations, inherited conditions predominate; such conditions can be divided into those with structurally normal hearts and those associated with structural heart disease. Conditions associated with structurally normal hearts include channelopathies such as long QT syndrome (LQTS),[9] short QT syndrome, Brugada syndrome, and catecholaminergic polymorphic VT (CPVT). Inherited conditions associated with structural heart disease include hypertrophic cardiomyopathy (HCM),[10] lamin A/C dilated cardiomyopathy,[11] and arrhythmic right ventricular cardiomyopathy (ARVC). Despite significant advances, however, the majority of arrhythmias occur in patients not identified by current criteria.[12]

CLINICAL PRESENTATION

The presentation of VT and VF can vary from resuscitated sudden death and highly symptomatic conscious patients to individuals with mild-to-moderate symptoms in the setting of slower VT or a ventricular arrhythmia and left ventricular assist device.[13] Symptoms depend upon tachycardia rate, duration, and extent of structural or ischemic heart disease. Episodes can be nonsustained VT (NSVT; <30 s), sustained with hemodynamic stability, or unstable potentially resulting in severe palpitations, chest pain, syncope, and arrest. Electrical storm, defined as three or more episodes of VT occurring within 24 hours, is a severe presentation of VT with a poor prognosis.[14]

CLINICAL EVALUATION

History and Physical Examination

Workup for patients with VT and VF is presented in flowchart 1.

Central to this workup is a thorough history and physical examination. Important elements of the history include the presence of chest pain, chest pressure, arm or jaw pain, nausea, or shortness of breath suggesting ischemia. Such patients should be evaluated for myocardial ischemia and undergo revascularization, if possible. Other important elements of the history include precipitating factors and severity of symptoms—particularly symptoms suggesting hemodynamic instability such as syncope or presyncope.

Pertinent past medical problems include history of coronary heart disease or prior myocardial infarction, prior cardiac procedures or surgery, congestive heart failure, and associated risk factors such as hypertension

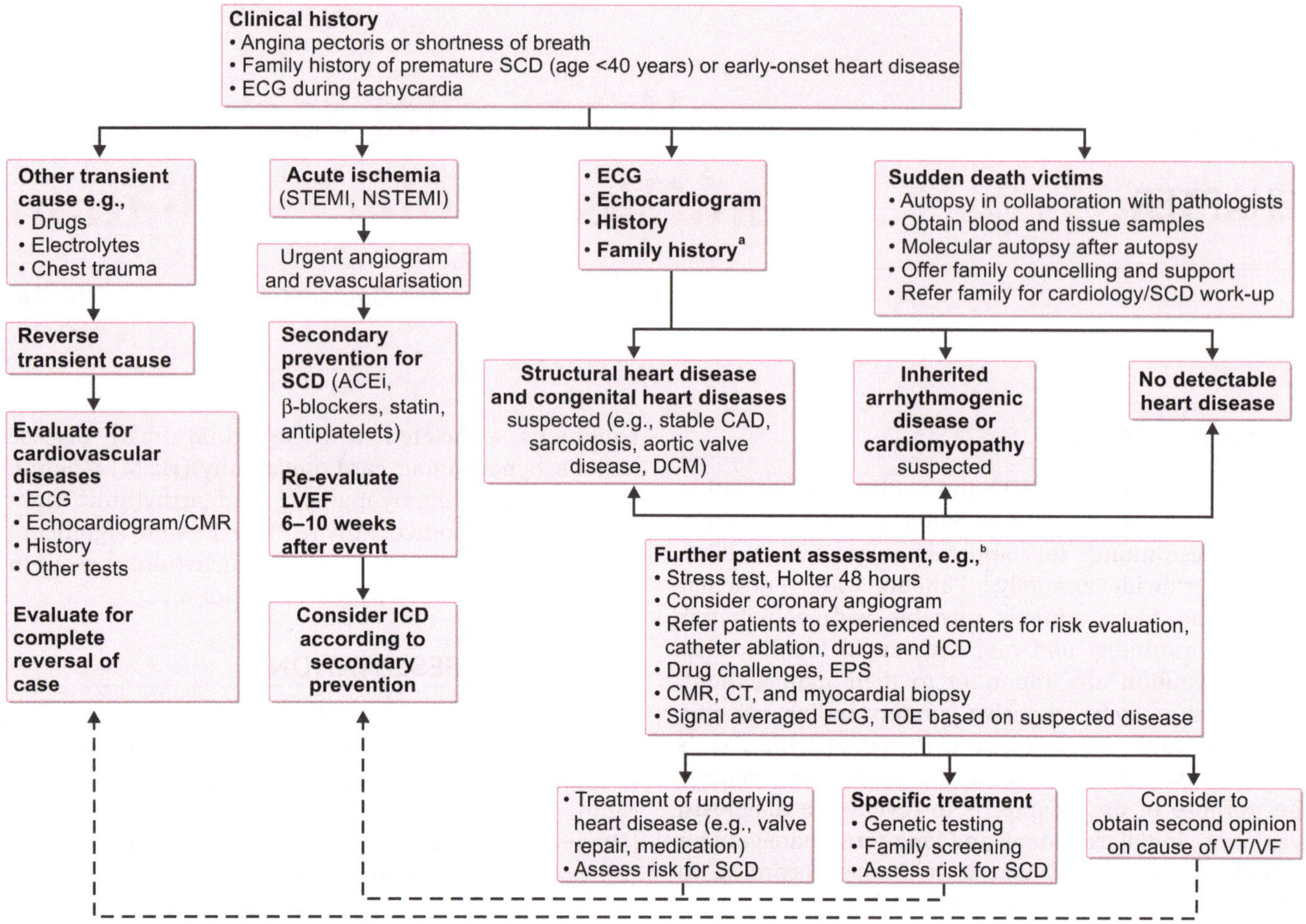

[a]Clinical history of chest pain, dyspnea, and symptoms associated with certain cardiac conditions and family tree.

[b]The need for further tests and evaluations will be guided by the initial assessment and by suspected cardiovascular diseases.

ACEIs, angiotensin-converting enzyme inhibitors; CAD, coronary artery disease; CMR, cardiac magnetic resonance; CT, computed tomography; DCM, dilated cardiomyopathy; ECG, electrocardiogram; EPS, electrophysiological study; ICD, implantable cardioverter; LVEF, left ventricular ejection fraction; NSTEMI, non-ST segment elevation myocardial infarction; SCD, sudden cardiac death; STEMI, ST segment elevation myocardial infarction; TOE, transoesophageal echocardiography; VF, ventricular fibrillation; VT, ventricular tachycardia.

FLOWCHART 1: Diagnostic evaluation of patients presenting with sustained ventricular tachycardia or ventricular fibrillation

With permission from: Priori SG, Blomstrom-Lundqvist C, Mazzanti A, et al. 2015 ESC Guidelines for the management of patients with ventricular arrhythmias and the prevention of sudden cardiac death: The Task Force for the Management of Patients with Ventricular Arrhythmias and the Prevention of Sudden Cardiac Death of the European Society of Cardiology (ESC). Endorsed by: Association for European Paediatric and Congenital Cardiology (AEPC). Eur Heart J. 2015;36(41):2793-867.

and diabetes mellitus. A family history should be obtained including history of syncope and sudden death. Patients should be asked about inherited syndromes associated with VT and VF such as LQTS, HCM, ARVC, CPVT, Brugada syndrome, and others.

A complete physical examination, including vital signs, with thorough cardiac assessment should also be performed. Particular attention should be given to signs of heart failure including assessment for cardiac enlargement, a positive 3rd heart sound, jugular venous distension, pulmonary rales, and lower extremity edema. Other physical findings associated with ventricular arrhythmias include the presence of a jerky pulse and midsystolic ejection murmur suggestive of hypertrophic cardiomyopathy. A patient with woolly hair and plantar keratosis may have Naxos disease,[15] a form of ARVC. Nerve deafness in a patient with prolonged QT on the electrocardiogram (ECG) may indicate Jervell and Lange-Nielsen syndrome,[16] while craniofacial abnormalities may suggest Noonan syndrome and HCM;[17] such patients are also at increased risk for ventricular arrhythmias.

Laboratory Testing

Comprehensive metabolic testing should be performed at baseline to assess for electrolyte abnormalities, renal dysfunction, liver dysfunction, and thyroid abnormalities. Additionally, biomarkers should be drawn to evaluate for myocardial infarction and ventricular overload.

Deceased victims of SCD in whom an inherited arrhythmia syndrome is suspected should have blood samples sent for molecular autopsy if the diagnosis cannot be ascertained by family history.[1] A diagnosis can be determined in approximately 50% of such cases,[18] which may provide significant benefit to surviving family members.[19]

Electrocardiogram

The electrocardiogram is the most important tool in establishing the diagnosis of ventricular tachycardia. The diagnosis of VT requires three or more consecutive ventricular beats which exceeds an average rate of 100 bpm. An ECG of VT is shown in figure 1.

The ECG during VT may show a single QRS morphology (monomorphic VT, Fig. 2) or may continuously change overtime (polymorphic VT). For monomorphic VT, an important aspect of ECG interpretation is differentiating the arrhythmia from other wide complex tachycardias such as supraventricular tachycardias (SVT) with

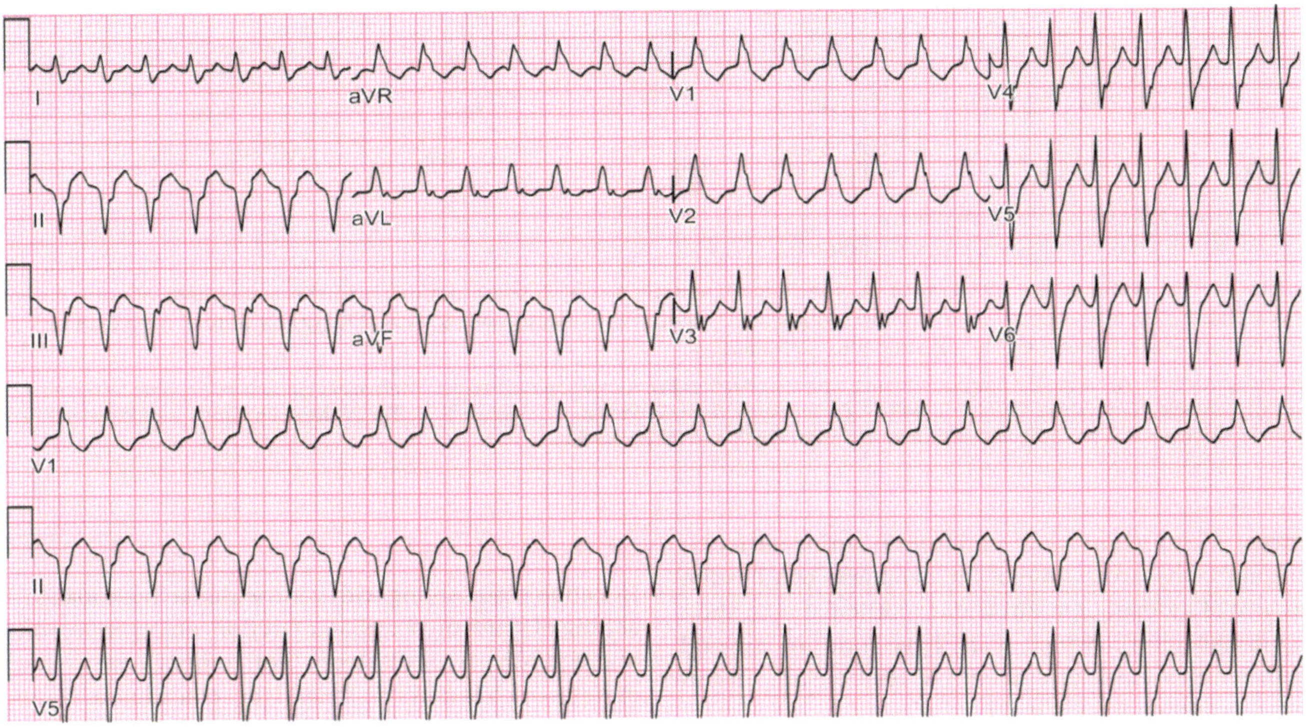

FIG. 1. Electrocardiogram of ventricular tachycardia. This electrocardiogram from a 66-year-old male with ischemic cardiomyopathy shows VT at a rate of 170 bpm

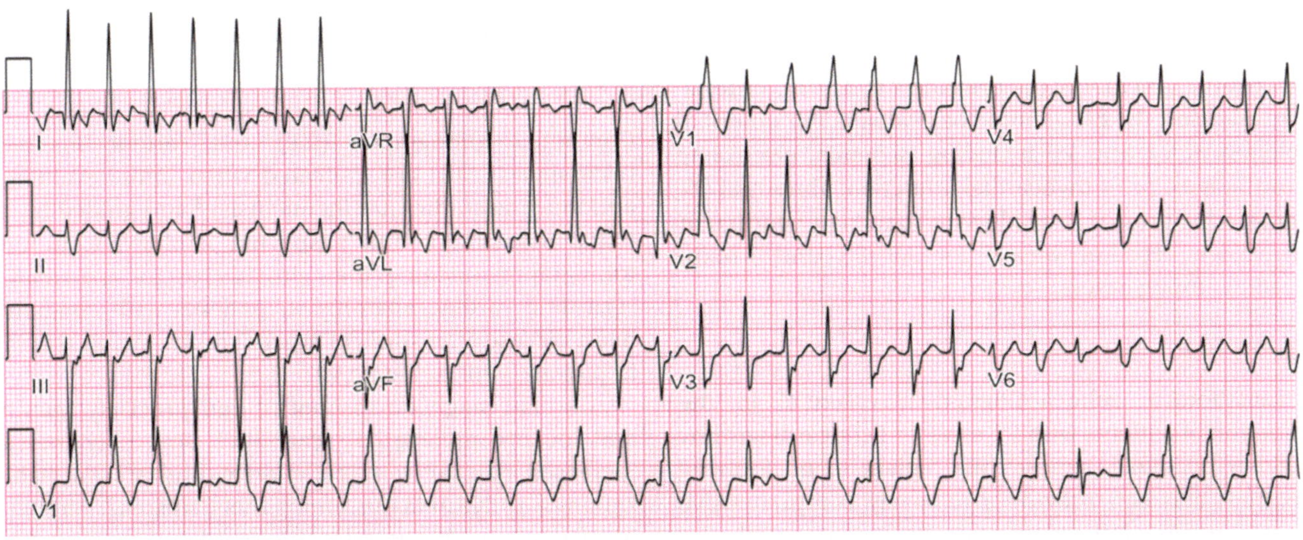

FIG. 2: Ventricular tachycardia (VT) with capture beats. Complexes 4, 17, and 25 are narrower than others, and represent capture beats, consistent with AV dissociation and VT in this wide complex tachycardia in a 26-year-old patient with severe palpitations and presyncope and a preserved ejection fraction. Due to the morphology and axis of the VT, fascicular VT (discussed later) was suspected, and VT was successfully suppressed with verapamil

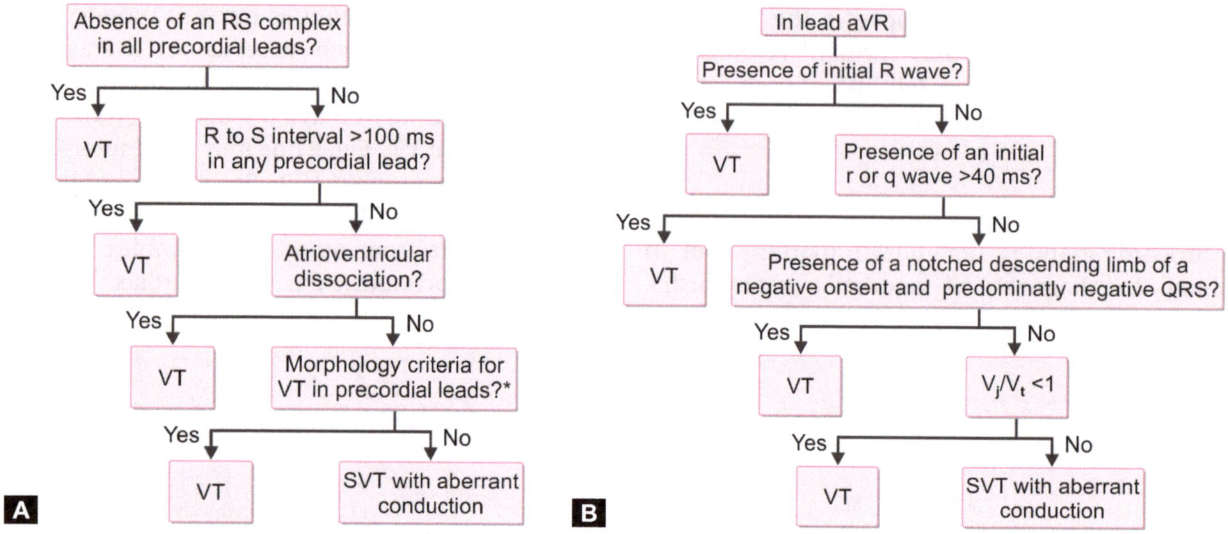

*Refer to reference 20 for complete morphology criteria.
VT, ventricular tachycardia;ms,millisecond;SVT, supraventricular.

FLOWCHART 2: Brugada and aVR Criteria. **A,** The Brugada criteria has a stepwise approach to the assessment of wide complex tachycardias. If any of the criteria are satisfied, ventricular tachycardia is diagnosed. **B,** The aVR criteria utilizes only lead aVR in a sequential approach to differentiate wide complex tachycardias

With permissions from: **A,** Brugada P, Brugada J, Mont L, Smeets J, Andries EW. A new approach to the differential diagnosis of a regular tachycardia with a wide QRS complex. Circulation. 1991;83(5):1649-59. **B,** Vereckei A, Duray G, Szenasi G, Altemose GT, Miller JM. New algorithm using only lead aVR for differential diagnosis of wide QRS complex tachycardia. Heart Rhythm. 2008;5(1):89-98.

aberrant conduction and antidromic atrioventricular reentrant tachycardia. One of the hallmarks of VT is the evidence of independent atrial and ventricular activation (AV dissociation), which can have one of several manifestations—lack of a fixed A-V relationship, fusion beats, or capture beats (Fig. 2).

However, there can be 1:1 retrograde ventricular arrhythmia conduction or no discernable P-waves during rapid tachycardia, which makes the diagnosis more difficult. Several algorithms have been developed to assist in the differentiation between VT and SVT with aberrancy (Flowchart 2), including the Brugada[20] and aVR[21] criteria.

In all cases, the ECG should be evaluated for potential etiologies of VT and VF including ischemia, electrolyte abnormalities, prior myocardial infarction, abnormal QT intervals, features of Brugada syndrome, left ventricular hypertrophy, epsilon waves (for ARVC), and J-point elevation among others.

Echocardiography

A transthoracic echocardiogram is essential in the evaluation of patients with VT or VF.[1,2] Echocardiography is widely available, exposes the patient to no ionizing radiation, and can provide a relatively comprehensive assessment for left ventricular dysfunction, valvular disease, hypertrophy, and the presence of congenital abnormalities in most patients.[23]

Ischemic Evaluation

In patients presenting with ventricular arrhythmias in the setting of acute myocardial infarction, emergent coronary angiography is indicated.[1] For others, an ischemic etiology of VT and VF should be considered. Patients suspected of ischemia-triggered arrhythmias should undergo ischemic evaluation, either by exercise stress testing, stress echocardiography, perfusion imaging, or coronary angiography. Identified ischemia may then be referred for potential revascularization.

Advanced Imaging

Computed tomography (CT) and cardiac magnetic resonance (CMR) are indicated when initial evaluation and imaging studies are inconclusive[2] and guided by the initial assessment and suspected etiology. Computed tomography imaging may provide useful information regarding cardiac anatomy in patients with congenital heart disease after surgical repair[24] or the location of scar in patients with ischemic VT.[25]

Cardiac magnetic resonance can precisely quantify and localize myocardial scar. Such scar may indicate increased risk for ventricular arrhythmias[26] via stabilization of arrhythmia-sustaining mechanisms.[27] Similarly, in patients with hypertrophic cardiomyopathy, CMR identification of ventricular scar may help determine eligibility for implantable cardioverter (ICD) therapy.[28]

Cardiac magnetic resonance may also assist in the diagnosis of conditions such as ARVC,[29] and may help risk stratify mutation carriers.[30]

Outpatient Electrocardiogram Monitoring

Ambulatory ECG monitoring is increasingly used to diagnose and assess ventricular arrhythmias. There are four types of ambulatory ECG monitors—continuous recorders (Holter monitors), event monitors, outpatient telemetry, and implantable (insertable) cardiac monitors.

Holter monitors are optimal in two settings—frequent arrhythmias and in the assessment of arrhythmia burden [such as premature ventricular complexes (PVCs)].[31] They are not well suited for rare arrhythmias or in life-threatening arrhythmias, as analysis typically occurs *post hoc*.

Event monitors are typically worn for 7–30 days, and are well suited to detect arrhythmias during symptoms. They also have autotrigger detection based upon predefined parameters (heart rate). They are suboptimal for asymptomatic arrhythmias or in the quantification of arrhythmia burden.

Continuous outpatient telemetry is suitable for detecting symptomatic and asymptomatic arrhythmias with intermittent frequency (weekly to monthly episodes). Data are transmitted wirelessly, analyzed automatically, and over-read by a technician. Such systems have been shown to be more effective than standard event recorders.[32]

Technical improvements have miniaturized implantable loop recorders such that they now may be injected in a simple outpatient procedure. Such devices improve the diagnosis of arrhythmias compared with other modalities in patients with palpitations or syncope due to supraventricular or ventricular arrhythmias.[33]

Notably, in patients with suspected ventricular arrhythmias who may be considered at increased risk for syncope or sudden death, the wearable cardioverter-defibrillator is a potential device which event monitoring capabilities in addition to defibrillation capability, and may be useful in the workup of such patients.[34]

Additional Testing

Electrophysiology study (EPS) involves the insertion of pacing catheters into the heart and stimulating the heart in an attempt to induce the ventricular arrhythmia. Electrophysiology study is typically performed to determine whether syncope was due to a ventricular arrhythmia or to risk stratify patients for ICD implantation.[35] Presently, EPS is used in patients with an intermediate ejection fraction (EF) between 35 and 40%.[36] Induction of a stable, monomorphic VT is considered a positive response and ICD therapy may be indicated.

The signal averaged ECG (SAECG) records the ECG over multiple beats in order to increase the signal-to-noise ratio for small electrical potentials at the end of the QRS complex.[37] It is particularly useful in identifying ARVC as a positive test is a minor diagnostic criterion for this condition. In other settings, SAECG testing is adjunctive.[38]

Finally, T-wave alternans is a measure of oscillations in the T wave which have been linked to increased arrhythmia risk. A negative T-wave alternans in patients with an EF less than 35% have a relatively low risk for sudden cardiac arrest. Additionally, patients with an EF of 35–40% have an increased risk of ventricular arrhythmias,[39] such testing has a class II indication in patients at risk for ventricular arrhythmias.[40]

MANAGEMENT

Acute Management of Monomorphic Ventricular Tachycardia

In the acute setting of sustained VT, the most important determinant of treatment strategy is patient stability (Flowchart 3). In stable patients, initial medical therapy strategy should be implemented. In contrast, if there is any evidence of hemodynamic instability, patient should proceed directly to direct current (DC) cardioversion, which can be followed with an antiarrhythmic medication to prevent recurrence.

In the hemodynamically stable setting, amiodarone, procainamide, and lidocaine are first-line medical therapy for VT conversion.[1] Amiodarone is the most commonly used antiarrhythmic medication in this setting and is usually administered as a 150 mg intravenous bolus over 10 minutes, followed by a continuous infusion over the next 24 hours. Procainamide may also be effective, but should not be used in patients with severe congestive heart failure or acute myocardial infarction. Lidocaine can also be effective as an adjunctive agent in refractory VT, particularly in the setting of ischemia.

If medication is ineffective in terminating the VT, DC cardioversion should be applied to convert the patient into normal rhythm. Synchronized shock at 200 J with biphasic waveform is the usual starting energy. Although lower energy is often effective, the risks and discomfort of multiple shocks must be considered if initial attempts are unsuccessful.

Acute Medical Therapy for Specific Types of Ventricular Tachycardia

Fascicular VT (Flowchart 2), characterized by right bundle branch block with a narrower QRS complex and a superior axis, may be particularly responsive to verapamil.[41]

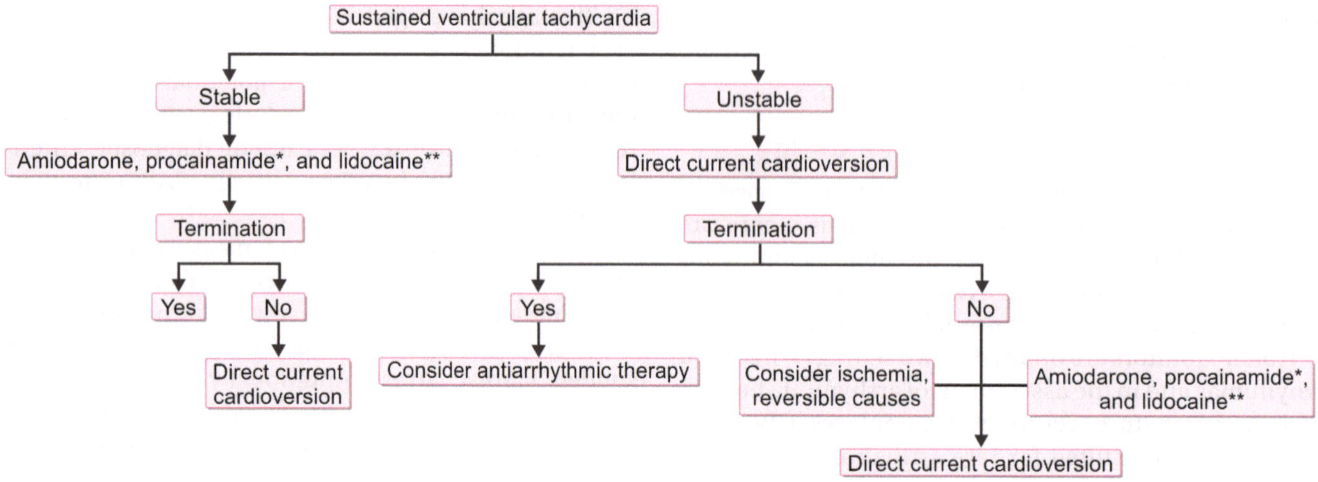

*In the absence of severe heart failure and myocardial infarction.
**Only moderately effective in monomorphic ventricular tachycardia.

FLOWCHART 3: Stepwise approach the acute treatment of sustained ventricular tachycardia

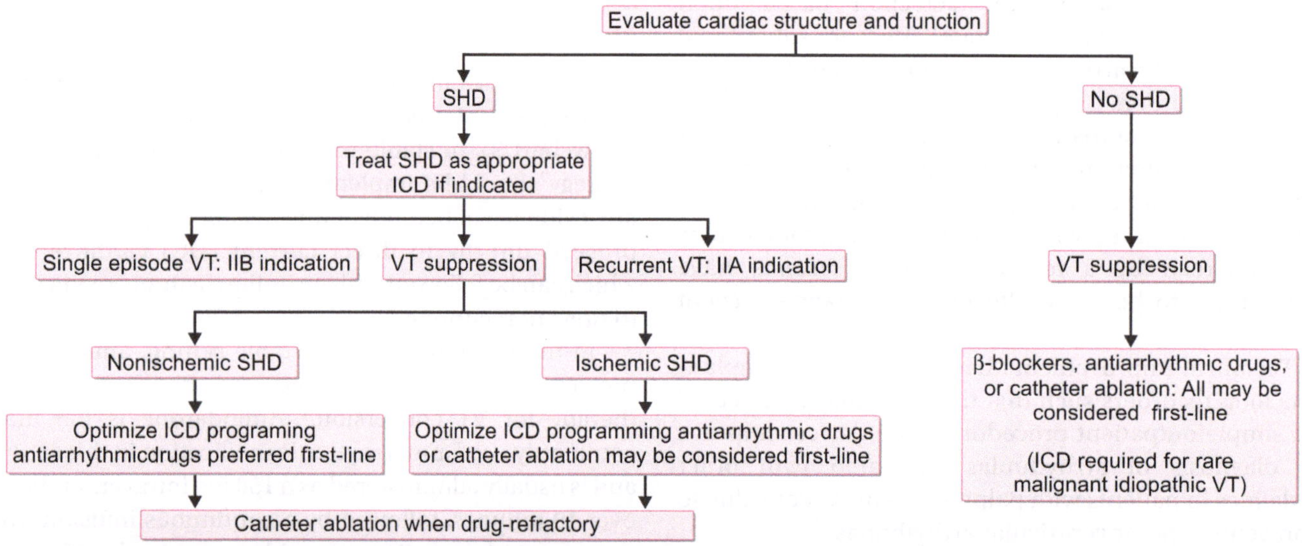

ICD, implantable cardioverter-defibrillator; SHD, structural heart disease; VT, ventricular tachycardia.

FLOWCHART 4: Chronic management of monomorphic ventricular tachycardia

With permission from: Pedersen CT, Kay GN, Kalman J, et al. EHRA/HRS/APHRS expert consensus on ventricular arrhythmias. Heart Rhythm. 2014;11(10):e166-96.

Ablation in the Acute Setting

Patients in electrical storm who fail medical management may be taken to emergency ablation in experienced centers.[42] Ablation may also be considered first-line therapy for incessant sustained monomorphic VT in the setting of ischemic cardiomyopathy. In incessant sustained monomorphic VT in the setting of nonischemic VT, ablation should be considered after a trial of medical therapy.[2]

Chronic Management of Monomorphic Ventricular Tachycardia

As shown in flowchart 4, long-term treatment strategies are directed at preventing arrhythmic recurrence and are largely dependent on the presence or absence of structural heart disease.

Presence of Structural Heart Disease

The first step for managing monomorphic VT in the setting of structural heart disease is initiation of appropriate neurohormonal therapy, including β-blockers and angiotensin-converting enzyme inhibitors/angiotensin II receptor blockers. The second step is to determine whether an ICD is indicated.

Simplifying this decision, an ICD is indicated for most patients with SHD and sustained VT.[43] Prior work has demonstrated that ICDs improve survival in patients with VT and reduced systolic function.[44-46] Furthermore, current guidelines[47] and expert consensus papers[2] note that ICDs are indicated for patients with sustained monomorphic VT (MMVT) and myocardial scar, even when systolic function is normal or near-normal.

Implantable cardioverter therapy itself has adverse effects on patients' psychologic and physical health, and patients with recurrent ICD shocks benefit from suppression of their ventricular arrhythmias with antiarrhythmics or ablation.[48] If ventricular arrhythmias recur and patients receive ICD shocks, the next step is to both reprogram ICD settings in the hope to terminate VT with antitachycardia pacing and consider antiarrhythmic drug therapy for VT suppression. For patients with ischemic cardiomyopathy, VT ablation may also be considered as first-line therapy for recurrent VT. In patients with nonischemic cardiomyopathy, ablation should be considered after a trial of antiarrhythmic drug therapy.

Specifically, β-blockers, sotalol, dofetilide, and amiodarone are commonly used in this setting, tailored to patients' response, tolerance, and side effects. Sotalol in particular should be used with caution in patients with depressed LV function. Patients who are not responsive to medical therapy or ablation with frequent ventricular arrhythmias may be considered for sympathectomy[49,50] or cardiac transplant.

Absence of Structural Heart Disease

In the absence of structural heart disease, treatment should be focused at VT suppression. In this setting, medical therapy and VT ablation are both first-line interventions.[2]

The first choice for medical therapy of VT without structural heart disease is often β-blockade. When ineffective or not tolerated, antiarrhythmic therapy with sotalol or dofetilide may be considered in patients with preserved renal function. These medications require baseline renal function assessment and frequent monitoring for QTc prolongation, both at initiation and at regular follow-up. In other patients without structural heart disease, flecainide, mexilitine, or propafenone may be used, with consideration of potential proarrhythmic risk.[51] In others, amiodarone may be effective, although it requires baseline and yearly thyroid function, liver function, pulmonary function, and ophthalmologic testing to monitor for adverse effects. Ablation is also considered first-line therapy for MMVT without structural heart disease (see below). In rare cases of malignant idiopathic VT, an ICD may be required.[2]

Tailored Chronic Medical Therapy for Specific Types of Monomorphic Ventricular Tachycardia

In fascicular VT, verapamil may be considered for long-term suppression of fascicular VT[41] in patients in whom ablation is not an option or is not desired.

Ablation in the Chronic Management of Monomorphic Ventricular Tachycardia

Studies have shown the utility of ablation for the chronic management of VT,[48] including reducing appropriate ICD shocks. Consultation with emergency physicians is recommended to allow a thorough discussion with the patient of all the risks, benefits, and probability of success in each case.

Classically, VT associated with ischemic heart disease is more amenable to ablation. Ventricular tachycardia in nonischemic cardiomyopathy classically has a lower ablation success rate. However, newer techniques, such as endocardial-epicardial homogenization of proarrhythmic substrate,[52] and new technologies, such as bipolar and needle[53] ablation, have shown promise.

Frequently, idiopathic VT subtypes such as left or right ventricular outflow tract VTs are amenable to ablation, which may be considered early in the treatment strategy. A cardiac electrophysiology consultation should be obtained for a detailed discussion of all treatment options.

Acute Management of Polymorphic Ventricular Tachycardia or Ventricular Fibrillation

The acute management of polymorphic VT or VF consists of defibrillation. For patients in torsades de pointes (polymorphic VT in the setting of a rate-corrected, sinus rhythm QT interval greater than 440 ms in males or 460 ms in females, commonly seen in patients with long-QT syndrome), atrial pacing at a rate 90 bpm or intravenous isoproterenol may provide effective arrhythmia suppression.[2]

Patients with refractory arrhythmias related to either Brugada syndrome or idiopathic VF related to inferolateral early repolarization[54] may also benefit from intravenous isoproterenol in the acute setting.

Chronic Management of Polymorphic Ventricular Tachycardia or Ventricular Fibrillation

The chronic management of polymorphic VT or VF is illustrated in flowchart 5.

The first step in management of polymorphic VT or VF following stabilization is to determine whether acute coronary syndrome (ACS) is present.

Management of Polymorphic Ventricular Tachycardia/Ventricular Fibrillation with Acute Coronary Syndrome

Patients with ACS should be referred for potential revascularization. Patients who are not revascularized should be considered for ICD therapy and started on guideline directed neurohormonal therapy.

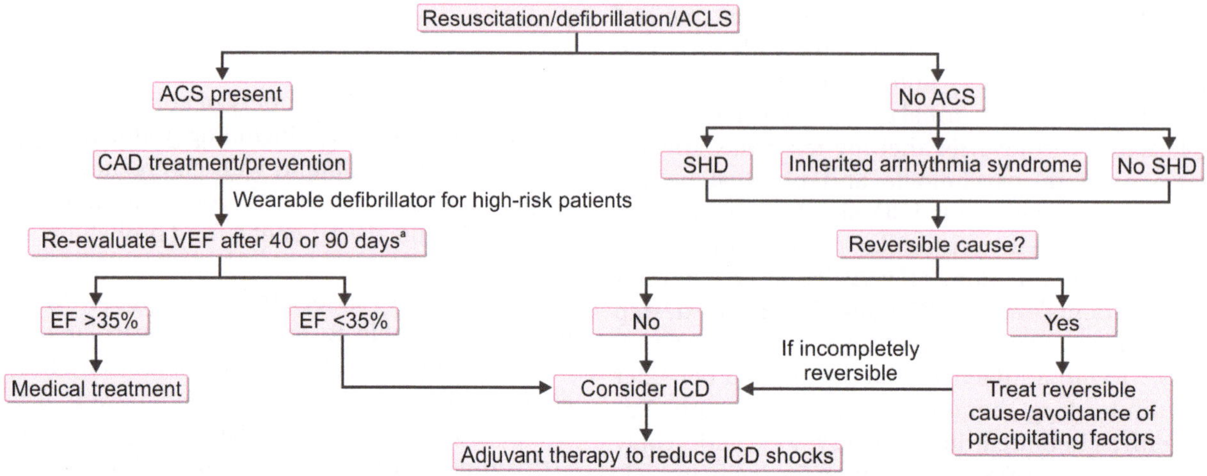

ACLS, advanced cardiovascular life support; ACS, acute coronary syndrome; CAD, coronary artery disease; SHD, structural heart disease; LVEF, left ventricular ejection fraction; EF, ejection fraction; ICD, implantable cardioverter.

FLOWCHART 5: Chronic management of polymorphic ventricular tachycardia or ventricular fibrillation

With permission from: Pedersen CT, Kay GN, Kalman J, et al. EHRA/HRS/APHRS expert consensus on ventricular arrhythmias. Heart Rhythm. 2014;11(10):e166-96.

Patient who are revascularized should be considered for a wearable cardioverter-defibrillator[34] and their EF evaluated after 3 months. If the EF is more than 35%, medical therapy should be continued. However, if the EF is below 35%, an ICD should be considered.

Management of Polymorphic Ventricular Tachycardia/Ventricular Fibrillation without Acute Coronary Syndrome

For patients without ACS, the next step is to attempt to determine the specific etiology of the arrhythmia; directed care based on the underlying cause may then be started. In all cases, an assessment should be made whether the etiology is completely reversible or not.[2] For patients without a completely reversible cause, ICD therapy should be considered. Otherwise, treatment of the reversible cause or avoidance of precipitating factors is indicated.

Tailored Chronic Medical Therapy for Specific Types of Polymorphic Ventricular Tachycardia/Ventricular Fibrillation

Recently, quinidine (class IA) has been shown to be useful long-term arrhythmia suppression in patients with early repolarization syndrome and idiopathic VF.[54]

Management of Frequent Premature Ventricular Complexes and Nonsustained Ventricular Tachycardia

Premature ventricular complexes may be benign in the majority of patients with a low burden, however, a high burden of PVCs (>10,000 PVCs per 24 h) may be a risk factor for the development of cardiomyopathy,[55] and should be managed as represented in flowchart 6.

In patients without structural heart disease, patients should be reassured, particularly if asymptomatic. Highly symptomatic patients may benefit from medical suppression; β-blockers are typically used as first-line agents in this setting.[2] Nondihydropyridine calcium antagonists may also be considered. If ineffective, flecainide, propafenone, sotalol, dofetilide, or amiodarone may be considered, although the risk of proarrhythmia and side effects are greater than for β-blockers or calcium channel blockers.[56] Alternatively, PVC ablation may be considered.

For patients with structural heart disease, an assessment of PVC burden should be performed, typically with a 24 hour Holter monitor or similar ambulatory ECG technology. If the burden of PVCs is greater than 10,000 PVCs per 24 hours, tailored medical suppression may be considered using β-blockers as first-line, followed by trials of sotalol, dofetilide, or amiodarone. Premature ventricular complex ablation has shown effectiveness in several trials,[57] with subsequent recovery of ventricular function.

Management of Nonsustained Ventricular Tachycardia

Nonsustained VT is defined as self-limited beats of ventricular origin lasting from 3 beats to 30 seconds with a rate greater than 100 bpm. In general, therapy for the underlying cardiac disease is indicated rather than for NSVT. However, NSVT may be an important marker for

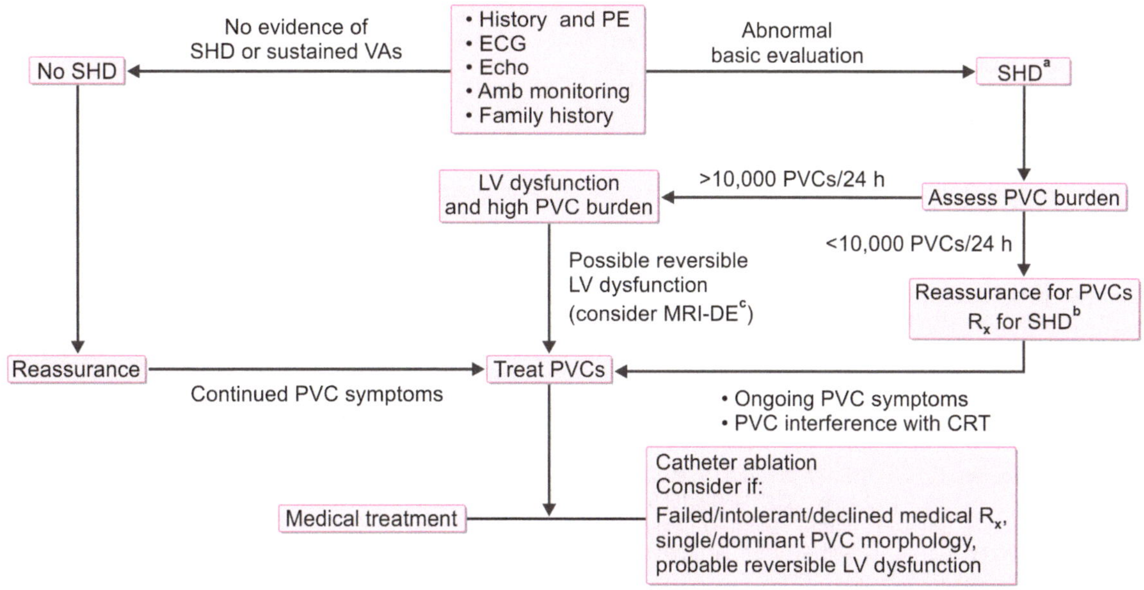

PE, physical examination; ECG, electrocardiogram; Amb, ambulatory; SHD, structural heart disease; VAs, ventricular arrhythmias; LV, left ventricular; PVC, premature ventricular complexes; CRT, cardiac resynchronization therapy.

FLOWCHART 6: Management of frequent premature ventricular complexes

With permission from: Pedersen CT, Kay GN, Kalman J, et al. EHRA/HRS/APHRS expert consensus on ventricular arrhythmias. Heart Rhythm. 2014;11(10):e166-96.

increased risk of morbidity and mortality, and should trigger a workup similar to patients with VT (Flowchart 1).[2]

Management of NSVT may be broadly classified according to the presence or absence of apparent structural heart disease; readers are, therefore, directed to recent guidelines[2] for a full discussion of the evaluation and management of PVCs in specific situations.

One important aspect of care for patients with NSVT to note regards patients with ischemic cardiomyopathy and an ejection fraction between 35 and 40%. In these patients, the presence of NSVT potentially signifies increased risk for sudden death, and should prompt referral for electrophysiology study.[36] Induction of a sustained VT or VF in such patients is a positive result, and ICD implantation is recommended.[47]

PROGNOSIS OF PATIENTS WITH VENTRICULAR ARRHYTHMIAS

The prognosis for patients with ventricular arrhythmias is dependent upon both the specific etiology and the presence of structural heart disease. For patients with idiopathic VT and normal ventricular function, the prognosis is relatively benign. In contrast, patients with inherited channelopathies such as LQTS, or those with VT and structural heart disease, may be at higher risk and require further stratification and ICD implantation, based upon current guidelines.[40,47]

CONCLUSION

The presentation of VT can vary from asymptomatic, non-sustained episodes to unstable events precipitating VF. Initial evaluation should focus on hemodynamic stability, with immediate intervention in unstable patients. Once suppressed, further diagnostics are required for determining the correct identification of the arrhythmia and etiology. Long-term management is directed at both arrhythmia elimination via antiarrhythmic drugs or ablation, and risk reduction with ICD implantation, as required. With the advent of advanced electrophysiology care, timely initiation of optimal management has the potential to dramatically improve the survival of patients with VT.

REFERENCES

1. Priori SG, Blomstrom-Lundqvist C, Mazzanti A, Blom N, Borggrefe M, Camm J, et al. 2015 ESC Guidelines for the management of patients with ventricular arrhythmias and the prevention of sudden cardiac death: The Task Force for the Management of Patients with Ventricular Arrhythmias and the Prevention of Sudden Cardiac Death of the European Society of Cardiology (ESC). Endorsed by: Association for European Paediatric and Congenital Cardiology (AEPC). Eur Heart J. 2015;36(41):2793-867.
2. Pedersen CT, Kay GN, Kalman J, Borggrefe M, Della-Bella P, Dickfeld T, et al. EHRA/HRS/APHRS expert consensus on ventricular arrhythmias. Heart Rhythm. 2014;11(10):e166-96.
3. Zipes DP, Camm AJ, Borggrefe M, Buxton AE, Chaitman B, Fromer M, et al. ACC/AHA/ESC 2006 Guidelines for Management of Patients With Ventricular Arrhythmias and the Prevention of Sudden Cardiac Death: A report of the American College of Cardiology/American Heart Association Task Force and

the European Society of Cardiology Committee for Practice Guidelines (writing committee to develop Guidelines for Management of Patients With Ventricular Arrhythmias and the Prevention of Sudden Cardiac Death): Developed in collaboration with the European Heart Rhythm Association and the Heart Rhythm Society. Circulation. 2006;114(10):e385-484.
4. Eckart RE, Shry EA, Burke AP, McNear JA, Appel DA, Castillo-Rojas LM, et al. Sudden death in young adults: An autopsy-based series of a population undergoing active surveillance. J Am Coll Cardiol. 2011;58(12):1254-61.
5. Scheinman MM, Huang S. The 1998 NASPE prospective catheter ablation registry. Pacing Clin Electrophysiol. 2000;23(6):1020-8.
6. Myerburg RJ, Kessler KM, Castellanos A. Sudden cardiac death. Structure, function, and time-dependence of risk. Circulation. 1992;85(1 Suppl):I2-10.
7. Moss AJ, Zareba W, Hall WJ, Klein H, Wilber DJ, Cannom DS, et al. Prophylactic implantation of a defibrillator in patients with myocardial infarction and reduced ejection fraction. N Engl J Med. 2002;346(12):877-83.
8. Bardy GH, Lee KL, Mark DB, Poole JE, Packer DL, Boineau R, et al. Amiodarone or an implantable cardioverter-defibrillator for congestive heart failure. N Engl J Med. 2005;352(3):225-37.
9. Priori SG, Schwartz PJ, Napolitano C, Bloise R, Ronchetti E, Grillo M, et al. Risk stratification in the long-QT syndrome. N Engl J Med. 2003;348(19):1866-74.
10. Spirito P, Bellone P, Harris KM, Bernabo P, Bruzzi P, Maron BJ. Magnitude of left ventricular hypertrophy and risk of sudden death in hypertrophic cardiomyopathy. New Engl J Med. 2000;342(24):1778-85.
11. van Rijsingen IA, Arbustini E, Elliott PM, Mogensen J, Hermans-van Ast JF, van der Kooi AJ, et al. Risk factors for malignant ventricular arrhythmias in lamin a/c mutation carriers a European cohort study. J Am Coll Cardiol. 2012;59(5):493-500.
12. Myerburg RJ, Mitrani R, Interian A, Jr., Castellanos A. Interpretation of outcomes of antiarrhythmic clinical trials: Design features and population impact. Circulation. 1998;97(15):1514-21.
13. Fitzgibbon J, Kman NE, Gorgas D. Asymptomatic sustained polymorphic ventricular tachycardia in a patient with a left ventricular assist device: Case report and what the emergency physician should know. J Emerg Med. 2016;50(3):e135-41.
14. Gao D, Sapp JL. Electrical storm: Definitions, clinical importance, and treatment. Curr Opin Cardiol. 2013;28(1):72-9.
15. McKoy G, Protonotarios N, Crosby A, Tsatsopoulou A, Anastasakis A, Coonar A, et al. Identification of a deletion in plakoglobin in arrhythmogenic right ventricular cardiomyopathy with palmoplantar keratoderma and woolly hair (Naxos disease). Lancet. 2000;355(9221):2119-24.
16. Duggal P, Vesely MR, Wattanasirichaigoon D, Villafane J, Kaushik V, Beggs AH. Mutation of the gene for IsK associated with both Jervell and Lange-Nielsen and Romano-Ward forms of long-QT syndrome. Circulation. 1998;97(2):142-6.
17. Burch M, Sharland M, Shinebourne E, Smith G, Patton M, McKenna W. Cardiologic abnormalities in Noonan syndrome: phenotypic diagnosis and echocardiographic assessment of 118 patients. J Am Coll Cardiol. 1993;22(4):1189-92.
18. Behr ER, Dalageorgou C, Christiansen M, Syrris P, Hughes S, Tome Esteban MT, et al. Sudden arrhythmic death syndrome: Familial evaluation identifies inheritable heart disease in the majority of families. Eur Heart J. 2008;29(13):1670-80.
19. Christiaans I, van Langen IM, Birnie E, Bonsel GJ, Wilde AA, Smets EM. Quality of life and psychological distress in hypertrophic cardiomyopathy mutation carriers: A cross-sectional cohort study. Am J Med Genet A. 2009;149A(4):602-12.
20. Brugada P, Brugada J, Mont L, Smeets J, Andries EW. A new approach to the differential diagnosis of a regular tachycardia with a wide QRS complex. Circulation. 1991;83(5):1649-59.
21. Feld GK, Nademanee K, Stevenson W, Weiss J, Klitzner T, Singh BN. Clinical and electrophysiologic effects of amiodarone in patients with atrial fibrillation complicating the Wolff-Parkinson-White syndrome. Am Heart J. 1988;115 (1 Pt 1):102-7.
22. Vereckei A, Duray G, Szenasi G, Altemose GT, Miller JM. New algorithm using only lead aVR for differential diagnosis of wide QRS complex tachycardia. Heart Rhythm. 2008;5(1):89-98.
23. Cheitlin MD, Armstrong WF, Aurigemma GP, Beller GA, Bierman FZ, Davis JL, et al. ACC/AHA/ASE 2003 guideline update for the clinical application of echocardiography--summary article: A report of the American College of Cardiology/American Heart Association Task Force on Practice Guidelines (ACC/AHA/ASE Committee to Update the 1997 Guidelines for the Clinical Application of Echocardiography). J Am Coll Cardiol. 2003;42(5):954-70.
24. Tops LF, de Groot NM, Bax JJ, Schalij MJ. Fusion of electroanatomical activation maps and multislice computed tomography to guide ablation of a focal atrial tachycardia in a fontan patient. J Cardiovasc Electrophysiol. 2006;17(4):431-4.
25. Bello D, Kipper S, Valderrabano M, Shivkumar K. Catheter ablation of ventricular tachycardia guided by contrast-enhanced cardiac computed tomography. Heart Rhythm. 2004;1(4):490-2.
26. Kwong RY, Chan AK, Brown KA, Chan CW, Reynolds HG, Tsang S, et al. Impact of unrecognized myocardial scar detected by cardiac magnetic resonance imaging on event-free survival in patients presenting with signs or symptoms of coronary artery disease. Circulation. 2006;113(23):2733-43.
27. Krummen DE, Hayase J, Morris DJ, Ho J, Smetak MR, Clopton P, et al. Rotor stability separates sustained ventricular fibrillation from self-terminating episodes in humans. J Am Coll Cardiol. 2014;63(24):2712-21.
28. O'Hanlon R, Grasso A, Roughton M, Moon JC, Clark S, Wage R, et al. Prognostic significance of myocardial fibrosis in hypertrophic cardiomyopathy. J Am Coll Cardiol. 2010;56(11):867-74.
29. Borgquist R, Haugaa KH, Gilljam T, Bundgaard H, Hansen J, Eschen O, et al. The diagnostic performance of imaging methods in ARVC using the 2010 Task Force criteria. Eur Heart J Cardiovasc Imaging. 2014;15(11):1219-25.
30. te Riele AS, Bhonsale A, James CA, Rastegar N, Murray B, Burt JR, et al. Incremental value of cardiac magnetic resonance imaging in arrhythmic risk stratification of arrhythmogenic right ventricular dysplasia/cardiomyopathy-associated desmosomal mutation carriers. J Am Coll Cardiol. 2013;62(19):1761-9.
31. Boudoulas H, Schaal SF, Lewis RP, Robinson JL. Superiority of 24-hour outpatient monitoring over multi-stage exercise testing for the evaluation of syncope. J Electrocardiol. 1979;12(1):103-8.
32. Rothman SA, Laughlin JC, Seltzer J, Walia JS, Baman RI, Siouffi SY, et al. The diagnosis of cardiac arrhythmias: A prospective multi-center randomized study comparing mobile cardiac outpatient telemetry versus standard loop event monitoring. J Cardiovasc Electrophysiol. 2007;18(3):241-7.
33. Farwell DJ, Freemantle N, Sulke N. The clinical impact of implantable loop recorders in patients with syncope. Eur Heart J. 2006;27(3):351-6.
34. Klein HU, Goldenberg I, Moss AJ. Risk stratification for implantable cardioverter defibrillator therapy: the role of the wearable cardioverter-defibrillator. Eur Heart J. 2013;34(29):2230-42.
35. Rahimtoola SH, Zipes DP, Akhtar M, Burchell H, Mason J, Myerburg R, et al. Consensus statement of the conference on the state of the art of electrophysiologic testing in the diagnosis and treatment of patients with cardiac arrhythmias. Circulation. 1987;75(4 Pt 2):III3-11.
36. Buxton AE, Lee KL, Fisher JD, Josephson ME, Prystowsky EN, Hafley G. A randomized study of the prevention of sudden death in patients with coronary artery disease. Multicenter Unsustained Tachycardia Trial Investigators. N Engl J Med. 1999 ;341(25):1882-90.
37. Marcus FI, McKenna WJ, Sherrill D, Basso C, Bauce B, Bluemke DA, et al. Diagnosis of arrhythmogenic right ventricular cardiomyopathy/dysplasia: Proposed modification of the task force criteria. Circulation. 2010;121(13):1533-41.
38. Goldberger JJ, Basu A, Boineau R, Buxton AE, Cain ME, Canty JM Jr., et al. Risk stratification for sudden cardiac death: A plan for the future. Circulation. 2014;129(4):516-26.
39. Verrier RL, Klingenheben T, Malik M, El-Sherif N, Exner DV, Hohnloser SH, et al. Microvolt T-wave alternans physiological basis, methods of measurement, and clinical utility--consensus guideline by International Society for Holter and Noninvasive Electrocardiology. J Am Coll Cardiol. 2011;58(13):1309-24.
40. Epstein AE, DiMarco JP, Ellenbogen KA, Estes NA 3rd, Freedman RA, Gettes LS, et al. 2012 ACCF/AHA/HRS focused update incorporated into the ACCF/AHA/HRS 2008 guidelines for device-based therapy of cardiac rhythm abnormalities: A report of the American College of Cardiology Foundation/American Heart Association Task Force on Practice Guidelines and the Heart Rhythm Society. J Am Coll Cardiol. 2013;61(3):e6-75.
41. Belhassen B, Rotmensch HH, Laniado S. Response of recurrent sustained ventricular tachycardia to verapamil. Br Heart J. 1981;46(6):679-82.
42. Aliot EM, Stevenson WG, Almendral-Garrote JM, Bogun F, Calkins CH, Delacretaz E, et al. EHRA/HRS Expert Consensus on Catheter Ablation of Ventricular Arrhythmias: developed in a partnership with the European Heart Rhythm Association (EHRA), a Registered Branch of the European Society of Cardiology (ESC), and the Heart Rhythm Society (HRS); in collaboration with the American College of Cardiology (ACC) and the American Heart Association (AHA). Europace. 2009;11(6):771-817.
43. Russo AM, Stainback RF, Bailey SR, Epstein AE, Heidenreich PA, Jessup M, et al. ACCF/HRS/AHA/ASE/HFSA/SCAI/SCCT/SCMR 2013 appropriate use

criteria for implantable cardioverter-defibrillators and cardiac resynchronization therapy: A report of the American College of Cardiology Foundation appropriate use criteria task force, Heart Rhythm Society, American Heart Association, American Society of Echocardiography, Heart Failure Society of America, Society for Cardiovascular Angiography and Interventions, Society of Cardiovascular Computed Tomography, and Society for Cardiovascular Magnetic Resonance. J Am Coll Cardiol. 2013;61(12):1318-68.

44. A comparison of antiarrhythmic-drug therapy with implantable defibrillators in patients resuscitated from near-fatal ventricular arrhythmias. The Antiarrhythmics versus Implantable Defibrillators (AVID) Investigators. N Engl J Med. 1997;337(22):1576-83.
45. Kuck KH, Cappato R, Siebels J, Ruppel R. Randomized comparison of antiarrhythmic drug therapy with implantable defibrillators in patients resuscitated from cardiac arrest: the Cardiac Arrest Study Hamburg (CASH). Circulation. 2000;102(7):748-54.
46. Connolly SJ, Gent M, Roberts RS, Dorian P, Roy D, Sheldon RS, et al. Canadian implantable defibrillator study (CIDS): A randomized trial of the implantable cardioverter defibrillator against amiodarone. Circulation. 2000;101(11):1297-302.
47. Epstein AE, Dimarco JP, Ellenbogen KA, Estes NA 3rd, Freedman RA, Gettes LS, et al. ACC/AHA/HRS 2008 guidelines for device-based therapy of cardiac rhythm abnormalities: Executive summary. Heart Rhythm. 2008;5(6):934-55.
48. Reddy VY, Reynolds MR, Neuzil P, Richardson AW, Taborsky M, Jongnarangsin K, et al. Prophylactic catheter ablation for the prevention of defibrillator therapy. N Engl J Med. 2007;357(26):2657-65.
49. Hayase J, Patel J, Narayan SM, Krummen DE. Percutaneous stellate ganglion block suppressing VT and VF in a patient refractory to VT ablation. J Cardiovasc Electrophysiol. 2013;24(8):926-8.
50. Vaseghi M, Gima J, Kanaan C, Ajijola OA, Marmureanu A, Mahajan A, et al. Cardiac sympathetic denervation in patients with refractory ventricular arrhythmias or electrical storm: intermediate and long-term follow-up. Heart Rhythm. 2014;11(3):360-6.
51. Hoffmayer KS, Gerstenfeld EP. Diagnosis and management of idiopathic ventricular tachycardia. Curr Probl Cardiol. 2013;38(4):131-58.
52. Di Biase L, Burkhardt JD, Lakkireddy D, Carbucicchio C, Mohanty S, Mohanty P, et al. Ablation of stable VTs versus substrate ablation in ischemic cardiomyopathy: The VISTA randomized multicenter trial. J Am Coll Cardiol. 2015;66(25):2872-82.
53. Sapp JL, Beeckler C, Pike R, Parkash R, Gray CJ, Zeppenfeld K, et al. Initial human feasibility of infusion needle catheter ablation for refractory ventricular tachycardia. Circulation. 2013;128(21):2289-95.
54. Haissaguerre M, Sacher F, Nogami A, Komiya N, Bernard A, Probst V, et al. Characteristics of recurrent ventricular fibrillation associated with inferolateral early repolarization role of drug therapy. J Am Coll Cardiol. 2009;53(7):612-9.
55. Baman TS, Lange DC, Ilg KJ, Gupta SK, Liu TY, Alguire C, et al. Relationship between burden of premature ventricular complexes and left ventricular function. Heart Rhythm. 2010;7(7):865-9.
56. Stec S, Sikorska A, Zaborska B, Krynski T, Szymot J, Kulakowski P. Benign symptomatic premature ventricular complexes: Short- and long-term efficacy of antiarrhythmic drugs and radiofrequency ablation. Kardiol Pol. 2012;70(4):351-8.
57. Yarlagadda RK, Iwai S, Stein KM, Markowitz SM, Shah BK, Cheung JW, et al. Reversal of cardiomyopathy in patients with repetitive monomorphic ventricular ectopy originating from the right ventricular outflow tract. Circulation. 2005;112(8):1092-7.

30 CHAPTER

Emergency Bradycardias

Amir A Schricker, David E Krummen

INTRODUCTION

Bradycardia is not a common presentation in patients seeking emergency care, however, those with hemodynamically significant bradycardia require prompt attention. While its overall prevalence is not known, one series found 6 per 10,000 patients presenting to the emergency department had compromising bradycardia.[1]

Bradycardia is defined as a ventricular rate of less than 60 beats/min. However, patients with symptomatic bradycardia typically have rates less than 50 beats/min. Furthermore, while in some people, particularly well-trained athletes, a resting heart rate less than 50 beats/min may be physiologically normal and not cause symptoms, for others a heart rate more than 50 beats/min may be insufficient.

APPROACH TO BRADYCARDIC PATIENT

Initial Evaluation

Emergency providers must quickly identify any symptoms or signs of hemodynamic instability in the bradycardic patient. Instability refers to a patient in whom diminished cardiac output results in insufficient end-organ perfusion or impaired function (e.g., altered mental status, acute kidney injury, acute liver injury, etc.), hypotension, or debilitating symptoms. Common symptoms due to bradycardia include shortness of breath, lightheadedness, dizziness, palpitations, decreased exercise capacity, or syncope. Bradycardia may also occasionally lead to chest pain. In an unstable bradycardic patient, immediate interventions are indicated (described within "treatment of the unstable patient").

Because hypoxia is often a cause of bradycardia, a patient's oxygenation status should quickly be evaluated, as should their work of breathing. If oxygenation is insufficient or the patient has increased work of breathing, supplemental oxygen should be provided immediately.

Diagnostic Workup

In the hemodynamically stable patient, a thorough history and physical examination should be performed. In additional for evaluating for any of the previously mentioned symptoms, relevant elements of the history include prior cardiac history, including congestive heart failure, myocardial infarction (MI), prior arrhythmias, or prior cardiac surgery; active or prior illnesses such as hypothyroidism, obstructive sleep apnea, malignancy, or sarcoidosis and other inflammatory conditions; and medications including β-blockers, calcium channel blockers, digoxin/digitalis, and certain antiarrhythmic medications.

The physical examination should include vital signs, a thorough cardiac and pulmonary examination to evaluate for valvular heart disease, myocardial ischemia, and volume status (jugular venous distension, peripheral edema, and pulmonary congestion). The remainder of the examination should assess for level of consciousness, pallor, cyanosis, and signs of poor perfusion.

Laboratory blood tests, including comprehensive metabolic panel, complete blood count, and thyroid function tests, are essential to rule out both etiologies and sequelae of bradycardia, such as hypokalemia, acute kidney injury, acute liver injury, hypoglycemia, anemia, infection, and hypothyroidism. Specialized blood tests to evaluate for toxic ingestions should be performed depending on clinical suspicion.

TREATMENT OF THE UNSTABLE PATIENT

An unstable bradycardic patient is one in whom persistent bradycardia causes hypotension, signs of shock, and/or acutely altered level of consciousness. These patients require immediate treatment with cardiopulmonary resuscitation and are oftentimes guided by algorithms such as Basic Life Support or Advanced Cardiac Life Support. Examples of such algorithms are demonstrated in flowchart 1.

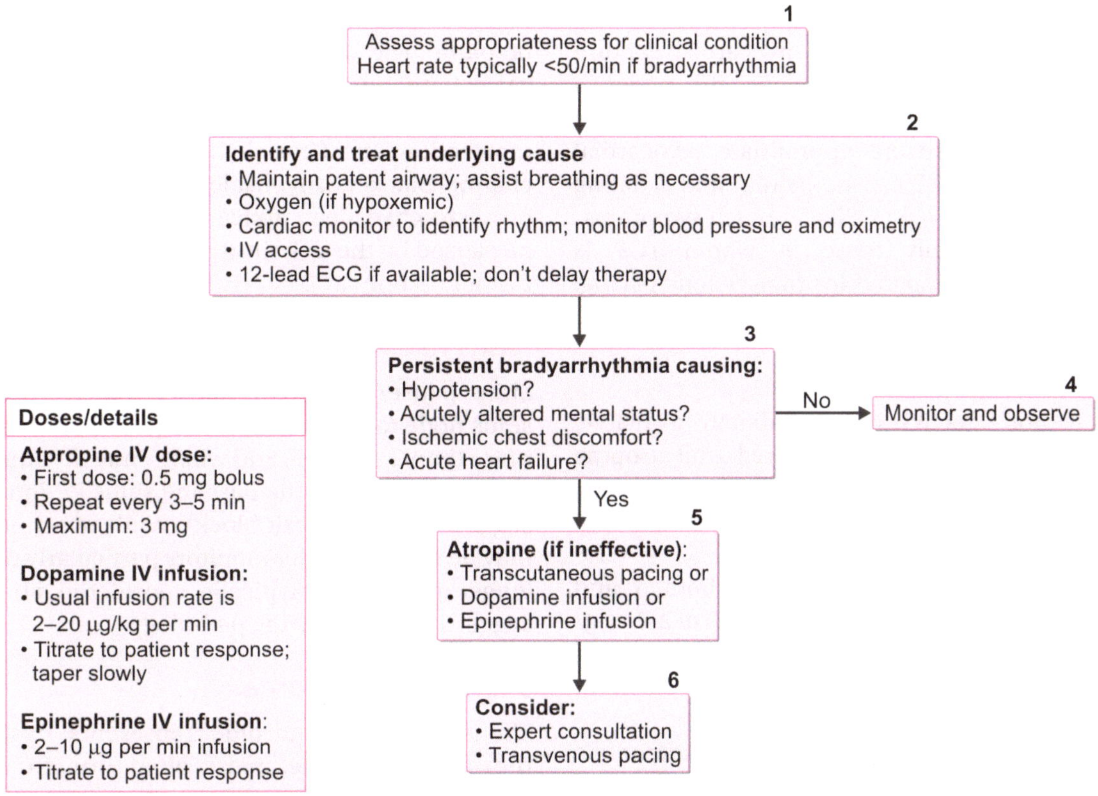

IV, intravenous; ECG, electrocardiogram.

FLOWCHART 1: Advanced Cardiac Life Support algorithm for bradycardic adults with a pulse

Reprinted with permission from Web-based Integrated 2010 & 2015 American Heart Association Guidelines for CPR and ECC. Part 7: ACLS. ©2015 American Heart Association, Inc.

Hemodynamically stable patients who are not exhibiting any symptoms due to bradycardia may be closely monitored without necessarily requiring intervention.

Therapy

Atropine

Atropine sulfate remains the first line therapy for any patient with acute and symptomatic bradycardia in the absence of reversible causes and is a class IIa indication.[2] Atropine inhibits the parasympathetic nervous system by acting as a muscarinic blocker (i.e., anticholinergic) and is useful for treating sinus bradycardia and atrioventricular (AV) block at the level of the AV node.

Several clinical trials have demonstrated that atropine is effective at improving heart rate, signs, and symptoms due to bradycardia.[3,4] The recommended atropine dosing for adults is 0.5 mg intravenous every 3-5 minutes, with maximum total dose of 3 mg. Several doses are often necessary.

Atropine should be used with caution in patients with higher grade AV block where the anatomic level of block is below the AV node (e.g., bundle of His or more distal Purkinje system), such as second degree Mobitz type II and third degree block. In such rhythms, atropine could cause a paradoxical worsening of the ventricular rate by increasing the sinoatrial rate, which further worsens AV conduction to the ventricles. Atropine should also be used cautiously in patients with active myocardial ischemia, as the higher heart rate could increase myocardial oxygen demand, and thus exacerbate ischemia. Furthermore, in cardiac transplantation patients, atropine is not useful and may even have paradoxic effects as the donor heart lacks vagal innervation.[5]

Atropine should be used as a temporizing measure in patients with significant bradycardia until transcutaneous pacing (TCP) can be initiated, and atropine administration should not delay TCP.

Pacing

Transcutaneous pacing is a class IIa indication for symptomatic bradycardia unresponsive to atropine.[2] It should be initiated immediately if atropine is ineffective at increasing heart rate, and should be considered if multiple doses of atropine are needed. Transcutaneous pacing is a noninvasive bedside procedure, and when capturing properly, it is effective at treating symptoms and signs caused by bradycardia.

Care must be taken to ensure that consistent myocardial capture is occurring. The pacing pads often stimulate the pectoral muscles, and thus muscle twitching may give the false impression that myocardial capture is occurring when it is not. Therefore, the patient's pulse must be palpated and/or an arterial waveform must be displayed to ensure appropriate myocardial capture. Furthermore, TCP can be painful and sedating medications should be given to alleviate such symptoms.

All patients—especially those in whom TCP is ineffective—should be prepared for transvenous pacing, whether temporary or permanent.

Other Medications

If atropine is not effective or immediately available, alternative medications may be considered until atropine or TCP becomes available.[2] Most of the following medications are adrenergic agonists with the exception of glucagon.

- Dopamine: A catecholamine that has both α and β-adrenergic activity. Dopamine infusions of 2–10 μg/kg/min infusion are useful at increasing contractility and chronotropy. At higher doses (>10 μg/kg/min), vasoconstriction occurs
- Epinephrine: Also possesses α and β-adrenergic activity. It may useful for patients with bradycardia induced hypotension. Recommended infusion doses are 2–10 μg/min and may be added to dopamine
- Isoproterenol: A nonselective β-adrenergic agonist that is useful for increasing heart rate. The recommended dose is 1–20 μg/min infusion
- Glucagon: While not an adrenergic agonist, glucagon may be appropriate in situations where β-blocker or calcium channel blocker overdose is suspected and atropine is not effective. The recommended dose is 3 mg followed by infusion at 3 mg/h if needed.

In general, cardioversion/defibrillation has no role in any bradycardia and is strongly discouraged.

COMMON BRADYARRHYTHMIAS

It is important to make the correct diagnosis in order to provide correct therapy. Incorrect therapy could be ineffective or even deleterious. A 12-lead electrocardiogram (ECG) is the preferred method of evaluating the rhythm, although a single-lead telemetry strip is the most commonly available modality and usually sufficient. The following describes common rhythms resulting in bradycardia. Therapy is detailed in further sections (treatment of the unstable patient).

Sinus Bradycardia

Sinus bradycardia is sinus rhythm with a resting heart rate less than 60 beats/min, however, patients typically do not become symptomatic until the heart rate decreases to less than 50 beats/min. It is often an incidental finding, and causes of sinus bradycardia can be either physiologic or pathologic. Physiologic etiologies include increased vagal tone, typically in athletes or during sleep. Pathologic etiologies include hypothyroidism, hypothermia, medication effect/toxicity (e.g., β-blockers or calcium channel blockers), hypokalemia, hypoglycemia, infection, or obstructive sleep apnea. Sinus bradycardia may also be caused by the sick sinus syndrome (SSS) (discussed in further sections).

Sinus Pause/Arrest

Sinus pause/arrest represents a transient failure of the sinus node to form impulses (Fig. 1). Pauses are typically more than 2 seconds, and when sinus rhythm resumes, it is not a multiple of the baseline sinus PP interval (which suggests sinoatrial exit block). While short pauses (<3 s) may be seen on Holter monitors particularly during sleep, longer pauses are typically considered abnormal and suggestive of underlying pathology.

Sick Sinus Syndrome

The sick sinus syndrome represents dysfunction of the sinoatrial node, most often due to aging. It is characterized by inappropriate sinus bradycardia, sinus pause/arrest, and sinoatrial exit block. If it is accompanied by supraventricular tachycardias, such as atrial fibrillation (AF) or atrial tachycardia, it is referred to as the tachycardia-bradycardia syndrome (Fig. 2). The SSS is a common arrhythmia in the elderly with a prevalence of approximately 1 in 600 cardiac patients over 65 years old.[6]

Atrioventricular Block

Atrioventricular blocks are classified as first, second, or third degree depending on the severity of the block. First degree AV block is characterized by a prolonged PR interval of more than 200 ms, and thus itself not a cause of bradycardia.

Second Degree Atrioventricular Block

Second degree AV block is characterized by one or more nonconducted P waves. In type I AV block (also known as Wenckebach block), there is gradual prolongation of the PR interval until a single P wave is not conducted to the ventricles; there is associated shortening of the RR interval, and the QRS is often narrow complex (Fig. 3A). The level of block is typically within the AV node and above the His bundle, although less commonly it may be infranodal. Type II AV block is characterized by a sudden nonconducted P wave without prolongation of the PR interval (Fig. 3B). The QRS complexes are typically not narrow, and the site of block is usually below the level of the AV node.

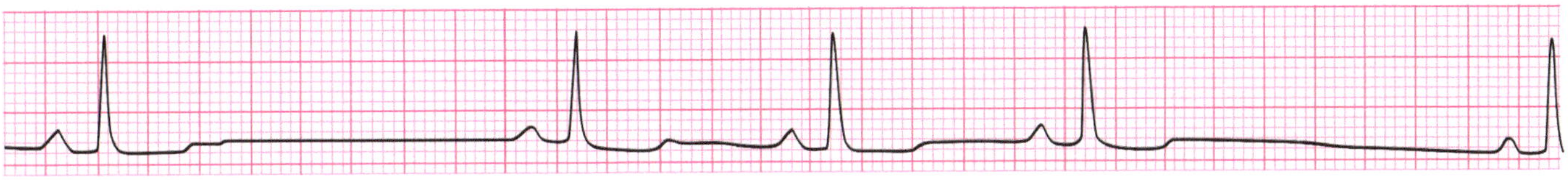

FIG. 1: Sinus pause. Rhythm strip demonstrating two sinus pauses of nearly 2 seconds each, punctuated by normal sinus rhythm

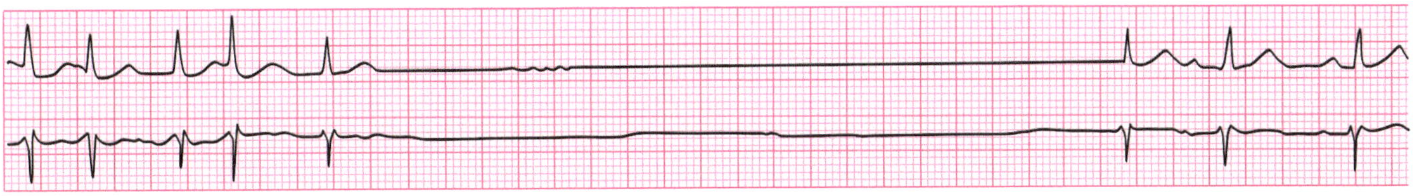

FIG. 2: Tachycardia-bradycardia syndrome. Rhythm strip demonstrating atrial fibrillation (AF) with rapid ventricular response, with termination of AF but very delayed resumption of sinus rhythm. This is characteristic of the tachycardia-bradycardia syndrome, a manifestation of the sick sinus syndrome

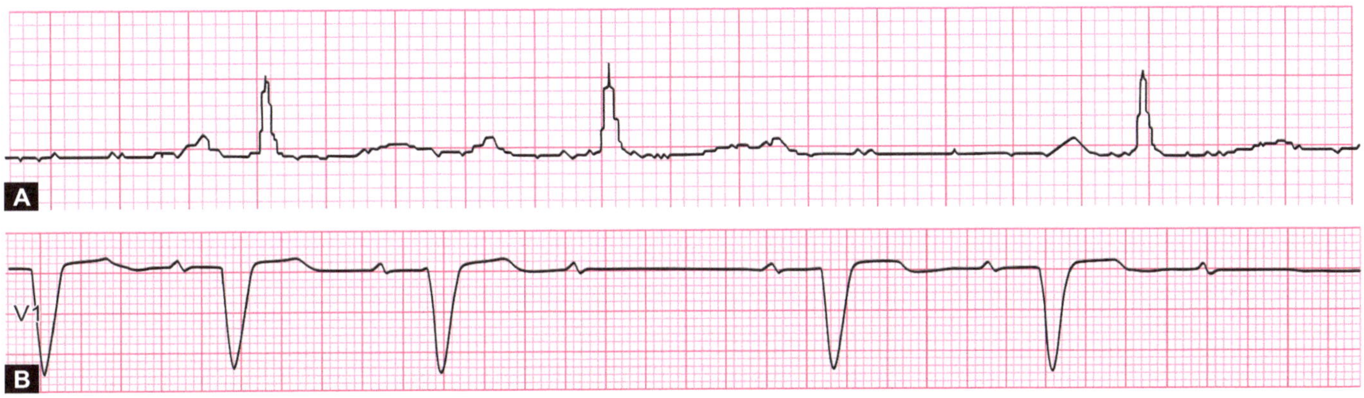

FIG. 3: Second degree atrioventricular (AV) block. **A,** Sinus rhythm with second degree type I (Wenckebach) AV block and 3:2 conduction; **B,** sinus rhythm with second degree type II AV block. Note the fixed PR intervals

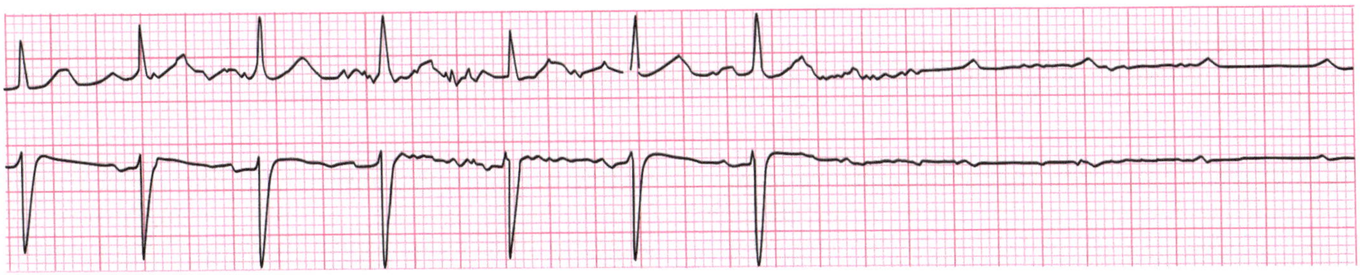

FIG. 4: High grade atrioventricular (AV) block. Sinus rhythm with sudden AV block as demonstrated by multiple nonconducted P waves

High grade AV block is a term used when there is more than one consecutive nonconducted P wave (Fig. 4).

Third Degree Atrioventricular Block

In third degree AV block, or complete heart block (CHB), there is complete absence of conduction through the AV node (Fig. 5). None of the atrial impulses reach the ventricles, and a perfusing rhythm is maintained by either a junctional or ventricular escape. On the ECG, CHB is characterized by AV dissociation, whereby P waves march out independently of the QRS complexes. The anatomic origin of the escape rhythm typically determines the ventricular rate, with more proximal sites such as the AV junction leading to rates of 40–60 beats/min and more distal ventricular sites demonstrating slower rates, 20–40 beats/min.

Nearly all patients with CHB will present with symptoms of reduced cardiac output, although they may be of varying severity. Fatigue and shortness of breath are common, as is presyncope or syncope.

In most cases, the cause is not identified and is attributed to idiopathic progressive conduction system disease (Lenegre's or Lev's disease). Identifiable etiologies of CHB may be acquired or congenital. Common causes

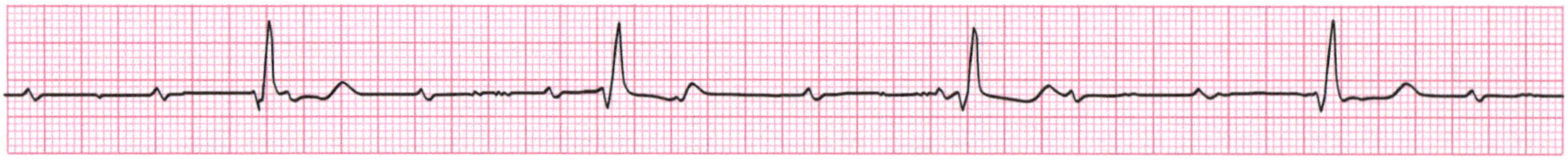

FIG. 5: Third degree (complete) atrioventricular block. Sinus rhythm with complete heart block and right bundle branch block. The progression of P waves can be marched out independent of the escape rhythm, with sinus rate 85 beats/min and ventricular rate approximately 30 beats/min

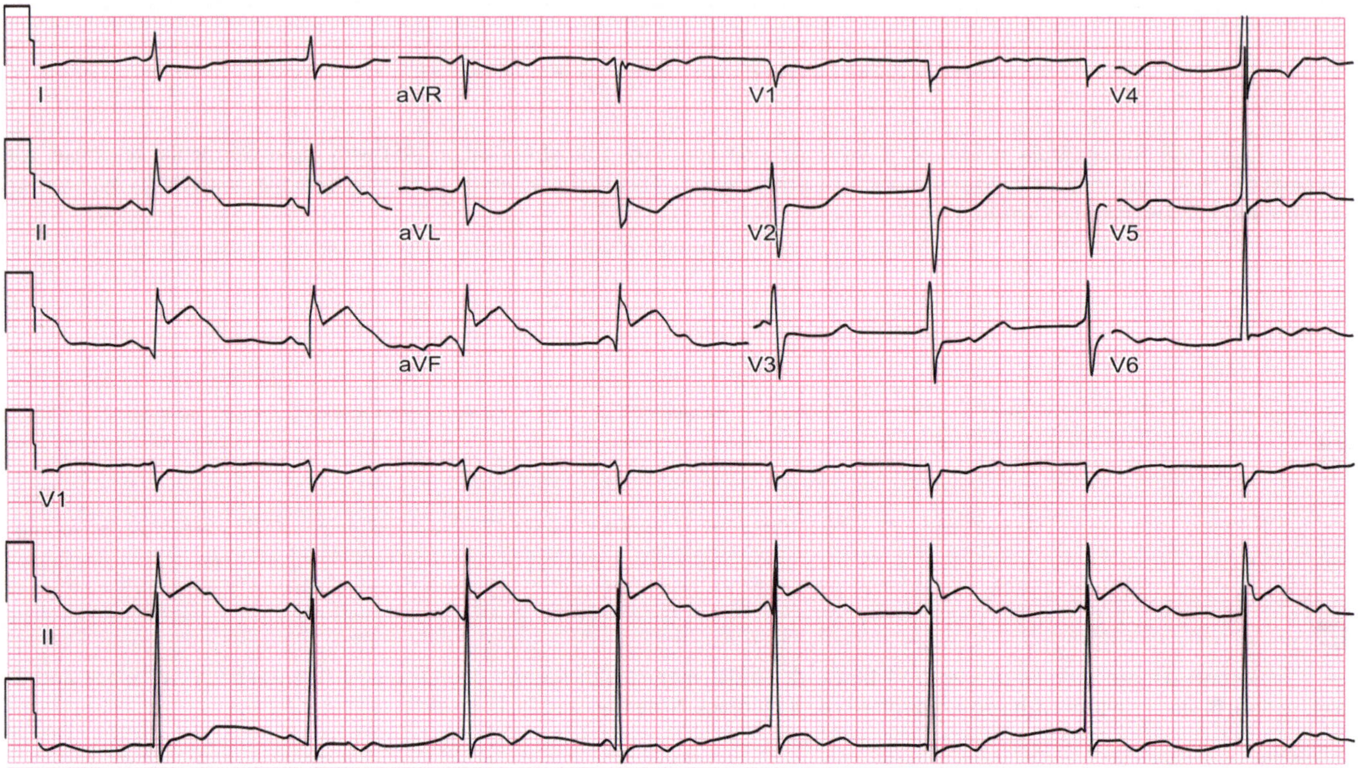

FIG. 6: Complete atrioventricular (AV) block complicating acute myocardial infarction. This 12-lead electrocardiogram demonstrates underlying sinus rhythm with complete AV block during an acute inferior myocardial infarction. After appropriate revascularization, the AV block resolved

of acquired CHB include myocardial ischemia, cardiomyopathy, endocarditis, post-cardiac surgery, and medication related, in particular AV nodal blocking agents. Congenital CHB is an uncommon and irreversible cause, occurring in 1 in 15,000 to 1 in 22,000 infants, and 70–90% can be linked to maternal/neonatal lupus.[7]

Atrioventricular block is an important and well-recognized complication of acute myocardial infarction (AMI), and thus should be evaluated for in the patient with new AV block. The incidence of high grade or complete AV block in AMI is 7–10%.[8,9] High grade or complete AV block occurs in 4–9% of inferior MI and 0.9–3% of anterior MI, and typically occur within the first 24 hours. The AV block associated with anterior MI is less common but more serious, and the severity of the arrhythmia depends on the extent of the infarction. The natural history of patients with AV block as a complication of AMI depends on the type of MI. Atrioventricular block that occurs after inferior MI (Fig. 6) is typically transient if timely revascularization is performed, however, AV block complicating any acute MI reduces inhospital mortality.[10,11] Of note, a particularly worrisome finding is AV block associated with either left bundle branch or with right bundle branch block plus left anterior or posterior fascicular block. In these circumstances, the association of intraventricular conduction delay with AV block, regardless of location of MI, is more reflective of more extensive infarction rather than an isolated electrical problem.[12]

Acute treatment of AV block in the setting of MI is the same as described above, with initial stabilization being followed immediately by revascularization, as indicated.

Pulseless Electrical Activity

Pulseless electrical activity (PEA) is defined as the absence of a measureable pulse despite organized electrical activity in the heart. Pulseless electrical activity typically occurs in the setting of profound systemic illness that prevents the cardiac muscle cells to generate a sufficient force of contraction. Common causes include hypovolemia, hypoxia, pulmonary embolism, cardiac tamponade, toxic ingestions, tension pneumothorax, and severe metabolic disturbances, namely, hyper- or hypokalemia. The prognosis for PEA is poor, and therapy is directed at the underlying etiology. Adjunctive therapies also include cardiopulmonary resuscitation, airway support, epinephrine, and atropine if the rhythm is bradycardic.

CONCLUSION

In this chapter, an overview of management of bradycardia is presented, focusing on the hemodynamically unstable patient. A comprehensive discussion of all aspects of the remainder of current guidelines is beyond the scope of this chapter. For additional resources, the reader should direct attention to the guidelines for advanced cardiac life support by Neumar, et al.[2]

REFERENCES

1. Sodeck GH, Domanovits H, Meron G, Rauscha F, Losert H, Thalmann M, et al. Compromising bradycardia: management in the emergency department. Resuscitation. 2007;73:96-102.
2. Neumar RW, Otto CW, Link MS, Kronick SL, Shuster M, Callaway CW, et al. Part 8: adult advanced cardiovascular life support: 2010 American Heart Association Guidelines for Cardiopulmonary Resuscitation and Emergency Cardiovascular Care. Circulation. 2010;122:S729-67.
3. Swart G, Brady WJ Jr., DeBehnke DJ, Ma OJ, Aufderheide TP. Acute myocardial infarction complicated by hemodynamically unstable bradyarrhythmia: prehospital and ED treatment with atropine. Am J Emerg Med. 1999;17:647-52.
4. Brady WJ, Swart G, DeBehnke DJ, Ma OJ, Aufderheide TP. The efficacy of atropine in the treatment of hemodynamically unstable bradycardia and atrioventricular block: prehospital and emergency department considerations. Resuscitation. 1999;41:47-55.
5. Bernheim A, Fatio R, Kiowski W, Weilenmann D, Rickli H, Brunner-La Rocca HP. Atropine often results in complete atrioventricular block or sinus arrest after cardiac transplantation: an unpredictable and dose-independent phenomenon. Transplantation. 2004;77:1181-5.
6. Rodriguez RD, Schocken DD. Update on sick sinus syndrome, a cardiac disorder of aging. Geriatrics. 1990;45:26-30, 33-6.
7. Michaelsson M, Engle MA. Congenital complete heart block: an international study of the natural history. Cardiovasc Clin. 1972;4:85-101.
8. Meine TJ, Al-Khatib SM, Alexander JH, Granger CB, White HD, Kilaru R, et al. Incidence, predictors, and outcomes of high-degree atrioventricular block complicating acute myocardial infarction treated with thrombolytic therapy. Am Heart J. 2005;149:670-4.
9. An international randomized trial comparing four thrombolytic strategies for acute myocardial infarction. The GUSTO investigators. N Engl J Med. 1993;329: 673-82.
10. Nicod P, Gilpin E, Dittrich H, Polikar R, Henning H, Ross J Jr. Long-term outcome in patients with inferior myocardial infarction and complete atrioventricular block. J Am Coll Cardiol. 1988;12:589-94.
11. Goldberg RJ, Zevallos JC, Yarzebski J, Alpert JS, Gore JM, Chen Z, et al. Prognosis of acute myocardial infarction complicated by complete heart block (the Worcester Heart Attack Study). Am J Cardiol. 1992;69:1135-41.
12. Domenighetti G and Perret C. Intraventricular conduction disturbances in acute myocardial infarction: short- and long-term prognosis. Eur J Cardiol. 1980;11:51-9.

31

CHAPTER

ABC of Pacing: Temporary and Permanent

Kay-Won Chang, Boris Arbit, Alan S Maisel

INTRODUCTION

Pathologic cardiac arrhythmias are some of the most critical conditions that emergency department (ED) providers encounter. When faced with severely symptomatic and hemodynamically unstable patients, appropriate and timely diagnosis, triage, and management are crucial. There are certain clinical scenarios when a pacemaker, temporary or permanent, is indicated. In the ED setting, it is imperative to know when to initiate temporary pacing, as this can be lifesaving. It is also important for ED providers to know the indications for a permanent pacemaker (PPM), as there are circumstances when this is a better solution than temporary pacing. This chapter will cover an in-depth review on the cardiac conduction pathway, indications for pacemaker implantation in the ED setting, types of pacing techniques, complications of pacemakers, and clinical approach to patients with pacemakers.

CARDIAC CONDUCTION

A brief review of the native cardiac conduction pathway will be helpful for our review. The cardiac conduction pathway consists of three major components: (i) sinus node, (ii) atrioventricular (AV) junctional area, and (iii) bundle branches.[1] The sinus node consists of nodal cells, which normally generate periodic electrical impulses.[1] This electrical impulse then travels to the AV junctional area, which consists of the transitional cell zone, AV node, and His bundle in sequential order.[2] The AV node serves as a filter between the sinus node and the bundle branches. When referring to pathology in the His bundle, it is commonly referred to as "intra-His." The conduction pathway distal to the His bundle is commonly referred to as "infra-His." Conduction degeneration in the infra-His region may be most hazardous in terms of hemodynamics and symptoms, requiring pacemaker support. The His bundle courses through the membranous septum and separates into the right and left bundle branches.[3] The left bundle branch then bifurcates into anterior and posterior fascicles. The distal ends of these bundle branches connect with Purkinje fibers, which then form networks on the endocardial surfaces of both ventricles and allow for ventricular contraction in response to an electrical impulse.[2]

INDICATIONS FOR PACING

Temporary versus Permanent

Pacing is typically indicated when a patient is severely symptomatic (e.g., severe chest pain, dyspnea, syncope, presyncope, altered mental status, hypotension, shock, pulmonary edema, etc.) secondary to an underlying arrhythmia and is refractory to pharmacologic therapy. Pathologic arrhythmias can lead to diminished cardiac output, which can be due to decreased heart rate (HR), decreased stroke volume, or both. Clinically, it can manifest as hypotension, altered mental status (cerebral hypoperfusion), oliguria (renal hypoperfusion), cool extremities (skin hypoperfusion), significant transaminitis (shock liver), and/or lactic acidosis (anaerobic metabolism). It will be up to the treatment provider as well as consultant cardiologist to establish the acuity and reversibility of the underlying arrhythmia. The American College of Cardiology Foundation and American Heart Association (ACCF/AHA) has an updated, evidence based guideline that delineates indications for PPM, illustrated in box 1.[4] While the ACCF/AHA guideline on ST segment elevation myocardial infarction (STEMI) recommends temporary pacing for refractory bradycardia in the setting of STEMI, there are no evidence based guidelines on other indications for temporary pacing.[5,6] Overall, the indications for temporary pacing appear to overlap with the indications for PPM, but the key clinical questions are urgency of pacing and reversibility of arrhythmia.[4,5] A temporary pacemaker is reasonable if a PPM cannot be implanted in a timely fashion. Another scenario when temporary cardiac pacing is indicated, is an acute but reversible condition where the arrhythmia is expected to resolve. Examples of acute reversible conditions are listed in box 2. An algorithmic approach to bradycardia in the ED setting is shown in flowchart 1.

BOX 1 Indications for permanent pacemaker based on the American College of Cardiology Foundation and American Heart Association device based therapy guidelines

Bradyarrhythmias

- Symptomatic sinus node dysfunction
  - Persistent sinus bradycardia
  - Chronotropic incompetence
  - Sinus arrest
  - Tachy-brady syndrome
- AV block
  - Symptomatic
  - Asymptomatic 3rd degree AV block
  - Asymptomatic 2nd degree AV block Mobitz type II
- Bifascicular block
  - Alternating bundle branch block
- Carotid sinus hypersensitivity syndrome
- Neurocardiogenic syncope

Tachyarrhythmias

- Refractory supraventricular tachycardia
- Sustained pause dependent ventricular tachycardia
- Long QT syndrome

AV, atrioventricular.

BOX 2 Indications for temporary pacemaker

- Acute myocardial infarction
- Cardiac trauma
- Repetitive monomorphic ventricular tachycardia
- Electrolyte disturbances (e.g., hyperkalemia)
- Aortic valve abscess
- Myocarditis
- Lyme disease
- Chagas disease

Some recent work has supported earlier PPM placement.[7] A retrospective study in Denmark examined patients requiring hospitalization while waiting for a PPM, and it showed that the mean time interval between acute indication for pacemaker and PPM implantation was 4.5 days.[7] Of these patients, 32% experienced at least one adverse event [e.g., infection, syncope, asystole, nonsustained ventricular tachycardia (VT), cardiac arrest, death] during this waiting period.[7] Furthermore, two out of 30 patients (6.6%) suffered complications related to a temporary transvenous pacemaker (lead displacements), and one of these patients had a cardiac arrest due to pace failure.[7] This study suggested that a 24-hour PPM implantation service is necessary for better clinical outcomes. As an ED provider, for patients who may have an acute indication for PPM, it is important to consult colleagues from cardiology and/or electrophysiology (EP) in a timely manner.

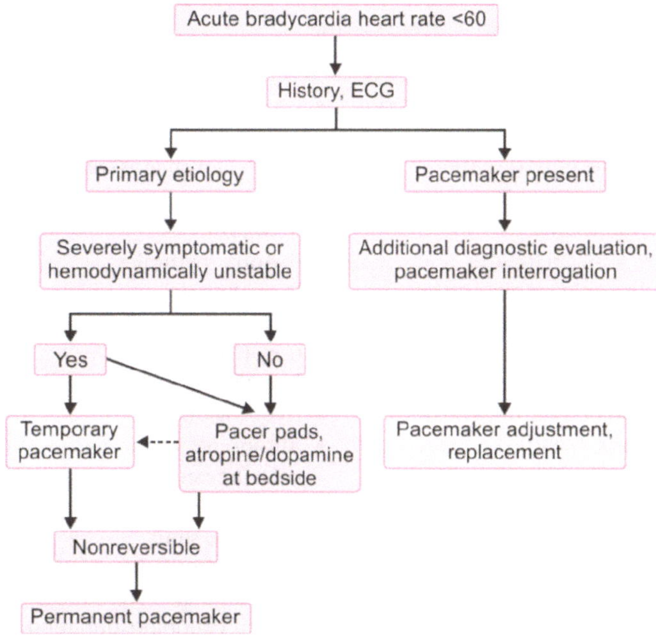

ECG, electrocardiogram.

FLOWCHART 1: Algorithmic approach to bradycardia

Bradyarrhythmias

When a patient presents to the ED with a HR less than 60 beats/min, it is important to obtain/interpret an electrocardiograph (ECG) and to distinguish between physiologic and pathologic bradycardia.[4] Symptomatic bradycardia is defined as a documented bradyarrhythmia that is directly responsible for development of syncope or near syncope, transient dizziness or lightheadedness, or altered mental status secondary to cerebral hypoperfusion.[4] Before making a diagnosis of symptomatic bradycardia, it is important to rule out intrinsic and extrinsic causes of bradycardia, listed in box 3.[3]

Bradyarrhythmias can be further classified into the following subgroups:

- Sinus node dysfunction (SND)
- Acquired AV block in adults
- Chronic bifascicular block
- Atrioventricular block associated with acute myocardial infarction
- Carotid sinus hypersensitivity
- Neurocardiogenic syncope.

Sinus node dysfunction, also known as sick sinus syndrome, is a heterogeneous term that encompasses persistent sinus bradycardia, chronotropic incompetence (unable to increase HR adequately), paroxysmal or persistent sinus arrest with replacement by escape rhythms, and tachy-brady syndrome (oscillate between sinus bradyarrhythmia and paroxysmal atrial fibrillation).[4] Electrocardiographic examples of various types of SND are shown in figures 1–3. The natural history of SND is highly variable.[4] For SND patients with a history of syncope, the

BOX 3 Causes of bradycardia

Intrinsic causes
- Myocardial ischemia and/or infarction
- Infectious diseases
  - Endocarditis
  - Chagas
- Surgical trauma
  - Valve replacement
  - Correction of congenital heart disease
  - Heart transplantation
- Idiopathic degeneration (ex. Aging)
- Infiltrative diseases
  - Sarcoidosis
  - Amyloidosis
  - Hemochromatosis
- Collagen vascular diseases
  - Systemic lupus erythematosus
  - Rheumatoid arthritis
  - Scleroderma
- Myotonic muscular dystrophy
- Familial diseases

Extrinsic causes
- Drugs
  - Beta blockers
  - Calcium channel blockers
  - Clonidine
  - Digoxin
  - Antiarrhythmics
- Hypothermia
- Electrolyte disturbances (e.g., hypo- or hyperkalemia)
- Hypothyroidism
- Autonomic syndromes
  - Neurocardiogenic syncope
  - Carotid sinus hypersensitivity
  - Situational disturbances (e.g., coughing, urinating, defecating, vomiting)

risk of recurrent syncope is significantly higher compared to those without a history of syncope.[8] However, the overall mortality rate in SND is quite low, comparable to that of the normal population.[9,10] Therefore, the main purpose of PPM implantation in SND is to improve symptoms rather than to improve survival, which is why PPM implantation is only reserved for patients with symptomatic SND.[11] Chronotropic incompetence is defined as the inability of the heart to increase its rates in response to exercise (increased sympathetic tone and metabolic workload).[12] Unfortunately, no single metric has been established as a gold standard for diagnosis of chronotropic incompetence.[4,12] If a patient has symptoms secondary to suspected chronotropic incompetence, a PPM can be implanted for symptom relief. Finally, if a patient has symptomatic bradycardia due to treatment of a rapid rhythm (e.g., β-blocker for rate control of rapid atrial fibrillation), a PPM is also indicated.[4]

Atrioventricular block refers to abnormalities in the cardiac conduction system and is classified into the following groups. Electrocardiographic examples are shown in figures 4–7.

- First degree AV block: PR interval more than 0.2 seconds
- Second degree AV block

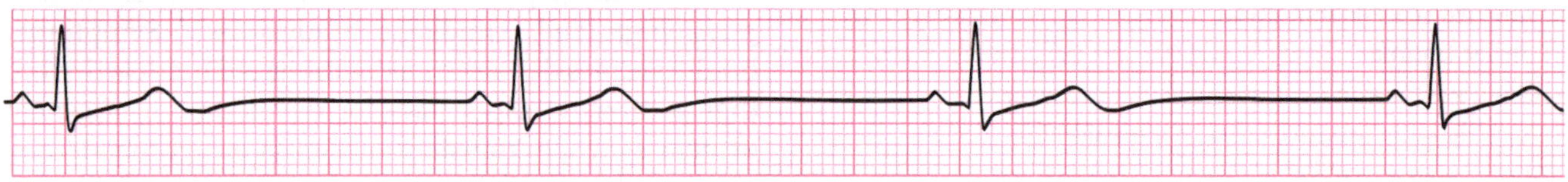

FIG. 1: Sinus bradycardia

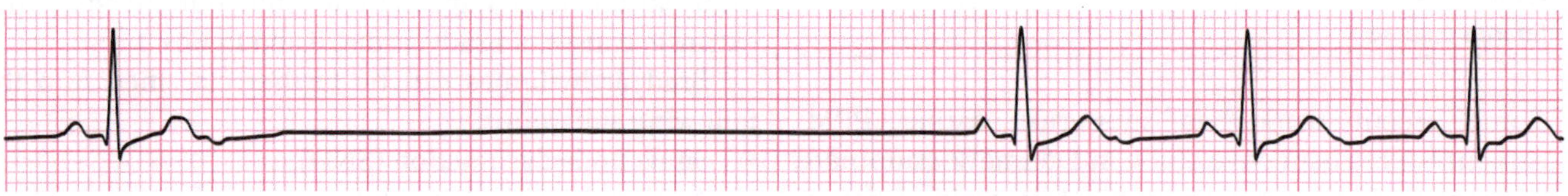

FIG. 2: Sinus arrest

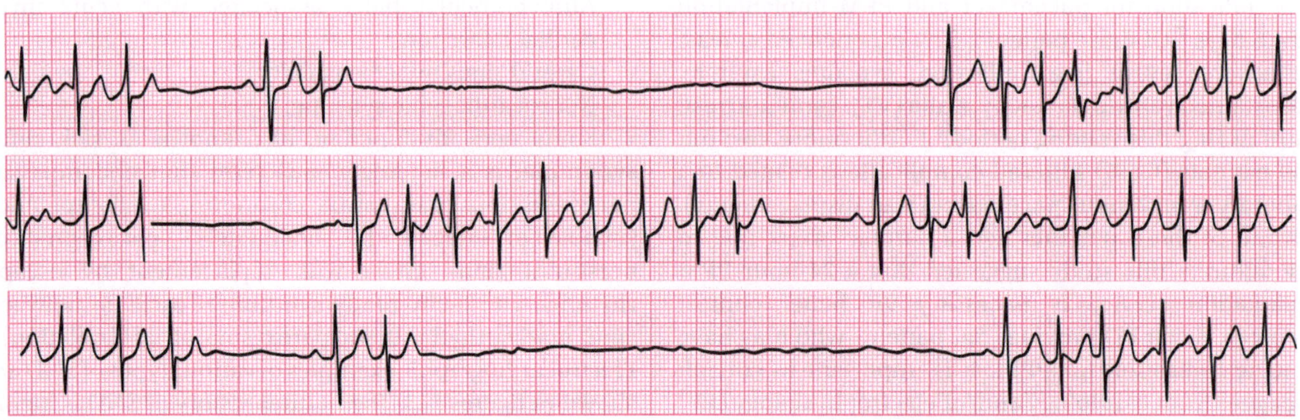

FIG. 3: Tachy-brady syndrome

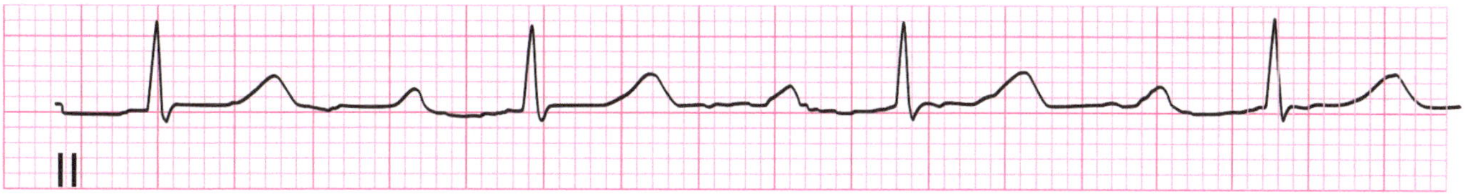

FIG. 4: First degree atrioventricular block

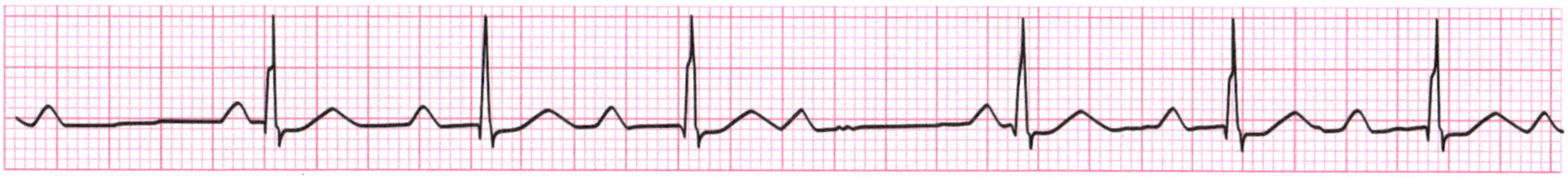

FIG. 5: Second degree atrioventricular block Mobitz type I

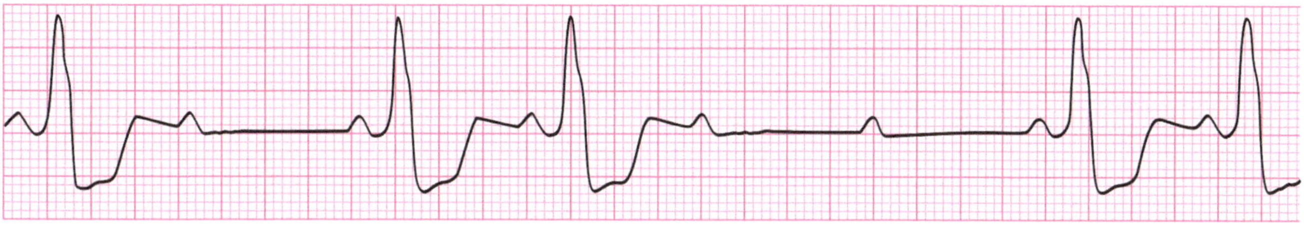

FIG. 6: Second degree atrioventricular block Mobitz type II

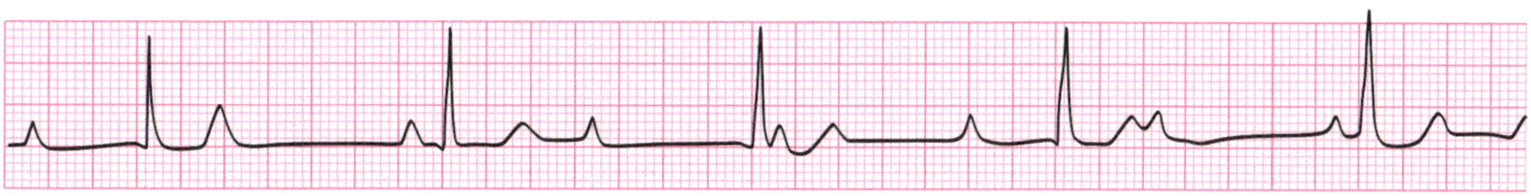

FIG. 7: Third degree atrioventricular block

  - Mobitz type I: Progressive prolongation of PR interval before a nonconducted beat
  - Mobitz type II: Fixed PR intervals before and after nonconducted beats.
- Third degree AV block: P waves and QRS complexes independent of each other.

The indications for pacing in AV block have evolved over the last 40 years based on small-scale case series and clinical experience.[4] Unfortunately, there are no randomized controlled trials (RCTs) to support the use of pacemakers for AV block, mainly because no acceptable alternative options exist to treat symptomatic bradycardia in the setting of AV block.[4]

The 1st degree AV block with moderate PR prolongation has long been considered to be a benign condition given rare progression to more advanced AV block.[13] However, in a patient with 1st degree AV block and marked PR prolongation (i.e., PR interval >300 ms), the close proximity of atrial systole to prior ventricular systole can compromise hemodynamics due to inadequate timing of atrial and ventricular contractions.[14]

With regards to 2nd degree AV block, traditional teaching conveyed that while Mobitz type I block affects the AV node and is well-tolerated, Mobitz type II block is distal to the AV node and potentially more hazardous. This anatomic concept of Mobitz type I versus type II was supported by an EP study that examined 15 patients with 2nd degree AV block, both Mobitz type I and II, and bundle branch block on surface ECG, which showed that patients with Mobitz type I had a block proximal to the His bundle, whereas patients with Mobitz type II had a block distal to the His bundle.[15] All nine patients with a block distal to the His bundle eventually required PPM implantation, and three out of four patients with a block proximal to the His bundle required PPM.[15] However, a different EP study showed that Mobitz type I block can also affect the bundle branches, challenging the notion that Mobitz type I block is always proximal to the His bundle.[16] Therefore, certain forms of Mobitz type I block can be intra- or even infra-His, and this can only be confirmed by a dedicated EP study.[17] For patients with no evidence of organic heart disease, Mobitz type I block is relatively benign, but it may be pathologic in the setting of underlying coronary artery disease (CAD).[18] In a prospective case series of 56 patients with Mobitz type I block (proximal to His bundle proven by EP study), only one out of 19 patients without organic heart disease, defined as prior myocardial infarction and/or exertional angina, required a PPM due to symptomatic bradycardia.[18] On the other hand, of the 37 patients with organic heart disease, 10 required PPM implantation (eight for congestive heart failure, two for syncope), and 16 out of 37 patients died.[18]

In the 3rd degree AV block, also known as complete heart block (CHB), electrical impulses are unable to traverse from the sinus node to the ventricles, so the atria and ventricles contract independently of each other. In other words, there is no AV conduction.[4] In patients with syncope and CHB, mortality rate after surgical implantation of internal electric pacemakers was 17% at 37 months, which was significantly better than previously published data that revealed 50% mortality at 42 months in patients who were medically managed, suggesting that PPM improves survival in patients with syncope due to CHB.[19,20] The prognosis of CHB is poor. A different cohort study, reported a 1-year mortality rate of 50% in patients with symptomatic CHB who were only paced when severely symptomatic.[21] Experts have consistently maintained that asymptomatic patients with CHB warrant PPM placement.[22]

Based on the available evidence, it appears that for symptomatic patients with any degree of irreversible AV block, a PPM is indicated. For asymptomatic patients with Mobitz type II or 3rd degree AV block, a PPM is indicated given poor prognosis without a pacemaker. There is no indication for a PPM in asymptomatic Mobitz type I block unless an EP study confirms that the block is either intra- or infra-His, which is suggestive of more advanced AV block and poor prognosis.[4] There is no indication for a PPM in asymptomatic 1st degree AV block.

The ACCF/AHA guidelines define bifascicular block (BFB) as ECG evidence of impaired conduction in both left and right bundle branches distal to the AV node, meaning both left bundle branch block (LBBB) and right bundle branch block (RBBB).[4] Alternating bundle branch block (BBB), also known as bilateral BBB, refers to successive ECG evidence of impaired conduction in all three fascicles: RBBB, left anterior fascicular block (LAFB), and left posterior fascicular block (LPFB).[4] Numerous BFB studies have defined BFB more literally as impaired conduction in two (bilateral) fascicles, rather than three fascicles.[23-27] Therefore, we will define BFB as ECG evidence of impaired conduction in two fascicles (RBBB and LPFB, RBBB and LAFB, or LBBB) rather than all three.

Syncope is a common presentation of BFB, but patients with syncope or even recurrent syncope are not at higher risk of death.[27-29] In the ED setting, if a patient presents with syncope and is found to have alternating BBB on serial ECGs, a PPM is indicated.[4] Otherwise, most management of chronic BFB can be addressed as an outpatient. There is thought that BFB is a precursor to CHB, which theoretically makes sense.[4] However, a prospective cohort study of 554 patients with chronic bifascicular and trifascicular blocks showed that the risks of CHB (3.4%) and death from bradyarrhythmia (0.4%) were low.[29] It must be noted that there were 160 deaths (28.9%) in this study population, mainly due to tachyarrhythmia and myocardial infarction, and predictors of death included increased age, congestive heart failure, and CAD.[29] A different cohort study that examined patients with incidental ECG findings of chronic RBBB and LAFB confirmed rare progression to advanced 2nd degree AV block (8.4%) and CHB (2.4%), suggesting that prophylactic pacing in this patient population is not warranted.[30] It may be concluded that BFB alone, in the absence of significant cardiac risk factors, does not warrant emergent therapy and may be addressed as an outpatient.

When a patient presents to the ED with chest pain, prompt ECG with cardiac biomarkers is typically obtained to assess for acute myocardial infarction (AMI). Cardiac arrhythmias secondary to ischemia may complicate the disease course of AMI. A retrospective analysis of a large database showed that patients with an inferior or posterior AMI were more likely to develop AV node conduction abnormalities compared to those with anterior or lateral AMI [3.7% vs. 1.0%, hazard ratio (HR) 3.9, $p < 0.001$] but less likely to develop ventricular fibrillation (VF) (8.1% vs. 9.0%, HR 0.89, $p = 0.02$).[31] In addition to location of AMI, it is important to assess for BBB on ECG, since it portends a high mortality rate.[32-34] Progression to Mobitz type II and/or CHB occurs more frequently in patients with RBBB + LAFB, RBBB + LPFB, or alternating BBB as opposed to isolated LBBB or RBBB, and patients with transient high degree AV block (Mobitz type II or CHB) had a 28% incidence of sudden cardiac death or recurrent high degree AV block in 1-year follow-up.[32] Patients who underwent temporary cardiac pacing had significantly decreased incidence of sudden cardiac death or recurrent high degree AV block compared to those who were not paced (10 vs. 65%, $p < 0.001$).[32] A recent meta-analysis showed that admission ECG for patients with AMI had prognostic value, namely that 2nd or 3rd degree AV block and QRS more than or equal to 0.10 second were strong predictors of increased short-term mortality, and LBBB was a strong predictor of long-term mortality.[34] Robust data does not exist for PPM implantation in this patient population, but temporary cardiac pacing is currently recommended for symptomatic bradycardia in setting of STEMI.[6]

Carotid sinus hypersensitivity (CSH) syndrome and neurocardiogenic syncope (also known as vasovagal syncope) should always be on the differential diagnosis for syncope, especially recurrent syncope, in the ED. For patients over age of 50 years who present to the ED with nonaccidental fall, it is also important to consider CSH.[35] Carotid sinus hypersensitivity syndrome is defined as syncope or presyncope secondary to an extreme reflex response to carotid sinus stimulation.[4] An extreme reflex response to carotid sinus stimulation is defined as asystole more than 3 seconds due to either sinus arrest or AV block, substantial symptomatic hypotension, or both.[4] Carotid sinus hypersensitivity can be further classified into three types: (i) cardioinhibitory, (ii) vasodepressor, and (iii) mixed.[4,35] The cardioinhibitory type refers to increased parasympathetic (or vagal) tone that results in slowing of HR, PR interval prolongation, and/or advanced AV block.[4] The vasodepressor type refers to reduced sympathetic tone, resulting in loss of vascular tone and hypotension but no change in HR.[4] Mixed type refers to clinical features of both cardioinhibitory and vasodepressor types. By observing changes in HR and blood pressure in response to carotid sinus stimulation, it is important to decipher between cardioinhibitory and vasodepressor types, since a PPM has been shown to reduce syncopal episodes in cardioinhibitory type.[36,37] In addition, a PPM has been shown to reduce nonaccidental falls in adults over an age of 50 years with cardioinhibitory type of CSH, suggesting a potential role for PPM even in patients without syncope.[35] To date, there is no data to support pacing in vasodepressor type of CSH.[38] Therefore, a PPM is only indicated for patients with recurrent syncope secondary to cardioinhibitory type of CSH.

Neurocardiogenic, also known as vasovagal, syncope refers to a variety of clinical scenarios in which triggering of a neural reflex results in an episode of systemic hypotension characterized by both bradycardia and peripheral vasodilation.[4] It tends to occur in younger patients and usually exhibits three distinct phases: (i) prodrome of lightheadedness, nausea, diaphoresis, or visual changes; (ii) sudden loss of consciousness; and (iii) rapid recovery.[39] Possible triggers include pain, anxiety, stress, urination, defecation, or crowded conditions.[4] The primary diagnostic modality for vasovagal syncope has been tilt table testing.[40] For patients with recurrent vasovagal syncope, it remains unclear whether a PPM is beneficial in decreasing recurrence of syncope.[4] The Vasovagal Pacemaker Study (VPS) I and Vasovagal Syncope International Study (VASIS) trials were both unblinded RCTs that showed reduced recurrence of syncope in paced patients compared to those who received no therapy.[41,42] The Syncope Diagnosis and Treatment (SYDIT) trial was an unblinded RCT that showed reduced recurrence of syncope in paced patients compared to those who received atenolol.[43] However, the VPS II trial was a single blinded RCT in which patients received a PPM that was switched off, and it showed no difference in recurrence of syncope between paced and unpaced patients.[44] In summary, PPM implantation is controversial for recurrent vasovagal syncope, and it is important to discuss these complex cases with colleagues from cardiology and/or EP.

Tachyarrhythmias

The role of pacing alone in tachyarrhythmias is limited, especially in the current age of implantable cardioverter defibrillators. There is potential utility in refractory supraventricular tachycardia, pause-dependent VT, and congenital long QT syndrome, but these issues are not relevant to the ED setting.[4] In summary, there is minimal role for temporary or permanent cardiac pacing for tachyarrhythmias in the ED setting.

TYPES OF PACING TECHNIQUES

There are four methods of temporary pacing: transcutaneous pacing, transvenous pacing, epicardial pacing, and transesophageal pacing.[45] Epicardial pacing is usually performed after cardiac surgery since it requires direct access to the external surface of the myocardium.[45] Transesophageal pacing is not commonly used since it is uncomfortable, unreliable, and extremely invasive. Therefore, these two temporary pacing modalities will not be covered, as they are impractical and irrelevant in the ED setting. Transcutaneous pacing is the least invasive and can be achieved rapidly with minimal training.[45] Transcutaneous pacing electrodes, commonly known as "pacer pads," are placed in an anteroposterior or anterolateral configuration.[45] The idea is to configure the pacer pads such that the heart is in between the two pacing electrodes, but due to variations in patient heart anatomies, this can be challenging. The major pitfalls with transcutaneous pacing are adequate capture and discomfort to the patient. Due to the impedance of the chest wall between the heart and pacer pads, there can be difficulty with the myocardium capturing the electrical signal from the pacer pads. Furthermore, more energy from the pacemaker may be required for adequate capture of the electrical signal, and this can be very uncomfortable to an awake patient. Therefore, transcutaneous pacing is preferable in an unconscious or sedated patient.

Transvenous pacing involves placing a catheter based electrode into the right side of the heart.[5] The equipment required includes a central venous access kit, introducer sheath, pacing catheter, and external pacing generator. After gathering all of the necessary equipments, setting up in an organized fashion, and creating a sterile field, the provider must perform two procedures. First, the provider establishes central venous access, ideally via the right internal jugular or left subclavian vein, since these two sites have demonstrated the highest rates of proper placement in code situations.[5] Next, the provider introduces and directs the electrode through the venous system into the right ventricular wall. Overall, transvenous pacing is significantly more invasive and technically challenging compared to transcutaneous pacing, but it offers a more comfortable and stable temporary pacing solution. If the ED provider is uncomfortable performing this procedure, it is reasonable to consult colleagues from cardiology and/or EP.

COMPLICATIONS

As discussed above, transcutaneous pacemaker is the least invasive pacing modality with minimal complications other than failure to capture (myocardium unable to receive electrical signal) and patient discomfort. Transvenous pacemakers, on the other hand, are quite invasive and carry numerous risks. With relation to central venous access, the usual complications apply, including risk of bleeding, infection, and damage to nearby structures. Damage to nearby structures include risk of pneumothorax (particularly with a subclavian approach) and accidental arterial puncture.[5] More serious but rare complications include risk of air embolism, venous thromboembolism and thrombophlebitis, and catheter/guidewire looping and entrapment.[5] With regards to the right heart catheterization, the risks include inducing pathologic arrhythmias, failure to pace, failure to capture, failure to sense, and most seriously, ventricular free wall perforation.[5] Failure to pace, failure to capture, and failure to sense will be discussed in the next section. Signs and symptoms suggestive of ventricular free wall perforation include loss of capture, chest pain, pacing of thoracic chest wall, and/or new pericardial friction rub.[5] Serious downstream consequences of free wall perforation include hemopericardium, pericardial tamponade, and death.[5] Therefore, it is good practice to obtain an echocardiogram on a patient after placing a temporary transvenous pacemaker.

APPROACH TO PATIENT WITH PACEMAKER

In any patient who presents to the ED with a pacemaker, it is important to consider pacemaker complication or malfunction on the differential diagnosis. First and foremost, the patient should be assessed for hemodynamic stability. If patient is hemodynamically unstable, clinical stabilization is more important than thorough evaluation of PPM. If there is suspicion for PPM failure (e.g., symptomatic bradycardia despite PPM), initial management should include transcutaneous pacing. If patient is hemodynamically stable, then the ED provider can proceed with a more thorough evaluation that consists of history, physical examination, ECG, laboratory data, chest X-ray, and application of a magnet.[46] History should focus on symptoms that could relate to the pacemaker system, including palpitations, weakness, fatigue, shortness of breath, hiccups (diaphragmatic stimulation), muscle twitches, presyncope, syncope, dizziness, and pain or erythema around the implant.[46] In addition, symptoms of upper extremity deep venous thrombosis (erythema, edema, pain, facial swelling), infection (fever, chills, malaise, weight loss, fatigue), and bleeding should be elicited.[46] It is also important to obtain the model number, manufacturer, and program code associated with a patient's PPM, since this information allows the ED provider to interrogate the device.[46] Physical examination should focus on vital signs, mental status, jugular venous pressure, cardiopulmonary examination, and inspection of PPM site (erythema, edema, tenderness, trauma).[46] The chest wall should be examined for extracardiac stimulation, including pectoralis muscles and diaphragmatic twitching or fasciculations.[46] After a baseline ECG is obtained, it is of diagnostic utility to repeat an ECG while applying a magnet over the generator, which converts the pacemaker to asynchronous (fixed, nondemand) pacing and allows the ED provider to assess for capture on ECG.[46]

For any patient with a PPM, the ED provider must be aware of the complications of PPM implantation, which can be divided into three geographic areas: (i) the "pocket" where the PPM is implanted, (ii) transvenous lead placement, and (iii) electrode-myocardium interface.[46] The so-called "pocket" is a submuscular or subcutaneous space created by the implanting physician where the PPM is implanted.[46] Pocket complications include hematoma, infection, wound dehiscence, migration of pacemaker, and erosion of the pocket wall.[46] If there is a palpable hematoma, patient needs surgical exploration.[46] If there is suspicion for pocket infection, obtaining cultures from the pocket itself may have diagnostic value.[46] Transvenous lead complications are similar to those encountered in temporary transvenous pacemaker implantation, but there is a higher risk of infection given chronicity of PPM. Electrode-myocardium interface complications are also similar to those encountered in temporary transvenous pacemaker implantation, but there is higher risk of lead dislodgement and migration given chronicity of PPM. Lead dislodgement and migration usually present as pacemaker malfunction, and the diagnosis can be confirmed with a chest X-ray.[46] If there is concern for lead infection, at least two sets of blood cultures and transesophageal, not transthoracic, echocardiogram should be obtained urgently to evaluate for vegetations.[47]

If device infection is confirmed, then the PPM and leads need to be removed.[47]

Pacemaker malfunction can be divided into the following areas:

- Failure to pace
- Failure to capture
- Failure to sense
- Pacemaker mediated arrhythmia.[48]

Failure to pace means the pacemaker is unsuccessful at delivering an electrical signal to the heart.[48] The most common cause of failure to pace is oversensing.[48] In oversensing, the pacemaker is inappropriately inhibited because it senses signals that it should not normally detect.[48] For example, the pacemaker may misinterpret an artifact electrical signal as a QRS complex, inhibiting ventricular pacing. Electrocardiographic example of oversensing is illustrated in figure 8. Other causes are related to pacemaker malfunction, such as battery failure, lead dislodgement, and lead migration.[48] To distinguish between oversensing and pacemaker malfunction, the ED provider should place a magnet over the PPM, which disables sensing function.[48] If the etiology is oversensing, pacemaker spikes should appear on ECG after the magnet is applied. If the etiology is pacemaker malfunction, pacemaker spikes will not appear even with a magnet.

Failure to capture means the electrical signal from the pacemaker fails to trigger myocardial depolarization, shown in figure 9.[48] Typically, this is related to pacemaker malfunction, but there are organic causes of elevated voltage threshold.[48] An elevated voltage threshold refers to needing a higher voltage electrical signal in order to trigger a myocardial depolarization. Organic causes include myocardial ischemia, antiarrhythmic agents, external defibrillation, acidemia, hyperkalemia, hypoxemia, and hypothyroidism.[48]

Failure to sense, also known as undersensing, means the pacemaker fails to sense or detect native cardiac activity, shown in figure 10.[48] In addition to usual pacemaker malfunction issues, other causes include AMI, VF, VT, premature ventricular complexes, atrial fibrillation, atrial flutter, and new bundle branch blocks.[48] Management is aimed at correcting the underlying cause.[48]

Occasionally, a pacemaker itself can be the source of an arrhythmia.[48] Examples include pacemaker mediated tachycardia, runaway pacemaker, arrhythmias secondary to lead dislodgement, and sensor induced tachycardias.[48] Pacemaker mediated tachycardia is a re-entry arrhythmia where a dual chamber pacemaker itself acts as part of the re-entry circuit.[48] The tachycardia cannot exceed the programmed upper limit of the PPM.[48] Applying a magnet is both diagnostic and therapeutic, since it will terminate the

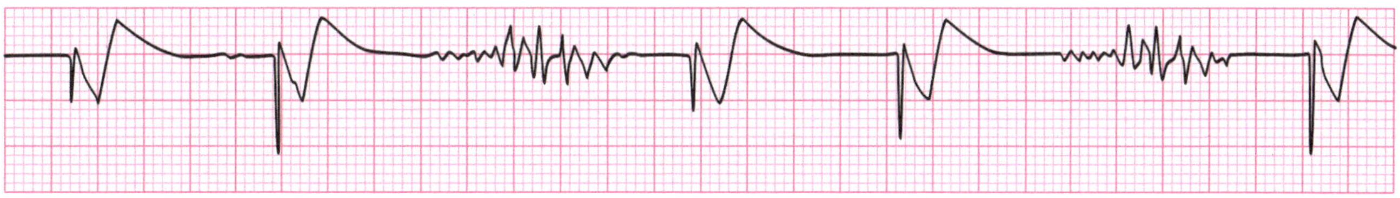

FIG. 8: Oversensing

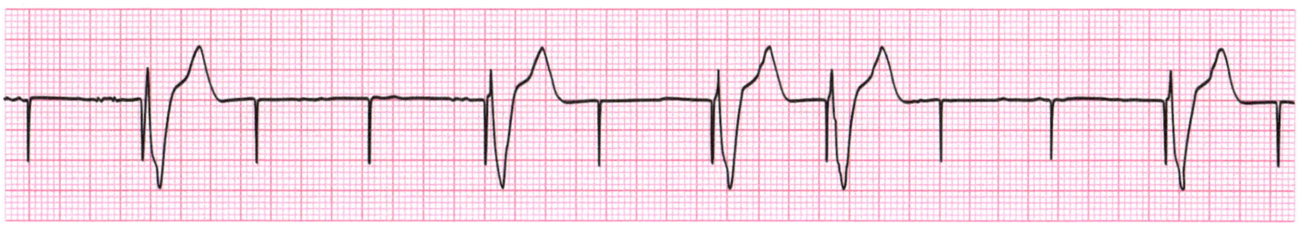

FIG. 9: Failure to capture

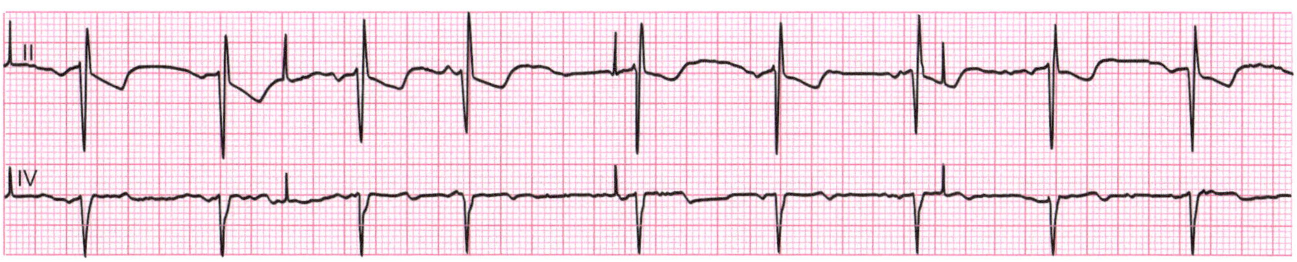

FIG. 10: Failure to sense

sensing function of the PPM and consequently terminate the tachyarrhythmia.[48] Alternative management options include vagal maneuvers and adenosine, which block both retrograde and anterograde conduction through the AV node.[48] Runaway pacemaker is a rare but true medical emergency that occurs secondary to inappropriately rapid discharges from the PPM, potentially inducing VT or VF.[48] Modern pacemakers are programmed to prevent discharges beyond a set limit, usually 180 beats/min.[48] Management options include magnet, emergency reprogramming, and if all else fails, surgical intervention to disconnect the leads.[48] Lead dislodgement, depending on where the lead is displaced, can act as a focus for ventricular arrhythmias.[48] Sensor induced tachycardias refer to scenarios where the PPM senses exterior activity such as loud noises, strong vibrations, or temperature extremes and consequently increases the pacing rate.[48] This is easily addressed with a magnet, which disables sensing.[48]

Pacemaker syndrome is a complex process that is thought to involve suboptimal AV synchrony or AV dyssynchrony, which then decreases cardiac output.[48] Clinically, the symptoms are similar to that of symptomatic bradycardia with manifestations of hypoperfusion. Management involves switching the pacing mode to one that restores AV synchrony, often from a single chamber pacing system to a dual chamber pacemaker, and this can usually be addressed as an outpatient.[48]

Finally, there are two life-threatening clinical scenarios which must be discussed—AMI and cardiac arrest. The ECG diagnosis of AMI is more complex in patients with PPM, since right ventricular pacing manifests as a LBBB pattern with discordant ST segment abnormalities, meaning the ST segment and T wave complex point in the opposite direction of the QRS complex (figure 11).[48] There are three criteria, defined by Sgarbossa, that are used to predict AMI:

1. ST segment elevation more than or equal to 5 mm discordant with QRS polarity (sensitivity 53%, specificity 88%)[49]
2. ST segment elevation more than or equal to 1 mm concordant with QRS polarity (sensitivity 18%, specificity 94%)[49]
3. ST segment depression more than or equal to 1 mm in leads V1, V2, or V3 (sensitivity 29%, specificity 82%).[49]

The limitations of Sgarbossa's criteria should be kept in mind, especially the criterion of ST segment elevation more than or equal to 5 mm discordant with QRS polarity, since there are instances when ST segment elevation is less than or equal to 5 mm, but the uphill convex elevation of the ST segment suggests AMI.[50] Electrocardiographic examples are illustrated in figures 12–14.[50] When there is concern for AMI in a patient with PPM, it is important to consult colleagues from cardiology for assistance with ECG interpretation. If a patient presents with cardiac arrest, it is reasonable to follow advanced cardiac life

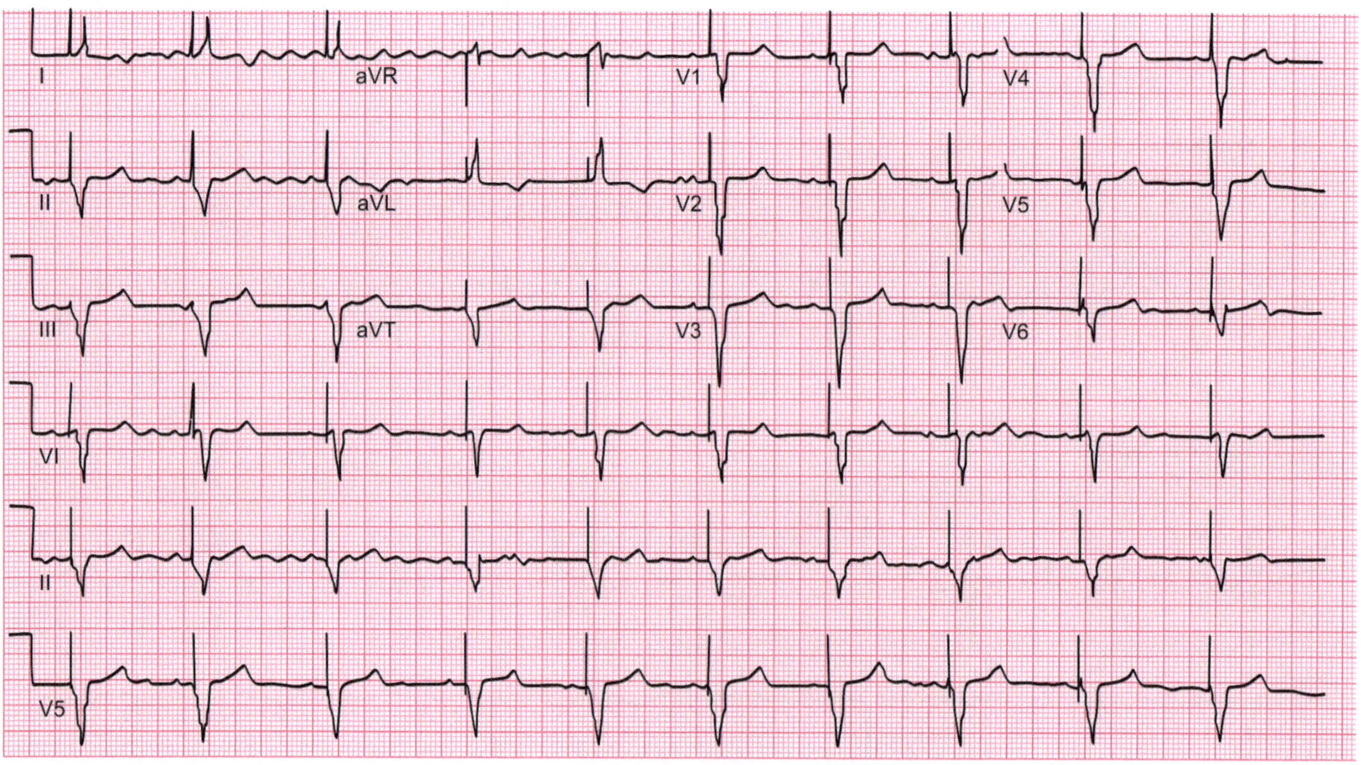

FIG. 11: Left bundle branch block pattern in ventricular pacing

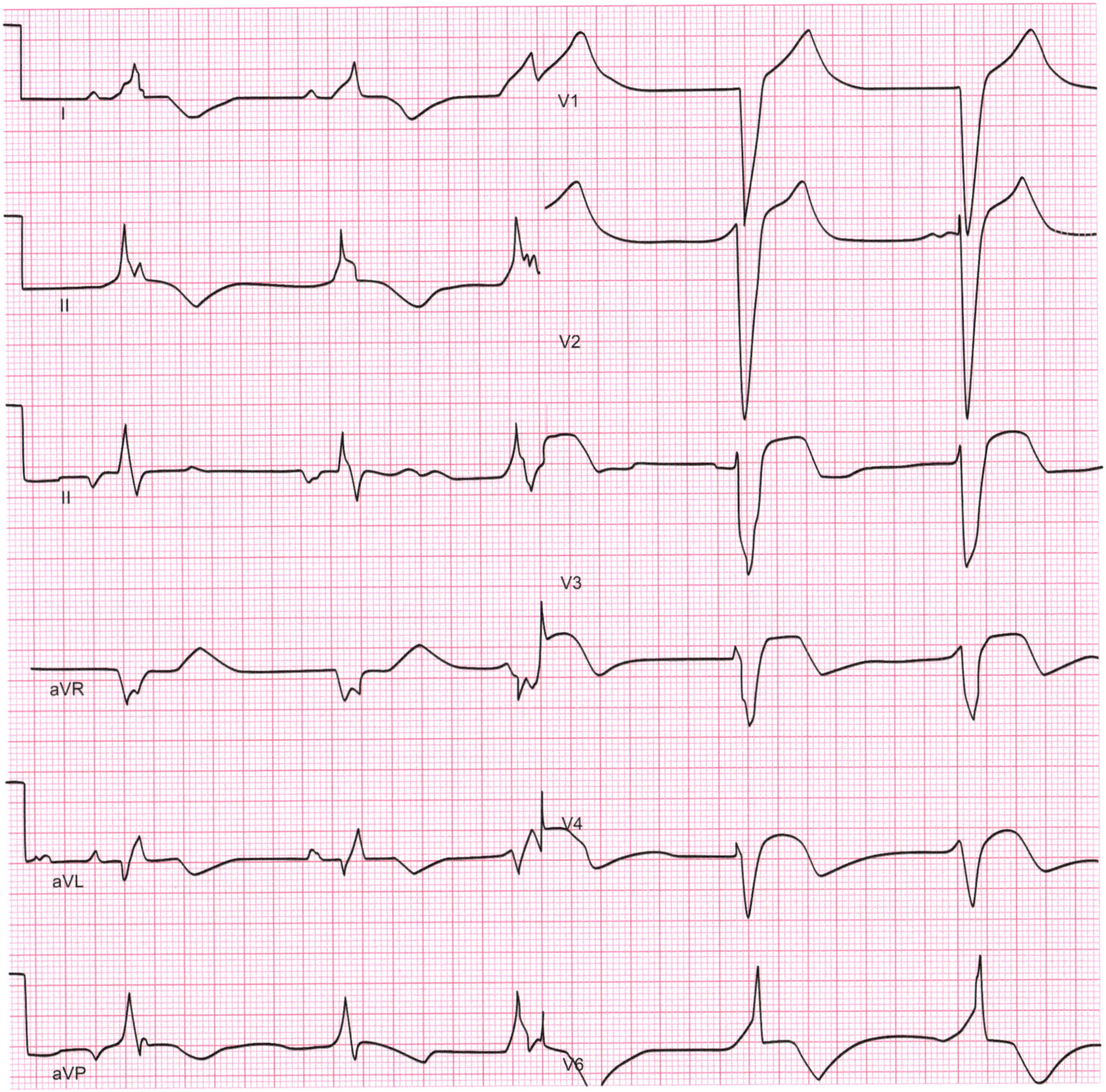

FIG. 12: ST segment elevation ≥5 mm with discordant QRS

support algorithms to aggressively resuscitate the patient with high quality chest compressions, since clinical stabilization is more important than the effects of external defibrillation and antiarrhythmics on the existing PPM.[48] The problems associated with pacemakers are summarized in table 1.

CONCLUSION

There are specific indications for pacing in patients with pathologic arrhythmias. Since there are no alternatives to pacing for symptomatic bradycardia that is refractory to other interventions, RCT data are limited. Most importantly to the ED provider, it is important to ensure clinical stability of bradycardic patients with medications and if necessary, temporary cardiac pacing with pacer pads, before consulting colleagues from cardiology and/or EP for PPM implantation. For asymptomatic patients, the ED provider must use clinical judgment to decide on the urgency of arrhythmia management. Finally, the ED provider must be able to recognize and manage pacemaker malfunction and complications.

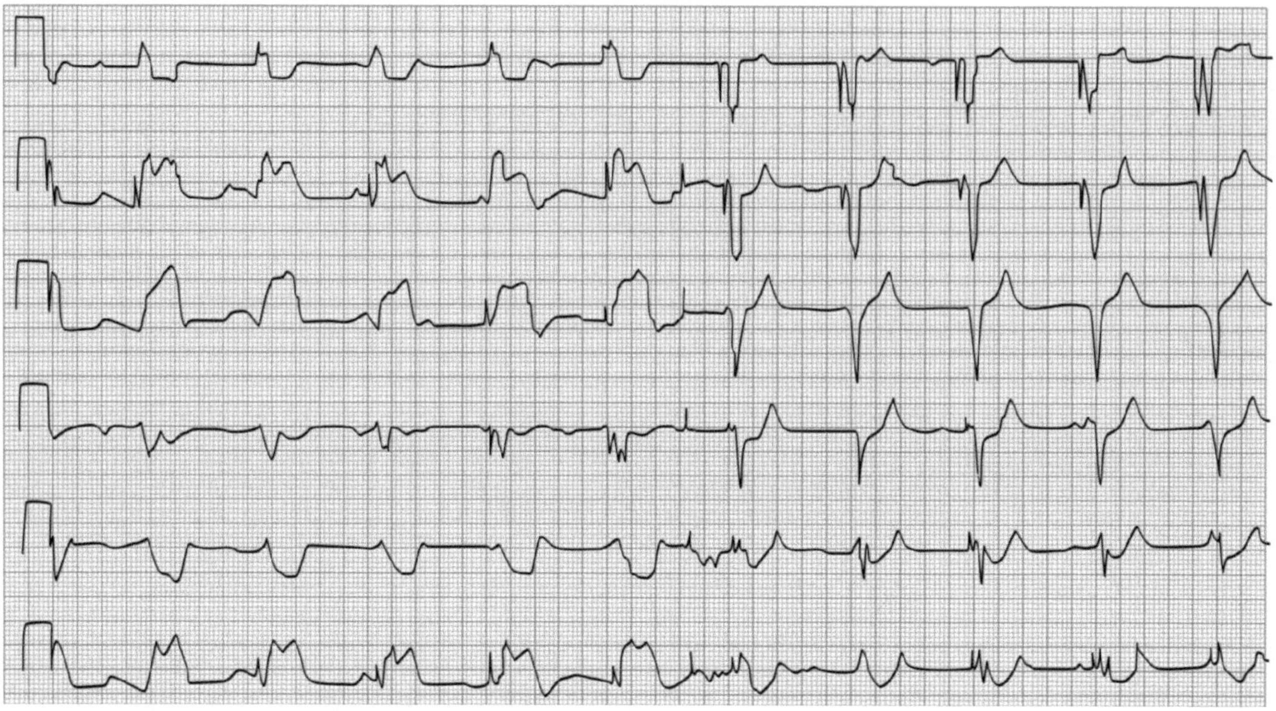

FIG. 13: ST segment elevation ≥1 mm with concordant QRS

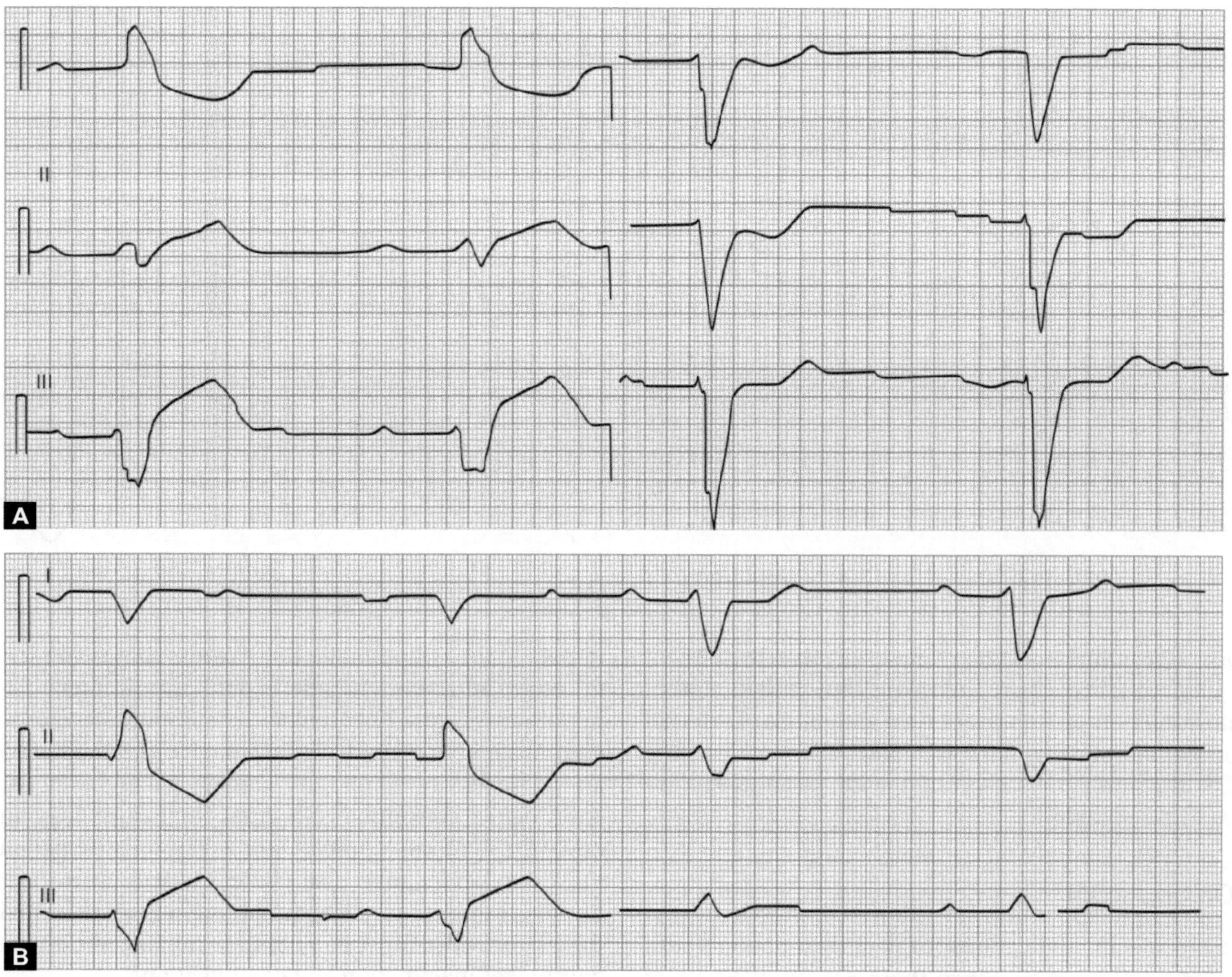

FIG. 14: ST segment depression ≥1 mm in leads V_1, V_2, and V_3

TABLE 1: Workup and management of pacemaker problems[46]

Pacemaker problems	Workup and management
Acute myocardial infarction	• ECG, troponin • Consult cardiology for assistance with ECG interpretation
Cardiac arrest	• Advanced cardiac life support algorithm
Lead infection	• More than 2 sets of blood cultures • Transesophageal echocardiogram • Broad spectrum antibiotics (e.g., intravenous vancomycin) • If diagnosis confirmed, remove PPM and leads
Bleeding	• Complete blood count • Packed red blood cell transfusion if hemoglobin is less than 7 • If palpable hematoma, surgical exploration
Upper extremity deep venous thrombosis	• Bilateral upper extremity Doppler ultrasound • Anticoagulation
Failure to pace	• Apply magnet over PPM and repeat ECG ○ If new pacemaker spikes appear on ECG → oversensing → adjust pacemaker settings ○ If no change in ECG → pacemaker malfunction → new PPM
Failure to capture	• Rule out myocardial ischemia, antiarrhythmic agents, external defibrillation, acidemia, hyperkalemia, hypoxemia, and hypothyroidism • If above workup negative → pacemaker malfunction → new PPM
Failure to sense	• Rule out acute myocardial infarction, ventricular fibrillation; ventricular tachycardia, premature ventricular complexes, atrial fibrillation, atrial flutter, and new bundle branch blocks • If above workup negative → pacemaker malfunction → new PPM
Pacemaker mediated tachycardia	• Apply magnet over PPM → should terminate tachyarrhythmia ○ If refractory or magnet unavailable → vagal maneuvers, intravenous adenosine
Runaway pacemaker	• Apply magnet over PPM → should slow down rate • Reprogram PPM • If above interventions fail → surgery to disconnect leads
Sensor induced tachycardia	• Apply magnet over PPM → disable sensing

ECG, electrocardiogram; PPM, permanent pacemaker.

REFERENCES

1. Waller BF, Gering LE, Branyas NA, Slack JD. Anatomy, histology, and pathology of the cardiac conduction system: Part I. Clin Cardiol. 1993;16:249-52.
2. Waller BF, Gering LE, Branyas NA, Slack JD. Anatomy, histology, and pathology of the cardiac conduction system: Part II. Clin Cardiol. 1993;16:347-52.
3. Mangrum JM, DiMarco JP. The evaluation and management of bradycardia. N Engl J Med. 2000;342:703-9.
4. Epstein AE, DiMarco JP, Ellenbogen KA, Estes NA 3rd, Freedman RA, Gettes LS, et al. 2012 ACCF/AHA/HRS focused update incorporated into the ACCF/AHA/HRS 2008 guidelines for device-based therapy of cardiac rhythm abnormalities: a report of the American College of Cardiology Foundation/American Heart Association Task Force on Practice Guidelines and the Heart Rhythm Society. Circulation. 2013;127:e283-352.
5. Harrigan RA, Chan TC, Moonblatt S, Vilke GM, Ufberg JW. Temporary transvenous pacemaker placement in the Emergency Department. J Emerg Med. 2007;32:105-11.
6. O'Gara PT, Kushner FG, Ascheim DD, Casey DE Jr., Chung MK, de Lemos JA, et al. 2013 ACCF/AHA guideline for the management of ST-elevation myocardial infarction: a report of the American College of Cardiology Foundation/American Heart Association Task Force on Practice Guidelines. Circulation. 2013;127:e362-425.
7. Risgaard B, Elming H, Jensen GV, Johansen JB, Toft JC. Waiting for a pacemaker: is it dangerous? Europace. 2012;14:975-80.
8. Menozzi C, Brignole M, Alboni P, Boni L, Paparella N, Gaggioli G, et al. The natural course of untreated sick sinus syndrome and identification of the variables predictive of unfavorable outcome. Am J Cardiol. 1998;82:1205-9.
9. Shaw DB, Holman RR, Gowers JI. Survival in sinoatrial disorder (sick-sinus syndrome). Br Med J. 1980;280:139-41.
10. Alt E, Volker R, Wirtzfeld A, Ulm K. Survival and follow-up after pacemaker implantation: a comparison of patients with sick sinus syndrome, complete heart block, and atrial fibrillation. Pacing Clin Electrophysiol. 1985;8:849-55.
11. Rubenstein JJ, Schulman CL, Yurchak PM, DeSanctis RW. Clinical spectrum of the sick sinus syndrome. Circulation. 1972;46:5-13.
12. Katritsis D, Camm AJ. Chronotropic incompetence: a proposal for definition and diagnosis. Br Heart J. 1993;70:400-2.
13. Mymin D, Mathewson FA, Tate RB, Manfreda J. The natural history of primary first-degree atrioventricular heart block. N Engl J Med. 1986;315:1183-7.
14. Barold SS. Indications for permanent cardiac pacing in first-degree AV block: class I, II, or III? Pacing Clin Electrophysiol. 1996;19:747-51.
15. Dhingra RC, Denes P, Wu D, Chuquimia R, Rosen KM. The significance of second degree atrioventricular block and bundle branch block. Observations regarding site and type of block. Circulation. 1974;49:638-46.
16. Ranganathan N, Dhurandhar R, Phillips JH, Wigle ED. His Bundle electrogram in bundle-branch block. Circulation. 1972;45:282-94.
17. Zipes DP. Second-degree atrioventricular block. Circulation. 1979;60:465-72.
18. Strasberg B, Amat YLF, Dhingra RC, Palileo E, Swiryn S, Bauernfeind R, et al. Natural history of chronic second-degree atrioventricular nodal block. Circulation. 1981;63:1043-9.
19. Gadboys HL, Wisoff G, Litwak RS. Surgical treatment of complete heart block. An analysis of 36 cases. Jama. 1964;189:97-102.
20. Penton GB, Miller H, Levine SA. Some clinical features of complete heart block. Circulation. 1956;13:801-24.
21. Friedberg CK, Donoso E, Stein WG. Nonsurgical acquired heart block. Ann N Y Acad Sci. 1964;111:835-47.

22. Kastor JA. Atrioventricular block (second of two parts). N Engl J Med. 1975;292:572-4.
23. Denes P, Dhingra RC, Wu D, Wyndham CR, Amat-y-Leon F, Rosen KM. Sudden death in patients with chronic bifascicular block. Arch Intern Med. 1977;137:1005-10.
24. Dhingra RC, Wyndham C, Amat-y-Leon F, Denes P, Wu D, Sridhar S, et al. Incidence and site of atrioventricular block in patients with chronic bifascicular block. Circulation. 1979;59:238-46.
25. Dhingra RC, Wyndham C, Bauernfeind R, Swiryn S, Deedwania PC, Smith T, et al. Significance of block distal to the His bundle induced by atrial pacing in patients with chronic bifascicular block. Circulation. 1979;60:1455-64.
26. Dhingra RC, Palileo E, Strasberg B, Swiryn S, Bauernfeind RA, Wyndham CR, et al. Significance of the HV interval in 517 patients with chronic bifascicular block. Circulation. 1981;64:1265-71.
27. Dhingra RC, Denes P, Wu D, Chuquimia R, Amat-y-Leon F, Wyndham C, et al. Syncope in patients with chronic bifascicular block. Significance, causative mechanisms, and clinical implications. Ann Intern Med. 1974;81:302-6.
28. McAnulty JH, Kauffman S, Murphy E, Kassebaum DG, Rahimtoola SH. Survival in patients with intraventricular conduction defects. Arch Intern Med. 1978;138:30-5.
29. McAnulty JH, Rahimtoola SH, Murphy E, DeMots H, Ritzmann L, Kanarek PE, et al. Natural history of "high-risk" bundle-branch block: final report of a prospective study. N Engl J Med. 1982;307:137-43.
30. DePasquale NP, Bruno MS. Natural history of combined right bundle branch block and left anterior hemiblock (bilateral bundle branch block). Am J Med. 1973;54:297-303.
31. Hreybe H, Saba S. Location of acute myocardial infarction and associated arrhythmias and outcome. Clin Cardiol. 2009;32:274-7.
32. Hindman MC, Wagner GS, JaRo M, Atkins JM, Scheinman MM, DeSanctis RW, et al. The clinical significance of bundle branch block complicating acute myocardial infarction. 2. Indications for temporary and permanent pacemaker insertion. Circulation. 1978;58:689-99.
33. Col JJ, Weinberg SL. The incidence and mortality of intraventricular conduction defects in acute myocardial infarction. Am J Cardiol. 1972;29:344-50.
34. Petrina M, Goodman SG, Eagle KA. The 12-lead electrocardiogram as a predictive tool of mortality after acute myocardial infarction: current status in an era of revascularization and reperfusion. Am Heart J. 2006;152:11-8.
35. Kenny RA, Richardson DA, Steen N, Bexton RS, Shaw FE, Bond J. Carotid sinus syndrome: a modifiable risk factor for nonaccidental falls in older adults (SAFE PACE). J Am Coll Cardiol. 2001;38:1491-6.
36. Sugrue DD, Gersh BJ, Holmes DR Jr., Wood DL, Osborn MJ, Hammill SC. Symptomatic "isolated" carotid sinus hypersensitivity: natural history and results of treatment with anticholinergic drugs or pacemaker. J Am Coll Cardiol. 1986;7:158-62.
37. Brignole M, Menozzi C, Lolli G, Bottoni N, Gaggioli G. Long-term outcome of paced and nonpaced patients with severe carotid sinus syndrome. Am J Cardiol. 1992;69:1039-43.
38. Brignole M. Randomized clinical trials of neurally mediated syncope. J Cardiovasc Electrophysiol. 2003;14:S64-9.
39. Grubb BP. Neurocardiogenic syncope and related disorders of orthostatic intolerance. Circulation. 2005;111:2997-3006.
40. Benditt DG, Sutton R. Tilt-table testing in the evaluation of syncope. J Cardiovasc Electrophysiol. 2005;16:356-8.
41. Connolly SJ, Sheldon R, Roberts RS, Gent M. The North American Vasovagal Pacemaker Study (VPS). A randomized trial of permanent cardiac pacing for the prevention of vasovagal syncope. J Am Coll Cardiol. 1999;33:16-20.
42. Sutton R, Brignole M, Menozzi C, Raviele A, Alboni P, Giani P, et al. Dual-chamber pacing in the treatment of neurally mediated tilt-positive cardioinhibitory syncope: pacemaker versus no therapy: a multicenter randomized study. The Vasovagal Syncope International Study (VASIS) Investigators. Circulation. 2000;102:294-9.
43. Ammirati F, Colivicchi F, Santini M. Permanent cardiac pacing versus medical treatment for the prevention of recurrent vasovagal syncope: a multicenter, randomized, controlled trial. Circulation. 2001;104:52-7.
44. Connolly SJ, Sheldon R, Thorpe KE, Roberts RS, Ellenbogen KA, Wilkoff BL, et al. Pacemaker therapy for prevention of syncope in patients with recurrent severe vasovagal syncope: Second Vasovagal Pacemaker Study (VPS II): a randomized trial. Jama. 2003;289:2224-9.
45. Gammage MD. Temporary cardiac pacing. Heart. 2000;83:715-20.
46. Cardall TY, Chan TC, Brady WJ, Perry JC, Vilke GM, Rosen P. Permanent cardiac pacemakers: issues relevant to the emergency physician, Part I. J Emerg Med. 1999;17:479-89.
47. Baddour LM, Epstein AE, Erickson CC, Knight BP, Levison ME, Lockhart PB, et al. Update on cardiovascular implantable electronic device infections and their management: a scientific statement from the American Heart Association. Circulation. 2010;121:458-77.
48. Cardall TY, Brady WJ, Chan TC, Perry JC, Vilke GM, Rosen P. Permanent cardiac pacemakers: issues relevant to the emergency physician, part II. J Emerg Med. 1999;17:697-709.
49. Sgarbossa EB, Pinski SL, Gates KB, Wagner GS. Early electrocardiographic diagnosis of acute myocardial infarction in the presence of ventricular paced rhythm. GUSTO-I investigators. Am J Cardiol. 1996;77:423-4.
50. Klimczak A, Wranicz JK, Cygankiewicz I, Chudzik M, Goch JH, Baranowski R. Electrocardiographic diagnosis of acute coronary syndromes in patients with left bundle branch block or paced rhythm. Cardiol J. 2007;14:207-13.

32 CHAPTER

Supraventricular Tachycardia

David E Krummen, Amir A Schricker

INTRODUCTION

Supraventricular tachycardias (SVTs) are common arrhythmia etiologies in the emergency department (ED), resulting in over 50,000 ED visits in the United States annually.[1] The SVTs may cause serious symptoms, lost productivity, morbidity and rarely mortality. The major types of SVTs, subtypes and arrhythmia characteristics are listed in table 1. The term SVT itself typically does not refer to atrial fibrillation; atrial fibrillation and atrial flutter are discussed separately in chapter 34 (Atrial Fibrillation and Atrial Flutter). Paroxysmal SVTs are a subset of SVT and are characterized by an abrupt onset and offset. Paroxysmal SVTs typically include atrioventricular (AV)

TABLE 1: Supraventricular tachycardia types

Arrhythmia	Subtypes	General characteristics
Sinus tachycardia	• Physiologic sinus tachycardia • Inappropriate sinus tachycardia (IST)	• Physiologic sinus tachycardia is a response to pathologic stimuli • IST is characterized by heart rate 120–140 mm Hg, in the absence of physiologic stimuli
Atrioventricular nodal re-entrant tachycardia (AVNRT)	• Typical AVNRT • Atypical AVNRT	• Heart rate commonly 180–220 mm Hg • Typical AVNRT may display pseudo R in lead V1
Atrioventricular re-entrant tachycardia (AVRT)	• Orthodromic AVRT ○ Permanent junctional reciprocating tachycardia • Antidromic AVRT • Pre-excited atrial fibrillation	• Orthodromic AVRT shows a regular, narrow QRS complex or wide QRS complex consistent with right or left bundle branch block without pre-excitation • Antidromic AVRT exhibits wide QRS complex inconsistent with right or left bundle branch block, and may be difficult to separate from ventricular tachycardia
Atrial tachycardia (AT)	• Focal AT • Multifocal atrial tachycardia (MAT)	• Focal AT may continue despite atrioventricular block during vagal maneuvers or adenosine • MAT exhibits ≥3 distinct P wave morphologies
Junctional tachycardia (JT)	• Paroxysmal JT • Nonparoxysmal JT	• Paroxysmal JT is due to abnormal automaticity in the atrioventricular node or His-Purkinje system • Nonparoxysmal JT is associated with digoxin toxicity or myocardial ischemia
Atrial flutter (AFL)	• Typical AFL • Atypical AFL	• Typical AFL characterized by stereotypical sawtooth flutter waves in leads II, III, and aVF • Atypical AFL is characterized by re-entry not involving the cavotricuspid isthmus • See chapter 28 (Atrial Fibrillation and Atrial Flutter) for additional details
Atrial fibrillation (AF)	• Paroxysmal AF • Persistent AF	• AF is characterized by continuously varying atrial activation with an atrial cycle length often ≤220 milliseconds (heart rate >270 beats/min) and irregularly irregular ventricular activation • Paroxysmal AF terminates spontaneously in <7 days • See chapter 28 (Atrial Fibrillation and Atrial Flutter) for additional details

nodal re-entrant tachycardia (AVNRT), AV re-entrant tachycardia (AVRT), and focal atrial tachycardia (AT).

SUPRAVENTRICULAR TACHYCARDIA PRESENTATION AND DIAGNOSIS

Incidence and Prevalence

Supraventricular tachyarrhythmias affect approximately 2.3 per 1,000 persons.[2] Annually, there are approximately 80,000 new cases of SVT in the United States, and 570,000 individuals with ongoing paroxysmal SVT.[2] The majority of new cases present to the ED for initial management. Thus, a working knowledge of SVTs and their associated diagnostic and therapeutic strategies are essential.

Clinical Presentation

Symptoms are common in patients with SVT and include palpitations, chest pain, lightheadedness, dizziness, presyncope, and syncope.[3] The diagnosis of SVT is typically made in the ED with the electrocardiogram (ECG) and the arrhythmia response to vagal and pharmacologic interventions. Diagnosis may be assisted with patient characteristics and symptom qualities.

Age may help to separate SVT types with younger patients more likely to have AVRT. Prior work reports the average age for patients with AVRT was 23 years versus 32 years for AVNRT.[4] Older patients (>50 years) with SVT are more likely to have atrial flutter.[5] While many patients with SVT have no associated structural heart disease, patients with pulmonary disease occasionally present with multifocal atrial tachycardia (MAT). Patients with AVNRT are more likely to be female[6] and describe symptoms of neck pounding, due to right atrial contraction while the tricuspid valve is closed.[7]

Electrocardiogram

In patients presenting during tachycardia, the 12-lead ECG can frequently identify the arrhythmia mechanism. For tachycardias with a narrow QRS morphology, the first objective is to determine whether the tachycardia is regular (Flowchart 1).[8]

An irregular tachycardia is typically seen in four arrhythmias: (i) atrial fibrillation, (ii) rapid focal AT, or (iii) atrial flutter with irregular AV nodal conduction,[9] and (iv) MAT.

For a regular tachycardia, the next step in ECG interpretation is to determine (if possible) the relationship between atrial and ventricular activation. If the atrial rate is greater than the ventricular rate, then atrial flutter or AT is likely. Rarely, AVNRT with 2:1 conduction may be present.

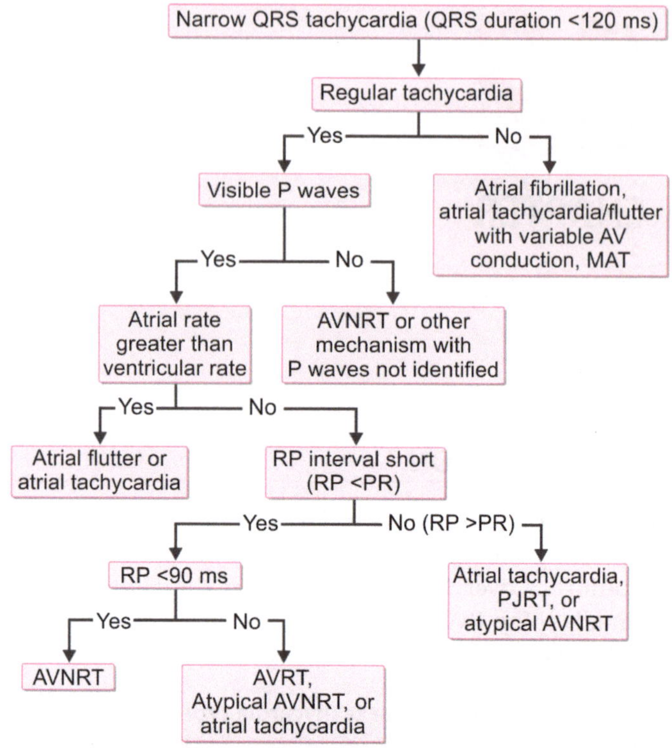

MAT, multifocal atrial tachycardia; AVNRT, atrioventricular nodal re-entrant tachycardia; AVRT, atrioventricular re-entrant tachycardia; PJRT, permanent junctional reciprocating tachycardia.

FLOWCHART 1: Electrocardiogram diagnosis of supraventricular tachycardia. This flowchart illustrates the analysis process for patients presenting with supraventricular tachycardia

With permission from: Page RL, Joglar JA, Caldwell MA, et al. 2015 ACC/AHA/HRS Guideline for the Management of Adult Patients With Supraventricular Tachycardia: A Report of the American College of Cardiology/American Heart Association Task Force on Clinical Practice Guidelines and the Heart Rhythm Society. J Am Coll Cardiol. 2016;67(13):e27-115.

If the atrial and ventricular rates are similar, the next goal in ECG interpretation is to determine whether the interval from ventricular activation to atrial activation (the RP interval) is less than the interval from atrial activation to the subsequent ventricular activation (PR interval). If yes and the RP interval is less than 90 ms, typical AVNRT is probable. An illustration of typical AVNRT is shown in figure 1, showing atrial activation and ventricular activation, which are nearly simultaneous, leading to an inverted P wave at the end of the QRS complex in lead V1 (pseudo R-prime).

If the RP interval is shorter than the PR, but the RP interval is more than 90 ms, AVRT, atypical AVNRT, and focal AT are likely. An illustration of orthodromic AVRT is shown in figure 2, with an RP interval of 120 ms.

Finally, if the RP interval is greater than the PR interval, focal AT, permanent junctional reciprocating tachycardia, and atypical AVNRT are likely. An example of focal AT is shown in figure 3.

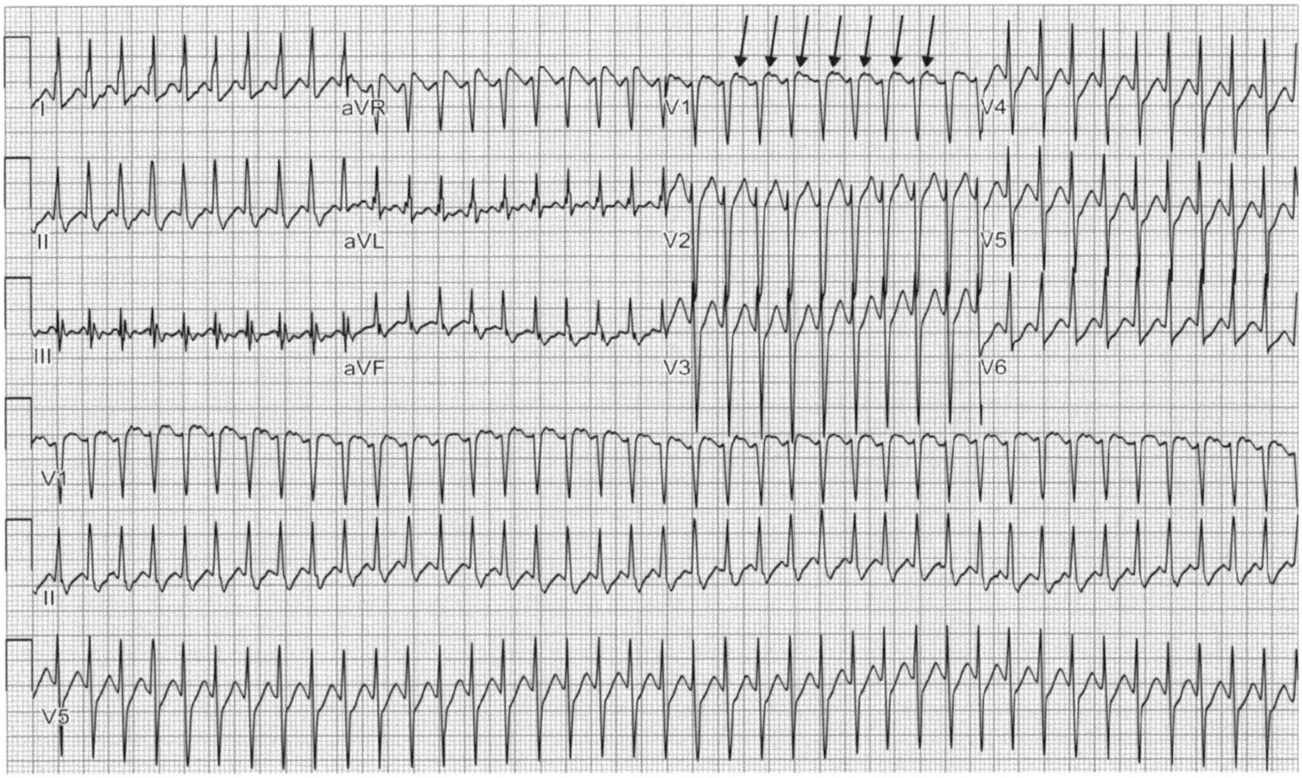

FIG. 1: ECG of typical atrioventricular nodal re-entrant tachycardia. 12-lead ECG of a 36-year-old male patient with atrioventricular nodal reentrant tachycardia, with atrial activation occurring during the terminal portion of the QRS complex (arrows), termed pseudo R-prime waves. Patient underwent successful ablation of the atrioventricular nodal slow pathway, with 3 years of subsequent arrhythmia-free follow-up.

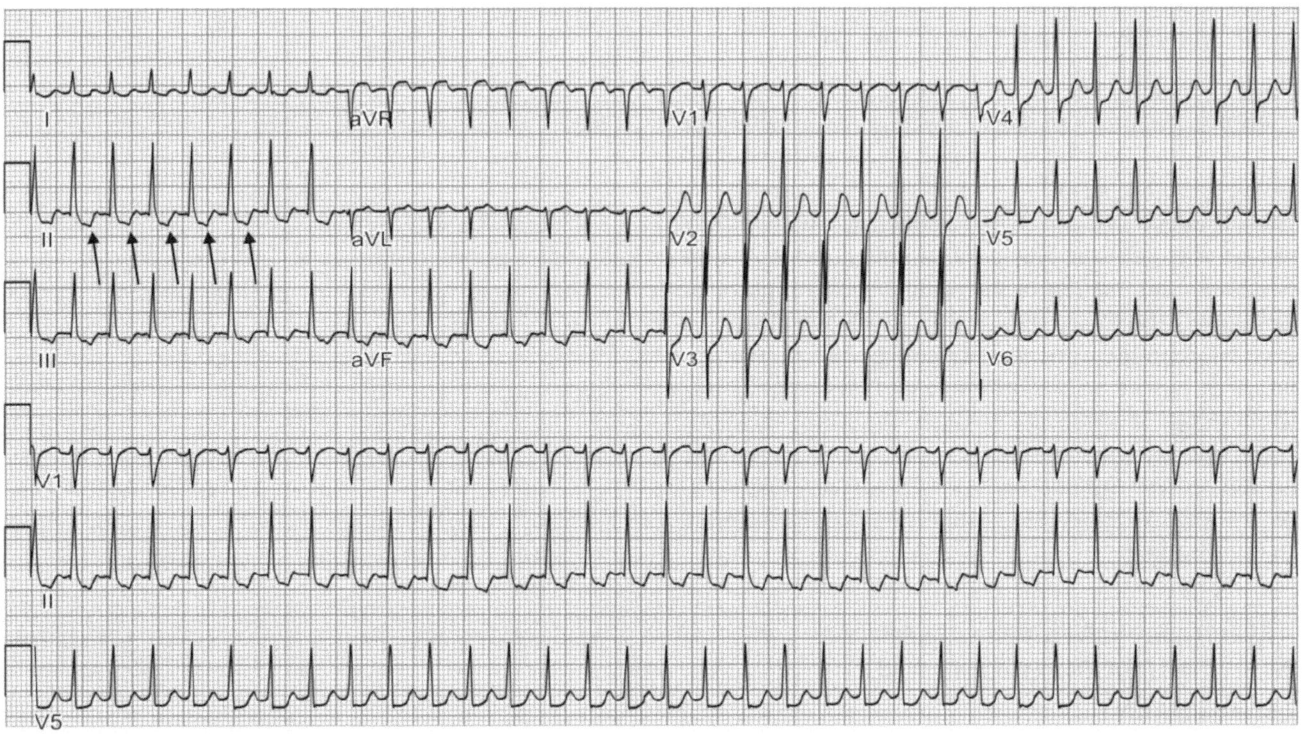

FIG. 2: ECG of orthodromic atrioventricular re-entrant tachycardia. This ECG illustrates orthodromic atrioventricular re-entrant tachycardia with a heart rate of 193 beats/min displaying a short-RP interval measuring more than 90 ms (arrows). The accessory pathway was localized to the posterolateral left atrium during successful catheter ablation

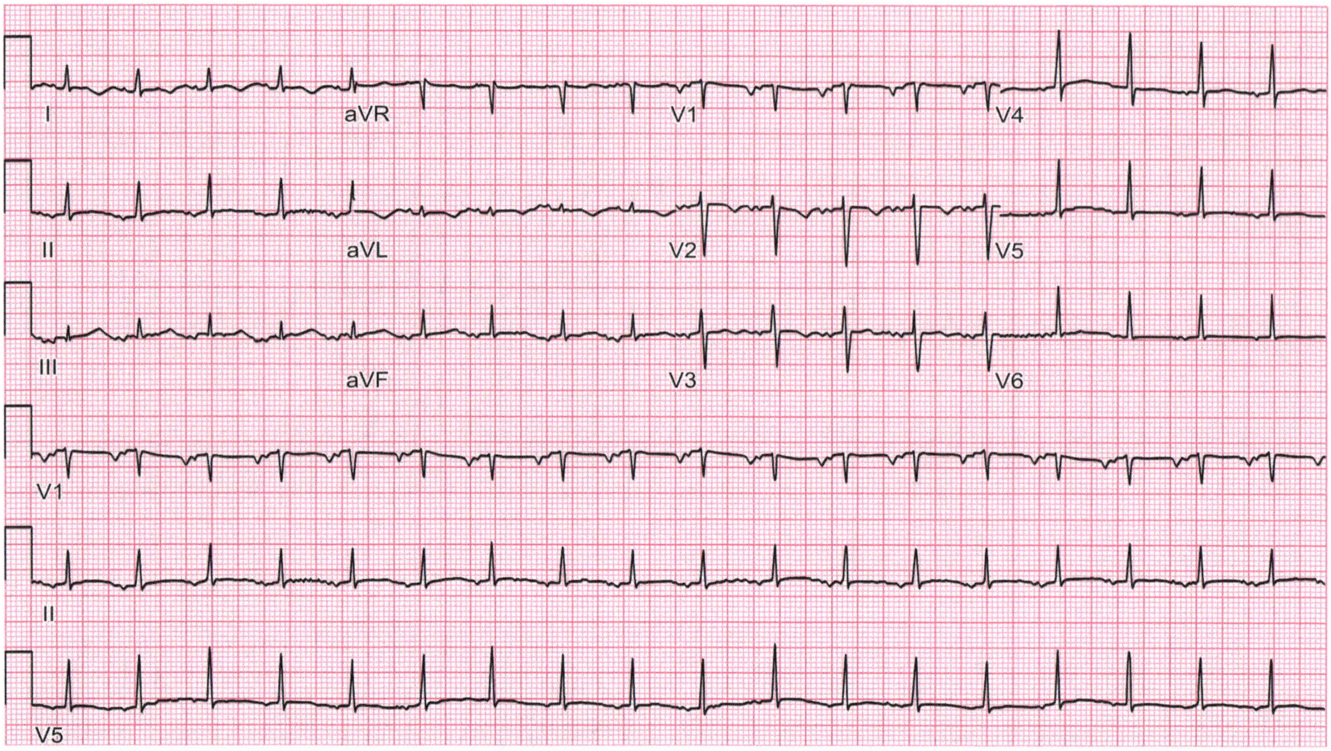

FIG. 3: Focal atrial tachycardia. This ECG shows focal atrial tachycardia at a rate of 110 beats/min. The source was localized to the inferolateral tricuspid valve during successful catheter ablation

INITIAL MANAGEMENT IN UNDIFFERENTIATED SUPRAVENTRICULAR TACHYCARDIA

The initial management of a regular SVT with an undifferentiated mechanism (Flowchart 2) consists of vagal maneuvers and intravenous (IV) adenosine while recording a rhythm strip.[8]

These interventions, when effective, will either terminate the SVT or block AV nodal conduction to allow better visualization of the atrial activation pattern. If ineffective, the next step is to assess whether the patient is hemodynamically stable. If the patient is stable, IV β-blockers, IV diltiazem, or IV verapamil are recommended. If these are ineffective or not feasible, cardioversion is recommended. Conversely, if the patient is unstable, current guidelines recommend cardioversion. A caveat is that for arrhythmias that break spontaneously and recur frequently, cardioversion is not appropriate.

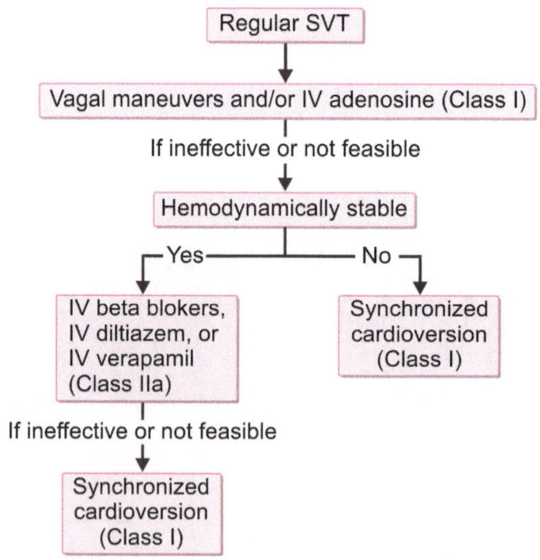

SVT, supraventricular tachycardia; IV, intravenous

FLOWCHART 2: Initial treatment of a regular supraventricular tachycardia

With permission from: Page RL, Joglar JA, Caldwell MA, et al. 2015 ACC/AHA/HRS Guideline for the Management of Adult Patients With Supraventricular Tachycardia: A Report of the American College of Cardiology/American Heart Association Task Force on Clinical Practice Guidelines and the Heart Rhythm Society. J Am Coll Cardiol. 2016;67(13):e27-115.

SPECIFIC SUPRAVENTRICULAR TACHYCARDIA DIAGNOSIS AND MANAGEMENT

Sinus Tachycardia

Physiologic sinus tachycardia is not a pathologic arrhythmia, but is a normal physiologic reaction to physiologic stressors, such as infection, dehydration, blood loss, heart failure, hyperthyroidism, drugs, pain, or anxiety. As such, physiologic sinus tachycardia does not require specific therapy; therapy for physiologic sinus tachycardia involves management of the underlying cause.

Inappropriate sinus tachycardia (IST) is a rare form of sinus tachycardia not due to underlying extrinsic pathophysiologic stressor. Inappropriate sinus tachycardia is a diagnosis of exclusion since underlying causes must be ruled out prior to making the diagnosis. Treatment of IST is challenging due to incomplete responses to standard medications, such as β-blockers or calcium-channel blockers, and side effects of such therapies. Ivabradine has recently been investigated for the treatment of symptomatic IST with promising results.[10]

Radiofrequency ablation of the sinoatrial node is typically not recommended. In this setting, ablation is frequently ineffective and carries a high risk for significant harm, including dependence upon a permanent pacemaker. As such, it is reserved for highly symptomatic patients refractory to medical management willing to accept pacemaker therapy.

Atrioventricular Nodal Re-entrant Tachycardia

Atrioventricular nodal re-entrant tachycardia is the most common SVT, typically occurring in younger-to-middle age, predominantly female[11] patients without structural heart disease. As its name implies, it involves re-entry in the compact AV node and perinodal tissue. In AVNRT, the perinodal pathways include a rapidly conducting pathway with a long-refractory period (e.g., fast pathway) and a slowly conducting pathway with a short-refractory period (e.g., slow pathway). In typical AVNRT, the re-entrant impulse travels down the slow pathway to the AV node, and then concurrently down the His-Purkinje system to the ventricles and retrograde up the fast pathway to the atria. The cycle then repeats resulting in a regular tachycardia with a rate often between 180 beats/min to 220 beats/min, but occasionally as slow at 120 beats/min or as fast as 280 beats/min. In atypical AVNRT, the impulse may travel down the fast pathway to the AV node, and then retrograde through the slow pathway. Alternatively, atypical AVNRT may use two separate slow pathways.

Because AVNRT conducts down the His-Purkinje system, the QRS complex is often narrow, but may be wide due to pre-existing or rate-related bundle branch block. In approximately 10% of patients, AVNRT may conduct in a 2:1 ratio to the ventricles[12] because of functional block in the His bundle.

Symptoms during AVNRT commonly include palpitations, dizziness, dyspnea, and chest pain.[13] As noted earlier, the symptom of neck pounding is somewhat specific for AVNRT due to atrial contraction while the tricuspid valve is closed. Syncope is uncommon during AVNRT, but may be related to a high-heart rate or to associated neurocardiogenic syncope. Cardiac arrest associated with AVNRT has been described as a rare complication.[14]

For patients in whom AVNRT is suspected, acute management consists of vagal maneuvers or IV adenosine in attempt to terminate tachycardia.[8] If unsuccessful then IV β-blockers, diltiazem, or verapamil can be used in hemodynamically stable patients to slow the heart rate. Intravenous amiodarone may also be considered for rate control or termination of AVNRT. If ineffective or the patient is unstable, cardioversion is indicated.

The diagnosis of AVNRT may be made by 12-lead ECG during tachycardia. Near-simultaneous ventricular and atrial activation (the pseudo R-prime) is uncommon in other SVT mechanisms (but may rarely be seen in focal AT with a long-AV interval or even more rarely in AVRT with a decremental retrograde accessory pathway). Thus a very short-RP tachycardia (<90 ms) is most likely typical AVNRT (Fig. 1). In atypical AVNRT, the RP interval is longer and is difficult, to distinguish from AVRT on 12-lead ECG.

Successful long-term management of AVNRT requires an assessment of symptoms. Because of the low-risk nature of AVNRT, asymptomatic or minimally symptomatic patients can be managed without therapy, or using a pill-in-the-pocket strategy in which patients are prescribed β-blockers, diltiazem or verapamil to take during episodes of AVNRT.

Symptomatic patients have the option of electing ablation therapy or medications. For patients who are candidates for ablation and wish to undergo the procedure, catheter ablation in experienced centers provides a high rate of success and low rate of complications.[11] In symptomatic patients, ablation has also been shown to be cost effective[12] compared with medical therapy.

In patients, who are not candidates for ablation or prefer to take medications, first-line therapy consists of AV nodal blocking agents, such as diltiazem or metoprolol. Flecainide or propafenone may be added in patients without structural heart disease, while amiodarone, sotalol, or dofetilide may be considered in patients with existing structural heart disease.[8] If medications are ineffective or not tolerated, ablation may be reconsidered.

Atrioventricular Re-entrant Tachycardia

Atrioventricular re-entrant tachycardia is also a re-entrant arrhythmia using the normal conduction system and a separate accessory pathway connecting the atria and ventricles. Differences in the conduction properties between the AV node and accessory pathway allow conduction block to occur in either the AV node or accessory pathway, initiating re-entry.

The most common form (90–95%) of AVRT is orthodromic AVRT,[15] and consists of conduction down the AV node, through the ventricular tissue, retrograde up the accessory pathway, through atrial tissue and repeating the cycle. Orthodromic AVRT may display a narrow QRS complex or a wide complex QRS with a stereotypical bundle branch block pattern. A type of orthodromic AVRT presenting in early childhood is permanent junctional reciprocating tachycardia (PJRT), discussed separately below.

Less commonly (<10% of cases[15]) antidromic AVRT is seen with the reverse pattern of re-entry in which conduction proceeds down the accessory pathway and from ventricles to atria using the AV node and His-Purkinje system. The ECG in patients with antidromic AVRT is wide and typically does not conform to a classic right of left bundle branch block pattern.

Symptoms during either orthodromic or antidromic AVRT include palpitations, lightheadedness, chest pain and syncope. Sudden death has been reported in patients with AVRT,[16] most commonly in children with rapidly-conducting accessory pathways (refractory periods ≤240 ms at baseline).

Orthodromic Atrioventricular Re-entrant Tachycardia

Initial therapy of orthodromic AVRT consists of vagal maneuvers and/or IV adenosine (Flowchart 3).

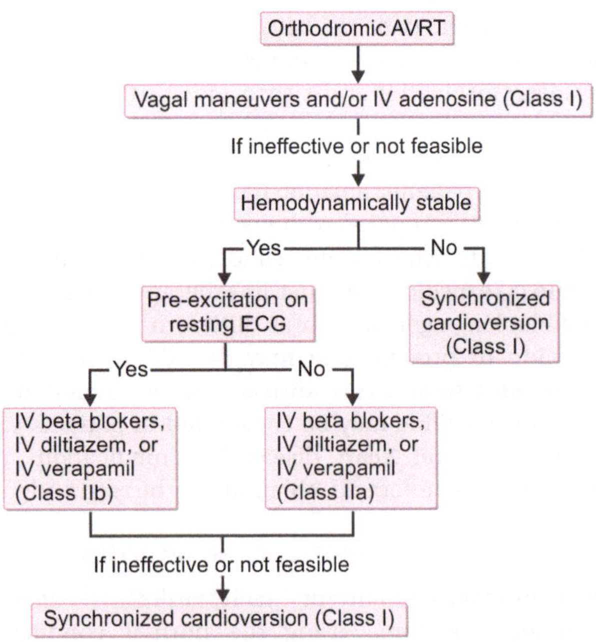

AVRT, atrioventricular re-entrant tachycardia; IV, intravenous; ECG, electrocardiogram

FLOWCHART 3: Initial treatment of atrioventricular re-entrant tachycardia

With permission from: Page RL, Joglar JA, Caldwell MA, et al. 2015 ACC/AHA/HRS Guideline for the Management of Adult Patients With Supraventricular Tachycardia: A Report of the American College of Cardiology/American Heart Association Task Force on Clinical Practice Guidelines and the Heart Rhythm Society. J Am Coll Cardiol. 2016;67(13):e27-115.

If ineffective or not feasible, the next step is to assess hemodynamic stability. If unstable, synchronized cardioversion is recommended. If stable, IV β-blockers, diltiazem, or verapamil may be administered. If ineffective or not feasible, synchronized cardioversion is recommended.

For long-term management, patients with orthodromic AVRT should be assessed regarding their willingness and suitability for catheter ablation of the accessory pathway. Overall procedural success rates are favorable with a low rate of complications in experienced centers.[17]

In patients, who do not wish to have ablation or are not candidates for the procedure, medical therapy for orthodromic AVRT in patients without structural heart disease consists of oral flecainide[18] or propafenone.[19] In patients with structural heart disease, oral dofetilide, sotalol, or amiodarone are recommended.[8] In patients without pre-excitation or with accessory pathways with a longer refractory periods, β-blockers, diltiazem, or verapamil may be considered.[8] If medical therapy is ineffective, patients should be reconsidered for catheter ablation.

Antidromic Atrioventricular Re-entrant Tachycardia

Antidromic AVRT is characterized by conduction from atrial to ventricles using an accessory pathway, then through ventricular tissue, up either the AV node or another accessory pathway, through atrial tissue and then repeating the cycle. In antidromic AVRT, therapy is different than orthodromic AVRT due to a number of issues. First, antidromic AVRT and ventricular tachycardia may have similar appearances on the 12-lead ECG. Patients with VT can become unstable if administered AV nodal blocking agents as in orthodromic AVRT. Second, there may be multiple accessory pathways present. In this setting, administration of AV nodal blocking agents may paradoxically increase the rate of tachycardia and lead to clinical deterioration.

Diagnosis of AVRT is made with the 12-lead ECG and often other factors, such as a prior ECG showing pre-excitation. Subtle findings such as a constant relationship between the QRS complex and P wave despite changes in the tachycardia rate may also be helpful.

Because of the potential for clinical deterioration with AV nodal blocking agents, the acute management of antidromic AVRT consists of IV procainamide. Procainamide slows conduction in the accessory pathway, slowing the tachycardia and improving hemodynamics and frequently terminating AVRT.

Long-term therapy for antidromic AVRT is similar to orthodromic AVRT with the exception that AV nodal blocking agents are not recommended. Thus, patients with antidromic AVRT should be assessed regarding their willingness and suitability for catheter ablation of the accessory pathway. Overall procedural success is high with a low rate of complications.[17]

In patients, who are not ablation candidates or who do not desire ablation, oral flecainide[2] or propafenone[1] are recommended in the absence of structural heart disease. Oral dofetilide, sotalol, or amiodarone can be used in patients with structural heart disease. Like in orthodromic AVRT, catheter ablation should be reconsidered, if medical therapy is ineffective or not tolerated.

Permanent Junctional Reciprocating Tachycardia

Permanent junctional reciprocating tachycardia (PJRT) is a rare form of orthodromic AVRT typically seen in pediatric patients most commonly due to a slowly conducting posteroseptal accessory pathway. For such patients, the arrhythmia is incessant and often difficult to control with medications.[20] Ablation of the accessory pathway is, therefore, the primary therapeutic option in PJRT. As a temporizing agent, flecainide can be used for rate control in symptomatic patients.

Pre-excited Atrial Fibrillation

Atrial fibrillation in the presence of an accessory pathway is a potentially hazardous condition because conduction of the rapid atrial activity to the ventricles via the accessory pathway can lead to ventricular tachycardia or ventricular fibrillation. Importantly, drugs, which block the AV node, can paradoxically increase the ventricular activation rate via preferential conduction down the accessory pathway. Therefore, AV nodal blocking agents are contraindicated in this situation. Instead, urgent cardioversion should be used in hemodynamically unstable patients. For hemodynamically stable patients, IV ibutilide[21] or IV procainamide should be used.

Such patients should be considered for catheter ablation of the accessory pathway with or without catheter ablation of atrial fibrillation. Medical therapy in patients who are not candidates for ablation includes flecainide and propafenone in patients without structural heart disease. In patients with structural heart disease, sotalol, dofetilide or amiodarone[22,23] may be considered.

Asymptomatic Pre-excitation

Electrocardiograms showing pre-excitation of the QRS complex, or delta waves, are frequently seen in the ED. A recent review,[24] performed for the current SVT guidelines,[8] suggests that such patients should undergo ambulatory monitoring and/or ECG stress testing. Patients without SVT on these studies in whom loss of pre-excitation is seen may be considered low risk (class I). In patients without such findings, an electrophysiology study is reasonable (class IIa) for risk stratification. Catheter ablation is reasonable in patients with high-risk pathways or for patients with particular occupations (e.g., operators of heavy machinery or pilots).[25]

Focal Atrial Tachycardia

Focal AT is a less common type of SVT, accounting for approximately 10% of patients referred for SVT ablation.[26] As the name implies, focal AT is characterized by rapid activation from a specific location, or locations within the atria with an outward spread of activation. Prior work has shown that focal AT may be due to automatic, triggered or micro-re-entrant activity. However, strategies to separate these mechanisms are suboptimal.

Initial treatment for known or suspected focal AT is shown in flowchart 4. The first step is to assess hemodynamic stability.

In patients, who are hemodynamic unstable, IV adenosine is recommended while preparing for urgent cardioversion. If adenosine is ineffective, not feasible or would significantly delay cardioversion, treatment should proceed to urgent cardioversion.

In patients, who are hemodynamically stable, IV adenosine can be useful if the diagnosis of focal AT is uncertain. Once focal AT has been diagnosed then IV AV nodal blocking agents, such as β-blockers, diltiazem or verapamil, are recommended. If ineffective, IV amiodarone or IV ibutilide may be considered.

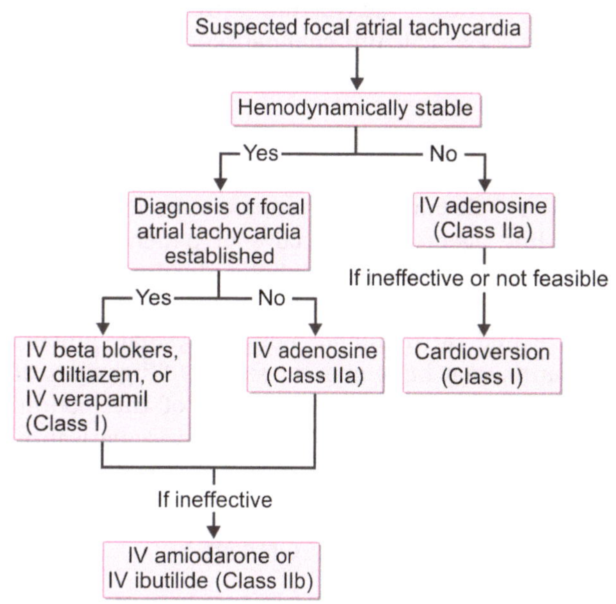

FLOWCHART 4: Initial management of known or suspected focal atrial tachycardia

With permission from: Page RL, Joglar JA, Caldwell MA, et al. 2015 ACC/AHA/HRS Guideline for the Management of Adult Patients With Supraventricular Tachycardia: A Report of the American College of Cardiology/American Heart Association Task Force on Clinical Practice Guidelines and the Heart Rhythm Society. J Am Coll Cardiol. 2016;67(13):e27-115.

Current guidelines recommend catheter ablation in an experienced center as a Class I recommendation for long-term management of focal AT.[26] In patients, who are not candidates or prefer not to pursue ablation, AV nodal blocking agents are recommended, supplemented by flecainide or propafenone in patients without structural heart disease. In patients with structural heart disease, oral amiodarone or sotalol is reasonable.[8] If medications are ineffective, catheter ablation may be reconsidered.

Multifocal Atrial Tachycardia

Multifocal atrial tachycardia is an uncommon arrhythmia most often seen in patients with advanced pulmonary or cardiopulmonary disease. Therapeutic options for MAT remain suboptimal; antiarrhythmic drugs and cardioversion are typically not useful for this arrhythmia. First-line therapy involves administration of IV magnesium in patients with low-serum levels. IV metoprolol or verapamil can be useful in acutely.

For long-term management of MAT, oral verapamil, diltiazem, or metoprolol are reasonable options. Catheter ablation has no clear role in MAT.

Junctional Tachycardia

Paroxysmal junctional tachycardia is an uncommon arrhythmia in adults caused by abnormal automaticity from the AV node or His-Purkinje system.[27] In adult patients, junctional tachycardia is treated acutely with IV β-blockers or calcium channel blockers. Intravenous procainamide is also reasonable for refractory arrhythmias in the acute setting.

Long-term management consists of oral β-blockers, diltiazem, or verapamil as first-line therapy. In non-responders, flecainide or propafenone are preferred second-line agents. If ineffective or patients unable to tolerate these medications, catheter ablation may be reasonable.[28]

A related arrhythmia, nonparoxysmal junctional tachycardia, may be seen in the setting of digoxin toxicity or myocardial infarction. Treatment of this condition focuses on reducing digoxin levels or revascularization.

SUPRAVENTRICULAR TACHYCARDIA IN PREGNANCY

Supraventricular tachycardia is common in pregnancy and carries an increased risk to mother and fetus both from arrhythmia and from pharmacologic effects. Management of such patients is challenging; goals include use of established medications[8] at the lowest effective dose with frequent monitoring of treatment efficacy and for side effects. In drug-refractory arrhythmias, ablation may be reasonable in pregnant patients[29] with the goal of reducing or eliminating[30,31] radiation exposure. Readers are encouraged to consult current guidelines[8] for additional information.

CONCLUSION

SVTs are commonly encountered in emergency medicine. In this chapter an overview of SVT evaluation, diagnosis and management has been presented. For issues not covered in this work, consultation of the recent SVT guidelines by Page et al.[8] is recommended.

REFERENCES

1. Murman DH, McDonald AJ, Pelletier AJ, Camargo CA Jr. U.S. emergency department visits for supraventricular tachycardia, 1993-2003. Acad Emerg Med. 2007;14(6):578-81.
2. Orejarena LA, Vidaillet H Jr, DeStefano F, Nordstrom DL, Vierkant RA, Smith PN, et al. Paroxysmal supraventricular tachycardia in the general population. J Am Coll Cardiol. 1998;31(1):150-7.
3. Cain N, Irving C, Webber S, Beerman L, Arora G. Natural history of Wolff-Parkinson-White syndrome diagnosed in childhood. Am J Cardiol. 2013;112(7):961-5.
4. Goyal R, Zivin A, Souza J, Shaikh SA, Harvey M, Bogun F, et al. Comparison of the ages of tachycardia onset in patients with atrioventricular nodal reentrant tachycardia and accessory pathway-mediated tachycardia. Am Heart J. 1996;132(4):765-7.
5. Rahman F, Wang N, Yin X, Ellinor PT, Lubitz SA, LeLorier PA, et al. Atrial flutter: Clinical risk factors and adverse outcomes in the Framingham Heart Study. Heart Rhythm. 2016;13(1):233-40.
6. Porter MJ, Morton JB, Denman R, Lin AC, Tierney S, Santucci PA, et al. Influence of age and gender on the mechanism of supraventricular tachycardia. Heart Rhythm. 2004;1(4):393-6.
7. Gonzalez-Torrecilla E, Almendral J, Arenal A, Atienza F, Atea LF, del Castillo S, et al. Combined evaluation of bedside clinical variables and the electrocardiogram for the differential diagnosis of paroxysmal atrioventricular reciprocating tachycardias in patients without pre-excitation. J Am Coll Cardiol. 2009;53(25):2353-8.
8. Page RL, Joglar JA, Caldwell MA, Calkins H, Conti JB, Deal BJ, et al. 2015 ACC/AHA/HRS Guideline for the Management of Adult Patients With Supraventricular Tachycardia: A Report of the American College of Cardiology/American Heart Association Task Force on Clinical Practice Guidelines and the Heart Rhythm Society. J Am Coll Cardiol. 2016;67(13):e27-115.
9. Krummen DE, Feld GK, Narayan SM. Diagnostic accuracy of irregularly irregular RR intervals in separating atrial fibrillation from atrial flutter. Am J Cardiol. 2006;98(2):209-14.
10. Benezet-Mazuecos J, Rubio JM, Farre J, Quinones MA, Sanchez-Borque P, Macia E. Long-term outcomes of ivabradine in inappropriate sinus tachycardia patients: appropriate efficacy or inappropriate patients. Pacing Clin Electrophysiol. 2013;36(7):830-6.
11. Liuba I, Jonsson A, Safstrom K, Walfridsson H. Gender-related differences in patients with atrioventricular nodal reentry tachycardia. Am J Cardiol. 2006;97(3):384-8.
12. Man KC, Brinkman K, Bogun F, Knight B, Bahu M, Weiss R, et al. 2:1 atrioventricular block during atrioventricular node reentrant tachycardia. J Am Coll Cardiol. 1996;28(7):1770-4.
13. Wood KA, Drew BJ, Scheinman MM. Frequency of disabling symptoms in supraventricular tachycardia. Am J Cardiol. 1997;79(2):145-9.
14. Wang YS, Scheinman MM, Chien WW, Cohen TJ, Lesh MD, Griffin JC. Patients with supraventricular tachycardia presenting with aborted sudden death: incidence, mechanism and long-term follow-up. J Am Coll Cardiol. 1991;18(7):1711-9.
15. Ceresnak SR, Tanel RE, Pass RH, Liberman L, Collins KK, Van Hare GF, et al. Clinical and electrophysiologic characteristics of antidromic tachycardia in children with Wolff-Parkinson-White syndrome. Pacing Clin Electrophysiol. 2012;35(4):480-8.
16. Pappone C, Vicedomini G, Manguso F, Saviano M, Baldi M, Pappone A, et al. Wolff-Parkinson-White syndrome in the era of catheter ablation: insights from a registry study of 2169 patients. Circulation. 2014;130(10):811-9.

17. Scheinman MM, Huang S. The 1998 NASPE prospective catheter ablation registry. Pacing Clin Electrophysiol. 2000;23(6):1020-8.
18. Kim SS, Lal R, Ruffy R. Treatment of paroxysmal reentrant supraventricular tachycardia with flecainide acetate. Am J Cardiol. 1986;58(1):80-5.
19. Ludmer PL, McGowan NE, Antman EM, Friedman PL. Efficacy of propafenone in Wolff-Parkinson-White syndrome: electrophysiologic findings and long-term follow-up. J Am Coll Cardiol. 1987;9(6):1357-63.
20. Kang KT, Potts JE, Radbill AE, La Page MJ, Papagiannis J, Garnreiter JM, et al. Permanent junctional reciprocating tachycardia in children: a multicenter experience. Heart Rhythm. 2014;11(8):1426-32.
21. Glatter KA, Dorostkar PC, Yang Y, Lee RJ, Van Hare GF, Keung E, et al. Electrophysiological effects of ibutilide in patients with accessory pathways. Circulation. 2001;104(16):1933-9.
22. Feld GK, Nademanee K, Stevenson W, Weiss J, Klitzner T, Singh BN. Clinical and electrophysiologic effects of amiodarone in patients with atrial fibrillation complicating the Wolff-Parkinson-White syndrome. Am Heart J. 1988;115(1 Pt 1):102-7.
23. Kappenberger LJ, Fromer MA, Steinbrunn W, Shenasa M. Efficacy of amiodarone in the Wolff-Parkinson-White syndrome with rapid ventricular response via accessory pathway during atrial fibrillation. Am J Cardiol. 1984;54(3):330-5.
24. Al-Khatib SM, Arshad A, Balk EM, Das SR, Hsu JC, Joglar JA, et al. Risk Stratification for Arrhythmic Events in Patients With Asymptomatic Pre-Excitation: A Systematic Review for the 2015 ACC/AHA/HRS Guideline for the Management of Adult Patients With Supraventricular Tachycardia: A Report of the American College of Cardiology/American Heart Association Task Force on Clinical Practice Guidelines and the Heart Rhythm Society. Circulation. 2016;133(14):e575-86.
25. Epstein AE, Miles WM, Benditt DG, Camm AJ, Darling EJ, Friedman PL, et al. Personal and public safety issues related to arrhythmias that may affect consciousness: implications for regulation and physician recommendations. A medical/scientific statement from the American Heart Association and the North American Society of Pacing and Electrophysiology. Circulation. 1996;94(5):1147-66.
26. Medi C, Kalman JM, Haqqani H, Vohra JK, Morton JB, Sparks PB, et al. Tachycardia-mediated cardiomyopathy secondary to focal atrial tachycardia: long-term outcome after catheter ablation. J Am Coll Cardiol. 2009;53(19): 1791-7.
27. Ruder MA, Davis JC, Eldar M, Abbott JA, Griffin JC, Seger JJ, et al. Clinical and electrophysiologic characterization of automatic junctional tachycardia in adults. Circulation. 1986;73(5):930-7.
28. Scheinman MM, Gonzalez RP, Cooper MW, Lesh MD, Lee RJ, Epstein LM. Clinical and electrophysiologic features and role of catheter ablation techniques in adult patients with automatic atrioventricular junctional tachycardia. Am J Cardiol. 1994;74(6):565-72.
29. Szumowski L, Szufladowicz E, Orczykowski M, Bodalski R, Derejko P, Przybylski A, et al. Ablation of severe drug-resistant tachyarrhythmia during pregnancy. J Cardiovasc Electrophysiol. 2010;21(8):877-82.
30. Fernandez-Gomez JM, Morina-Vazquez P, Morales Edel R, Venegas-Gamero J, Barba-Pichardo R, Carranza MH. Exclusion of fluoroscopy use in catheter ablation procedures: six years of experience at a single center. J Cardiovasc Electrophysiol. 2014;25(6):638-44.
31. Bigelow AM, Crane SS, Khoury FR, Clark JM. Catheter ablation of supraventricular tachycardia without fluoroscopy during pregnancy. Obstet Gynecol. 2015;125(6):1338-41.

33 CHAPTER

Use of Anticoagulation in Arrhythmias

Nicholas Phreaner, Jonathan Harrison, Alex Pearce

INTRODUCTION

Atrial fibrillation (AF) is the most common clinically significant cardiac arrhythmia. Atrial fibrillation increases with age. Approximately 1% of patients with AF are less than 60 years of age, whereas up to 12% of patients with AF are within 75-84 years of age.[1] Atrial fibrillation is a potent risk factor for stroke and overall increases the risk of ischemic stroke by fivefold.[2] The risk of stroke is reduced by use of anticoagulation. Due to high morbidity, mortality, and prevalence of this arrhythmia, a thorough knowledge of AF, the indications and subtleties of anticoagulation treatment are necessary knowledge for physicians.

Traditionally, anticoagulation in AF has been accomplished through vitamin K antagonists (VKAs), most commonly warfarin. Recently, approval of new oral anticoagulants, including direct thrombin inhibitors (DTIs) and factor Xa inhibitors, has expanded the therapeutic management options for AF. The new oral anticoagulants are appealing because they eliminate the need for frequent monitoring and dietary restrictions. However, there remain concerns about the lack of quick and effective reversal agents in the setting of severe bleeding. In this chapter, the risks and benefits of anticoagulation in AF, utilization of risk classification schemes, and details of antiplatelet therapy, VKAs as well as the direct oral anticoagulants (DOACs) will be discussed in detail. In addition, a general approach to anticoagulation in AF as well as anticoagulation management in the setting of surgery and cardioversion will also be discussed.

ATRIAL FIBRILLATION

Thromboembolic Risk in Atrial Fibrillation

Patients with AF, regardless of episode duration are at increased risk of thromboembolic ischemic stroke.[3] In general, the risk of stroke in nonvalvular AF is five times that of the general population, while risk of stroke is increased twenty times in patients with AF and mitral stenosis.[4,5] Thromboembolism in AF is one of the leading causes of morbidity and mortality in these patients.

The anatomy of the left atrium (LA) and the pathophysiologic changes associated with AF contribute to thrombus formation. Atrial fibrillation leads to a lack of coordinated contractility within the atria, impaired emptying, and associated blood stasis. The low flow state promotes formation of thrombi consisting of red blood cells and fibrin. Atrial fibrillation also causes dilation of the LA and left atrial appendage (LAA), leading to pathologic changes associated with thrombus formation in AF.[6] The LAA, a blind-ended passage attached to the LA, is at particularly high risk for thrombus formation. The LAA is long, with a narrow inlet, thereby predisposing to blood stasis.[7] In a review of echocardiographic, autopsy, and operative findings, 91% of nonvalvular AF associated thrombi were isolated to, or originated from the LAA.[8] There is also evidence to suggest AF is associated with changes in the atrial endothelium and increased inflammation which further promotes a prothrombotic state in AF and contributes to thrombosis formation and thromboembolic sequelae.[7]

Although VKAs have been used to reduce the risk of thromboembolic events associated with AF since the 1950s, a large scale randomized controlled trial (RCT) did not take place until the 1980s. Investigators undertook the Stroke Prevention in Atrial Fibrillation (SPAF) study to evaluate the use of anticoagulation and antiplatelet agents to ameliorate the thromboembolic risk associated with AF. This study established both warfarin and aspirin as superior to placebo, supporting the practice of using antithrombotic agents in the setting of AF.[9] Several studies have since confirmed a significant reduction in stroke in patients with AF when treated with warfarin or aspirin, with a relative risk reduction of 60% and 20%, respectively.[10]

An understanding of the types of AF, atrial flutter (AFL), the distinction between valvular and nonvalvular AF is important in order to make appropriate clinical decisions regarding therapy. Several classification schemes have been developed to help clinicians identify which patients

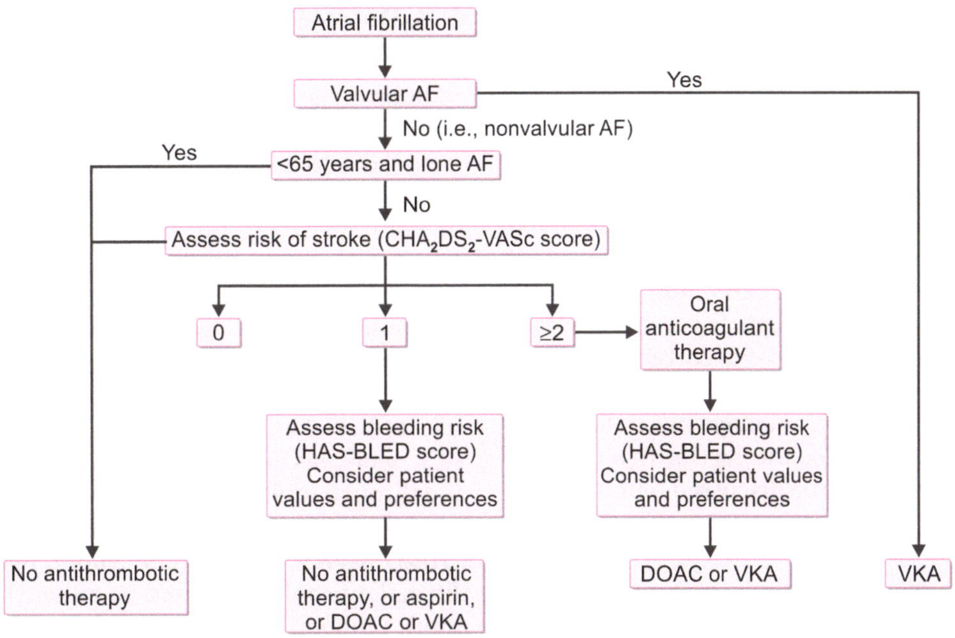

AF, atrial fibrillation; HAS-BLED, Hypertension, Abnormal renal/liver function, Stroke, Bleeding history predisposition, Labile international normalized ratio (INR), Elderly, Drugs/Alcohol concomitantly; DOAC, direct oral anticoagulant; VKA, vitamin K antagonist.

FLOWCHART 1: Algorithm for the management of antithrombotic therapy based on risk stratification schemes[4]

are high risk and will benefit from oral anticoagulation (OAC) and which patients are low risk and could refrain from OAC use. With the increased risk of major bleeding with OAC use, schema to assess bleeding risk has also been developed.

Classification of Atrial Fibrillation

Atrial fibrillation can be described in terms of episode duration. First, AF can be divided into paroxysmal or persistent. In paroxysmal AF, episodes resolve spontaneously or with intervention within 7 days of onset. Persistent AF is continuous and lasts for more than 7 days. Persistent AF can further be defined as "long-standing persistent AF", in which the patient has had continuous AF for more than 12 months. Permanent AF is a term that describes a situation where physician and patient have come to an agreement to stop attempting to restore sinus rhythm. Lone AF is used to describe a younger patient that does not have the clinical or imaging evidence indicative of cardiopulmonary disease, hypertension, or diabetes mellitus.[4]

Although terminology of AF can be used to define AF type in a clinical setting, these definitions do not always change management. Patients with AF, regardless of episode duration are at increased risk of thromboembolic ischemic stroke.[3] Studies show that both paroxysmal and persistent AF have similar annual risk of stroke.[3] Thus, although described differently, paroxysmal and persistent AF should be anticoagulated the same, based on stroke risk profiling and not on AF duration. Studies have shown that despite guidelines recommending anticoagulation for patients at high risk of stroke, the duration of AF still influences how providers prescribe anticoagulation.[11]

Valvular versus Nonvalvular Atrial Fibrillation

The definition of valvular disease in terms of AF anticoagulation can differ between guidelines.[12] As per 2014 American Heart Association/American College of Cardiology/Heart Rhythm Society (AHA/ACC/HRS) guidelines, valvular disease is defined as rheumatic mitral stenosis, a previous mitral valve repair, or valve replacement with mechanical valve or bioprosthesis.[4] Early studies identified the increased risk of thromboembolism in patients with valvular disease from rheumatic heart disease.[13] This increased risk of thromboembolism is compounded when valvular disease, such as mitral stenosis, is coupled with AF.[13] Although large scale RCTs have never been conducted, observational studies indicate that anticoagulation results in a large reduction in thromboembolism risk for patients with concomitant AF and rheumatic valvular disease.[13,14]

It is important to note that not all forms of valvular disease confer the same degree of increased thromboembolism risk when associated with AF. For instance, patients with aortic stenosis and AF do not have an increased risk of thromboembolism beyond the risk solely attributed to AF.[12] Current guidelines recommend long-term VKA therapy for patients with valvular AF. However, if the patient is intolerant of VKA, then clopidogrel and acetylsalicylic acid (ASA) together are recommended over ASA alone.[15]

Atrial Fibrillation versus Atrial Flutter

Atrial fibrillation and AFL are the only two arrhythmias for which guidelines currently recommend routine anticoagulation. Atrial flutter is less common than AF, but this population also appears to be at an increased risk of thromboembolism.[16,17] Also, AFL can often coexist with AF in the same patient.[18] Although fewer studies exist concerning thromboembolism in AFL, current European Society of Cardiology (ESC) guidelines recommend approaching antithrombotic management for AFL in a similar way as AF.[4,19] For the rest of this chapter, anticoagulation will primarily be discussed in the context of AF.

SELECTING ANTITHROMBOTIC THERAPY: EXAMINATION OF RISKS AND BENEFITS

Prevention of thromboembolic phenomenon in patients with AF is effectively accomplished through routine anticoagulant use. However, the use of anticoagulants is associated with an increased risk of bleeding. The use of risk stratification scoring systems is essential to evaluate the risks and benefits of anticoagulation on an individual basis and to determine the most appropriate use of anticoagulation. The CHA_2DS_2-VASc score, which improved upon the original $CHADS_2$ scoring system, is the most commonly used scoring system to assess stroke risk in nonvalvular AF.[20-22]

Stroke Risk Stratification Schemes

$CHADS_2$

The $CHADS_2$ score attributes 1 point for each of the following risk factors: hypertension, congestive heart failure (CHF), age more than or equal to 75 years and diabetes mellitus and 2 points for a prior stroke, transient ischemic attack (TIA), or thromboembolism (Table 1).[21] In the $CHADS_2$ scoring system, a score of 0 is low risk, 1–2 is intermediate risk, and 3–6 is defined as high risk. Each point is associated with approximately 1–2% increase stroke risk per year.[21]

TABLE 1: $CHADS_2$ score[21]

Definition and Scores for CHADS^2	Score
Congestive heart failure	1
Hypertension	1
Age ≥75 years	1
Diabetes mellitus	1
Stroke/transient ischemic attack/thromboembolism	2
Maximum score	6

CHA_2DS_2-VASc

CHA_2DS_2-VASc is similar to $CHADS_2$ but also includes an additional age category (65–74 years), history of vascular disease (including myocardial infarction, peripheral arterial disease, and aortic plaque), and also incorporates female gender into risk stratification (Table 2).[23-25]

For CHA_2DS_2-VASc, a score of 0 defines a patient as low risk for thromboembolism. A score of 1 indicates the patient is at intermediate risk and a score of 2 or greater suggests that the patient is at high risk for thromboembolism. Similar to $CHADS_2$, an increasing CHA_2DS_2-VASc score correlates with an increasing adjusted stroke rate per year (Table 3). The CHA_2DS_2-VASc score has been validated in multiple patient cohorts and through multiple nationwide studies.[26,27]

Guidelines for intermediate risk ($CHADS_2$ or CHA_2DS_2-VASc of 1) are ambiguous, recommending that the patient could be started on either OAC, aspirin or no antithrombotic therapy.[4] CHA_2DS_2-VASc is better able to distinguish individuals into high risk or low risk, leaving fewer patients in the intermediate category. Under the classic $CHADS_2$ scoring system a large percentage (61.9%)

TABLE 2: $CHADS_2$ score and stroke rate[22]

Adjusted stroke rate (% per year)	$CHADS_2$ score
0	1.9
1	2.8
2	4.0
3	5.9
4	8.5
5	12.5
6	18.2

TABLE 3: CHA_2DS_2-VASc score and stroke rate[4]

CHA_2DS_2-VASc	
Congestive heart failure/left ventricular dysfunction	1
Hypertension	1
Age ≥75 years	2
Diabetes mellitus	1
Stroke/transient ischemic attack/ thromboembolism	2
Vascular disease (previous myocardial infarction, peripheral arterial disease, or aortic plaque)	1
Age 65–74 years	1
Sex category (i.e., female sex)	1
Maximum score	9

Continued

Continued

CHA_2DS_2-VASc	Adjusted stroke rate (% per year)
0	0
1	1.3
2	2.2
3	3.2
4	4.0
5	6.7
6	9.8
7	9.6
8	6.7
9	15.2

TABLE 4: HAS-BLED bleeding risk score[29]

HAS-BLED Bleeding risk score		
Letter	**Clinical characteristics**	**Points awarded**
H	Hypertension	1
A	Abnormal renal and liver function (1 point each)	1 or 2
S	Stroke	1
B	Bleeding	1
L	Labile international normalized ratios	1
E	Elderly (>65 years)	1
D	Drugs or alcohol (1 point each)	1 or 2

of patients were defined as intermediate risk, while 20.4 and 17.7% of individuals were categorized as low risk and high risk, respectively.[22] Under CHA_2DS_2-VASc, only 15.1% of subjects were considered intermediate risk, 9.2% were low risk, and 75.7% were classified as high risk.[22] CHA_2DS_2-VASc is also better at identifying patients truly at low risk, as no patients with a score of 0 had a thromboembolic event during follow-up for the initial study compared to a thromboembolism rate of 1.9% per year with a $CHADS_2$ score of 0.[21,22]

Bleeding Risk Scheme

Several scores to assess bleeding risk exist. The HAS-BLED score [Hypertension, Abnormal renal/liver function, Stroke, Bleeding history predisposition, Labile international normalized ratio (INR), Elderly, Drugs/alcohol concomitantly] is the simplest of these scoring systems and has been validated in several studies.[28] The HAS-BLED criteria evaluate the risk of major bleeding within 1 year. Major bleeding is defined as an intracranial bleed, hospitalization, hemoglobin decrease more than 2 g/L, and/or transfusion.[29] In the HAS-BLED schema, one point is awarded for each of the following risk factors—hypertension (uncontrolled, >160 mm Hg systolic), abnormal renal/liver function, previous stroke (especially lacunar), bleeding history or predisposition (i.e., anemia), labile INR (therapeutic time in range <60%), elderly (age >65 years), drugs (antiplatelet agents, nonsteroidal anti-inflammatory drugs), and alcohol excess (see Table 4). A score of 0 indicates that the patient is low risk, 1–2 is moderate risk, and 3 or greater indicates a patient at high risk of major bleed. In follow-up validation studies of HAS-BLED, the risk of major bleed in the low risk cohort was less than 1% per year.[28]

The HAS-BLED scoring schema exhibited good predictive accuracy in patients who were not on antithrombotic therapy as well as patients already on antiplatelet or antithrombotic therapy.[28,29] Compared to other bleeding risk schemes, HAS-BLED most accurately predicts intracerebral hemorrhage, which may be the most feared complication of anticoagulant therapy.[30] The HAS-BLED score can be used as an additional tool in risk assessment, however, current guidelines do not recommend excluding a patient from OAC therapy because of a predicted high bleeding risk.[4] Instead, HAS-BLED should be used to identify modifiable bleeding risk factors in a patient and help correct them where possible.[31]

Decisions Regarding Therapy

Current 2014 AHA/ACC/HRS guidelines recommend OAC in patients with a CHA_2DS_2-VASc score of more than or equal to 2. For patients considered intermediate risk, CHA_2DS_2-VASc of 1, either aspirin, warfarin, or no therapy is recommended. Forgoing oral anticoagulation is recommended if the patient is low risk, CHA_2DS_2-VASc of 0.[4]

European Society of Cardiology guidelines are similar to AHA/ACC/HRS guidelines and emphasize assessment of stroke risk factors utilizing CHA_2DS_2-VASc (Table 5). The ESC recommends against anticoagulation in patients with lone AF and age less than 65 years. The ESC guidelines also highlight how to utilize female gender as a risk factor. If female gender is the sole reason for a patient receiving a score of 1 and the patient has lone AF and age less than 65 years, they do not recommend anticoagulation. Otherwise, the guidelines recommend avoiding anticoagulation with a CHA_2DS_2-VASc score of 0 and recommend either DOAC or VKA in patients with scores of 1 or more than or equal to 2.[19]

In the end, the ultimate decision to use antithrombotic therapy should be based on a discussion between provider and patient, taking into account the individual patient's risks, benefits, and preferences. Risk schemes and published consensus guidelines should be used to inform this decision-making process.

TABLE 5: Antithrombotic therapy recommendations by risk score[4,19]

CHA_2DS_2-VASc score	2014 AHA/ACC/HRS guidelines	2012 ESC guidelines
0	No therapy	No therapy
1	No therapy/oral anticoagulant/aspirin	If point is only due to female sex, then no therapy. Otherwise, oral anticoagulant should be considered
≥2	Oral anticoagulant	Oral anticoagulant

AHA, American Heart Association; ACC, American College of Cardiology; HRS, Heart Rhythm Society; ESC, European Society of Cardiology.

ANTITHROMBOTIC OPTIONS

Antiplatelet Therapy

The utility of aspirin for AF thromboprophylaxis has been debated. In a meta-analysis by Hart et al., aspirin was shown to reduce the risk of stroke by 22% [confidence interval (CI) 2–38%] when compared with placebo.[32] However, in the meta-analysis, the positive effects of aspirin monotherapy was largely attributed to a single trial, SPAF-1.[9] The other six trials examined showed trends toward stroke risk reduction but they were not statistically significant.[32] Also, aspirin monotherapy did not cause a significant reduction in all-cause mortality.[32]

In a comparison of aspirin alone versus clopidogrel plus aspirin, the combination antiplatelet therapy reduced the risk of stroke by 28%.[33] However, clopidogrel plus aspirin are inferior to warfarin in terms of stroke prevention.[34]

For low risk AF patients, aspirin does not appear to be effective and may be unsafe. One prospective trial evaluating aspirin in AF patients with low thromboembolism risk showed aspirin therapy increased bleeding risk while also increasing the risk of combined endpoint events which included cardiovascular death, symptomatic brain infarction, and TIA.[35] Current guideline recommendations state that aspirin should be considered in patients with an intermediate risk for thromboembolism (CHA_2DS_2-VASc of 1) although no antithrombotic therapy or OAC can also be considered.[4] In summary, the data to support the use of aspirin to reduce stroke in AF is limited but can be considered in patients with intermediate risk of stroke.

Oral Anticoagulants

Warfarin

Warfarin is a VKA that has been used as an oral anticoagulant for stroke prevention in AF since the 1950s. Warfarin produces its anticoagulant effect by interfering with cyclic interconversion of vitamin K by inhibiting vitamin K epoxide reductase (VKORC1), modulating g-carboxylation of regions of the vitamin K dependent coagulation factors II, VII, IX, X, protein C and S. Treatment with warfarin results in hepatic production of partially carboxylated and decarboxylated proteins with reduced coagulant activity.[36,37]

There have been several large RCTs regarding warfarin use in nonvalvular AF. In a meta-analysis combining 2,900 participants between 6 RCTs, adjusted dose warfarin resulted in a relative risk reduction of 64% and an absolute risk reduction of 2.7% per year for ischemic and hemorrhagic stroke compared to placebo.[10] Overall, the number needed to treat for 1 year to prevent one stroke was 37. In patients who had a prior history of TIA or stroke, the number needed to treat was 12. For primary prevention of stroke in AF, warfarin was associated with a statistically significant reduction in all strokes, ischemic stroke, disabling or fatal stroke, and death when compared to placebo.[38] Warfarin is currently the only oral anticoagulant approved for use in valvular AF, and has been shown to be superior to dabigatran with significantly decreased rates of stroke and major bleeding in patients with mechanical heart valves.[39]

Despite strong evidence for reducing stroke risk in AF, there are several factors that limit warfarin use. These factors include risk of major or fatal bleeding, need for frequent INR monitoring, and the potential for drug and dietary interactions.

Dosing

The initial starting dose for warfarin is typically 5 mg daily, or in healthy individuals, 10 mg daily for 2 days.[40] However, a starting dose less than 5 mg may be appropriate in elderly patients or patients with other comorbid conditions such as CHF, nutritional deficiencies, or liver disease.[36] Warfarin dosing should be individualized for each patient according to their INR response. The standard goal INR is 2–3 for warfarin use in AF.[41] The relative risk of thromboembolism increases strikingly at INR less than 1.8 and odds of intracranial hemorrhage increases markedly at INR values more than 3.5.[41] A higher INR goal is recommended for certain patients with mechanical heart valves based on prosthesis thrombogenicity and patient-related risk factors.[42]

Renal Dosing

No dosage adjustment necessary. However, caution should be used in patients with renal failure due to increased risk of bleeding complications.[43]

Hepatic Dosing

No dosage adjustments necessary. However, caution should be used in patients with decreased liver function regardless of cause as coagulation factor synthesis may be impaired, leading to increased sensitivity to warfarin.[44]

Monitoring

When initiating warfarin therapy inpatient, INR levels are evaluated daily until therapeutic range is achieved and maintained for at least 2 days.[36] Once steady state INR is achieved, then testing can occur every 4–6 weeks.[36]

Pharmacokinetics

Warfarin is highly water soluble, rapidly absorbed from the gastrointestinal tract, has high bioavailability, and reaches maximal blood concentrations about 90 minutes after oral administration.[45,46] The half-life of warfarin is 36–42 hours.[47] The half-life of prothrombin (factor II) is relatively long, 60–72 hours, compared to the short half-life of the other vitamin K dependent factors, whose half-lives are 6–24 hours. Because the protective effect of warfarin is mostly attributed to lowering prothrombin levels, whose half-life is relatively long, time to therapeutic level after initiating warfarin is often more than or equal to 4 days.[48-50]

Pharmacodynamics of warfarin are affected by both genetic and environmental factors. Genomic variants in cytochrome P450 2C9 (CYP2C9) and/or VKORC1 (C1 subunit of vitamin K 2,3 epoxide reductase complex) may impact warfarin metabolism and dosing. Patients with CYP2C9 variant allele have increased risk of major bleeding complications.[51] Polymorphisms of VKORC1 are also associated with a need for decreased warfarin dose.[52]

Warfarin has a significant number of drug and food interactions. Warfarin is primarily metabolized by several specific cytochrome P450 isoenzymes, drugs that induce or inhibit these enzymes can affect warfarin metabolism, decreasing or increasing warfarin's potency, respectively.[53] A critical analysis of possible interactions between food, drugs, and warfarin found strong evidence of interaction in 39 of 81 drugs and food appraised.[54] Many other drugs have been reported to affect warfarin and over 131 drug interactions are listed in the drug information packet.[44] Close monitoring while initiating a new medication is recommended for nearly all prescription medications or herbal supplements.[37] Alterations in vitamin K consumption can also affect warfarin.[55] Drastic changes in dietary habits, such as eating large amounts of leafy green vegetables, should be avoided.[44]

Surgery

In general, warfarin can be discontinued 5 days prior to the planned procedure. An INR should be obtained 24 hours prior to the procedure and if it is above the desired value, this can be corrected with fresh frozen plasma or vitamin K.[56] An INR less than or equal to 1.5 is considered safe for high risk procedure.[57] However, some clinicians recommend an INR of less than or equal to 1.2 for procedures with a risk of bleeding into high risk spaces, such as closed spaces during intracranial or spinal surgery.[58] It is further discussed in the sections titled "Perioperative Management of Anticoagulation" and "Using Heparin as Perioperative Bridge for Warfarin".

Cost

The wholesale cost per 5 mg pill of generic warfarin is $0.68, with a 30-day supply costing $20.04.[59] This price does not take into account the cost of monitoring therapy, including clinic and lab fees.

Major Adverse Events

The primary complication associated with taking warfarin is bleeding. When the INR is greater than 3.5–4, the likelihood of bleed significantly increases.[41,60,61] Odds of extracranial hemorrhage were found to be significantly elevated when using warfarin for secondary stroke prevention when compared to placebo.[62] In several studies comparing warfarin to DOACs, the annual rate of major bleeding, intracranial hemorrhage, and gastrointestinal bleed on warfarin therapy were 3.09–3.4%, 0.7–0.8%, and 0.86–1.02%, respectively.[33,63,64]

In addition to bleeding risk, patients on warfarin can also experience acute thrombotic complications such as skin necrosis. Although rare (<0.1%), this complication occurs early during the initiation of therapy, typically within 3-8 days.[36,44,65] This complication is attributed to an abrupt fall in protein C levels before levels of factors II, XII, IX, and X have also decreased, and an exaggerated procoagulant effect can be seen in patients with protein C deficiency.[66,67]

"Purple toe syndrome" is another distinct syndrome associated with warfarin therapy. It is caused by embolization of cholesterol microthrombi, released from atheromatous plaques, and usually occurs 3–8 weeks after starting therapy.[68] Systemic atheroemboli and cholesterol microemboli can also occur in other locations, most commonly kidneys, pancreas, spleen, and liver.[44]

Warfarin also contributes to abnormal fetal bone formation if taken by a mother during pregnancy.[36,69,70] Other major congenital malformations, as well as fetal hemorrhage, and increased risk of spontaneous abortion are also attributed to the use of warfarin during pregnancy.[44] For these reasons, warfarin should be avoided during pregnancy.

Recommendations for Warfarin Reversal

In patients that have an elevated INR (INR >4.5–10) but no bleeding, guidelines recommend against giving vitamin K.[71] Studies show that there is no benefit to giving vitamin K over holding anticoagulation in these patients.[71] However, if INR is more than 10, then giving oral vitamin K is recommended.[71]

In patients that have anticoagulant related bleeding, there are several products that can be utilized for hemostasis including vitamin K, prothrombin complex concentrate (PCC), fresh frozen plasma (FFP), and

TABLE 6: Anticoagulant major trials and results[9,63,78,64,131,187]

	Warfarin	Dabigatran	Rivaroxaban	Apixaban	Edoxaban
Trial name	**SPAF-I**	**RE-LY**	**ROCKET AF**	**ARISTOTLE**	**ENGAGE AF-TIMI 48**
Support	United States Agency for Healthcare Policy and Research	Boehringer Ingelheim	J&J and Bayer	Bristol-Myers Squibb/Pfizer	Daiichi Sankyo Pharma
Patient number enrolled	1,330 patients; 627 anticoagulation candidates, 703 nonanticoagulation candidates	18,113	14,264	18,201	21,105
Pertinent inclusion criteria	- AF on ECG within 12 months - Age >18 years	• AF on ECG within 6 months • Age >75 or 65–74 years with DMII, HTN, or CAD • One of following: ○ Prior stroke/TIA ○ LVEF <40% or ○ NYHA class II–IV within 6 months	• AF on ECG • $CHADS_2 \geq 2$ • Age ≥18 years	• AF or flutter at enrollment or ≥2 episodes of AF or flutter on ECG, at least 2 weeks apart within 12 months of enrollment • ≥1 of the following: • Age ≥75 years • Prior stroke/TIA or embolism • Symptomatic heart failure within 3 months or LVEF <40% • DMII or • HTN requiring pharmacologic treatment	• AF on ECG within 12 months • $CHADS_2 \geq 2$ • Anticoagulation therapy planned for the duration of the trial • Age ≥21 years
Exclusion criteria	• Prosthetic heart valve • Mitral stenosis • Stroke or TIA within 24 months • Age <60 years without overt cardiovascular disease	• Severe valvular disease • Stroke within 14 days • CrCl <30 mL/min • Severe stroke within 6 months • Active liver disease	• Hemodynamically significant mitral valve disease • Prosthetic valve • Atrial myxoma • LV thrombus • Platelets <90 K/uL • Hb <10 g/dL • Stroke within 14 days (TIA within 3 days) • ASA >100 mg/day within 5 days • HIV • CrCl <30 mL/min • Liver disease or ALT >3X ULN	• Cr >2.5 or CrCl <25 mL/min • Moderate or severe mitral stenosis • ASA >165 mg/day or ASA and clopidogrel use • Stroke within 7 days	• AF due to reversible disorder • CrCl <30 mL/min • High risk of bleeding • Use of DAPT • Moderate-to-severe mitral stenosis • Other indications for anticoagulation therapy • ACS • Coronary revascularization • Stroke within 30 days • Inability to adhere to study procedures

Continued

Continued

	Warfarin	Dabigatran	Rivaroxaban	Apixaban	Edoxaban
Trial name	**SPAF-I**	**RE-LY**	**ROCKET AF**	**ARISTOTLE**	**ENGAGE AF-TIMI 48**
% of time with therapeutic INR in the coumadin group	NA	64%	55%	62%	68%
Study design	Two parallel randomized controlled trials; aspirin or coumadin vs. placebo	Open label coumadin vs. double blind; D110 vs. D150	Double blind vs. coumadin	Double blind vs. coumadin	Double blind vs. coumadin
Primary efficacy outcome	Ischemic stroke or SE	Stroke or SE	Stroke or SE	Stroke or SE	Stroke or SE
Primary safety outcome	Major bleeding, intracranial hemorrhage	Major bleeding	Major bleeding and clinically relevant bleeding	Major bleeding	Major bleeding
Outcome, relative risk (95% confidence interval)					
Stroke/SE	0.33* (NA)	D110: 0.91 (0.74–1.11); D150: 0.66 (0.53–0.82)	0.79 (0.65–0.95)	0.79 (0.66–0.95)	E30: 1.07 (0.87–1.31); E60: 0.79 (0.63–0.99)
Hemorrhagic stroke	NA	D110: 0.31 (0.17–0.56); D150: 0.26 (0.14–0.49)	0.59 (0.37–0.93)	0.51 (0.35–0.75)	E30: 0.33 (0.22–0.50); E60: 0.54 (0.38–0.77)
Intracranial bleeding	NA (annual rate of 1.2% per year)	D110: 0.30 (0.19–0.45); D150: 0.41 (0.28–0.60)	0.67 (0.47–0.93)	0.42 (0.38–0.58)	E30: 0.30 (0.21–0.43); E60: 0.47 (0.34–0.63)
Ischemic stroke	0.35* (NA)	D110: 1.11 (0.89–1.40); D150: 0.76 (0.59–0.97)	0.94 (0.75–1.17)	0.92 (0.74–1.13)	E30: 1.41 (1.19–1.67); E60: 1.00 (0.83–1.19)
Total mortality	0.75* (NA)	D110: 0.91 (0.80–1.03); D150: 0.88 (0.77–1.00)	0.85 (0.7–1.02)	0.89 (0.80–0.998)	E30: 0.87 (0.79–0.96); E60: 0.92 (0.83–1.01)
Major bleeding	0.995* (NA)	D110: 0.80 (0.69–0.93); D150: 0.93 (0.81–1.07)	1.04 (0.90–1.20)	0.57 (0.46–0.70)	E30: 0.47 (0.41–0.55); E60: 0.80 (0.71–0.91)
Gastrointestinal bleeding	NA	D110: 1.10 (0.86–1.41); D150: 1.50 (1.19–1.89)	1.39 (1.19–1.61)	0.89 (0.70–1.15)	E30: 0.67 (0.53–0.83); E60: 1.23 (1.02–1.50)

ACS, acute coronary syndrome; AF, atrial fibrillation; ALT, alanine aminotransferase; ASA, aspirin; CrCl, creatinine clearance; Cr, creatinine; D110, dabigatran 110 mg dose; D150, dabigatran 150 mg dose; DAPT, dual antiplatelet therapy; E30, edoxaban 30 mg dose; E60, edoxaban 60 mg dose; ECG, electrocardiogram; SE, status epilepticus; Hb, hemoglobin; HIV, human immunodeficiency virus; TIA, transient ischemic attack; ULN,upper limit of normal; NA, not available; RE-LY, Randomized Evaluation of Long-term anticoagulation therapy; ARISTOTLE, Apixaban for Reduction in Stroke and other Thromboembolic Events in atrial fibrillation; ENGAGE AF-TIMI 48, Effective Anticoagulation with Factor Xa Next Generation in Atrial Fibrillation-Thrombolysis in Myocardial Infarction 48; ROCKET AF, Rivaroxaban Once Daily Oral Direct Factor Xa Inhibitor Compared with Vitamin K Antagonism for Prevention of Stroke and Embolism Trial in Atrial Fibrillation; SPAF-I, Stroke Prevention in Atrial Fibrillation; LVEF, left ventricular ejection fraction.

*Coumadin RR compared to placebo.

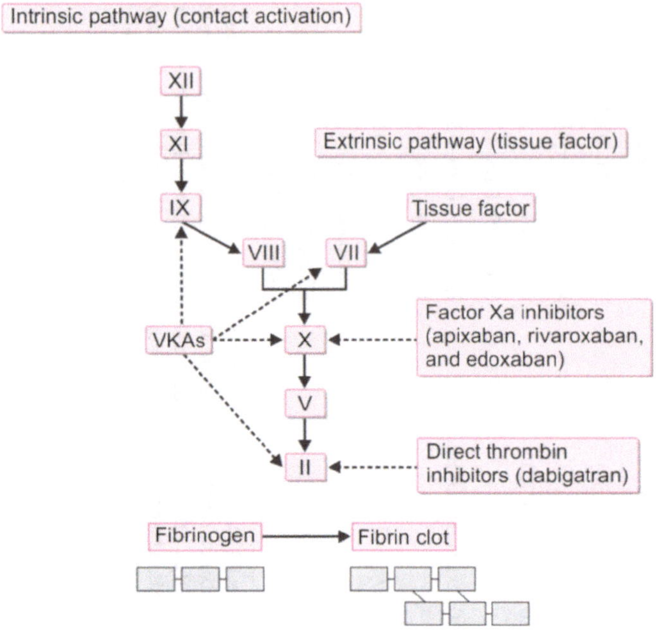

FLOWCHART 2: Coagulation pathway and anticoagulant mechanism of action

recombinant factor VIIa (rFVIIa). In patients with warfarin associated major bleeding, current guidelines recommend giving 5 or 10 mg vitamin K by intravenous injection and rapid reversal with four-factor PCC.[71] Prothrombin complex concentrate and rFVIIa are recommended over FFP because there is less potential for allergic reaction, infection, volume overload, and PCC has a shorter preparation time.[71]

Summary

Warfarin is more effective in stroke prevention in AF compared to placebo or aspirin. In addition, VKAs are the only oral medications approved for use in valvular AF and mechanical heart valves. Concern for adverse events has limited the use and prescribing of warfarin. Several studies have suggested that warfarin is underused in patient populations that would benefit from treatment and that prescribing practices do not always follow current guideline recommendations.[11,72,73] Efficacy of warfarin is further limited by a tight therapeutic window and difficulty maintaining a therapeutic INR. In research studies, patients were found to have a therapeutic INR 63.6% of the time, while in general, United States patients have a therapeutic INR only about one-half of the time.[74,75] Due to these limitations, several newer medications (discussed below) could be preferred over warfarin for use in nonvalvular AF.

Direct Oral Anticoagulants

Introduction

Various terms have been used to describe the 'new' class of oral anticoagulants including novel/new oral anticoagulants, DOACs, and target-specific oral anticoagulants. Currently, the International Society on Thrombosis and Hemostasis recommends using the term "direct oral anticoagulant".[76]

There are four Food and Drug Administration (FDA) approved DOACs for use in patients with nonvalvular AF. These are divided into two different pharmacological classes, DTIs and factor Xa (FXa) inhibitors. These medications contain a more predictable set of pharmacokinetics than warfarin, and therefore require only baseline laboratory monitoring (Table 7). Although more expensive than warfarin, decreased need for monitoring, lack of dietary limitations, and fewer drug interactions make DOACs attractive.[77] Two major limitations for the DOACs include reversibility concerns as well as expense when compared to warfarin. This chapter will evaluate each individual DOAC. In addition, options for reversibility will be discussed together at the end.

Direct Thrombin Inhibitors

Direct thrombin inhibitors function by preventing thrombin from cleaving fibrinogen to fibrin and can inhibit both active clot-bound and circulating thrombin.

Dabigatran etexilate

Dabigatran is the first, and currently, only FDA approved DOAC for the prevention of stroke and systemic embolism associated with AF. The major trial leading to the FDA approval of dabigatran was the Randomized Evaluation of Long-term anticoagulation therapy (RE-LY) trial.[78] Patients randomized into three groups, dabigatran dosed at 110 or 150 mg or therapeutic warfarin.[78] The RE-LY study found that dabigatran administered at a dose of 150 mg twice daily, as compared with warfarin, was associated with lower rates of stroke and systemic embolism but similar rates of major hemorrhage.[78] It should be noted that in the warfarin group, the mean time with a therapeutic INR (INR 2–3) was 64%.[78] The primary outcome of stroke or systemic embolism occurred at a rate of 1.53% per year in the 110 mg dabigatran group, 1.11% per year in the 150 mg dabigatran group, and 1.69% per year in the warfarin group (both doses of dabigatran were noninferior to warfarin with $p < 0.001$, the 150 mg dose of dabigatran was superior to warfarin with $p < 0.001$).[78]

Dosing: Standard dosing for a patient with atrial fibrillation for the prevention of stroke and systemic embolism for dabigatran is 150 mg twice daily with or without food.

P-glycoprotein (P-gp) inhibitors are associated with increased plasma concentration of dabigatran to a modest extent.[78] However, the risk of major bleeding and stroke are not significantly changed when P-gp inhibitors are used concomitantly with dabigatran.[78] Therefore, as discussed below, only in patients with creatinine clearance (CrCl) less than 50 and high risk bleeding

TABLE 7: Anticoagulation dosing and monitoring[77, 80, 83-88, 91, 109, 110, 118, 125, 127, 133]

	Warfarin	Dabigatran	Rivaroxaban	Apixaban	Edoxaban
Mechanism of action	**Vitamin K antagonist**	**Direct thrombin inhibitor**	**Direct factor Xa inhibitor**	**Direct factor Xa inhibitor**	**Direct factor Xa inhibitor**
Dosing	2–5 mg once daily (can start 10 mg once daily for 2 days in healthy outpatient)	150 mg twice daily with or without food	20 mg once daily with largest meal	5 mg twice daily with or without food (unless two of the following: Age >80 years, weight <60 kg, or creatinine >1.5 then 2.5 mg twice daily)	60 mg once daily
Renal dosing	No adjustment (caution)	• CrCl 30–50 mL/min: no adjustment unless on dronedarone or oral ketoconazole then 75 mg twice daily • CrCl 15–30 mL/min: 75 mg twice daily • CrCl <15 mL/min: not defined and HD not defined (CrCl <30 mL/min excluded from RE-LY trial)	• If CrCl 15–50 mL/min: 15 mg daily; • If CrCl <15 mL/min: Avoid use	• 2.5 mg twice daily if two or more: • Age >80 years • Weight <60 kg or • Cr >1.5 • HD: 5 mg twice daily except if age >80 or <60 kg, then 2.5 mg twice daily	• CrCl >95 mL/min: avoid use; • CrCl 51–95 mL/min: No adjustment • CrCl 15–50 mL/min: 30 mg once daily • CrCl <15 mL/min: Avoid use
Hepatic dosing	No adjustment (caution)	No adjustment	• Child Pugh A: No adjustment; • Child Pugh B or C: Avoid use	• Child Pugh A: No adjustment • Child Pugh B: No adjustment • Child Pugh C: Not recommended	• Child Pugh A: No adjustment • Child Pugh B or C: Not recommended
Monitoring	• INR • PT • Hematocrit	At baseline: • Thrombin time (most sensitive) • PT/PTT • Creatinine • After initiating based on patients' characteristics: • CrCl 30–60 mL/min, and age >75 years: renal function every 6 months; • CrCl 15–30 mL/min renal function every 3 months • If condition changes, check renal and/or liver function	At baseline: • Creatinine occasionally • Antifactor Xa • Complete blood count • Blood pressure	At baseline: • Antifactor Xa • PT/PTT/INR (expected to prolong after use) • Hepatic function • Creatinine	At baseline: • Antifactor Xa • PT/PTT (expected to prolong after use) • Creatinine
Pharmaco-kinetics	• Metabolism: Liver (CYP450, primarily CYP2C9) • Excretion: Urine 92%, half-life 20–60 h (highly variable)	• Metabolism: Liver (CYP450 none) • Excretion: Urine 80%, half-life 12–14 h (14–17 h in elderly)	• Metabolism: Liver (CYP450, CYP2J2 and CYP3A4/5) • Excretion: Urine 66%, feces 28%, half-life 5–11 h (11–13 h in elderly)	• Metabolism: Liver (CYP450, primarily CYP3A4) • Excretion: Urine 27%, feces 56%, half-life 12 h	• Metabolism: Minimal liver (CYP450, primary CYP3A4) • Excretion: Urine 50%, biliary secretion 50%, half-life 10–14 h

Continued

Continued

	Warfarin	Dabigatran	Rivaroxaban	Apixaban	Edoxaban
Mechanism of action	**Vitamin K antagonist**	**Direct thrombin inhibitor**	**Direct factor Xa inhibitor**	**Direct factor Xa inhibitor**	**Direct factor Xa inhibitor**
Hold time prior to low bleeding risk surgery	5–6 days; can use LMWH at therapeutic or intermediate dose as bridging	24–48 h before surgery; unless CrCl 30–50 mL/min and then 3–5 days before surgery	At least 24 h before surgery; unless CrCl 15–29.9 mL/min and then 3 days before surgery	At lease 24 h before surgery; unless CrCl 30-50 mL/min then 3 days	At least 24 h prior to surgery
Hold time prior to high bleeding risk surgery	5–6 days; can use LMWH at therapeutic or intermediate dose as bridging	3 days before surgery; unless CrCl 30–50 mL/min and then 4–5 days before surgery	3 days before surgery; unless CrCl 15–29.9 mL/min and then 4 days before surgery	At least 2–3 days before surgery; unless CrCl 30–50 mL/min then 4 days before surgery	At least 24 h prior to surgery

CrCl, creatinine clearance; CYP450, cytochrome P450 enzymes; INR, international normalized ratio; LMWH, low molecular weight heparin; PT, prothrombin time; PTT, partial thromboplastin time.

patients, is there need for dose adjustment of dabigatran etexilate when P-gp inhibitors are coadministered.

Renal dosing: Based on the RE-LY trial data, when CrCl drops between 30 and 50 mL/min, it is recommended to decrease dabigatran only if the patient is also using certain P-gp inhibitors.[78] When the CrCl drops to 15-30 mL/min, the recommended dose is 75 mg twice daily. Dabigatran dosing is not defined when the CrCl is less than 15 mL/min.

Hepatic dosing: No adjustment necessary.

Monitoring: Patients taking dabigatran require baseline laboratory testing.[81] Initial testing should include baseline laboratory assessment including hemoglobin/hematocrit, liver function, renal function, and coagulation studies (PT/INR). At each subsequent visit, medication adherence, signs/symptoms of bleeding or thromboembolism, side effects, and medications should be reviewed.[77] Annual laboratory assessment should be completed including hemoglobin/hematocrit, renal function, and liver function.[77] More frequent laboratory testing is recommended in certain patient populations. For patients with CrCl 30-60 mL/min, and age more than 75 years, renal function should be checked every 6 months. If CrCl is 15-30 mL/min, then renal function should be checked every 3 months. Dabigatran does not require routine coagulation monitoring; however, studies, such as activated partial thromboplastin time (aPTT), thrombin clotting time, and ecarin clotting time, can be used to assess the degree of anticoagulation.[82]

Pharmacokinetics: Dabigatran etexilate is a prodrug that is rapidly absorbed and quickly hydrolyzed by nonspecific ubiquitous esterases in the gut, plasma, and liver to its active form, dabigatran.[78,80] Dabigatran plasma concentrations and anticoagulation effects are dose dependent and predictable, peaking within 0.5-2 hours (mean 1.5 h) of oral administration.[83-85] Time to reach steady-state is relatively short (approximately 3 days), and thus dabigatran typically does not require bridging during initiation of therapy.[83] Notably, the mean terminal half-life of dabigatran after oral administration is approximately 8 hours after a single dose and ranges from 12 to 14 hours after multiple doses.[80,83-88] However, in older healthy volunteers, the half-life is about 13 hours and in patients with CrCL of less than 30 mL/min, the half-life increased to more than 24 hours.[80,84,89] Renal excretion is the predominant elimination pathway for dabigatran, removing up to 80% of circulating dabigatran while about 20% of dabigatran is excreted via the biliary system.[80,90]

Surgery: In patients with CrCl more than or equal to 50 mL/min, the manufacturer recommends that dabigatran be held 24-48 hours prior to planned procedure.[91] However, in patients with CrCl less than 50 mL/min, it is recommended that dabigatran be held for 3-5 days before planned procedure.[91] With major surgeries or spinal/epidural procedures, longer drug-free periods may be considered.

Major adverse events: As described in the RE-LY trial, the rate of major bleeding was 3.36% per year in the warfarin group, as compared to 2.71% per year in the 110 mg dabigatran group ($p = 0.003$) and 3.11% per year in the 150 mg dabigatran group ($p = 0.31$). Intracranial bleeding rates were higher with the warfarin group (0.74%), when compared to both the 110 mg dose of dabigatran (0.23%) and the 150 mg dose of dabigatran (0.30%).[78,79] However, the rate of gastrointestinal bleeding (GIB) was significantly higher in the 150 mg dabigatran group (1.50% per year, $p < 0.001$) compared to warfarin, but was similar in the 110 mg dabigatran group (1.12% per year, $p = 0.43$).[78,79]

Subsequent studies have shown varying results regarding major bleeding on dabigatran compared to warfarin. The RE-LY RCT and observational studies (all using Medicare populations) failed to observe an increased incidence of major bleeding on dabigatran.[78,92,93] However, further subgroup analysis of older patients found there was a higher incidence of major bleeding and particularly increased risk of GIB.[94-96] Previous studies document an increased risk of bleeding in the first 90 days of warfarin treatment in elderly patients, however, these patients were excluded from the studies, and therefore, could have overestimated the bleeding risk of dabigatran in the elderly.[94]

A study out of Hong Kong showed a potential reduction of associated GIB in dabigatran when using gastroprotective agents such as proton pump inhibitors or H2-receptor antagonists.[97] Further studies are warranted to assess the potential risk and benefits of gastroprotection in patients on dabigatran by quantifying the risk of thromboembolism versus the benefit of preventing GIB.

Cost: The wholesale cost of dabigatran has been quoted as $6.75 for two 150 mg capsules or approximately $200 for a 30-day supply.[91,98] Although it is convenient that dabigatran does not require regular laboratory monitoring for dose adjustment, the drug cost of dabigatran therapy appears to be more than the cost of warfarin and INR monitoring combined.[91,99]

Summary: The RE-LY trial demonstrated dabigatran had a lower rate of intracranial hemorrhage, but a higher rate of major and GIB compared to warfarin. As discussed above, the major bleeding risk is largely associated with patients older than 75 years,[78,96] and therefore, improved prescribing practices and patient selection could help reduce the bleeding risk.[78] In addition, the development and approval of newer and potentially safer anticoagulants has raised the question of whether dabigatran will ultimately be considered a second or third line therapy for prophylaxis in patients with AF.[100, 101]

Direct Factor Xa Inhibitors

Direct factor Xa inhibitors function by preventing factor Xa from cleaving prothrombin to thrombin. One major benefit to these direct FXa inhibitors is they can provide more consistent and predictable anticoagulation compared to warfarin.[102, 103] The three currently FDA approved direct FXa inhibitors for the treatment of nonvalvular AF include rivaroxaban, apixaban, and edoxaban.

Rivaroxaban

Rivaroxaban was the first FDA approved direct FXa inhibitor for the prevention of stroke and systemic thromboembolism associated with AF. Rivaroxaban is dosed once daily in nonvalvular AF patients and has no requirement for routine coagulation monitoring and has few drug-drug interactions.[102,104-106]

The major trial leading to the FDA approval of rivaroxaban was the Rivaroxaban Once Daily Oral Direct Factor Xa Inhibitor Compared with Vitamin K Antagonism for Prevention of Stroke and Embolism Trial in Atrial Fibrillation (ROCKET AF) trial, comparing rivaroxaban to warfarin.[107] In this study, rivaroxaban was noninferior to warfarin for the prevention of stroke or systemic embolism. The primary outcome of stroke or systemic embolism occurred at a rate of 1.7% per year in the rivaroxaban group and 2.2% per year in the warfarin group ($p < 0.001$ for noninferiority and $p = 0.01$ for superiority of rivaroxaban).[64] There was no significant between-group difference in the risk of major bleeding, although intracranial and fatal bleeding occurred less frequently in the rivaroxaban group.[64] However, there is some controversy concerning the faulty point-of-care device used to measure INR values during the trial. The faulty device may have given falsely low INR readings, raising the question of whether rivaroxaban may have appeared safer because the warfarin cohort received higher doses than necessary.[108]

Dosing: Standard dosing for a patient with AF for the prevention of stroke and systemic embolism for rivaroxaban is 20 mg once a day. The liver is the main route of elimination and concomitant administration with strong CYP3A4 and P-gp inhibitors and inducers should be avoided, and caution should be exercised with weak CYP3A4 inhibitors and inducers.[109]

Renal dosing: Renal impairment results in modest increases in drug exposure, with a more pronounced effect on factor Xa inhibition.[110] Periodic renal function monitoring is recommended in patients with rivaroxaban as clinically indicated.[19] Patients with moderate renal impairment (creatinine clearance of 30–49 mL/min) have been found to experience the same exposure if the dose of rivaroxaban was reduced to 15 mg once daily.[107,111,112] Patients with CrCl of 15–20 mL/min were excluded from clinical trials and recommendations for these patients are based on pharmacokinetic data.[64,109,113-115] Rivaroxaban should be avoided in patients with CrCl of less than 15 mL/min.[109]

Hepatic dosing: With the liver as the main route of elimination for rivaroxaban, this medication should be avoided in patients with Child-Pugh B or C hepatic impairment and in those with liver disease associated with coagulopathy as exposure is increased and has been associated with prolongation of prothrombin time.[109]

Monitoring: Although routine monitoring is not required, laboratory testing may be considered in cases of severe bleeding, renal failure, need for urgent surgery, or in patients at extremes of body weight.[109] The prothrombin time is influenced by rivaroxaban in a dose dependent manner but only with some but not all reagents.[116] Activated partial thromboplastin time and antifactor Xa activity are also affected by rivaroxaban but a standard for calibration for this agent is currently lacking.[109]

Pharmacokinetics: Rivaroxaban is an oral, direct, reversible, and dose dependent inhibitor of factor Xa, blocking free and bound factor Xa.[109, 117] Rivaroxaban is in an active form upon ingestion and does not require conversion. It has a half-life of 5–11 hours in healthy younger individuals and 11–13 hours in elderly individuals.[109] It has a shallow dose-response curve for effectiveness but a steeper dose-response curve for safety; thus, small increases in dose have a limited effect on improving efficacy but may be accompanied by sharp rise in bleeding risk.[109] The liver is a main route of elimination for rivaroxaban and it is extensively metabolized by the cytochrome P450 (CYP) enzyme system.[118] Excretion is primarily in the urine (~68%) and feces (~28%).[118]

Surgery: Rivaroxaban should be discontinued at least 24 hours before a planned procedure and 3 days in patients with CrCl 15–29.9 mL/min. However, risk of bleeding should always be weighed against the urgency of the intervention and rivaroxaban should be restarted as soon as hemostasis is established.[109]

Major adverse effects: As described in the ROCKET-AF Trial, major bleeding occurred at a rate of 3.6% per year in the rivaroxaban group and 3.4% per year in the warfarin group ($p = 0.58$).[64] Rates of intracranial hemorrhage were significantly lower in the rivaroxaban group than in the warfarin group (0.5 vs. 0.7% per year, $p = 0.02$). However, major bleeding from a gastrointestinal site was more common in the rivaroxaban group compared to warfarin (3.2 vs. 2.2%, $p <0.001$).[64, 119] Factors, such as age (>65 years), female sex, elevated diastolic blood pressure, history of chronic obstructive pulmonary disease, prior GIB, prior aspirin use, and anemia were associated with increased risk of major bleeding.[119]

Cost: The wholesale cost of rivaroxaban is around $10 for a 20 mg tablet or approximately $300 for a 30-day supply.[120] While the cost of rivaroxaban may be greater than warfarin, decision-analytic models suggest that it is cost-effective in AF.[109] Specifically, an economic analysis based on the ROCKET-AF study, in which drug and monitoring costs were excluded, there was a reduction in costs with rivaroxaban associated with primary and secondary events such as stroke and myocardial infarction, in addition to decreased cost associated with bleeding events.[109, 121]

Summary: Rivaroxaban was the first FDA direct FXa inhibitor approved for anticoagulation in AF. Standard dosing is once daily, with a lower dose recommended for moderate renal impairment. Avoiding rivaroxaban is recommended for moderate-to-severe liver impairment. The ROCKET-AF study showed that rivaroxaban was noninferior to warfarin for prevention of stroke or systemic embolism. There was no significant difference in major bleeding, although the rivaroxaban group had less intracranial hemorrhage compared to the warfarin group.

Apixaban

Apixaban was the second FDA approved direct FXa inhibitor for the prevention of stroke and systemic thromboembolism associated with AF. The major trial leading to the FDA approval of apixaban was the Apixaban for Reduction in Stroke and other Thromboembolic Events in atrial fibrillation (ARISTOTLE) trial.[122] The trial compared apixaban to warfarin.[122] Apixaban was found to be superior to warfarin for the prevention of stroke or systemic embolism, and was associated with less overall bleeding and lower mortality.[122] Stroke or systemic embolism occurred at a rate of 1.27% per year in the apixaban group as compared to 1.60% per year in the warfarin group ($p <0.001$ for noninferiority and $p = 0.01$ for superiority of apixaban compared to warfarin).[122] Another important trial[123] in the evaluation of apixaban was the Apixaban Versus Acetylsalicylic Acid to prevent Strokes (AVERROES) trial that studied patients considered 'unsuitable' for VKAs. This study was stopped short due to the clear superiority of apixaban over aspirin, with similar rates of major bleeding, including intracerebral hemorrhage.[123, 124]

Dosing: Standard dosing for a patient with AF for the prevention of stroke and systemic embolism for apixaban is 5 mg twice a day with or without food, unless the patient meets two of the following criteria: (i) age more than or equal to 80 years, body weight less than or equal to 60 kg, or (ii) serum creatinine more than or equal to 1.5 mg/dL, then the dose is decreased to 2.5 mg twice a day.[125]

Strong inhibitors of CYP3A4 and P-gp (e.g., ketoconazole, itraconazole, ritonavir, clarithromycin) are associated with increased plasma concentration of apixaban. Patients should have their apixaban dose reduced by 50% when coadministered with strong CYP450 3A4 inhibitors.[125] In patients taking the lowest dose of apixaban (2.5 mg twice daily), strong CYP450 3A4 inhibitors should be avoided.[125] Furthermore, strong inducers of CYP3A4 and P-gp (e.g., rifampin, carbamazepine, phenytoin, or St. John's wort) should also be avoided because such drugs will decrease exposure to apixaban.[125]

Renal dosing: Although renal impairment results in modest increases in drug exposure with a more pronounced effect on factor Xa inhibition,[110] apixaban does not require dose adjustment for patients with renal impairment alone. Dose adjustment should occur if patient meets more than two of the criteria listed above or if the patient has end-stage renal disease (ESRD) maintained on hemodialysis.[125] Of note, studies did not look at patients with CrCl less than 15 mL/min not receiving dialysis, thus the dosing is based on pharmacokinetic and pharmacodynamic data in subjects with ESRD maintained on dialysis only.[125] Apixaban is currently the preferred direct factor Xa inhibitor in patients with renal impairment.

Hepatic dosing: No dosage adjustment is required in patients with mild hepatic impairment (Child-Pugh Class A). Due to limited clinical experience in patients with moderate hepatic impairment (Child-Pugh Class B), there is no dosing recommendations. However, caution should be exercised due to the possibility that patients have intrinsic coagulation abnormalities.[125] Apixaban is not recommended in patients with severe hepatic impairment (Child-Pugh Class C).[125]

Monitoring: As with rivaroxaban discussed above, routine monitoring for apixaban is not required, although it may be considered in cases of severe bleeding, renal failure, need for urgent surgery, or in patients at extremes of body weight. The dilute Russell's viper venom time (DRVVT) is a sensitive test to determine the anticoagulant effect of apixaban, but has a low specificity.[126] Chromogenic anti-Xa assay is a sensitive assay to determine the inhibition of factor Xa by apixaban and provide estimates of plasma concentration of the drug, however, it is time-consuming and not routinely used.[126]

Pharmacokinetics: Apixaban is an oral, selective, direct, reversible inhibitor of the coagulation factor Xa (FXa). Apixaban is rapidly absorbed and maximum concentration is achieved at 1 hour, on average, after oral dose administration.[127] Average half-life is 12.7 hours in healthy individuals. Pharmacokinetic data suggest that the apixaban elimination profile is approximately 56% via feces, 27% via urine, with minor biliary excretion.[127] Overall, apixaban and its metabolites are excreted by multiple elimination pathways, thus patients with hepatic or renal impairments may be treated with apixaban and the likelihood of significant drug-drug interactions may be low.[127,128]

Surgery: Apixaban should be discontinued at least 24 hours prior to elective surgery or invasive procedure with a low risk of bleeding and 48 hours prior to procedures with a moderate-to-high risk of unacceptable or clinically significant bleeding.[125] Generally, anticoagulation bridging is not required while holding apixaban. It is safe to initiate apixaban when adequate hemostasis has been achieved unless oral therapy cannot be administered, then administration of a parenteral anticoagulant should be considered.[125]

Major adverse events: Apixaban has significantly less major bleeding as compared to warfarin.[122] In the ARISTOTLE trial, major bleeding occurred in 2.13% per year in the apixaban group compared to 3.09% per year in the warfarin group ($p < 0.001$). Furthermore, there was a significant reduction in the rate of intracranial hemorrhage for the apixaban group compared to the warfarin group (0.33 vs. 0.80% per year, $p < 0.001$). However, there were similar rates of GIB in the apixaban group compared to the warfarin group, 0.76% per year and 0.86% per year, respectively.[122]

Cost: The wholesale cost of apixaban is around $6.92 for a 5 mg tablet or approximately $400 for a 30-day supply.[129] Studies have shown that apixaban was projected to result in fewer recurrent venous thromboembolism (VTE) and bleeding events in comparison to rivaroxaban, low molecular weight heparin (LMWH)/dabigatran, and LMWH/VKA.[130] Therefore, it is projected that apixaban will be a more cost-effective alternative to warfarin and other DOACs.[130]

Summary: Apixaban is a factor Xa inhibitor with twice daily dosing. Dose adjustment is recommended if a patient meets two of the stated criteria (age ≥80 years, body weight ≤60 kg, or serum creatinine ≥1.5 mg/dL). Avoidance is recommended in moderate-to-severe liver impairment. In the ARISTOTLE study, apixaban was found to be superior to warfarin in preventing stroke or systemic embolism, and had significantly less overall bleeding and decreased overall mortality. In addition, apixaban is clearly superior to ASA in patients who are intolerant of VKAs.

Edoxaban

The latest FDA approved direct factor Xa inhibitor for the prevention of stroke and systemic thromboembolism associated with AF is edoxaban. Edoxaban was compared to warfarin in the Effective Anticoagulation with Factor Xa Next Generation in Atrial Fibrillation-Thrombolysis in Myocardial Infarction 48 (ENGAGE AF-TIMI 48) trial.[131] Results showed both edoxaban regimens were noninferior to warfarin with respect to stroke or systemic embolism and were associated with significantly lower rates of bleeding and death from cardiovascular causes.[131] The lower dose of edoxaban (30 mg) was used if the estimated creatinine clearance was 30–50 mL/min, body weight less than or equal to 60 kg, or the concomitant use of verapamil, quinidine, or dronedarone (potent P-gp inhibitors). The primary outcome of stroke or systemic embolism occurred at a rate of 1.18% per year in the high dose edoxaban group ($p < 0.001$ for noninferiority and $p = 0.02$ for superiority compared to warfarin), 1.61% per year in the low dose edoxaban group ($p = 0.005$ for noninferiority and $p = 0.44$ for superiority compared to warfarin) compared to 1.50% per year in the warfarin group.[131]

Dosing: Standard edoxaban dosing for a patient with AF for the prevention of stroke and systemic embolism is 60 mg once a day.

Although intestinal transport of edoxaban occurs through the P-gp efflux transporter mechanism, no dose adjustment is recommended in patients also on P-gp inhibitors.[132, 133] The ENGAGE AF-TIMI 48 study showed dose reduction in patients concomitantly receiving P-gp inhibitors resulted in edoxaban blood levels that were lower than in patients who were given the full dose.[132, 133] Concomitant use of edoxaban with P-gp inducers, such as rifampin, should be avoided.[133]

Renal dosing: Renal clearance accounts for approximately 50% of the total clearance of edoxaban. Blood levels of edoxaban are increased in patients with poor renal function.[133] Therefore, when CrCl is 15–50 mL/min, the recommended dose is 30 mg once daily.[133] Limited clinical data exists in patients with CrCl less than 15 mL/min, therefore, edoxaban is not recommended in these patients.[133]

Hepatic dosing: No dosage reduction is required in patients with mild hepatic impairment (Child-Pugh Class A).[133] Edoxaban is not recommended in patients with moderate or severe hepatic impairment (Child-Pugh Class B and C) due to the risk of patients having intrinsic coagulation abnormalities.[133]

Monitoring: Like other DOACs, routine monitoring for edoxaban is not required, although it may be considered in cases of severe bleeding, renal failure, need for urgent surgery, or in patients at extremes of body weight. The DRVVT, HepTest, and prothrombinase induced clotting time methods demonstrate linear dose-response to edoxaban and may potentially have applications for drug monitoring.[134, 135] Overall, use of prothrombin time is limited to excluding high levels of edoxaban and aPTT does not appear to be helpful.[135]

Pharmacokinetics: Edoxaban is an oral, selective, direct, reversible inhibitor of the coagulation factor Xa. Peak plasma concentration is achieved within 1–2 hours of edoxaban administration and steady state is achieved after 3 days.[136] Elimination half-life ranges from 10 to 14 hours and clearance is half via the renal pathway and half via biliary secretion.[136] A limited proportion of edoxaban (<4%) is metabolized by CYP450.[132]

Surgery: Edoxaban should be discontinued at least 24 hours prior to elective surgery or invasive procedures.[133] It is safe to restart edoxaban when adequate hemostasis has been achieved unless oral therapy cannot be administered, then administration of a parenteral anticoagulant should be considered.[133]

Major adverse events: In the ENGAGE AF-TIMI 48 trial, the annual rate of major bleeding events was 3.43% with the warfarin group compared to 2.75% with high dose edoxaban (p >0.001) and 1.61% with low dose edoxaban (p <0.001). Similarly, reductions in life-threatening bleeding with high and low dose edoxaban as compared to warfarin were seen with rates of 0.4% (high dose), 0.25% (low dose), and 0.78% (warfarin).[131] Intracranial bleeding rates for high dose, low dose, and warfarin were 0.39%, 0.26%, and 0.85%, respectively (p <0.001 for comparison of warfarin with each dose of edoxaban).[131] Interestingly, the rate of major GIB was higher with high dose edoxaban than with warfarin (1.51 vs. 1.23%).[131] The GIB rate was lowest with low dose edoxaban (0.82%).[131]

Cost: The wholesale cost of edoxaban is around $11.65 for a 60 mg tablet or approximately $350 for a 30-day supply.[137] Further studies are required for the cost-effectiveness of edoxaban versus warfarin and the other DOACs.

Summary: Edoxaban is the latest FDA approved factor Xa inhibitor for anticoagulation in AF. It is dosed once daily, with a lower dose recommended in patients with moderate renal impairment. Avoiding edoxaban is recommended for moderate-to-severe hepatic impairment. In the ENGAGE AF-TIMI 48 trial, edoxaban was found to be noninferior to warfarin in preventing stroke or systemic emboli and had less major bleeding, intracranial hemorrhage, life-threatening bleeding, and death from cardiovascular cause.

Reversal Strategies for Direct Oral Anticoagulants

Overview and general recommendation for reversal strategies

A major concern among prescribing clinicians includes the ability to reverse DOACs. Initially, specific reversal agents for non-vitamin K antagonist anticoagulants were lacking; however, over the last few years, new specific and nonspecific reversal agents have emerged. Table 8 shows the current published research on the major forms of reversal agents and their effects/timing on the FDA approved oral anticoagulants for AF.

Initial management

When there is a concern for bleeding or OAC overdose, the anticoagulant should be discontinued and supportive care should include fluid resuscitation, red blood cell transfusions, maintenance of renal function, identification of bleeding source, or surgical intervention as needed. As these new oral anticoagulants have relatively short half-lives, this will likely be sufficient for many patients.[138-140]

Activated charcoal

Activated charcoal prevents drug absorption and should be considered if ingestion occurred within 2–3 hours of presentation.[141] *In vitro* studies showed that activated charcoal can absorb up to 99.9% of dabigatran.[142-144] Similarly, the use of charcoal in factor Xa overdose may reduce absorption if given early.[138]

Hemodialysis

Due to dabigatran's low protein binding, hemodialysis should be considered as a viable strategy for treating patients with dabigatran overdose.[89, 143] Studies have shown that dialysis can remove 40–68% of dabigatran in a 2–4 hour session, however, dabigatran levels can rebound up to 87%, 2 hours after removal and therefore continuous renal replacement therapy has been suggested as an alternative.[145]

In contrast to dabigatran, factor Xa inhibitors (particularly rivaroxaban and apixaban) have high plasma protein binding. Thus, hemodialysis is not expected to have significant ability to remove factor Xa inhibitors.[138, 146]

Prothrombin complex concentrate

Prothrombin complex concentrates are purified products derived from plasma. Prothrombin complex concentrates can be divided into 3 or 4 factor concentrates. The 3 factor concentrates contain factors II, IX, and X, while the 4 factor concentrates also include factor VII. In the event of major or life-threatening DOAC associated bleeding or when emergency surgery is necessary, recommendations suggest administering PCC, with preference for activated prothrombin complex concentrates.[139, 141, 147, 148] Despite recommendations, both animal studies and human trials have yielded mixed results concerning the utility of PCC in DOAC reversal.

For DTI reversal, initial animal studies suggested inactivated PCC may reduce bleeding with dabigatran, however, this has not been replicated in human or *ex vivo* studies.[149-152] In contrast, PCCs are promising candidates for reversal of all factor Xa inhibitors.[153] A small human study showed the complete reversal of rivaroxaban with PCC.[151] Although results are promising, a major concern with PCCs is their potential to induce thrombosis at doses used to treat bleeding. The safety and efficacy in treating DOAC associated bleeding with PCC has not been validated in large prospective clinical trials and further studies are warranted.

Fresh frozen plasma

Compared to PCC, reversal of the new anticoagulants with FFP would require a high volume transfusion in order to overwhelm the direct effect of the drugs.[138] High volume transfusions come with increased risk of complications such as volume overload, allergic reaction, infection, and other transfusion side effects.[141] Multiple studies have shown no benefit when FFP is used for dabigatran related bleeding.[142] In summary, there is little data for the use of FFP for emergent reversal of DOACs.[138]

Recombinant factor VIIa

Currently, there is no data to support the use of rFVIIa in DOAC associated bleeding. There are also risks associated with administering rFVIIa such as thrombosis, volume overload, and transfusion reactions. There have been reported cases of negligible benefit with dabigatran associated bleeding, and limited studies show a decrease in bleeding time in dabigatran treated rats, however, it does not reverse the anticoagulant effect.[138, 143] Similar results have been seen in using rFVIIa to reverse effects of factor Xa inhibitors.[138]

Recent and in-development specific reversal agents

Currently, there is one FDA approved selective reversal agent for dabigatran, idarucizumab. Two other DOAC reversal agents are in development, adrexanet-α, a recombinant altered human factor Xa targeted towards

TABLE 8: Anticoagulant reversal strategies[82,149,151,154,160,188-193]

Reversal agents	Warfarin	Dabigatran	Rivaroxaban	Apixaban	Edoxaban
Oral activated charcoal	-	Slow ****	Slow	Slow	- ****
Fresh frozen plasma	Fast	-	- (*)	- *	- *
Recombinant factor VIIa	Prompt	Fast	Rapid	Rapid	Rapid ***
Prothrombin complex concentrate	Rapid	-	Rapid	Rapid	Fast***
Activated prothrombin complex concentrate	Rapid	Rapid	Rapid	Rapid**	Fast**
Hemodialysis	-	Prompt@	-	-	-
Intravenous vitamin K	Prompt	-	-	-	-
Oral vitamin K	Slow	-	-	-	-
Idarucizumab	-	Fast	-	-	-
Andexanet alfa	-	-	Rapid	Rapid@@	Rapid**

Rapid, 10–15 min; Fast, >15 min–4 h; Prompt, 4–6 h; Slow, within 24 h; -, no effect;
*No published data exist to support the use of fresh frozen plasma for reversal during acute hemorrhage
**Currently, no published studies or case reports are available regarding utilization for apixaban reversal. However, having the same mechanism of action as rivaroxaban, extrapolation of data
****In vivo* - Fukuda T et al, Thromb Haemost, 2012
****Limited studies, consider helpful if given within ~2 h of ingestion;
@May take more than 4 h depending on initial dabigatran levels
@@, dose dependent effect.

direct and indirect Xa inhibitors, and ciraparantag, a small molecule with activity towards all DOACs as well as indirect Xa inhibitors.

Reversal of Direct Thrombin Inhibitors

Idarucizumab

The FDA recently approved idarucizumab, a humanized monoclonal antibody fragment (Fab) and the first specific reversal agent for the DTI, dabigatran. Dabigatran has very high affinity for idarucizumab, a greater affinity than that of dabigatran for thrombin.[155-157] *In vivo* studies showed that at 4 hours post-treatment with idarucizumab, 96.5% of the patients had free dabigatran levels near the lower limit of quantification.[158] In some patients, a subsequent increase in dabigatran concentration 12–24 hours after administration of idarucizumab was observed, which may reflect the redistribution of extravascular dabigatran into the intravascular compartment.[158] The medication has been well-tolerated with minimal thrombotic events and minimal side effects.[159]

Reversal of Factor Xa Inhibitors

Andexanet alfa

Andexanet alfa is a recombinant modified human factor Xa decoy protein that is designed to neutralize the anticoagulant effects of both direct and indirect factor Xa inhibitors.[160] Current research on adrexanet include two parallel trials to establish efficacy and safety: Andexanet alfa a Novel Antidote to the Anticoagulant Effects of Apixaban (ANNEXA-A) and Rivaroxaban (ANNEXA-R).[160] Initial results of phase III trials show rapid reduction (within 2–5 min) of anti-factor Xa activity with andexanet compared to placebo for both apixaban and rivaroxaban with reversal activity persisting 1–2 hours after infusion completion.[160] There were no serious adverse events, no thrombotic events, and the medication was well-tolerated. Further studies are warranted, however, the initial data shows promise for andexanet in the reversal of rivaroxaban and apixaban, and similar effectiveness is expected with other factor Xa inhibitors.

Reversal of Factor IIa and Xa Inhibitors

Ciraparantag/aripazine

Ciraparantag/aripazine is a synthetic small molecule that works as a nonspecific reversal agent.[161] Initially designed to bind unfractionated heparin through noncovalent hydrogen bonding and charge-charge interactions, ciraparantag binds in a similar way to all DOACs.[161-164] In thromboelastographic studies and animal studies, ciraparantag has been shown to reverse anticoagulation with each of the new oral agents.[161, 163, 164] The first small human study, involving 80 healthy persons given a single intravenous dose of ciraparantag, showed whole-blood clotting time decreased to within 10% of baseline values in 10 min or less.[161] Further studies are necessary before FDA approval and release can be expected.

SPECIAL CONSIDERATIONS

Perioperative Management of Anticoagulation

Interruption for a planned or elective procedure is common and affects 1 in 6 people on chronic anticoagulation for AF yearly.[165,166] The decision to use bridging therapy can be based on risk stratifying both the surgery type and the patient. Although, the ultimate decision should be based on the discussion between the prescribing physician, the operating physician, and the patient, taking into account the individual patient and procedural risks.

For patients undergoing low-risk surgeries, bridging is not necessary and anticoagulation can be continued throughout the procedure. For example, in patients undergoing pacemaker or defibrillator placement, a strategy of continued warfarin treatment markedly reduced the incidence of clinically significant device-pocket hematomas without a statistical difference in major surgical or thromboembolic complications compared to bridging therapy with heparin.[167] For surgeries that have moderate-to-high bleeding risk, the decision to bridge should be determined by the patient's risk for thromboembolism. In patients at low risk for thromboembolism, anticoagulation can be held preoperatively without bridging therapy.

Recent literature questions the utility of bridging for surgical procedures. Data from a prospective, observational study (ORBIT-AF) showed that bridging anticoagulation was used in 25% of procedures and was associated with higher risk for bleeding and adverse events.[168] While bridging with a parenteral agent such as unfractionated heparin (UFH) or LMWH is common, the data on prevention of embolic events are limited and the rate of bleeding is significantly increased.[169] Similarly, the recently published Perioperative Bridging Anticoagulation in Patients with Atrial Fibrillation (BRIDGE) trial showed no reduction in the incidence of thromboembolism with bridging versus no bridging.[170] However, bridging was associated with 1.9% absolute risk increase in major bleeding.[170] Several caveats should be considered in analysis of the BRIDGE trial. Most of the patients included were not at high risk of thromboembolism (about 3% of the patients included had $CHADS_2$ score of 5–6). Patients with mechanical heart valves, previously diagnosed VTE, or cerebral vascular accident or TIA within 12 weeks were excluded from the study. In addition, the BRIDGE study did not include patients on therapy with DOACs.

Although there is building evidence against bridging therapy, it is still reasonable to use bridging therapy in patients that are high risk of thrombosis. This includes patients with nonvalvular AF at high risk by thromboembolic risk calculators ($CHADS_2$ ≥4) and patients at high risk due to the presence of additional diagnoses that independently require anticoagulation, such as mechanical mitral valve, two or more mechanical valves, VTE diagnosed within previous 3 months, or severe thrombophilia.[171] Additional studies are needed to further assess perioperative interruption of anticoagulation with DOACs and management of DOAC interruption should be individualized, with emphasis on the type of procedure as well as individual thromboembolic risk.[77]

Using Heparin as Perioperative Bridge for Warfarin

In patients on warfarin where bridging anticoagulation is appropriate, the most commonly used anticoagulant is LMWH followed by UFH. Warfarin should be stopped 5 days prior to the procedure and when the INR falls below a therapeutic level, LMWH or UFH should be initiated. Once the procedure is completed and hemostasis obtained, warfarin and LMWH or UFH can be resumed and should be continued until the INR is again therapeutic, usually 5 days after restarting warfarin.

Anticoagulation in Setting of Pharmacological and Electrical Cardioversion

Atrial fibrillation causes stasis in the atria and increases the risk of thrombus formation. In electrical or pharmacological cardioversion, the return of sinus rhythm and atrial activity acutely places the patient at risk for a cardioembolic event. Echocardiographic studies have shown that return of atrial mechanical activity can be delayed for up to 4 weeks after restoration of sinus rhythm.[172-175] Thus, anticoagulation strategies are aimed at minimizing the risk of thromboembolism during these high risk timeframes.

Embolic risk is highest in the hours to days after cardioversion. In a review, it was found that 98% of embolic events in patients with AF who underwent cardioversion occurred within 10 days and 82% were within 72 hours.[172] The overall risk of thromboembolism within 30 days of cardioversion is low (<1%). Commonly used risk assessment tools (i.e., CHA_2DS_2-VASc) are highly predictive for thromboembolism in this acute (<30 days) setting.[176] Risks with cardioversion of AFL are similar and requires the same anticoagulation management as AF.[177]

Determining anticoagulation management surrounding electrical cardioversion is largely dependent on the duration of AF prior to presentation, hemodynamic stability, and thromboembolic risk (Flowchart 3). For patients that are unstable, immediate electrical cardioversion is recommended and should not be delayed to start anticoagulation.

For stable patients experiencing AF for less than 48 hours, electrical or pharmacological cardioversion can be completed without immediate initiation of anticoagulation. Weigner et al. showed that in low risk patients with AF episode duration less than 48 hours, the incidence of thromboembolism was low (0.8–0.9%)

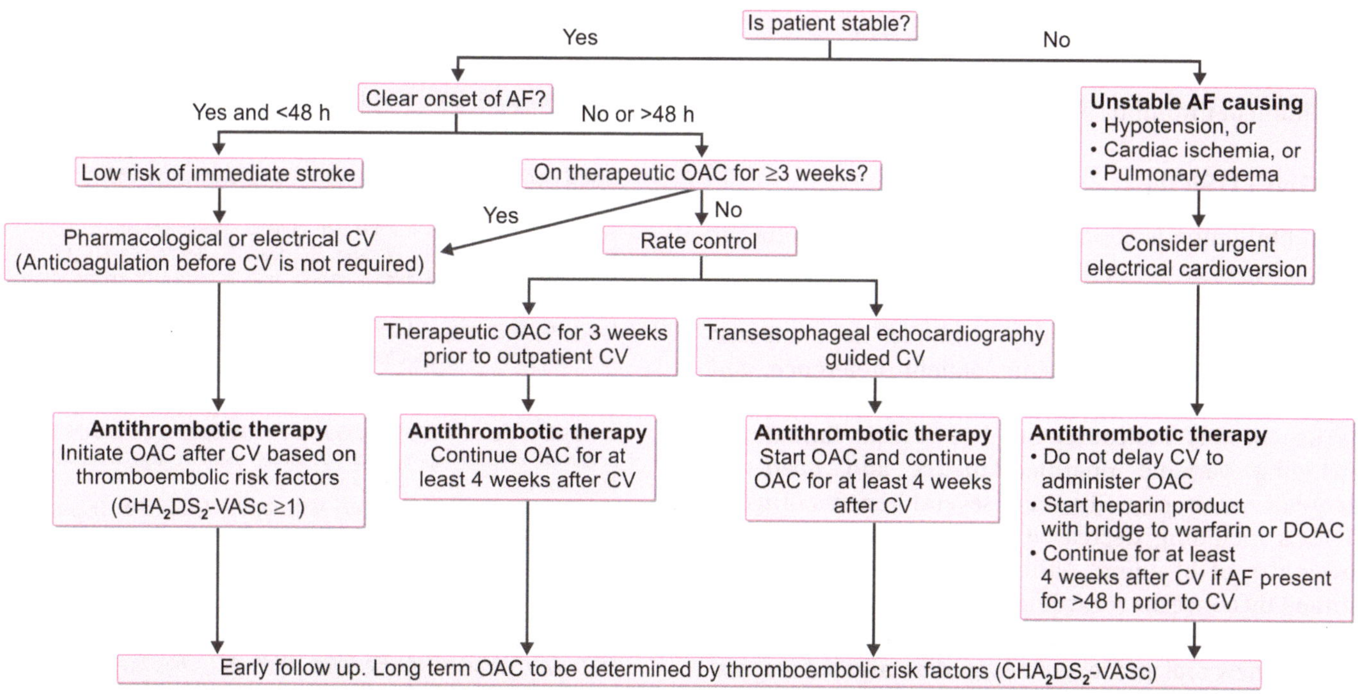

AF, atrial fibrillation; OAC, oral anticoagulant; CV, cardioversion; DOAC, direct oral anticoagulant.

FLOWCHART 3: Algorithm for anticoagulation management in setting of cardioversion[4] and that initiation of anticoagulation therapy did not significantly reduce thromboembolism risk in this patient subset.[178] The decision to start and continue anticoagulation after cardioversion should be based on the individual's thromboembolic and bleeding risk profile.

For stable patients with AF of 48 hours duration or longer, or where the duration of AF is unknown, guidelines recommend therapeutic anticoagulation for at least 3 weeks before cardioversion. This recommendation is based on observational studies that showed 3 weeks of anticoagulation with warfarin resulted in high rates of atrial thrombi resolution.[179] Similar use of DOACs in patients who were receiving long-term anticoagulation (>3 weeks) prior to cardioversion is supported by data from ROCKET AF, RE-LY, and ARISTOTLE trials and a subsequent meta-analysis.[180-183]

In patients with AF of 48 hours duration or longer, an alternative strategy to 3 weeks of anticoagulation would be to perform a transesophageal echocardiogram guided cardioversion.

In a large randomized study, there was no significant difference in the rate of embolic events between transesophageal echocardiography (TEE) guided therapy or conventional therapy with empiric anticoagulation with warfarin for 3 weeks prior to electrical cardioversion.[184] Although, patients in the TEE guided group had shorter time to direct current cardioversion and improved rate of successful restoration of sinus rhythm compared to the conventional therapy group.[184] In patients where an atrial thrombus is identified on TEE, cardioversion should be delayed and anticoagulation should be initiated if it has not already been started. A follow-up TEE should be repeated after 3–4 weeks of anticoagulation to ensure resolution of thrombus prior to cardioversion.[185]

CONCLUSION

Atrial fibrillation is common and a potent risk factor for stroke. Use of anticoagulation in the setting of AF reduces the risk of stroke. The decision to use anticoagulation should be based on thromboembolic risk assessed using the CHA_2DS_2-VASc score, patient preference, and bleeding risk. Warfarin has strong evidence to support its use in this indication but has several limitations, including variable pharmacokinetics and need for frequent monitoring. There are several benefits of using DOACs including decreased need for monitoring and lower risk of bleeding. Although, DOAC use has been limited by concerns regarding reversibility and the novel nature of these drugs. As clinicians become more familiar with the new oral anticoagulants, and as targeted reversal agents are developed, the use of DOACs will likely become more commonplace. Due to the high prevalence and the morbidity associated with thromboembolic events in the setting of AF, detailed knowledge of anticoagulant use will become increasingly necessary for all clinicians.

REFERENCES

1. Wolf PA, Benjamin EJ, Belanger AJ, Kannel WB, Levy D, D'Agostino RB. Secular trends in the prevalence of atrial fibrillation: The Framingham Study. Am Heart J. 1996 Apr;131(4):790-5.
2. Risk factors for stroke and efficacy of antithrombotic therapy in atrial fibrillation. Analysis of pooled data from five randomized controlled trials. Arch Intern Med. 1994;154(13):1449-57.
3. Hohnloser SH, Pajitnev D, Pogue J, Healey JS, Pfeffer MA, Yusuf S, et al. Incidence of stroke in paroxysmal versus sustained atrial fibrillation in patients taking oral anticoagulation or combined antiplatelet therapy: an ACTIVE W Substudy. J Am Coll Cardiol. 2007;50(22):2156-61.
4. January CT, Wann LS, Alpert JS, Calkins H, Cigarroa JE, Cleveland JC Jr, et al. 2014 AHA/ACC/HRS guideline for the management of patients with atrial fibrillation: a report of the American College of Cardiology/American Heart Association Task Force on Practice Guidelines and the Heart Rhythm Society. J Am Coll Cardiol. 2014;64(21):e1-76.
5. Wolf PA, Abbott RD, Kannel WB. Atrial fibrillation as an independent risk factor for stroke: the Framingham Study. Stroke. 1991;22(8):983-8.
6. Pollick C, Taylor D. Assessment of left atrial appendage function by transesophageal echocardiography. Implications for the development of thrombus. Circulation. 1991;84(1):223-31.
7. Watson T, Shantsila E, Lip GY. Mechanisms of thrombogenesis in atrial fibrillation: Virchow's triad revisited. Lancet. 2009;373(9658):155-66.
8. Blackshear JL, Odell JA. Appendage obliteration to reduce stroke in cardiac surgical patients with atrial fibrillation. Ann Thorac Surg. 1996;61(2):755-9.
9. Stroke Prevention in Atrial Fibrillation Study. Final results. Circulation. 1991; 84(2):527-39.
10. Hart RG, Pearce LA, Aguilar MI. Meta-analysis: antithrombotic therapy to prevent stroke in patients who have nonvalvular atrial fibrillation. Ann Intern Med. 2007;146(12):857-67.
11. Waldo AL, Becker RC, Tapson VF, Colgan KJ, NABOR Steering Committee. Hospitalized patients with atrial fibrillation and a high risk of stroke are not being provided with adequate anticoagulation. J Am Coll Cardiol. 2005;46(9):1729-36.
12. De Caterina R, Camm AJ. What is 'valvular' atrial fibrillation? A reappraisal. Eur Heart J. 2014;35(47):3328-35.
13. SZEKELY P. Systemic Embolism and Anticoagulant Prophylaxis in Rheumatic Heart Disease. Br Med J. 1964;1(5392):1209-12.
14. Fleming HA. Anticoagulants in rheumatic heart-disease. Lancet. 1971;2(7722):486.
15. You JJ, Singer DE, Howard PA, Lane DA, Eckman MH, Fang MC, et al. Antithrombotic therapy for atrial fibrillation: Antithrombotic Therapy and Prevention of Thrombosis, 9th ed: American College of Chest Physicians Evidence-Based Clinical Practice Guidelines. Chest. 2012;141(2 Suppl):e531S-75S.
16. Seidl K, Hauer B, Schwick NG, Zellner D, Zahn R, Senges J. Risk of thromboembolic events in patients with atrial flutter. Am J Cardiol. 1998;82(5):580-3.
17. Vadmann H, Nielsen PB, Hjortshoj SP, Riahi S, Rasmussen LH, Lip GY, et al. Atrial flutter and thromboembolic risk: a systematic review. Heart. 2015;101(18):1446-55.
18. Tunick PA, McElhinney L, Mitchell T, Kronzon I. The alternation between atrial flutter and atrial fibrillation. Chest. 1992;101(1):34-6.
19. Camm AJ, Lip GY, De Caterina R, Savelieva I, Atar D, Hohnloser SH, et al. 2012 focused update of the ESC Guidelines for the management of atrial fibrillation: an update of the 2010 ESC Guidelines for the management of atrial fibrillation. Developed with the special contribution of the European Heart Rhythm Association. Eur Heart J. 2012;33(21):2719-47.
20. Hart RG, Pearce LA, Rothbart RM, McAnulty JH, Asinger RW, Halperin JL. Stroke with intermittent atrial fibrillation: incidence and predictors during aspirin therapy. Stroke Prevention in Atrial Fibrillation Investigators. J Am Coll Cardiol. 2000;35(1):183-7.
21. Gage BF, Waterman AD, Shannon W, Boechler M, Rich MW, Radford MJ. Validation of clinical classification schemes for predicting stroke: results from the National Registry of Atrial Fibrillation. JAMA. 2001;285(22):2864-70.
22. Lip GY, Nieuwlaat R, Pisters R, Lane DA, Crijns HJ. Refining clinical risk stratification for predicting stroke and thromboembolism in atrial fibrillation using a novel risk factor-based approach: the euro heart survey on atrial fibrillation. Chest. 2010;137(2):263-72.

23. Dagres N, Nieuwlaat R, Vardas PE, Andresen D, Levy S, Cobbe S, et al. Gender-related differences in presentation, treatment, and outcome of patients with atrial fibrillation in Europe: a report from the Euro Heart Survey on Atrial Fibrillation. J Am Coll Cardiol. 2007;49(5):572-7.
24. Schmitt J, Duray G, Gersh BJ, Hohnloser SH. Atrial fibrillation in acute myocardial infarction: a systematic review of the incidence, clinical features and prognostic implications. Eur Heart J. 2009;30(9):1038-45.
25. Conway DS, Lip GY. Comparison of outcomes of patients with symptomatic peripheral artery disease with and without atrial fibrillation (the West Birmingham Atrial Fibrillation Project). Am J Cardiol. 2004;93(11):1422-5, A10.
26. Coppens M, Eikelboom JW, Hart RG, Yusuf S, Lip GY, Dorian P, et al. The CHA2DS2-VASc score identifies those patients with atrial fibrillation and a CHADS2 score of 1 who are unlikely to benefit from oral anticoagulant therapy. Eur Heart J. 2013;34(3):170-6.
27. Olesen JB, Torp-Pedersen C, Hansen ML, Lip GY. The value of the CHA2DS2-VASc score for refining stroke risk stratification in patients with atrial fibrillation with a CHADS2 score 0-1: a nationwide cohort study. Thromb Haemost. 2012;107(6):1172-9.
28. Lip GY, Frison L, Halperin JL, Lane DA. Comparative validation of a novel risk score for predicting bleeding risk in anticoagulated patients with atrial fibrillation: the HAS-BLED (Hypertension, Abnormal Renal/Liver Function, Stroke, Bleeding History or Predisposition, Labile INR, Elderly, Drugs/Alcohol Concomitantly) score. J Am Coll Cardiol. 2011;57(2):173-80.
29. Pisters R, Lane DA, Nieuwlaat R, de Vos CB, Crijns HJ, Lip GY. A novel user-friendly score (HAS-BLED) to assess 1-year risk of major bleeding in patients with atrial fibrillation: the Euro Heart Survey. Chest. 2010;138(5):1093-100.
30. Lip GY. Assessing bleeding risk with the HAS-BLED score: Balancing simplicity, practicality, and predictive value in bleeding-risk assessment. Clin Cardiol. 2015;38(9):562-4.
31. Lane DA, Lip GY. Use of the CHA(2)DS(2)-VASc and HAS-BLED scores to aid decision making for thromboprophylaxis in nonvalvular atrial fibrillation. Circulation. 2012;126(7):860-5.
32. Hart RG, Benavente O, McBride R, Pearce LA. Antithrombotic therapy to prevent stroke in patients with atrial fibrillation: a meta-analysis. Ann Intern Med. 1999;131(7):492-501.
33. ACTIVE Investigators, Connolly SJ, Pogue J, Hart RG, Hohnloser SH, Pfeffer M, et al. Effect of clopidogrel added to aspirin in patients with atrial fibrillation. N Engl J Med. 2009;360(20):2066-78.
34. ACTIVE Writing Group of the ACTIVE Investigators, Connolly S, Pogue J, Hart R, Pfeffer M, Hohnloser S, et al. Clopidogrel plus aspirin versus oral anticoagulation for atrial fibrillation in the Atrial fibrillation Clopidogrel Trial with Irbesartan for prevention of Vascular Events (ACTIVE W): a randomised controlled trial. Lancet. 2006;367(9526):1903-12.
35. Sato H, Ishikawa K, Kitabatake A, Ogawa S, Maruyama Y, Yokota Y, et al. Low-dose aspirin for prevention of stroke in low-risk patients with atrial fibrillation: Japan Atrial Fibrillation Stroke Trial. Stroke. 2006;37(2):447-51.
36. Ageno W, Gallus AS, Wittkowsky A, Crowther M, Hylek EM, Palareti G, et al. Oral anticoagulant therapy: Antithrombotic Therapy and Prevention of Thrombosis, 9th ed: American College of Chest Physicians Evidence-Based Clinical Practice Guidelines. Chest. 2012;141(2 Suppl):e44S-88S.
37. Hirsh J, Fuster V, Ansell J, Halperin JL, American Heart Association/American College of Cardiology Foundation. American Heart Association/American College of Cardiology Foundation guide to warfarin therapy. J Am Coll Cardiol. 2003;41(9):1633-52.
38. Aguilar MI, Hart R. Oral anticoagulants for preventing stroke in patients with non-valvular atrial fibrillation and no previous history of stroke or transient ischemic attacks. Cochrane Database Syst Rev. 2005;20(3):CD001927.
39. Eikelboom JW, Connolly SJ, Brueckmann M, Granger CB, Kappetein AP, Mack MJ, et al. Dabigatran versus warfarin in patients with mechanical heart valves. N Engl J Med. 2013;369(13):1206-14.
40. Guyatt GH, Akl EA, Crowther M, Gutterman DD, Schuunemann HJ, American College of Chest Physicians Antithrombotic Therapy and Prevention of Thrombosis Panel. Executive summary: Antithrombotic Therapy and Prevention of Thrombosis, 9th ed: American College of Chest Physicians Evidence-Based Clinical Practice Guidelines. Chest. 2012;141(2 Suppl):7S-47S.
41. Singer DE, Chang Y, Fang MC, Borowsky LH, Pomernacki NK, Udaltsova N, et al. Should patient characteristics influence target anticoagulation intensity for stroke prevention in nonvalvular atrial fibrillation?: the ATRIA study. Circ Cardiovasc Qual Outcomes. 2009;2(4):297-304.
42. Vahanian A, Alfieri O, Andreotti F, Antunes MJ, Baron-Esquivias G, Baumgartner H, et al. Guidelines on the management of valvular heart disease (version 2012): the Joint Task Force on the Management of Valvular Heart Disease of the European Society of Cardiology (ESC) and the European Association for Cardio-Thoracic Surgery (EACTS). Eur J Cardiothorac Surg. 2012;42(4):S1-44.
43. Grand'Maison A, Charest AF, Geerts WH. Anticoagulant use in patients with chronic renal impairment. Am J Cardiovasc Drugs. 2005;5(5):291-305.
44. Coumadin (warfarin sodium) [package insert]. Princeton, New Jersey: Bristol-Myers Squibb Complany; 2015.
45. Breckenridge A. Oral anticoagulant drugs: pharmacokinetic aspects. Semin Hematol. 1978;15(1):19-26.
46. Kelly JG, O'Malley K. Clinical pharmacokinetics of oral anticoagulants. Clin Pharmacokinet. 1979;4(1):1-15.
47. O'Reilly RA. Warfarin metabolism and drug-drug interactions. Adv Exp Med Biol. 1987;214:205-12.
48. Patel P, Weitz J, Brooker LA, Paes B, Mitchell L, Andrew M. Decreased thrombin activity of fibrin clots prepared in cord plasma compared with adult plasma. Pediatr Res. 1996;39(5):826-30.
49. Furie B, Diuguid CF, Jacobs M, Diuguid DL, Furie BC. Randomized prospective trial comparing the native prothrombin antigen with the prothrombin time for monitoring oral anticoagulant therapy. Blood. 1990;75(2):344-9.
50. Zivelin A, Rao LV, Rapaport SI. Mechanism of the anticoagulant effect of warfarin as evaluated in rabbits by selective depression of individual procoagulant vitamin K-dependent clotting factors. J Clin Invest. 1993;92(5):2131-40.
51. Aithal GP, Day CP, Kesteven PJ, Daly AK. Association of polymorphisms in the cytochrome P450 CYP2C9 with warfarin dose requirement and risk of bleeding complications. Lancet. 1999;353(9154):717-9.
52. Rieder MJ, Reiner AP, Gage BF, Nickerson DA, Eby CS, McLeod HL, et al. Effect of VKORC1 haplotypes on transcriptional regulation and warfarin dose. N Engl J Med. 2005;352(22):2285-93.
53. Miners JO, Birkett DJ. Cytochrome P4502C9: an enzyme of major importance in human drug metabolism. Br J Clin Pharmacol. 1998;45(6):525-38.
54. Wells PS, Holbrook AM, Crowther NR, Hirsh J. Interactions of warfarin with drugs and food. Ann Intern Med. 1994;121(9):676-83.
55. O'Reilly RA, Rytand DA. "Resistance" to warfarin due to unrecognized vitamin K supplementation. N Engl J Med. 1980;303(3):160-1.
56. Woods K, Douketis JD, Kathirgamanathan K, Yi Q, Crowther MA. Low-dose oral vitamin K to normalize the international normalized ratio prior to surgery in patients who require temporary interruption of warfarin. J Thromb Thrombolysis. 2007;24(2):93-7.
57. Dzik WS. Reversal of drug-induced anticoagulation: old solutions and new problems. Transfusion. 2012;52(Suppl 1):45S-55S.
58. Douketis JD, Spyropoulos AC, Spencer FA, Mayr M, Jaffer AK, Eckman MH, et al. Perioperative management of antithrombotic therapy: Antithrombotic Therapy and Prevention of Thrombosis, 9th ed: American College of Chest Physicians Evidence-Based Clinical Practice Guidelines. Chest. 2012;141(2 Suppl):e326S-50S.
59. Warfarin. Lexicomp Online®, Medi-Span®, Hudson, Ohio: Lexi-Comp, Inc.; January 29, 2016.
60. van der Meer FJ, Rosendaal FR, Vandenbroucke JP, Briet E. Bleeding complications in oral anticoagulant therapy. An analysis of risk factors. Arch Intern Med. 1993;153(13):1557-62.
61. Hylek EM, Singer DE. Risk factors for intracranial hemorrhage in outpatients taking warfarin. Ann Intern Med. 1994;120(11):897-902.
62. Saxena R, Koudstaal P. Anticoagulants versus antiplatelet therapy for preventing stroke in patients with nonrheumatic atrial fibrillation and a history of stroke or transient ischemic attack. Cochrane Database Syst Rev. 2004;18(4):CD000187.
63. Granger CB, Alexander JH, McMurray JJ, Lopes RD, Hylek EM, Hanna M, et al. Apixaban versus warfarin in patients with atrial fibrillation. N Engl J Med. 2011;365(11):981-92.
64. Patel MR, Mahaffey KW, Garg J, Pan G, Singer DE, Hacke W, et al. Rivaroxaban versus warfarin in nonvalvular atrial fibrillation. N Engl J Med. 2011;365(10):883-91.
65. DeFranzo AJ, Marasco P, Argenta LC. Warfarin-induced necrosis of the skin. Ann Plast Surg. 1995;34(2):203-8.
66. Broekmans AW, Bertina RM, Loeliger EA, Hofmann V, Klingemann HG. Protein C and the development of skin necrosis during anticoagulant therapy. Thromb Haemost. 1983;49(3):251.

67. Samama M, Horellou MH, Soria J, Conard J, Nicolas G. Successful progressive anticoagulation in a severe protein C deficiency and previous skin necrosis at the initiation of oral anticoagulant treatment. Thromb Haemost. 1984;51(1):132-3.
68. Feder W, Auerbach R. "Purple toes": an uncommon sequela of oral coumarin drug therapy. Ann Intern Med. 1961;55:911-7.
69. Hall JG, Pauli RM, Wilson KM. Maternal and fetal sequelae of anticoagulation during pregnancy. Am J Med. 1980;68(1):122-40.
70. Pettifor JM, Benson R. Congenital malformations associated with the administration of oral anticoagulants during pregnancy. J Pediatr. 1975;86(3):459-62.
71. Holbrook A, Schulman S, Witt DM, Vandvik PO, Fish J, Kovacs MJ, et al. Evidence-based management of anticoagulant therapy: Antithrombotic Therapy and Prevention of Thrombosis, 9th ed: American College of Chest Physicians Evidence-Based Clinical Practice Guidelines. Chest. 2012;141(2 Suppl):e152S-84S.
72. Zimetbaum P. Antiarrhythmic drug therapy for atrial fibrillation. Circulation. 2012;125(2):381-9.
73. Ogilvie IM, Newton N, Welner SA, Cowell W, Lip GY. Underuse of oral anticoagulants in atrial fibrillation: a systematic review. Am J Med. 2010;123(7):638-45.e4.
74. Baker WL, Cios DA, Sander SD, Coleman CI. Meta-analysis to assess the quality of warfarin control in atrial fibrillation patients in the United States. J Manag Care Pharm. 2009;15(3):244-52.
75. van Walraven C, Jennings A, Oake N, Fergusson D, Forster AJ. Effect of study setting on anticoagulation control: a systematic review and metaregression. Chest. 2006;129(5):1155-66.
76. Barnes GD, Ageno W, Ansell J, Kaatz S, Subcommittee on the Control of Anticoagulation of the International Society on Thrombosis and Haemostasis. Recommendation on the nomenclature for oral anticoagulants: communication from the SSC of the ISTH. J Thromb Haemost. 2015;13(6):1154-6.
77. Kovacs RJ, Flaker GC, Saxonhouse SJ, Doherty JU, Birtcher KK, Cuker A, et al. Practical management of anticoagulation in patients with atrial fibrillation. J Am Coll Cardiol. 2015;65(13):1340-60.
78. Connolly SJ, Ezekowitz MD, Yusuf S, Eikelboom J, Oldgren J, Parekh A, et al. Dabigatran versus warfarin in patients with atrial fibrillation. N Engl J Med. 2009;361(12):1139-51.
79. Reilly PA, Lehr T, Haertter S, Connolly SJ, Yusuf S, Eikelboom JW, et al. The effect of dabigatran plasma concentrations and patient characteristics on the frequency of ischemic stroke and major bleeding in atrial fibrillation patients: the RE-LY Trial (Randomized Evaluation of Long-Term Anticoagulation Therapy). J Am Coll Cardiol. 2014;63(4):321-8.
80. Hankey GJ, Eikelboom JW. Dabigatran etexilate: a new oral thrombin inhibitor. Circulation. 2011;123(13):1436-50.
81. Heidbuchel H, Verhamme P, Alings M, Antz M, Hacke W, Oldgren J, et al. EHRA practical guide on the use of new oral anticoagulants in patients with non-valvular atrial fibrillation: executive summary. Eur Heart J. 2013;34(27):2094-106.
82. Pollack CV Jr. Coagulation assessment with the new generation of oral anticoagulants. Emerg Med J. 2016;33(6):423-30.
83. Stangier J, Rathgen K, Stahle H, Gansser D, Roth W. The pharmacokinetics, pharmacodynamics and tolerability of dabigatran etexilate, a new oral direct thrombin inhibitor, in healthy male subjects. Br J Clin Pharmacol. 2007;64(3):292-303.
84. Stangier J. Clinical pharmacokinetics and pharmacodynamics of the oral direct thrombin inhibitor dabigatran etexilate. Clin Pharmacokinet. 2008;47(5):285-95.
85. Troconiz IF, Tillmann C, Liesenfeld KH, Schafer HG, Stangier J. Population pharmacokinetic analysis of the new oral thrombin inhibitor dabigatran etexilate (BIBR 1048) in patients undergoing primary elective total hip replacement surgery. J Clin Pharmacol. 2007;47(3):371-82.
86. Wolowacz SE, Roskell NS, Maciver F, Beard SM, Robinson PA, Plumb JM, et al. Economic evaluation of dabigatran etexilate for the prevention of venous thromboembolism after total knee and hip replacement surgery. Clin Ther. 2009;31(1):194-212.
87. Wolowacz SE, Roskell NS, Plumb JM, Clemens A, Noack H, Robinson PA, et al. Economic evaluation of dabigatran etexilate for the prevention of venous thromboembolism in patients aged over 75 years or with moderate renal impairment undergoing total knee or hip replacement. Thromb Haemost. 2010;103(2):360-71.
88. Freeman JV, Zhu RP, Owens DK, Garber AM, Hutton DW, Go AS, et al. Cost-effectiveness of dabigatran compared with warfarin for stroke prevention in atrial fibrillation. Ann Intern Med. 2011;154(1):1-11.
89. Stangier J, Rathgen K, Stahle H, Mazur D. Influence of renal impairment on the pharmacokinetics and pharmacodynamics of oral dabigatran etexilate: an open-label, parallel-group, single-centre study. Clin Pharmacokinet. 2010;49(4):259-68.
90. Ebner T, Wagner K, Wienen W. Dabigatran acylglucuronide, the major human metabolite of dabigatran: in vitro formation, stability, and pharmacological activity. Drug Metab Dispos. 2010;38(9):1567-75.
91. Tran A, Cheng-Lai A. Dabigatran etexilate: the first oral anticoagulant available in the United States since warfarin. Cardiol Rev. 2011;19(3):154-61.
92. Graham DJ, Reichman ME, Wernecke M, Zhang R, Southworth MR, Levenson M, et al. Cardiovascular, bleeding, and mortality risks in elderly Medicare patients treated with dabigatran or warfarin for nonvalvular atrial fibrillation. Circulation. 2015;131(2):157-64.
93. Klil-Drori A, Azoulay L. The role of selection in the risk of bleeding with dabigatran in patients with atrial fibrillation. JAMA Intern Med. 2015;175(7):1243-4.
94. Hernandez I. Time to reconsider dabigatran 110 mg in the USA. Am J Cardiovasc Drugs. 2015;15(5):307-9.
95. Lauffenburger JC, Rhoney DH, Farley JF, Gehi AK, Fang G. Predictors of gastrointestinal bleeding among patients with atrial fibrillation after initiating dabigatran therapy. Pharmacotherapy. 2015;35(6):560-8.
96. Romanelli RJ, Nolting L, Dolginsky M, Kym E, Orrico KB. Dabigatran Versus Warfarin for Atrial Fibrillation in Real-World Clinical Practice: A Systematic Review and Meta-Analysis. Circ Cardiovasc Qual Outcomes. 2016;9(2):126-34.
97. Chan EW, Lau WC, Leung WK, Mok MT, He Y, Tong TS, et al. Prevention of Dabigatran-Related Gastrointestinal Bleeding With Gastroprotective Agents: A Population-Based Study. Gastroenterology. 2015;149(3):586-95.e3.
98. Dabigatran etexilate (Pradaxa) [package insert]. Ridgefield, CT: Boehringer Ingelheim Pharmaceuticals, Inc.; 2014.
99. Menzin J, Boulanger L, Hauch O, Friedman M, Marple CB, Wygant G, et al. Quality of anticoagulation control and costs of monitoring warfarin therapy among patients with atrial fibrillation in clinic settings: a multi-site managed-care study. Ann Pharmacother. 2005;39(3):446-51.
100. Miyares MA. One-Year Risk of Bleeding With Dabigatran in Patients With Atrial Fibrillation: Placing Real-World Results Into Perspective. JAMA Intern Med. 2015;175(7):1242-3.
101. Pink J, Pirmohamed M, Hughes DA. Comparative effectiveness of dabigatran, rivaroxaban, apixaban, and warfarin in the management of patients with nonvalvular atrial fibrillation. Clin Pharmacol Ther. 2013;94(2):269-76.
102. Kubitza D, Becka M, Wensing G, Voith B, Zuehlsdorf M. Safety, pharmacodynamics, and pharmacokinetics of BAY 59-7939—an oral, direct Factor Xa inhibitor—after multiple dosing in healthy male subjects. Eur J Clin Pharmacol. 2005;61(12):873-80.
103. Kubitza D, Becka M, Roth A, Mueck W. Dose-escalation study of the pharmacokinetics and pharmacodynamics of rivaroxaban in healthy elderly subjects. Curr Med Res Opin. 2008;24(10):2757-65.
104. Mueck W, Becka M, Kubitza D, Voith B, Zuehlsdorf M. Population model of the pharmacokinetics and pharmacodynamics of rivaroxaban—an oral, direct factor xa inhibitor--in healthy subjects. Int J Clin Pharmacol Ther. 2007;45(6):335-44.
105. Perzborn E, Roehrig S, Straub A, Kubitza D, Misselwitz F. The discovery and development of rivaroxaban, an oral, direct factor Xa inhibitor. Nat Rev Drug Discov. 2011;10(1):61-75.
106. Kubitza D, Becka M, Voith B, Zuehlsdorf M, Wensing G. Safety, pharmacodynamics, and pharmacokinetics of single doses of BAY 59-7939, an oral, direct factor Xa inhibitor. Clin Pharmacol Ther. 2005;78(4):412-21.
107. ROCKET AF Study Investigators. Rivaroxaban-once daily, oral, direct factor Xa inhibition compared with vitamin K antagonism for prevention of stroke and Embolism Trial in Atrial Fibrillation: rationale and design of the ROCKET AF study. Am Heart J. 2010;159(3):340-7.e1.
108. Cohen D. Rivaroxaban: can we trust the evidence? BMJ. 2016;352:i575.
109. Reddy P, Giugliano RP. The role of rivaroxaban in atrial fibrillation and acute coronary syndromes. J Cardiovasc Pharmacol Ther. 2014;19(6):526-32.
110. Kubitza D, Becka M, Mueck W, Halabi A, Maatouk H, Klause N, et al. Effects of renal impairment on the pharmacokinetics, pharmacodynamics and safety of rivaroxaban, an oral, direct Factor Xa inhibitor. Br J Clin Pharmacol. 2010; 70(5):703-12.
111. Camm AJ, Amarenco P, Haas S, Hess S, Kirchhof P, van Eickels M, et al. XANTUS: rationale and design of a noninterventional study of rivaroxaban for the prevention of stroke in patients with atrial fibrillation. Vasc Health Risk Manag. 2014;10:425-34.

112. Mega JL, Braunwald E, Mohanavelu S, Burton P, Poulter R, Misselwitz F, et al. Rivaroxaban versus placebo in patients with acute coronary syndromes (ATLAS ACS-TIMI 46): a randomised, double-blind, phase II trial. Lancet. 2009;374(9683):29-38.
113. Mega JL. A new era for anticoagulation in atrial fibrillation. N Engl J Med. 2011;365(11):1052-4.
114. EINSTEIN-PE Investigators, Buller HR, Prins MH, Lensin AW, Decousus H, Jacobson BF, et al. Oral rivaroxaban for the treatment of symptomatic pulmonary embolism. N Engl J Med. 2012;366(14):1287-97.
115. EINSTEIN Investigators, Bauersachs R, Berkowitz SD, Brenner B, Buller HR, Decousus H, et al. Oral rivaroxaban for symptomatic venous thromboembolism. N Engl J Med. 2010;363(26):2499-510.
116. Favaloro EJ, Lippi G, Koutts J. Laboratory testing of anticoagulants: the present and the future. Pathology. 2011;43(7):682-92.
117. Perzborn E, Strassburger J, Wilmen A, Pohlmann J, Roehrig S, Schlemmer KH, et al. *In vitro* and *in vivo* studies of the novel antithrombotic agent BAY 59-7939—an oral, direct Factor Xa inhibitor. J Thromb Haemost. 2005;3(3):514-21.
118. Scaglione F. New oral anticoagulants: comparative pharmacology with vitamin K antagonists. Clin Pharmacokinet. 2013;52(2):69-82.
119. Goodman SG, Wojdyla DM, Piccini JP, White HD, Paolini JF, Nessel CC, et al. Factors associated with major bleeding events: insights from the ROCKET AF trial (rivaroxaban once-daily oral direct factor Xa inhibition compared with vitamin K antagonism for prevention of stroke and embolism trial in atrial fibrillation). J Am Coll Cardiol. 2014;63(9):891-900.
120. Rivaroxaban. Lexicomp Online®, Medi-Span®, Hudson, Ohio: Lexi-Comp, Inc.; January 29, 2016.
121. Deitelzweig S, Amin A, Jing Y, Makenbaeva D, Wiederkehr D, Lin J, et al. Medical cost reductions associated with the usage of novel oral anticoagulants vs warfarin among atrial fibrillation patients, based on the RE-LY, ROCKET-AF, and ARISTOTLE trials. J Med Econ. 2012;15(4):776-85.
122. Granger CB, Alexander JH, McMurray JJ, Lopes RD, Hylek EM, Hanna M, et al. Apixaban versus warfarin in patients with atrial fibrillation. N Engl J Med. 2011;365(11):981-92.
123. Connolly SJ, Eikelboom J, Joyner C, Diener HC, Hart R, Golitsyn S, et al. Apixaban in patients with atrial fibrillation. N Engl J Med. 2011;364(9):806-17.
124. Morais J, De Caterina R. Stroke Prevention in Atrial Fibrillation: A Clinical Perspective on Trials of the Novel Oral Anticoagulants. Cardiovasc Drugs Ther. 2016;30(2):201-14.
125. Eliquis (apixaban) [prescribing information]. Princeton, NJ: Bristol-Myers Squibb; June 2015.
126. Ramos-Esquivel A. Monitoring anticoagulant therapy with new oral agents. World J Methodol. 2015;5(4):212-5.
127. Raghavan N, Frost CE, Yu Z, He K, Zhang H, Humphreys WG, et al. Apixaban metabolism and pharmacokinetics after oral administration to humans. Drug Metab Dispos. 2009;37(1):74-81.
128. Wang X, Tirucherai G, Marbury TC, Wang J, Chang M, Zhang D, et al. Pharmacokinetics, pharmacodynamics, and safety of apixaban in subjects with end-stage renal disease on hemodialysis. J Clin Pharmacol. 2016;56(5):628-36.
129. Apixaban. Lexicomp Online®, Medi-Span®, Hudson, Ohio: Lexi-Comp, Inc.; January 29, 2016.
130. Lanitis T, Leipold R, Hamilton M, Rublee D, Quon P, Browne C, et al. Cost-effectiveness of Apixaban Versus Other Oral Anticoagulants for the Initial Treatment of Venous Thromboembolism and Prevention of Recurrence. Clin Ther. 2016;38(3):478-93.e16.
131. Giugliano RP, Ruff CT, Braunwald E, Murphy SA, Wiviott SD, Halperin JL, et al. Edoxaban versus warfarin in patients with atrial fibrillation. N Engl J Med. 2013;369(22):2093-104.
132. Bounameaux H, Camm AJ. Edoxaban: an update on the new oral direct factor Xa inhibitor. Drugs. 2014;74(11):1209-31.
133. Savaysa (edoxaba) [prescribing information]. Pasippany, NJ: Daiichi Sankyo: January 2015.
134. Samama MM, Mendell J, Guinet C, Le Flem L, Kunitada S. In vitro study of the anticoagulant effects of edoxaban and its effect on thrombin generation in comparison to fondaparinux. Thromb Res. 2012;129(4):e77-82.
135. Dale BJ, Chan NC, Eikelboom JW. Laboratory measurement of the direct oral anticoagulants. Br J Haematol. 2016;172(3):315-36.
136. Parasrampuria DA, Truitt KE. Pharmacokinetics and pharmacodynamics of edoxaban, a non-vitamin K antagonist oral anticoagulant that inhibits clotting factor Xa. Clin Pharmacokinet. 2016;55(6):641-55.
137. Edoxaban. Lexicomp Online®, Medi-Span®, Hudson, Ohio: Lexi-Comp, Inc.; January 29, 2016.
138. Kaatz S, Kouides PA, Garcia DA, Spyropolous AC, Crowther M, Douketis JD, et al. Guidance on the emergent reversal of oral thrombin and factor Xa inhibitors. Am J Hematol. 2012;87 Suppl 1:S141-5.
139. Burness CB. Idarucizumab: First Global Approval. Drugs. 2015;75(18): 2155-61.
140. Siegal DM. Managing target-specific oral anticoagulant associated bleeding including an update on pharmacological reversal agents. J Thromb Thrombolysis. 2015;39(3):395-402.
141. Ansell JE. Reversing the effect of oral anticoagulant drugs: Established and newer options. Am J Cardiovasc Drugs. 2016;16(3):163-70.
142. King AE, Szarlej DK, Rincon F. Dabigatran-Associated Intracranial Hemorrhage: Literature Review and Institutional Experience. Neurohospitalist. 2015;5(4):234-44.
143. Harinstein LM, Morgan JW, Russo N. Treatment of dabigatran-associated bleeding: case report and review of the literature. J Pharm Pract. 2013;26(3): 264-9.
144. Suryanarayan D, Schulman S. Potential antidotes for reversal of old and new oral anticoagulants. Thromb Res. 2014;133 Suppl 2:S158-66.
145. Singh T, Maw TT, Henry BL, Pastor-Soler NM, Unruh ML, Hallows KR, et al. Extracorporeal therapy for dabigatran removal in the treatment of acute bleeding: a single center experience. Clin J Am Soc Nephrol. 2013;8(9):1533-9.
146. Xarelto (rivaroxaban) [package insert]. Titusville, NJ: Janssen Pharmaceutical; 2013.
147. Steiner T, Bohm M, Dichgans M, Diener HC, Ell C, Endres M, et al. Recommendations for the emergency management of complications associated with the new direct oral anticoagulants (DOACs), apixaban, dabigatran and rivaroxaban. Clin Res Cardiol. 2013;102(6):399-412.
148. Costin J, Ansell J, Laulicht B, Bakhru S, Steiner S. Reversal agents in development for the new oral anticoagulants. Postgrad Med. 2014;126(7):19-24.
149. Kalus JS. Pharmacologic interventions for reversing the effects of oral anticoagulants. Am J Health Syst Pharm. 2013;70(10 Suppl 1):S12-21.
150. Zhou W, Schwarting S, Illanes S, Liesz A, Middelhoff M, Zorn M, et al. Hemostatic therapy in experimental intracerebral hemorrhage associated with the direct thrombin inhibitor dabigatran. Stroke. 2011;42(12):3594-99.
151. Eerenberg ES, Kamphuisen PW, Sijpkens MK, Meijers JC, Buller HR, Levi M. Reversal of rivaroxaban and dabigatran by prothrombin complex concentrate: a randomized, placebo-controlled, crossover study in healthy subjects. Circulation. 2011;124(14):1573-9.
152. Marlu R, Hodaj E, Paris A, Albaladejo P, Cracowski JL, Pernod G. Effect of non-specific reversal agents on anticoagulant activity of dabigatran and rivaroxaban: a randomised crossover ex vivo study in healthy volunteers. Thromb Haemost. 2012;108(2):217-24.
153. Fukuda T, Honda Y, Kamisato C, Morishima Y, Shibano T. Reversal of anti-coagulant effects of edoxaban, an oral, direct factor Xa inhibitor, with haemostatic agents. Thromb Haemost. 2012;107(2):253-9.
154. Eikelboom JW, Quinlan DJ, van Ryn J, Weitz JI. Idarucizumab: The Antidote for Reversal of Dabigatran. Circulation. 2015;132(25):2412-22.
155. van Ryn J, Stangier J, Haertter S, Liesenfeld KH, Wienen W, Feuring M, et al. Dabigatran etexilate--a novel, reversible, oral direct thrombin inhibitor: interpretation of coagulation assays and reversal of anticoagulant activity. Thromb Haemost. 2010;103(6):1116-27.
156. Schiele F, van Ryn J, Canada K, Newsome C, Sepulveda E, Park J, et al. A specific antidote for dabigatran: functional and structural characterization. Blood. 2013;121(18):3554-62.
157. Pollack CV,Jr, Reilly PA, Eikelboom J, Glund S, Verhamme P, Bernstein RA, et al. Idarucizumab for Dabigatran Reversal. N Engl J Med. 2015;373(6):511-20.
158. Glund S, Moschetti V, Norris S, Stangier J, Schmohl M, van Ryn J, et al. A randomised study in healthy volunteers to investigate the safety, tolerability and pharmacokinetics of idarucizumab, a specific antidote to dabigatran. Thromb Haemost. 2015;113(5):943-51.
159. Siegal DM, Curnutte JT, Connolly SJ, Lu G, Conley PB, Wiens BL, et al. Andexanet Alfa for the Reversal of Factor Xa Inhibitor Activity. N Engl J Med. 2015;373(25):2413-24.
160. Ansell JE, Bakhru SH, Laulicht BE, Steiner SS, Grosso M, Brown K, et al. Use of PER977 to reverse the anticoagulant effect of edoxaban. N Engl J Med. 2014;371(22):2141-2.
161. Sarich TC, Seltzer JH, Berkowitz SD, Costin' J, Curnutte JT, Gibson CM, et al. Novel oral anticoagulants and reversal agents: Considerations for clinical development. Am Heart J. 2015;169(6):751-7.

162. Laulicht B, Bakhru S, Steiner S, Brown K, Grosso M, Lanz H, et al. PER977 (ciraparantag) reverses edoxaban anticoagulation at steady state and has no effect on re-anticoagulation at the next scheduled dose [Abstract No. 4971]. Eur Heart J. 2015;36(abstract supplement):859-60.
163. Laulicht B, Bakhru S, Lee C, Baker C, Jiang X, Mathiowitz E, et al. Small molecule antidote for anticoagulants. Circulation. 2012;126(A11395).
164. Healey JS, Eikelboom J, Douketis J, Wallentin L, Oldgren J, Yang S, et al. Periprocedural bleeding and thromboembolic events with dabigatran compared with warfarin: results from the Randomized Evaluation of Long-Term Anticoagulation Therapy (RE-LY) randomized trial. Circulation. 2012;126(3):343-8.
165. Garcia D, Alexander JH, Wallentin L, Wojdyla DM, Thomas L, Hanna M, et al. Management and clinical outcomes in patients treated with apixaban vs warfarin undergoing procedures. Blood. 2014;124(25):3692-8.
166. Birnie DH, Healey JS, Wells GA, Verma A, Tang AS, Krahn AD, et al. Pacemaker or defibrillator surgery without interruption of anticoagulation. N Engl J Med. 2013;368(22):2084-93.
167. Steinberg BA, Peterson ED, Kim S, Thomas L, Gersh BJ, Fonarow GC, et al. Use and outcomes associated with bridging during anticoagulation interruptions in patients with atrial fibrillation: findings from the Outcomes Registry for Better Informed Treatment of Atrial Fibrillation (ORBIT-AF). Circulation. 2015; 131(5):488-94.
168. Siegal D, Yudin J, Kaatz S, Douketis JD, Lim W, Spyropoulos AC. Periprocedural heparin bridging in patients receiving vitamin K antagonists: systematic review and meta-analysis of bleeding and thromboembolic rates. Circulation. 2012;126(13):1630-9.
169. Douketis JD, Spyropoulos AC, Kaatz S, Becker RC, Caprini JA, Dunn AS, et al. Perioperative Bridging Anticoagulation in Patients with Atrial Fibrillation. N Engl J Med. 2015;373(9):823-33.
170. Baron TH, Kamath PS, McBane RD. Management of antithrombotic therapy in patients undergoing invasive procedures. N Engl J Med. 2013;368(22):2113-24.
171. Berger M, Schweitzer P. Timing of thromboembolic events after electrical cardioversion of atrial fibrillation or flutter: a retrospective analysis. Am J Cardiol. 1998;82(12):1545-7, A8.
172. O'Neill PG, Puleo PR, Bolli R, Rokey R. Return of atrial mechanical function following electrical conversion of atrial dysrhythmias. Am Heart J. 1990;120(2): 353-9.
173. Grimm RA, Stewart WJ, Maloney JD, Cohen GI, Pearce GL, Salcedo EE, et al. Impact of electrical cardioversion for atrial fibrillation on left atrial appendage function and spontaneous echo contrast: characterization by simultaneous transesophageal echocardiography. J Am Coll Cardiol. 1993;22(5):1359-66.
174. Black IW, Fatkin D, Sagar KB, Khandheria BK, Leung DY, Galloway JM, et al. Exclusion of atrial thrombus by transesophageal echocardiography does not preclude embolism after cardioversion of atrial fibrillation. A multicenter study. Circulation. 1994;89(6):2509-13.
175. Airaksinen KE, Gronberg T, Nuotio I, Nikkinen M, Ylitalo A, Biancari F, et al. Thromboembolic complications after cardioversion of acute atrial fibrillation: the FinCV (Finnish CardioVersion) study. J Am Coll Cardiol. 2013;62(13):1187-92.
176. Gallagher MM, Hennessy BJ, Edvardsson N, Hart CM, Shannon MS, Obel OA, et al. Embolic complications of direct current cardioversion of atrial arrhythmias: association with low intensity of anticoagulation at the time of cardioversion. J Am Coll Cardiol. 2002;40(5):926-33.
177. Weigner MJ, Caulfield TA, Danias PG, Silverman DI, Manning WJ. Risk for clinical thromboembolism associated with conversion to sinus rhythm in patients with atrial fibrillation lasting less than 48 hours. Ann Intern Med. 1997;126(8):615-20.
178. Collins LJ, Silverman DI, Douglas PS, Manning WJ. Cardioversion of nonrheumatic atrial fibrillation. Reduced thromboembolic complications with 4 weeks of precardioversion anticoagulation are related to atrial thrombus resolution. Circulation. 1995;92(2):160-3.
179. Piccini JP, Stevens SR, Lokhnygina Y, Patel MR, Halperin JL, Singer DE, et al. Outcomes after cardioversion and atrial fibrillation ablation in patients treated with rivaroxaban and warfarin in the ROCKET AF trial. J Am Coll Cardiol. 2013;61(19):1998-2006.
180. Nagarakanti R, Ezekowitz MD, Oldgren J, Yang S, Chernick M, Aikens TH, et al. Dabigatran versus warfarin in patients with atrial fibrillation: an analysis of patients undergoing cardioversion. Circulation. 2011;123(2):131-6.
181. Flaker G, Lopes RD, Al-Khatib SM, Hermosillo AG, Hohnloser SH, Tinga B, et al. Efficacy and safety of apixaban in patients after cardioversion for atrial fibrillation: insights from the ARISTOTLE Trial (Apixaban for Reduction in Stroke and Other Thromboembolic Events in Atrial Fibrillation). J Am Coll Cardiol. 2014;63(11):1082-7.
182. Sen P, Kundu A, Sardar P, Chatterjee S, Nairooz R, Amin H, et al. Outcomes After Cardioversion in Atrial Fibrillation Patients Treated with Non-Vitamin K Antagonist Oral Anticoagulants (NOACs): Insights from a Meta-Analysis. Am J Cardiovasc Drugs. 2016;16(1):33-41
183. Klein AL, Grimm RA, Murray RD, Apperson-Hansen C, Asinger RW, Black IW, et al. Use of transesophageal echocardiography to guide cardioversion in patients with atrial fibrillation. N Engl J Med. 2001;344(19):1411-20.
184. Jaber WA, Prior DL, Thamilarasan M, Grimm RA, Thomas JD, Klein AL, et al. Efficacy of anticoagulation in resolving left atrial and left atrial appendage thrombi: A transesophageal echocardiographic study. Am Heart J. 2000; 140(1):150-6.
185. Nutescu EA, Shapiro NL, Chevalier A, Amin AN. A pharmacologic overview of current and emerging anticoagulants. Cleve Clin J Med. 2005;72 (Suppl 1): S2-6.
186. Arbit B, Hsu JC. Non-Vitamin K Antagonist Oral Anticoagulant Use in Patients With Atrial Fibrillation and Associated Intracranial Hemorrhage: A Focused Review. Clin Cardiol. 2015;38(11):684-91.
187. van Ryn J, Schurer J, Kink-Eiband M, Clemens A. Reversal of dabigatran-induced bleeding by coagulation factor concentrates in a rat-tail bleeding model and lack of effect on assays of coagulation. Anesthesiology. 2014;120(6):1429-40.
188. Hanley JP. Warfarin reversal. J Clin Pathol. 2004;57(11):1132-9.
189. Freeman WD, Brott TG, Barrett KM, Castillo PR, Deen HG,Jr, Czervionke LF, et al. Recombinant factor VIIa for rapid reversal of warfarin anticoagulation in acute intracranial hemorrhage. Mayo Clin Proc. 2004;79(12):1495-500.
190. Babilonia K, Trujillo T. The role of prothrombin complex concentrates in reversal of target specific anticoagulants. Thromb J. 2014;12:8.
191. Perzborn E, Heitmeier S, Laux V, Buchmuller A. Reversal of rivaroxaban-induced anticoagulation with prothrombin complex concentrate, activated prothrombin complex concentrate and recombinant activated factor VII in vitro. Thromb Res. 2014;133(4):671-81.
192. Straznitskas A, Giarratano M. Emergent reversal of oral anticoagulation: review of current treatment strategies. AACN Adv Crit Care. 2014;25(1):5-12.

34 CHAPTER Cardiac Toxicity Due to Drugs

Spencer C Greene, Stephen Sanders

INTRODUCTION

Improper use of medication, whether intentional or accidental, is a major public health threat. Poisonings are the leading causes of unintentional injury death in the United States, particularly in adults between the ages of 25 and 64 years.[1] Suicide is the second most common cause of death in the age range of 15–35 years, with overdoses ranking first for females and third for males.[2,3] Many of these ingestions directly or indirectly affected the heart and/or vasculature. Cardiovascular medications were involved in 3.91% of all human exposures reported to United States poison centers in 2013, ranked seventh behind analgesics, cosmetics and other personal care products, household cleaning substances, antipsychotics and sedatives, antidepressants, and foreign bodies such as toys.[4] Cardiovascular drugs were the fourth most commonly implicated substances in "serious" exposures and in exposures in adults greater than or equal to 20 years old.

Cardiotoxicity is not restricted to medications intended to treat various cardiovascular conditions. A host of xenobiotics can produce a variety of manifestations such as conduction disturbances, dysrhythmias, abnormally elevated or depressed blood pressure, and impaired inotropy. The mechanisms responsible for these signs are as numerous as the toxicants that can cause them.

The onset and duration of cardiotoxic signs and symptoms depend on both patient factors and properties of the medication. It is essential to consider pharmacokinetics when evaluating a patient with suspected or known poisoning. While intravenous exposure should produce toxicity rapidly, ingestions are much more variable. Some xenobiotics are rapidly absorbed and produce clinical features within the first hours; others have delayed and prolonged absorption. Toxicity may not manifest for up to 24 hours and may not peak for 1 or more days.

CLINICAL FEATURES

Cardiovascular Toxicity

Tachycardia is arguably the most common cardiovascular manifestation following overdose and innumerable toxicants can cause it (Table 1). Stimulants, including medications such as caffeine and theophylline and illicit substances such as amphetamines, synthetic cathinones, cocaine, and phencyclidine raise the heart rate by directly stimulating myocardial β1-adrenergic receptors. Stimulation of myocardial β1-adrenergic receptors causes activation of adenylyl cyclase and formation of cyclic adenosine monophosphate (cAMP) through a second-messenger system. Intracellular cAMP then enhances calcium influx which subsequently enhances calcium release from the sarcoplasmic reticulum. The resultant increase in intracellular calcium enhances inotropy and chronotropy. A great number of medications and naturally occurring substances antagonize muscarinic receptors, producing tachycardia by reducing the vagal stimulation that serves to lower heart rate. Drugs with antimuscarinic, or, more commonly, anticholinergic properties include atropine, benztropine, tricyclic antidepressants (TCAs), first-generation histamine (H1) antagonists, low-potency typical and some atypical antipsychotics, phenothiazines, carbamazepine, oxcarbazepine, orphenadrine, cyclobenzaprine, amantadine, tolterodine, oxybutynin, dicyclomine, scopolamine, and glycopyrrolate. Plants, such as *Atropa belladonna*, *Datura stramonium*, and *Hyoscyamus niger*, also contain atropine and other tropane alkaloids that produce antimuscarinic toxicity.

Tachycardia may also be observed as a reflex phenomenon following hypotension due to vasodilation. Drugs that antagonize peripheral α1-adrenergic receptors include prazosin, doxazosin, terazosin, TCAs, and some low-potency and atypical antipsychotics to some low-potency and atypical antipsychotics, e.g., chlorpromazine and risperidone. Calcium channel antagonists of the

TABLE 1: Xenobiotics affecting heart rate and blood pressure

Finding	Hypotension	Hypertension
Bradycardia	• β-adrenergic receptor antagonists • Calcium channel antagonists • Cholinesterase inhibitors • Clonidine • MAO inhibitors • Opioids • Trazodone	• Phenylephrine • Phenylpropanolamine
Tachycardia	• ACE inhibitors • Amitriptyline and other TCAs • Dihydropyridine calcium channel antagonists • Diuretics • Doxazosin • Hydralazine • Lithium • Minoxidil • Nitrates • Paliperidone • Phenothiazines • Prazosin • Risperidone	• Amphetamines • Bupropion • Caffeine and other methylxanthines • Cathinones • Cocaine • MAO inhibitors

ACE, angiotensin-converting-enzyme; MAO, monoamine oxidase; TCA, tricyclic antidepressant.

dihydropyridine class cause vasodilation, though in significant overdose the vasculature selectivity is lost, and myocardial toxicity results in bradycardia. Other vasodilators include minoxidil, hydralazine, sodium nitroprusside, and various nitrites and nitrates.

Tachycardia can also accompany hypotension caused by intravascular volume depletion. This can result from sensible water loss secondary to vomiting, diarrhea and/or urination, and may occur from overdoses of iron, salicylates, and diuretics. It may also follow ingestions of poisonous mushrooms such as *Omphalotus olearius* and *Chlorophyllum molybdites*. Muscarine-containing mushrooms, such as *Clitocybe dealbata*, will cause similar gastrointestinal signs and symptoms, but will often be accompanied by bradycardia. Volume depletion resulting in hypotension with reflex tachycardia may also result from third-spacing of fluids, which is observed in colchicine, iron and arsenic ingestions, among others.

Bradycardia may be observed in poisoning and overdose and is generally due to decreased activity at the sinoatrial (SA) node. The most common bradydysrhythmia is sinus bradycardia, but all types of atrioventricular (AV) blocks have been reported. Sympatholytics such as β-adrenergic antagonists and clonidine can cause bradycardia even after minor exposures. Blockade of myocardial β1-adrenergic receptors antagonizes the adenylyl cyclase cascade previously described. Calcium channel antagonists—particularly nondihydropyridines such as verapamil and diltiazem—produce bradycardia by preventing the calcium-mediated calcium release in myocytes. Opioids and other central nervous system (CNS) depressants may lower heart rate in overdose by indirectly reducing CNS sympathetic stimulation. Certain medications cause significant bradycardia when combined. It has been shown that when sofosbuvir, with or without ledipasvir, is combined with amiodarone, serious and potentially fatal bradycardia may ensure.[5] Cholinesterase inhibitors, such as pyridostigmine and neostigmine, cause bradycardia by indirectly enhancing the vagal stimulation that results from elevated levels of circulating acetylcholine. Bradycardia has also been observed following overdoses from trazodone, lithium, and propoxyphene and may be a preterminal finding following ingestion of TCAs and other membrane-stabilizing xenobiotics.

Digoxin toxicity can be associated with bradycardia or tachycardia. Acute poisonings are more often associated with the former, while chronic toxicity presents with the latter, but there is wide variability. Digoxin inhibits the Na^+/K^+ ATPase in myocardial cells. Under normal conditions, the pump exchanges 3 Na^+ ions extracellularly for every 2 K^+ ions that move intracellularly, creating a resting potential of approximately –85 mV. When digoxin inhibits this pump function, Na^+ export is hampered and the cell becomes more positively charged. This in turn facilitates Na^+/Ca^{2+} exchange at the Na^+/Ca^{2+} antiporter, raising intracellular and sarcoplasmic reticulum Ca^{2+}

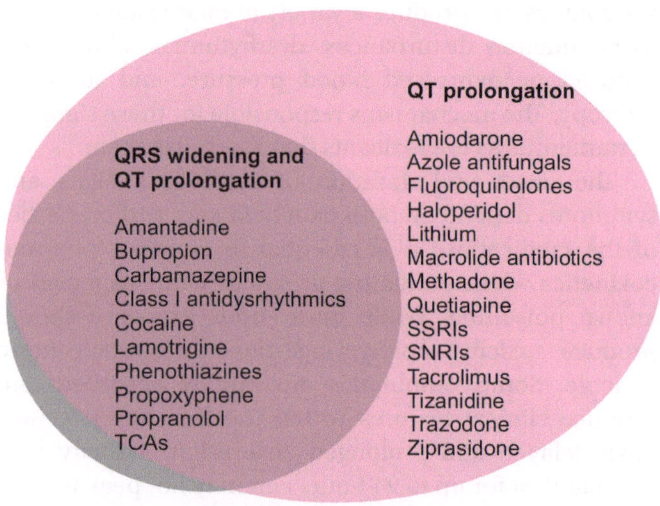

SNRIs, serotonin norepinephrine reuptake inhibitors; SSRIs, selective serotonin reuptake inhibitors; TCAs, tricyclic antidepressants.

FIG. 1: Drugs that prolong the QT interval ± widen the QRS complex concentrations. Contractility is improved as more calcium becomes available to the contractile proteins, and the excitability of the cell increases, enhancing automaticity and the potential for tachycardia.[6]

The seemingly paradoxical effect of controlling atrial dysrhythmias results from the digoxin's indirect effects. Digoxin-mediated Na^+/K^+ ATPase inhibition indirectly causes stimulation of the parasympathetic autonomic nervous system, with resulting vagal effects on the AV node and, to a lesser degree, the SA node.[7]

A similar clinical picture may be observed following exposure to plant- and animal-derived cardioactive steroids. Examples of plants containing cardenolides include lily of the valley, *Convallaria majalis*; poison milkweed, *Asclepias subverticillata*; sea onion, *Urginea maritima*; *Nerium oleander*; Peruvian oleander, *Thevetia peruviana*; dogbane, *Apocynum cannabinum*; and various *Adonis* and *Adenium* species.[8]

Though variations in heart rate are the most common cardiovascular manifestations of drug toxicity, blood pressure may also be affected. Both hypertension and hypotension may be observed, with the latter generally requiring more immediate intervention. There are several mechanisms that can cause hypotension in the overdose patient, and oftentimes, there is a synergistic effect. When a patient presents with hypotension, it is wise to evaluate all three components of the cardiovascular system: (i) the heart, (ii) the blood, and (iii) the blood vessels. Hypotension may be secondary to decreased cardiac output, which in turn may be due to any of the aforementioned xenobiotics that cause bradycardia. Cardiac output is determined by both stroke volume and heart rate. A low heart rate, even when the heart is pumping well, may result in hypotension.

It was previously noted that hypotension may cause a reflex tachycardia, but in some instances severe tachycardia can cause hypotension. When the heart rate is significantly elevated, diastole is so brief that there is insufficient time for the ventricles to fill with blood. In this case, cardiac output is decreased despite the high heart rate because stroke volume is so compromised.

Intoxications that diminish myocardial inotropy can produce hypotension irrespective of the heart rate. Blockade of myocardial L-type calcium channels results in diminished calcium-mediated calcium release as previously described. Antagonism of the sodium channels involved in phase 0 of the myocardial action potential causes a less vigorous depolarization, resulting in impaired inotropy and dromotropy. This manifests clinically as hypotension and electrocardiographically as a widened QRS interval, and may be observed in poisonings from TCAs and similar xenobiotics.

Cardiomyopathy has also been observed following toxicity from anthracyclines, antimony, cobalt, and syrup of ipecac, among others.[9-12] Oftentimes, the mechanism cannot be elucidated. Clozapine has been implicated in cases of myocarditis and cardiomyopathy.[13,14]

Hypotension may also be the result of generalized vasodilation or intravascular depletion as described earlier. Most intoxications in which hypotension is attributed to either of these mechanisms will be associated with tachycardia as previously described, though carvedilol, which antagonizes β-adrenergic receptors in addition to α-adrenergic receptors, may be associated with bradycardia.[15]

Hypertension is generally a less emergent manifestation of cardiovascular toxicity, though there are some situations in which severe hypertension can produce significant cardiac and extracardiac manifestations. Blood pressure is proportional to cardiac output and systemic vasculature resistance, so any xenobiotic that can increase one or both of these can produce hypertension. Stimulation of myocardial β1-adrenergic receptors will enhance both chronotropy and inotropy, while agonism of peripheral α1-adrenergic receptors will raise systemic vascular resistance. If a xenobiotic agonizes both β1-adrenergic and β2-adrenergic receptors, hypertension may not be present because of the β2-mediated smooth vascular muscle relaxation. Indirect agonism of α1-adrenergic receptors may result when a xenobiotic inhibits the reuptake of norepinephrine or other catecholamines, which may be observed in poisonings from monoamine oxidase inhibitor (MAOI), amphetamines, cocaine, and phencyclidine.

Electrocardiographic Manifestations

Electrocardiographic abnormalities frequently precede clinical findings following poisonings. The QRS duration, which represents ventricular depolarization, is determined by the influx of sodium ions during phase 0 of the myocardial action potential. The QRS widening may reflect poisoning from TCAs and other sodium channel antagonists, such as type I antidysrhythmics, bupropion, propranolol and other membrane-stabilizing β-adrenergic receptor antagonists, propoxyphene, amantadine, venlafaxine, diphenhydramine, and lamotrigine.[16-23] Nonpharmaceutical substances that can poison sodium channels include taxine, from the yew, *Taxus brevifolia* and tetrodotoxin, which can be found in a large number of animals, including some species of newts, toads, pufferfish, and the blue-ringed octopus.

The QT interval, which represents the entire duration of ventricular systole, may be prolonged indirectly by a widened QRS or can be affected directly by xenobiotics that prolong ventricular repolarization. The QT prolongation is observed in intoxications from a variety of medicinal and nonmedicinal substances, including class III antidysrhythmics, antipsychotics, fluoroquinolone and macrolide antibiotics, cesium, arsenic, organophosphorus compounds, ethylene glycol, cocaine, trazodone, tizanidine, and methadone.[24-28] Patients with prolonged QT intervals must be identified and treated to prevent the development of torsades des pointes (TdP), a form of polymorphic ventricular tachycardia with significant mortality. Xenobiotics may indirectly cause QT prolongation by inducing hypokalemia, as is seen in toxicity from soluble barium salts and from glycyrrhizic acid, which is found in natural licorice and causes pseudohyperaldosteronism.[29,30]

A number of xenobiotics can cause bradycardia in overdose. Sinus bradycardia is most common, but junctional escape rhythms and a variety of AV heart blocks have been reported.[31] First-degree heart block has been observed in toxicity from trazodone.[25] Second-degree heart block has been ascribed to overdoses from fingolimod.[32] Complete (third-degree) heart block has been attributed to pregabalin, lithium, and flecainide toxicity as well as following overdoses of diltiazem and lamotrigine.[17,33-36]

Other electrocardiographic findings secondary to xenobiotic cardiotoxicity may include transient ST elevation, which has been observed in the absence of coronary artery stenosis following carbon monoxide toxicity and atenolol ingestion.[37]

Electrocardiographic stigmata of the "digoxin effect" include downsloping ST-segment depression, flat, inverted or biphasic T-waves, and a short QT interval (Figs 2 and 3). Other signs may include an increased PR interval, U waves, J point depression, or peaked terminal portion of the T-waves. It is essential to recognize that these findings suggest the presence of digoxin but are not indicative of toxicity.[38] Electrocardiographically, digoxin toxicity may masquerade as nearly any arrhythmia with the exceptions of rapidly conducted atrial fibrillation or atrial flutter. Consistent with its mechanism of action, typical arrhythmias associated with digoxin toxicity include junctional tachycardia, paroxysmal atrial tachycardia with a 2:1 block, bidirectional ventricular tachycardia and atrial fibrillation with slow ventricular response.

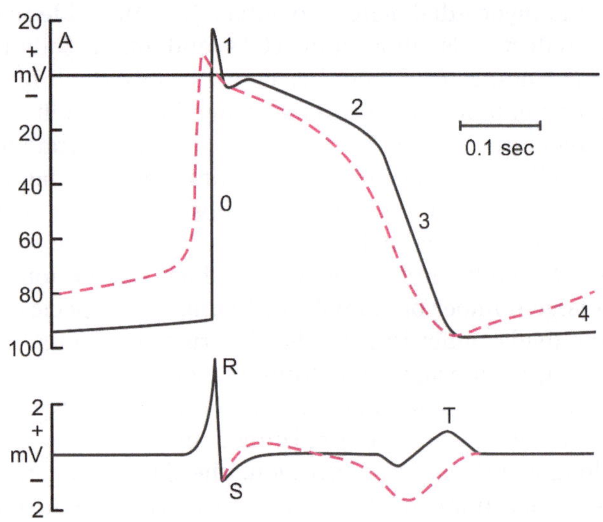

FIG. 2: Digoxin effect on the cardiac action potential. Unipolar recording of a transmembrane action potential from a Purkinje fiber. Control conditions are traced with a solid line, digitalized tissue with dashed line.

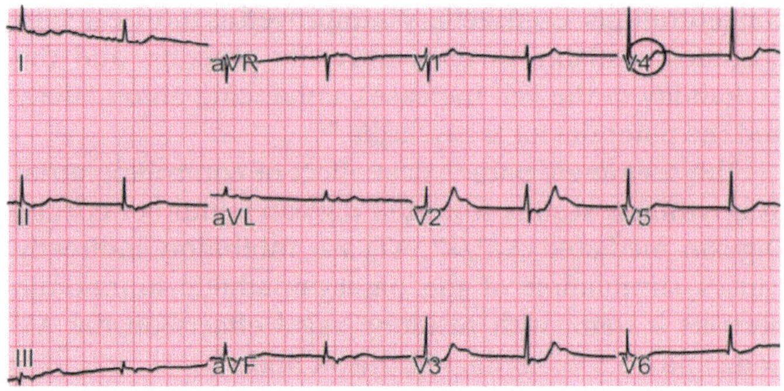

FIG. 3: Digoxin effect on electrocardiogram

Noncardiac Clinical Features

Extracardiac manifestations often provide clues that help identify the agent responsible for cardiotoxicity. Hyperglycemia, e.g., often accompanies the hypotension and bradycardia observed in calcium channel antagonist poisonings. The presence of elevated blood sugar in someone with no history of diabetes mellitus may help the physician distinguish a calcium channel antagonist overdose from a β-adrenergic receptor antagonist overdose, which may present with similar cardiotoxicity. Hyperglycemia and even diabetic ketoacidosis (DKA) may be observed following exposure to a number of atypical antipsychotics, including olanzapine, clozapine, and risperidone.[39]

Hyperkalemia is observed following acute digoxin overdoses and provides both diagnostic and prognostic information. It has been shown that patients with potassium greater than 5.5 in the setting of acute digoxin toxicity have a 100% mortality rate, if they go untreated. Conversely, patients whose potassium is less than 5.0 following digoxin overdoses have a survival rate of 100%.[40] Angioedema is a well-documented complication of ACE-inhibitor use, particularly in the African-American population, with a relative risk of 3.0 compared to non-Black patients.[41]

Mydriasis is common after overdose. Sympathomimetics, antimuscarinic substances, and drugs which agonize serotonin receptors may all produce dilated pupils, although it should be noted that some drugs have effects at other receptors that can confound the diagnosis. Many atypical antipsychotics as well as low-potency typical antipsychotics, e.g., cause the altered mental status, tachycardia, mumbling speech, and ileus commonly observed in antimuscarinic toxicity, but miosis, not mydriasis, is observed because of the antagonism at peripheral α1-adrenergic receptors. Miosis also frequently accompanies intoxications from opioids, direct-acting and indirect-acting muscarinic agonists, and centrally acing sympatholytics such as clonidine. Again, it should be noted that miosis may be conspicuously absent. Meperidine produces an opioid intoxication, but miosis is rarely observed because of concomitant muscarinic antagonism.

Neuropsychiatric manifestations are common in overdose, so the presence of altered mental status, seizures, malaise, or weakness does little to narrow the differential diagnosis. Normal mentation, however, in the setting of significant vital sign abnormalities may reflect poisoning from a substance with little ability to cross the blood-brain barrier. This is commonly observed following overdoses of calcium channel antagonists, in which CNS depression reflects hypoperfusion of the brain more than direct neurotoxicity. There are some neuropsychiatric clinical features that suggest a particular intoxication. However, digoxin and other cardiac glycosides may cause the ocular phenomena photopsia and chromatopsia.[42]

Extrapyramidal side effects (EPSE) may accompany toxicity from antipsychotics. Patients may present with dystonia, akathisia, Parkinsonism, or tardive dyskinesia. High-potency typical antipsychotics are most frequently implicated, all antipsychotics except clozapine can cause them.

Serotonin toxicity may present with some combination of clonus, hyperreflexia, altered mental status, rigidity, and diaphoresis along with tachycardia and labile blood pressure.

The physical examination may also reveal findings which may occasionally accompany intoxications from cardiotoxic substances but are not consistent enough to aide in the diagnosis. Paralytic ileus has been reported in the setting of chronic amlodipine toxicity[43] and nonocclusive colonic and mesenteric ischemias have been observed in acute verapamil[44] and chronic atenolol[45] toxicity, respectively.

EVALUATION

The evaluation of any patient presenting with substance-induced cardiotoxicity must start with a comprehensive history, when possible. It is essential to determine what medications the patient is prescribed or can access. Recent adjustments in dosages and formulations should also be acknowledged, as should any use of complementary, alternative, and homeopathic therapies. Comorbid medical conditions should be identified, and the potential for substance abuse, including alcohol, tobacco, and illicit drugs must be investigated.

Because the patient or someone in proximity may initiate treatment prior to evaluation in the hospital, it is important to inquire about this, as some prehospital interventions may be more dangerous than the exposure that warranted them.

A physical examination may identify conditions requiring immediate intervention and can provide clues to the offending agent. The presence of a toxidrome may help narrow the differential diagnosis and allow the clinician to initiate specific antidotal therapy.

An electrocardiogram (ECG) and continuous telemetry are recommended on all ingestions and are especially important in cases of actual or potential cardiotoxicity. The frequency of serial ECGs is determined by the pharmacokinetics of the substance and the severity of the toxicity. In addition to the electrocardiographic findings described previously, an ECG may yield indirect evidence of xenobiotic-induced toxicity. The prognostic significance of the serum potassium level in the setting of digoxin toxicity was previously identified, and the ECG may demonstrate one or more findings of significant hyperkalemia, including peaked T-waves, widening and eventual loss of P waves, QRS widening, high-grade AV blocks, bundle branch block morphology, and a preterminal sinusoidal pattern.[46]

Laboratory testing is essential in cases of xenobiotic-induced cardiotoxicity. In some circumstances, specific drug levels may confirm the diagnosis, though when patients are unstable, empiric treatment may be required. Medications for which quantitative serum levels are readily available include carbamazepine, theophylline, lithium, phenobarbital, valproic acid, phenytoin, iron, acetaminophen, and salicylates. Digoxin will not be completely distributed for up to 6 hours, and early measurement of digoxin concentration will suggest a higher body burden than may be present, which can lead to unnecessarily aggressive treatment. In contrast, steady-state digoxin concentration is a reliable indicator of body stores of digoxin, but because of individual susceptibility and variable specificity and sensitivity of analytical methods for nondigoxin cardiac glycosides, digoxin concentration should not be used as the sole measure of cardiac glycoside intoxication.[47] Tricyclic antidepressants levels may be available in some healthcare facilities, but the utility of this test has been questioned, because TCA toxicity is ultimately a clinical and electrocardiographic diagnosis. The urine drug screen is available in nearly all emergency departments, but the necessity of this test has also been challenged.[48]

The results of urine and blood tests may help narrow the differential diagnosis. In addition to the previously mentioned significance of hyperkalemia and hyperglycemia, laboratory studies may identify wide-gap acidosis, acute kidney injury, and other electrolyte abnormalities such as hypocalcemia. Troponin should be measured with clinical findings of or risk factors for infarction. B-type natriuretic peptide should be obtained on patients with unexplained hypotension or evidence of heart failure. Creatine phosphokinase is recommended in patients with possible rhabdomyolysis or unexplained acute kidney injury. Liver function tests are also recommended in significant poisonings.

Radiographic studies have a limited role in the assessment of a poisoned patient. A chest radiograph should be obtained in patients with chest pain, dyspnea, or increased work of breathing. Computed tomography of the head should be reserved for patients with unexplained altered mental status, focal neurological deficits, or increased risk of intracranial bleeding, or if there is evidence of trauma.

MANAGEMENT

Treatment of cardiotoxic effects from xenobiotics consists of initial resuscitation, preventing absorption when possible, providing supportive care, use of toxicant-specific therapies, and enhancing elimination of the causative agents when applicable.

Initial Resuscitation

Life-threatening conditions must be immediately identified and stabilized. Patients with unprotected airways due to CNS depression or anatomic or physiologic abnormalities should be intubated. Hypoxic patients should receive 100% oxygen. Mechanical ventilation is necessary for hypercarbic patients.

Hypotension should initially be managed with fluid resuscitation. If hypotension is the result of volume loss or vasodilation, intravenous fluids may be sufficient treatment. Fluid is the initial intervention for tachycardic patients with signs of tissue hypoperfusion, even if the patients are normotensive. Normal saline is the most commonly used crystalloid solution and is generally acceptable. Lactated Ringer's solution may be more appropriate when acidosis must be avoided, because normal saline can contribute to a hyperchloremic acidosis.[49] Euglycemia must be ensured in patients with altered mental status and/or focal neurological deficits. Naloxone may be administered in the setting of CNS and respiratory depression. The potential for concomitant trauma must always be considered in patients "found down".

Preventing Absorption

Cardioactive xenobiotics can only exert their toxicity following systemic absorption. For many years, various methods of gastrointestinal decontamination were used to prevent absorption with varying degrees of success. More recently, their utility has been questioned.[50] In 1997, the American Academy of Clinical Toxicology and the European Association of Poison Centres and Clinical Toxicologists first published position statements on five of these methods: (i) single-dose activated charcoal, (ii) gastric lavage, (iii) ipecac, (iv) cathartics, and (v) whole-bowel irrigation (WBI).[51-55] These have since been updated, but the recommendations have changed little. In general, gastrointestinal decontamination is rarely indicated. Ipecac and cathartics have no role in the poisoned patient, and the most recent position statement suggests that gastric lavage "should not be performed routinely, if at all, for the treatment of poisoned patients". In specific circumstances, single-dose activated charcoal or WBI may be considered.

Single-dose Activated Charcoal

Although single-dose activated charcoal was once considered a standard treatment for all ingestions, its role has declined substantially, as evidence suggests it rarely confers a benefit. At this time, it can only be recommended in situations in which the ingestion has a high likelihood of toxicity and when the potential benefits outweigh the risks. Charcoal should be administered shortly after the ingestion in order to prevent absorption. In most situations, the acceptable time frame is within 1 hour, though some toxicants, such as extended-release products, will remain in the gastrointestinal tract longer. Others will be absorbed in less than 1 hour, and the presence of signs and symptoms suggests that a significant amount of the xenobiotic has already been absorbed. Charcoal is unlikely to benefit the patient at that point. If giving charcoal, the patient should be awake and alert enough to protect his or her airway. Central nervous system depression should be considered a contraindication to charcoal because of the risk of pulmonary aspiration. There should be no evidence of emergent gastrointestinal tract pathology such as obstruction or perforation. Finally, activated charcoal should not be used when the ingestant is known not to be adsorbable by charcoal. While the overwhelming majority of substances are adsorbable, certain toxicants are not. These include alcohols such as methanol, ethanol, and ethylene glycol, and elements, i.e., lithium and iron. Charcoal is also contraindicated following ingestion of a caustic agent, both because many are not adsorbable and because charcoal obscures the view on endoscopy, which is often necessary to evaluate the severity of the ingestion. If there are no contraindications to the use of activated charcoal, a single dose of 50–100 g (1 g/kg in pediatric patients) should be given per os as close to the time of ingestion as possible. Charcoal may also be given via nasogastric tube, but this will increase patient's discomfort and may increase the risk of complications.

Whole-Bowel Irrigation

Whole-bowel irrigation consists of the installation of high molecular weight polyethylene glycol (PEG) orally or via a nasogastric tube in an effort to decrease the transit time of a xenobiotic through the gastrointestinal tract. It has supplanted the use of cathartics because, unlike the latter, the high molecular weight PEG causes no net secretion or absorption of fluids or ions. Its use is limited to toxicants that remain in the gastrointestinal tract for several hours or longer, such as transdermal patches or sustained-release or extended-release products. It is also useful in the setting of asymptomatic body packers who have large volumes of well-sealed material, i.e., cocaine, sitting throughout the intestines. Although volunteer studies suggest that WBI may reduce the bioavailability of xenobiotics, there are no data that indicate improved outcomes. This method decreases transit time of ingested substances through the gastrointestinal tract and may prevent absorption of all or part of such ingestions. If WBI is to be performed, the PEG should be given at 1,500–2,000 mL/h in adults or 1,000 mL/h in children aged 6–12 years. Children form 9 months to 6 years old are treated at 500 mL/h. Irrigation is continued until the rectal effluent is clear.

Antidotal Therapy

Standard cardiopulmonary resuscitation drugs are often effective in the management of xenobiotic-induced cardiotoxicity. It is important to determine which patients require intervention and which treatments are likely to be beneficial. For example, isolated bradycardia rarely requires intervention, and atropine is often ineffective when bradycardia is accompanied by more serious signs of toxicity.[56]

Vasopressors

A number of different vasopressors have been used to treat xenobiotic-induce cardiotoxicity with varying degrees of success. Norepinephrine primarily stimulates α-adrenergic receptors, increasing systemic vascular resistance and improving venous return to the heart. Its agonist effect at myocardial β1-adrenergic receptors can also raise the heart rate and improve contractility. In cases of hypotension with reflex tachycardia due to profound vasodilation, phenylephrine is an effective treatment that will not raise the heart rate further. Epinephrine works similarly to norepinephrine but will also agonize smooth muscle β2-adrenergic receptors. Its use is more common in pediatric patients and in the settings of cardiac arrest or anaphylaxis. Although dopamine is commonly used to treat hypotension due to a variety of etiologies, its use is not recommended following overdoses. Dopamine relies on the presence of endogenous norepinephrine stores to exert its pressor effect and may be ineffective and possibly harmful in poisonings by substances that inhibit the reuptake of norepinephrine, i.e., MAOI. The roles of vasopressin, milrinone, dobutamine, and isoproterenol are less well-established in the setting of xenobiotic-induced cardiotoxicity.

Glucagon

Glucagon is the initial antidote in cases of significant hypotension with bradycardia following cardiac β-adrenergic receptor antagonism. When β-adrenergic receptors are blocked, the cascade leading to increased intracellular calcium cannot commence, leading to impaired chronotropy and inotropy. Glucagon stimulates G proteins that can initiate the same cascade and improve cardiac function.[57-59] Unlike its indication for hypoglycemia, glucagon should be administered intravenously when treating cardiotoxicity. Variable dosing recommendations exist; it is reasonable to start with a bolus of 2–10 mg (0.15 mg/kg in children) followed by an infusion of 2–10 mg/h (0.05–0.1 mg/kg/h). Tachyphylaxis is common, so the patient may develop recurrence of toxicity. Profound nausea may also be observed, and prophylactic administration of an antiemetic should be considered. Glucagon may also be helpful in the setting of hypotension and bradycardia due to calcium channel antagonist toxicity, though in these situations, because there is no antagonism at the β1-adrenergic receptors, glucagon confers no advantage over traditional vasopressors.

Calcium

Calcium can be used as an initial therapy in cases of calcium channel blockade. Bolus 10% calcium gluconate 10–20 mL (0.2–0.3 mL/kg in children) every 10–20 minutes as needed to achieve hemodynamic stability.[60] Calcium chloride contains three times the elemental calcium per gram as calcium gluconate, but because of its caustic effect on veins and soft tissues, it should only be administered via central venous line except in perimortem patients.[61]

Hyperinsulinemia-euglycemia Therapy

High-dose insulin can improve inotropy following poisonings from calcium channel antagonists and β-adrenergic receptor antagonists by transporting glucose into myocytes. Under normal circumstances, myocardial cells rely on lipids as the primary energy source. Under physiologic stress, however, glucose is used preferentially. This hyperinsulinemia euglycemia (HIE) therapy consists of doses much higher than those used in more common conditions such as DKA. The current recommended insulin dosing for DKA is 0.12 unit/kg/h. When treating poisonings with HIE, the recommended starting dose is a bolus of 0.51 unit/kg followed by an infusion of 1 unit/kg/h with titration to 10 units/kg/h.[62] Because healthcare providers may not be familiar or comfortable with the use of such large doses of insulin, consultation with a medical toxicologist is strongly recommended. Close monitoring of blood glucose is necessary when administering such large doses of insulin, and it is recommended that blood sugar be checked every 15 minutes while the dose is being titrated upward, then hourly once at a stable infusion rate. Careful monitoring of potassium, magnesium, and phosphorus is also suggested. For greatest efficacy, high-dose insulin should be instituted as early as possible in cases of moderate-to-severe cardiovascular poisoning because there is often a delay in its action.

Other Antidotes

Naloxone antagonizes μ-opioid receptors and can rapidly reverse the CNS and respiratory depression that accompanies opioid intoxication. There is anecdotal evidence of benefit in the treatment of hypotension following clonidine and ACE-inhibitor poisoning.[63-65] Because of the minimal risk of naloxone administration, its use should be considered in these poisonings. It should be noted that patients may require higher doses of naloxone than those used to treat opioid intoxication. We recommend 2 mg every minute as needed to a maximum of 10 mg. For recurrent hypotension, patients should be placed on a naloxone infusion using two-thirds of arousal dose hourly.

Methylene blue has been shown to correct hypotension secondary to amlodipine toxicity. Though more commonly used as the antidote for methemoglobinemia, methylene blue can antagonize endothelial nitric oxide synthase activity and may scavenge nitric oxide and inhibit guanylate cyclase. These effects synergistically inhibit vasodilation, making the vasculature more responsive to standard vasoconstrictors.[66]

Sodium Bicarbonate

Poisoning of myocardial sodium channels manifests clinically as hypotension and electrocardiographically as a widened QRS interval. Sodium bicarbonate can overcome the sodium channel blockade when given in sufficient doses.[67,68] The QRS width warranting treatment has been debated by toxicologists.[69] The most commonly accepted QRS width requiring treatment is 120 ms. Conversely, the majority of poison center medical directors agree that QRS durations less than 100 ms do not require sodium bicarbonate unless there is concomitant hypotension attributed to decreased inotropy. The suggested initial dose is 50–100 mEq of sodium bicarbonate, and may be repeated every 15 minutes as needed until there is clinical improvement or the pH exceeds 7.55. Many patients will require several boluses, and there are reports of patients requiring several dozen boluses.[70] The utility of a sodium bicarbonate infusion is questionable. Even an aggressive bicarbonate drip made with 150 mEq of sodium bicarbonate per liter and administered at 250 mL/h provides only 37.5 mEq hourly, which does little to overcome a sodium channel blockade. Serum alkalinization may provide some benefit by reducing the receptor binding of cardioactive medications and promote greater binding to serum proteins, but the significance of this is unknown.

Digoxin Fab Fragments

Administration of D-Fab is the standard of care for significant toxicity from digoxin and may be helpful in poisonings from other cardioactive glycosides. D-Fab are ovine derived, so an allergy to sheep products must be excluded prior to use. The fragments bind rapidly to digoxin, producing clinical benefit in minutes following completion of infusion. Free (toxic) digoxin levels have been shown to drop rapidly after administration of D-Fab, and modified dosing guidelines to improve efficacy and reduce cost have been proposed.[71-72]

Indications for D-Fab administration include any life-threatening dysrhythmia; serum potassium concentration in excess of 5 mEq/L in the setting of acute digoxin intoxication; serum digoxin concentration in excess of 15 ng/mL at any time before D-Fab administration or in excess of 10 ng/mL 6 hours after ingestion; subacute elevation of digoxin serum concentration in excess of 5 mEq/L in patients with dysrhythmias, uncontrolled nausea, vomiting, abdominal pain, or altered mental status; and acute ingestion of 10 mg or more in an adult or 4 mg or more in a child. It should be noted that once D-Fab is administered, total serum digoxin levels will rise dramatically as the drug leaves the cells, and clinical decision cannot be based on the total serum digoxin concentration.

Dosing of D-Fab may be determined empirically in the absence of history or laboratory information or can be calculated based upon amount ingested or upon serum digoxin concentration, ideally at steady state or 6 or more hours after ingestion. Empiric dosing in acute digoxin overdose is 10–20 vials; for chronic poisoning the dose is 3–6 vials for adults and 1–2 vials for children. Dose for digoxin poisoning may be calculated using the following formula and rounded up to the nearest whole number of vials:[73]

$$\text{Dose (in number of vials)} = \frac{(\text{serum digoxin concen-tration in ng/mL}) \times (\text{patient weight in kg})}{100}$$

The cost of D-Fab is sometimes considered a barrier to the use of this potentially life-saving treatment. It can be argued that treatment with D-Fab, both for critically ill patients and for those with less serious toxicity, is cost-effective when compared to the cost of prolonged hospitalization, the required serial laboratory testing and the need for critical care, e.g., pacemaker insertion in cases where D-Fab is not used.[74,75]

Digoxin Fab fragments may bind cardiac glycosides other than digoxin and may potentially ameliorate poisoning, but the affinity of the antibody fragments for nondigoxin glycosides may be variable and dosing therefore uncertain. It may be best to underestimate the binding affinity and overestimate the dose for D-Fab in such cases.[76]

Antiarrhythmics

Magnesium has been long recognized for its beneficial effect in the setting of cardiotoxicity. It is the drug of choice in the setting of QT prolongation because it prevents the progression to torsades de pointes. Magnesium is beneficial even in the absence of hypomagnesemia, so supplementation should proceed irrespective of serum magnesium levels. Potassium supplementation is recommended in the setting of hypokalemia.

Vaughan Williams class IA antiarrhythmic drugs are contraindicated in cardiac glycoside poisoning due to their suppression of cardiac conduction and their proarrhythmic effects. When considering the use of a class IB agent, phenytoin may offer advantages over lidocaine. Phenytoin may effectively improve AV nodal conduction impaired by digoxin and inhibit ectopic tachydysrhythmias promoted by the increased automaticity.[77]

Lipid Rescue Therapy

Lipid resuscitation therapy consists of the intravenous infusion of a soybean oil emulsion commonly used for total parenteral nutrition as a treatment for poisonings by lipid-soluble medications. Its benefits were first demonstrated in the setting of local anesthetic toxicity and has since been shown to reverse the toxicity following β-blocker and calcium channel blocker poisoning.[78-82] Poisonings from other lipid-soluble xenobiotics, including amitriptyline, bupropion and olanzapine, among others, have since been published.[83-85]

Several theories regarding the mechanism of lipid rescue therapy exist. The prevailing thought is the "lipid sink" theory, which postulates that injection of this compound creates an additional lipid compartment within the bloodstream into which lipid-soluble toxicants are drawn, thereby reducing their intracellular concentrations. Other postulated mechanisms include:

- The "metabolic effect", which suggests that lipid infusion enhances mitochondrial fatty acid uptake
- The "membrane effect", in which the lipid interferes with the binding of local anesthetics at sodium channels
- The "cytoprotective effect", which activates a cascade that minimizes ischemia and reperfusion injury
- The "inotropic effect", by which lipid promotes calcium entry into the cell
- The "pharmacokinetic effect", in which intravenous lipid exerts its effects by enhancing the elimination of the fat-soluble xenobiotics.[86]

Lipid rescue therapy should be initiated at the earliest sign of impending cardiovascular collapse. The suggested dose is a bolus of 1.5 mL/kg of a 20% lipid solution given over 2–3 minutes followed by an infusion of 0.25 mL/kg/min.[87] The bolus may be repeated and the infusion rate may be increased to 0.5 mL/kg/min. The ideal duration of therapy is unknown and various protocols exist. The American College of Medical Toxicology recommends limiting lipid emulsion therapy to 1 hour when possible. The American Society of Regional Anesthesia and Pain Medicine advocates maintaining the infusion for an additional 10 minutes after hemodynamic stability has been achieved.[88]

Treatment of Hypertension

Hypertension following poisoning is generally the result of increased sympathetic tone at the myocardial cells and/or the vasculature. Because the increased tone is often secondary to central neuroexcitation, the initial intervention is sedation. Benzodiazepines are very effective in the management of hypertension due to sympathomimetic toxicity, gamma-aminobutyric acid (GABA) withdrawal, and serotonin syndrome. Alternative GABA agonists, such as phenobarbital, may also be considered when there is evidence of benzodiazepine resistance or in the case of drug shortages.

Hypertension that is at least partially mediated by increased vascular tone may be treated with a peripheral α1-antagonist such as phentolamine. Beta-adrenergic antagonists should not be used as monotherapy because of the theoretical concern of unopposed α-adrenergic stimulation causing severe hypertension. Additionally, there is concern that they may contribute to delirium in the setting of drug-induced cardiotoxicity. Alternatively, sodium nitroprusside can be used as a titratable, short-acting agent.

Electrical Therapy

Poisonings are best managed with supportive care and appropriate antidotal therapy. Overdrive pacing may induce dysrhythmias in the setting of cardiac glycoside toxicity.[89] Life-threatening ventricular arrhythmias have been associated with transthoracic electrical cardioversion for digoxin-induced atrial tachydysrhythmias.[90] Ventricular pacing may even exacerbate hypotension by interfering with ventricular relaxation or due to the loss of a coordinated atrial contraction.[91] Defibrillation is still indicated for patients in ventricular fibrillation or pulseless ventricular tachycardia, and cardioversion is recommended for tachydysrhythmias accompanied by hemodynamic instability.

Enhancing Elimination

There are several methods of eliminating toxicants from the body, though most xenobiotics are not amenable to these techniques. Elimination via the urine can be enhanced through alkalinization. Resins and multiple doses of activated charcoal (MDAC) can increase the elimination from the gastrointestinal tract and toxicants can be removed from the blood using one or more variants of hemodialysis.

Urinary Alkalinization

In addition to its utility in overcoming poisoned sodium channels, sodium bicarbonate can effectively alkalinize the serum and the urine. Urinary alkalinization has proved to effectively enhance the elimination of a number of xenobiotics, including salicylates, phenobarbital, methotrexate, diflunisal, fluoride, chlorpropamide, and the herbicides mecoprop and 2,4-dichlorophenoxyacetate.[92] It has been our experience that many healthcare providers mistakenly believe that urinary alkalinization is helpful in the setting of TCA toxicity. Alkalinization will not enhance the elimination of TCAs and other sodium channel poisoners. There is some concern that alkaluria will actually decrease the elimination of flecainide, though this is not consistently observed.[93-94]

An effective way to alkalinize the urine is to prepare a liter of D5W (5% dextrose in water) and add 150 mEq of sodium bicarbonate and 40 mEq of potassium chloride and infuse at a rate of 200–250 mL/h with a goal urine output of 2–3 mL/kg/h. Potassium can be held if the situation warrants, but it is essential to prevent hypokalemia. When serum potassium levels drop, the kidneys will reabsorb potassium in exchange for hydrogen, thus, preventing successful alkalinization.

Multiple-dose Activated Charcoal

Giving MDAC may help eliminate toxicants with long elimination half-lives by interrupting enteroenteric recirculation and, occasionally, enterohepatic and enterogastric recirculation. There is evidence that digoxin can be eliminated more quickly with repeat dosing of activated charcoal, and its use may be especially helpful in the setting of renal insufficiency or if D-Fab are unavailable.[95,96] A position statement issued jointly by the American Academy of Clinical Toxicology and the European Association of Poison Centres and Clinical Toxicologists recommends considering the use of MDAC in significant intoxications due to carbamazepine, phenobarbital, theophylline, quinine, or dapsone.[97] They caution that there is not strong evidence of clinical improvement. The position statement also acknowledges that there are conflicting data regarding the use of MDAC in the setting of digoxin, disopyramide, nadolol, phenytoin, sotalol, and amitriptyline toxicity. The use of MDAC is contraindicated in patients lacking a protected airway and when there is evidence of intestinal obstruction or anatomic abnormalities.

Resins

Toxicants can also be eliminated from the gastrointestinal tract using binding resins. The elimination of cardiac glycosides may be enhanced by cholestyramine or colestipol.[98] Sodium polystyrene sulfonate has been used to treat hyperkalemia and is an option for lithium toxicity.[99,100] Prussian blue can enhance the elimination of both thallium and cesium.[101]

Hemodialysis

Hemodialysis can effectively enhance the elimination of toxicants with specific physical characteristics: small size, typically less than 500 daltons; minimal protein binding; high polarity, and water-solubility; and low volume of distribution, ideally less than 1 L/kg. Xenobiotics that satisfy these criteria include, but are not limited to, salicylates, ethylene glycol, phenobarbital, and lithium. Substances that would not be considered easily dialyzable in therapeutic use may become candidates for hemodialysis in overdose because the free concentration rises once maximal protein binding has occurred. This may be observed in poisonings from carbamazepine, valproic acid, phenytoin, and disopyramide, among others (Table 2).

Because hemodialysis is an invasive procedure with potential, albeit rare, complications, the decision to dialyze the patient should be based on the clinical appearance of the patient and in consultation with a medical toxicologist.

Albumin dialysis is increasingly becoming an alternative to standard hemodialysis. This technique of extra-

TABLE 2: Dialyzable medications

Drug	Volume of distribution	% protein binding
Acyclovir	0.66–0.8	15
Aspirin	0.1–0.3	50–80
Carbamazepine	1.4–3	75
Lithium	0.7–1.4	0
Phenobarbital	0.5–0.9	20–50
Phenytoin	0.5–1.0	>90
Procainamide	1.5–2.5	15
Theophylline	0.5	40

corporeal elimination combines traditional continuous venovenous hemofiltration with a 20% human serum albumin dialysate. Several products currently exist, including the molecular adsorbent recirculating system (MARS), Prometheus, plasma-exchange with hemodialysis (PE/HD), and single pass albumin dialysis (SPAD). By providing the albumin, this technique can remove highly protein-bound xenobiotics along with traditionally dialyzable substances simultaneously. Great success has been attributed to albumin dialysis in cases of poisonings from calcium channel antagonists, TCAs, valproic acid, carbamazepine, acetaminophen, lamotrigine, phenytoin, theophylline, and *Amanita phalloides* mushrooms.[102-108]

CONCLUSION

Cardiovascular toxicity may result from accidental or intentional overdose of various pharmaceutical agents and other xenobiotics. Idiosyncratic reactions may also occur in therapeutic use. Mainstays of treatment include airway management, circulatory support with intravenous fluids and/or traditional and non-traditional vasopressors, control of dysrhythmias, and, when appropriate, specific antidotal therapy. Gastrointestinal decontamination and extracorporeal elimination may be indicated in specific situations. Physicians caring for these patients should consider consulting with a medical toxicologist for expert guidance.

REFERENCES

1. Centers for Disease Control and Prevention. (2016). 10 leading causes of injury death by age group highlighting unintentional injury death, United States - 2013. [online] Available from: http://www.cdc.gov/injury/images/lc-charts/leading_causes_of_injury_deaths_highlighting_unintentional_injury_2013-a.gif. [Accessed April, 2016].
2. Centers for Disease Control and Prevention. (2016). 10 leading causes of death by age group, United States - 2013. [online] Available from: http://www.cdc.gov/injury/wisqars/pdf/leading_causes_of_death_by_age_group_2013-a.pdf. [Accessed April, 2016].
3. Centers for Disease Control and Prevention. (2015). National suicide statistics at a glance. [online] Available from: http://www.cdc.gov/violenceprevention/pdf/suicide-datasheet-a.pdf. [Accessed April, 2016].
4. Mowry JB, Spyker DA, Cantilena LR, McMillan N, Ford M. 2013 Annual Report of the American Association of Poison Control Centers' National Poison Data System (NPDS): 31st Annual Report. Clin Toxicol. 2014;52(10):1032-283.
5. The Medical Letter. The Medical Letter on Drugs and Therapeutics. 2015; 57(1466):52-8.
6. Smith TW, Antman EM, Friedman PL, Blatt CM, Marsh JD. Digitalis glycosides: mechanisms and manifestations of toxicity: Part I. Prog Cardiovasc Dis. 1984;26(5):495-530.
7. Ferguson DW, Berg WJ, Sanders JS, Roach PJ, Kempf JS, Kienzle MG. Sympathoinhibitory responses to digitalis glycosides in heart failure patients: Direct evidence from sympathetic neural recordings. Circulation. 1989;80(1):65-77.
8. Oerther SE. Plant poisonings: common plants that contain cardiac glycosides. J Emerg Nurs. 2011;37(1):102-3.
9. Alexander CS. Cobalt-beer cardiomyopathy. A clinical and pathologic study of twenty-eight cases. Am J Med. 1972;53(4):395-417.
10. Dresser LP, Massey EW, Johnson EE, Bossen E. Ipecac myopathy and cardiomyopathy. J Neurol Neurosurg Psychiatry. 1993;56(5):560-62.
11. Husten L. Trace elements linked to cardiomyopathy. Lancet. 1999; 353(9164): 1594.
12. Giantris A, Abdurrahman L, Hinkle A, Asselin B, Lipshultz SE. Anthracycline-induced cardiotoxicity in children and young adults. Crit Rev Oncol Hematol. 1998;27(1):53-68.
13. Munshi TA, Volochniouk D, Hassan T, Mazhar N. Clozapine-induced myocarditis: is mandatory monitoring warranted for its early recognition? Case Rep Psychiatry. 2014;2014: 513108.
14. Layland JJ, Liew D, Prior DL. Clozapine-induced cardiotoxicity: a clinical update. Med J Aust. 2009;190(4):190-2.
15. Bouchard NC, Forde J, Hoffman RS. Carvedilol overdose with quantitative confirmation. Basic Clin Pharmacol Toxicol. 2008;103(1):102-3.
16. Jovic-Stosic J, Gligic B, Putic V, Brajkovic G, Spasic R. Severe propranolol and ethanol overdose with wide complex tachycardia treated with intravenous lipid emulsion: a case report. Clin Toxicol. 2011;49(5):426-30.
17. French LK, McKeown NJ, Hendrickson RG. Complete heart block and death following lamotrigine overdose. Clin Toxicol (Phila). 2011;49(4):330-3.
18. Stork CM, Redd JT, Fine K, Hoffman RS. Propoxyphene-induced wide QRS complex dysrhythmia responsive to sodium bicarbonate—a case report. J Toxicol Clin Toxicol. 1995;33(2):179-83.
19. Herold TJS. Lamotrigine as a possible cause of QRS prolongation in a patient with known seizure disorder. CJEM. 2006;8(5):361-4.
20. Caillier B, Pilote S, Castonguay A, Patoine D, Ménard-Desrosiers V, Vigneault P, et al. QRS and QT prolongation under bupropion: a unique cardiac electrophysiological profile. Fundam Clin Pharmacol. 2012;26(5):599-608.
21. Kuo CC, Huang RC, Lou BS. Inhibition of Na(+) current by diphenhydramine and other diphenyl compounds: molecular determinants of selective binding to the inactivated channels. Mol Pharmacol. 2000;57:135-43.
22. Dick IE, Brochu RM, Purohit Y, Kaczorowski GJ, Martin WJ, Priest BT. Sodium channel blockade may contribute to the analgesic efficacy of antidepressants. J Pain. 2007;8(4):315-24.
23. Brugada J, Boersma L, Kirchhof C, Allessie M. Proarrhythmic effects of flecainide. Experimental evidence for increased susceptibility to reentrant arrhythmias. Circulation. 1991;84(4):1808-18.
24. Jolly K, Gammage MD, Cheng KK, Bradburn P, Banting MV, Langman MJ. Sudden death in patients receiving drugs tending to prolong the QT interval. Br J Clin Pharmacol. 2009;68(5):743-51.
25. Service JA, Waring WS. QT Prolongation and delayed atrioventricular conduction caused by acute ingestion of trazodone. Clin Toxicol. 2008; 46:71-3.
26. Kaddar N, Vigneault P, Pilote S, Patoine D, Simard C, Drolet B. Tizanidine (Zanaflex): a muscle relaxant that may prolong the QT interval by blocking IKr. J Cardiovasc Pharmacol Ther. 2012;17(1):102-9.
27. Manini AF, Raspberry D, Hoffman RS, Nelson LS. QT prolongation and Torsades de Pointes following overdose of ziprasidone and amantadine. J Med Toxicol. 2007;3(4):178-81.
28. BB Alipour A, Cruz R, Lott RS. Torsade de pointes after ziprasidone overdose with coingestants. J Clin Psychopharmacol. 2010;30(1):76-7.
29. Panduranga P, Al-Rawahi N. Licorice-induced severe hypokalemia with recurrent torsade de pointes. Ann Noninvasive Electrocardiol. 2013;18(6):593-6.
30. Roza O, Berman LB. The pathophysiology of barium: hypokalemic and cardiovascular effects. J Pharmacol Exp Ther. 1971;177(2):433-9.
31. Connolly PT, Harris C. Unusual ECG findings mimicking complete heart block in an unrecognized calcium antagonist overdose. Resuscitation. 2006;68(3):429-32.
32. Hojer J, Olsson E. AV block II in a toddler after ingestion of a single tablet fingolimod. Clin Toxicol (Phila). 2014;52(6):644.
33. Aksakal E, Bakirci EM, Emet M, Uzkeser M. Complete atrioventricular block due to overdose of pregabalin. Am J Emerg Med. 2012;30(9):2101.e1-4.
34. Seriken M, Karcioglu O, Korkmaz A. Rarely seen cardiotoxicity of lithium overdose: complete heart block. Int J Cardiol. 2009;132(2):276-8.
35. Lloyd T, Zimmerman J, Griffin GD. Irreversible third-degree heart block and pacemaker implant in a case of flecainide toxicity. Am J Emerg. 2013;31(9): 1418.e1-2.
36. Wills BK, Liu JM, Wahl M. Third-degree AV block from extended-release diltiazem ingestion in a nine-month old. J Emerg Med. 2010;38(3):328-31.
37. Petrov D, Sardowski S, Gesheva M. 'Silent' Prinzmetal's ST elevation related to atenolol overdose. J Emerg Med. 2007;33:123-6.
38. Pick A. Digitalis and the electrocardiogram. Circulation. 1957;15(4):603-8.
39. Ramaswamy K, Kozma CM, Nasrallah H. Risk of diabetic ketoacidosis after exposure to risperidone or olanzapine. Drug Saf. 2007;30(7):589-99.

40. Bismuth C, Gaultier M, Conso F, Efthymiou ML. Hyperkalemia in acute digitalis poisoning: prognostic significance and therapeutic implications. Clin Toxicol. 1973;6(2):153-62.
41. McDowell SE, Coleman JJ, Ferner RE. Systematic review and meta-analysis of ethnic differences in risks of adverse reactions to drugs used in cardiovascular medicine. BMJ. 2006;332(7551):1177-81.
42. Arnold WN, Loftus LS. Xanthopsia and van Gogh's yellow palette. Eye (Lond). 1991;5(Pt 5):503-10.
43. Devasahayam J, Pillai U, Uppaluri C. Acute severe intestinal obstruction secondary to amlodipine toxicity. QJM. 2012;105(5):467-9.
44. Perbet S, Constantin JM, Guerin R, Faure M, Brugere C, Da Ines D, et al. Non-occlusive colonic ischemia induced by verapamil ER overdose. Intensive Care Med. 2009;35(5):956-7.
45. Hoot NR, Benitez JG, Palm KH. Hemodynamically unstable: accidental atenolol toxicity? J Emerg Med. 2013;45(3):355-7.
46. Life in the Fast Lane. (2016). Hyperkalaemia. [online] Available from: http://lifeinthefastlane.com/ecg-library/basics/hyperkalaemia/. [Accessed April, 2016].
47. Selzer A. Role of serum digoxin assay in patient management. J Am Coll Cardiol. 1985;5(5 Suppl A):106A-110A.
48. Tenenbein M. Do you really need that emergency drug screen? Clin Toxicol (Phila). 2009;47(4):286-91.
49. Scheingraber S, Rehm M, Sehmisch C, Finsterer U. Rapid saline infusion produces hyperchloremic acidosis in patients undergoing gynecologic surgery. Anesthesiology. 1999;90(5):1265-70.
50. Greene S, Harris C, Singer J. Gastrointestinal decontamination of the poisoned patient. Pediatr Emerg Care. 2008;24(3):176-89.
51. Krenzelok EP, McGuigan M, Lheur P. Position statement: ipecac syrup. American Academy of Clinical Toxicology and European Association of Poisons Centres and Clinical Toxicologists. J Toxicol Clin Toxicol. 1997;35(7):699-709.
52. Chyka PA, Seger D. Position statement: single dose activated charcoal. American Academy of Clinical Toxicology and European Association of Poisons Centres and Clinical Toxicologists. J Toxicol Clin Toxicol. 1997; 35(7):721-41.
53. Vale JA. Position statement: gastric lavage. American Academy of Clinical Toxicology and European Association of Poisons Centres and Clinical Toxicologists. J Toxicol Clin Toxicol. 1997;35(7):711-9.
54. Barceloux D, McGuigan M, Hartigan-Go K. Position statement: cathartics. American Academy of Clinical Toxicology and European Association of Poisons Centres and Clinical Toxicologists. J Toxicol Clin Toxicol. 1997;35(7):743-52.
55. Tenenbein M. Position statement: whole bowel irrigation. American Academy of Clinical Toxicology and European Association of Poisons Centres and Clinical Toxicologists. J Toxicol Clin Toxicol. 1997;35(7):753-62.
56. Kerns W. Management of beta-adrenergic blocker and calcium channel antagonist toxicity. Emerg Med Clin North Am. 2007;25(2):309-31.
57. Doyon S, Roberts JR. The use of glucagon in a case of calcium channel blocker overdose. Ann Emerg Med. 1993;22(7):1229-33.
58. Glick G, Parmley WW, Wechsler AS, Sonnenblick EH. Glucagon: Its enhancement of cardiac performance in the cat and dog and persistence of its inotropic action despite beta receptor blockade with propranolol. Circ Res. 1968;22(6):789-99.
59. Peterson CD, Leeder JS, Sterner S. Glucagon therapy for beta blocker overdose. Drug Intell Clin Pharm. 1984;18(5):394-8.
60. Henry M, Kay MM, Viccellio P. Cardiogenic shock associated with calcium-channel and beta blockers: Reversal with intravenous calcium chloride. Am J Emerg Med. 1985;3(4):334-6.
61. Gault DT. Extravasation injuries. Br J Plast Surg. 1993;46(2):91-6.
62. Engebretsen KM, Kaczmarek KM, Morgan J, Holger JS. High-dose insulin therapy in beta-blocker and calcium channel-blocker poisoning. Clin Toxicol. 2011;49(4):277-83.
63. Kulig K, Duffy J, Rumack BH, Mauro R, Gaylord M. Naloxone for treatment of clonidine overdose. JAMA. 1982;247(12):1697.
64. Botero M, Enneking FK. Reversal of prolonged unconsciousness by naloxone after an intravascular injection of a local anesthetic and clonidine. Anesth Analg. 1999;88(5):1185-6.
65. Varon J, Duncan SR. Naloxone reversal of hypotension due to captopril overdose. Ann Emerg Med. 1991;20(10):1125-7.
66. Jang DH, Nelson LS, Hoffman RS. Methylene blue in the treatment of refractory shock from an amlodipine overdose. Ann Emerg Med. 2011;58(6):565-7.
67. Kerr GW, McGuffie AC, Wilkie S. Tricyclic antidepressant overdose: a review. Emerg Med J. 2001;18(4):236-41.
68. Bradberry SM, Thanacoody HK, Watt BE, Thomas SH, Vale JA. Management of the cardiovascular complications of tricyclic antidepressant poisoning: role of sodium bicarbonate. Toxicol Rev. 2005;24(3):195-204.
69. Seger DL, Hantsch C, Zavoral T, Wrenn K. Variability of recommendations for serum alkalinization in tricyclic antidepressant overdose: a survey of U.S. Poison Center medical directors. Toxicol Clin Toxicol. 2003;41(4):331-8.
70. Pierog JE, Kane KE, Kane BG, Donovan JW, Helmick T. Tricyclic antidepressant toxicity treated with massive sodium bicarbonate. Am J Emerg Med. 2009;27(9):1168.e3-7.
71. Chan BS, Buckley NA. Digoxin-specific antibody fragments in the treatment of digoxin toxicity. Clin Toxicol (Phila). 2014;52(8):824-36.
72. Eyer F, Steimer W, Müller C, Zilker T. Free and total digoxin in serum during treatment of acute digoxin poisoning with Fab fragments: case study. Am J Crit Care. 2010;19(4):387-91.
73. Hack JB. Cardioactive steroids. In: Nelson LS, Lewin NA, Howland MA, Hoffman R, Goldfrank L, Flomenbaum N (Eds). Goldfrank's Toxicologic Emergencies, 9th edition. New York: McGraw-Hill; 2011. p. 941.
74. Mauskopf JA, Wenger TL. Cost-effectiveness analysis of the use of digoxin immune Fab (ovine) for treatment of digoxin toxicity. Am J Cardiol. 1991;68(17):1709-14.
75. DiDomenico RJ, Walton SM, Sanoski CA, Bauman JL. Analysis of the use of digoxin immune Fab for the treatment of non-life-threatening digoxin toxicity. J Cardiovasc Pharmacol Ther. 2000;5(2):77-85.
76. Flanagan RJ, Jones AL. Fab antibody fragments: some applications in clinical toxicology. Drug Saf. 2004;27(14):1115-33.
77. Rumack BH, Wolfe RR, Gilfinch H. Phenytion (diphenylhydantoin) treatment of massive digoxin overdose. Br Heart J. 1974;36(4):405-8.
78. Weinberg GL, VadeBoncouer T, Ramaraju GA, Garcia-Amaro MF, Cwik MJ. Pretreatment or resuscitation with a lipid infusion shifts the dose-response to bupivicaine-induced asystole in rats. Anesthesiology. 1998;88(4):1071-5.
79. Bania TC, Chu J, Perez E, Su M, Hahn IH. Hemodynamic effects of intravenous fat emulsion in an animal model of severe verapamil toxicity resuscitated with atropine, calcium, and saline. Acad Emerg Med. 2007; 14(2):105-11.
80. Doepker B, Healy W, Cortez E, Adkins EJ. High-dose insulin and intravenous lipid emulsion therapy for cardiogenic shock induced by intentional calcium-channel blocker and beta-blocker overdose: a case series. J Emerg Med. 2014;46(4):486-90.
81. Liang CW, Diamond SJ, Hagg DS. Lipid rescue of massive verapamil overdose: a case report. J Med Case Rep. 2011;5:399.
82. Litz RJ, Roessel T, Heller AR, Stehr SN. Reversal of central nervous system and cardiac toxicity after local anesthetic intoxication bylined emulsion therapy. Anesth Analg. 2008;106(5):1575-7.
83. Kiberd M, Minor S. Lipid therapy for the treatment of a refractory amitriptyline overdose. CJEM. 2012;14(3):194-7.
84. Sirianni AJ, Osterhout KC, Callelo DP, Muller AA, Waterhouse MR, Goodkin MB, et al. Use of lipid emulsion in the resuscitation of a patient with prolonged cardiovascular collapse after overdose of buproprion and lamotrigine. Ann Emerg Med. 2008;51(4):412-5.
85. McAllister RK, Tutt CD, Colvin CS. Lipid 20% emulsion ameliorates the symptoms of olanzapine toxicity in a 4-year-old. Am J Emerg Med. 2012;30(6):1012.e1-2.
86. Weinbrg GL. Lipid emulsion infusion: resuscitation for local anesthetic and other drug overdose. Anesthesiology. 2012;117(1):180-7.
87. American College of Medical Toxicology. ACTM position statement: interim guidance for the use of lipid resuscitation therapy. J Med Toxicol. 2011;7(1):81-2.
88. American Society of Regional Anesthesia and Pain Medicine. (2014). Checklist for treatment of local anesthesia systemic toxicity. [online] Available from: https://www.asra.com/advisory-guidelines/article/3/checklist-for-treatment-of-local-anesthetic-systemic-toxicity. [Accessed April, 2016].
89. Taboulet P, Baud FJ, Bismuth C, Vicaut E. Acute digitalis intoxication—is pacing still appropriate? J Toxicol Clin Toxicol. 1993;31(2):261-73.
90. Sarubbi B, Ducceschi V, D'Antonello A, Liccardo B, Santangelo L, Iacono A. Atrial fibrillation: what are the effects of drug therapy on the effectiveness and complications of electrical cardioversion? Can J Cardiol. 1998;14(10):1267-73.
91. Taboulet P, Cariou, A, Berdeaux A, Bismuth C. Pathophysiology and management of self-poisoning with beta-blockers. J Toxicol Clin Toxicol. 1993;31(4):531-51.
92. Proudfoot AT, Krenzelok EP, Vale JA. Position paper on urinary alkalinization. J Toxicol Clin Toxicol. 2004;42(1):1-26.
93. Devin R, Garrett P, Anstey C. Managing cardiovascular collapse in severe flecainide overdose without recourse to extracorporeal therapy. Emerg Med Australas. 2007;19(2):155-9.

94. Van Reet B, Dens J. Auto-intoxication with flecainide and quinapril: ECG-changes, symptoms, and treatment. Acta Cardiol. 2006;61(6):669-72.
95. Lalonde RL, Deshpande R, Hamilton PP, McLean WM, Greenway DC. Acceleration of digoxin clearance by activated charcoal. Clin Pharmacol Ther. 1985;37(4):367-71.
96. Critchley JA, Critchley LA. Digoxin toxicity in chronic renal failure: treatment by multiple dose activated charcoal intestinal dialysis. Hum Exp Toxicol. 1997;16(12):733-5.
97. Position statement and practice guidelines on the use of multi-dose activated charcoal in the treatment of acute poisoning. American Academy of Clinical Toxicology and European Association of Poisons Centres and Clinical Toxicologists. J Toxicol Clin Toxicol. 1999;37(6):731-51.
98. Henderson RP, Solomon CP. Use of cholestyramine in the treatment of digoxin intoxication. Arch Intern Med. 1988;148(3):745-6.
99. Kessler C, Ng J, Valdez K, Xie H, Geiger B. The use of sodium polystyrene sulfonate in the inpatient management of hyperkalemia. J Hosp Med. 2011;6(3):136-40.
100. Roberge RJ, Martin TG, Schneider SM. Use of sodium polystyrene sulfonate in a lithium overdose. Ann Emerg Med. 1993;22(12):1911-5
101. Ries NL, Dart RC. New developments in antidotes. Med Clin N Am. 2005;89(6): 1379-97.
102. Ash SR, Levy H, Akmal M, Mankus RA, Sutton JM, Emery DR, et al. Treatment of severe tricyclic antidepressant overdose with extracorporeal sorbent detoxification. Adv Ren Replace Ther. 2002;9(1):31-41
103. Narayan R, Rizzo M, Cole M. Successful treatment of severe carbamazepine toxicity with 5% albumin-enhanced continuous venovenous hemodialysis. J Artif Organs. 2014;17(2):206-9.
104. Pichon N, Dugard A, Clavel M, Amiel JB, Francois B, Vignon P. Extracorporeal albumin dialysis in three cases of acute calcium channel blocker poisoning with life-threatening refractory cariogenic shock. Ann Emerg Med. 2012;59(6):540-4.
105. Belleflamme M, Hantson P, Gougnard T, Minon JM, Wittebole X, Laterre PF, et al. Survival despite extremely high plasma diltiazem level in a case of acute poisoning treated by the molecular-adsorbent recirculation system. Eur J Emerg Med. 2012;19(1):59-61.
106. Wittebole X, Hantson P. Use of the molecular adsorbent recirculating system (MARS) for the management of acute poisoning with or without liver failure. Clin Toxicol (Phila). 2011;49(9):782-93.
107. Bunchman TE, Ferris ME. Management of toxic ingestions with the use of renal replacement therapy. Pediatr Nephrol. 2011;26(4):535-41.
108. Korsheed S, Selby NM, Fluck RJ. Treatment of severe theophylline poisoning with the molecular adsorbent recirculating system (MARS). Nephrol Dial Transplant. 2007;22(3):969-70.

35 CHAPTER

Acute Pulmonary Embolism

Adam J Singer

INTRODUCTION

Venous thromboembolism (VTE) is a spectrum of diseases that begins with asymptomatic deep vein thrombosis (DVT) and can progress to fulminant and fatal pulmonary embolism (PE). Deep vein thrombosis is a condition in which a thrombus forms in one of the deep veins of the calf or thigh, such as the popliteal or femoral vein. While generally non-life-threatening, DVT can sometimes lead to PE which can be life-threatening, and results when a thrombus in a deep vein detaches from the vessel wall and travels as an embolus through the inferior vena cava into the right side of the heart, ultimately obstructing blood flow in the pulmonary arteries.

Autopsy studies have shown that PE is diagnosed prior to death in less than half of all patients.[1] In contrast, contemporary studies indicate that most patients diagnosed with a PE have a good prognosis when managed appropriately.[2] The evaluation of patients with suspected PE can be streamlined using clinical risk stratification, biomarkers such as D-dimer, and selective use of definitive tests such as a computed tomography (CT) pulmonary angiography.[3,4] Traditionally, PE was managed exclusively in the hospital using bridging therapy with a parenteral agent such as unfractionated heparin or low molecular weight heparin, followed by a prolonged course of an oral vitamin K antagonist. The development of PE risk stratification tools and novel oral anticoagulants have resulted in a paradigm shift whereby low risk patients may be considered for early discharge without the need for bridging therapy.[5] Additionally, recent studies have helped to clarify which patient subpopulations benefit most from more intensive therapy such as intravenous thrombolytics.

EPIDEMIOLOGY

According to the Centers for Disease Control and Prevention, it is estimated that VTE is the cause of approximately 100,000–300,000 deaths each year, which is more than the number of deaths attributed to breast cancer, human immunodeficiency virus, and traffic accidents combined.[6] The precise number of patients affected by VTE is not known. However, estimates range from 350,000 to 600,000, while modeling suggests greater than 900,000 people are affected by VTE annually.[7,8] Approximately 550,000 people are hospitalized annually in the United States with DVT and/or PE,[9] with annual healthcare costs up to $10 billion.[10]

Of patients diagnosed with PE, 10–30% of people will die within 1 month of diagnosis. Sudden death is the first symptom in about one-fourth (25%) of people who have a PE. Among people who have had a DVT, one-half will have long-term complications such as swelling, pain, discoloration, and scaling in the affected limb (the post-thrombotic syndrome). One-third of the people with DVT/PE will have a recurrence within 10 years. Approximately 5–8% of the United States population has one of several genetic risk factors, also known as inherited thrombophilias, in which a genetic defect can be identified that increases the risk for thrombosis.[10]

PATHOPHYSIOLOGY

Nearly all PEs arise from thrombi in the lower extremity or pelvic veins and the risk of embolization is higher with thrombi proximal to the calf veins. Venous thromboembolism results when there is an imbalance between prothrombotic and anticoagulant/fibrinolytic systems aimed at maintaining homeostasis. This generally occurs when one or more of the three components of Virchow's triad are involved—damage to the vessel wall, stasis, or hypercoagulability. Regardless of the underlying cause of pulmonary embolism, the clinical severity of pulmonary embolism in any individual patient is usually the result of acute pulmonary hypertension and determined by the size and location of the clot as well as the presence of patient comorbidities such as underlying cardiac or pulmonary disease. The severity of the PE cannot be predicted by the size of the clot alone.[11]

It is generally thought that development of acute pulmonary hypertension occurs with obstruction of greater than 30–50% of the pulmonary bed in otherwise healthy individuals.[12] A rise in pulmonary artery pressure leads to an increase in right ventricular afterload and right ventricular dilation resulting in right sided heart failure. A sudden drop in right ventricular cardiac output can also result in a subsequent drop in left ventricular output leading to syncope or even pulseless electrical activity and cardiac arrest in extreme cases. Activation of the sympathetic nervous system together with the Frank-Starling mechanism increases pulmonary artery pressure crucial to maintaining pulmonary and systemic circulation. The release of local and systemic mediators further contribute to pulmonary vasoconstriction and pulmonary hypertension. Respiratory insufficiency may develop as a result of a reduction in local or regional pulmonary blood flow leading to a mismatch of ventilation and perfusion (V/Q). In addition, low cardiac output leads to a low mixed venous oxygen saturation further contributing to pulmonary insufficiency. Loss of surfactant also leads to atelectasis and alveolar hypoventilation further contributing to V/Q mismatch.

RISK FACTORS

While PE may occur in patients with underlying conditions, many are unprovoked. Patient risk factors include age more than 60 years, personal history of VTE, active malignancy, or another disabling condition such as cardiac or respiratory failure, congenital or acquired coagulation disorders, hormonal replacement therapy, or oral contraception. The British Thoracic Society has classified the risk factors into major and minor ones based on their associated risks.[13] Risk factors for PE may also be classified based on whether they are permanent (such as age) or temporary (such as after major surgery or immobilization). A summary of risk factors is presented in table 1. Critically injured or ill patients are also at considerable risk of VTE. Immobility has often been cited as predictive of PE, however, risk may vary by type of immobility. Limb, whole body, or neurologic immobility, but not travel greater than 8 hours, were associated with a higher risk of PE.[14] A systematic review of epidemiologic and pathophysiologic studies about the association between travel and venous thrombosis (VT) concluded that long-distance travel increases the risk of VT approximately two- to fourfold.[15] The absolute risk of a symptomatic event within 4 weeks of flights longer than 4 hours was estimated to be 1/4,600 flights. The risk of severe PE occurring immediately after air travel increased with duration of travel, up to 4.8 per million in flights longer than 12 hours.[15]

CLINICAL PRESENTATION

Over the years, the clinical presentation of PE has drastically changed. Once frequently diagnosed only on

TABLE 1: Risk factors of venous thromboembolism

	Permanent	Temporary
Major	• Active malignancies • History of venous thromboembolism • Thrombophilias (factor V Leiden, protein C, S, antithrombin III deficiency)	• Postoperative state • Obstetrics • Lower limb fractures/ varicosities • Limited mobility
Mild	• Congenital heart disease • Heart failure • Hypertension • Superficial venous thrombosis • Chronic obstructive pulmonary disease • Latent malignancy • Obesity • Inflammatory bowel disease • Nephrotic syndrome • Chronic dialysis • Myeloproliferative diseases	• Central venous catheter • Estrogen use • Long distance travel

autopsy, thanks to widespread use of advanced testing and imaging, less severe cases are being diagnosed more frequently. The mortality rate in a large United States sample of 1,880 patients with confirmed PE enrolled at 22 emergency departments (EDs) was only 1% [95% confidence interval (CI), 0–1.6%].[2] Classically, patients present with sudden onset of shortness of breath, pleuritic chest pain, hemoptysis, and syncope. However, this presentation is quite rare. The most common symptoms at presentation were dyspnea at rest (50.1%), pleuritic chest pain (39.4%), dyspnea with exertion (27.0%), cough with hemoptysis (22.9%), and substernal chest pain (15.2%).[2] The most common physical findings were extremity swelling suggestive of DVT (23.5%), respiratory distress (16.4%), rales (8.4%), and diaphoresis (7.1%). Chest plain films were normal 40% of the time; the most common radiographic abnormalities were atelectasis (16.9%), pleural effusion (16.2%), infiltrate (13.5%), and cardiomegaly (11.9%).

A prospective study of 7,940 ED patients with suspected PE found that out of 25 potential predictor variables, only 3 were associated with VTE—noncancer related thrombophilia [odds ratio (OR) 1.99], pleuritic chest pain (OR 1.53), and family history of VTE (OR 1.51).[16] In contrast, the three variables that were associated with reduced risk of VTE were female gender (OR 0.60), current smoking (OR 0.60), and substernal chest pain (OR 0.60). Tachypnea (a respiratory rate >24 breath/min) and patient perception of dyspnea were also associated with VTE (OR 1.26 for both); however, the lower boundaries of the 95% CIs were 1.02 and 1.00, respectively.

PREDICTION RULES FOR PULMONARY EMBOLISM

Due to difficulty in diagnosing PE and the consequences of missing a PE, a large number of clinical prediction rules have been developed to help predict the risk of PE. The Pulmonary Embolism Rule Out Criteria (PERC) rule was developed by Kline et al to identify a low risk population that would have a very low mortality rate (<2%) in whom even a D-dimer would not be necessary.[17] A combination of gestalt estimate of low suspicion for PE, age less than 50, pulse less than 100 beats/min, oxygen saturation (SaO_2) more than or equal to 95%, no hemoptysis, no estrogen use, no surgery or trauma requiring hospitalization within 4 weeks, no prior VTE, and no unilateral leg swelling yielded a false-negative rate of only 1% (95% CI, 0.6–1.6%). Of all clinical prediction aids, the most commonly used are the ones based on Wells' criteria and the Geneva score.[18,19] A study by Klok et al. validated a simplified version of the Geneva score, which was found to be as accurate as the original score [the areas under the receiver-operating characteristic curve for a 3 level risk classification were 0.68 (95% CI, 0.64–0.72) and 0.70 (95% CI, 0.66–0.74), respectively].[20]

A summary of the Wells' score and the Revised Geneva score for PE is presented in table 2. An advantage of the Revised Geneva score is that it does not rely on practitioner gestalt, which is a major component of the Wells' score. Of note, the Wells' score was validated in patients admitted to the hospital while the Revised Geneva score was validated in ED patients with a PE prevalence greater than 20%, which is much higher than reported in most United States ED based studies. A recent study comparing clinical gestalt and a validated computer-derived method for estimating the pretest probability of PE found that clinicians overestimated pretest probability but on receiver operating curve analysis were as accurate as the computerized technique.[21]

DIAGNOSTIC APPROACH

Pulmomary embolism should be suspected in any patient presenting with dyspnea, chest pain, or shock without any other obvious cause. Patients who present hemodynamically stable should be classified based on one of a number of clinical prediction rules such as the Wells', Geneva, or Revised Geneva scores (Table 2). In patients at low to intermediate risk, a sensitive D-dimer (a fibrin degradation product) test should be ordered.[22] A normal D-dimer result in these patients essentially excludes pulmonary embolism since the risk of developing a PE within the next 3 months is only 0.14% (95% CI, 0.05–0.41).[23] Patients at high risk of PE, as well as those with low-to-intermediate risk with an elevated D-dimer (without an obvious cause for the elevation such as infection) should proceed to multidetector pulmonary computed tomography angiography (Flowchart 1).[23,24] Recent data suggest that the threshold for a positive D-dimer (generally 500 µg/L) should be raised by age ×10 for patients 50 years and older.[25]

TABLE 2: Clinical prediction rules for diagnosing pulmonary embolism

Wells' score for PE	
Previous PE or DVT	+1.5
Heart rate >100/min	+1.5
Recent surgery or immobilization	+1.5
Clinical signs of DVT	+3
Alternative diagnosis less likely than PE	+3
Hemoptysis	+1
Cancer	+1
PE unlikely if score ≤4 (3%)	
Revised Geneva score for PE	
Age >65	+1
Previous DVT or PE	+3
Surgery (under general anesthesia) or fracture (of lower limb) within 1 month	+2
Active malignancy (solid or hematological malignancy currently active or cured within 1 year)	+2
Unilateral leg pain	+3
Hemoptysis	+2
Heart rate 75–94/min	+3
Heart rate >95/min	+5
Pain on deep palpation in leg and unilateral edema	+4
0–3 points indicates low probability of PE (8%)	
4–10 points indicates intermediate probability of PE (28%)	
11 points or more indicates high probability of PE (74%)	

PE, pulmonary embolism; DVT, deep vein thrombosis.

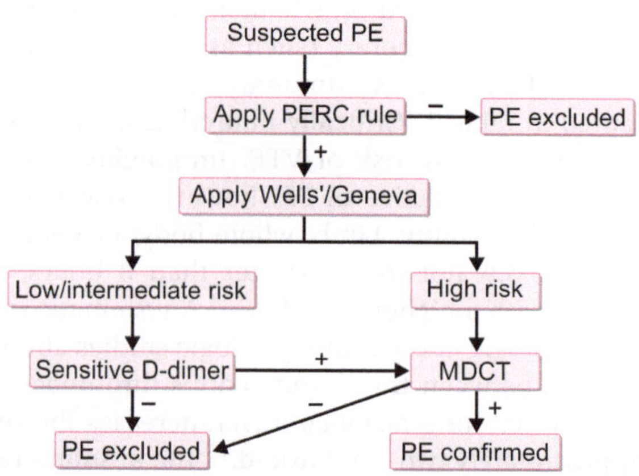

PE, pulmonary embolism;PERC, pulmonary embolism rule-out criteria;MDCT, multiple detector computed tomography.

FLOWCHART 1: Diagnostic approach in patients with suspected pulmonary embolism

When CT angiography is contraindicated (renal insufficiency or contrast allergy), ventilation-perfusion scanning or bilateral compression ultrasonography should be considered. The presence of a normal perfusion scan can be used to exclude PE, while the presence of a high probability V/Q scan or ultrasonographic finding of a DVT can be used to determine the need for anticoagulation in a patient with suspected PE. Magnetic resonance angiography should also be considered in patients with contraindications to CT pulmonary angiography.[26]

PULMOMARY EMBOLISM SEVERITY RISK STRATIFICATION

Clinical Scoring Systems

As with many other medical conditions, prognosis and management are best determined by assessing the patients' risk of adverse events. Identification of low risk patients may allow early discharge from the ED or hospital with standard treatment alone. In contrast, high-risk patients often require more aggressive therapies such as thrombolytics or embolectomy and are best managed in an intensive care setting. In some patients, such as those in shock or with severe respiratory distress, risk stratification is obvious. In others, a number of clinical scoring systems can be used to help classify patients into low- and high-risk groups.[27] The Pulmonary Embolism Severity Index (PESI) was developed and validated in over 16,000 patients.[28] In validation studies, a PESI score less than 66 predicted a 30-day mortality rate of less than 3%.[29] The simplified PESI (sPESI) score is a more simple score that can be used instead of the full PESI score to estimate risk.[30] The Geneva score may also be used (Table 3).[31]

Biomarkers

The presence of right ventricular strain, as evidenced by an elevation in either troponin I or T, brain natriuretic peptide (BNP), or N-terminal proBNP, helps identify a subset of patients at higher risk of mortality.[27] An elevated troponin level has been associated with a sevenfold increase in the rate of adverse events in patients with PE.[32] Elevations in BNP (>90 pg/mL) or proBNP (>900 pg/mL) have also been associated with a five- to seven-fold increase in the risk of adverse events.[33,34] While BNP or proBNP levels appear to be more predictive of risk than troponin levels, the combination of a natriuretic peptide with troponin has the highest predictive value of poor outcomes. The rates of PE-related death, all-cause death, and any serious adverse events were 0%, 0.2%, and 1.6%, respectively, in PE patients in whom both natriuretic peptides and troponin were within the normal range identifying a very low risk group that should be considered for standard therapy and outpatient management or early discharge.[35]

TABLE 3: Pulmonary embolism severity scoring systems

Variable	Score		
	PESI	sPESI	Geneva
Age >80 years	Age in years	1	–
Male sex	10	0	–
History of cancer	30	1	2
History of heart failure	10	1	1
History of chronic lung disease	10	1	–
Pulse ≥110 bpm	20	1	–
Systolic BP <100 mm Hg	30	1	2
Respiratory rate ≥30/min	20	0	–
Temperature <36°C	20	0	–
Altered mental status	60	0	–
SaO_2 <90%	20	1	1
Prior DVT	–	–	1
Current DVT	–	–	1
Low score	<66	0	<3

PESI, Pulmonary Embolism Severity Index; sPESI, simplified Pulmonary Embolism Severity Index; bpm, beats per minute; BP, blood pressure; SaO_2, arterial oxygen saturation; DVT, deep vein thrombosis.

Advanced Imaging

Other methods for assessing the presence of right ventricular strain, and thus the physiological consequences of PE, include echocardiography and CT pulmonary angiography.[36,37] A dilated or hypokinetic right ventricle or leftward shifting of the intraventricular septum towards the left ventricle on echocardiography are evidence for right ventricular strain and are associated with increased mortality.[38] Similarly, an elevated ratio of short axes of right ventricular diameter/left ventricular diameter on CT pulmonary angiography (Fig. 1), as well as inferior vena cava (IVC) contrast reflux, suggests right ventricular strain.

MANAGEMENT OF PULMONARY EMBOLISM

Patients with confirmed PE as well as those at high risk of PE should be immediately started on anticoagulation therapy, even prior to confirmation.[5,39] Options for initial therapy include intravenous unfractionated heparin (80 U/kg bolus followed by a continuous drip of 18 U/kg adjusted to achieve a partial thromboplastin time of 1.5–2 times normal), subcutaneous low molecular weight heparin (1 mg/kg enoxaparin every 12 h), or one of the novel oral anticoagulants (NOACs). Concomitant initiation of therapy with an oral vitamin K antagonist (e.g., warfarin at a dose of 2–10 mg/day) should occur in patients

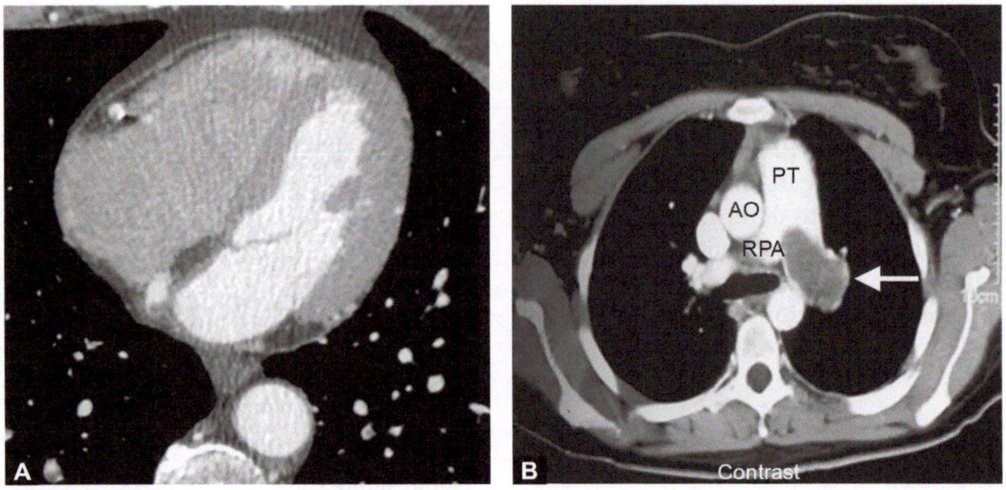

FIG. 1: Computed tomography pulmonary angiography **A,** Evidence of right ventricular overload; **B,** Image of central pulmonary embolism
Courtesy: Dr Michael Poon.

treated with heparin. Hemodynamically unstable patients and those with significant right ventricular strain should probably be started on unfractionated heparin since its effects can be rapidly reversed when the heparin drip is discontinued. Use of unfractionated heparin also does not preclude more advanced therapies such as thrombolytics or embolectomy. Patients at high risk of bleeding should also probably be started on unfractionated heparin (if the benefits of anticoagulation outweigh the risks of bleeding) since the effects of unfractionated heparin wear off rapidly when discontinued if significant bleeding ensues. Patients with significant renal impairment should be treated with unfractionated heparin. According to the American College of Clinical Pharmacy (ACCP) guidelines, patients with active cancer should be treated with low molecular weight heparin.[5] Low risk PE patients can be started on either a low molecular weight heparin together with a vitamin K antagonist such as warfarin or one of the novel oral anticoagulants. When using warfarin, bridging therapy with low molecular weight heparin should be continued until a therapeutic International Normalized Ratio (INR) of 2–3 is achieved and maintained for at least 24 hours.[5] With the oral factor Xa inhibitors rivaroxaban and apixaban, no bridging or lead in therapy with heparin is required.[40,41] In contrast, both dabigatran (an oral thrombin inhibitor) and edoxaban (an oral factor Xa inhibitor) require lead in therapy with heparin.[42,43] The advantages of the novel oral agents are their predictable pharmacokinetic and pharmacodynamic properties that result in rapid onset (within 1–4 h), a relatively short half-life (generally under 12 h), no food-drug interactions, and fewer drug-drug interactions than warfarin. The novel agents also do not require routine therapeutic monitoring. A summary of the NOAC trials is presented in table 4. In general, the NOACs are noninferior at preventing recurrent venothrombotic events and have a greater safety profile (lower risk of major life-threatening bleeds) than traditional therapy with heparin and warfarin. A pooled meta-analysis concluded that the NOACs were noninferior to enoxaparin/vitamin K antagonist (VKA) [relative risk (RR) 0.91 (95% CI, 0.79–1.06)] and had superior safety [RR 0.59 (95% CI, 0.41–0.87)].[44] Another meta-analysis concluded that the combination of unfractionated heparin/VKA had inferior efficacy compared to all other therapies and less bleeding was noted with rivaroxaban/apixaban.[45] Selection of a specific NOAC should be based on patient and physician preferences (e.g., once vs. twice daily administration) as well as local availability and coverage.

While more expensive, NOACs may be cost effective due to a reduction in costs associated with parenteral administration of heparin, routine monitoring of INR, and management of major bleeding episodes. Contra-indications to the NOACs include hemodynamic instability, significant hepatic or renal impairment, pregnancy and the concomitant use of combined P-glycoprotein, and strong inducers or inhibitors of the cytochrome CYP3A4 isoenzymes. Patients with contraindications to anticoagulation (such as active pathological bleeding or recent hemorrhagic stroke) as well as those who have failed anticoagulation should be considered candidates for placement of an IVC filter.[5,46] Patients with a reversible cause of PE should be treated for at least 3–6 months while those with a permanent risk factor or with unprovoked PE should receive extended therapy with an anticoagulant as long as the risk benefit ratio favors treatment.[5] Frequent reevaluations will be required to determine whether the risk benefit ratio changes over time.

A Cochrane review of eight trials with a total of 679 patient that compared thrombolytics with heparin to

TABLE 4: Comparison of novel oral anticoagulant trials

	Rivaroxaban	Dabigatran	Apixaban	Edoxaban
Name of study	**EINSTEIN**	**RECOVER**	**AMPLIFY**	**HOKUSAI**
Study design	Open label	Double blind	Double blind	Double blind
No. of patients	8,281	2,539	5,244	8,240
Lead in heparin	No	Yes	No	Yes
No. of daily doses	Twice daily × 21 days then once daily	Twice daily	Twice daily	Once daily
Efficacy	Noninferior	Noninferior	Noninferior	Noninferior, superior with right ventricular dysfunction
Safety	Less major bleeds	Less total bleeds	Less major bleeds	Less major bleeds
Lowest creatinine clearance	30 mL/min	30 mL/min	25 mL/min	30 mL/min
Duration	3, 6, 12 months	6 months	6 months	3–12 months
FDA approved	Yes	Yes	Yes	Yes

heparin alone in patients with acute PE found similar rates of death [odds ratio (OR) 0.89 (95% CI, 0.45–1.78)], recurrence of PE [OR 0.63 (95% CI, 0.33–1.20)], and major bleeding [OR 1.61 (9% CI, 0.91–2.86)].[47] As a result, the use of thrombolytics is not recommended for low risk patients. Whether all patients with small subsegmental PE should be anticoagulated is the subject of intense debate.[48] However, a study comparing the outcomes of patients with symptomatic subsegmental and more proximal PE demonstrated similar VTE recurrence rates and mortality.[49]

Management of High- and Intermediate-risk Pulmonary Embolism

High-risk PE is characterized by overt hemodynamic instability warranting immediate aggressive therapy with heparin and consideration of fibrinolysis.[5] A prospective observational study of 1,875 patients, of whom 58 (3.1%) had massive PE found that mortality was fourfold higher in patients with massive PE, yet only 12% received fibrinolytic therapy suggesting poor adherence to guidelines.[50] Importantly, mortality was lower in those patients with massive PE who received fibrinolytics compared to those treated with heparin alone (2.6% vs. 14%, p <0.001).

While most experts agree that thrombolytics should be given to hemodynamically unstable patients,[5] there is considerable debate regarding its use in patients with right ventricular dysfunction. A recent randomized controlled trial (RCT) of 1,006 patients with intermediate-risk PE (normotensive patients with right ventricular dysfunction on echocardiography or CT together with a positive troponin) found that fibrinolytic therapy with tenecteplase prevented hemodynamic decompensation but increased the risk of major stroke compared with heparin alone, further complicating the decision to initiate thrombolytic therapy in massive PE.[51] A subsequent

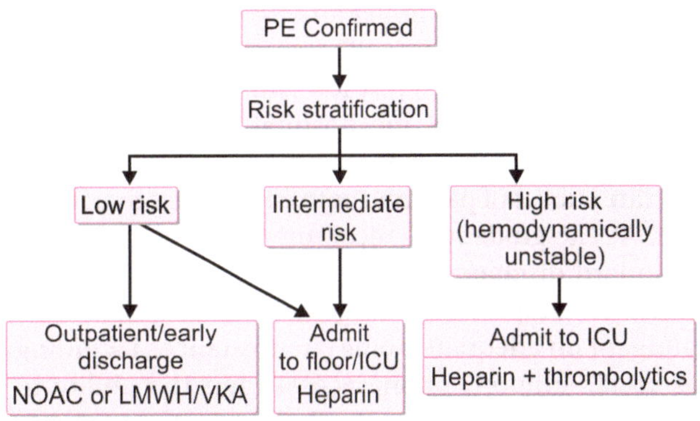

PE, pulmonary embolism; ICU, intensive care unit; NOAC, novel oral anticoagulants; LMWH, low molecular weight heparins; VKA, vitamin K antagonists.

FLOWCHART 2: Therapeutic approach to patients with confirmed pulmonary embolism

meta-analysis of 11 studies with 1,833 patients found that the number needed to harm (27 to cause one major bleeding) outweighed the number needed to treat (125 to prevent one fatality).[52] As a result, thrombolytics should not be given to intermediate high risk PE unless there is hemodynamic deterioration.[53] Flowchart 2 summarizes a proposed therapeutic approach to patients with acute PE.

OUTPATIENT MANAGEMENT OF PULMOMARY EMBOLISM

Outpatient management of low risk PE patients offers many potential advantages over hospital admission including a reduction in hospital admissions, substantial cost savings, an improvement in health-related quality of life, and an increase in physical activity and social functioning. Considerable evidence supports outpatient management of patients with DVT. In contrast, the evidence supporting outpatient management or early discharge of patients with low risk PE is less compelling.[54]

A single RCT of 339 low risk PE patients compared outpatient treatment with enoxaparin 1 mg/kg twice daily (n = 171) to similar inpatient treatment (n = 168).[55] All participants also received an oral VKA. There were no significant differences between the groups in 30-day mortality [RR 0.33 (95% CI, 0.01–7.98), p = 0.49], 90-day mortality [RR 0.98 (95% CI, 0.06–15.58), p = 0.99], major bleeding within 14 days [RR 4.91 (95% CI, 0.24–101.57), p = 0.30], and major bleeding within 90 days [RR 6.88, (95% CI, 0.36–134.14), p = 0.20]. One death due to pneumonia and cancer occurred at day 17 in the inpatient group, while one death due to trauma-related aortic rupture occurred at day 34 in the outpatient group. Another meta-analysis of 3 studies including 1,657 patients discharged within 24 hours found a pooled incidence of recurrent VTE of 1.7% in outpatients, 1.1% in patients discharged between 24 and 72 hours after admission, and 1.2% in inpatients.[56] The pooled incidence of major bleeding and mortality were also similar among the groups. While roughly half of all low risk PE patients in Canada are managed as outpatients,[57] very few United States patients are managed outside of the hospital.[2] The availability of the NOACs has made outpatient management in the appropriate subset of patients more convenient than ever. Current ACCP guidelines recommend early discharge over standard discharge (grade 2B) in appropriately low risk patients.[5] Outpatient management or early discharge is contingent on adequate home circumstances including strong social support, phone access, and the ability to return to the hospital promptly. Patients with comorbid illnesses requiring hospitalization, active or high risk of bleeding, severe hypertension, catheter associated thromboembolism, recent surgery, morbid obesity, hypercoagulable state, or pregnancy should be admitted for standard inpatient treatment. Patients without significant pain or discomfort, normal blood pressure and oxygen saturation, and without thrombocytopenia, severe liver or kidney disease may all be candidates for outpatient therapy. A PESI score of less than 66, a sPESI score of 0, normal troponin and BNP levels, and no evidence of right sided heart strain on CT or echocardiography further support outpatient management. If patients are to be discharged from the ED, adequate follow-up with a primary care physician or a physician specializing in VTE within a timely period must be arranged for as well as an adequate supply of medications. Patients should be told to return immediately to the hospital if they are short of breath, dizzy, have severe pain, or any evidence of bleeding.

MANAGEMENT OF BLEEDING EPISODES IN PATIENTS RECEIVING ANTICOAGULATION

Patients with minor bleeds (such as epistaxis and mild menorrhagia) may not require any adjustments in their anticoagulation. In contrast, patients with life-threatening bleeding will require local measures to control bleeding and supportive care including hemodynamic resuscitation, fluid and blood product resuscitation, and surgical or advanced radiological interventions such as arterial embolization. In patients on an oral VKA with major bleeding (such as intracranial hemorrhage or life-threatening gastro-intestinal or retroperitoneal bleeding) the ACCP recommends 4-factor prothrombin complex concentrate (PCC) in addition to vitamin K 10 mg intravenously (although the latter may take 6–24 hours to be effective).[5] The management of patients on NOACs is unclear; while dabigatran is dialyzable, other NOACs are not a specific antidote for dabigatran has recently been approved.[58] While the evidence for 4-factor PCC, as well as other agents such as 3-factor PCC, activated PCC, or recombinant factor VIIa is weak, 4-factor PCC should be strongly considered with life-threatening bleeding.[59,60] Ongoing trials are currently evaluating several specific antidotes for the various NOACs.

PREVENTION OF PULMOMARY EMBOLISM

As always, prevention of PE is preferred to management of already established PE. For patients undergoing total hip or knee replacement thromboprophylaxis with warfarin, heparins (low molecular weight heparin or low-dose unfractionated heparin two or three times daily), fondaparinux (2.5 mg/day), or one of the NOACs is both safe and effective.[61] Venous thromboembolism prophylaxis with one of the above treatment should also be used for a minimum of 10–14 days in moderate and high-risk medical patients (e.g., heart failure, respiratory failure, and sepsis) admitted to the hospital.[5,62]

CONCLUSION

Pulmonary embolism is still a common and potentially fatal disease. The availability of clinical prediction rules that help predict the likelihood of PE as well as the risk of complications in patients with confirmed PE allow a systematic approach to diagnosing and managing PE. The introduction of novel oral anticoagulants has further simplified the treatment of PE, especially in patients suitable for outpatient management. An antidote to one of these agents is already approved with further agents in development.

REFERENCES

1. Pineda LA, Hathwar VS, Grant BJ. Clinical suspicion of fatal pulmonary embolism. Chest. 2001;120:791-5.
2. Pollack CV, Schreiber D, Goldhaber SZ, Slattery D, Fanikos J, O'Neil BJ, et al. Clinical characteristics, management, and outcomes of patients diagnosed with acute pulmonary embolism in the emergency department: initial report of

EMPEROR (Multicenter Emergency Medicine Pulmonary Embolism in the Real World Registry). J Am Coll Cardiol. 2011;57:700-6.

3. Goldhaber SZ, Bounameaux H. Pulmonary embolism and deep vein thrombosis. Lancet. 2012;379:1835-46.
4. Agnelli G, Becattini C. Acute pulmonary embolism. N Engl J Med. 2010;363:266-74.
5. Kearon C, Akle EA, Comerota AJ, Prandoni P, Bounameaux H, Goldhaber SZ, et al. Antithrombotic therapy for VTE disease: Antithrombotic therapy and prevention of thrombosis, 9th ed: American College of Chest Physicians Evidence-Based Clinical Practice Guidelines. Chest. 2012;141(2 Suppl):e419S-e496S.
6. Centers for Disease Control and Prevention. Available from: http://www.cdc.gov/ncbddd/dvt/data.html [Accessed January 5, 2015].
7. Heit JA. The epidemiology of venous thromboembolism in the community. Arterioscler Thromb Vasc Biol. 2008;28:370-2.
8. Cohen AT, Agnelli G, Anderson FA, Arcelus JI, Bergqvist D, Brecht JG, et al. Venous thromboembolism (VTE) in Europe. The number of VTE events and associated morbidity and mortality. Thromb Haemost. 2007;98(4):756-64.
9. Centers for Disease Control and Prevention. Venous thromboembolism in adult hospitalizations—United States, 2007–2009. MMWR Morb Mortal Wkly Rep. 2012;61(22):401-4.
10. Beckman MG, Hooper WC, Critchley SE, Ortel TL. Venous thromboembolism: a public health concern. Am J Prev Med. 2010;38(4 Suppl):S495-501.
11. Kline JA, Zeitouni R, Hernandez-Nino J, Rose GA. Size isn't everything. J Thromb Haemost. 2008;6:397-399.
12. McIntyre KM, Sasahara AA. The hemodynamic response to pulmonary embolism in patients without prior cardiopulmonary disease. Am J Cardiol. 1971;28:288-94.
13. British Thoracic Society Standards of Care Committee Pulmonary Embolism Guideline Development Group. British Thoracic Society guidelines for the management of suspected acute pulmonary embolism. Thorax. 2003;58:470-83.
14. Beam DM, Courtney DM, Kabrhel C, Moore CL, Richman PB, Kline JA. Risk of thromboembolism varies, depending on category of immobility in outpatients. Ann Emerg Med. 2009;54:147-52.
15. Kuipers S, Schreijer AJ, Cannegieter SC, Büller HR, Rosendaal FR, Middeldorp S. Travel and venous thrombosis: a systematic review. J Intern Med. 2007;262(6):615-34.
16. Courtney DM, Kline JA, Kabrhel C, Moore CL, Smithline HA, Nordenholz KE, et al. Clinical features from the history and physical examination that predict the presence or absence. Ann Emerg Med. 2010;55:307-15.
17. Kline JA, Courtney DM, Kabrhel C, Moore CL, Smithline HA, Plewa MC, et al. Prospective multicenter evaluation of the pulmonary embolism rule-out criteria. J Thromb Haemost. 2008;6:772-80.
18. Wells PS, Anderson DR, Rodger M, Ginsberg JS, Kearon C, Gent M, et al. Derivation of a simple clinical model to categorize patients probability of pulmary embolism: increasing the models utility with SimpliRED D-dimer. Thromb Haemost. 2000;83:416-20.
19. Le Gal G, Righini M, Roy PM, Sanchez O, Aujesky D, Bounameaux H, et al. Prediction of pulmonary embolism in the emergency department: the revised Geneva score. Ann Int Med. 2006;144:165-71.
20. Klok FA, Mos IC, Nijkeuter M, Righini M, Perrier A, Le Gal G, et al. Simplification of the revised Geneva score for assessing clinical probability of pulmonary embolism. Arch Intern Med. 2008;168(19):2131-6.
21. Kline JA, Stubblefield WB. Clinician gestalt estimate of pretest probability of acute coronary syndrome and pulmonary embolism in patients with chest pain and dyspnea. Ann Emerg Med. 2014;63:275-80.
22. Carrier M, Righini M, Djurabi RK, Huisman MV, Perrier A, Wells PS, et al. VIDAS D-dimer in combination with clinical pre-test probability to rule out pulmonary embolism - A systematic review of management outcome studies. Thromb Haemost. 2009;101:886-92.
23. Agnelli G, Becattini C. Acute pulmonary embolism. N Engl J Med. 2010; 363:266-74.
24. Goldhaber SZ, Bounameaux H. Pulmonary embolism and deep vein thrombosis. Lancet. 2012;379:1835-46.
25. Righini M, Van Es J, Den Exeter PL, Roy PM, Verschuren F, Ghuysen A, et al. Age-adjusted D-dimer cutoff levels to rule out pulmonary embolism: The ADJUST-PE study. JAMA. 2014;311:1117-24.
26. Ersoy H, Goldhaber SZ, Cai T, Luu T, Rosebrook J, Mulkern R, et al. Time-resolve MR angiography: a primary screening examination in patients with suspected pulmonary embolism and contraindications to administration of iodinated contrast material. Am J Roentgenol. 2007;188:1245-54.
27. Kline JA, Miller DW. Risk stratification for acute pulmonary embolism. J Natl Compr Canc Netw. 2011;9:800-10.
28. Aujesku D, Obrosky DS, Stone AA, Auble TE, Perrier A, Cornuz J, et al. Derivation and validation of a prognostic model for pulmonary embolism. Am J Crit Care Med. 2005;172:1041-6.
29. Chan CM, Woods C, Shorr AF. The validation and reproducibility of the pulmonary embolism severity index. J Thromb Haemost. 2010;8:1509-14.
30. Jiminez D, Aujesky D, Moores L, Gómez V, Lobo JL, Uresandi F, et al. Simplification of the pulmonary embolism severity index for prognostication in patients with acute symptomatic pulmonary embolism. Arch Intern Med. 2010;170:1383-9.
31. Wicki J, Perrier A, Perneger TV, Bounameaux H, Junod AF. Predicting adverse outcome in patients with acute pulmonary embolism: a risk score. Thromb Haemost. 2000;84:548-52.
32. Bova C, Pesavento R, Marchiori A, Palla A, Enea I, Pengo V, et al. Risk stratification and outcomes in hemodynamically stable patients with acute pulmonary embolism. A prospective, muticentre, cohort study with three months follow up. J Thromb Haemost. 2009;7:938-44.
33. Klok FA, Mos IC, Huisman MV. Brain-type natriuretic peptide levels in the prediction of adverse outcome in patients with pulmonary embolism: a systematic review and meta-analysis. Am J Respir Crit Care Med. 2008;178:425-30.
34. Sanchez O, Trinquart L, Colombet I, Durieux P, Huisman MV, Chatellier G, et al. Prognostic value of right ventricular dysfunction in patients with haemodynamically stable pulmonary embolism: a systematic review. Eur Heart J. 2008;29:1569-77.
35. Lega JC, Lacasse Y, Lakhal L, Provencher S. Natriuretic peptides and troponins in pulmonary embolism: a meta-analysis. Thorax. 2009;64:869-875.
36. Kucher N, Rossi E, De RM, Goldhaber SZ. Pronostic role of echocardiography among patients with acute pulmonary embolism and a systolic arterial pressure of 90 mmHg or higher. Arch Intern Med. 2005;165:1777-81.
37. Subramaniam RM, Mandrekar J, Chang C, , Blair D, Gilbert K, Peller PJ, et al. Pulmonary embolism outcome: a prospective evaluation of CT pulmonary clot burden score and ECG score. Am J Roentgenol. 2008;190:1599-1604.
38. Khemasuwan D, Yingchoncharoen T, Tunsupon P, Kusunose K, Moghekar A, Klein A, et al. Right ventricular echocardiographic parameters are associated with mortality after acute pulmonary embolism. J Am Soc Echocardiogr. 2015;28(3):355-62.
39. Kline JA, Mrchick MR, Khrhel C, Courtney, DM. Prospective study of the frequency and outcomes of patients with suspected pulmonary embolism administered heparin prior to confirmatory imaging. Thromb Res. 2012;129:e25-e28.
40. EINSTEIN–PE Investigators, Büller HR, Prins MH, Lensin AW, Decousus H, Jacobson BF, et al. Oral rivaroxaban for the treatment of symptomatic pulmonary embolism. N Engl J Med. 2012;366(14):1287-97.
41. Agnelli G, Buller HR, Cohen A, Curto M, Gallus AS, Johnson M, et al; AMPLIFY Investigators. Oral apixaban for the treatment of acute venous thromboembolism. N Engl J Med. 2013;369(9):799-808.
42. Schulman S, Kearon C, Kakkar AK, Mismetti P, Schellong S, Eriksson H, et al; RE-COVER Study Group. Dabigatran versus warfarin in the treatment of acute venous thromboembolism. N Engl J Med. 2009;361(24):2342-52.
43. Hokusai-VTE Investigators, Büller HR, Décousus H, Grosso MA, Mercuri M, Middeldorp S, et al. Edoxaban versus warfarin for the treatment of symptomatic venous thromboembolism. N Engl J Med. 2013;369(15):1406-15.
44. Hirschl M, Kundi M. New oral anticoagulants in the treatment of acute venous thromboembolism—a systematic review with indirect comparisons. Vasa. 2014;43(5):353-64.
45. Castellucci LA, Cameron C, Le Gal G, Rodger MA, Coyle D, Wells PS, et al. Clinical and safety outcomes associated with treatment of acute venous thromboembolism: a systematic review and meta-analysis. JAMA. 2014;312(11):1122-35.
46. Dalen JE, Stein PD. Are vena cava filters effective in the treatment of pulmonary embolism? Am J Med. 2013;126:851-2.
47. Dong BR, Hao Q, Yue J, Wu T, Liu GJ. Thrombolytic therapy for pulmonary embolism. Cochrane Database Syst Rev. 2009;(3):CD004437.
48. Den Exter PL, Van Roosmalen MJ, Van Den Hoven P, Klok FA, Monreal M, Jiminez D, et al. Physician's management approach to an incidental pulmonary embolism: an international survey. J Throm Haemost. 2013; 11:208-13.

49. Den Exter PL, van Es J, Klok FA, Kroft LJ, Kruip MJ, Kamphuisen PW, et al. Risk profile and clinical outcome of symptomatic subsegmental acute pulmonary embolism. Blood. 2013;122:1144-9.
50. Lin BW, Schreiber DH, Liu G, Briese B, Hiestand B, Slattery D, et al. Therapy and outcomes in massive pulmonary embolism in the real world registry. Am J Emerg Med. 2012;30:1774-81.
51. Meyer G, Vicaut E, Danays T, Agnelli G, Becattini C, et al. Fibrinolysis for patients with intermediate-risk pulmonary embolism. N Eng J Med. 2014;370:1402-11.
52. Riera-Mestre A, Becattinin C, Giustozzi M, Agnelli G. Thrombolysis in hemodynamically stable patients with acute pulmonary embolism: a meta-analysis. Thromb Res. 2014;311:2414-21.
53. Klok FA, Huisman MV. Thrombolysis for hemodynamically stable pulmonary embolism: time to close the book? Thromb Res. 2104;134:1169-70.
54. Yoo HH, Queluz TH, El Dib R. Outpatient versus inpatient treatment for acute pulmonary embolism. Cochrane Database Syst Rev. 2014;(11):CD010019.
55. Aujesky D, Roy PM, Verschuren F, Righini M, Osterwalder J, Egloff M, et al. Outpatient versus inpatient treatment for patients with acute pulmonary embolism: an international open-label, randomized, non-inferiority trial. Lancet. 2011;378:41-8.
56. Zodag W, Kooima J, Klok FA, Dekkers OM, Huisman MV. Outpatient versus inpatient treatment in patients with pulmonary embolism: a meta-analysis. Eur Respir J. 2013;42(1):134-44.
57. Baglin T. Fifty percent of patients with pulmonary embolism can be treated as outpatients. J Thromb Haemost. 2010;8:2404-5.
58. Pollack CV Jr, Reilly PA, van Ryn J, et al. Idarucizumab for dabigatran reversal--Full cohort analysis. N Engl J Med. 2017;377:431-41.
59. Veltkamp R, Horstmann S. Treatment of intracerebral hemorrhage associated with new oral anticoagulant use: the neurologist's view. Clin Lab Med. 2014;34(3):587-94.
60. Majeed A, Schulman S. Bleeding and antidotes in new oral anticoagulants. Best Pract Res Clin Haematol. 2013;26(2):191-202.
61. Chan NC, Siegal D, Lauw MN, Ginsberg JS, Eikelboom JW, Guyatt GH, et al. A systematic review of contemporary trials of anticoagulants in orthopaedic thromboprophylaxis: suggestions for a radical reappraisal. J Thromb Thrombolysis. 2015 Aug;40(2):231-9.
62. Dentali F, Douketis JD, Gianni M, Lim W, Crowther MA. Meta-analysis: anticoagulant prophylaxis to prevent symptomatic venous thromboembolism in hospitalized medical patients. Ann Intern Med. 2007;146:278-88.

36 CHAPTER

Kidney Injury in the Face of Heart Disease

Nicholas W Wettersten, Sutton R Fox

INTRODUCTION

The importance of the interaction between the heart and kidney has been known for more than 25 years.[1] Each organ is vital to the other's appropriate functioning. While the kidney maintains homeostasis of electrolytes, acid-base, and fluid balance, which all have direct impact on cardiac function, the heart provides adequate renal perfusion and influences intrarenal hemodynamics. This interaction is involved in multiple cardiac diseases including hypertension, coronary artery disease (CAD), and heart failure (HF).

During the management of these cardiac conditions, acute kidney injury (AKI) can occur with significant implications on outcomes. Acute kidney injury can arise from contrast induced nephropathy during cardiac catheterization, inflammatory and hemodynamic factors during cardiac surgery, and by the complex pathophysiology of cardiorenal syndrome during treatment of acute decompensated heart failure (AHF). Diagnosis of AKI is based on measurement of serum creatinine, but novel biomarkers are being studied that may change the diagnostic criteria and management of AKI. These novel biomarkers are greatly needed, as major goals of management are prevention and early recognition. The focus of this chapter is on the impact and potential management of acute kidney dysfunction in cardiac diseases, many of which are acute cardiac disorders, but this chapter will also touch on the relevance of chronic kidney disease in the management of cardiac disease.

INCIDENCE AND PROGNOSIS

The incidence and implications of AKI in heart disease vary based on the cardiac condition being treated, procedure being performed, and the pathophysiologic processes involved. However, regardless of the cardiac disease or the cause of AKI, AKI has repeatedly been shown to increase morbidity and mortality.[2-5] In a meta-analysis of hospitalized patients who developed AKI, long-term mortality was 2.6 times greater and myocardial infarction (MI) was 2.2 times greater compared to patients who did not have AKI.[2] In addition, the incidence of developing chronic kidney disease (CKD) and end-stage renal disease (ESRD) were 7.8 events/100 patient-years and 4.9 events/100 patient-years in patients with AKI, respectively.[2] Specific cardiac conditions in which AKI is commonly encountered include acute coronary syndromes (ACS), cardiac catheterization, cardiac surgery, and during treatment of AHF.

Acute Coronary Syndrome

The exact incidence of AKI in ACS is unknown because of a variety of different definitions of AKI used in studies as well as the heterogeneity in clinical presentation of ACS. The incidence has been reported to be anywhere from 5 to 55%.[6] Based on reports from registries, single center studies, and retrospective review of ACS trials, the incidence is more likely close to between 15 and 20%,[7-10] though this may be an underestimate because of an underappreciation of AKI events.

Although the exact incidence of AKI in ACS is unknown, kidney injury in ACS is clearly associated with increased morbidity and mortality.[6-8,10] With increasing severity of AKI, inhospital mortality also increases. In an analysis of almost 60,000 patients in the Acute Coronary Treatment and Intervention Outcomes Network (ACTION) registry, the rates of inhospital mortality were 6.6%, 14.2%, and 31.8% for patients with mild, moderate, and severe AKI, respectively, compared to 2.1% in patients without AKI.[7] Mild, moderate, and severe AKI were found to have odd ratios of 2.4, 4.5, and 12.6, respectively, for inhospital mortality.[7] Inhospital complications and bleeding are increased in patients with AKI.[7,11] Acute kidney injury in ACS also increases long-term mortality.[9,12] An important factor to be considered is whether the AKI is transient or persistent. Patients with transient AKI have an intermediate risk of mortality while those with persistent AKI experience the highest mortality.[8,13] Acute kidney injury also contributes to long-term renal dysfunction, CKD, and ESRD.[13,14]

Cardiac Catheterization and Cardiac Surgery

Potential causes of AKI in ACS are the cardiac procedures performed for management including cardiac catheterization with percutaneous coronary intervention (PCI) and cardiac surgery. The most common and recognized cause of AKI after cardiac catheterization is contrast induced nephropathy. The incidence of contrast induced nephropathy has been reported to occur in between 3.3 and 18.7% of cardiac catheterizations.[4,9,15-18] This broad incidence range is a result of varying populations studied and different definitions used to define contrast induced AKI. Contrast induced nephropathy has also been linked to a doubling of adverse events and a 2–5 times higher short- and long-term mortality.[4,13,15,19] Even after controlling for confounders and competing comorbidities, which are frequently present in patients who develop contrast induced nephropathy, contrast induced nephropathy is still associated with an increased rate of death.[15,20]

A less common cause of AKI during cardiac catheterization, which can also occur after cardiac surgery, is atheroembolism. This process is likely under-recognized as it usually presents subacutely a week or later after cardiac catheterization or surgery. In a study of over 1,700 patients undergoing cardiac catheterization, 0.9% developed kidney dysfunction from atheroembolism.[21] The inhospital mortality was markedly higher (16%) in patients with atheroemboli than in those without (0.5%).[21]

Acute kidney injury after cardiac surgery has a very high incidence; 30–50% of patients develop postoperative AKI, depending on the definition of AKI used and cardiac procedure performed.[3,22-24] Coronary artery bypass grafting tends to have the lowest incidence, while valvular and combined surgeries have higher incidences.[25] Acute kidney injury in the setting of cardiac surgery is associated with significant morbidity and mortality. Mortality varies based on the severity of AKI, but if patients require dialysis, mortality has been reported as high as 60–70%.[23] Risk of inhospital mortality can increase 3–18-fold based on severity of AKI.[23] Long-term mortality increases as well, with a similar increase in mortality rate based on the severity of AKI, regardless of whether the AKI resolves during the hospital stay or not.[24] Patients with AKI suffer more often from postoperative infections and are at increased risk to develop CKD.[23,24]

Heart Failure

The heart and kidneys have a special and important interaction in HF. Both underlying renal dysfunction and AKI are common in HF patients. Between 20 and 57% of patients with chronic HF and 30–67% of patients with AHF have CKD.[26] Acute kidney injury develops in 18–40% of patients hospitalized for AHF; the different diagnostic criteria used in studies partially explains this variability in incidence.[26] A large meta-analysis by Damman et al. in 2014 looked at the incidence and prognosis of CKD and AKI in HF.[5] The prevalence of CKD and AKI was 32% over 57 studies and 23% over 28 studies, respectively.[5] The significant prevalence of CKD and AKI emphasizes the importance of evaluating renal function in patients with HF.

There is little debate about the impact of CKD on morbidity and mortality in both acute and chronic HF. In the Damman et al. meta-analysis, having CKD yielded an odds ratio of 2.34 [95% confidence interval (CI) 2.20–2.50] for all-cause mortality (with no publication bias found).[5] The association between CKD and mortality has been seen in studies of both acute and chronic HF.[27,28] Chronic kidney disease has also been associated with increased length of hospital stay and risk of HF hospitalization.[29-32] As might be expected, patients with CKD are at increased risk of developing AKI.

The impact of AKI on morbidity and mortality in AHF has become an area of debate. Though the term "acute kidney injury" is commonly used to describe a rise in serum creatinine (and this term will continue to be used in the text), the classic pathophysiologic changes associated with renal injury have not been clearly shown to occur in AHF.[33] The term worsening renal function (WRF) is often favored to describe a rise in creatinine during AHF as renal filtration function may be altered during AHF, but without tubular injury.[34] Regardless of the terminology debate, early studies showed an increased mortality with AKI in AHF.[35,36] The meta-analysis by Damman et al. confirmed an increased risk of mortality with an odds ratio of 1.81 (95% CI 1.55–2.12); however, a publication bias was noted.[5] More recent studies have begun to question the significance of a rise in creatinine and WRF in AHF.

The clinical impact of a rising creatinine depends on the clinical status of the patient and the characteristics of the rise such as the severity and duration.[34] As discussed, preexisting renal dysfunction is associated with worse outcomes in patients with AHF. While these patients are at increased risk of AKI and experience AKI at greater rates, the patient's renal function at admission and discharge is more prognostic of adverse outcomes than a rise in creatinine.[37,38] Thus, preexisting CKD is a more important risk factor in AHF than the increased frequency of AKI events experienced by this population.

Simply defining AKI as a rise in creatinine by a certain percentage or absolute value or by a percentage decrease in estimated glomerular filtration rate (eGFR) fails to recognize the variability in degree of AKI that can occur and the clinical context in which it occurs. One study closely followed 299 patients hospitalized with AHF for the development of AKI and evaluated the context in which AKI occurred.[39] After excluding patients who experienced major complications that would be expected to cause AKI (such as sepsis or cardiogenic shock), patients who developed AKI had the same risk of adverse outcomes as patients without AKI.[39] Another study highlighted the importance of considering the degree and duration of AKI. Patients who experienced transient AKI during AHF had a similar mortality rate at 6 months as patients without AKI, while patients with persistent AKI at 30 days had an increased mortality.[40] Diuretics are believed to be a major cause of AKI and have been shown to more likely cause AKI; however, the rise in creatinine as a result of diuretic therapy did not persist at 60 days after treatment or lead to worse outcomes[41]. With so many conflicting results on the relevance of AKI in AHF, what factors might explain the difference in outcomes and when AKI is relevant for adverse outcomes?

As mentioned, persistent AKI or AKI as the result of a major complication, such as ACS, shock, or sepsis, will adversely affect prognosis. Acute kidney injury frequently occurs during treatment of AHF when therapies decrease blood pressure; however, this combination was shown not to portend a worse prognosis, while AKI occurring without a decrease in blood pressure did lead to increased adverse outcomes.[42] Potentially the most important factor in determining the significance of AKI in AHF is persistent congestion (volume overload). Multiple studies have now shown that patients who experience AKI but also have effective diuresis as evidenced by hemoconcentration and resolution of signs and symptoms of congestion, have no difference in outcomes than patients without AKI.[43-45] In fact, one of these studies showed that patients with AKI and no congestion had better outcomes than subjects without AKI but persistent signs of congestion.[43] Even in studies showing worse outcomes with AKI, concurrent hemoconcentration has been shown to attenuate the significance of AKI.[46] A recent study has used B-type natriuretic peptide (BNP) as a measure of congestion.[47] In this study, patients with AKI (defined as a decrease in eGFR ≥20%) and significant declines in BNP (a decrease of ≥40%) had better long-term outcomes than patients with AKI and no significant decline in BNP.[47] In total, these studies highlight the need to consider the clinical context and status of the patient when AKI occurs in AHF.

Therefore, in a patient with AHF and a rising creatinine, but improving symptoms and signs of congestion, AKI may not increase the risk of adverse outcomes. This has been termed by some as "pseudo-worsening renal function."[34] However, in patients with AKI and worsening clinical status, worsening renal function predicts a worse prognosis and increased morbidity and mortality. While many recent studies have questioned the clinical significance of a rise in creatinine and whether true kidney injury occurs, other recent studies continue to demonstrate the increase in mortality with AKI highlighting the need for further research.[48]

PATHOPHYSIOLOGY

The pathophysiology of AKI in cardiac diseases is complicated by the numerous different factors contributing to injury. While contrast induced nephropathy and cardiac surgery have a specific inciting event (i.e., the administration of intravenous contrast and performing surgery), ACS and AHF occur over a more prolonged period of time and do not necessarily have a single specific insult that triggers the development of AKI. Furthermore, these cardiac conditions occur over a spectrum of disease severity, preexisting renal dysfunction, and renal insult—from the small contrast volume needed for a diagnostic coronary angiogram in an elective outpatient to the large amount needed in patients with an anterior ST elevation MI with cardiogenic shock. However, regardless of the condition, similar pathophysiologic processes of hemodynamic perturbations, neurohormonal activation, nephrotoxic agents, inflammation, and oxidative stress play a role.[3,6,49-53]

Acute Coronary Syndrome

Because the presentation of ACS is so heterogeneous, the pathophysiologic processes contributing to AKI in ACS also vary widely.[6,11,50] As PCI has become the primary means for treating ACS, contrast induced nephropathy and/or atheroembolism can be the cause or significant contributing factors to AKI.[9,11,54] Hemodynamic instability from myocardial injury and reduced cardiac output can result in reduced renal blood flow and venous congestion, altering renal hemodynamics.[6] In addition, during ACS, there is significant neurohormonal activation of the renin-angiotensin-aldosterone system (RAAS) and sympathetic nervous system (SNS) that creates an imbalance in endogenous vasoconstrictors and vasodilators, which in turn affects renal hemodynamics.[6,55,56] Acute coronary syndromes is a highly inflammatory state with increased oxidative stress that can also contribute to AKI.[57] Bleeding, hypoxia, acidosis, and medications administered during treatment of ACS may also contribute to renal injury.[6] In critically ill patients, often with cardiogenic shock, percutaneous assist devices may be used to correct hemodynamic abnormalities, but these may also be the cause of renal injury. Intra-aortic balloon pumps, if positioned too low, can directly block renal blood flow, and percutaneous left ventricular assist devices may cause hemolysis, contributing to AKI.[6] While these are some of the key pathophysiologic processes that may cause or contribute to AKI in ACS, the pathophysiology is not fully understood and will vary by patient.

Contrast-induced Nephropathy

The cause of AKI in percutaneous cardiac procedures such as coronary angiography and PCI is most often a result of contrast induced nephropathy. Contrast induced nephropathy is a complex pathophysiologic process that is not fully understood; however, the driving factor is believed to be vasoconstriction.[4,54] Iodinated contrast is believed to cause perturbations in vasoactive hormones. Potent renal vasoconstrictors, like endothelin and adenosine, are increased while vasodilatory hormones, like prostaglandin and nitrous oxide, are reduced.[54] The osmolarity of the contrast media may exacerbate these effects; higher osmolar contrast causes a greater insult.[54] Furthermore, iodinated contrast may be directly toxic to the renal tubular cells and decreased flow through the kidney can exacerbate injury.[4] These factors lead to sustained hypoxia, resultant oxidative stress, and inflammation.[4,52] Any other concurrent insults, such as hypotension or atheroemboli, will potentiate the injury.

Atheroembolism

As discussed earlier, another cause of renal injury that could masquerade as contrast induced nephropathy or occur concurrently is atheroembolism.[54] Catheters used for intra-arterial procedures have a chance of disrupting and dislodging atheroma that embolize to the kidney. This can also occur during cardiac surgery involving vessel manipulation and clamping. The emboli are not thrombi, but instead usually consist of cholesterol laden plaque. When they embolize, they become lodged in the small arterial beds of the kidney (and other organs of the body as well) and usually only partially obstruct blood flow, leading to ischemia.[58] Subsequent immune activation and inflammation leads to further ischemia and subsequent kidney atrophy in the region supplied.[59] So, while atheroembolic processes present subacutely a week or two after the procedure, the injury and damage continue for weeks, leading to a progressive decline in kidney function.

Cardiac Surgery

The pathophysiology of AKI with cardiac surgery is multifactorial.[3,25] Many factors are similar to other cardiac conditions, but a unique feature is cardiopulmonary bypass (CPB). Intraoperative hemodynamic instability can lead to renal ischemia. Cardiopulmonary bypass may alter renal blood flow, contributing to renal ischemia. These episodes of renal ischemia can lead to oxidative stress and reperfusion injury. The operation itself and CPB can promote inflammation and neurohormonal activation, exacerbating injury, and ischemia. Surgery and CPB can also lead to atheroembolism. Cardiopulmonary bypass can cause hemolysis, leading to pigment nephropathy and the generation of free radicals. There are likely other unknown factors that contribute as well.

Heart Failure and the Cardiorenal Syndrome

Heart failure is the final pathologic state of many of the diseases described above and thus shares many of the same pathophysiologic processes during AKI. Yet, AKI in HF has received significant attention over the years because of its complex pathophysiology that is not fully understood, which has been dubbed the cardiorenal syndrome (CRS).[50] The CRS has been divided into five subtypes to recognize the significant interaction that occurs between the two organs (Fig. 1). Type 1 CRS refers to AHF leading to acute or acute on chronic renal dysfunction. Type 2 CRS denotes chronic HF leading to chronic renal dysfunction. Type 3 CRS is acute renal dysfunction leading to acute or acute on chronic cardiac dysfunction. Type 4 CRS represents chronic renal dysfunction leading to chronic HF. Type 5 is the acute dysfunction of both the heart and kidney from another process, most classically seen in sepsis. While all five CRS subtypes are important in HF and their different pathophysiologies have been described recently, this section will focus on type 1 CRS, which is the most often seen and studied, yet still not well-understood (Fig. 2).[51,60-63]

The pathophysiology of CRS is complex and believed to involve the interplay of hemodynamic mechanisms, neurohormonal activation, inflammation, oxidative stress, hypothalamic-pituitary stress, anemia, and iatrogenic causes.[34,49,51,64] The hemodynamic factors thought to

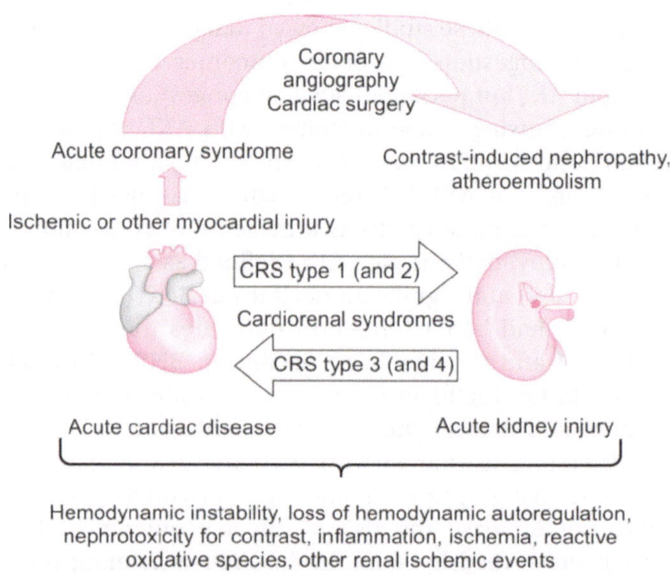

FIG. 1: General pathophysiology of the heart and kidney. Modes of renal injury or loss of function may occur via extrinsic (as in cardiac surgery) or intrinsic (as in Cardiorenal syndrome). Generally, kidney pathophysiology is divided into three categories: pre-renal, renal or tubular, and postrenal

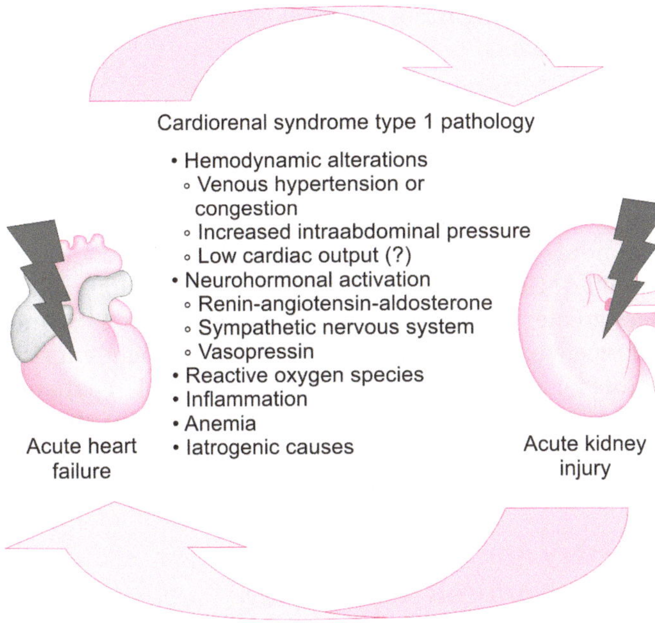

FIG. 2: Cardiorenal syndrome (CRS) type 1. In CRS type 1, an acute cardiac event leads to acute kidney injury. Multiple pathophysiological processes are speculated to contribute to renal insult in response to an acute cardiac events

be involved are impaired intrarenal hemodynamics, decreased cardiac output, and venous congestion; all contributing to reduced renal blood flow.[49,51] Though not fully understood, the state of HF itself leads to an impairment in renal autoregulation out of proportion to the severity of cardiac impairment.[34] This may result from concurrent pathophysiologic process such as neurohormonal activation, inflammation, oxidative stress, and endothelial dysfunction.

The concept that reduced cardiac output leads to a decrease in effective circulating volume and thus reduced renal blood flow with subsequent tubular ischemia, hypoxia, fibrosis, and reduced glomerular filtration makes sense as a plausible mechanism of CRS.[51] However, numerous studies have found no correlation between ejection fraction, cardiac output, or cardiac index and AKI.[65,66] It is unclear why cardiac output has not been found to predict AKI and CRS, as reduced cardiac output has been shown to result in reduced renal blood flow and glomerular filtration.[64] While these studies cast doubt on the role of decreased cardiac output in CRS, they likely did not capture all the different phenotypes of AHF, especially those with cardiogenic shock requiring inotropic or mechanical circulatory support.

Unlike reduced cardiac output, multiple studies have clearly shown that increased venous congestion contributes to AKI and CRS.[38,66-68] Similarly, elevated intra-abdominal pressure also contributes to AKI and CRS.[69,70] A likely mechanism explaining how increased venous pressure leads to AKI is the resulting decrease in the transrenal gradient (the difference in arterial and venous pressure across the kidney) from elevated venous pressure.[64] As the kidney is an encapsulated organ, the backward pressure of venous hypertension translates to increased renal interstitial and tubule pressure. With a rise in intratubular pressure, ultrafiltration pressure drops, leading to a decrease in glomerular filtration. Though this mechanism is plausible, it is only theoretical and has not been directly proven in HF, especially in light of the several other concomitant pathological pathways.[64]

Aside from the hemodynamic mechanisms, numerous nonhemodynamic factors contribute to CRS. Activation of the RAAS and SNS both contribute to CRS by causing vasoconstriction, increased salt retention, renal hypertrophy and fibrosis, and decreased responsiveness to natriuretic peptides.[34,49] Another neurohormone activated in CRS is arginine vasopressin in the hypothalamic-pituitary adrenal axis.[49] Increased production leads to increased salt and water retention exacerbating venous congestion.[49] The multitude of activated neurohormonal systems synergistically increases cardiac stress and venous congestion, which further disrupts intrarenal hemodynamics. Simultaneously, these disruptions also drive another potential pathophysiologic mechanism of CRS—immune activation and inflammation.[71]

Venous congestion and neurohormonal activation lead to increased production of inflammatory markers such as tumor necrosis factor-α and -β, interleukin-1, interleukin-6, and nuclear factor-κB.[49,71] These further contribute to renal inflammation, dysfunction, and fibrosis with further salt and water reabsorption.[49,71] Another important driver of inflammation is congestion of abdominal organs, specifically the gut. Intestinal congestion can lead to bacterial translocation and the release of endotoxins.[49,70] With cytokine activation and possible bacterial translocation, immune cell activation increases and contributes to CRS. Defective regulation of the immune system, possibly with macrophages in particular, exacerbates the CRS.[51] Activation of the immune system and cytokines, as well as other ongoing pathophysiologic processes, contributes to oxidative stress.

A shared pathophysiologic process amongst hemodynamic mechanisms, neurohormonal activation, and inflammation is oxidative stress. The formation of reactive oxidative species (ROS) occurs in both the heart and kidney leading to further injury of both organs and exacerbates the state of CRS.[49,71] The generation of ROS also leads to endothelial dysfunction, compromising intrarenal hemodynamic autoregulatory mechanisms. Reactive oxygen species, such as superoxide, directly inactivate nitric oxide, an important vasodilator and moderator of blood vessel tone.[71] The extent to which ROS and endothelial dysfunction contribute to CRS is not known, but as a shared pathophysiologic process, it is likely an important component of the disease process.

Anemia is very common in patients with HF and portends a worse prognosis.[71] The kidney is the primary endocrine organ for production of erythropoietin to stimulate red blood cell production. Heart failure patients have both decreased production and sensitivity of erythropoietin.[71] Anemia in HF could be a marker of renal dysfunction or cardiac dysfunction. While anemia may not directly contribute to AKI, it may worsen HF and exacerbate the cardiorenal interaction.[71]

A final potential pathologic cause, critical to consider due to its potentially modifiable nature, is iatrogenic contributions to AKI and CRS.[49] The implications of contrast induced nephropathy have been discussed and HF is a risk factor for the development of contrast induced nephropathy, so the information obtained from iodinated contrast studies should be carefully weighed against the risks of contrast induced nephropathy. Nephrotoxic drugs, such as antibiotics, should be avoided if possible. Nonsteroidal anti-inflammatory medications impair renal autoregulation and contribute to salt and water retention. Loop diuretics are the main treatment for congestion and volume overload in AHF; they also increase neurohormonal activation and risk of AKI.[49] However, as discussed earlier, rises in creatinine with aggressive diuretic therapy and effective decongestion have not been associated with adverse outcomes.[41] Angiotensin converting enzyme (ACE) inhibitors and angiotensin receptor blockers (ARBs) alter renal hemodynamics by decreasing vasoconstriction of the efferent arteriole (and the afferent arteriole to a lesser extent) in the glomerulus leading to a reduction in glomerular filtration rate (GFR). When AKI develops, holding these medications is often considered; however, withholding them has been associated with worse outcomes while continuing them increases the rate of AKI, but without worse outcomes.[49,72] While the current data on diuretics, ACE inhibitors, and ARBs are conflicting with regards to the harm they pose, other potential causes of iatrogenic AKI should be avoided if possible.

RISK FACTORS FOR ACUTE KIDNEY INJURY

Numerous risk factors have been identified for developing AKI in different cardiac conditions (Table 1). Some risk factors are unique to the condition, such as iodinated contrast administration with coronary angiography. Many others are shared between conditions. Among these, two conditions that are always risk factors for AKI in any cardiac condition are underlying CKD and diabetes mellitus (DM). These two factors have repeatedly been shown to increase the risk of AKI and should be recognized comorbidities when managing cardiac patients.

Acute Coronary Syndrome

As stated, CKD and DM are two common risk factors for AKI in ACS.[7,8] Older age, male gender, hypertension, and prior myocardial infarction are other risk factors commonly seen.[7,8] In a multivariate analysis, age, baseline eGFR, hypertension, anterior infarction, Killip class greater than 1, ejection fraction less than 45%, and not receiving reperfusion therapy were independent risk factors for AKI.[8] Another possible cause of AKI in patients with ACS is iodinated contrast (discussed below), though as just mentioned, lack of revascularization is associated with an increased risk of AKI as well.[8]

Coronary Angiography and Contrast-induced Nephropathy

Aside from CKD and DM, multiple other risk factors predispose to contrast induced nephropathy.[4,73] Older age and female gender increase the risk of contrast induced nephropathy.[16] Another important risk factor is dehydration because this is a potentially modifiable risk factor.[74] Hemodynamic instability, HF, anemia, and the volume of contrast have also been identified as risk factors for contrast induced nephropathy.[11,75,76] These risk factors are additive for increasing the risk of contrast induced nephropathy.[75] Aside from contrast induced nephropathy, atheroembolism could also be a cause for AKI. Risk factors for this include older age, atherosclerosis, hypertension, and an elevated C-reactive protein.[21]

Cardiac Surgery

Preoperative, intraoperative, and postoperative risk factors for AKI have been identified in patients undergoing cardiac surgery. As with other cardiac conditions, preoperative CKD and DM are two important risk factors for AKI.[3,25,77,78] Other pre-operative risk factors include advanced age, female gender, hypertension, hyperlipidemia, peripheral vascular disease, prior stroke, smoking, anemia, reduced left ventricular systolic function, HF, and prior cardiac surgery.[3,25,77] Of these, age, CKD, DM, and prior cardiac surgery are most commonly seen in different predictive models.[3] Intraoperative risk factors include on-pump surgery, duration of cardiopulmonary bypass, hypotension, hypovolemia, venous congestion, inotrope use, and aortic cross clamp time.[3,25,77] Postoperative risk factors include vasopressor and inotrope use, anemia, hypovolemia, blood transfusion, venous congestion, sepsis, and cardiogenic shock.[3,25] The majority of these risk factors are not modifiable (age, DM, CKD), so it is critical to manage the few that are modifiable, such as volume status.

TABLE 1: Risk factors for kidney injury in different cardiac diseases

Acute coronary syndrome	Coronary angiography: Contrast-induced nepropathy and/or atheroembolism	Cardiac surgery	Heart failure
• Advanced age • Male gender • Hypertension • Prior myocardial infarction • Low baseline estimated glomerular filtration rate • Hypertension • Anterior infarction • Killip class >1 • Ejection fraction <45% • Not receiving reperfusion therapy	• ***Advanced age*** • **Female gender** • **Dehydration** • **Hemodynamic instability** • **Congestive heart failure** • **Anemia** • **Volume of contrast administered** • *Atherosclerosis* • *Hypertension* • *Elevated C-reactive protein*	Preoperative • Advanced age • Female gender • Hypertension • Hyperlipidemia • Peripheral vascular disease • Prior stroke • Smoking • Anemia • Reduced left ventricular systolic function • Heart failure • Prior cardiac surgery Intraoperative • On-pump surgery • Duration of cardiopulmonary bypass • Hypotension • Hypovolemia • Venous congestion • Use of inotropes • Increased aortic cross clamp time Postoperative • Vasopressor and inotrope use • Anemia • Hypovolemia • Transfusion • Venous congestion • Sepsis • Cardiogenic shock	• Hypertension • Male gender • History of heart failure • Hyponatremia • Atrial fibrillation • Obesity • Cardiometabolic changes • Cachexia • Proteinuria • Uremia • Anemia • Bone and mineral disorders • Recurrence of subclinical acute kidney injury
• Chronic kidney disease and diabetes mellitus			

Note that chronic kidney disease and diabetes mellitus predispose to acute kidney injuries/worsening renal function in the face of all types of acute cardiac insults. For cardiac surgery, **bold** text indicates risk factors for contrast-induced nephropathy, italicized text indicates risk factors for atheroembolism, and ***bold italicized*** text indicates risk factors for both conditions.

Heart Failure

Again, DM and CKD are common risk factors for AKI in patients with AHF.[26,79] Other risk factors identified include hypertension, male gender, history of HF, hyponatremia, and atrial fibrillation.[26,79] More novel risk factors being explored include obesity, cardiometabolic changes, cachexia, proteinuria, uremia, anemia, bone and mineral disorders, and recurrence of subclinical AKI.[49] These latter risk factors reflect that HF is a systemic condition influencing multiple organs, including the kidney. Many of these risk factors are not directly modifiable because they are a result of HF; therefore, optimal care of HF itself is important for managing concurrent diseases and risk factors.

DIAGNOSIS AND NOVEL BIOMARKERS

One of the complicating matters for evaluating AKI in heart disease is the lack of a standardized definition. Some of the most commonly used cutoffs for determining AKI are a rise in creatinine of 0.3 mg/dL from baseline, an increase in creatinine by 25% above baseline, or a decrease in eGFR by 25%.[26,34] Other criteria used include a creatinine increase of 0.5 mg/dL from baseline or an increase in creatinine by 50% above baseline. Contrast-induced nephropathy has used a variety of different definitions, but the most commonly used is a rise in creatinine by 0.5 mg/dL or 25% from baseline within 48 hours of being given contrast.[4] The variability of these definitions partially explains the variability in reported incidences of AKI and, likely, the prognostic outcomes observed.

A variety of standardized definitions have been proposed. One of the first criteria, proposed in 2004, was the Risk, Injury, Failure, Loss of Kidney Function (RIFLE) criteria (Table 2).[80] Notable characteristics of the RIFLE criteria include defining AKI as a percentage rise in creatinine or drop in eGFR that occurs over 7 days and is sustained for at least 24 hours. In 2007, the Acute Kidney Injury Network (AKIN) criteria were proposed.[81] These criteria did not use eGFR but rather an absolute increase or percentage increase in creatinine. Also, the creatinine increase must be rapid, occurring within 48 hours. In 2012, the Kidney Disease Improving Global Outcomes (KDIGO) criteria were released.[82] These criteria melded the RIFLE and AKIN criteria to include an absolute creatinine increase over 48 hours or a percentage increase over 7 days. The criteria did not include a decline in eGFR that the RIFLE criteria used. All three criteria also use urine output for defining AKI, but this is not commonly used in studies, given the difficulties with accurate urine collection. Additionally, patients in cardiology studies are frequently given diuretics, which may make urine output criteria less accurate.

A difficulty with these varied criteria is they have not been specifically validated in different cardiac conditions such as ACS or AHF. Only a few studies have compared the criteria in cardiac conditions. The RIFLE and KDIGO criteria have been compared in acute myocardial infarction and the KDIGO criteria had better prognostic value.[83] All three criteria were compared in cardiac surgery patients and again the KDIGO criteria were found to be superior.[84] A comparison of the three criteria in AHF did not find a significant difference in prognostic value.[85] These data would argue that the KDIGO criteria should be used as the preferred diagnostic criteria. However, it should be remembered that these criteria have not been rigorously tested in different cardiac conditions to confirm they are appropriate definitions of AKI in each condition.

A weakness of all AKI definitions is the reliance on creatinine, which is an imperfect biomarker of renal function. Creatinine is a byproduct of muscle breakdown and produced at a relatively constant rate.[86] It is largely freely filtered at the glomerulus, though a small portion is actively secreted by the proximal tubule as well.[86] This assumed steady state has allowed the creation of equations that use creatinine to calculate an eGFR. However, creatinine has shortcomings that influence its use as a biomarker for AKI. The relationship between creatinine and GFR is not linear but exponential. This means small changes in creatinine at values in the normal range reflect large changes in GFR while small changes in creatinine at high values reflect minimal changes in GFR. Creatinine

TABLE 2: Criteria for renal injury

Risk, Injury, Failure, Loss of Kidney Function (RIFLE)		
Level	**Based on (1) sCr or (2) eGFR***	**Based on urine output**
Risk	1. ↑sCr = 1.5–2 × baseline 2. eGFR↓ 25%	<0.5 mL/kg/h within 6 h
Injury	1. ↑sCr = 2–3 × baseline 2. eGFR↓ 50%	<0.5 mL/kg/h in more than 12 h
Failure	1a. ↑sCr = 3 × baseline 1b. sCr ≥4 mg/dL* 2. eGFR↓ 75%	<0.3 mL/kg/h in more than 24 h or anuria 12 h
Loss of function (LOF)	Ongoing acute failure requiring dialysis >4 weeks	–
ESRD	Loss of function requiring dialysis >3 months	–
Acute Kidney Injury Network (AKIN)		
Stage	**Based on Δ sCr**	**Based on urine output**
1	↑sCr 0.3 mg/dL or more, or 1.5–2 × baseline within 48 h	<0.5 mL/kg/h within 6 h
2	↑sCr 2–3 × baseline	<0.5 mL/kg/h in more than 12 h
3	1. ↑sCr >3 × baseline or 2. ↑sCr ≥0.5 mg/dL if baseline sCr ≥4 mg/dL or 3. LOF requiring renal replacement therapy	<0.3 mL/kg/h in more than 24 h or anuria 12 h
Kidney Disease: Improving Global Outcomes (KDIGO)		
Stage	**Based on sCr or eGFR**	**Based on urine output**
1	1. ↑sCr = 1.5–1.9 × baseline (within prior 7 days) or 2. ↑≥0.3 mg/dL in sCr (prior 48 h)$	Identical to AKIN
2	↑sCr = 2.0–2.9 × baseline	
3	1. sCr = 3 × baseline or 2. sCr ≥4 mg/dL or 3. LOF requiring renal replacement therapy or 4. If <18 years old, ↓eGFR to <35 mL/min/1.73 m²	

Note: Class of injury should be based on the worst observed alternative in each category. In the RIFLE criteria, the previous 7 days should be used to examine creatinine, whereas AKIN and KDIGO (in the designated instances) should utilize sCr in the past 48 hours.

sCr, serum creatinine; eGFR, estimated glomerular filtration rate.
*Change over 7 days.
#With short-term rise of ≥0.5 mg/dL.
$Short-term rise (≤48 k).
Note: Conversion to SI units is 1 mg/dL = 88.4 μmol/L.

is influenced by patient age, muscle mass, and gender, and its production may not be constant.[86,87] Creatinine reflects glomerular filtration and renal function, but not kidney injury.[88] Lastly, creatinine has a delayed rise in AKI with the value not rising until 24–48 hours after the injury has occurred significantly hampering timely diagnosis and treatment.[88]

Given these shortcomings, there has been significant interest in finding novel biomarkers of renal function and injury. In addition, there has been a paradigm shift in the evaluation of AKI whereby kidney injury could be secondary to functional change, renal damage, or both (Fig. 3).[89] This new definition implies that there could be a clinical scenario where a novel biomarker detects renal injury without a change in renal function. Thus, creatinine values would not change even though the novel injury biomarker values would change. This scenario would be analogous to a rise in troponin during a myocardial infarction, but no change in left ventricular ejection fraction or cardiac function. Given the numerous novel biomarkers being explored in different cardiac conditions, especially HF, a brief overview of the more studied biomarkers will be provided (Table 3).

Cystatin C

Cystatin C is a small protein produced by all nucleated cells in the body and is freely filtered at the glomerulus.[86] Thus, similar to creatinine, plasma cystatin C serves as a marker of renal filtration and function. It does not seem to have the same problems as creatinine in regards

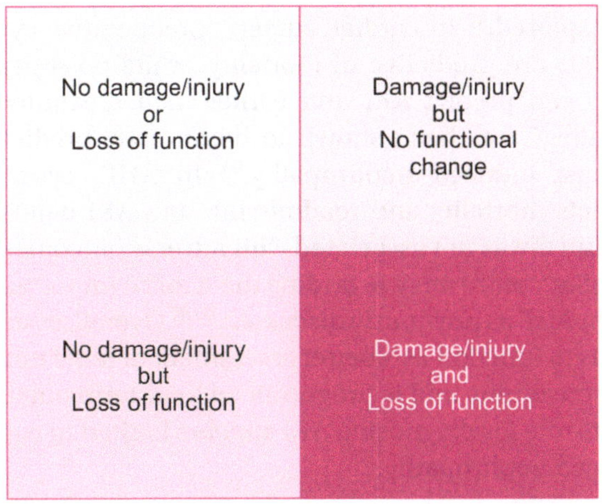

FIG. 3: The new paradigm of acute kidney injury. While serum creatinine is the standard biomarker for assessing kidney injury, serum creatinine reflects functional loss. With the rise of novel biomarkers reflecting kidney injury/damage that can occur even without functional loss, this new paradigm of kidney injury has been proposed

TABLE 3: Biomarkers of cardiac and/or kidney dysfunction

Biomarker	Utility/elevated in
Serum creatinine	Kidney injury, risk, failure (RIFLE, AKIN, or KDIGO); in cases of lower glomerular filtration but not in renal cell injury (function); dependent on age, race, gender, muscle mass
Cystatin C	Prognostic value in ACS; preoperative predictor of mortality; postoperative AKI; CIN; AHF, though not AKI in AHF (controversial)
Blood urea nitrogen	Mortality in AHF (BUN:sCr ratio); differentiates between CRS and intrinsic dysfunction when used with BNP; neurohormonal activation
Albuminuria	Mortality in CHF; limited data in AHF; evidence of AKI during cardiac surgery (urinary albumin: sCr ratio); potentially AKI in ACS (one study)
Neutrophil gelatinase-associated lipocalin	AKI and other risk stages of CKD (strong evidence); AKI due to cardiac surgery (strong evidence); limited data for diagnosing CRS, but can predict pooled adverse outcomes; poor prognosis in AHF at discharge, prognostic more than diagnostic
Kidney injury molecule 1	AKI; limited value in cardiac surgery (moderate prognostic utility in CIN); strong prognosis in chronic HF prognosis and worsening renal function
N-acetyl-beta-d-glucosaminidase	ACS (renal ischemia-reperfusion); AKI in surgery (not strongly predictive); mortality; HF hospitalization; more data needed on all
Fatty acid binding proteins (L-FABP and H-FABP)	Contrast induced nephropathy precontrast (L-FABP); cardiac surgery (both); AKI in AHF and mortality (H-FABP, one study); more data needed on all
Interleukin 18	Confounded in AKI and ACS together; fair in CIN; fair in AKI in cardiac surgery; AKI in AHF (IL-18:sCr ratio, one small study
Insulin-like growth factor-binding protein 7 and tissue inhibitor of metalloproteinase-2	Critically ill patients with AKI; AKI after cardiac surgery (small studies, more data needed)

Note: This list reflects a select few established, reapplied, and/or novel biomarkers of kidney function. Listed in the right-hand column are indications and/or level of evidence shown for each marker in various cardiac or cardiorenal conditions such as cardiorenal syndrome, acute coronary syndrome, acute heart failure, contrast-induced nephropathy, and acute kidney injury.

RIFLE, risk, injury, failure, loss of kidney function, and end-stage kidney disease; AKIN, acute kidney injury network; KDIGO, kidney disease improving global outcomes; ACS, acute coronary syndrome; AKI, acute kidney injury; AHF, acute heart failre; BUN, blood urea nitrogen; sCr, serum creatinine; CRS, cardiorenal syndrome; BNP, brain natriuretic peptide; CHF, chronic heart failure; CKD, chronic kidney disease.

to age, race, gender, or muscle mass.[88] Cystatin C is superior to creatinine in estimating GFR, but its role in diagnosing AKI in cardiac disease is less well-defined.[90] In ACS, cystatin C levels were found to predict future cardiovascular events, but its use for diagnosing AKI was not explored.[91] In cardiac surgery, preoperative cystatin C levels are predictive of mortality, while postoperative levels can predict AKI and earlier than creatinine.[92-94] Cystatin C has been shown to be an early predictor of contrast induced nephropathy.[95] In AHF, cystatin C predicts mortality and readmission, but AKI defined by cystatin C was not associated with adverse outcomes with a similar controversy regarding the clinical importance of AKI in AHF as previously discussed.[96,97] Overall, cystatin C seems to function as a better assessment of renal function than creatinine and is prognostic of long-term outcomes, but its role for diagnosing AKI appears limited to contrast induced nephropathy.

Blood Urea Nitrogen

While not a novel biomarker for renal function, blood urea nitrogen (BUN) has had a reappraisal for importance in cardiac disease, specifically in HF. The BUN correlates not only with renal function but also with neurohormonal activation.[86] Elevated and rising BUN is a powerful prognostic marker for mortality in AHF.[98,99] Other studies have focused on the BUN to creatinine ratio. This has been argued to be a better predictor of mortality in AHF and, when used in conjunction with BNP, it can discern when AKI originates from CRS versus intrinsic renal dysfunction.[100,101] Given the renewed interest in BUN, especially with its relation to neurohormonal activation, an old biomarker may once again become novel.

Albuminuria

Albumin is a large protein that is normally not filtered by the glomerulus. The presence of albumin in the urine (albuminuria) identifies renal dysfunction at the level of the glomerulus. In the absence of cardiovascular disease, albuminuria is a well-described risk factor for the development of cardiovascular disease, especially HF.[102,103] Albuminuria strongly predicts mortality in chronic HF.[104-106] There is limited data in AHF, but one small study noted urine albumin excretion decreased with treatment of AHF and this correlated with decreasing natriuretic peptide levels and bilirubin levels.[107] Further research is needed to determine if albuminuria can be used for monitoring in AHF and thus potentially aid in the diagnosis of CRS. In cardiac surgery, proteinuria and urinary albumin to creatinine ratio have been shown to identify patients at increased risk of developing AKI.[108,109] In a study evaluating ACS patients, a spot urine albumin to creatinine ratio was the most predictive biomarker for the development of AKI.[110] Further studies are needed to confirm these findings and see if albuminuria is a modifiable risk factor.

Neutrophil Gelatinase-associated Lipocalin

Of all the novel renal injury biomarkers, neutrophil gelatinase-associated lipocalin (NGAL) has shown the most promise. It has been found to be a powerful predictor of AKI in a variety of conditions. Neutrophil gelatinase associated lipocalin is a member of the lipocalin family and believed to be primarily involved in iron transport.[111] It exists in both a monomeric and dimeric form, can be detected in both the serum and urine, and is produced in the kidney, lung, stomach, colon, and potentially heart and other organs.[87] NGAL is reabsorbed in the proximal tubule with increased reabsorption during periods of injury believed to contribute to the elevated serum levels detected in AKI.[111] Urine NGAL is thought to come primarily from increased production in the distal tubule during kidney injury, though some may also come from inhibited reabsorption because of injury to the proximal tubule.[111]

In a general population of patients presenting to the emergency department with AKI, urinary NGAL was shown to distinguish between normal function, prerenal azotemia, and CKD, and predict worse inpatient outcomes.[112] NGAL has been extensively studied in cardiac surgery, and a meta-analysis showed both urine and serum NGAL to be highly predictive of AKI after cardiac surgery.[113] A different meta-analysis also confirmed serum and urine NGAL to be prognostic for AKI in cardiac surgery as well as in contrast induced nephropathy and critical illness.[114] The data for NGAL in HF is not as robust.

Small studies have shown serum NGAL to be prognostic for AKI and CRS.[115,116] One study showed urine NGAL to be associated with AKI in AHF.[117] While data for NGAL's diagnostic utility for AKI and CRS is limited, its prognostic utility is notable. In a pooled analysis of studies that had a significant number of patients with CRS, NGAL (both serum and urine) was found to be prognostic for mortality, renal replacement therapy, and duration of hospital stay.[118] This study was notable in that patients with (i) only elevated creatinine, (ii) only elevated NGAL, or (iii) elevation of both markers had worse outcomes than patients with neither marker elevated, supporting the new paradigm for evaluating AKI with both functional and injury markers. Serum NGAL measured at discharge is also prognostic for mortality and readmission in patients hospitalized for AHF.[119,120] Currently, the data more strongly supports NGAL's prognostic utility for poor outcomes in AHF than its diagnostic utility for AKI.

Kidney Injury Molecule-1

Kidney injury molecule-1 (KIM-1) is a glycoprotein that is expressed in proximal renal tubular cells during injury and regeneration.[121] It can be detected in both serum and urine, but studies have primarily focused on urine KIM-1. Kidney injury molecule-1 is best studied in cardiac surgery. A meta-analysis of 11 studies involving 2,979 patients found KIM-1 to have excellent predictive value for AKI with a 74% sensitivity and 86% specificity for AKI.[122] Kidney injury molecule-1 is less studied in HF, ACS, and contrast induced nephropathy. One study evaluating KIM-1 in ACS focused on contrast induced nephropathy after coronary angiography for ACS.[123] In this study, KIM-1 showed good predictive value, but less so than NGAL.[123] Another study of KIM-1 in contrast induced nephropathy suggested a potential role as an early marker of AKI.[124] Overall though, the data for KIM-1 for contrast induced nephropathy is limited. In chronic HF, elevated KIM-1 levels were slightly prognostic for increased mortality and HF hospitalization, but strongly prognostic for worsening renal function.[125,126] The data for KIM-1 in AHF is mixed with one study showing no predictive value, and another study showing the combination of cystatin C and KIM-1 to predict AKI.[127,128] Further studies are needed to define KIM-1's role in ACS, contrast induced nephropathy, and HF, but current data is promising for KIM-1 as an early marker of AKI after cardiac surgery.

N-acetyl-β-d-glucosaminidase

N-acetyl-β-d-glucosaminidase (NAG) is a lysosomal enzyme found in the proximal tubules of the kidney and detected in the urine when there is breakdown of lysosomes.[121] Studies of NAG in ACS have not focused on AKI but have rather viewed NAG as a biomarker for ischemia and reperfusion.[129,130] Few studies have evaluated NAG in contrast induced nephropathy, but one study suggested it is potentially useful.[131] NAG has been shown to have fair predictive value for AKI in cardiac surgery, but not significantly better than other biomarkers except when used in conjunction with liver-type fatty acid binding protein (L-FABP), which enhanced its predictive ability.[132,133] NAG has not been found to diagnose AKI and CRS in AHF.[134] In chronic HF, NAG was prognostic for worsening renal function in univariate analysis, but not multivariate analysis. Notwithstanding, it is predictive for mortality and HF hospitalization.[126,135] Overall, initial data suggests NAG has some prognostic utility, though not necessarily more than other biomarkers; yet, further studies in larger cohorts are needed to better determine a role, if any, for NAG.

Fatty Acid Binding Proteins

Fatty acid binding proteins (FABPs) are involved in fatty acid metabolism and found in many tissues of the body.[86] Two types have been found in the kidney. Liver-type fatty acid binding protein is found in the proximal tubule and heart-type fatty acid binding protein (H-FABP) is found in the distal tubule.[86] Similar to NAG, FABPs have been largely studied for their diagnostic and prognostic utility in ACS rather than for AKI in ACS.[136] Liver-type FABP has been found to help risk stratify patients for the development of contrast induced nephropathy after contrast administration, but only has fair predictive value for contrast induced nephropathy after contrast has been administered.[123,137] Both L-FABP and H-FABP have been evaluated in cardiac surgery. In a small study of children undergoing cardiac surgery, early postoperative L-FABP levels were highly predictive of AKI.[138] In a much larger study, both pre- and postoperative levels of H-FABP were found to be predictive of AKI.[139] One study has looked at H-FABP in AHF, and it found higher levels measured shortly after admission predicted the development of AKI and mortality.[140] While these findings are promising, data is overall limited for FABPs use in diagnosing AKI.

Interleukin-18

Interleukin-18 (IL-18) is a cytokine produced by immune cells in response to inflammation and/or ischemia.[121] In the kidney, it is released in the urine during periods of injury.[121] Though IL-18 is measured in the urine when evaluating for AKI, its association with ischemia likely confounds its ability to predict AKI in ACS because concurrent coronary ischemia could potentially alter urinary levels of IL-18. A few studies have looked at IL-18 for contrast induced nephropathy. Some found good prognostic value, though others find it does not perform as well as other biomarkers.[141-143] Two meta-analyses have looked at IL-18 in cardiac surgery and found it to have fair to good predictive value for AKI.[132,144] One small study looked at IL-18 for diagnosing AKI in AHF and found the ratio of urinary IL-18 to urinary creatinine was the strongest predictor for a persistently elevated creatinine at 6 months.[127] Like other novel biomarkers, further studies are needed to determine a role for IL-18 in cardiac diseases.

Insulin-like Growth Factor-binding Protein 7 and Tissue Inhibitor of Metalloproteinase-2

Insulin-like growth factor-binding protein 7 (IGFBP-7) and tissue inhibitor of metalloproteinase-2 (TIMP-2) are both inducers of cell cycle arrest and were found to be the top candidate biomarkers for AKI in critically ill patients with AKI.[145] In a separate cohort of critically ill patients, the combination of these two biomarkers maintained their predictive value for diagnosing AKI.[145] Only recently studies have started to examine these candidate biomarkers in cardiovascular diseases. Two small studies have shown promising results for the early diagnosis of

AKI after cardiac surgery.[146,147] Further studies are needed in large cohorts and other cardiovascular diseases to see if the same promising results found in critically ill patients can be reproduced in different cardiovascular diseases.

MANAGEMENT

Regardless of the cardiac condition, management is directed at the underlying pathophysiologic causes. Unfortunately, most pharmacotherapies and procedures investigated to treat or prevent AKI have had disappointing results. As such, one of the most important steps is predicting which patient is at heightened risk for AKI and attempting to prevent or mitigate risk while closely monitoring for AKI. Additionally, after an episode of AKI, close follow-up is important not only for continued management and stabilization of the provoking cardiac condition but also for the ongoing management of AKI.

Other general principles for the management of AKI have been proposed by the 2012 KDIGO guidelines (Table 4).[148] This working group has made recommendations based on the severity of AKI. For high risk patients, nephrotoxic agents should be discontinued if possible, volume status should be optimized, renal perfusion pressure should be optimized, functional hemodynamic monitoring should be considered, creatinine and urine output should be closely monitored, and both hyperglycemia and iodinated contrast should be avoided. Once AKI develops, a noninvasive workup should be performed, and invasive evaluation should be considered. As AKI progresses to more severe stages, medication doses should be adjusted, the patient may need admission to the intensive care unit, renal replacement therapy should be considered, and subclavian catheters should be avoided to preserve these vessels for future dialysis access.

TABLE 4: Risk-lowering, management, and follow-up recommendations for addressing acute kidney injury in acute cardiac conditions

General measures for managing acute kidney injury		
Predict and prevent risk	**During injury**	**Close postinjury follow-up**
1. Discontinue nephrotoxic agents 2. Optimize volume status 3. Optimize renal perfusion pressure 4. Avoid hyperglycemia 5. Avoid iodinated contrast	1. Non-invasive workup (consider invasive evaluation) 2. Functional hemodynamics 3. Monitor creatinine and urine output	1. Adjust medications 2. Admit to ICU if necessary 3. Consider renal replacement therapy 4. Avoid subclavian catheters in case dialysis needed
Acute kidney injury in acute coronary syndrome		
Predict and prevent risk	**During injury**	**Close postinjury follow-up**
1. Risk stratify for CIN	1. As above	1. As above
Contrast-induced nephropathy and cardiac catheterization		
Predict and prevent risk	**During injury**	**Close postinjury follow-up**
1. National Cardiovascular Data Registry Cath-PCI Registry risk score 2. Use low-osmolal or isomolal agents 3. Avoid dehydration (prehydrate with saline) 4. Use of statins	1. Continue statins 2. As above	1. As above
Cardiac surgery		
Predict and prevent risk	**During injury**	**Close postinjury follow-up**
1. Stratify with Cleveland Clinic Model 2. Avoid: NSAIDs, iodinated contrast, nephrotoxic antibiotics 3. Carefully consider potentially-protective ACE inhibitors 4. Avoid statins 5. No benefit to vasodilatory meds (e.g. dopamine and fenoldopam) 6. Tight postoperative glycemic control	1. Intensive/invasive hemodynamic monitoring to ensure hydration 2. As above	1. Maintain good nutrition 2. Glycemic control 3. Early initiation of renal replacement therapies (consider experimental: stem-cell therapy or alkaline phosphatase)

Continued

Continued

Heart failure		
Predict and prevent risk	**During injury**	**Close postinjury follow-up**
1. Difficult to predict risk 2. Manage volume and pressure with appropriate dosing of loop diuretics and vasodilators (preferred over inotropic support) 3. Consider serelaxin as novel vasodilator and potential protector of renal function 4. Use inotropes in patients with signs of systemic hypoperfusion	1. As above 2. Can use ultrafiltration if refractory to diuretics	1. Control volume status as in risk prevention 2. Generally continue ACE-Is and ARBs 3. Withhold medications with low blood pressure, volume contraction, hyponatremia, and severe AKI

Note: While general guideline recommendations for the management of AKI exist, evidence has pointed towards specialized actions for minimizing risk of AKI, managing the patient when AKI occurs, and ameliorating effects after an episode of injury. Though more comprehensive treatments should be sought from guidelines and more comprehensive resources, we underscore here the differential pathology of AKI in various cardiac settings, with a particular emphasis on special preventative actions in controlled conditions such as cardiac surgery

ICU, intensive care unit; PCI, percutaneous coronary intervention; NSAID, non-steroidal anti-inflammatory drug; ACE, angiotensin converting enzyme; ARB, angiotensin receptor blocker; AKI, acute kidney injury.

Acute Coronary Syndrome

There are no specific recommendations or studies focusing on the management of AKI in patients with ACS; therefore, recommendations are generalized from other forms of AKI. As the causes of AKI in ACS are multifactorial, management should be directed at the presumed pathophysiologic processes driving AKI. The general management recommendations of the KDIGO Working Group listed above should be implemented. In addition, as contrast induced nephropathy is one of the major causes of AKI in ACS, risk stratification and preventive strategies detailed below should be performed if possible. As ACS is an unpredictable event with many risk factors for AKI unable to be modified, attempts at preventing AKI are limited to preventing contrast induced nephropathy.

Cardiac Catheterization and Contrast Nephropathy

As the implications of AKI after cardiac catheterization are significant, there is increasing interest on predicting and mitigating risks. In 2014, a risk score for AKI was developed using the National Cardiovascular Data Registry CathPCI Registry.[149] The score was developed using almost 950,000 procedures and showed good predictive value (C statistic of 0.71). While this score provides potential risk factors and an estimated risk of AKI, it does not necessarily help one determine how to mitigate risk. An area where prediction and measures should be taken to mitigate risk is contrast induced nephropathy.[4] Risk scores have also been developed to specifically predict contrast induced nephropathy after angiography.[17,75] Identifying high risk patients may help with selecting patients to pretreat and choice of contrast agent.

High osmolar agents are believed to cause more potent vasoconstriction and increase the risk of contrast induced nephropathy; therefore, low osmolar or iso-osmolar agents, such as iodixanol, iohexol, and iopamidol, are recommended. Some studies suggest that iodixanol has the best outcomes, though this is an area of significant debate.[4,18,150-153] Dehydration is a significant risk factor for contrast induced nephropathy, and prehydration with isotonic saline has been shown to reduce the risk of contrast induced nephropathy; this approach may be contraindicated in patients with HF.[154] Intravenous bicarbonate has also been advocated to possibly protect against free radicals; however, results from studies have been mixed regarding benefit, and no studies have shown significant improvements in outcomes over saline.[155] Another agent commonly used is acetylcysteine because of its potential vasodilatory and antioxidant properties. Results of a meta-analysis are mixed on benefit, and the largest randomized trial showed no benefit.[155-157] Statins have been shown to decrease the risk of contrast induced nephropathy.[158-160] At this time, prehydration with intravenous isotonic saline or sodium bicarbonate, if appropriate, appears to be the most reasonable protective measure. In addition, most patients with cardiac conditions will be on a statin, which should be continued.

Cardiac Surgery

As with other conditions, it is critical to identify high risk patients and implement preventive measures to mitigate risk for management. Numerous different risk scores have been developed. A meta-analysis showed that the Cleveland Clinic Model is the most widely used and has the highest discrimination.[78] Maintaining adequate hydration while avoiding over-resuscitation is important;

therefore, often, invasive hemodynamic monitoring is performed.[3,25,77,161] Nephrotoxic agents, such as non-steroidal anti-inflammatories, iodinated contrast, and nephrotoxic antibiotics, should be avoided pre-operatively.[3,25] Angiotensin-converting enzyme inhibitors used to be considered harmful, but recent studies have not supported this; in fact, it has been shown that they may be protective.[162] Conversely, statins were thought to prevent AKI, but a recent study did not find this effect and actually showed increased AKI.[25,161,163] Vasodilatory medications, like dopamine and fenoldopam, have not shown benefit.[3,164] As cardiopulmonary bypass is a major contributor to AKI, off-pump procedures are preferable, if possible.[3,77] Postoperatively, tight glycemic control can help prevent AKI.[3,77,161]

If postoperative AKI does develop, maintenance of good nutrition and glycemic control is important.[3] Early initiation of renal replacement therapies may reduce mortality and adverse outcomes.[3,165] Experimental therapies include stem cell technologies and alkaline phosphatase.[3] Overall, care should be focused on avoiding complications and supporting the patient until renal recovery.

Heart Failure

Determining effective management strategies for AKI/CRS in AHF has been a clinical challenge. As with all other cardiac conditions, identifying high risk patients is key and the risk factors for CRS should be considered when treating patients. There is a paucity of risk scores to predict CRS, with only one showing fair to poor predictive value.[166] Since hemodynamic derangements, mainly venous congestion and elevated intra-abdominal pressure, are major drivers of AKI and CRS, multiple studies have looked at different strategies and therapies to reduce volume overload and venous congestion.

Loop diuretics are the foundation of decongestive therapy in AHF. Loop diuretics provide powerful natriuresis and diuresis to relieve symptoms of congestion. However, as previously mentioned, loop diuretics are known to increase the RAAS and SNS, which could potentially exacerbate HF and are thought to contribute to diuretic resistance.[167] In addition, higher doses of diuretics are associated with increased electrolyte disturbances and rates of AKI; therefore, high doses were believed to be directly toxic. To overcome some of these issues, a continuous infusion of loop diuretics, compared to intermittent boluses, was thought to decrease the risk of renal injury and neurohormonal activation.[41] The largest study to test different dosing strategies was the Diuretic Strategies in Patients with Acute Decompensated Heart Failure (DOSE-AHF) trial.[41] Using a 2 × 2 design, patients were randomized to high dose or low dose loop diuretic and intermittent boluses or continuous infusions. In the end, no difference was found between boluses and continuous infusions.[41] Though patients in the study receiving high dose diuretics experienced more AKI, at 60 days, there was no difference in renal function or outcomes.[41] Ironically, in a subsequent study looking at activation of the RAAS in DOSE-AHF, there was no difference in the degree of RAAS activation between high and low dose diuretics, while continuous infusions were associated with greater RAAS activation than boluses.[168] These findings question the prior beliefs that high dose loop diuretics are harmful and bolster the argument that the use of high dose diuretics are a sign of HF severity and not the cause of poor outcomes.[71]

Another potential method for relieving congestion is with vasodilator therapies.[70,169,170] Theoretically, vasodilators can decrease venous pressure while increasing renal blood flow improving renal perfusion and hemodynamics. Commonly used vasodilators in AHF are nitroprusside, nitroglycerin, nesiritide (a recombinant BNP), and low dose dopamine. Unfortunately, some of these therapies have a paucity of data (nitroprusside), while others (nitroglycerin, dopamine, nesiritide) showed possible benefit in early small studies, but these findings were not confirmed in subsequent larger randomized controlled trials. For nesiritide, there was initial concern that the agent caused AKI, but a large multicenter study showed that nesiritide did not in fact cause AKI; however, it did not improve outcomes either.[171] Small studies have shown that both nitroglycerin and nesiritide do not worsen renal function and may reduce neurohormones; nesiritide potentially has a slightly greater benefit in preserving renal function and reducing inflammation.[172,173] In one of the few large randomized clinical trials evaluating different vasodilator therapies, both low dose dopamine and nesiritide were compared to diuretic therapy alone for AHF in the Renal Optimization Strategies Evaluation in Acute Heart Failure (ROSE-AHF) study.[174] Neither dopamine nor nesiritide improved diuresis or renal function.[174] While most vasodilator studies have failed to show harm or benefit, some studies have shown vasodilator therapy to reduce the risk of HF admission and the dose of diuretic needed for decongestion.[70] While the previously mentioned vasodilators have failed to show benefit, a new novel vasodilator, serelaxin, may finally show benefit.[175] Serelaxin is a recombinant form of the hormone relaxin-2, which is normally produced during pregnancy, and causes increased arterial compliance, cardiac output, and renal blood flow.[175] In the Efficacy, Safety and Tolerability of Serelaxin when Added to Standard Therapy in Acute Heart Failure (RELAX-AHF) study, treatment with serelaxin resulted in decreased worsening of HF, decreased mortality at 180 days, improved measures of renal function, and reduced rates of AKI.[175] These findings suggest there may finally be a vasodilator that improves renal function while reducing mortality and the incidence of AKI.

One therapy that often does lead to improvements in renal function is inotropic therapy.[71,170] The fact that inotropes improve renal function (presumably through increased cardiac output) is at conflict with other studies showing no association between cardiac output and worsening renal function. Though inotropes improve renal blood flow and function, they are associated with worse outcomes in AHF including arrhythmias and increased mortality.[170] Thus, inotropes should be reserved for patients with depressed cardiac output and signs of systemic hypoperfusion.

A method that initially showed promise as an alternative means of decongestion was extracorporeal volume removal through ultrafiltration. In the Ultrafiltration versus Intravenous Diuretics for Patients Hospitalized for Acute Decompensated Congestive Heart Failure (UNLOAD) study, ultrafiltration showed improved fluid removal with less renal impairment and reduced HF readmissions compared to diuretic therapy.[176] In the subsequent Ultrafiltration in Decompensated Heart Failure with Cardiorenal Syndrome (CARRESS-HF) study, specifically focusing on the prevention and treatment of CRS, ultrafiltration resulted in worse outcomes with increased rates of AKI in the ultrafiltration group as well as increased rates of adverse events largely from complications of vascular access.[177] A substudy showed that ultrafiltration increased RAAS activity more than diuretic therapy.[168] One possible reason that ultrafiltration failed to show benefit in CARRESS-HF is that the study had a strict and aggressive protocol for titrating diuretics, which may have led to more successful decongestion and improved outcomes compared to diuretic treatment in the UNLOAD study. Because of the findings of CARRESS-HF, the use of ultrafiltration has been tempered and is largely reserved for volume overloaded patients that are refractory to diuretics.[170]

While veno-venous ultrafiltration has not shown benefit, peritoneal dialysis has shown potential benefit. Small studies have shown peritoneal dialysis leads to effective decongestion with improvement in symptoms and quality of life.[70] As peritoneal dialysis allows for slow ultrafiltration, it is less likely to have a significant hemodynamic impact. At this time, studies are limited to small cohorts and single centers and larger randomized trials are needed.

While multiple different therapies have been used to prevent and treat AKI and CRS in AHF, most have failed to show any benefit. However, studies have shown the relative safety and efficacy of diuretic therapy, specifically the protocol in CARRESS-HF led to significant diuresis with good outcomes. Serelaxin is a promising new vasodilator shown to improve renal function and mortality. An area of clinical confusion is when to continue using ACE inhibitors and ARBs in the setting of renal dysfunction and AKI. In general, these medications should be continued even in the face of a rising creatinine as withdrawal is associated with worse outcomes.[26,49] Withholding these medications is reasonable in patients with low blood pressure, volume contraction, hyponatremia, and severe AKI. Interestingly, a study has shown that increasing neurohormonal therapy did not increase rates of AKI and in fact led to improved diuresis.[72] The initiation, maintenance, and uptitration of ACE inhibitors and ARBs in patients with AHF and AKI as well as their potential use as a therapy for CRS warrant further study.

CONCLUSION

Acute kidney injury in cardiac disease significantly increases morbidity and mortality. It is a critical condition to consider and recognize when managing a patient with cardiac disease. While steps have been taken forward in defining risk factors and the pathophysiologic processes involved in AKI, there are many unmet needs. Novel biomarkers are being explored to diagnose AKI earlier and improve prognostication. Studies have been performed to test methods to prevent and treat AKI during cardiac disease, but unfortunately most have not shown benefit. New therapies are critically needed. Until new therapies and preventive measures are developed, AKI will continue to significantly impact the outcomes of patients with cardiac disease.

REFERENCES

1. Ruilope LM, van Veldhuisen DJ, Ritz E, Luscher TF. Renal function: the Cinderella of cardiovascular risk profile. J Am Coll Cardiol. 2001;38:1782-7.
2. Coca SG, Yusuf B, Shlipak MG, Garg AX, Parikh CR. Long-term risk of mortality and other adverse outcomes after acute kidney injury: a systematic review and meta-analysis. Am J Kidney Dis. 2009;53:961-73.
3. O'Neal JB, Shaw AD, Billings FTt. Acute kidney injury following cardiac surgery: current understanding and future directions. Crit Care. 2016;20:187.
4. McCullough PA. Contrast-induced acute kidney injury. J Am Coll Cardiol. 2008;51:1419-28.
5. Damman K, Valente MA, Voors AA, O'Connor CM, van Veldhuisen DJ, Hillege HL. Renal impairment, worsening renal function, and outcome in patients with heart failure: an updated meta-analysis. Eur Heart J. 2014;35:455-69.
6. Marenzi G, Cosentino N, Bartorelli AL. Acute kidney injury in patients with acute coronary syndromes. Heart. 2015;101:1778-85.
7. Fox CS, Muntner P, Chen AY, Alexander KP, Roe MT, Wiviott SD. Short-term outcomes of acute myocardial infarction in patients with acute kidney injury: a report from the national cardiovascular data registry. Circulation. 2012;125:497-504.
8. Goldberg A, Kogan E, Hammerman H, Markiewicz W, Aronson D. The impact of transient and persistent acute kidney injury on long-term outcomes after acute myocardial infarction. Kidney Int. 2009;76:900-6.
9. Narula A, Mehran R, Weisz G, Dangas GD, Yu J, Généreux P, et al. Contrast-induced acute kidney injury after primary percutaneous coronary intervention: results from the HORIZONS-AMI substudy. Eur Heart J. 2014;35:1533-40.
10. Marenzi G, Cabiati A, Bertoli SV, Assanelli E, Marana I, De Metrio M, et al. Incidence and relevance of acute kidney injury in patients hospitalized with acute coronary syndromes. Am J Cardiol. 2013;111:816-22.

11. Marenzi G, Assanelli E, Campodonico J, Lauri G, Marana I, De Metrio M, et al. Contrast volume during primary percutaneous coronary intervention and subsequent contrast-induced nephropathy and mortality. Ann Intern Med. 2009;150:170-7.
12. Parikh CR, Coca SG, Wang Y, Masoudi FA, Krumholz HM. Long-term prognosis of acute kidney injury after acute myocardial infarction. Arch Intern Med. 2008;168:987-95.
13. Maioli M, Toso A, Leoncini M, Gallopin M, Musilli N, Bellandi F. Persistent renal damage after contrast-induced acute kidney injury: incidence, evolution, risk factors, and prognosis. Circulation. 2012;125:3099-107.
14. Chawla LS, Kimmel PL. Acute kidney injury and chronic kidney disease: an integrated clinical syndrome. Kidney Int. 2012;82:516-24.
15. Rihal CS, Textor SC, Grill DE, Berger PB, Ting HH, Best PJ, et al. Incidence and prognostic importance of acute renal failure after percutaneous coronary intervention. Circulation. 2002;105:2259-64.
16. Sidhu RB, Brown JR, Robb JF, Jayne JE, Friedman BJ, Hettleman BD, et al. Interaction of gender and age on post cardiac catheterization contrast-induced acute kidney injury. Am J Cardiol. 2008;102:1482-6.
17. Inohara T, Kohsaka S, Abe T, Miyata H, Numasawa Y, Ueda I, et al. Development and validation of a pre-percutaneous coronary intervention risk model of contrast-induced acute kidney injury with an integer scoring system. Am J Cardiol. 2015;115:1636-42.
18. Laskey W, Aspelin P, Davidson C, Rudnick M, Aubry P, Kumar S, et al. Nephrotoxicity of iodixanol versus iopamidol in patients with chronic kidney disease and diabetes mellitus undergoing coronary angiographic procedures. Am Heart J. 2009;158:822-8 e3.
19. Gruberg L, Mintz GS, Mehran R, Gangas G, Lansky AJ, Kent KM, et al. The prognostic implications of further renal function deterioration within 48 h of interventional coronary procedures in patients with pre-existent chronic renal insufficiency. J Am Coll Cardiol. 2000;36:1542-8.
20. Rudnick M, Feldman H. Contrast-induced nephropathy: what are the true clinical consequences? Clin J Am Soc Nephrol. 2008;3:263-72.
21. Fukumoto Y, Tsutsui H, Tsuchihashi M, Masumoto A, Takeshita A, Cholesterol Embolism Study I. The incidence and risk factors of cholesterol embolization syndrome, a complication of cardiac catheterization: a prospective study. J Am Coll Cardiol. 2003;42:211-6.
22. Lagny MG, Jouret F, Koch JN, Blaffart F, Donneau AF, Albert A, et al. Incidence and outcomes of acute kidney injury after cardiac surgery using either criteria of the RIFLE classification. BMC Nephrol. 2015;16:76.
23. Rosner MH, Okusa MD. Acute kidney injury associated with cardiac surgery. Clin J Am Soc Nephrol 2006;1:19-32.
24. Xu JR, Zhu JM, Jiang J, Ding XQ, Fang Y, Shen B, et al. Risk factors for long-term mortality and progressive chronic kidney disease associated with acute kidney injury after cardiac surgery. Medicine (Baltimore). 2015;94:e2025.
25. Mariscalco G, Lorusso R, Dominici C, Renzulli A, Sala A. Acute kidney injury: a relevant complication after cardiac surgery. Ann Thorac Surg. 2011;92:1539-47.
26. Cole RT, Masoumi A, Triposkiadis F, Giamouzis G, Georgiopoulou V, Kalogeropoulos A, et al. Renal dysfunction in heart failure. Med Clin North Am. 2012;96:955-74.
27. Heywood JT, Fonarow GC, Costanzo MR, Mathur VS, Wigneswaran JR, Wynne J; ADHERE Scientific Advisory Committee and Investigators. High prevalence of renal dysfunction and its impact on outcome in 118,465 patients hospitalized with acute decompensated heart failure: a report from the ADHERE database. J Card Fail. 2007;13:422-30.
28. Herzog CA, Muster HA, Li S, Collins AJ. Impact of congestive heart failure, chronic kidney disease, and anemia on survival in the Medicare population. J Card Fail. 2004;10:467-72.
29. Dries DL, Exner DV, Domanski MJ, Greenberg B, Stevenson LW. The prognostic implications of renal insufficiency in asymptomatic and symptomatic patients with left ventricular systolic dysfunction. J Am Coll Cardiol. 2000;35:681-9.
30. Akhter MW, Aronson D, Bitar F, Khan S, Singh H, Singh RP, et al. Effect of elevated admission serum creatinine and its worsening on outcome in hospitalized patients with decompensated heart failure. Am J Cardiol. 2004;94:957-60.
31. Hamaguchi S, Tsuchihashi-Makaya M, Kinugawa S, Yokota T, Ide T, Takeshita A, et al. Chronic kidney disease as an independent risk for long-term adverse outcomes in patients hospitalized with heart failure in Japan. Report from the Japanese Cardiac Registry of Heart Failure in Cardiology (JCARE-CARD). Circ J. 2009;73:1442-7.
32. Hillege HL, Nitsch D, Pfeffer MA, Swedberg K, McMurray JJ, Yusuf S, et al. Renal function as a predictor of outcome in a broad spectrum of patients with heart failure. Circulation. 2006;113:671-8.
33. Rosen S, Stillman IE. Acute tubular necrosis is a syndrome of physiologic and pathologic dissociation. J Am Soc Nephrol. 2008;19:871-5.
34. Damman K, Testani JM. The kidney in heart failure: an update. Eur Heart J. 2015;36:1437-44.
35. Gottlieb SS, Abraham W, Butler J, Forman DE, Loh E, Massie BM, et al. The prognostic importance of different definitions of worsening renal function in congestive heart failure. J Card Fail. 2002;8:136-41.
36. Smith GL, Vaccarino V, Kosiborod M, Lichtman JH, Cheng S, Watnick SG, et al. Worsening renal function: what is a clinically meaningful change in creatinine during hospitalization with heart failure? J Card Fail. 2003;9:13-25.
37. van Deursen VM, Hernandez AF, Stebbins A, Hasselblad V, Ezekowitz JA, Califf RM, et al. Nesiritide, renal function, and associated outcomes during hospitalization for acute decompensated heart failure: results from the Acute Study of Clinical Effectiveness of Nesiritide and Decompensated Heart Failure (ASCEND-HF). Circulation. 2014;130:958-65.
38. Nohria A, Hasselblad V, Stebbins A, Pauly DF, Fonarow GC, Shah M, et al. Cardiorenal interactions: insights from the ESCAPE trial. J Am Coll Cardiol. 2008;51:1268-74.
39. Cowie MR, Komajda M, Murray-Thomas T, Underwood J, Ticho B, Investigators P. Prevalence and impact of worsening renal function in patients hospitalized with decompensated heart failure: results of the prospective outcomes study in heart failure (POSH). Eur Heart J. 2006;27:1216-22.
40. Aronson D, Burger AJ. The relationship between transient and persistent worsening renal function and mortality in patients with acute decompensated heart failure. J Card Fail 2010;16:541-7.
41. Felker GM, Lee KL, Bull DA, Redfield MM, Stevenson LW, Goldsmith SR, et al. Diuretic strategies in patients with acute decompensated heart failure. N Engl J Med. 2011;364:797-805.
42. Testani JM, Coca SG, McCauley BD, Shannon RP, Kimmel SE. Impact of changes in blood pressure during the treatment of acute decompensated heart failure on renal and clinical outcomes. Eur J Heart Fail. 2011;13: 877-84.
43. Metra M, Davison B, Bettari L, Sun H, Edwards C, Lazzarini V, et al. Is worsening renal function an ominous prognostic sign in patients with acute heart failure? The role of congestion and its interaction with renal function. Circ Heart Fail. 2012;5:54-62.
44. Valente MA, Voors AA, Damman K, Van Veldhuisen DJ, Massie BM, O'Connor CM, et al. Diuretic response in acute heart failure: clinical characteristics and prognostic significance. Eur Heart J. 2014;35:1284-93.
45. Testani JM, Brisco MA, Chen J, McCauley BD, Parikh CR, Tang WH. Timing of hemoconcentration during treatment of acute decompensated heart failure and subsequent survival: importance of sustained decongestion. J Am Coll Cardiol. 2013;62:516-24.
46. Givertz MM, Postmus D, Hillege HL, Mansoor GA, Massie BM, Davison BA, et al. Renal function trajectories and clinical outcomes in acute heart failure. Circ Heart Fail. 2014;7:59-67.
47. Stolfo D, Stenner E, Merlo M, Porto AG, Moras C ,Barbati G, et al. Prognostic impact of BNP variations in patients admitted for acute decompensated heart failure with in-hospital worsening renal function. Heart Lung Circ. 2016;pii: S1443-9506(16)31507-4.
48. Metra M, Cotter G, Davison BA, Felker GM, Filippatos G, Greenberg BH, et al. Effect of serelaxin on cardiac, renal, and hepatic biomarkers in the Relaxin in Acute Heart Failure (RELAX-AHF) development program: correlation with outcomes. J Am Coll Cardiol. 2013;61:196-206.
49. Ronco C, Cicoira M, McCullough PA. Cardiorenal syndrome type 1: pathophysiological crosstalk leading to combined heart and kidney dysfunction in the setting of acutely decompensated heart failure. J Am Coll Cardiol. 2012;60:1031-42.
50. Ronco C, Haapio M, House AA, Anavekar N, Bellomo R. Cardiorenal syndrome. J Am Coll Cardiol. 2008;52:1527-39.
51. Haase M, Muller C, Damman K, Murray PT, Kellum JA, Ronco C, et al. Pathogenesis of cardiorenal syndrome type 1 in acute decompensated heart failure: workgroup statements from the eleventh consensus conference of the Acute Dialysis Quality Initiative (ADQI). Contrib Nephrol. 2013;182:99-116.
52. Kwasa EA, Vinayak S, Armstrong R. The role of inflammation in contrast-induced nephropathy. Br J Radiol 2014;87:20130738.

53. Bellomo R, Auriemma S, Fabbri A, D'Onofrio A, Katz N, McCullough PA, et al. The pathophysiology of cardiac surgery-associated acute kidney injury (CSA-AKI). Int J Artif Organs. 2008;31:166-78.
54. Tumlin J, Stacul F, Adam A, Becker CR, Davidson C, Lameire N, et al. Pathophysiology of contrast-induced nephropathy. Am J Cardiol. 2006;98:14K-20K.
55. Fujii T, Kurata H, Takaoka M, Muraoka T, Fujisawa Y, Shokoji T, et al. The role of renal sympathetic nervous system in the pathogenesis of ischemic acute renal failure. Eur J Pharmacol. 2003;481:241-8.
56. Brewster UC, Perazella MA. The renin-angiotensin-aldosterone system and the kidney: effects on kidney disease. Am J Med. 2004;116:263-72.
57. Anzai A, Anzai T, Naito K, Kaneko H, Mano Y, Jo Y, et al. Prognostic significance of acute kidney injury after reperfused ST-elevation myocardial infarction: synergistic acceleration of renal dysfunction and left ventricular remodeling. J Card Fail. 2010;16:381-9.
58. Mannesse CK, Blankestijn PJ, Man in 't Veld AJ, Schalekamp MA. Renal failure and cholesterol crystal embolization: a report of 4 surviving cases and a review of the literature. Clin Nephrol. 1991;36:240-5.
59. Thadhani RI, Camargo CA Jr., Xavier RJ, Fang LS, Bazari H. Atheroembolic renal failure after invasive procedures. Natural history based on 52 histologically proven cases. Medicine (Baltimore). 1995;74:350-8.
60. Bagshaw SM, Hoste EA, Braam B, Briguori C, Kellum JA, McCullough PA, et al. Cardiorenal syndrome type 3: pathophysiologic and epidemiologic considerations. Contrib Nephrol 2013;182:137-57.
61. Cruz DN, Schmidt-Ott KM, Vescovo G, House AA, Kellum JA, Ronco C, et al. Pathophysiology of cardiorenal syndrome type 2 in stable chronic heart failure: workgroup statements from the eleventh consensus conference of the Acute Dialysis Quality Initiative (ADQI). Contrib Nephrol 2013;182:117-36.
62. Mehta RL, Rabb H, Shaw AD, Singbartl K, Ronco C, McCullough PA, et al. Cardiorenal syndrome type 5: clinical presentation, pathophysiology and management strategies from the eleventh consensus conference of the Acute Dialysis Quality Initiative (ADQI). Contrib Nephrol. 2013;182:174-94.
63. Tumlin JA, Costanzo MR, Chawla LS, Herzog CA, Kellum JA, McCullough PA, et al. Cardiorenal syndrome type 4: insights on clinical presentation and pathophysiology from the eleventh consensus conference of the Acute Dialysis Quality Initiative (ADQI). Contrib Nephrol 2013;182:158-73.
64. Anand IS. Cardiorenal syndrome: a cardiologist's perspective of pathophysiology. Clin J Am Soc Nephrol. 2013;8:1800-7.
65. Hanberg JS, Sury K, Wilson FP, et al. Reduced cardiac index is not the dominant driver of renal dysfunction in heart failure. J Am Coll Cardiol. 2016;67:2199-208.
66. Mullens W, Abrahams Z, Francis GS, Sokos G, Taylor DO, Starling RC, et al. Importance of venous congestion for worsening of renal function in advanced decompensated heart failure. J Am Coll Cardiol. 2009;53:589-96.
67. Damman K, van Deursen VM, Navis G, Voors AA, van Veldhuisen DJ, Hillege HL. Increased central venous pressure is associated with impaired renal function and mortality in a broad spectrum of patients with cardiovascular disease. J Am Coll Cardiol. 2009;53:582-8.
68. Damman K, Voors AA, Hillege HL, Navis G, Lechat P, van Veldhuisen DJ, et al. Congestion in chronic systolic heart failure is related to renal dysfunction and increased mortality. Eur J Heart Fail. 2010;12:974-82.
69. Mullens W, Abrahams Z, Skouri HN, Francis GS, Taylor DO, Starling RC, et al. Elevated intra-abdominal pressure in acute decompensated heart failure: a potential contributor to worsening renal function? J Am Coll Cardiol. 2008;51:300-6.
70. Verbrugge FH, Dupont M, Steels P, Grieten L, Malbrain M, Tang WH, et al. Abdominal contributions to cardiorenal dysfunction in congestive heart failure. J Am Coll Cardiol. 2013;62:485-95.
71. Bock JS, Gottlieb SS. Cardiorenal syndrome: new perspectives. Circulation. 2010;121:2592-600.
72. Kula AJ, Hanberg JS, Wilson FP, Brisco MA, Bellumkonda L, Jacoby D, et al. Influence of titration of neurohormonal antagonists and blood pressure reduction on renal function and decongestion in decompensated heart failure. Circ Heart Fail. 2016;9:e002333.
73. Dangas G, Iakovou I, Nikolsky E, Aymong ED, Mintz GS, Kipshidze NN, et al. Contrast-induced nephropathy after percutaneous coronary interventions in relation to chronic kidney disease and hemodynamic variables. Am J Cardiol. 2005;95:13-9.
74. Krumlovsky FA, Simon N, Santhanam S, del Greco F, Roxe D, Pomaranc MM. Acute renal failure. Association with administration of radiographic contrast material. JAMA. 1978;239:125-7.
75. Mehran R, Aymong ED, Nikolsky E, Lasic Z, Iakovou I, Fahy M, et al. A simple risk score for prediction of contrast-induced nephropathy after percutaneous coronary intervention: development and initial validation. J Am Coll Cardiol. 2004;44:1393-9.
76. Nikolsky E, Mehran R, Lasic Z, Mintz GS, Lansky AJ, Na Y, et al. Low hematocrit predicts contrast-induced nephropathy after percutaneous coronary interventions. Kidney Int 2005;67:706-13.
77. Shaw A. Update on acute kidney injury after cardiac surgery. J Thorac Cardiovasc Surg. 2012;143:676-81.
78. Huen SC, Parikh CR. Predicting acute kidney injury after cardiac surgery: a systematic review. Ann Thorac Surg. 2012;93:337-47.
79. Forman DE, Butler J, Wang Y, Abraham WT, O'Connor CM, Gottlieb SS, et al. Incidence, predictors at admission, and impact of worsening renal function among patients hospitalized with heart failure. J Am Coll Cardiol. 2004;43:61-7.
80. Bellomo R, Ronco C, Kellum JA, Mehta RL, Palevsky P, Acute Dialysis Quality Initiative w. Acute renal failure—definition, outcome measures, animal models, fluid therapy and information technology needs: the Second International Consensus Conference of the Acute Dialysis Quality Initiative (ADQI) Group. Crit Care 2004;8:R204-12.
81. Mehta RL, Kellum JA, Shah SV, Molitoris BA, Ronco C, Warnock DG, et al. Acute Kidney Injury Network: report of an initiative to improve outcomes in acute kidney injury. Crit Care. 2007;11:R31.
82. Group IGOKAKIW. KDIGO Clinical Practice Guideline for Acute Kidney Injury. Kidney Int. 2012;2, Suppl:1-138.
83. Rodrigues FB, Bruetto RG, Torres US, Otaviano AP, Zanetta DM, Burdmann EA. Incidence and mortality of acute kidney injury after myocardial infarction: a comparison between KDIGO and RIFLE criteria. PLoS One. 2013;8:e69998.
84. Sampaio MC, Maximo CA, Montenegro CM, Mota DM, Fernandes TR, Bianco AC, et al. Comparison of diagnostic criteria for acute kidney injury in cardiac surgery. Arq Bras Cardiol. 2013;101:18-25.
85. Roy AK, Mc Gorrian C, Treacy C, Kavanaugh E, Brennan A, Mahon NG, et al. A comparison of traditional and novel definitions (RIFLE, AKIN, and KDIGO) of acute kidney injury for the prediction of outcomes in acute decompensated heart failure. Cardiorenal Med. 2013;3:26-37.
86. van Veldhuisen DJ, Ruilope LM, Maisel AS, Damman K. Biomarkers of renal injury and function: diagnostic, prognostic and therapeutic implications in heart failure. Eur Heart J. 2016;37(33):2577-85.
87. Damman K, Voors AA, Navis G, van Veldhuisen DJ, Hillege HL. Current and novel renal biomarkers in heart failure. Heart Fail Rev. 2012;17:241-50.
88. Cruz DN, Goh CY, Haase-Fielitz A, Ronco C, Haase M. Early biomarkers of renal injury. Congest Heart Fail 2010;16 Suppl 1:S25-31.
89. McCullough PA, Shaw AD, Haase M, Bouchard J, Waikar SS, Siew ED, et al. Diagnosis of acute kidney injury using functional and injury biomarkers: workgroup statements from the tenth Acute Dialysis Quality Initiative Consensus Conference. Contrib Nephrol. 2013;182:13-29.
90. Dharnidharka VR, Kwon C, Stevens G. Serum cystatin C is superior to serum creatinine as a marker of kidney function: a meta-analysis. Am J Kidney Dis. 2002;40:221-6.
91. Taglieri N, Fernandez-Berges DJ, Koenig W, Consuegra-Sanchez L, Fernandez JM, Robles NR, et al. Plasma cystatin C for prediction of 1-year cardiac events in Mediterranean patients with non-ST elevation acute coronary syndrome. Atherosclerosis. 2010;209:300-5.
92. Dardashti A, Nozohoor S, Algotsson L, Ederoth P, Bjursten H. The predictive value of s-cystatin C for mortality after coronary artery bypass surgery. J Thorac Cardiovasc Surg. 2016;152:139-46.
93. Zhu J, Yin R, Wu H, Yi J, Luo L, Dong G, et al. Cystatin C as a reliable marker of renal function following heart valve replacement surgery with cardiopulmonary bypass. Clin Chim Acta. 2006;374:116-21.
94. Haase M, Bellomo R, Devarajan P, Ma Q, Bennett MR, Möckel M, et al. Novel biomarkers early predict the severity of acute kidney injury after cardiac surgery in adults. Ann Thorac Surg. 2009;88:124-30.
95. Briquori C, Visconti G, Rivera NV, Focaccio A, Golia B, Giannone R, et al. Cystatin C and contrast-induced acute kidney injury. Circulation. 2010;121:2117-22.
96. Tang WH, Dupont M, Hernandez AF, Voors AA, Hsu AP, Felker GM, et al. Comparative assessment of short-term adverse events in acute heart failure with cystatin C and other estimates of renal function: results from the ASCEND-HF trial. JACC Heart Fail. 2015;3:40-9.
97. Campbell CY, Clarke W, Park H, Haq N, Barone BB, Brotman DJ. Usefulness of cystatin C and prognosis following admission for acute heart failure. Am J Cardiol. 2009;104:389-92.

98. Klein L, Massie BM, Leimberger JD, O'Connor CM, Piña IL, Adams KF Jr, et al. Admission or changes in renal function during hospitalization for worsening heart failure predict postdischarge survival: results from the Outcomes of a Prospective Trial of Intravenous Milrinone for Exacerbations of Chronic Heart Failure (OPTIME-CHF). Circ Heart Fail. 2008;1:25-33.
99. Fonarow GC, Adams KF, Jr., Abraham WT, Yancy CW, Boscardin WJ; ADHERE Scientific Advisory Committee, Study Group, and Investigators. Risk stratification for in-hospital mortality in acutely decompensated heart failure: classification and regression tree analysis. JAMA 2005;293:572-80.
100. Takaya Y, Yoshihara F, Yokoyama H, Kanzaki H, Kitakaze M, Goto Y, et al. Risk stratification of acute kidney injury using the blood urea nitrogen/creatinine ratio in patients with acute decompensated heart failure. Circ J. 2015;79:1520-5.
101. Testani JM, Damman K, Brisco MA, Chen S, Laur O, Kula AJ, et al. A combined-biomarker approach to clinical phenotyping renal dysfunction in heart failure. J Card Fail. 2014;20:912-9.
102. de Zeeuw D, Remuzzi G, Parving HH, Keane WF, Zhang Z, Shahinfar S, et al. Albuminuria, a therapeutic target for cardiovascular protection in type 2 diabetic patients with nephropathy. Circulation. 2004;110:921-7.
103. Hillege HL, Fidler V, Diercks GF, van Gilst WH, de Zeeuw D, van Veldhuisen DJ, et al. Urinary albumin excretion predicts cardiovascular and noncardiovascular mortality in general population. Circulation. 2002;106:1777-82.
104. Masson S, Latini R, Milani V, Moretti L, Rossi MG, Carbonieri E, et al. Prevalence and prognostic value of elevated urinary albumin excretion in patients with chronic heart failure: data from the GISSI-Heart Failure trial. Circ Heart Fail. 2010;3:65-72.
105. Anand IS, Bishu K, Rector TS, Ishani A, Kuskowski MA, Cohn JN. Proteinuria, chronic kidney disease, and the effect of an angiotensin receptor blocker in addition to an angiotensin-converting enzyme inhibitor in patients with moderate to severe heart failure. Circulation. 2009;120:1577-84.
106. Jackson CE, Solomon SD, Gerstein HC, Zetterstrand S, Olofsson B, Michelson EL, et al. Albuminuria in chronic heart failure: prevalence and prognostic importance. Lancet. 2009;374:543-50.
107. Koyama S, Sato Y, Tanada Y, Fujiwara H, Takatsu Y. Early evolution and correlates of urine albumin excretion in patients presenting with acutely decompensated heart failure. Circ Heart Fail. 2013;6:227-32.
108. Molnar AO, Parikh CR, Sint K, Coca SG, Koyner J, Patel UD, et al. Association of postoperative proteinuria with AKI after cardiac surgery among patients at high risk. Clin J Am Soc Nephrol. 2012;7:1749-60.
109. Koyner JL, Garg AX, Coca SG, Sint K, Thiessen-Philbrook H, Patel UD, et al. Biomarkers predict progression of acute kidney injury after cardiac surgery. J Am Soc Nephrol. 2012;23:905-14.
110. Tziakas D, Chalikias G, Kareli D, Tsigalou C, Risgits A, Kikas P, et al. Spot urine albumin to creatinine ratio outperforms novel acute kidney injury biomarkers in patients with acute myocardial infarction. Int J Cardiol. 2015;197:48-55.
111. Bolignano D, Donato V, Coppolino G, Campo S, Buemi A, Lacquaniti A, et al. Neutrophil gelatinase-associated lipocalin (NGAL) as a marker of kidney damage. Am J Kidney Dis. 2008;52:595-605.
112. Nickolas TL, O'Rourke MJ, Yang J, Sise ME, Canetta PA, Barasch N, et al. Sensitivity and specificity of a single emergency department measurement of urinary neutrophil gelatinase-associated lipocalin for diagnosing acute kidney injury. Ann Intern Med. 2008;148:810-9.
113. Zhou F, Luo Q, Wang L, Han L. Diagnostic value of neutrophil gelatinase-associated lipocalin for early diagnosis of cardiac surgery-associated acute kidney injury: a meta-analysis. Eur J Cardiothorac Surg. 2016;49:746-55.
114. Haase M, Bellomo R, Devarajan P, Schlattmann P, Haase-Fielitz A, Group NM-al. Accuracy of neutrophil gelatinase-associated lipocalin (NGAL) in diagnosis and prognosis in acute kidney injury: a systematic review and meta-analysis. Am J Kidney Dis. 2009;54:1012-24.
115. Aghel A, Shrestha K, Mullens W, Borowski A, Tang WH. Serum neutrophil gelatinase-associated lipocalin (NGAL) in predicting worsening renal function in acute decompensated heart failure. J Card Fail. 2010;16:49-54.
116. Alvelos M, Pimentel R, Pinho E, Gomes A, Lourenço P, Teles MJ, et al. Neutrophil gelatinase-associated lipocalin in the diagnosis of type 1 cardio-renal syndrome in the general ward. Clin J Am Soc Nephrol. 2011;6:476-81.
117. Collins SP, Hart KW, Lindsell CJ, Fermann GJ, Weintraub NL, Miller KF, et al. Elevated urinary neutrophil gelatinase-associated lipocalcin after acute heart failure treatment is associated with worsening renal function and adverse events. Eur J Heart Fail. 2012;14:1020-9.
118. Haase M, Devarajan P, Haase-Fielitz A, Bellomo R, Cruz DN, Wagener G, et al. The outcome of neutrophil gelatinase-associated lipocalin-positive subclinical acute kidney injury: a multicenter pooled analysis of prospective studies. J Am Coll Cardiol. 2011;57:1752-61.
119. Maisel AS, Mueller C, Fitzgerald R, Brikhan R, Hiestand BC, Iqbal N, et al. Prognostic utility of plasma neutrophil gelatinase-associated lipocalin in patients with acute heart failure: the NGAL EvaLuation Along with B-type NaTriuretic Peptide in acutely decompensated heart failure (GALLANT) trial. Eur J Heart Fail. 2011;13:846-51.
120. van Deursen VM, Damman K, Voors AA, van der Wal MH, Jaarsma T, van Veldhuisen DJ, et al. Prognostic value of plasma neutrophil gelatinase-associated lipocalin for mortality in patients with heart failure. Circ Heart Fail. 2014;7:35-42.
121. Brisco MA, Testani JM. Novel renal biomarkers to assess cardiorenal syndrome. Curr Heart Fail Rep. 2014;11:485-99.
122. Shao X, Tian L, Xu W, Zhang Z, Wang C, Qi C, et al. Diagnostic value of urinary kidney injury molecule 1 for acute kidney injury: a meta-analysis. PLoS One. 2014;9:e84131.
123. Torregrosa I, Montoliu C, Urios A, Andrés-Costa MJ, Giménez-Garzó C, Juan I, et al. Urinary KIM-1, NGAL and L-FABP for the diagnosis of AKI in patients with acute coronary syndrome or heart failure undergoing coronary angiography. Heart Vessels. 2015;30:703-11.
124. Akdeniz D, Celik HT, Kazanci F, Yilmaz H, Yalcin S, Bilgic MA, et al. Is kidney injury molecule 1 a valuable tool for the early diagnosis of contrast-induced nephropathy? J Investig Med. 2015;63:930-4.
125. Damman K, Van Veldhuisen DJ, Navis G, Vaidya VS, Smilde TD, Westenbrink BD, et al. Tubular damage in chronic systolic heart failure is associated with reduced survival independent of glomerular filtration rate. Heart. 2010;96:1297-302.
126. Damman K, Masson S, Hillege HL, Voors AA, van Veldhuisen DJ, Rossignol P, et al. Tubular damage and worsening renal function in chronic heart failure. JACC Heart Fail. 2013;1:417-24.
127. Verbrugge FH, Dupont M, Shao Z, Shrestha K, Singh D, Finucan M, et al. Novel urinary biomarkers in detecting acute kidney injury, persistent renal impairment, and all-cause mortality following decongestive therapy in acute decompensated heart failure. J Card Fail. 2013;19:621-8.
128. Yang CH, Chang CH, Chen TH, Fan PC, Chang SW, Chen CC, et al. Combination of urinary biomarkers improves early detection of acute kidney injury in patients with heart failure. Circ J. 2016;80:1017-23.
129. Iqbal MP, Kazmi K, Mehboobali N. N-acetyl-beta-D-glucosaminidase—a marker of reperfusion and a prognostic indicator in patients with acute myocardial infarction. Acta Cardiol. 2005;60:509-13.
130. Iqbal MP, Kazmi KA, Jafri HR, Mehboobali N. N-acetyl-beta-D-glucosaminidase in acute myocardial infarction. Exp Mol Med. 2003;35:275-8.
131. Ren L, Ji J, Fang Y, Jiang SH, Lin YM, Bo J, et al. Assessment of urinary N-acetyl-beta-glucosaminidase as an early marker of contrast-induced nephropathy. J Int Med Res. 2011;39:647-53.
132. Ho J, Tangri N, Komenda P, Kaushal A, Sood M, Brar R, et al. Urinary, plasma, and serum biomarkers' utility for predicting acute kidney injury associated with cardiac surgery in adults: A meta-analysis. Am J Kidney Dis. 2015;66:993-1005.
133. Katagiri D, Doi K, Honda K, Negishi K, Fujita T, Hisagi M, et al. Combination of two urinary biomarkers predicts acute kidney injury after adult cardiac surgery. Ann Thorac Surg. 2012;93:577-83.
134. Legrand M, De Berardinis B, Gaggin HK, Magrini L, Belcher A, Zancla B, et al. Evidence of uncoupling between renal dysfunction and injury in cardiorenal syndrome: insights from the BIONICS study. PLoS One. 2014;9:e112313.
135. Damman K, Masson S, Hillege HL, Maggioni AP, Voors AA, Opasich C, et al. Clinical outcome of renal tubular damage in chronic heart failure. Eur Heart J. 2011;32:2705-12.
136. Body R, Carley S, McDowell G, Pemberton P, Burrows G, Cook G, et al. The Manchester Acute Coronary Syndromes (MACS) decision rule for suspected cardiac chest pain: derivation and external validation. Heart. 2014;100:1462-8.
137. Manabe K, Kamihata H, Motohiro M, Senoo T, Yoshida S, Iwasaka T. Urinary liver-type fatty acid-binding protein level as a predictive biomarker of contrast-induced acute kidney injury. Eur J Clin Invest. 2012;42:557-63.
138. Portilla D, Dent C, Sugaya T, Nagothu KK, Kundi I, Moore P, et al. Liver fatty acid-binding protein as a biomarker of acute kidney injury after cardiac surgery. Kidney Int. 2008;73:465-72.
139. Schaub JA, Garg AX, Coca SG, Testani JM, Shlipak MG, Eikelboom J, et al. Perioperative heart-type fatty acid binding protein is associated with acute kidney injury after cardiac surgery. Kidney Int. 2015;88:576-83.
140. Shirakabe A, Hata N, Kobayashi N, Okazaki H, Shinada T, Tomita K, et al. Serum heart-type fatty acid-binding protein level can be used to detect acute kidney

injury on admission and predict an adverse outcome in patients with acute heart failure. Circ J. 2015;79:119-28.

141. Malyszko J, Bachorzewska-Gajewska H, Poniatowski B, Malyszko JS, Dobrzycki S. Urinary and serum biomarkers after cardiac catheterization in diabetic patients with stable angina and without severe chronic kidney disease. Ren Fail. 2009;31:910-9.
142. Ling W, Zhaohui N, Ben H, Leyi G, Jianping L, Huili D, et al. Urinary IL-18 and NGAL as early predictive biomarkers in contrast-induced nephropathy after coronary angiography. Nephron Clin Pract. 2008;108:c176-81.
143. He H, Li W, Qian W, Zhao X, Wang L, Yu Y, et al. Urinary interleukin-18 as an early indicator to predict contrast-induced nephropathy in patients undergoing percutaneous coronary intervention. Exp Ther Med. 2014;8:1263-6.
144. Liu Y, Guo W, Zhang J, Xu C, Yu S, Mao Z, et al. Urinary interleukin 18 for detection of acute kidney injury: a meta-analysis. Am J Kidney Dis. 2013;62:1058-67.
145. Kashani K, Al-Khafaji A, Ardiles T, Artigas A, Bagshaw SM, Bell M, et al. Discovery and validation of cell cycle arrest biomarkers in human acute kidney injury. Crit Care 2013;17:R25.
146. Meersch M, Schmidt C, Van Aken H, Martens S, Rossaint J, Singbartl K, et al. Urinary TIMP-2 and IGFBP7 as early biomarkers of acute kidney injury and renal recovery following cardiac surgery. PLoS One. 2014;9:e93460.
147. Pilarczyk K, Edayadiyil-Dudasova M, Wendt D, Demircioglu E, Benedik J, Dohle DS, et al. Urinary [TIMP-2]*[IGFBP7] for early prediction of acute kidney injury after coronary artery bypass surgery. Ann Intensive Care. 2015;5:50.
148. Group. KDIGOKAKIW. KDIGO Clinical Practice Guideline for Acute Kidney Injury. Kidney Int. 2012;Suppl:1-138.
149. Tsai TT, Patel UD, Chang TI, Kennedy KF, Masoudi FA, Matheny ME, et al. Validated contemporary risk model of acute kidney injury in patients undergoing percutaneous coronary interventions: insights from the National Cardiovascular Data Registry Cath-PCI Registry. J Am Heart Assoc. 2014;3:e001380.
150. Aspelin P, Aubry P, Fransson SG, et al. Nephrotoxic effects in high-risk patients undergoing angiography. N Engl J Med. 2003;348:491-9.
151. Dong M, Jiao Z, Liu T, Guo F, Li G. Effect of administration route on the renal safety of contrast agents: a meta-analysis of randomized controlled trials. J Nephrol. 2012;25:290-301.
152. Friedewald VE, Goldfarb S, Laskey WK, Vetrovec GW, Roberts WC. The editor's roundtable: contrast agents and risk for contrast-induced nephropathy. Am J Cardiol. 2011;107:1848-55.
153. King SB 3rd, Smith SC Jr., Hirshfeld JW Jr., Jacobs AK, Morrison DA, Williams DO, et al. 2007 Focused Update of the ACC/AHA/SCAI 2005 Guideline Update for Percutaneous Coronary Intervention: a report of the American College of Cardiology/American Heart Association Task Force on Practice Guidelines: 2007 Writing Group to Review New Evidence and Update the ACC/AHA/SCAI 2005 Guideline Update for Percutaneous Coronary Intervention, Writing on Behalf of the 2005 Writing Committee. Circulation. 2008;117:261-95.
154. Mueller C, Buerkle G, Buettner HJ, et al. Prevention of contrast media-associated nephropathy: randomized comparison of 2 hydration regimens in 1620 patients undergoing coronary angioplasty. Arch Intern Med 2002;162:329-36.
155. Subramaniam RM, Suarez-Cuervo C, Wilson RF, Turban S, Zhang A, Sherrod C, et al. Effectiveness of Prevention Strategies for Contrast-Induced Nephropathy: A Systematic Review and Meta-analysis. Ann Intern Med. 2016;164:406-16.
156. Fishbane S. N-acetylcysteine in the prevention of contrast-induced nephropathy. Clin J Am Soc Nephrol. 2008;3:281-7.
157. Investigators ACT. Acetylcysteine for prevention of renal outcomes in patients undergoing coronary and peripheral vascular angiography: main results from the randomized Acetylcysteine for Contrast-induced nephropathy Trial (ACT). Circulation. 2011;124:1250-9.
158. Han Y, Zhu G, Han L, Hou F, Huang W, Liu H, et al. Short-term rosuvastatin therapy for prevention of contrast-induced acute kidney injury in patients with diabetes and chronic kidney disease. J Am Coll Cardiol. 2014;63:62-70.
159. Leoncini M, Toso A, Maioli M, Tropeano F, Villani S, Bellandi F. Early high-dose rosuvastatin for contrast-induced nephropathy prevention in acute coronary syndrome: Results from the PRATO-ACS Study (Protective Effect of Rosuvastatin and Antiplatelet Therapy On contrast-induced acute kidney injury and myocardial damage in patients with Acute Coronary Syndrome). J Am Coll Cardiol. 2014;63:71-9.
160. Ukaigwe A, Karmacharya P, Mahmood M, Pathak R, Aryal MR, Jalota L, et al. Meta-analysis on efficacy of statins for prevention of contrast-induced acute kidney injury in patients undergoing coronary angiography. Am J Cardiol. 2014;114:1295-302.
161. Alsabbagh MM, Asmar A, Ejaz NI, Aiyer RK, Kambhampati G, Ejaz AA. Update on clinical trials for the prevention of acute kidney injury in patients undergoing cardiac surgery. Am J Surg. 2013;206:86-95.
162. Pretorius M, Murray KT, Yu C, Byrne JG, Billings FT 4th, Petracek MR, et al. Angiotensin-converting enzyme inhibition or mineralocorticoid receptor blockade do not affect prevalence of atrial fibrillation in patients undergoing cardiac surgery. Crit Care Med. 2012;40:2805-12.
163. Zheng Z, Jayaram R, Jiang L, Emberson J, Zhao Y, Li Q, et al. Perioperative rosuvastatin in cardiac surgery. N Engl J Med. 2016;374:1744-53.
164. Bove T, Zangrillo A, Guarracino F, Alvaro G, Persi B, Maglioni E, et al. Effect of fenoldopam on use of renal replacement therapy among patients with acute kidney injury after cardiac surgery: a randomized clinical trial. JAMA. 2014;312:2244-53.
165. Zarbock A, Kellum JA, Schmidt C, Van Aken H, Wempe C, Pavenstädt H, et al. Effect of early vs delayed initiation of renal replacement therapy on mortality in critically ill patients with acute kidney injury: The ELAIN Randomized Clinical Trial. JAMA. 2016;315:2190-9.
166. Cheng H, Chen YP. Clinical prediction scores for type 1 cardiorenal syndrome derived and validated in chinese cohorts. Cardiorenal Med. 2015;5:12-9.
167. Chiong JR, Cheung RJ. Loop diuretic therapy in heart failure: the need for solid evidence on a fluid issue. Clin Cardiol. 2010;33:345-52.
168. Mentz RJ, Stevens SR, DeVore AD, Lala A, Vader JM, AbouEzzeddine OF, et al. Decongestion strategies and renin-angiotensin-aldosterone system activation in acute heart failure. JACC Heart Fail. 2015;3:97-107.
169. Verbrugge FH, Dupont M, Steels P, Grieten L, Swennen Q, Tang WH, et al. The kidney in congestive heart failure: 'are natriuresis, sodium, and diuretics really the good, the bad and the ugly?' Eur J Heart Fail. 2014;16:133-42.
170. Jentzer JC, Chawla LS. A Clinical Approach to the Acute Cardiorenal Syndrome. Crit Care Clin. 2015;31:685-703.
171. O'Connor CM, Starling RC, Hernandez AF, Armstrong PW, Dickstein K, Hasselblad V, et al. Effect of nesiritide in patients with acute decompensated heart failure. N Engl J Med. 2011;365:32-43.
172. Chow SL, O'Barr SA, Peng J, Chew E, Pak F, Quist R, et al. Modulation of novel cardiorenal and inflammatory biomarkers by intravenous nitroglycerin and nesiritide in acute decompensated heart failure: an exploratory study. Circ Heart Fail. 2011;4:450-5.
173. Chow SL, O'Barr SA, Peng J, Chew E, Pak F, Quist R, et al. Renal function and neurohormonal changes following intravenous infusions of nitroglycerin versus nesiritide in patients with acute decompensated heart failure. J Card Fail. 2011;17:181-7.
174. Chen HH, Anstrom KJ, Givertz MM, Stevenson LW, Semigran MJ, Goldsmith SR, et al. Low-dose dopamine or low-dose nesiritide in acute heart failure with renal dysfunction: the ROSE acute heart failure randomized trial. JAMA. 2013;310:2533-43.
175. Teerlink JR, Cotter G, Davison BA, Felker GM, Filippatos G, Greenberg BH, et al. Serelaxin, recombinant human relaxin-2, for treatment of acute heart failure (RELAX-AHF): a randomised, placebo-controlled trial. Lancet. 2013;381: 29-39.
176. Costanzo MR, Guglin ME, Saltzberg MT, Jessup ML, Bart BA, Teerlink JR, et al. Ultrafiltration versus intravenous diuretics for patients hospitalized for acute decompensated heart failure. J Am Coll Cardiol. 2007;49:675-83.
177. Bart BA, Goldsmith SR, Lee KL, Givertz MM, O'Connor CM, Bull DA, et al. Ultrafiltration in decompensated heart failure with cardiorenal syndrome. N Engl J Med. 2012;367:2296-304.

Index

Page numbers followed by *b* refer to box, *f* refer to figure, *fc* refer to flowchart, and *t* refer to table.

B

D

E

I

J

K

L

Q

R

S

T